T0295051

ESSENTIALS OF

Osborn's Brain

A Fundamental Guide for Residents and Fellows

Anne G. Osborn

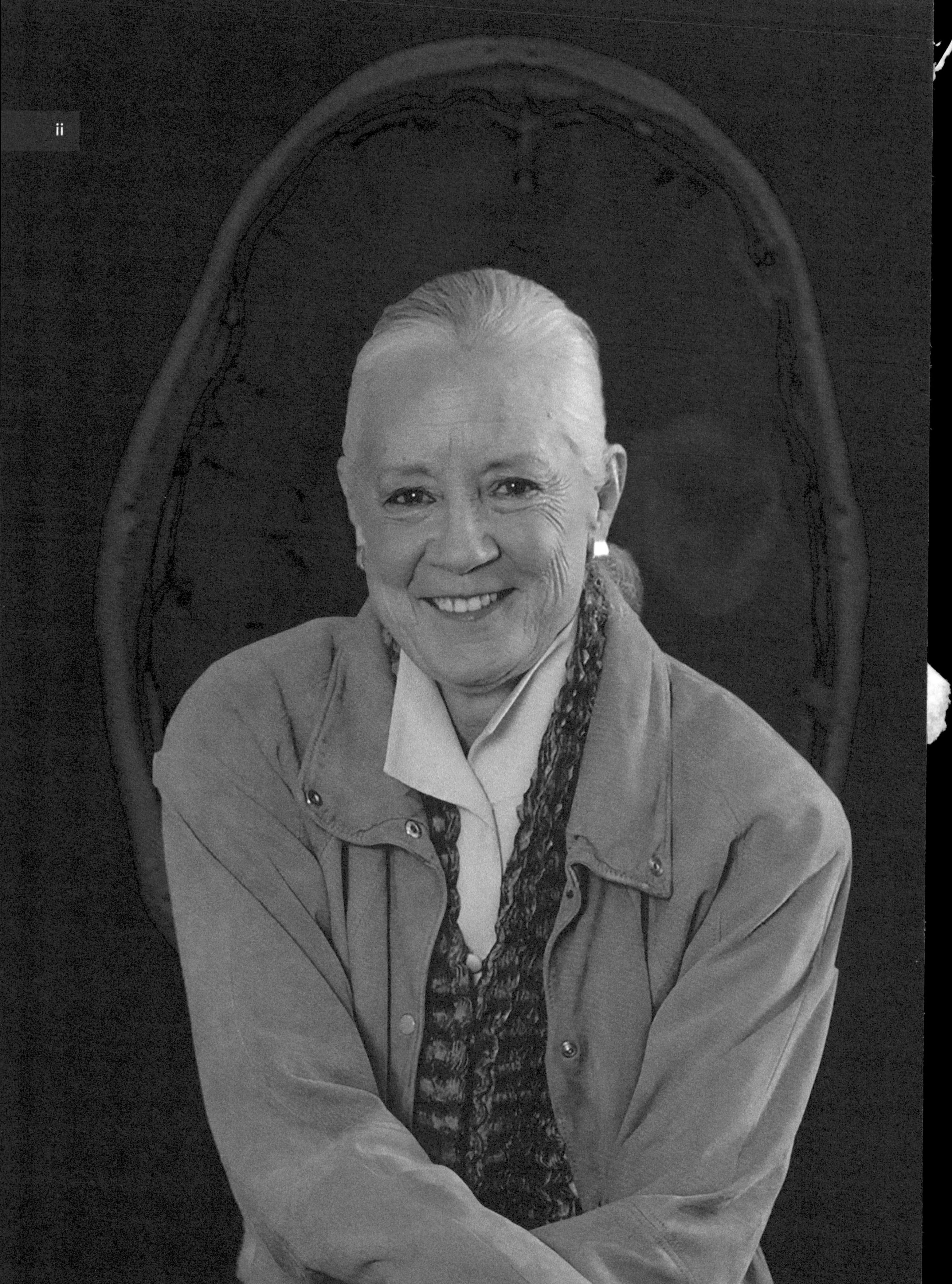

ESSENTIALS OF Osborn's Brain

A Fundamental Guide for Residents and Fellows

Anne G. Osborn, MD, FACR

University Distinguished Professor and
Professor of Radiology and Imaging Sciences
William H. and Patricia W. Child Presidential Endowed Chair in Radiology
University of Utah School of Medicine
Salt Lake City, Utah

ESSENTIALS OF OSBORN'S BRAIN: A FUNDAMENTAL GUIDE
FOR RESIDENTS AND FELLOWS

ISBN: 978-0-323-71320-7

Notices

Practitioners and researchers must always rely on their own experience and knowledge in evaluating and using any information, methods, compounds or experiments described herein. Because of rapid advances in the medical sciences, in particular, independent verification of diagnoses and drug dosages should be made. To the fullest extent of the law, no responsibility is assumed by Elsevier, authors, editors or contributors for any injury and/or damage to persons or property as a matter of products liability, negligence or otherwise, or from any use or operation of any methods, products, instructions, or ideas contained in the material herein.

Library of Congress Control Number: 2019941279

Cover Designer: Tom M. Olson, BA
Printed in the United States of America

Last digit is the print number: 9 8 7 6 5

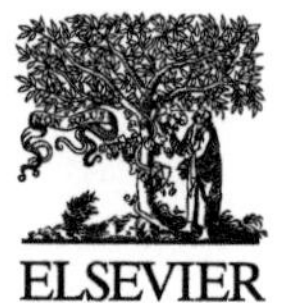

1600 John F. Kennedy Blvd.
Ste 1800
Philadelphia, PA 19103-2899

Contributing Authors

Gary L. Hedlund, DO
Adjunct Professor of Radiology
University of Utah School of Medicine
Salt Lake City, Utah

Karen L. Salzman, MD
Professor of Radiology and Imaging Sciences
Neuroradiology Section Chief and Fellowship Director
Leslie W. Davis Endowed Chair in Neuroradiology
University of Utah School of Medicine
Salt Lake City, Utah

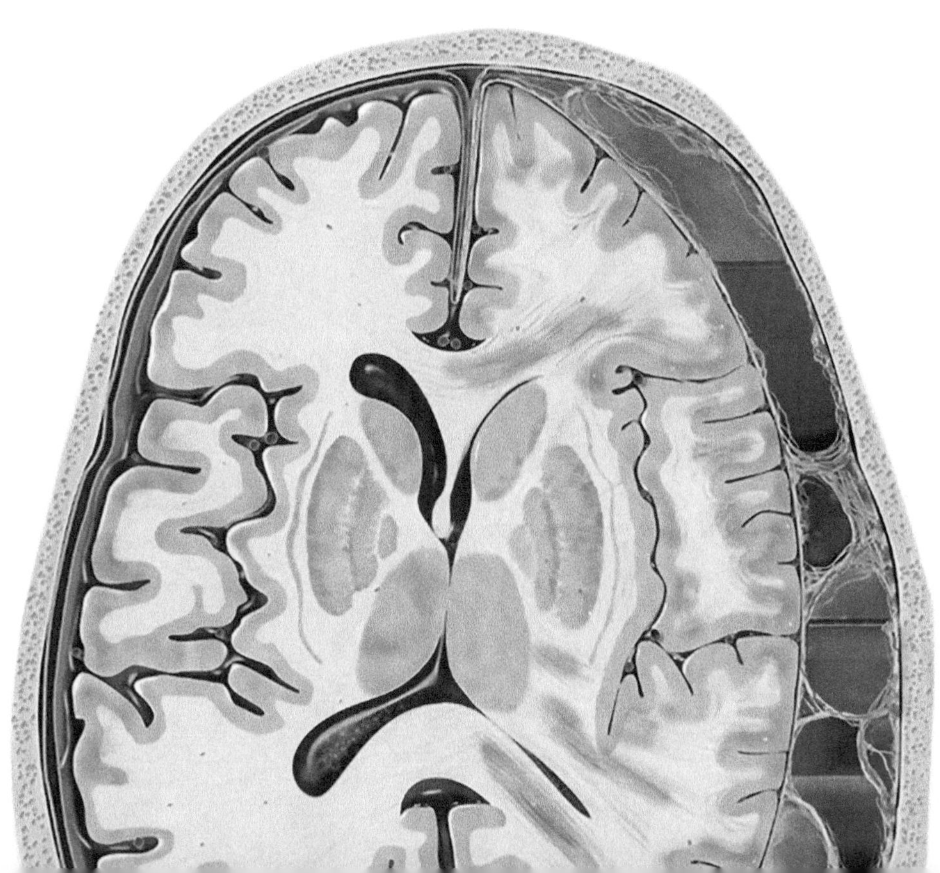

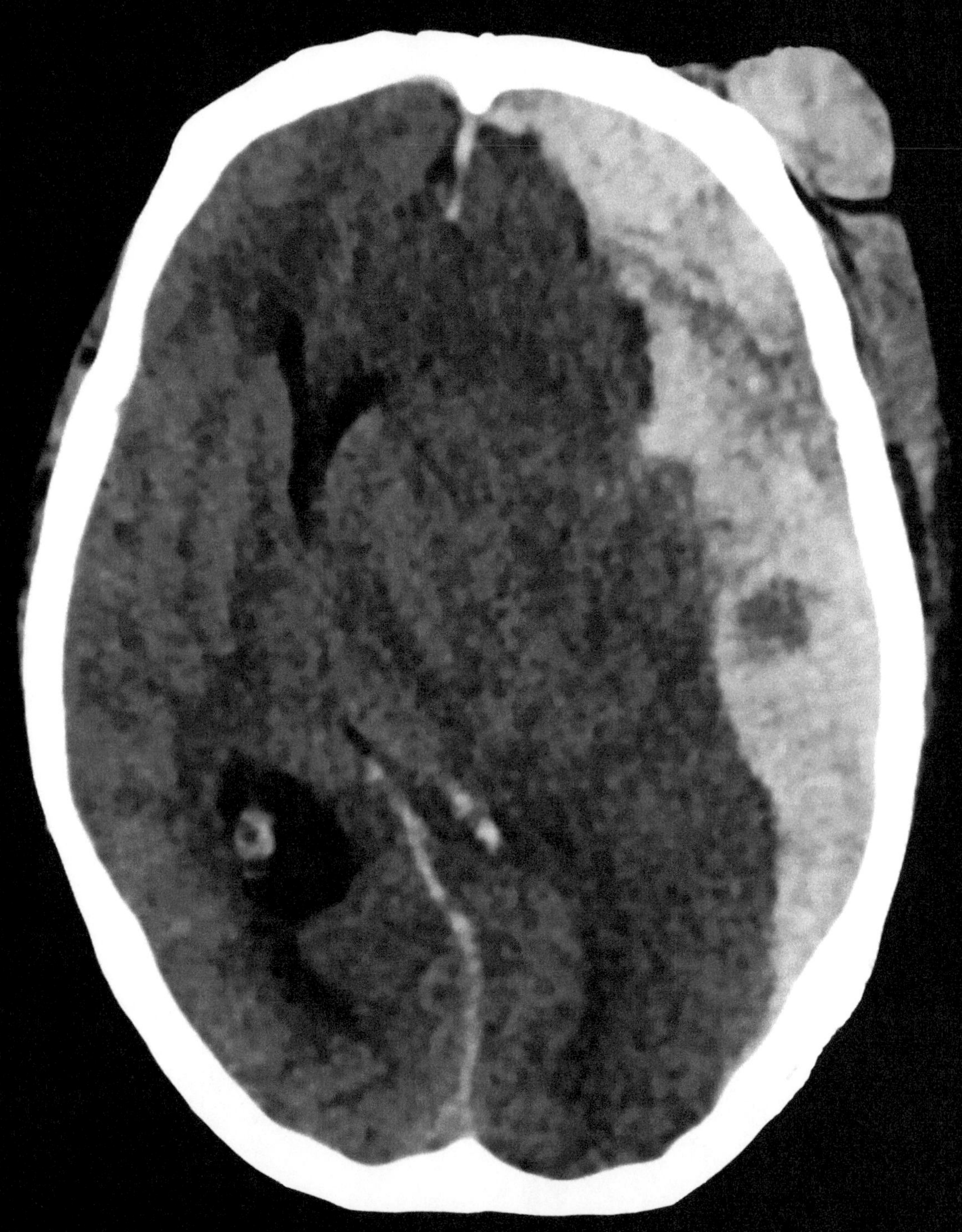

Introduction

Welcome to *Essentials of Osborn's Brain*! When I wrote the first edition of *Osborn's Brain* in 2013, it was written as a curriculum in neuroradiology with the "must know—now!" topics, such as brain trauma, strokes, and hemorrhage covered in the first few chapters of the text. At nearly 1,300 pages, the 2018 updated second edition was a comprehensive and very detailed delineation of brain pathology and imaging...more than even the most dedicated residents and fellows could absorb.

Hence the idea to edit and consolidate the most important concepts of *Osborn's Brain*, second edition into a shorter, more "digestible" text aimed at residents and fellows in radiology, neurology, and neurosurgery. We have constructed a year-by-year (or rotation-by-rotation) study guide that takes a trainee through the essentials but also enhances learning with complementary assignments from STATdx and RadPrimer, invaluable resources that are available through many institutional training programs. We've also scoured the web for free, universally accessible programs that supplement reading assignments and provide active links to the websites.

So let me be your guide to exploring the wonderful, fascinating world of brain anatomy, pathology, and imaging.

Anne G. Osborn, MD, FACR
University Distinguished Professor and Professor of Radiology and Imaging Sciences
William H. and Patricia W. Child Presidential Endowed Chair in Radiology
University of Utah School of Medicine
Salt Lake City, Utah

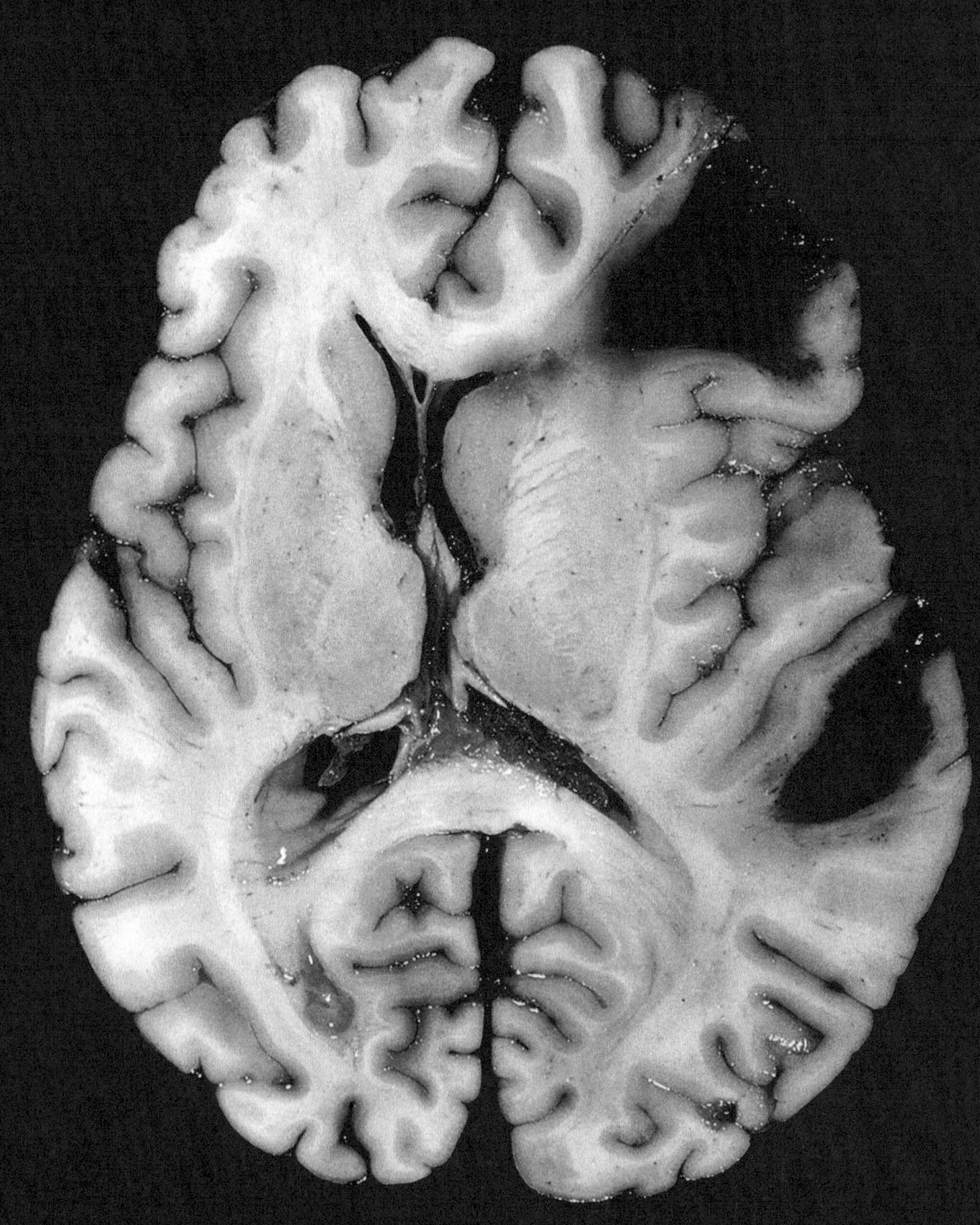

Image Contributors

AFIP Archives
D. P. Agamanolis, MD
N. Agarwal, MD
J. Ardyn, MD
M. Ayadi, MD
S. Aydin, MD
D. Bertholdo, MD
S. Blaser, MD
J. Boxerman, MD
M. Brant-Zawadski, MD
P. Burger, MD
S. Candy, MD
M. Castillo, MD
P. Chapman, MD
L. Chimelli, MD
S. Chung, MD
M. Colombo, MD
J. Comstock, MD
J. Curé, MD
B. Czerniak, MD
A. Datir, MD
B. N. Delman, MD
B. K. DeMasters, MD
K. Digre, MD
H. D. Dorfman, MD
M. Edwards-Brown, MD
D. Ellison, MD
H. Els, MD
A. Ersen, MD
W. Fang, MD
N. Foster, MD
C. E. Fuller, MD
S. Galetta, MD
C. Glastonbury, MBBS
S. Harder, MD
H. R. Harnsberger, MD
B. Hart, MD
E. T. Hedley-White, MD
G. Hedlund, DO
R. Hewlett, MD
P. Hildenbrand, MD
C. Y. Ho, MD
B. Horten, MD
C. Hsu, MD
M. Huckman, MD
P. Hudgins, MD
A. Illner, MD
B. Jones, MD
J. A. Junker, MD
E. C. Klatt, MD
D. Kremens, MD
W. Kucharczyk, MD
P. Lasjaunias, MD
S. Lincoff, MD
T. Markel, MD
M. Martin, MD
A. Maydell, MD
S. McNally, MD
T. Mentzel, MD
C. Merrow, MD
M. Michel, MD
K. Moore, MD
S. Nagi, MD
T. P. Naidich, MD
N. Nakase, MD
S. Narendra, MD
K. Nelson, MD
R. Nguyen, MD
G. P. Nielsen, MD
M. Nielsen, MS
K. K. Oguz, MD
J. P. O'Malley, MD
N. Omar, MD
J. Paltan, MD
G. Parker, MD
T. Poussaint, MD
R. Ramakantan, MD
C. Rambaud, MD
M. L. Rivera-Zengotita, MD
C. Robson, MBChB
F. J. Rodriguez, MD
P. Rodriguez, MD
A. Rosenberg, MD
E. Ross, MD
A. Rossi, MD
L. Rourke, MD
Rubinstein Collection, AFIP Archives
E. Rushing, MD
M. Sage, MD
B. Scheithauer, MD
P. Shannon, MD
A. Sillag, MD
E. T. Tali, MD
M. Thurnher, MD
T. Tihan, MD
K. Tong, MD
J. Townsend, MD
U. of Utah Dept. of Dermatology
S. van der Westhuizen, MD
M. Warmuth-Metz, MD
T. Winters, MD
A. T. Yachnis, MD
S. Yashar, MD

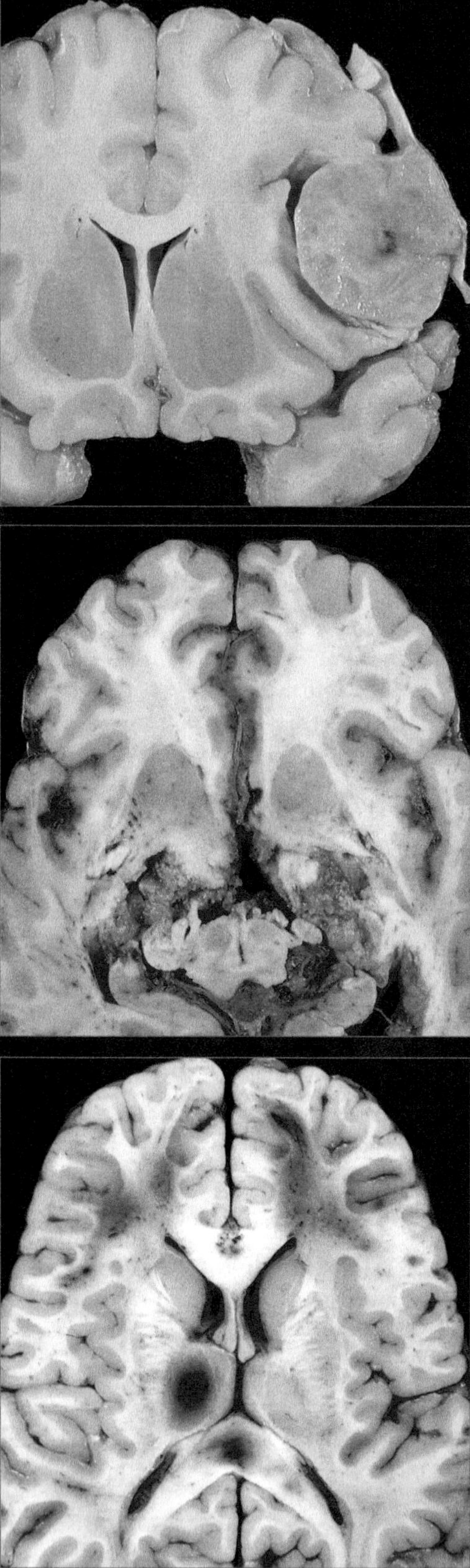

Acknowledgments

EDITOR IN CHIEF

Rebecca L. Bluth, BA

TEXT EDITORS

Arthur G. Gelsinger, MA
Nina I. Bennett, BA
Terry W. Ferrell, MS
Megg Morin, BA

IMAGE EDITORS

Jeffrey J. Marmorstone, BS
Lisa A. M. Steadman, BS

ILLUSTRATIONS

Richard Coombs, MS
Lane R. Bennion, MS
Laura C. Wissler, MA

ART DIRECTION AND DESIGN

Tom M. Olson, BA

PRODUCTION COORDINATORS

Emily C. Fassett, BA
John Pecorelli, BS

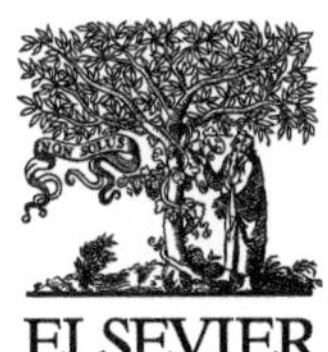

ELSEVIER

Table of Contents

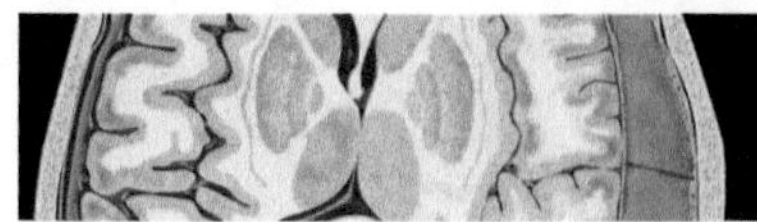

Section 1:

Trauma

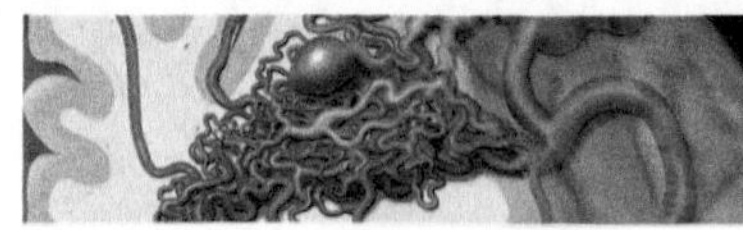

Section 2:

Nontraumatic Hemorrhage and Vascular Lesions

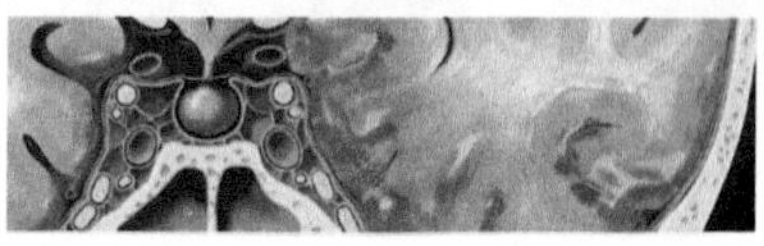

Section 3:

Infection, Inflammation, and Demyelinating Diseases

Table of Contents

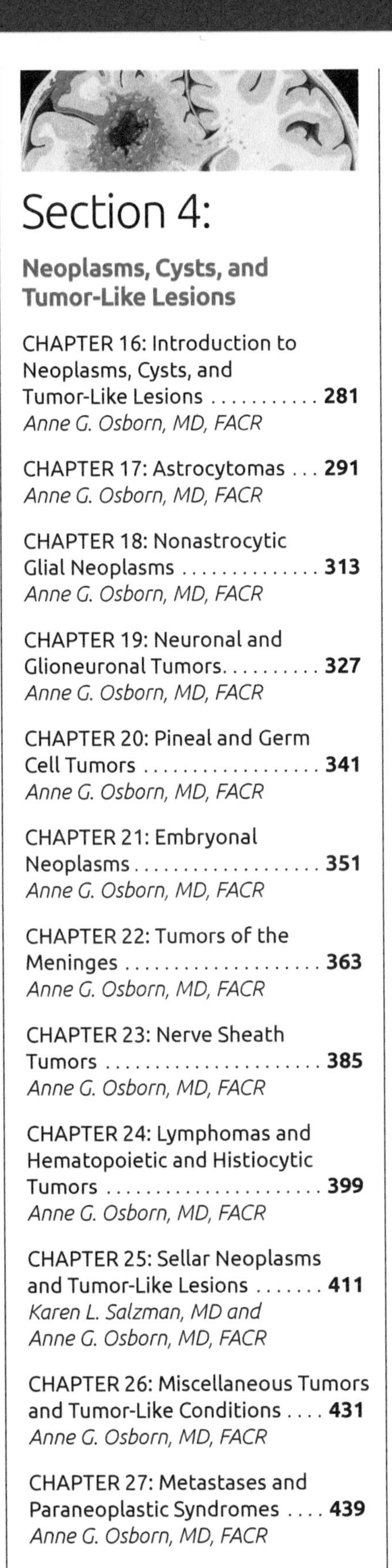

Section 4:

Neoplasms, Cysts, and Tumor-Like Lesions

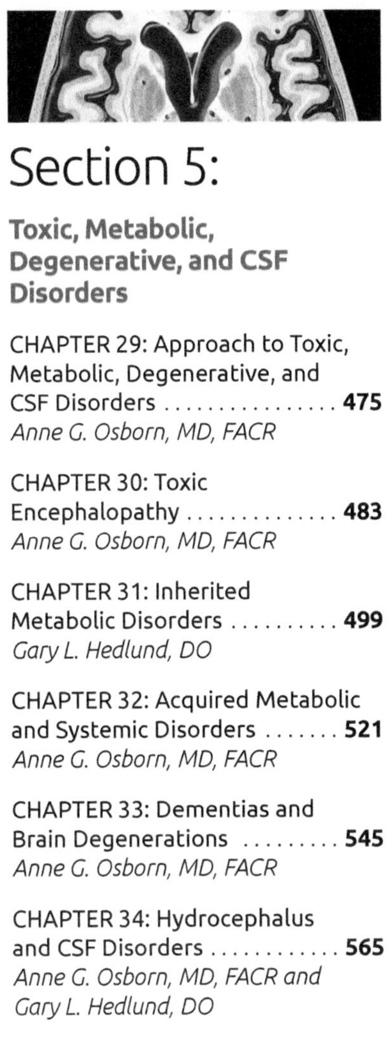

Section 5:

Toxic, Metabolic, Degenerative, and CSF Disorders

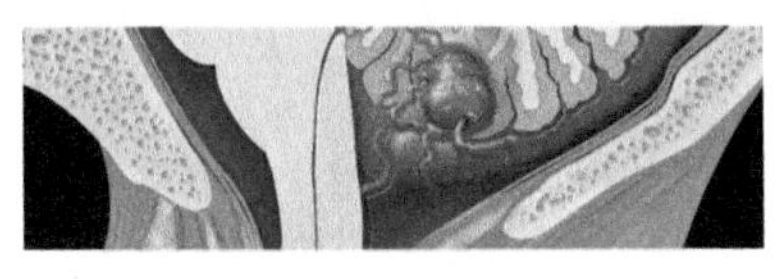

Section 6:

Congenital Malformations of the Skull and Brain

ESSENTIALS OF Osborn's Brain

A Fundamental Guide for Residents and Fellows

Anne G. Osborn

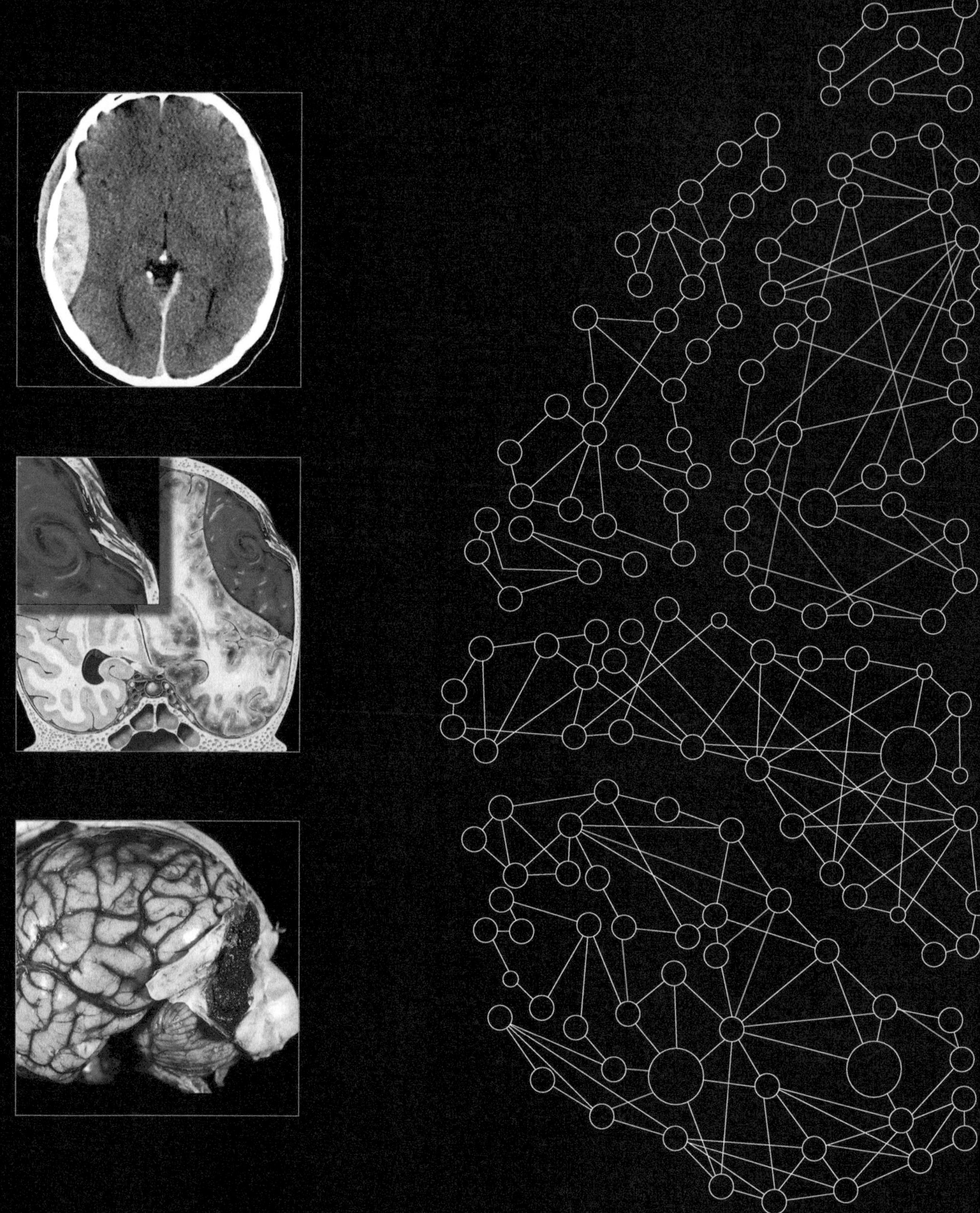

Section 1

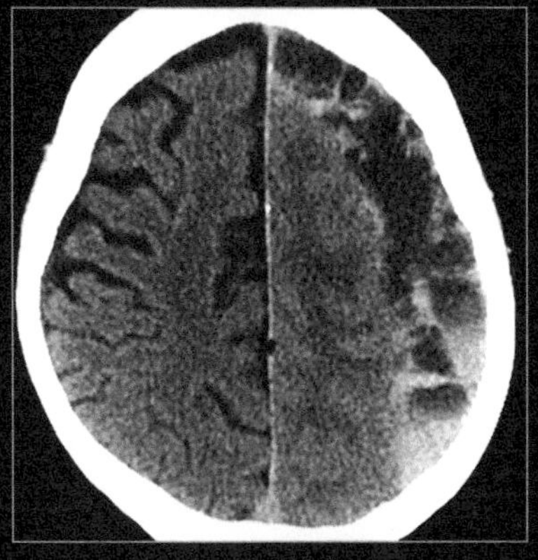

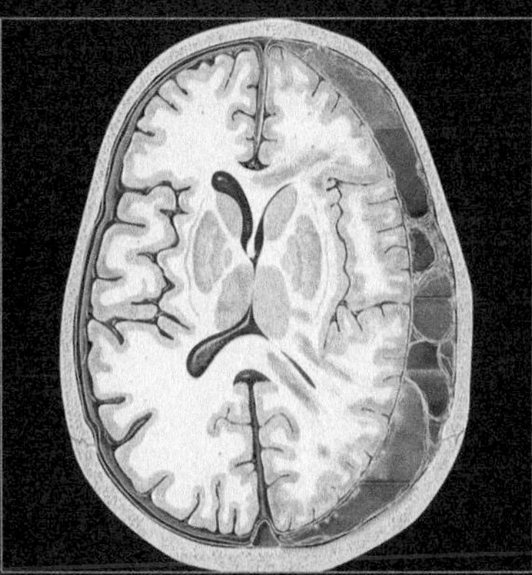

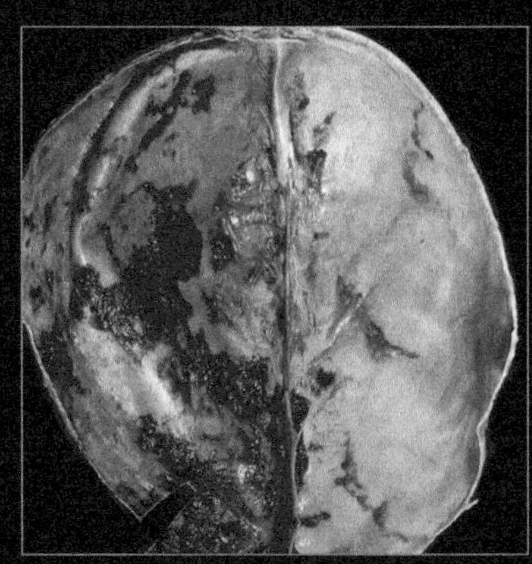

Section 1

Trauma

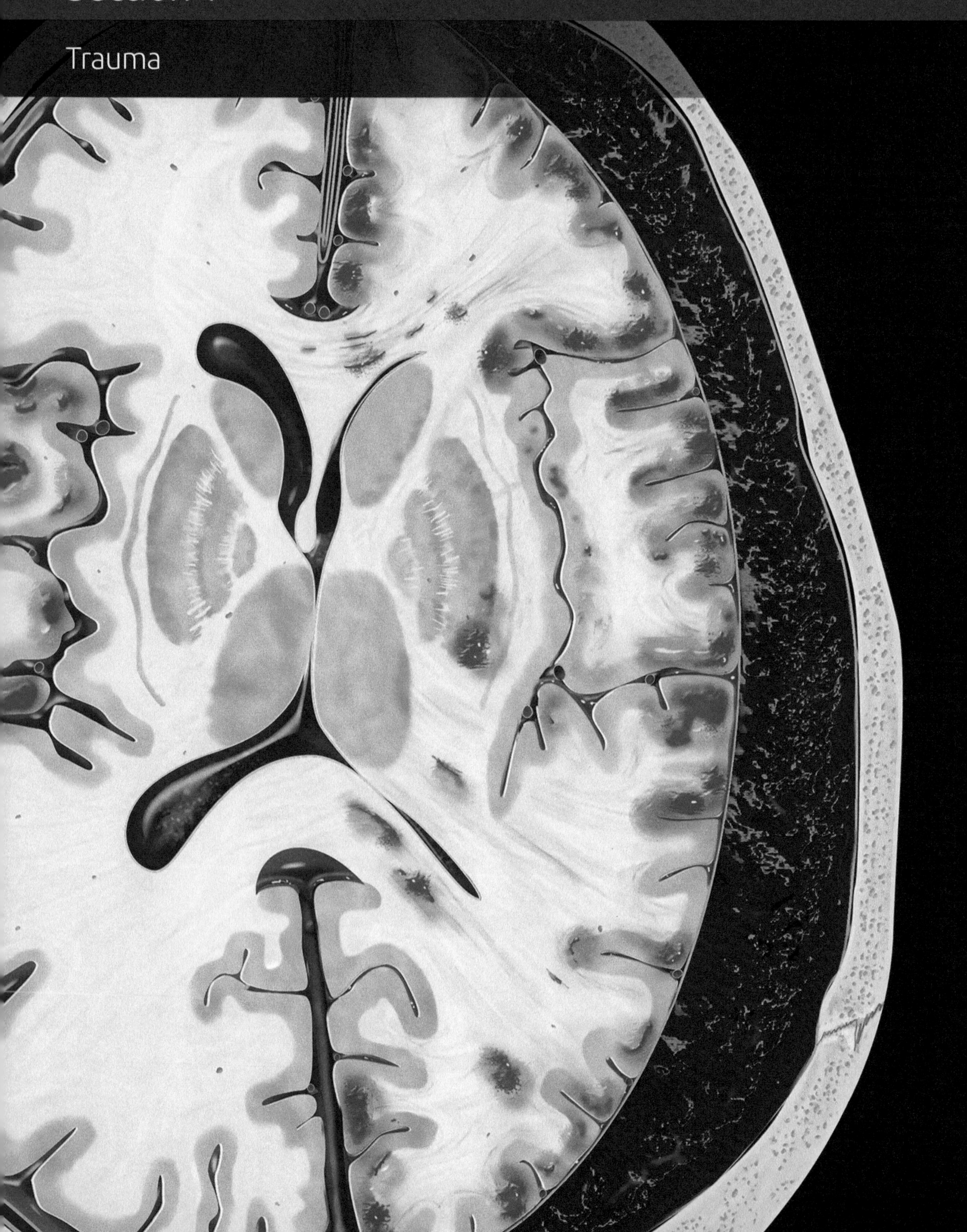

Trauma Overview

Trauma is one of the most frequent indications for emergent neuroimaging. Because imaging plays such a key role in patient triage and management, we begin this book by discussing skull and brain trauma.

We start with a brief consideration of epidemiology. Traumatic brain injury (TBI) is a critical public health and socioeconomic problem throughout the world. The direct medical costs of caring for acutely traumatized patients are huge. The indirect costs of lost productivity and long-term care for TBI survivors are even larger than the short-term direct costs.

We then briefly discuss the etiology and mechanisms of head trauma. Understanding the different ways in which the skull and brain can be injured provides the context for understanding the spectrum of findings that can be identified on imaging studies.

Introduction

Epidemiology of Head Trauma

At least 10 million people worldwide sustain TBI each year. Approximately 10% sustain fatal brain injury. Lifelong disability is common in those who survive. Between 5% and 10% of TBI survivors have serious permanent neurologic deficits, and an additional 20-40% have moderate disability. Even more have subtle deficits ("minimal brain trauma").

Etiology and Mechanisms of Injury

Trauma can be caused by missile or nonmissile injury. Nonmissile closed head injury (CHI) is a much more common cause of neurotrauma than missile injury. Falls have now surpassed road traffic incidents as the leading cause of TBI.

So-called "ground-level falls" (GLFs) are a common indication for neuroimaging in young children and older adults. In such cases, brain injury can be significant. With a GLF, a six-foot-tall adult's head impacts the ground at 20 MPH. Anticoagulated older adults are especially at risk for intracranial hemorrhages, even with minor head trauma.

Motor vehicle collisions occurring at high speed exert significant acceleration/deceleration forces, causing the brain to move suddenly within the skull. Forcible impaction of the brain against the unyielding calvarium and hard, knife-like dura results in gyral contusion. Rotation and sudden changes in angular momentum may deform, stretch, and damage long vulnerable axons, resulting in axonal injury.

Classification of Head Trauma

The most widely used *clinical* classification of brain trauma, the Glasgow Coma Scale (GCS), depends on the assessment of three features: Best eye, verbal, and motor responses. With the use of the GCS, TBI can be designated as a mild, moderate, or severe injury.

TBI can also be divided chronologically and *pathoetiologically* into primary and secondary injury, the system used in this text. **Primary injuries** occur at the time of initial trauma. Skull fractures, epi- and subdural hematomas, contusions, axonal injury, and brain lacerations are examples of primary injuries.

Secondary injuries occur later and include cerebral edema, perfusion alterations, brain herniations, and CSF leaks. Although vascular injury can be immediate (blunt impact) or secondary (vessel laceration from fractures, occlusion secondary to brain herniation), for purposes of discussion, it is included in the chapter on secondary injuries.

CLASSIFICATION OF HEAD TRAUMA

Primary Effects

- Scalp and skull injuries
- Extraaxial hemorrhage/hematomas
- Parenchymal injuries
- Miscellaneous injuries

Secondary Effects

- Herniation syndromes
- Cerebral edema
- Cerebral ischemia
- Vascular injury (can be primary or secondary)

Imaging Acute Head Trauma

Imaging is absolutely critical to the diagnosis and management of the patient with acute TBI. The goal of emergent neuroimaging is twofold: (1) Identify treatable injuries, especially emergent ones, and (2) detect and delineate the presence of secondary injuries, such as herniation syndromes and vascular injury.

How To Image

NECT

CT is now accepted as the "workhorse" screening tool for imaging acute head trauma. The reasons are simple: CT depicts both bone and soft tissue injuries. It is also widely accessible, fast, effective, and comparatively inexpensive.

Nonenhanced CT (NECT) scans (4 or 5 mm thick) from just below the foramen magnum through the vertex should be performed. Two sets of images should be obtained: One using brain and one with bone reconstruction algorithms. Viewing the brain images with a wider window width (150-200 HU, the so-called "subdural window") should be performed on PACS. The scout view should always be displayed as part of the study.

MDCT is now routine in trauma triage. Coronal and sagittal reformatted images using the axial source data improve the detection rate of acute traumatic subdural hematomas.

Three-dimensional shaded surface displays are helpful in depicting skull and facial fractures. If facial bone CT is also requested, a single MDCT acquisition can be obtained without overlapping radiation exposure to the eye and lower 1/2 of the brain.

Head trauma patients with acute intracranial lesions on CT have a higher risk for cervical spine fractures compared with patients with a CT-negative head injury. Because up to 1/3 of patients with moderate to severe head injury as determined by the GCS have concomitant spine injury, MDCT of the cervical spine is often obtained together with brain imaging. Soft tissue and bone algorithm reconstructions with multiplanar reformatted images of the cervical spine should be obtained.

CTA

CT angiography (CTA) is often obtained as part of a whole-body trauma CT protocol. Craniocervical CTA should also specifically be considered (1) in the setting of penetrating neck injury, (2) if a fractured foramen transversarium or facet subluxation is identified on cervical spine CT, or (3) if a skull base fracture traverses the carotid canal or a dural venous sinus. Arterial laceration or dissection, traumatic pseudoaneurysm, carotid-cavernous fistula, or dural venous sinus injury are nicely depicted on high-resolution CTA.

MR

Although MR can detect traumatic complications without radiation and is more sensitive for abnormalities, such as contusions and axonal injuries, there is general agreement that NECT is the procedure of choice in the initial evaluation of brain trauma. Limitations of MR include acquisition time, access, patient monitoring and instability, motion degradation of images, and cost.

With one important exception—suspected child abuse—using MR as a routine screening procedure in the setting of *acute* brain trauma is uncommon. Standard MR together with susceptibility-weighted imaging and DTI is most useful in the subacute and chronic stages of TBI. Other modalities, such as fMRI, are playing an increasingly important role in detecting subtle abnormalities, especially in patients with mild cognitive deficits following minor TBI.

Who and When To Image

Who to image and when to do it are paradoxically both well established and controversial. Patients with a GCS score indicating moderate (GCS = 9-12) or severe (GCS ≤ 8) neurologic impairment are invariably imaged. The real debate is about how best to manage patients with GCS scores of 13-15. In places with high malpractice rates, many emergency

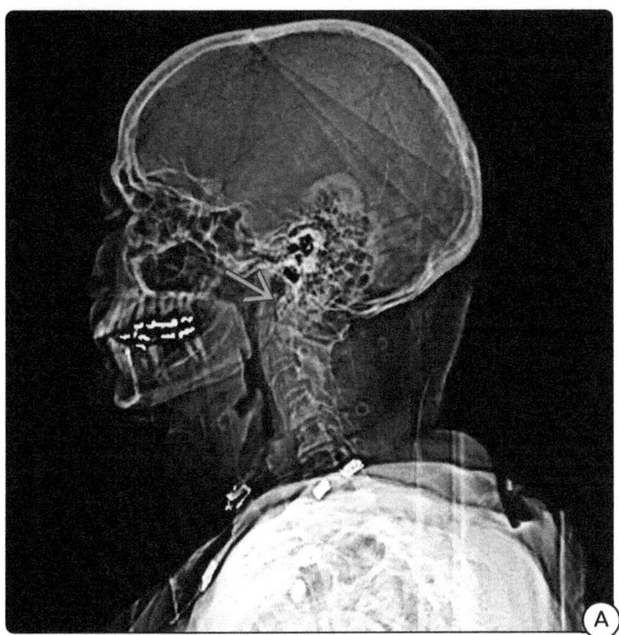

(1-1A) Scout view in a 66-year-old woman with a CT head requested to evaluate ground-level fall shows a posteriorly angulated C1-odontoid complex ⇒.

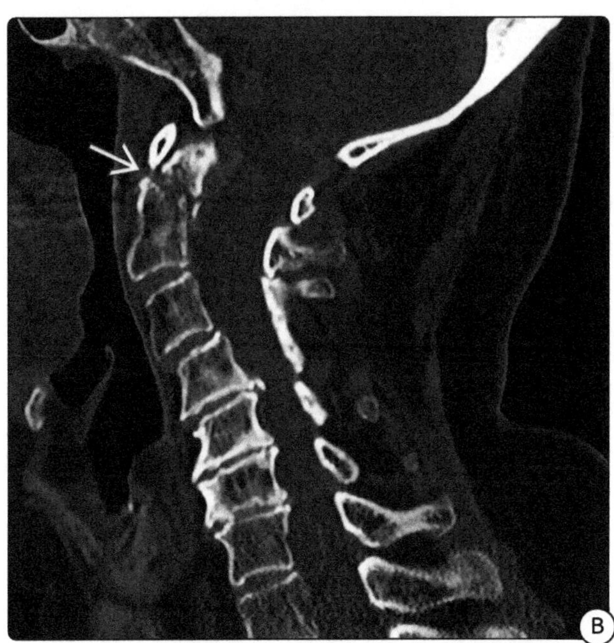

(1-1B) Head CT in the same case (not shown) was normal. Cervical spine CT was then performed. The sagittal image reformatted from the axial scan data shows a comminuted, posteriorly angulated dens fracture ➡.

physicians routinely order NECT scans on every patient with head trauma regardless of GCS score or clinical findings.

GLASGOW COMA SCALE

Best Eye Response (Maximum = 4)
- 1 = no eye opening
- 2 = eye opening to pain
- 3 = eyes open to verbal command
- 4 = eyes open spontaneously

Best Verbal Response (Maximum = 5)
- 1 = none
- 2 = incomprehensible sounds
- 3 = inappropriate words
- 4 = confused
- 5 = oriented

Best Motor Response (Maximum = 6)
- 1 = none
- 2 = extension to pain
- 3 = flexion to pain
- 4 = withdrawal to pain
- 5 = localizing to pain
- 6 = obedience to commands

Sum = "Coma Score" and Clinical Grading
- 13-15 = mild brain injury
- 9-12 = moderate brain injury
- ≤ 8 = severe brain injury

Trauma Imaging: Keys to Analysis

Four components are essential to the accurate interpretation of CT scans in patients with head injury: The scout image plus brain, bone, and subdural views of the NECT dataset. Critical information may be present on just one of these four components.

Suggestions on how to analyze NECT images in patients with acute head injury are delineated below.

Scout Image

Before you look at the NECT scan, examine the digital scout image! Look for cervical spine abnormalities, such as fractures or dislocations, jaw &/or facial trauma, and the presence of foreign objects **(1-1A)**. If there is a suggestion of cervical spine fracture or malalignment, MDCT of the cervical spine should be performed before the patient is removed from the scanner **(1-1B)**.

Brain Windows

Methodically and meticulously work your way from the outside in. First, evaluate the soft tissue images, beginning with the scalp. Look for scalp swelling, which usually indicates the impact point. Carefully examine the periorbital soft tissues.

Next, look for extraaxial blood. The most common extraaxial hemorrhage is traumatic subarachnoid hemorrhage (tSAH) followed by sub- and epidural hematomas. The prevalence of

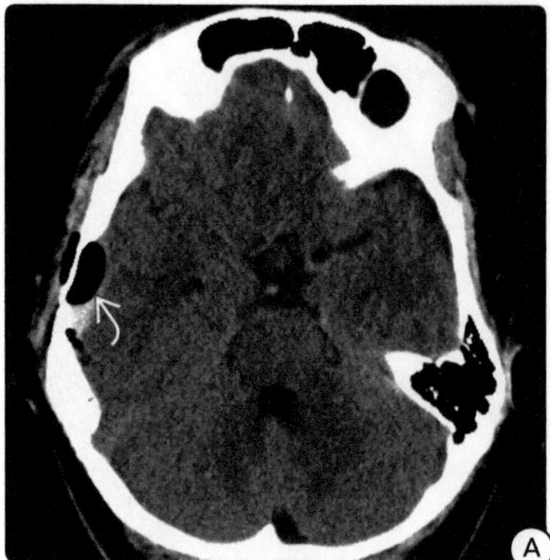

(1-2A) Axial NECT in an 18-year-old man who fell off his skateboard shows a small right epidural hematoma that also contains air ➡.

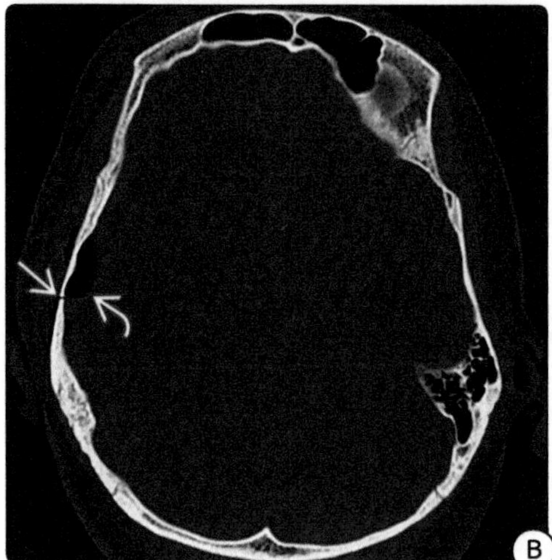

(1-2B) Bone algorithm reconstruction shows a nondisplaced linear fracture ➡ adjacent to the epidural blood and air ➡.

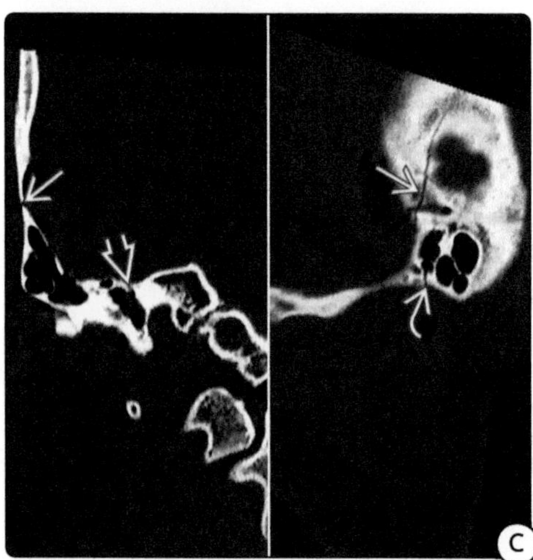

(1-2C) Reconstructed coronal (L) and sagittal (R) bone CTs show the fracture ➡ comminuted and crosses the mastoid ➡ and middle ear ➡.

tSAH in moderate to severe TBI approaches 100%. tSAH is usually found in the sulci adjacent to cortical contusions, along the sylvian fissures, and around the anteroinferior frontal and temporal lobes. The best place to look for subtle tSAH is the interpeduncular cistern, where blood collects when the patient is supine.

Any hypodensity within an extraaxial collection should raise suspicion of rapid hemorrhage with accumulation of unclotted blood or (especially in alcoholics or older patients) an underlying coagulopathy. This is an urgent finding that mandates immediate notification of the responsible clinician.

Look for intracranial air ("pneumocephalus"). Intracranial air is always abnormal and indicates the presence of a fracture that traverses either the paranasal sinuses or mastoid.

Now, move on to the brain itself. Carefully examine the cortex, especially the "high-yield" areas for cortical contusions (anteroinferior frontal and temporal lobes). If there is a scalp hematoma due to impact (a "coup" injury), look 180° in the opposite direction for a classic "contre-coup" injury. Hypodense areas around the hyperdense hemorrhagic foci indicate early edema and severe contusion.

Move inward from the cortex to the subcortical white and deep gray matter. Petechial hemorrhages often accompany axonal injury. If you see subcortical hemorrhages on the initial NECT scan, this is merely the "tip of the iceberg." There is usually *a lot* more damage than what is apparent on the first scan. A general rule: The deeper the lesion, the more severe the injury.

Finally, look inside the ventricles for blood-CSF levels and hemorrhage due to choroid plexus shearing injury.

Subdural Windows

Look at the soft tissue image with both narrow ("brain") and intermediate ("subdural") windows. Small, subtle subdural hematomas can sometimes be overlooked on standard narrow window widths (75-100 HU) yet are readily apparent when wider windows (150-200 HU) are used.

Bone CT

Bone CT refers to bone algorithm reconstruction viewed with wide (bone) windows. If you cannot do bone algorithm reconstruction from your dataset, widen the windows and use an edge-enhancement feature to sharpen the image. Three-dimensional shaded surface displays (3D SSDs) are especially helpful in depicting complex or subtle fractures **(1-2)**.

Even though standard head scans are 4-5 mm thick, it is often possible to detect fractures on bone CT. Look for basisphenoid fractures with involvement of the carotid canal, temporal bone fractures (with or without ossicular dislocation), mandibular dislocation ("empty" condylar fossa), and calvarial fractures. Remember: Nondisplaced linear skull fractures that do not cross vascular structures (such as a dural venous sinus or middle meningeal artery) are in and of themselves basically meaningless. The brain and blood vessels are what matter!

The most difficult dilemma is deciding whether an observed lucency is a fracture or a normal structure (e.g., suture line or vascular channel). Keep in mind: It is virtually unheard of for a calvarial fracture to occur in the absence of overlying soft tissue injury. If there is no scalp "bump," it is unlikely that the lucency represents a nondisplaced linear fracture.

Bone CT images are also very helpful in distinguishing low density from air vs. fat. Although most PACS stations have a region of interest (ROI) function that can measure attenuation, fat fades away on bone CT images, and air remains very hypodense.

CTA

CTA is generally indicated if (1) basilar skull fractures cross the carotid canal or a dural venous sinus **(1-3)**; (2) if a cervical spine fracture-dislocation is present, especially if the transverse foramina are involved; or (3) if the patient has stroke-like symptoms or unexplained clinical deterioration. Both the cervical and intracranial vasculature should be visualized.

Although it is important to scrutinize both the arterial and venous sides of the circulation, a CTA is generally sufficient. Standard CTAs typically show both the arteries and the dural venous sinuses well, whereas a CT venogram (CTV) often misses the arterial phase.

Examine the source images as well as the multiplanar reconstructions and maximum-intensity projection (MIP) reformatted scans. Traumatic dissection, vessel lacerations, intimal flaps, pseudoaneurysms, carotid-cavernous fistulas, and dural sinus occlusions can generally be identified on CTA.

HEAD TRAUMA: CT CHECKLIST

Scout Image
- Evaluate for
  - Cervical spine fracture-dislocation
  - Jaw dislocation, facial fractures
  - Foreign object

Brain Windows
- Scalp swelling (impact point)
- Extraaxial blood (focal hypodensity in clot suggests rapid bleeding)
  - Epidural hematoma
  - Subdural hematoma (SDH)
  - tSAH
- Pneumocephalus
- Cortical contusion
  - Anteroinferior frontal, temporal lobes
  - Opposite scalp laceration/skull fracture
- Hemorrhagic axonal injury
- Intraventricular hemorrhage

Subdural Windows
- 150-200 HU (for thin SDHs under skull)

Bone CT
- Bone algorithm reconstruction > bone windows
- Do any fractures cross a vascular channel?

Selected References: The complete reference list is available on the Expert Consult™ eBook version included with purchase.

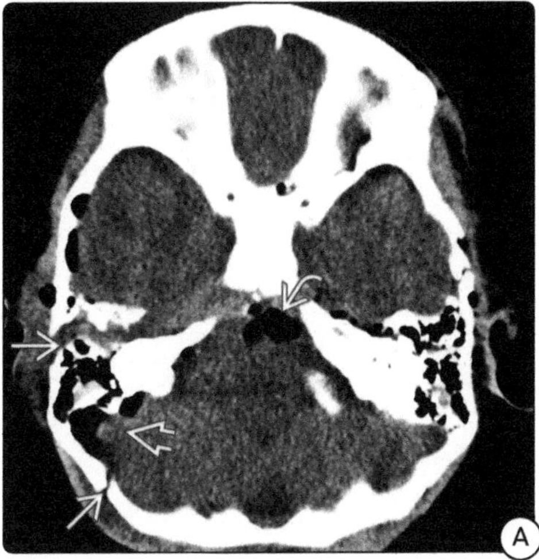

***(1-3A)** NECT shows pneumocephalus ➚, base of skull fractures ➡ adjacent to air, which seems to outline a displaced sigmoid sinus ➡.*

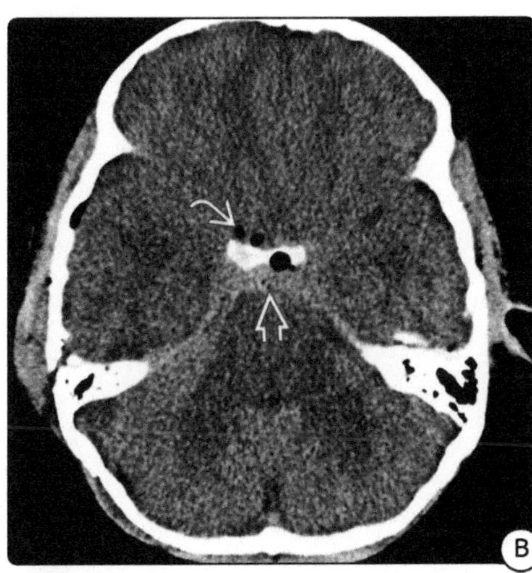

***(1-3B)** NECT in the same case shows diffuse brain swelling, pneumocephalus ➚, and traumatic subarachnoid hemorrhage ➡.*

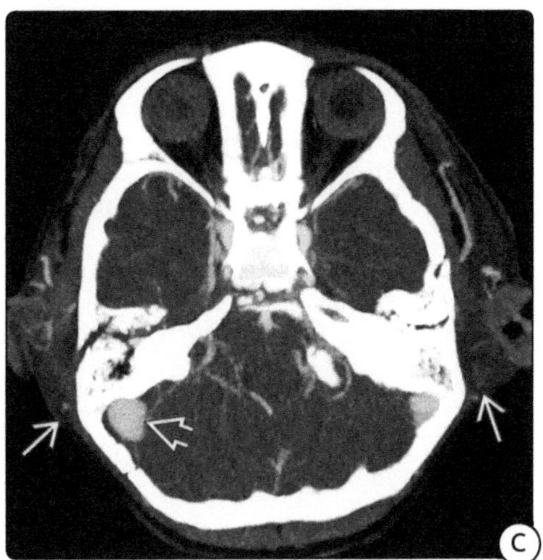

***(1-3C)** CTA in the same case shows that the sigmoid sinus ➡ is intact but displaced medially. Note rapidly enlarging subgaleal hematoma ➡.*

Primary Effects of CNS Trauma

Primary head injuries are defined as those that occur at the time of initial trauma, even though they may not be immediately apparent on initial evaluation.

Head injury can be caused by direct or indirect trauma. **Direct trauma** involves a blow to the head and is usually caused by automobile collisions, falls, or injury inflicted by an object, such as a hammer or baseball bat. Scalp lacerations, hematomas, and skull fractures are common. Associated intracranial damage ranges from none to severe.

Significant forces of acceleration/deceleration, linear translation, and rotational loading can be applied to the brain *without* direct head blows. Such **indirect trauma** is caused by angular kinematics and typically occurs in high-speed motor vehicle collisions (MVCs). Here, the brain undergoes rapid deformation and distortion. Depending on the site and direction of the force applied, significant injury to the cortex, axons, penetrating blood vessels, and deep gray nuclei may occur. Severe brain injury can occur in the absence of skull fractures or visible scalp lesions.

We begin our discussion with a consideration of scalp and skull lesions as we work our way from the outside to the inside of the skull. We then delineate the spectrum of intracranial trauma, starting with extraaxial hemorrhages. We conclude this chapter with a detailed discussion of injuries to the brain parenchyma (e.g., cortical contusion, diffuse axonal injury, and the serious deep subcortical injuries).

Scalp and Skull Injuries

Scalp and skull injuries are common manifestations of cranial trauma. Although brain injury is usually the most immediate concern in managing traumatized patients, superficial lesions, such as scalp swelling and focal hematoma, can be helpful in identifying the location of direct head trauma. On occasion, these initially innocent-appearing "lumps and bumps" can become life threatening. Before turning our attention to intracranial traumatic lesions, we therefore briefly review scalp and skull injuries, delineating their typical imaging findings and clinical significance.

Scalp Injuries

Scalp injuries include lacerations and hematomas. Scalp **lacerations** can occur in both penetrating and closed head injuries. Lacerations may extend partially or entirely through all five layers of the scalp (skin, subcutaneous fibrofatty tissue, galea aponeurotica, loose areolar connective tissue, and periosteum) to the skull **(2-1)**.

Focal discontinuity, soft tissue swelling, and subcutaneous air are commonly identified in scalp lacerations. Scalp lacerations should be carefully evaluated for the presence of any foreign bodies. If not removed during wound debridement, foreign bodies can be a potential source of substantial morbidity and are very important to identify on initial imaging studies. Wood fragments are often hypodense, whereas leaded glass, gravel, and metallic shards are variably hyperdense **(2-2)**.

Scalp lacerations may or may not be associated with scalp **hematomas**. There are two distinctly different types of scalp hematomas: Cephalohematomas and subgaleal hematomas. The former are usually of no clinical significance, whereas the latter can cause hypovolemia and hypotension.

Cephalohematomas are *subperiosteal* blood collections that lie in the potential space between the outer surface of the calvarium and the pericranium, which serves as the periosteum of the skull **(2-3)**. The pericranium continues medially into cranial sutures and is anatomically contiguous with the outer (periosteal) layer of the dura.

Cephalohematomas are the extracranial equivalent of an intracranial epidural hematoma. Cephalohematomas do not cross suture lines and are typically unilateral. Because they are anatomically constrained by the tough fibrous periosteum and its insertions, cephalohematomas rarely attain a large size.

Cephalohematomas occur in 1% of newborns and are more common following instrumented delivery. They are often diagnosed clinically but imaged only if they are unusually prominent or if intracranial injuries are suspected. NECT scans show a somewhat lens-shaped soft tissue mass that overlies a single bone (usually the parietal or occipital bone) **(2-4)**. If more than one bone is affected, the two collections are separated by the intervening suture lines.

Subgaleal hematomas are *subaponeurotic* collections and are common findings in traumatized patients of all ages. Here, blood collects under the aponeurosis (the "galea") of the occipitofrontalis muscle **(2-5)**. Because a subgaleal hematoma lies deep to the scalp muscles and galea aponeurotica but

(2-1) Coronal graphic depicts normal layers of the scalp. Skin, subcutaneous fibrofatty tissue overlie the galea aponeurotica, loose areolar connective tissue. The pericranium is the periosteum of the skull and continues into and through sutures to merge with the periosteal layer of the dura. (2-2) NECT shows scalp laceration, hyperdense foreign bodies, and subgaleal air.

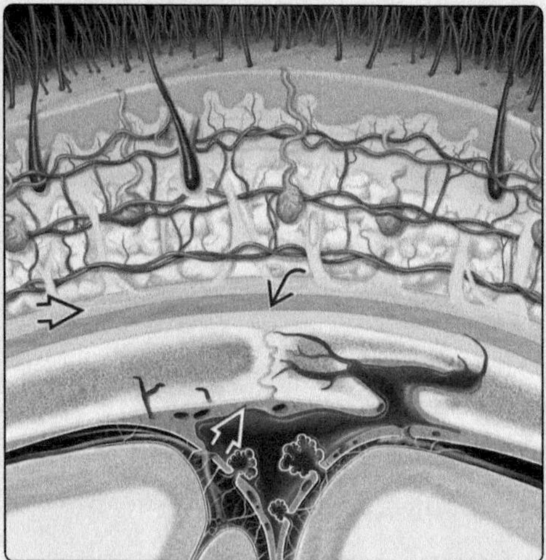

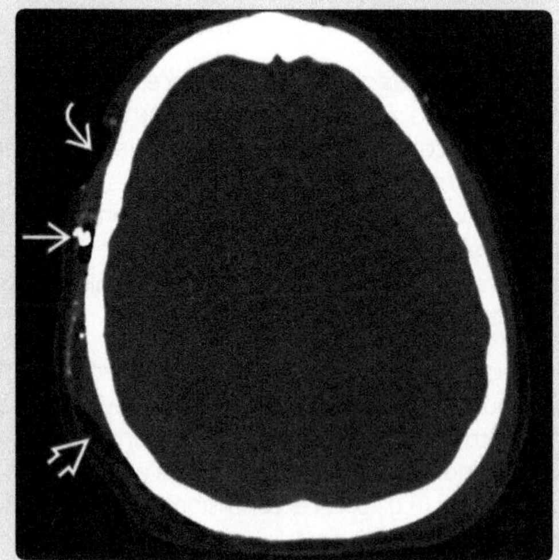

(2-3) Graphic shows the skull of a newborn, including the anterior fontanelle, coronal, metopic, sagittal sutures. Cephalohematoma is subperiosteal, limited by sutures. Subgaleal hematoma is under the scalp aponeurosis, not bounded by sutures. (2-4) NECT scan in a newborn shows a small right and a large left parietal cephalohematoma. Neither crosses the sagittal suture.

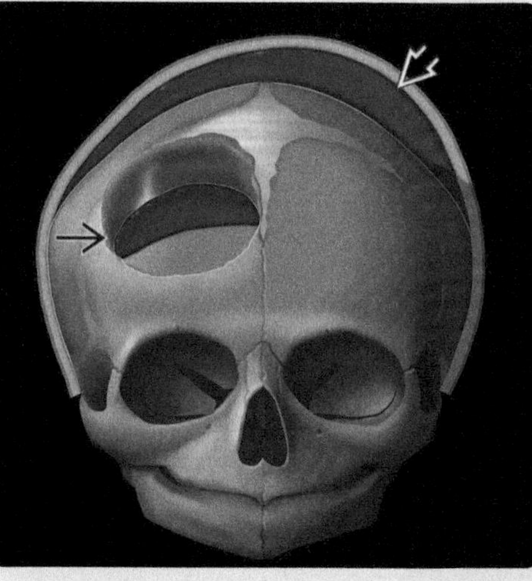

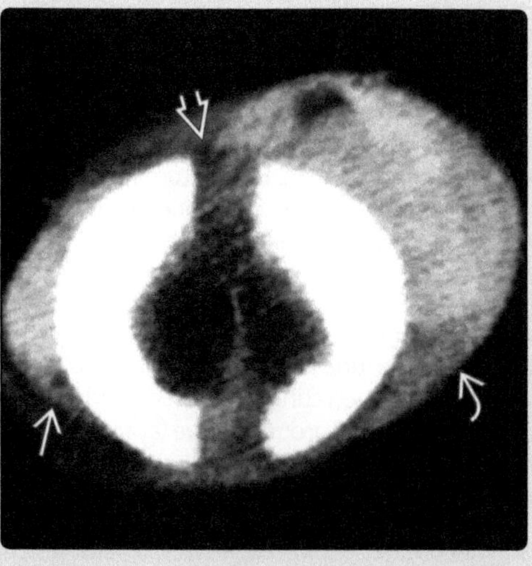

external to the periosteum, it is not anatomically limited by suture lines.

Bleeding into the subgaleal space can be very extensive. Subgaleal hematomas are usually bilateral lesions that often spread diffusely around the entire calvarium. NECT scans show a heterogeneously hyperdense crescentic scalp mass that crosses one or more suture lines **(2-6)**. In contrast to benign self-limited cephalohematomas, expanding subgaleal hematomas in infants and small children can cause significant blood loss.

Skull Fractures

Noticing a scalp "bump" or hematoma on initial imaging in head trauma is important, as calvarial fractures rarely—if ever—occur in the absence of overlying soft tissue swelling or scalp laceration. Skull fractures are present on initial CT scans in ~ 2/3 of patients with moderate head injury, although 25-35% of severely injured patients have no identifiable fracture, even with thin-section bone reconstructions.

Several types of acute skull fracture can be identified on imaging studies: Linear, depressed, and diastatic fractures **(2-7)**. Fractures can involve the calvarium, skull base, or both.

Linear Skull Fractures

A **linear skull fracture** is a sharply marginated linear defect that typically involves both the inner and outer tables of the calvarium **(2-8)**.

Most linear skull fractures are caused by relatively low-energy blunt trauma that is delivered over a relatively wide surface area. Linear skull fractures that extend into and widen a suture become diastatic fractures. When multiple complex fractures are present, 3D shaded surface display (SSD) can be very helpful in depicting their anatomy and relationships to cranial sutures.

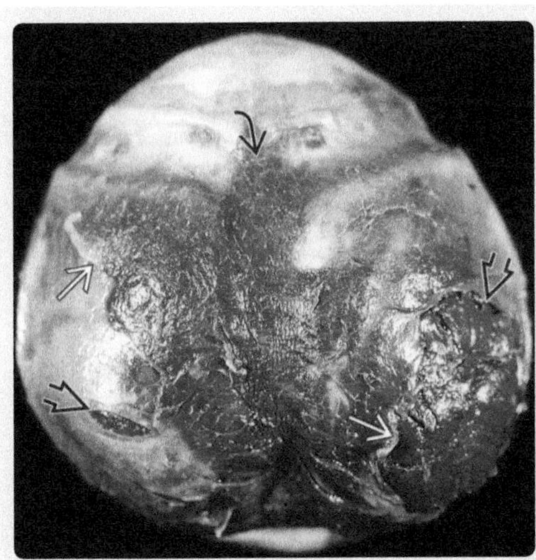

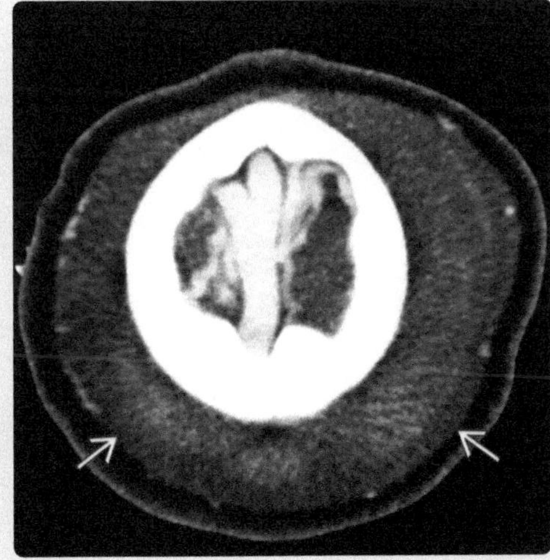

***(2-5)** Autopsy from a traumatized infant shows a massive biparietal subgaleal hematoma. The galea aponeurotica has been partially opened to show large biparietal hematoma that crosses the sagittal suture. **(2-6)** Axial CECT in 3y child shows massive subgaleal hematoma surrounding entire calvarium. Subgaleal hematomas cross sutures and can become life threatening, while cephalohematomas are anatomically limited.*

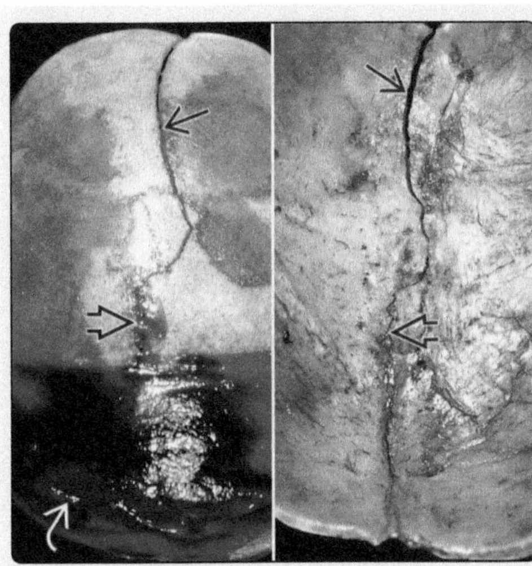

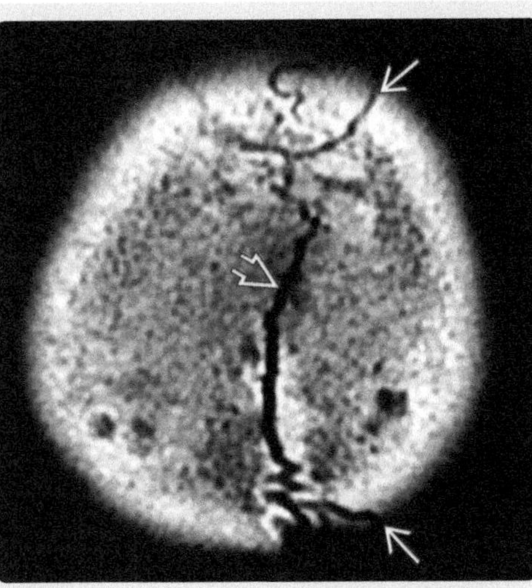

***(2-7)** Autopsied skull shows fatal trauma with exo- (L) and endocranial views (R). A linear fracture extends into the superior sagittal suture, causing diastasis and a subgaleal hematoma. **(2-8)** Bone CT through the top of the calvarium shows linear skull fractures extending into and widening the sagittal suture, causing a diastatic fracture.*

Patients with an isolated linear nondisplaced skull fracture (NDSF), no intracranial hemorrhage or pneumocephalus, normal neurologic examination, and absence of other injuries are at very low risk for delayed hemorrhage or other life-threatening complication. Hospitalization is not necessary for many children with NDSFs.

Depressed Skull Fractures

A **depressed skull fracture** is a fracture in which the fragments are displaced inward **(2-9)**. Comminution of the fracture fragments starts at the point of maximum impact and spreads centrifugally. Depressed fractures are most often caused by high-energy direct blows to a small surface with a blunt object (e.g., hammer, baseball bat, or metal pipe) **(2-10)**.

Depressed skull fractures typically tear the underlying dura and arachnoid and are often associated with cortical contusions and potential leakage of CSF into the subdural space. Fractures extending to a dural sinus or the jugular bulb are associated with venous sinus thrombosis in 40% of cases.

Diastatic Skull Fractures

A **diastatic skull fracture** is a fracture that widens ("diastases" or "splits open") a suture or synchondrosis. Diastatic skull fractures usually occur in association with a linear skull fracture that extends into an adjacent suture **(2-11)**.

Imaging

General Features. Both bone and soft tissue reconstruction algorithms should be used when evaluating patients with head injuries. Soft tissue reconstructions should be viewed with both narrow ("brain") and intermediate ("subdural") windows. Coronal and sagittal reformatted images obtained using the MDCT axial source data are helpful additions. SSDs can be useful in depicting complex and depressed fractures.

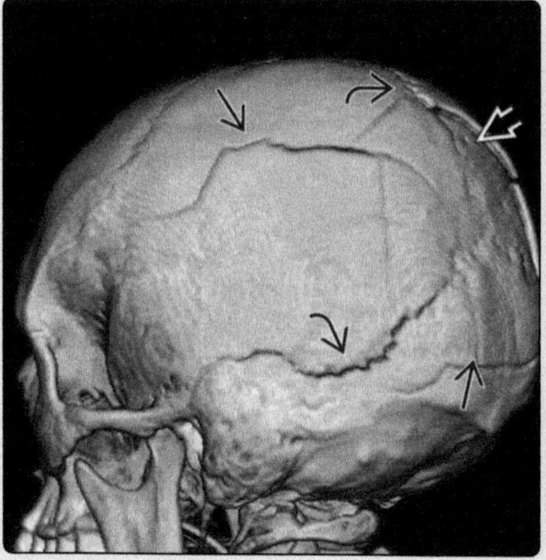

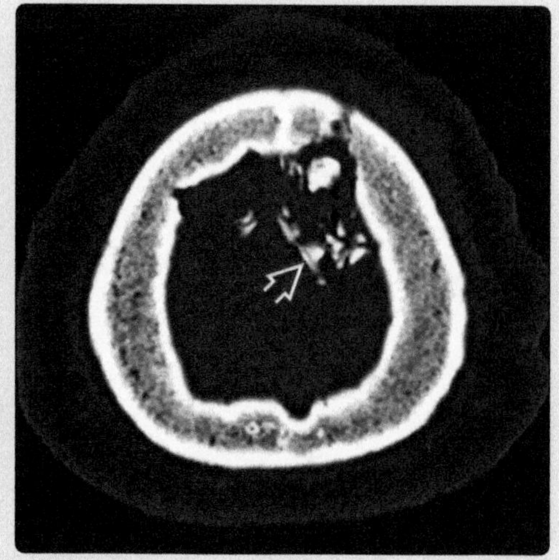

***(2-9)** 3D shaded surface display (SSD) in a patient with multiple linear ➙ and diastatic ➙ skull fractures shows utility of SSDs in depicting complex fracture anatomy. Note slight depression ➙ of the fractured parietooccipital calvarium. **(2-10)** Axial bone CT in a patient who was hit in the head with a falling ladder shows an extensively comminuted, depressed skull fracture ➙.*

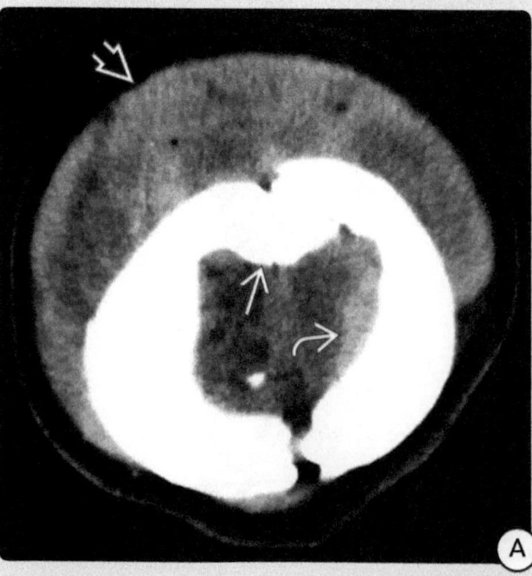

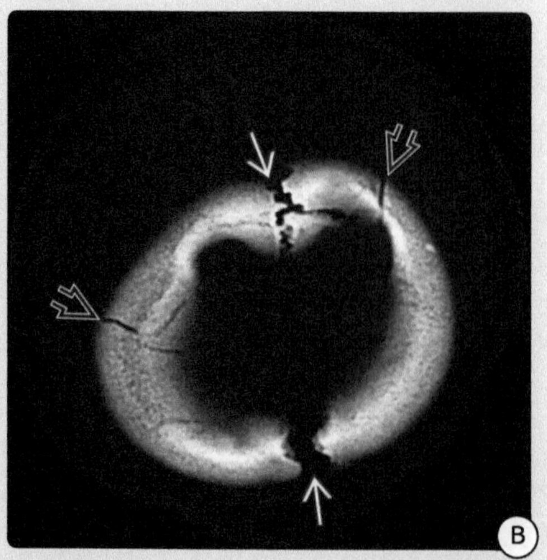

***(2-11A)** Axial NECT scan in a 20-year-old man who had a tree fall on his head shows a massive subgaleal hematoma ➙ crossing the anterior aspect of the sagittal suture ➙. A small extraaxial hematoma ➙, most likely a venous epidural hematoma (EDH), is present. **(2-11B)** Bone CT in the same case shows a diastatic fracture of the sagittal suture ➙. Nondisplaced linear fractures ➙ are also present.*

CT Findings. NECT scans demonstrate *linear* skull fractures as sharply marginated lucent lines. *Depressed* fractures are typically comminuted and show inward implosion of fracture fragments **(2-10)**. Diastatic fractures appear as widened sutures or synchondroses **(2-11)** **(2-13)** and are usually associated with linear skull fractures.

MR Findings. MR is rarely used in the setting of acute head trauma because of high cost, limited availability, and lengthy time required. Compared with CT, bone detail is poor, although parenchymal injuries are better seen. Adding T2* sequences, particularly SWI, is especially helpful in identifying hemorrhagic lesions.

Angiography. If a fracture crosses the site of a major vascular structure, such as the carotid canal or a dural venous sinus **(2-12)**, CT angiography is recommended. Sagittal, coronal, and MIP reconstructions help delineate the site and extent of vascular injuries.

Clival and skull base fractures are strongly associated with neurovascular trauma, and CTA should always be obtained in these cases **(2-13)**. Cervical fracture dislocations, distraction injuries, and penetrating neck trauma also merit further investigation. Uncomplicated asymptomatic soft tissue injuries of the neck rarely result in significant vascular injury.

SCALP AND SKULL INJURIES

Scalp Injuries
- Lacerations ± foreign bodies
- Cephalohematoma
  - Usually infants
  - Subperiosteal
  - Small, unilateral (limited by sutures)
- Subgaleal hematoma
  - Between galea, periosteum of skull
  - Circumferential, not limited by sutures
  - Can be very large, life threatening

Skull Fractures
- Linear
  - Sharp lucent line
  - Can be extensive and widespread
- Depressed
  - Focal
  - Inwardly displaced fragments
  - Often lacerates dura-arachnoid
- Diastatic
  - Typically associated with severe trauma
  - Usually caused by linear fracture that extends into suture
  - Widens, spreads apart suture or synchondrosis

Extraaxial Hemorrhages

Extraaxial hemorrhages and hematomas are common manifestations of head trauma. They can occur in any intracranial compartment, within any space (potential or actual), and between any layers of the cranial meninges. Only the subarachnoid spaces exist normally; all the other spaces are potential spaces and occur only under pathologic conditions.

Epidural hematomas (EDHs) arise between the inner table of the skull and outer (periosteal) layer of the dura. **Subdural hematomas (SDHs)** are located between the inner (meningeal) layer of the dura and the arachnoid.

***(2-12)** Autopsy shows multiple skull base fractures involving clivus, carotid canals, & jugular foramina. (E. T. Hedley-White, MD.)*

***(2-13A)** Linear, diastatic fractures of the skull base are present crossing the jugular foramen, both carotid canals.*

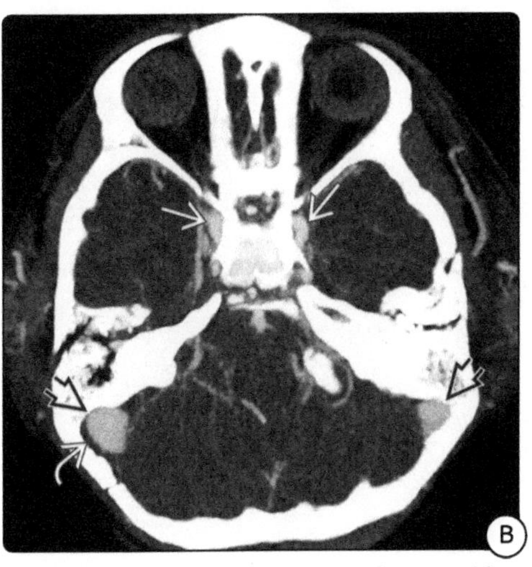

***(2-13B)** CT in the same case shows that carotid arteries and sigmoid sinuses are patent. A small right venous EDH is present.*

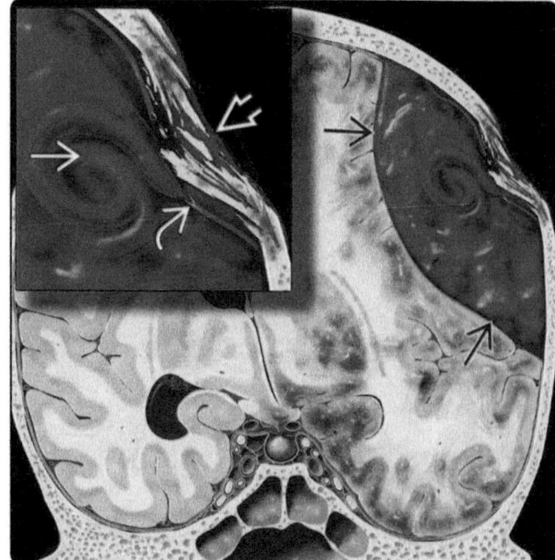

(2-14) *Graphic shows EDH ➔, depressed skull fracture ➔ lacerating middle meningeal artery ➔. Inset shows rapid bleeding, "swirl" sign ➔.*

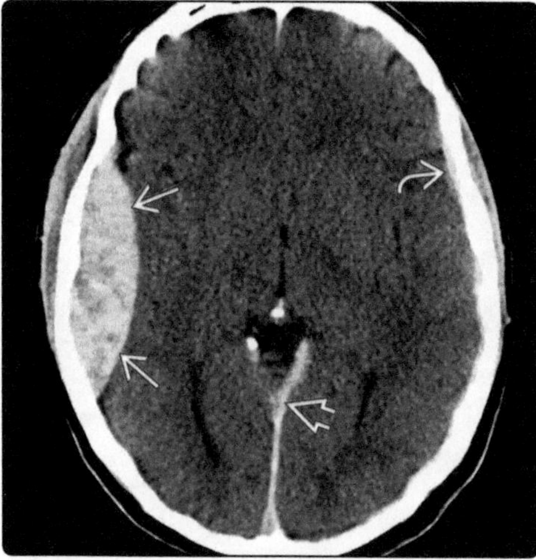

(2-15) *Biconvex aEDH ➔ is shown with a thin subdural blood collection along the tentorium, falx ➔, and left hemisphere ➔.*

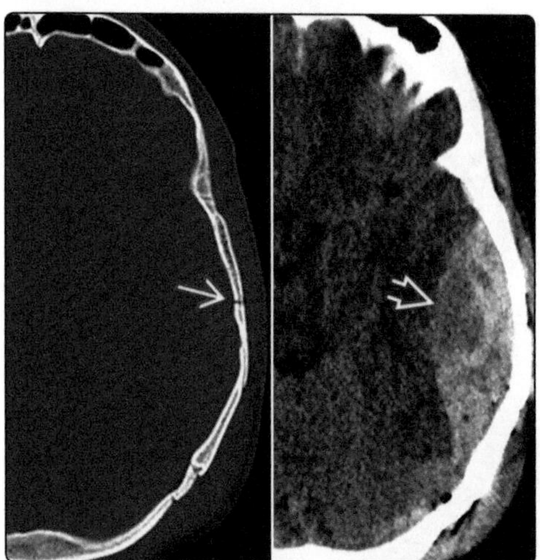

(2-16) *(L) Bone CT shows left temporal bone fracture ➔. (R) NECT shows mixed-density EDH with "swirl" sign ➔, rapid bleeding.*

Traumatic subarachnoid hemorrhage (tSAH) is found within the sulci and subarachnoid cisterns, between the arachnoid and the pia.

To discuss extraaxial hemorrhages, we work our way from the outside to inside. We therefore begin this section with a discussion of EDHs (both classic and variant), then move deeper inside the cranium to the more common SDHs. We conclude with a consideration of tSAH.

Arterial Epidural Hematoma

EDHs are uncommon but potentially lethal complications of head trauma. If an EDH is promptly recognized and appropriately treated, mortality and morbidity can be minimized.

Terminology

An EDH is a collection of blood between the calvarium and outer (periosteal) layer of the dura.

Etiology

Most EDHs arise from direct trauma to the skull that lacerates an adjacent blood vessel **(2-14)**. The vast majority (90%) are caused by arterial injury, most commonly to the middle meningeal artery. Approximately 10% of EDHs are venous, usually secondary to a fracture that crosses a dural venous sinus.

Pathology

Location. Over 90% of EDHs are unilateral and supratentorial. Between 90% and 95% are found directly adjacent to a skull fracture. The squamous portion of the temporal bone is the most common site.

Gross Pathology. EDHs are biconvex in shape. Adherence of the periosteal dura to the inner calvarium explains this typical configuration. As EDHs expand, they strip the dura away from the inner table of the skull, forming the classic lens-shaped hematoma **(2-14)**. Because the dura is especially tightly attached to sutures, EDHs in adults rarely cross suture lines (10% of EDHs in children *do* cross sutures, especially if a fracture traverses the suture or sutural diastasis is present).

The typical gross or intraoperative appearance of an acute EDH is a dark purple ("currant jelly") lentiform clot.

Clinical Issues

Epidemiology. EDHs are much less common than either tSAH or SDH. Although EDHs represent up to 10% of fatal injuries in autopsy series, they are found in only 1-4% of patients imaged for craniocerebral trauma.

Demographics. EDHs are uncommon in infants and the elderly. Most are found in older children and young adults. The M:F ratio is 4:1.

Presentation. The prototypical "lucid interval," during which a traumatized patient has an initial brief loss of consciousness followed by an asymptomatic period of various length prior to onset of coma &/or neurologic deficit, occurs in only 50% of EDH cases. Headache, nausea, vomiting, symptoms of intracranial mass effect (e.g., pupil-involving third cranial nerve palsy) followed by somnolence and coma are common.

Natural History. Outcome depends on size and location of the hematoma, whether the EDH is arterial or venous, and whether there is active bleeding. In the absence of other associated traumatic brain injuries, overall mortality rate with prompt recognition and appropriate treatment is under 5%.

Delayed development or enlargement of an EDH occurs in 10-15% of cases, usually within 24-36 hours following trauma.

Treatment Options. Many EDHs are now treated conservatively. Most traumatic EDHs are not surgical lesions at initial presentation, and the rate of conversion to surgery is low. Most venous and small classic hyperdense EDHs that do not exhibit a "swirl" sign and have minimal or no mass effect are managed conservatively with close clinical observation and follow-up imaging **(2-17)**. Significant clinical predictors of EDH progression requiring conversion to surgical therapy are coagulopathy and younger age.

Imaging

General Features. EDHs, especially in adults, typically do not cross sutures unless a fracture with sutural diastasis is present. In children, 10% of EDHs cross suture lines, usually the coronal or sphenosquamous suture.

Look for other comorbid lesions, such as "contre-coup" injuries, tSAH, and secondary brain herniations, all of which are common findings in patients with EDHs.

CT Findings. NECT scan is the procedure of choice for initial imaging in patients with head injury. Both soft tissue and bone reconstruction algorithms should be obtained. Multiplanar reconstructions are especially useful in identifying vertex EDHs, which may be difficult to detect if only axial images are obtained.

The classic imaging appearance of **classic (arterial) EDHs** is a hyperdense (60-90 HU) biconvex extraaxial collection **(2-15)**. Presence of a hypodense component ("swirl" sign) is seen in ~ 1/3 of cases and indicates active, rapid bleeding with unretracted clot **(2-14)**.

EDHs compress the underlying subarachnoid space and displace the cortex medially, "buckling" the gray matter-white matter interface inward.

Air in an EDH occurs in ~ 20% of cases and is usually—but not invariably—associated with a sinus or mastoid fracture.

Patients with mixed-density EDHs tend to present earlier than patients with hyperdense hematomas and have lower Glasgow Coma Scores (GCSs), larger hematoma volumes, and poorer prognosis.

Imaging findings associated with adverse clinical outcome are thickness > 1.5 cm, volume > 30 mL, pterional (lateral aspect of the middle cranial fossa) location, midline shift > 5 mm, and presence of a "swirl" sign within the hematoma on imaging.

MR Findings. Acute EDHs are typically isointense with underlying brain, especially on T1WI. The displaced dura can be identified as a displaced "black line" between the hematoma and the brain.

Angiography. DSA may show a lacerated middle meningeal artery with "tram-track" fistulization of contrast from the middle meningeal artery into the paired middle meningeal veins. Mass effect with displaced cortical arteries and veins is seen.

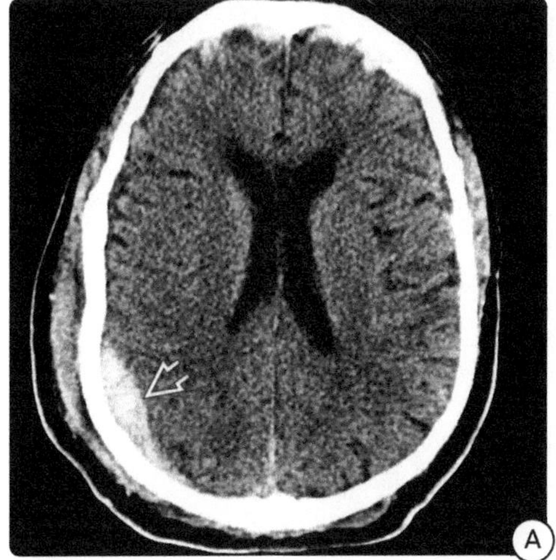

***(2-17A)** Serial imaging demonstrates temporal evolution of a small nonoperated EDH. Initial NECT scan shows a hyperdense biconvex EDH ➡.*

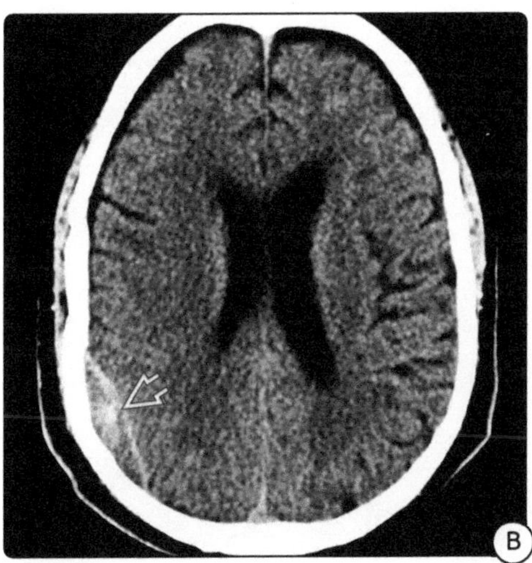

***(2-17B)** Repeat scan 10 days later reveals that density of the EDH ➡ has decreased significantly.*

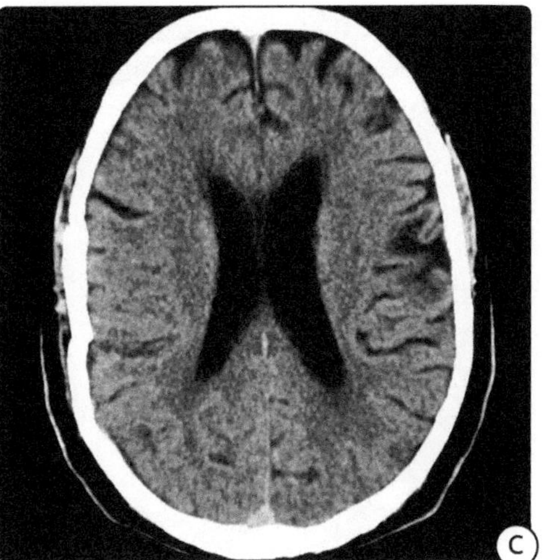

***(2-17C)** Repeat study 6 weeks after trauma reveals that the EDH has resolved completely.*

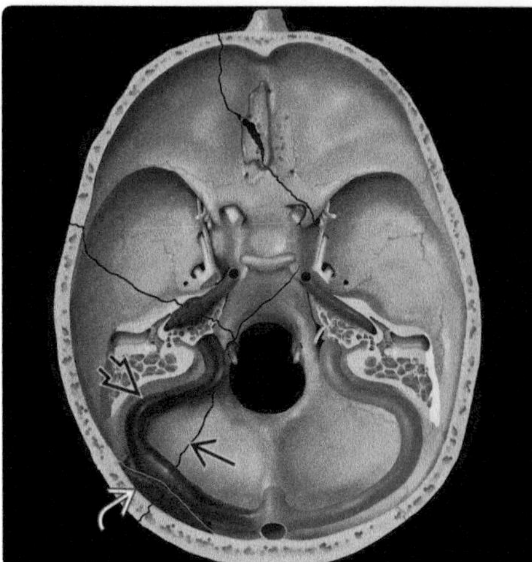

(2-18) Graphic shows basilar skull fracture ➡ with transverse sinus occlusion ➡ and posterior fossa venous EDH ➡.

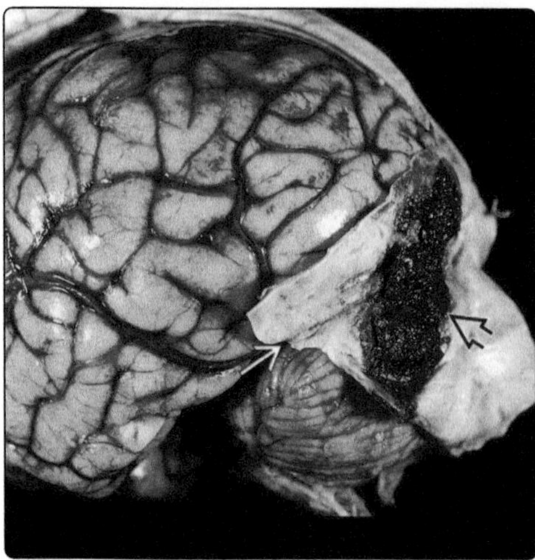

(2-19) Autopsy shows that venous EDH ➡ caused by transverse sinus injury "straddles" the tentorium ➡. (Courtesy R. Hewlett, MD.)

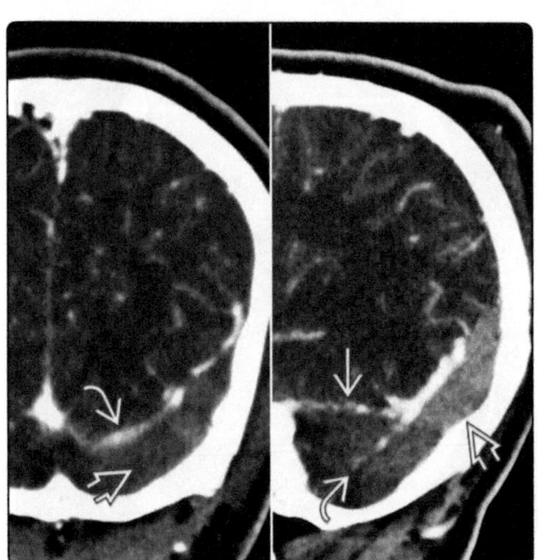

(2-20) (L) Coronal, (R) sagittal CTV shows venous EDH ➡ straddling the tentorium ➡, elevating the left transverse sinus ➡.

ACUTE ARTERIAL EPIDURAL HEMATOMA

Terminology
- EDH = blood between skull, dura

Etiology
- Associated skull fracture in 90-95%
- Arterial in 90%
  - Most often middle meningeal artery
- Venous in 10%

Pathology
- Unilateral, supratentorial (> 90%)
- Dura stripped away from skull → biconvex hematoma
- Usually does not cross sutures (exception = children, 10%)
- Does cross sites of dural attachment

Clinical
- Rare (1-4% of head trauma)
- Older children, young adults most common
- M:F = 4:1
- Classic "lucid interval" in only 50%
- Delayed deterioration common
- Low mortality if recognized, treated
- Small EDHs
  - If minimal mass, no "swirl" sign often managed conservatively

Imaging
- Hyperdense, lens-shaped
- "Swirl" sign (hypodensity) = rapid bleeding

Venous Epidural Hematomas

Not all EDHs are the same! **Venous EDHs** are often smaller, under lower pressure, and develop more slowly than their arterial counterparts. Most venous EDHs are caused by a skull fracture that crosses a dural venous sinus and therefore occur in the posterior fossa near the skull base (transverse/sigmoid sinus) **(2-18)** or the vertex of the brain [superior sagittal sinus (SSS)]. In contrast to their arterial counterparts, venous EDHs can "straddle" intracranial compartments, crossing both sutures and lines of dural attachment **(2-19)** and compressing or occluding the adjacent venous sinuses.

Venous EDHs can be subtle and easily overlooked. Coronal and sagittal reformatted images are key to the diagnosis and delineation of these variant EDHs **(2-20)**. Several anatomic subtypes of venous EDHs, each with different treatment implications and prognosis, are recognized.

Vertex EDH

"Vertex" EDHs are rare. Usually caused by a linear or diastatic fracture that crosses the SSS, they often accumulate over hours or even days with slow, subtle onset of symptoms. "Vertex" hematomas can be subtle and are easily overlooked unless coronal and sagittal reformatted images are obtained **(2-21)**.

Anterior Temporal EDH

Anterior temporal EDHs are a unique subgroup of hematomas that occur in the anterior tip of the middle cranial fossa **(2-22)**. Anterior temporal EDHs are caused either by an isolated fracture of the adjacent greater sphenoid wing or by an isolated zygomaticomaxillary complex ("tripod") facial fracture. The sphenoparietal dural venous sinus is injured as it curves medially along the undersurface of the lesser sphenoid wing, extravasating blood into the epidural space. Limited anatomically by the sphenotemporal suture laterally and the orbital fissure medially, anterior temporal EDHs remain stable in size and do not require surgical evacuation **(2-23)**.

Clival EDH

Clival EDHs usually develop after a hyperflexion or hyperextension injury to the neck and are possibly caused by stripping of the tectorial membrane from attachments to the clivus. Less commonly, they have been associated with basilar skull fractures that lacerate the clival dural venous plexus.

Clival EDHs most often occur in children and present with multiple cranial neuropathies. The abducens nerve is the most commonly affected followed by the glossopharyngeal and hypoglossal nerves. They are typically limited in size by the tight attachment of the dura to the basisphenoid and tectorial membrane **(2-24)**.

VENOUS EPIDURAL HEMATOMA

Not All EDHs Are the Same!
- Different etiologies in different anatomic locations
- Prognosis, treatment vary

Venous EDHs = 10% of All EDHs
- Skull fracture crosses dural venous sinus
  - Can cross sutures, dural attachments
- Often subtle, easily overlooked
  - Coronal, sagittal reformatted images key to diagnosis
- Usually accumulate slowly
- Can be limited in size; often treated conservatively

Subtypes
- Vertex EDH
  - Skull fracture crosses SSS
  - SSS can be lacerated, compressed, thrombosed
  - Hematoma under low pressure, develops gradually
  - Slow onset of symptoms
  - May become large, cause significant mass effect
- Anterior temporal EDH
  - Sphenoid wing or zygomaticomaxillary fracture
  - Injures sphenoparietal venous sinus
  - Hematoma accumulates at anterior tip of middle cranial fossa
  - Limited anatomically (laterally by sphenotemporal suture, medially by orbital fissure)
  - Benign clinical course
- Clival EDH
  - Most common = child with neck injury
  - May cause multiple cranial neuropathies (CNVI most common)
  - Hyperdense collection under clival dura
  - Limited by tight attachment of dura to basisphenoid, tectorial membrane
  - Usually benign course, resolves spontaneously

Management of a clival EDH is dictated by severity and progression of the neurologic deficits and stability of the atlantoaxial joint. In patients with minor cranial nerve involvement, the clinical course is usually benign, and treatment with a cervical collar is typical.

NECT scans show a hyperdense collection between the clivus and tectorial membrane. Sagittal MR of the craniocervical junction shows the hematoma elevating the clival dura and extending inferiorly between the basisphenoid and tectorial membrane anterior to the medulla.

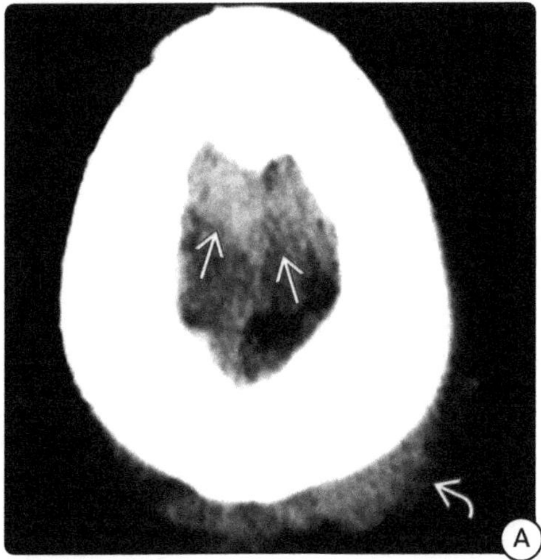

***(2-21A)** NECT shows scalp hematoma ➡, ill-defined hyperdensity extending anteriorly across the midline ➡.*

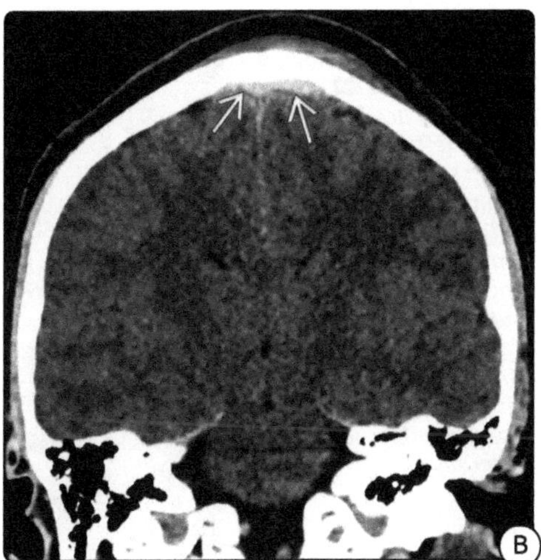

***(2-21B)** Coronal NECT reformatted from the axial source data shows the ill-defined hyperdensity ➡ crossing the midline.*

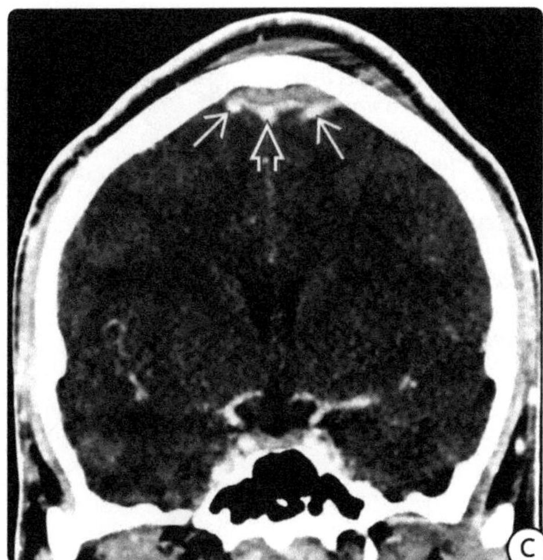

***(2-21C)** Coronal CTV shows a small venous vertex EDH that displaces the superior sagittal sinus ➡ and cortical veins ➡ inferiorly.*

(2-22) Graphic depicts benign anterior temporal EDH. Fracture ➡ disrupts the sphenoparietal sinus ➡. Low-pressure venous EDH ➡ is anatomically limited, medially by the orbital fissure ➡ and laterally by the sphenotemporal suture ➡. (2-23A) NECT shows a small biconvex left anterior middle cranial fossa EDH ➡.

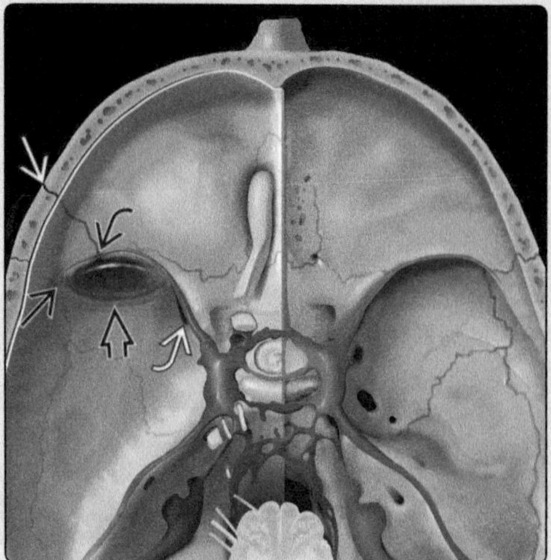

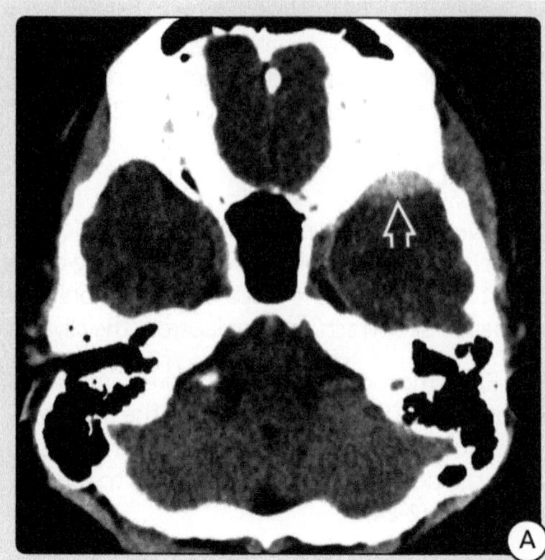

(2-23B) Bone CT shows a linear fracture ➡ extending across the floor of the left middle cranial fossa to the inferior orbital fissure. (2-23C) 3D SSD shows that the fracture ➡ extends across the sphenotemporal suture ➡. The middle fossa EDH is anatomically limited by the orbital fissure medially and the sphenotemporal suture laterally.

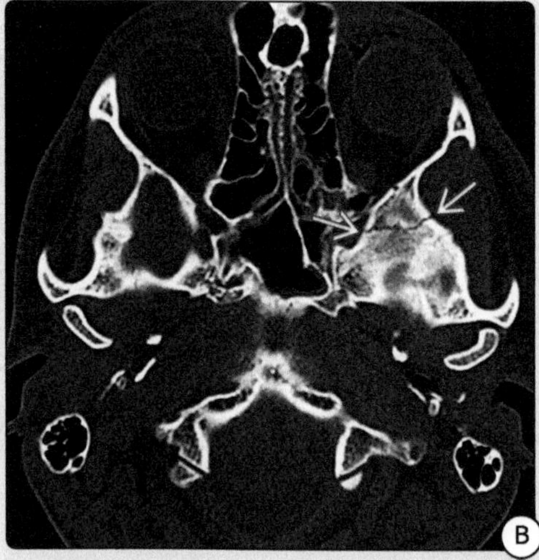

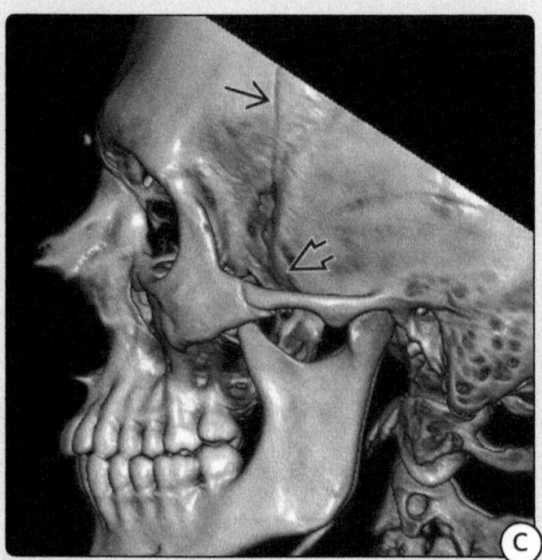

(2-24A) Axial CTA in a child with craniovertebral junction trauma shows a small clival EDH ➡. There was no evidence for vascular injury. (2-24B) Sagittal CTA reformatted from the axial source data nicely demonstrates the clival EDH ➡.

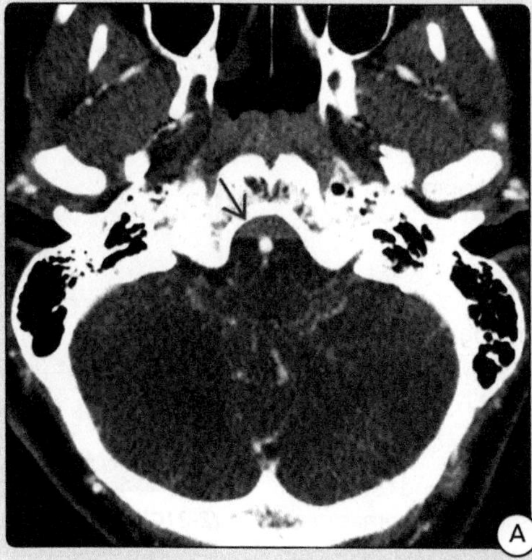

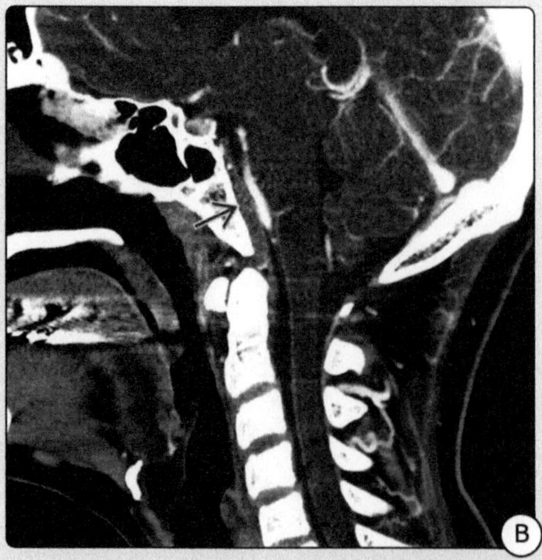

Acute Subdural Hematoma

Acute subdural hematomas (aSDHs) are one of the leading causes of death and disability in patients with severe traumatic brain injury (TBI). SDHs are much more common than EDHs. Most do not occur as isolated injuries; the vast majority of SDHs are associated with tSAH as well as significant parenchymal injuries, such as cortical contusions, brain lacerations, and diffuse axonal injuries.

Terminology

An aSDH is a collection of acute blood products that lies in or between the inner border cell layer of the dura and the arachnoid **(2-25)**.

Etiology

Trauma is the most common cause of aSDH. Both direct blows to the head and nonimpact injuries may result in formation of an aSDH. Tearing of bridging cortical veins as they cross the subdural space to enter a dural venous sinus (usually the SSS) is the most common etiology. Cortical vein lacerations can occur with either a skull fracture or the sudden changes in velocity and brain rotation that occur during nonimpact closed head injury (CHI).

Blood from ruptured vessels spreads quickly through the potential space between the dura and the arachnoid. Large SDHs may spread over an entire hemisphere, extending into the interhemispheric fissure and along the tentorium.

Tearing of cortical arteries from a skull fracture may also give rise to an aSDH. The arachnoid itself may also tear, creating a pathway for leakage of CSF into the subdural space, resulting in admixture of both blood and CSF.

Less common causes of aSDH include aneurysm rupture, skull/dura-arachnoid metastases from vascular extracranial primary neoplasms, and spontaneous hemorrhage in patients with severe coagulopathy.

Pathology

Gross Pathology. The gross appearance of an aSDH is that of a soft, purplish, "currant jelly" clot beneath a tense bulging dura. More than 95% are supratentorial. Most aSDHs spread diffusely over the affected hemisphere and are therefore typically crescent-shaped.

Clinical Issues

Epidemiology. An aSDH is the second most common extraaxial hematoma, exceeded only by tSAH. An aSDH is found in 10-20% of all patients with head injury and is observed in 30% of autopsied fatal injuries.

An aSDH may occur at any age from infancy to the elderly. There is no sex predilection.

Presentation. Even relatively minor head trauma, especially in elderly patients who are often anticoagulated, may result in an aSDH. In such patients, a definite history of trauma may be lacking.

Clinical findings vary from none to loss of consciousness and coma. Most patients with aSDHs have low GCSs on admission. Delayed deterioration, especially in elderly anticoagulated patients, is common.

Natural History. An aSDH may remain stable, grow slowly, or rapidly increase in size, causing mass effect and secondary brain herniations. Prognosis varies with hematoma thickness, midline shift, and the presence of

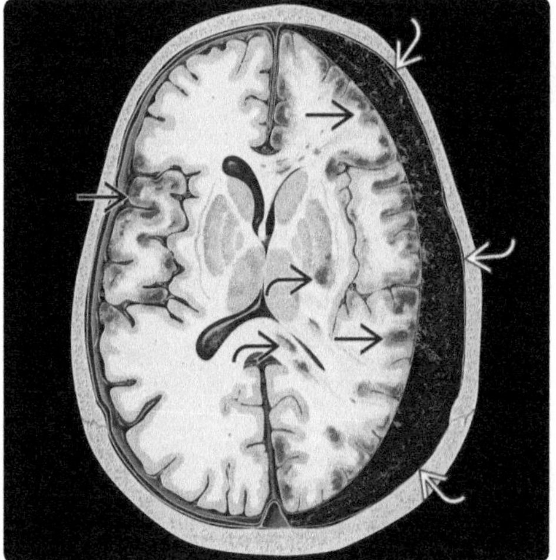

***(2-25)** Graphic depicts crescent-shaped acute SDH ➡ with contusions and "contre-coup" injuries ➡, diffuse axonal injuries ➡.*

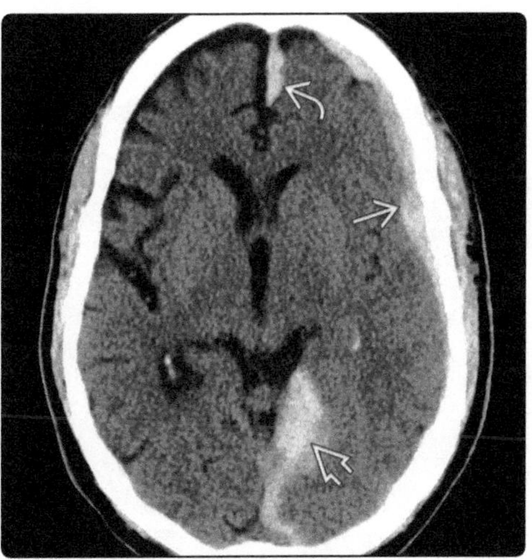

***(2-26)** Acute SDH spreads over left hemisphere ➡, along tentorium ➡, & into interhemispheric fissure ➡ but does not cross midline.*

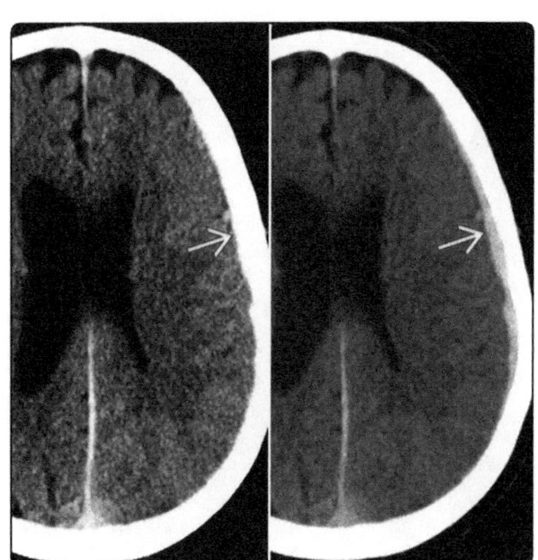

***(2-27)** NECT scan shows that a small SDH ➡ is easier to see with wider (R) compared with standard (L) windows.*

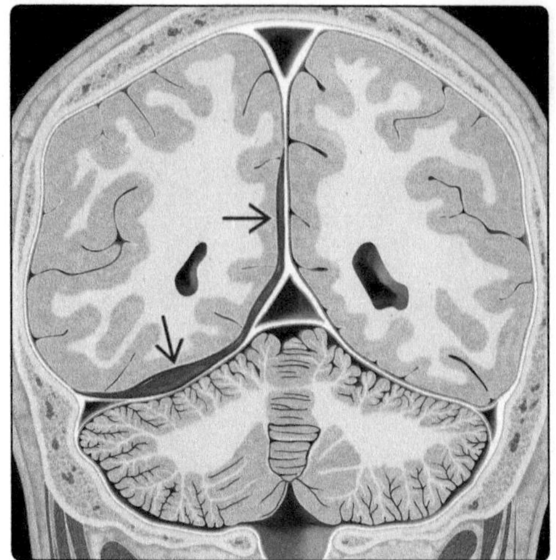

(2-28) Coronal graphic depicts thin aSDH layering along the tentorium and inferior falx cerebri ⇒.

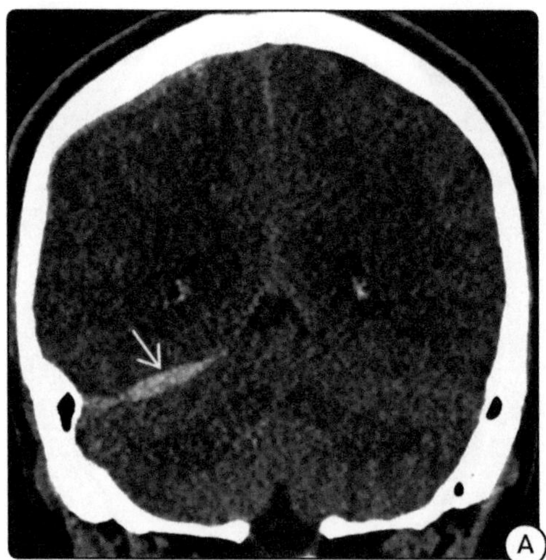

(2-29A) Reformatted coronal NECT scan using the axial source data shows a small right peritentorial aSDH ➡.

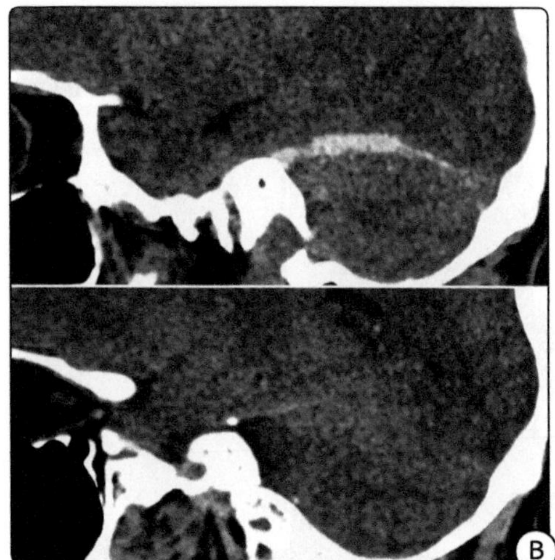

(2-29B) Sagittal scans in the same case show the right peritentorial aSDH (top) with normal left sagittal dura (bottom) for comparison.

associated parenchymal injuries. An aSDH that is thicker than 2 cm correlates with poor outcome (35-90% mortality). An aSDH that occupies more than 10% of the total available intracranial volume is usually lethal.

Treatment Options. The majority of patients with small SDHs are initially treated conservatively with close clinical observation and follow-up imaging. Small isolated falcine or tentorial SDHs typically do not increase in size and usually do not require short-term follow-up imaging.

Patients with larger SDHs, a lesion located at the convexity, alcohol abuse, and repetitive falls are at the greatest risk for deterioration. Surveillance with follow-up CT scans is recommended until the SDH resolves or at least up to five weeks following the initial trauma.

Imaging

General Features. The classic finding of an aSDH is a supratentorial crescent-shaped extraaxial collection that displaces the gray matter-white matter interface medially. SDHs are typically more extensive than EDHs, easily spreading along the falx, tentorium, and around the anterior and middle fossa floors **(2-26)**. SDHs may cross suture lines but generally do not cross dural attachments. Bilateral SDHs occur in 15% of cases. "Contre-coup" injuries, such as contusion of the contralateral hemisphere, are common.

Both standard soft tissue and intermediate ("subdural") windows as well as bone algorithm reconstructions should be used in all trauma patients, as small, subtle aSDHs can be obscured by the density of the overlying calvarium **(2-27)**. Coronal and sagittal reformatted images using the axial source data are especially helpful in visualizing small ("smear") peritentorial and parafalcine aSDHs **(2-28)** **(2-29)**.

CT Findings

NECT. Approximately 60% of aSDHs are hyperdense on NECT scans **(2-26)**. Mixed-attenuation lesions are found in 40% of cases. Pockets of hypodensity within a larger hyperdense aSDH usually indicate rapid bleeding **(2-30)**. "Dots" or "lines" of CSF trapped within compressed, displaced sulci are often seen underlying an SDH **(2-37)**.

Mass effect with an aSDH is common and expected. Subfalcine herniation should be proportionate to the size of the subdural collection. However, **if the difference between the midline shift and thickness of the hematoma is 3 mm or more, then mortality is very high.** This discrepancy occurs when underlying cerebral edema is triggered by the traumatic event. Early recognition and aggressive treatment for potentially catastrophic brain swelling are essential **(2-31)**.

In other cases, especially in patients with repeated head injury, severe brain swelling with unilateral hemisphere vascular engorgement occurs very quickly. Here, the mass effect is greatly disproportionate to the size of the SDH, which may be relatively small.

Occasionally, an aSDH is nearly isodense with the underlying cortex. This unusual appearance is found in extremely anemic patients (Hgb under 8-10 g/dL) **(2-32)** and sometimes occurs in patients with coagulopathy. In rare cases, CSF leakage through a torn arachnoid may mix with—and dilute—the acute blood that collects in the subdural space.

CECT/CTA. CECT scans are helpful in detecting small isodense aSDHs. The normally enhancing cortical veins are displaced inward by the extraaxial fluid collection. CTA may be useful in visualizing a cortical vessel that is actively bleeding into the subdural space.

MR Findings. MR scans are rarely obtained in acutely brain-injured patients. In such cases, aSDHs appear isointense on T1WI and hypointense on T2WI. Signal intensity on FLAIR scans is usually iso- to hyperintense compared with CSF but hypointense compared with the adjacent brain. aSDHs are hypointense on T2* scans.

DWI shows heterogeneous signal within the hematoma but may show patchy foci of restricted diffusion in the cortex underlying the aSDH.

Differential Diagnosis

In the setting of acute trauma, the major differential diagnosis is EDH. Shape is a helpful feature, as most aSDHs are crescentic, whereas EDHs are biconvex. EDHs are almost always associated with skull fracture; SDHs frequently occur in the absence of skull fracture. EDHs may cross sites of dural attachment; SDHs do not cross the falx or tentorium.

Subacute Subdural Hematoma

With time, SDHs undergo organization, lysis, and neomembrane formation. Within 2-3 days, the initial soft, loosely organized clot of an aSDH becomes organized. Breakdown of blood products and the formation of organizing granulation tissue change the imaging appearance of subacute and chronic SDHs.

Terminology

A subacute subdural hematoma (sSDH) is between several days and several weeks old.

Pathology

A collection of partially liquified clot with resorbing blood products is surrounded on both sides by a "membrane" of organizing granulation tissue **(2-33)**. The outermost

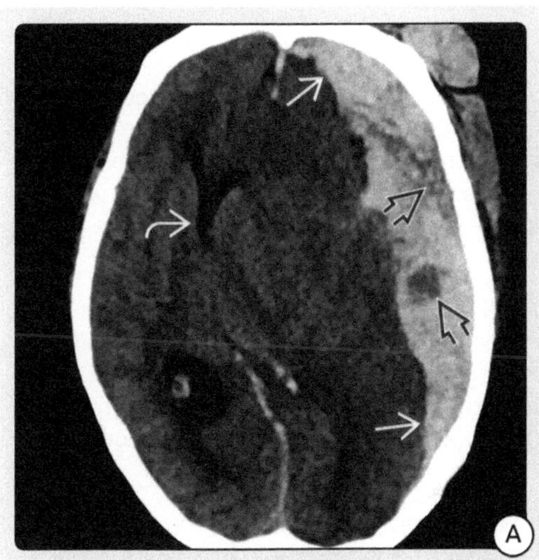

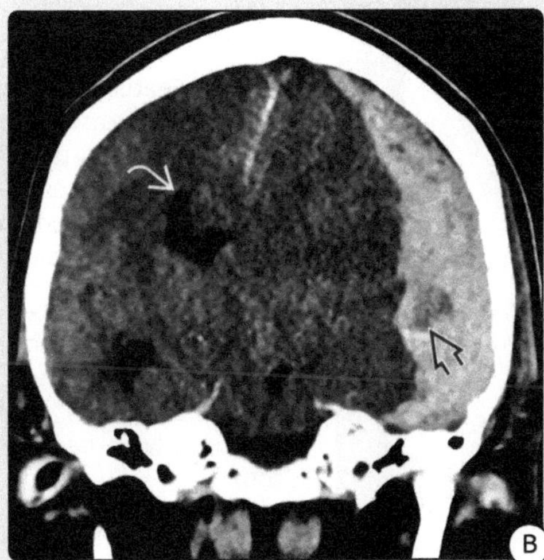

***(2-30A)** Axial NECT in a 74-year-old anticoagulated patient with a ground-level fall shows a huge, mixed-density aSDH with severe subfalcine herniation of the lateral ventricles. Low-density foci within the aSDH indicate rapid bleeding with unclotted blood. **(2-30B)** Coronal NECT shows the subfalcine herniation, mixed-density aSDH with hypodense foci. The patient expired shortly after the scan.*

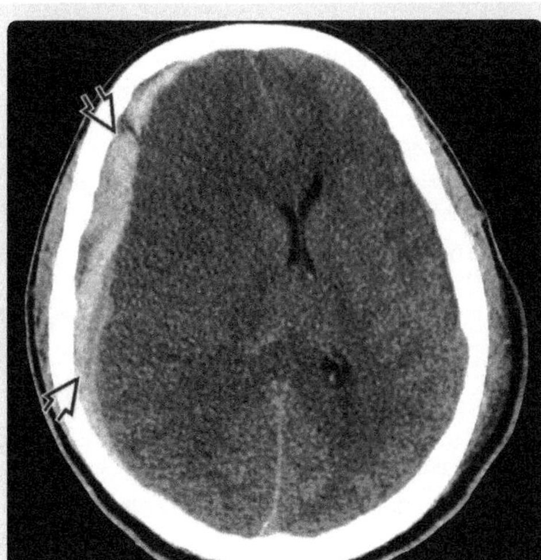

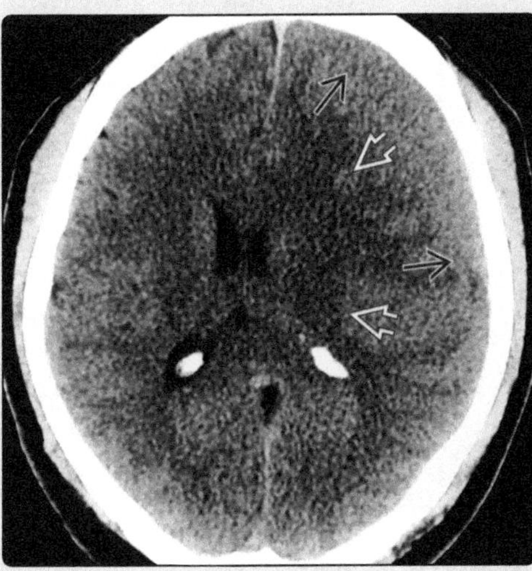

***(2-31)** NECT shows a mixed-density 12-mm aSDH with a disproportionately large subfalcine herniation of the lateral ventricles (17 mm), indicating that diffuse holohemispheric brain swelling is present. Subfalcine herniation ≥ 3 mm portends a poor prognosis. **(2-32)** NECT scan in a very anemic patient shows an isodense aSDH. The aSDH is almost exactly the same density as the underlying cortex. The gray-white interface is displaced inward.*

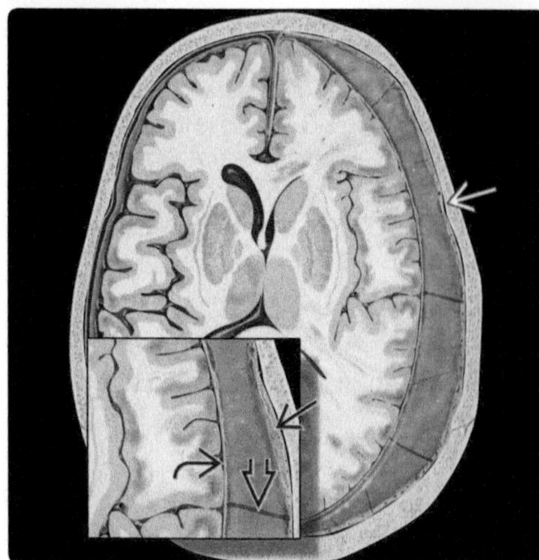

(2-33) Graphic depicts sSDH. Inset shows bridging vein and thin inner and thick outer membranes.

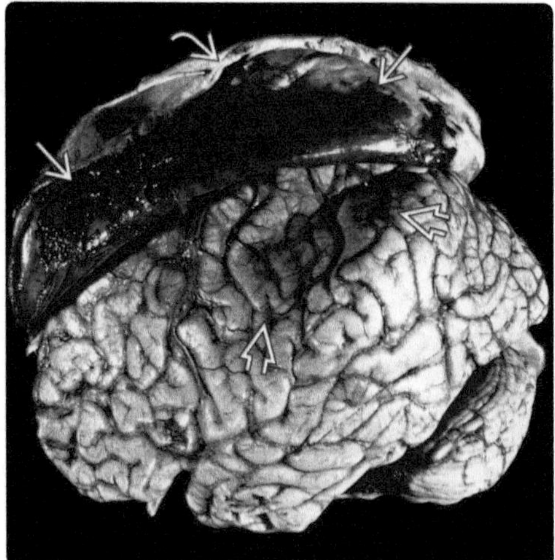

(2-34) Autopsy shows sSDH with organized hematoma, thick outer membrane, deformed brain. (Courtesy R. Hewlett, MD.)

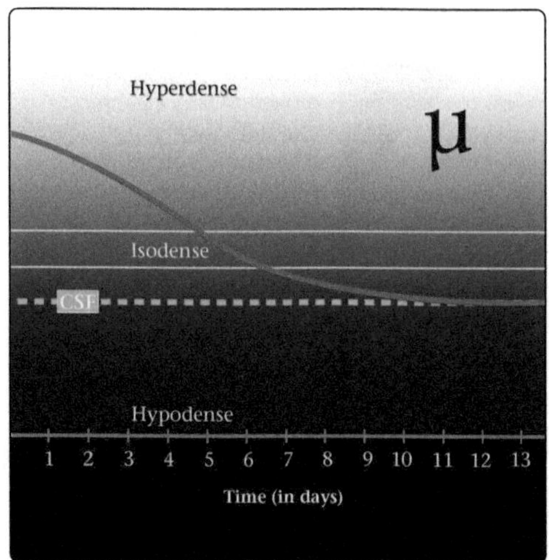

(2-35) SDHs decrease ~ 1.5 HU/day. By 7-10 days, blood in hematoma is isodense with cortex. By 10 days, it is hypodense.

membrane adheres to the dura and is typically thicker than the inner membrane, which abuts the thin, delicate arachnoid **(2-34)**.

In some cases, repetitive hemorrhages of different ages arising from the friable granulation tissue may be present. In others, liquefaction of the hematoma over time produces serous blood-tinged fluid.

Clinical Issues

Epidemiology and Demographics. SDHs are common findings at imaging and autopsy. In contrast to aSDHs, sSDHs show a distinct bimodal distribution with children and the elderly as the most commonly affected age groups.

Presentation. Clinical symptoms vary from asymptomatic to loss of consciousness and hemiparesis caused by sudden rehemorrhage into an sSDH. Headache and seizure are other common presentations.

Natural History and Treatment Options. Many sSDHs resolve spontaneously. In some cases, repeated hemorrhages may cause sudden enlargement and mass effect. Surgical drainage may be indicated if the sSDH is enlarging or becomes symptomatic.

Imaging

General Features. Imaging findings are related to hematoma age and the presence of encasing membranes. Evolution of an untreated, uncomplicated SDH follows a very predictable pattern on CT. Density of an extraaxial hematoma decreases ~ 1-2 HU each day **(2-35)**. Therefore, an SDH will become nearly isodense with the underlying cerebral cortex within a few days following trauma.

CT Findings. sSDHs are typically crescent-shaped fluid collections that are iso- to slightly hypodense compared with the underlying cortex on NECT **(2-36)**. Medial displacement of the gray-white interface ("buckling") is often present, along with "dot-like" foci of CSF in the trapped, partially effaced sulci underlying the sSDH **(2-37)** **(2-38)**. Mixed-density hemorrhages are common.

Bilateral sSDHs may be difficult to detect because of their "balanced" mass effect **(2-37)**. Sulcal effacement with displaced gray matter-white matter interfaces is the typical appearance.

CECT scans show that the enhanced cortical veins are displaced medially. The encasing membranes, especially the thicker superficial layer, may enhance.

MR Findings. MR can be very helpful in identifying sSDHs, especially small lesions that are virtually isodense with underlying brain on CT scans.

Signal intensity varies with hematoma age but is less predictable than on CT, making precise "aging" of subdural collections more problematic. In general, early subacute SDHs are isointense with cortex on T1WI and hypointense on T2WI but gradually become more hyperintense as extracellular methemoglobin increases **(2-39A)**. Most late-stage sSDHs are T1/T2 "bright-bright." A linear T2 hypointensity representing the encasing membranes that surround the SDH is sometimes present.

FLAIR is the most sensitive standard sequence for detecting sSDH, as the collection is typically hyperintense **(2-40)**. Because FLAIR signal intensity varies depending on the relative contribution of T1 and T2 effects, early sSDHs may initially appear hypointense due to their intrinsic T2 shortening.

T2* scans are also very sensitive, as sSDHs show distinct "blooming" **(2-39B)**.

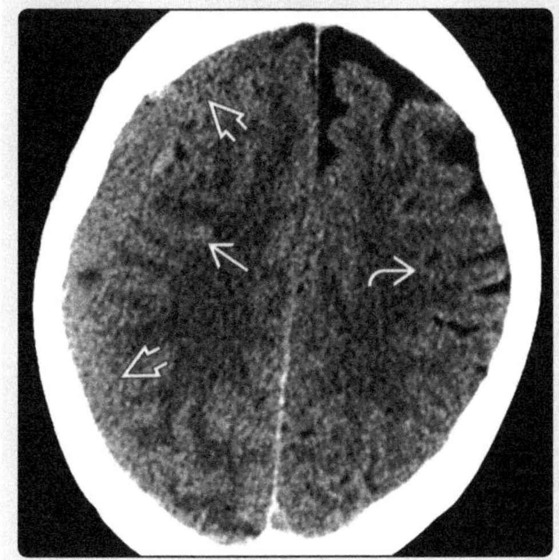

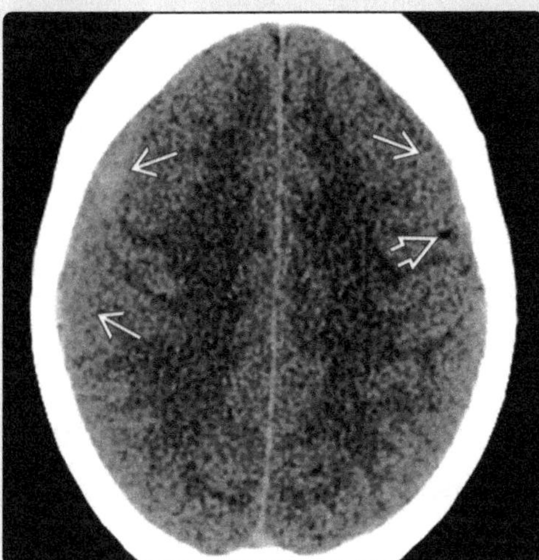

***(2-36)** Axial NECT scan shows right sSDH that is isodense with the underlying cortex. The right GM-WM interface is displaced and buckled medially compared with normal left side . **(2-37)** NECT scan in another patient shows bilateral "balanced" isodense subacute SDHs . Note that both GM-WM interfaces are inwardly displaced. A "dot" of CSF in the compressed subarachnoid space is seen under the left sSDH .*

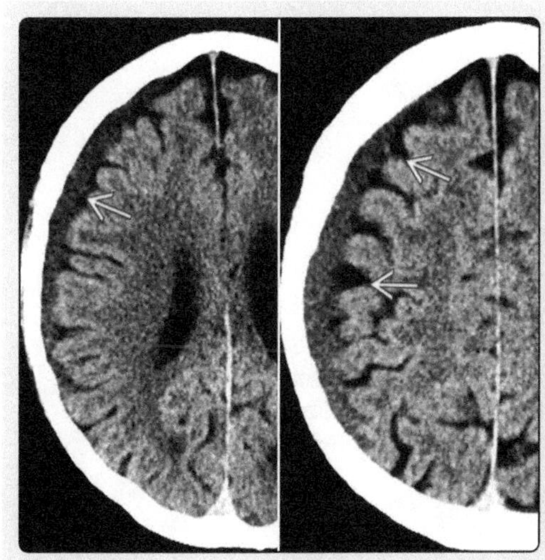

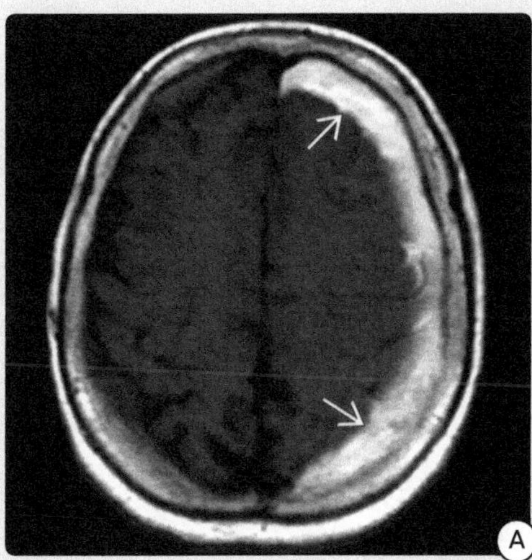

***(2-38)** NECT in an elderly patient with sSDH, moderate cortical atrophy shows difference between nearly isodense SDH and CSF in underlying compressed subarachnoid space, sulci . **(2-39A)** Axial T1WI in patient with a late-stage aSDH shows crescent-shaped hyperintense collection extending over entire surface of left hemisphere, gyral compression with almost obliterated sulci compared with normal right hemisphere.*

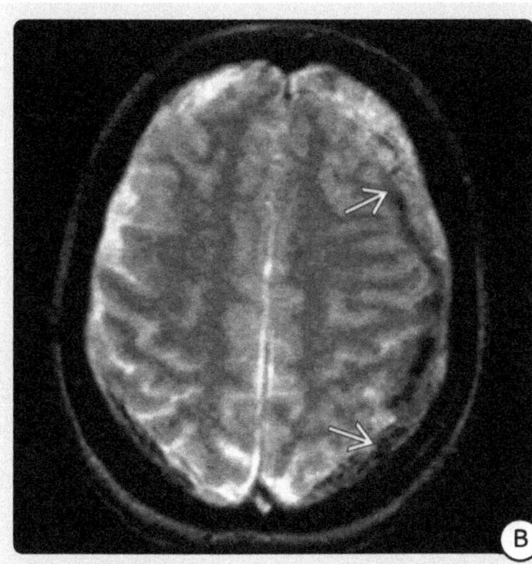

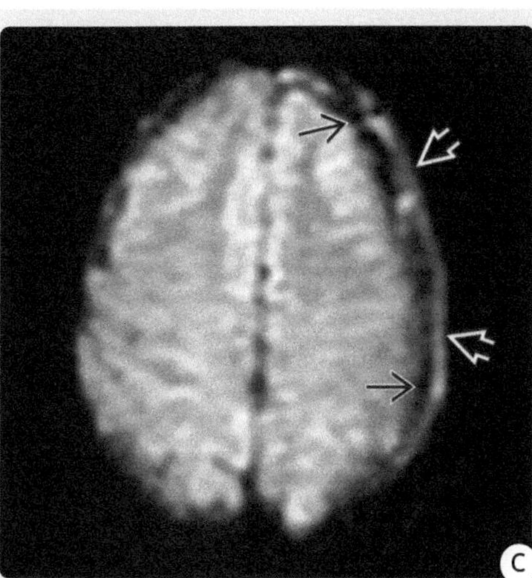

***(2-39B)** T2* GRE scan shows some "blooming" in the sSDH. **(2-39C)** DWI shows the classic double-layer appearance of an sSDH with hypointense rim on the inside and mildly hyperintense rim on the outside of the clot.*

Signal intensity on DWI also varies with hematoma age. DWI commonly shows a crescentic high-intensity area with a low-intensity rim closer to the brain surface (double-layer appearance) **(2-39C)**. The low-intensity area corresponds to a mixture of resolved clot and CSF, whereas the high-intensity area correlates with solid clot.

T1 C+ scans demonstrate enhancing, thickened, encasing membranes **(2-40D)**. The membrane surrounding an sSDH is usually thicker on the dural side of the collection. Delayed scans may show gradual "filling in" and increasing hyperintensity of the sSDH.

Differential Diagnosis

The major differential diagnosis of an sSDH is an **isodense aSDH**. These are typically seen only in an extremely anemic or anticoagulated patient. A **subdural effusion** that follows surgery or meningitis or that occurs as a component of intracranial hypotension can also mimic an sSDH. A **subdural hygroma** is typically isodense/isointense with CSF and does not demonstrate enhancing, encapsulating membranes.

Chronic/Mixed Subdural Hematoma

Terminology

A chronic subdural hematoma (cSDH) is an encapsulated collection of sanguineous or serosanguineous fluid confined within the subdural space. Recurrent hemorrhage(s) into a preexisting cSDH are common and produce a mixed-age or "acute on chronic" SDH (mSDH).

Etiology

With continued degradation of blood products, an SDH becomes progressively more liquified until it is largely serous fluid tinged with blood products **(2-41)**. Rehemorrhage, either from vascularized encapsulating membranes or rupture of stretched cortical veins crossing the expanded subdural

(2-40A) T1WI in a 59-year-old man with seizures shows bilateral subdural collections ➡ that are slightly hyperintense to CSF. (2-40B) T2WI shows that both collections ➡ are isointense with CSF in the underlying subarachnoid cisterns.

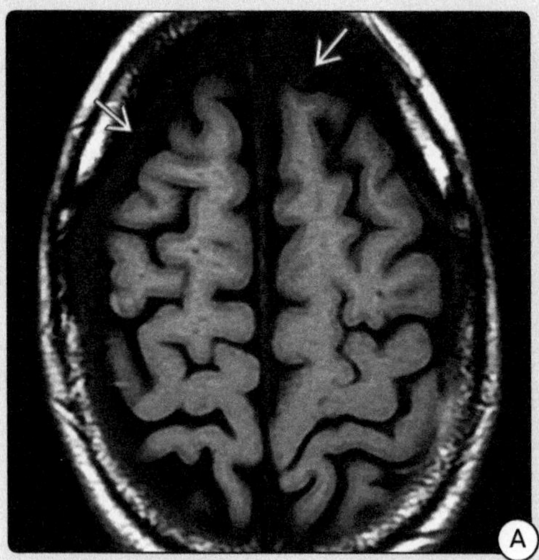

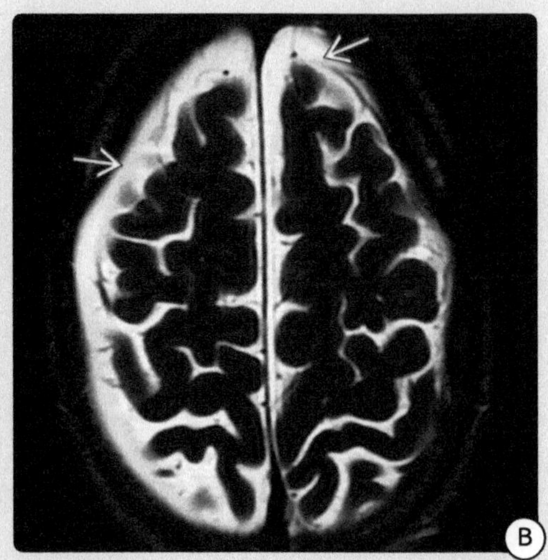

(2-40C) The fluid collections ➡ do not suppress on FLAIR and are hyperintense to CSF in the underlying cisterns. (2-40D) T1 C+ shows that the outer membrane of the SDH enhances ➡. Findings are consistent with late subacute/early chronic SDHs.

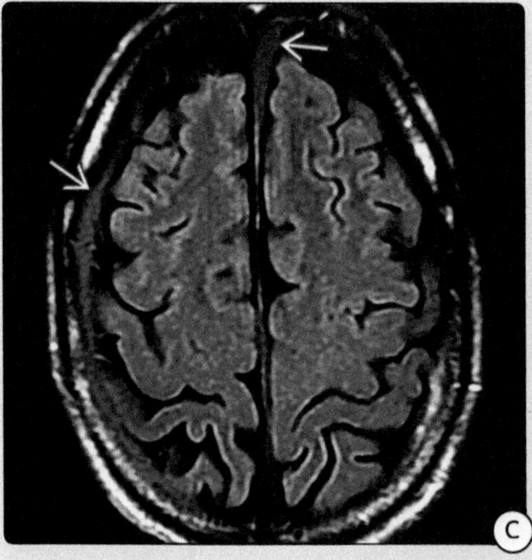

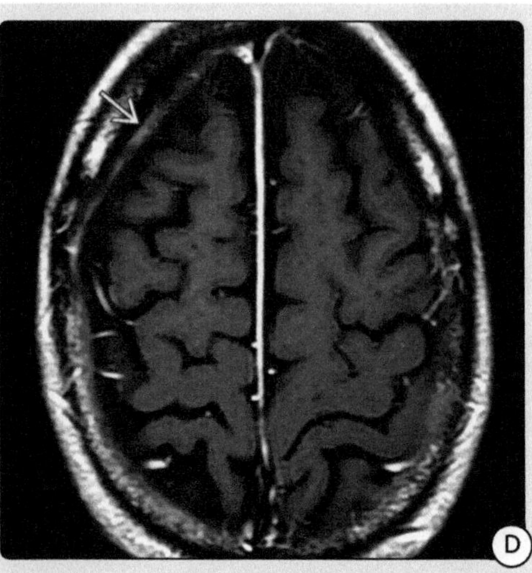

space, occurs in 5-10% of cSDHs and is considered "acute-on-chronic" SDH **(2-42)**.

Pathology

Gross Pathology. Blood within the subdural space incites tissue reaction around its margins. Organization and resorption of the hematoma contained within the "membranes" of surrounding granulation tissue continue. These neomembranes have fragile, easily disrupted capillaries and easily rebleed, creating an mSDH. Multiple hemorrhages of different ages are common in mSDHs **(2-43)**.

Eventually, most of the liquified clot in a cSDH is resorbed. Only a thickened dura-arachnoid layer remains with a few scattered pockets of old blood trapped between the inner and outer membranes.

Clinical Issues

Epidemiology. Unoperated, uncomplicated subacute SDHs eventually evolve into cSDHs. Approximately 5-10% will rehemorrhage, causing multiloculated mixed-age SDHs.

Demographics. cSDHs may occur at any age. Mixed-age SDHs are much more common in elderly patients.

Presentation. Presentation varies from no/mild symptoms (e.g., headache) to sudden neurologic deterioration if a preexisting cSDH rehemorrhages.

Natural History. In the absence of repeated hemorrhages, cSDHs gradually resorb and largely resolve, leaving a residue of thickened dura-arachnoid that may persist for months or even years. Older patients, especially those with brain atrophy, are subject to repeated hemorrhages.

Treatment Options. If follow-up imaging of a subacute SDH shows expected resorption and regression of the cSDH, no surgery may be required. Surgical drainage with evacuation of the cSDH and resection of its encapsulating membranes is performed if significant mass effect or repeated hemorrhages cause neurologic complications.

Imaging

General Features. cSDHs have a spectrum of imaging appearances. **Uncomplicated cSDHs** show relatively homogeneous density/signal intensity with slight gravity-dependent gradation of their contents ("hematocrit effect").

mSDHs with acute hemorrhage into a preexisting cSDH show a hematocrit level with distinct layering of the old (top) and new (bottom) hemorrhages. Sometimes, septated pockets that contain hemorrhages of different ages form. Dependent layering of blood within the loculated collections may appear quite bizarre.

Extremely old, **longstanding cSDHs** with virtually complete resorption of all liquid contents are seen as pachymeningopathies with diffuse dura-arachnoid thickening.

CT Findings

NECT. A hypodense crescentic fluid collection extending over the surface of one or both cerebral hemispheres is the classic finding in cSDH. Uncomplicated cSDHs approach CSF in density **(2-44)**. The hematocrit effect creates a slight gradation in density that increases from top to bottom.

Trabecular or loculated cSDHs show internal septations, often with evidence of repeated hemorrhages **(2-45A)**. With age, the encapsulating membranes

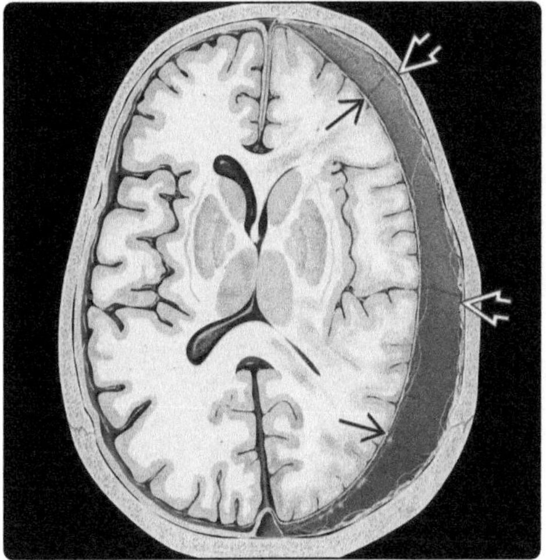

(2-41) Simple cSDHs contain serosanguineous fluid with hematocrit effect, thin inner ⇒, thick outer ➡ encapsulating membranes.

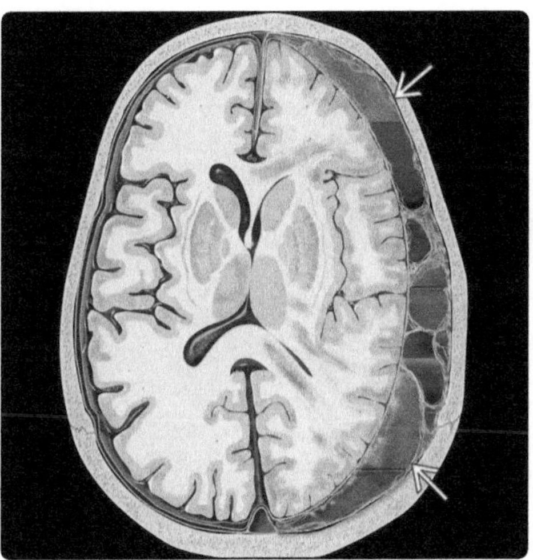

(2-42) Complicated cSDHs contain loculated pockets of old and new blood, seen as fluid-fluid levels ➡ within septated cavities.

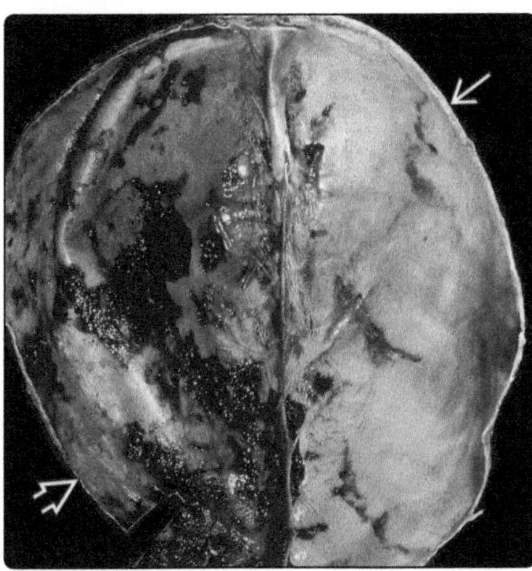

(2-43) cSDH autopsy: 1 side has thickened dura ➡, mixed acute, subacute, chronic hemorrhages on other ➡. (From DP: Hospital Autopsy.)

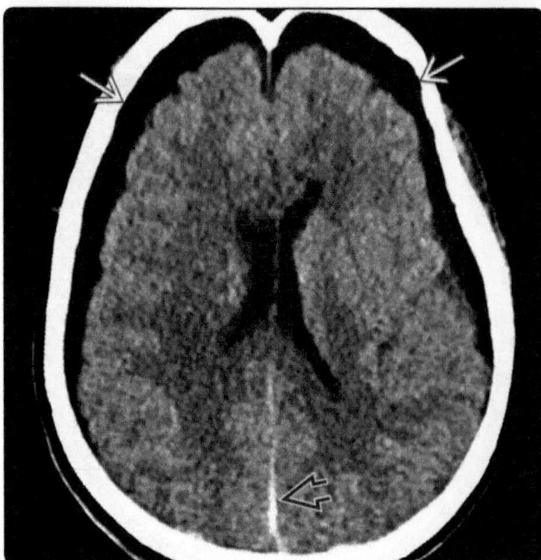

***(2-44)** NECT scan shows bilateral cSDHs ➡ causing mass effect on the underlying brain. A small left parafalcine aSDH is present ⇨.*

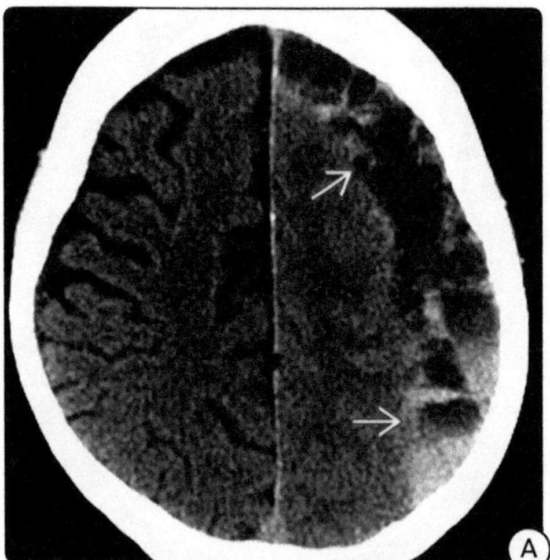

***(2-45A)** NECT shows mixed cSDH ➡ that features multiple loculated pockets of blood with old blood layered on top of recent hemorrhages.*

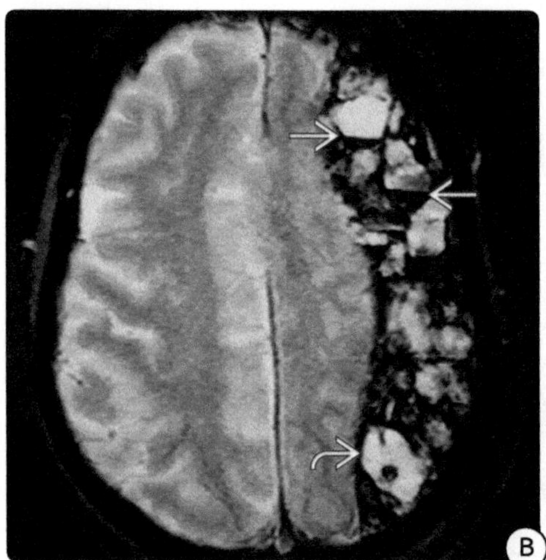

***(2-45B)** T2* GRE shows multiple loculated pockets of mixed-age blood ➡ with varying signal intensities and fluid-fluid levels ➡.*

surrounding the cSDH become thickened and may appear moderately hyperdense. Eventually, some cSDHs show peripheral calcifications that persist for many years. In rare cases, a cSDH may densely calcify or even ossify, a condition aptly termed "armored brain."

CECT. The encapsulating membranes around a cSDH contain fragile neocapillaries that lack endothelial tight junctions. Therefore, the membranes show strong enhancement following contrast administration.

MR Findings. As with all intracranial hematomas, signal intensity of a cSDH or mSDH is quite variable and depends on age of the blood products. On T1 scans, uncomplicated cSDHs are typically iso- to slightly hyperintense compared with CSF. Depending on the stage of evolution, cSDHs are iso- to hypointense compared with CSF on T2 scans.

Most cSDHs are hyperintense on FLAIR and may show "blooming" on T2* scans if subacute-chronic blood clots are still present **(2-45B)**. In ~ 1/4 of all cases, superficial siderosis can be identified over the gyri underlying a cSDH.

The encapsulating membranes of a cSDH enhance following contrast administration. Typically, the outer layer is thicker than the inner layer.

Uncomplicated cSDHs do not restrict on DWI. With cSDHs, a "double layer" effect—a crescent of hyperintensity medial to a nonrestricting fluid collection—indicates acute rehemorrhage.

Differential Diagnosis

An mSDH is difficult to mistake for anything else. In older patients, a small uncomplicated cSDH may be difficult to distinguish from simple **brain atrophy** with enlarged bifrontal CSF spaces. However, cSDHs exhibit mass effect; they flatten the underlying gyri, often extending around the entire hemisphere and into the interhemispheric fissure. The increased extraaxial spaces in patients with cerebral atrophy are predominantly frontal and temporal.

A traumatic **subdural hygroma** is an accumulation of CSF in the subdural space after head injury, probably secondary to an arachnoid tear. Subdural hygromas are sometimes detected within the first 24 hours after trauma; however, the mean time for appearance is nine days after injury. A subdural hygroma or a hematohygroma in an infant or young child should be considered highly suspicious for abusive head trauma (child abuse; see later discussion).

A classic uncomplicated subdural hygroma is a hypodense, CSF-like, crescentic extraaxial collection that consists purely of CSF, has no blood products, lacks encapsulating membranes, and shows no enhancement following contrast administration. CSF leakage into the subdural space is also present in the vast majority of patients with cSDH. Therefore, many—if not most—cSDHs contain a mixture of *both* CSF and blood products.

A **subdural effusion** is an accumulation of clear fluid over the cerebral convexities or in the interhemispheric fissure. Subdural effusions are generally complications of meningitis; a history of prior infection, not trauma, is typical.

A **subdural empyema** (SDE) is a hypodense extraaxial fluid collection that contains pus. Most SDEs are secondary to sinusitis or mastoiditis, have strongly enhancing membranes, and often coexist with findings of meningitis. A typical SDE restricts strongly and uniformly on DWI. Look for underlying sulcal/cisternal hyperintensity on FLAIR and enhancement on T1 C+.

Traumatic Subarachnoid Hemorrhage

tSAH is found in virtually all cases of moderate to severe head trauma. Indeed, trauma—*not* ruptured saccular aneurysm—is the most common cause of intracranial SAH.

Etiology

tSAH can occur with both direct trauma to the skull and nonimpact CHI. Tearing of cortical arteries and veins, rupture of contusions and lacerations into the contiguous subarachnoid space, and choroid plexus bleeds with intraventricular hemorrhage may all result in blood collecting within the subarachnoid cisterns.

Although tSAH occasionally occurs in isolation, it is usually accompanied by other manifestations of brain injury. Subtle tSAH *may be the only clue* on initial imaging studies that *more serious injuries lurk beneath the surface.*

Pathology

Location. tSAHs are predominantly found in the anteroinferior frontal and temporal sulci, perisylvian regions, and over the hemispheric convexities **(2-46)**. In very severe cases, tSAH spreads over most of the brain. In mild cases, blood collects in a single sulcus or the dependent portion of the interpeduncular fossa.

Gross Pathology. With the exception of location and associated parenchymal injuries, the gross appearance of tSAH is similar to that of aneurysmal SAH (aSAH). Curvilinear foci of bright red blood collect in cisterns and surface sulci **(2-47)**.

tSAH typically occurs adjacent to cortical contusions. tSAH is also commonly identified under acute epidural and subdural hematomas.

Clinical Issues

Epidemiology. tSAH is found in most cases of moderate trauma and is identified in virtually 100% of fatal brain injuries at autopsy.

Natural History. Breakdown and resorption of tSAH occurs gradually. Patients with isolated tSAH have very low rates of clinical or radiographic deterioration and typically do well.

Imaging

General Features. With the exception of location, the general imaging appearance of tSAH is similar to that of aSAH, i.e., sulcal-cisternal hyperdensity/hyperintensity **(2-48)**. tSAH is typically more focal or patchy than the diffuse subarachnoid blood indicative of aneurysmal hemorrhage.

CT Findings. Acute tSAH is typically peripheral, appearing as linear hyperdensities in sulci adjacent to cortical contusions or under epi- or subdural hematomas. Occasionally, isolated tSAH is identified within the interpeduncular fossa **(2-51)**.

MR Findings. As acute blood is isointense with brain, it may be difficult to detect on T1WI. "Dirty" sulci with "smudging" of the perisylvian cisterns is typical. Subarachnoid blood is hyperintense to brain on T2WI and appears similar in signal intensity to cisternal CSF. FLAIR scans show hyperintensity in the affected sulci.

"Blooming" with hypointensity can be identified on T2* scans, typically adjacent to areas of cortical contusion. tSAH is

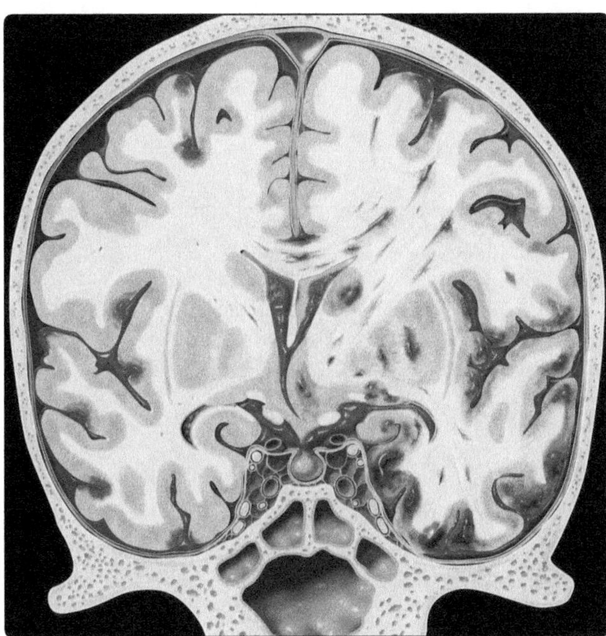

***(2-46)** Graphic depicts traumatic subarachnoid hemorrhage (tSAH). tSAH is most common around the sylvian fissures and in the sulci adjacent to contused gyri.*

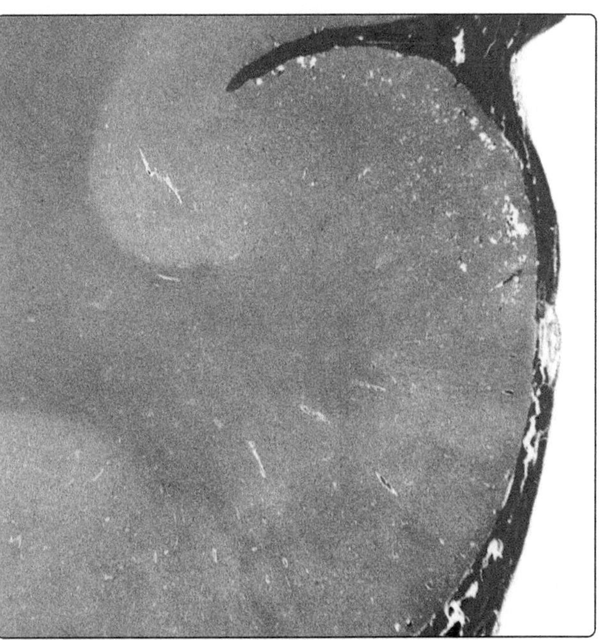

***(2-47)** Low-power photomicrograph shows an autopsied brain of a boxer who collapsed and expired after being knocked unconscious. Typical tSAH covers the gyri and extends into the sulci. (Courtesy J. Paltan, MD.)*

recognized on GRE or SWI sequences as hypointense signal intensity surrounded by hyperintense CSF.

Angiography. Emergent CTA is usually unnecessary in cases with typical peripheral tSAH on NECT. Patients with suprasellar ("central") SAH may harbor a ruptured aneurysm and should be screened with CTA regardless of mechanism of injury.

Differential Diagnosis

The major differential diagnosis of tSAH is **nontraumatic SAH** (ntSAH). Aneurysmal rupture causes 80-90% of all ntSAHs. In contrast to tSAH, aSAH is concentrated in the basal cisterns.

Sulcal-cisternal hyperintensity on FLAIR is nonspecific and can be caused by **meningitis, neoplasm, artifact** (incomplete CSF suppression), **contrast** leakage into the subarachnoid space (e.g., with renal failure), and **high inspired oxygen** during general anesthesia.

The term **pseudosubarachnoid hemorrhage** has been used to describe the CT appearance of a brain with severe cerebral edema. Hypodense brain makes circulating blood in arteries and veins look relatively hyperdense. The hyperdensity seen here is smooth and conforms to the expected shape of the vessels, not the subarachnoid spaces, and should not be mistaken for either tSAH or ntSAH.

(2-48) NECT shows sylvian fissure ➡, inferior frontal ➡, perimesencephalic ➡ tSAH, contusions ➡, and small left aSDH ➡. (2-49) Coronal NECT of tSAH shows hemorrhage in both lateral cerebral fissures ➡, while the basilar cisterns ➡ appear normal.

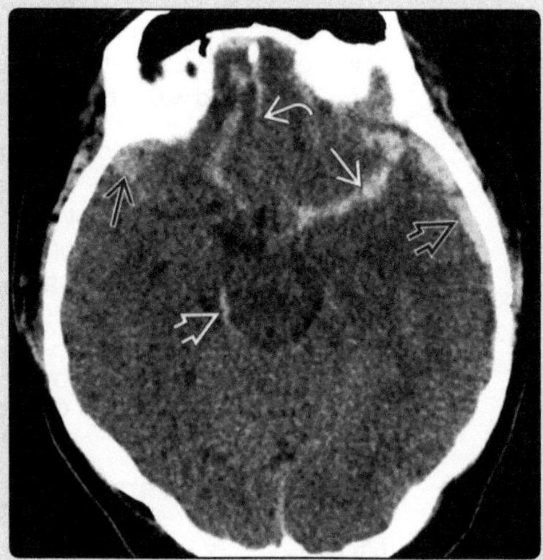

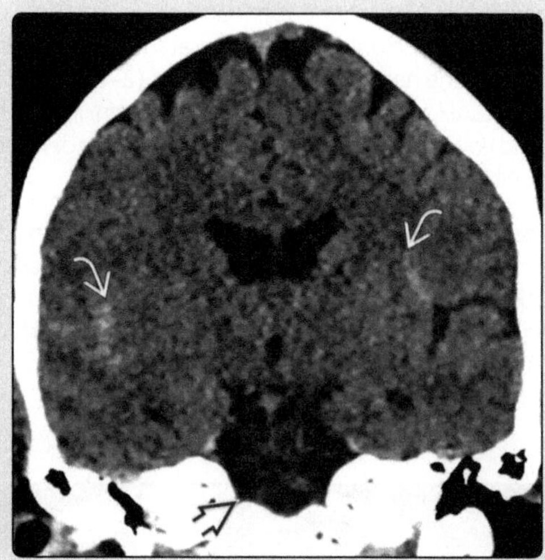

(2-50) NECT shows a small right SDH ➡ and multiple scattered foci of tSAH ➡ in the convexity sulci. (2-51) Axial NECT shows a small peritentorial aSDH ➡ and a small amount of subarachnoid blood in the interpeduncular cistern ➡.

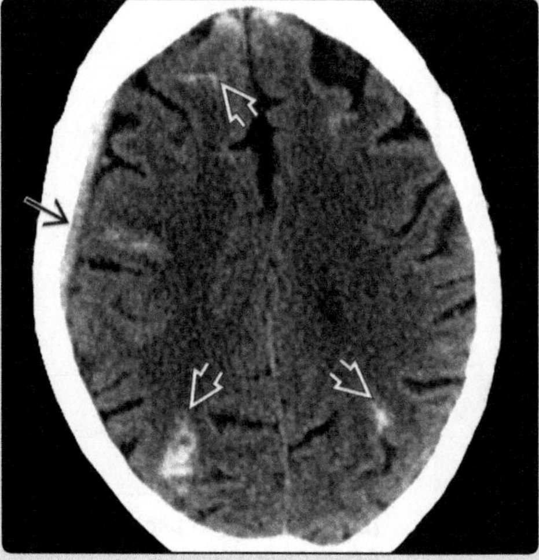

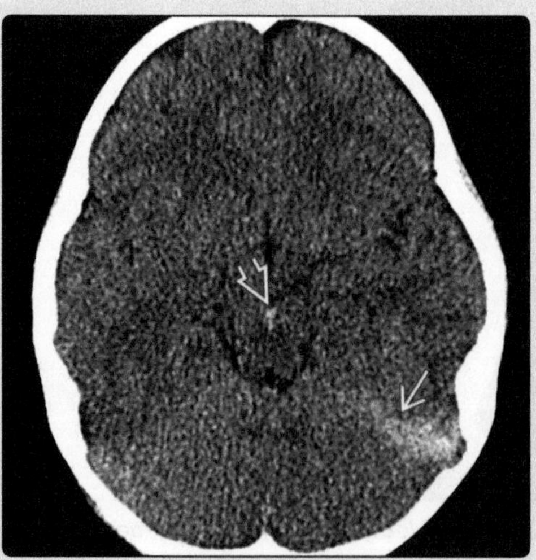

SUBDURAL AND SUBARACHNOID HEMORRHAGE

aSDH
- 2nd most common traumatic extraaxial hemorrhage
  - aSDH > > epidural hematoma
- Crescentic collection of blood between dura, arachnoid
  - Supratentorial (95%), bilateral (15%)
  - SDHs cross sutures
  - SDHs do not cross dural attachments
- CT
  - Hyperdense (60%)
  - Mixed (40%)
  - Isodense aSDH rare (anemia, coagulopathy, CSF mixture)

Subacute SDH (sSDH)
- Clot organizes, lyses, forms "neomembranes"
- CT
  - Density decreases 1-2 HU/day
  - Isodense with cortex in 7-10 days
  - Look for displaced "dots" of CSF under SDH
  - Gray-white interface "buckled" inward
  - Displaced cortical veins seen on CECT
- MR
  - Signal varies with clot age
  - T2* (GRE, SWI) shows "blooming"
  - T1 C+ shows clot inside enhancing membranes

Chronic/Mixed SDH (cSDH/mSDH)
- Serosanguineous fluid
  - Hypodense on NECT
  - Rehemorrhage (5-10%)
  - Loculated blood "pockets" with fluid-fluid levels common
- Differential diagnosis of uncomplicated cSDH
  - Subdural *hygroma* (arachnoid tear → subdural CSF)
  - Subdural *effusion* (clear fluid accumulates after meningitis)
  - Subdural *empyema* (pus)

tSAH
- Most common traumatic extraaxial hemorrhage
- tSAH > > aneurysmal SAH
- Adjacent to cortical contusions
- Superficial sulci > basilar cisterns

Parenchymal Injuries

Intraaxial traumatic injuries include cortical contusions and lacerations, diffuse axonal injury (DAI), subcortical injuries, and intraventricular hemorrhages. In this section, we again begin with the most peripheral injuries—cortical contusions—and work our way inward, ending with the deepest (subcortical) injuries. *In general, the deeper the abnormalities, the more serious the injury.*

Cerebral Contusions and Lacerations

Cerebral contusions are the most common of the intraaxial injuries. True brain lacerations are rare and typically occur only with severe (often fatal) head injury.

Terminology

Cerebral contusions are basically "brain bruises." They evolve with time and often are more apparent on delayed scans than at the time of initial imaging.

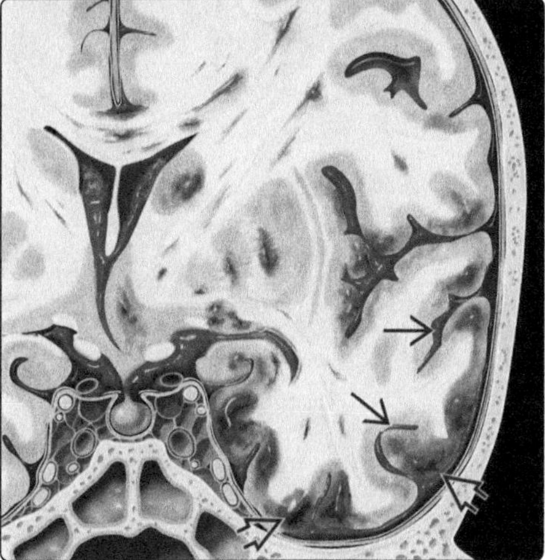

***(2-52)** Cortical contusions are located primarily along gyral crests ⇨, around a sylvian fissure. tSAH is common in adjacent sulci ⇨.*

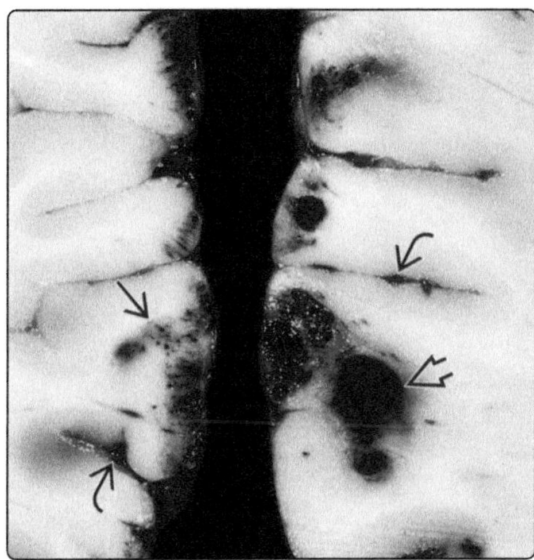

***(2-53)** Autopsy shows petechial ⇨ and larger confluent cortical contusions ⇨, tSAH in adjacent sulci ⇨. (Courtesy R. Hewlett, MD.)*

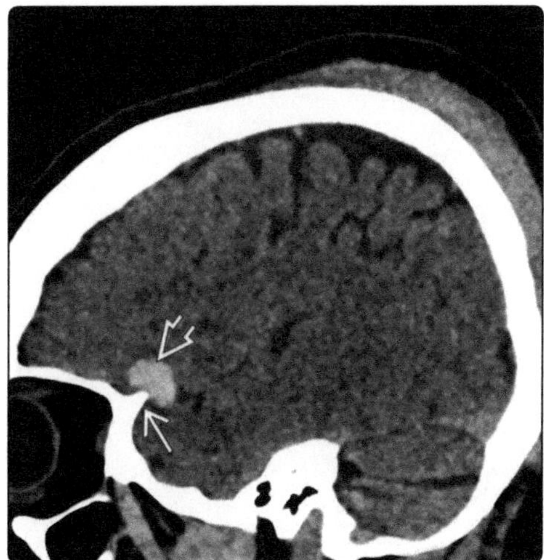

***(2-54)** Sagittal NECT in CHI shows cortical contusion ⇨ immediately adjacent to bony ridge of greater sphenoid wing ⇨.*

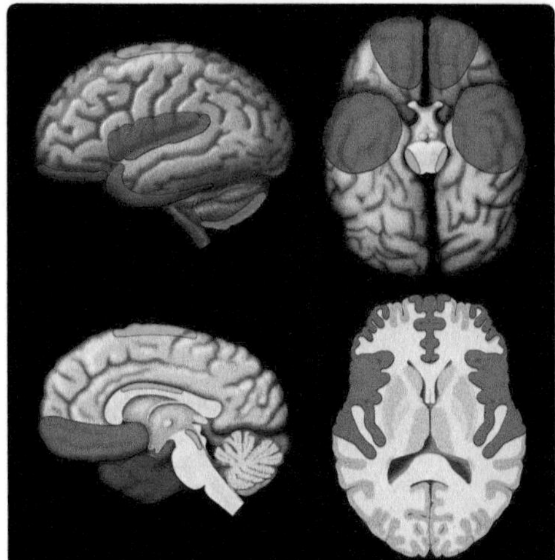

(2-55) Graphics depict the most common sites of cerebral contusions in red. Less common sites are shown in green.

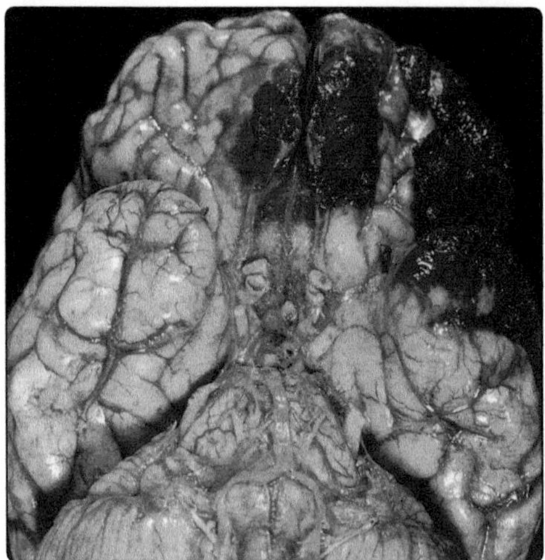

(2-56) Autopsied brain shows typical locations of contusions, i.e., the anteroinferior frontal and temporal lobes. (Courtesy R. Hewlett, MD.)

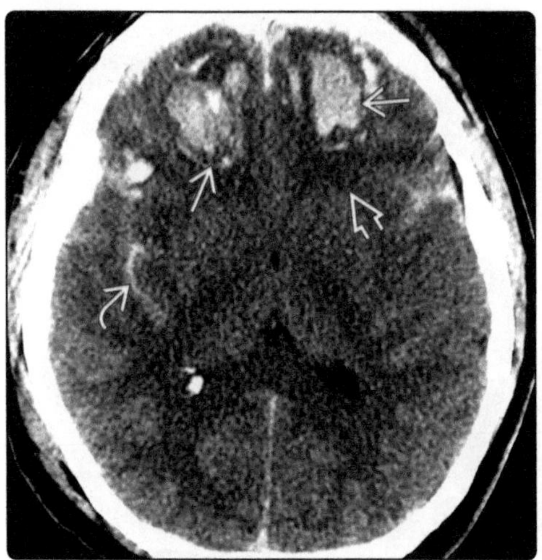

(2-57) NECT scan shows bilateral inferior frontal confluent contusions ⇒, perilesional edema ⇒, and traumatic SAH ⇒.

Cerebral contusions are also called gyral "crest" injuries **(2-52)**. The term "gliding" contusion is sometimes used to describe parasagittal contusions.

Etiology

Most cerebral contusions result from nonmissile or blunt head injury. CHI induces abrupt changes in angular momentum and deceleration. The brain is suddenly and forcibly impacted against an osseous ridge or the hard, knife-like edge of the falx cerebri and tentorium cerebelli. Less commonly, a depressed skull fracture directly damages the underlying brain.

Pathology

Location. Contusions are injuries of the brain surface that involve the gray matter and contiguous subcortical white matter **(2-52)** **(2-53)**. They occur in very characteristic, highly predictable locations. Nearly 1/2 involve the temporal lobes. The temporal tips, as well as the lateral and inferior surfaces and the perisylvian gyri, are most commonly affected **(2-55)**. The inferior (orbital) surfaces of the frontal lobes are also frequently affected **(2-56)**.

Convexity gyri, the dorsal corpus callosum body, dorsolateral midbrain, and cerebellum are less common sites of cerebral contusions. The occipital poles are rarely involved, even with relatively severe CHI.

Size and Number. Cerebral contusions vary in size from tiny lesions to large confluent hematomas. They are almost always multiple and often bilateral **(2-56)**. Contusions that occur at 180° opposite the site of direct impact (the "coup") are common and called "contre-coup" lesions.

Clinical Issues

Epidemiology and Demographics. Cerebral contusions account for ~ 1/2 of all traumatic parenchymal lesions. They occur at all ages, from infants to the elderly. The peak age is 15-24 years, and the M:F ratio is 3:1.

Imaging

CT Findings. Initial scans obtained soon after a CHI may be normal. The most frequent abnormality is the presence of focal or petechial hemorrhages along gyral crests immediately adjacent to the calvarium. A mixture of petechial hemorrhages surrounded by patchy ill-defined hypodense areas of edema is common **(2-57)** **(2-58)**.

A lesion "blooming" over time is frequent and seen with progressive increase in hemorrhage, edema, and mass effect **(2-59)**. Small lesions may coalesce, forming larger focal hematomas. Development of new lesions that were not present on initial imaging is also common.

MR Findings. MR is much more sensitive than CT in detecting cerebral contusions but is rarely obtained in the acute stage of TBI. T2 scans show patchy hyperintense areas (edema) surrounding hypointense foci of hemorrhage **(2-60A)**.

FLAIR scans are most sensitive for detecting cortical edema and associated tSAH, both of which appear as hyperintense foci on FLAIR. T2* (GRE, SWI) is the most sensitive sequence for imaging parenchymal hemorrhages. Significant "blooming" is typical in acute lesions **(2-60B)**.

Differential Diagnosis

The major differential diagnosis of cortical contusion is **DAI**. Both cerebral contusions and DAI are often present in patients who have sustained moderate to severe head injury. Contusions tend to be superficial, located along gyral crests. DAI is most commonly found in the corona radiata and

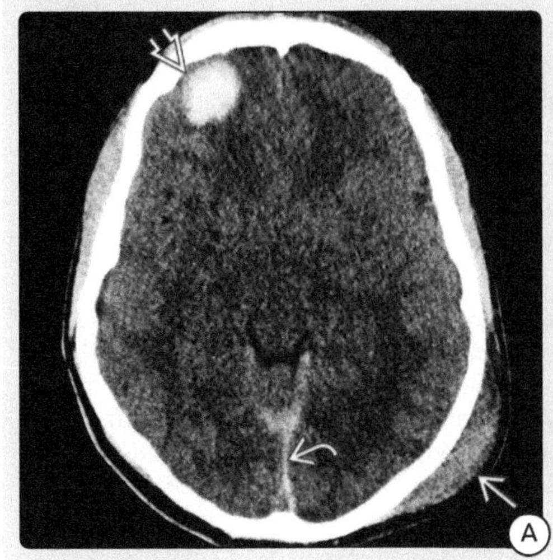
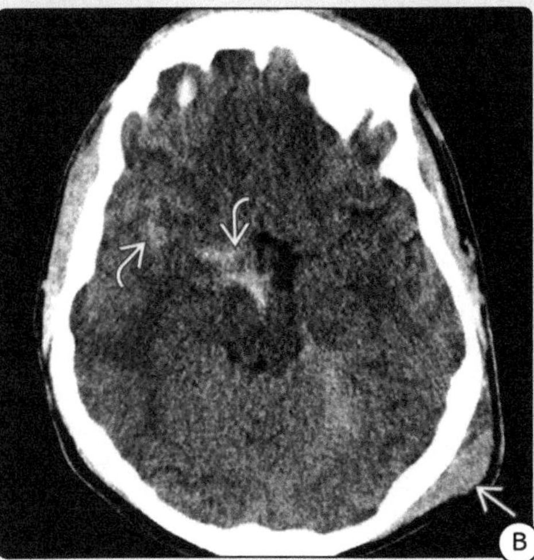

***(2-58A)** Contusions are a common "countre-coup" injury. In this case, the initial trauma was to the left parietooccipital region at the site of the scalp hematoma ➔. A large right frontal contusion ➔ is seen directly opposite the impact site. Note small ➔ peritentorial aSDH. **(2-58B)** Lower scan in the same case shows the scalp hematoma ➔ and traumatic SAH ➔, also opposite the impact site.*

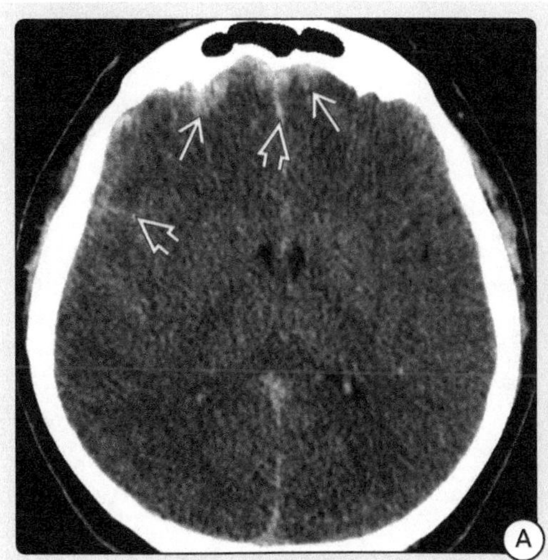
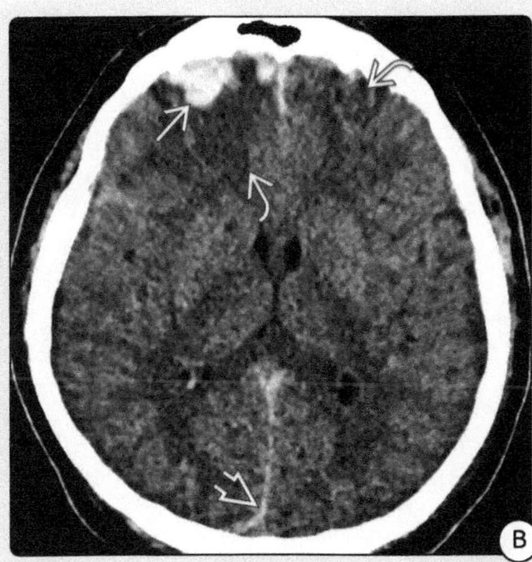

***(2-59A)** Series of NECT scans demonstrates expected interval evolution of cortical contusions. Admission imaging shows bilateral inferior frontal contusions ➔, some tSAH ➔. **(2-59B)** Follow-up NECT 6 hours later shows that the contusions have enlarged ➔ and bifrontal hypodensities around the contusions have become apparent ➔. Note small peritentorial aSDH ➔.*

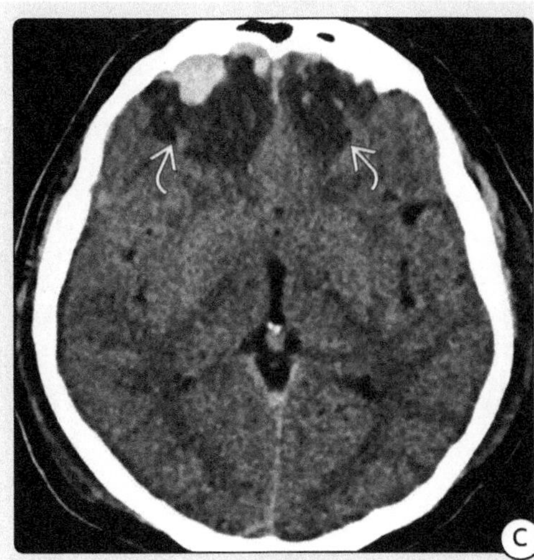
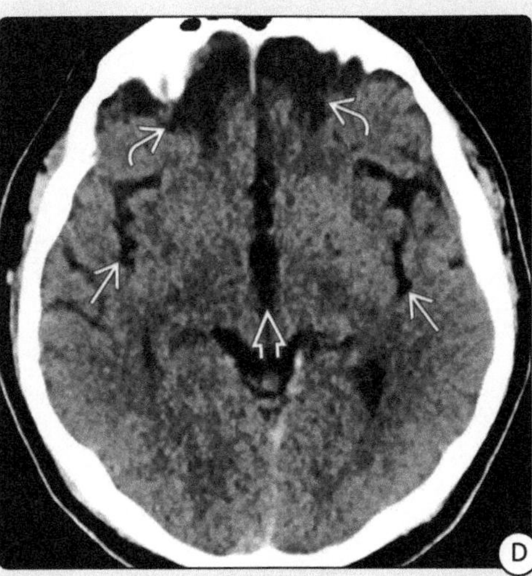

***(2-59C)** Repeat NECT at 48 hours shows that the bifrontal hypodensities ➔ have consolidated around the hemorrhages. The tSAH and peritentorial aSDH have largely resolved. **(2-59D)** NECT at 2 months shows bifrontal encephalomalacia ➔, enlarged sylvian fissures ➔, and prominent 3rd ventricle ➔. These changes are common following moderately severe head trauma.*

along compact white matter tracts, such as the internal capsule and corpus callosum.

Severe cortical contusion with confluent hematomas may be difficult to distinguish from brain laceration on imaging studies. **Brain laceration** occurs when severe trauma disrupts the pia and literally tears the underlying brain apart. Parenchymal brain laceration in infants and young children is typically associated with abusive head trauma.

A "burst lobe" is the most severe manifestation of frank brain laceration **(2-61)** **(2-62)**. Here, the affected lobe is grossly disrupted with large hematoma formation and adjacent tSAH. In some cases, especially those with depressed skull fracture, the arachnoid is also lacerated, and hemorrhage from the burst lobe extends to communicate directly with the subdural space, forming a coexisting SDH.

Diffuse Axonal Injury

DAI is the second most common parenchymal lesion seen in TBI, exceeded only by cortical contusions. Patients with DAI often exhibit an apparent discrepancy between clinical status (often moderately to severely impaired) and initial imaging findings (often normal or minimally abnormal).

Etiology

Most DAIs are caused by high-velocity MVCs and are dynamic, deformative, nonimpact injuries resulting from the inertial forces of rotation generated by sudden changes in acceleration/deceleration. The cortex moves at a different speed relative to underlying deep brain structures (white matter, deep gray nuclei). This results in axonal stretching, especially where brain tissues of different density intersect, i.e., the gray matter-white matter interface.

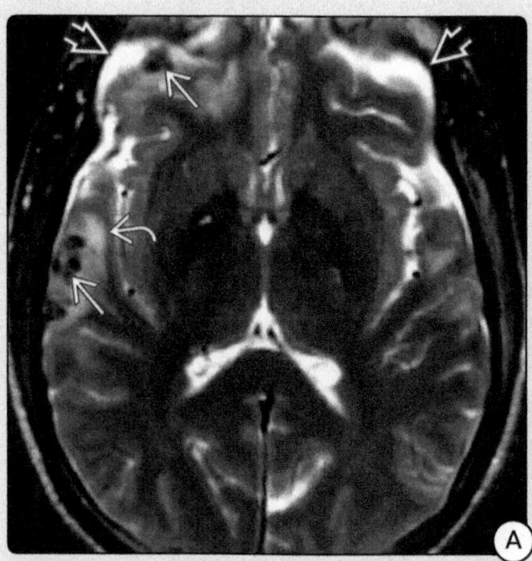

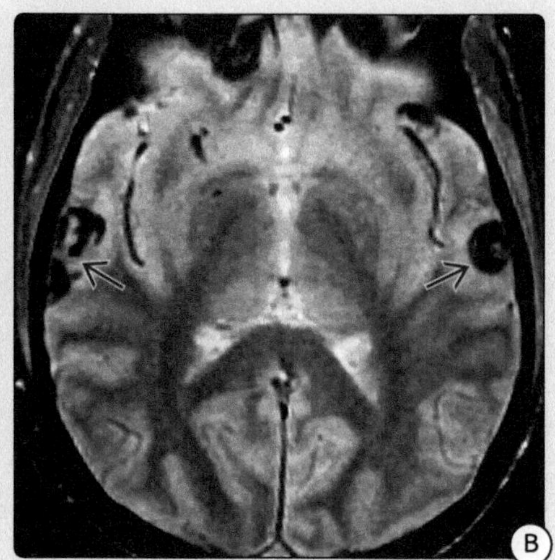

***(2-60A)** T2WI shows contusions ➡ with perilesional edema ➡ and bilateral subdural hygromas ➡. **(2-60B)** T2* GRE in the same case shows that the contusions "bloom" ➡.*

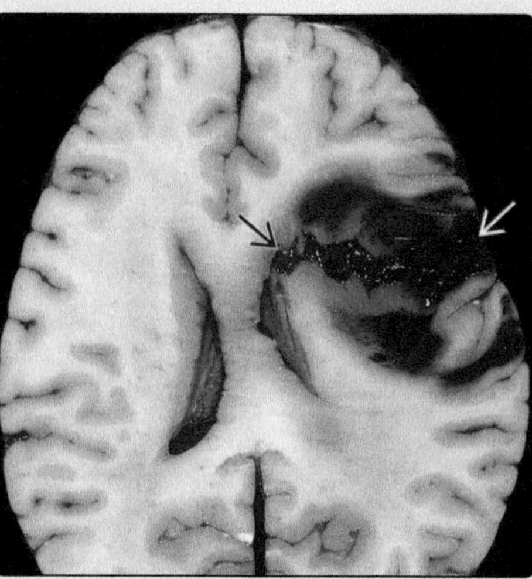

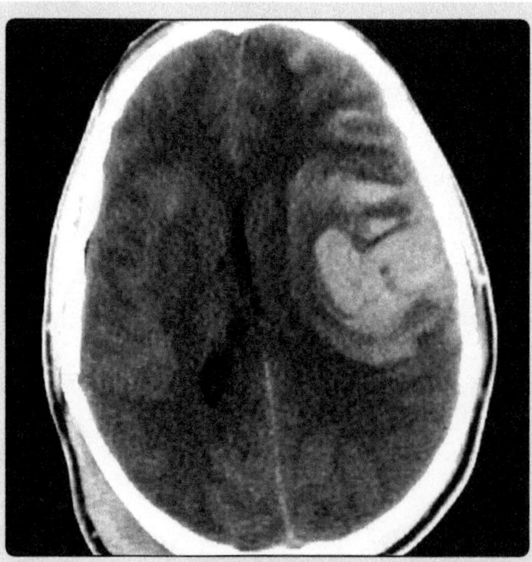

***(2-61)** Autopsy shows a "burst" lobe with a "full-thickness" laceration extending from the pial surface ➡ to the ventricle ➡. (Courtesy R. Hewlett, MD.) **(2-62)** NECT scan shows a "burst" lobe with rapid parenchymal hemorrhage extending deep into the brain. The patient died shortly after this scan was obtained.*

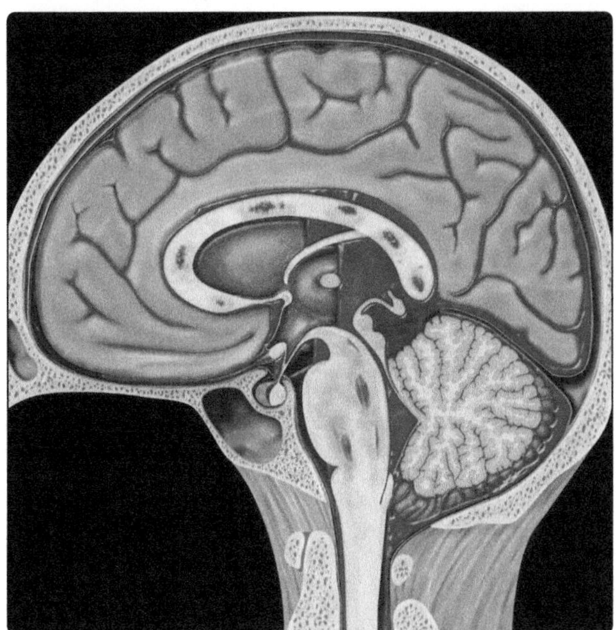

(2-63) Sagittal graphic depicts common sites of axonal injury in the corpus callosum and midbrain. Traumatic intraventricular and subarachnoid hemorrhage is present.

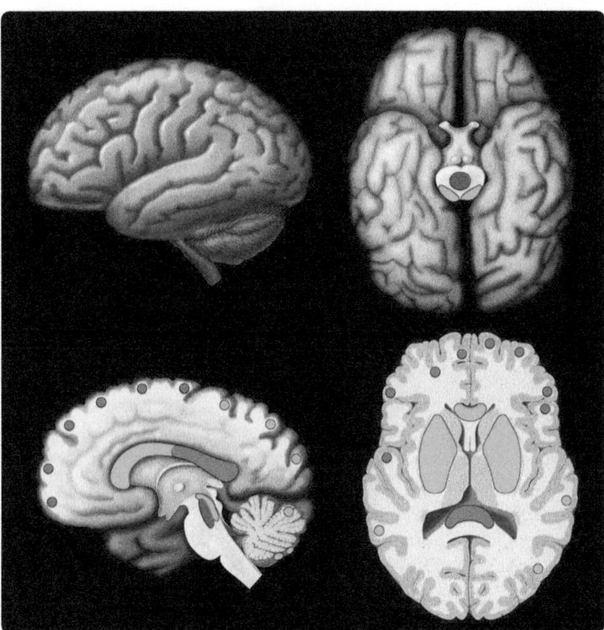

(2-64) Graphics depict the most common sites of axonal injury in red. Frequent but relatively less common locations are shown in green. Injury to the midbrain/upper pons (purple) is uncommon but often lethal.

Pathology

Location. DAI occurs in highly predictable locations. The cortex is typically spared; it is the subcortical and deep white matter that is most commonly affected. Lesions in compact white matter tracts, such as the corpus callosum, especially the genu and splenium, fornix, and internal capsule, are frequent. The midbrain and pons are less common sites of DAI **(2-63)** **(2-64)**.

Gross Pathology. The vast majority of DAIs are microscopic and nonhemorrhagic. Tears of penetrating vessels (diffuse vascular injury) may cause small round to ovoid or linear hemorrhages that sometimes are the only gross indications of underlying axonal injury **(2-65)**. These visible lesions are truly just the "tip of the iceberg."

Clinical Issues

Epidemiology and Demographics. DAI is present in virtually all fatal TBIs and is found in almost 3/4 of patients with moderate or severe injury who survive the acute stage.

DAI may occur at any age, but peak incidence is in young adults (15-24 years old). Male patients are at least twice as often afflicted with TBI as female patients.

Presentation. DAI typically causes much more significant impairment compared with extracerebral hematomas and cortical contusions. DAI often causes immediate loss of consciousness, which may be transient (in the case of mild TBI) or progress to coma (with moderate to severe injury).

Imaging

CT Findings. Initial NECT is often normal or minimally abnormal. Mild diffuse brain swelling with sulcal effacement may be present. A few small round or ovoid subcortical hemorrhages may be visible **(2-66)**, but the underlying damage is typically much more diffuse and much more severe than these relatively modest abnormalities would indicate.

MR Findings. MR is much more sensitive in detecting changes of DAI. T2WI and FLAIR may show hyperintense foci in the subcortical white matter and corpus callosum. Multiple lesions are the rule, and a combination of DAI and contusions or hematomas is very common.

T2* (GRE, SWI) scans are very sensitive to the microbleeds of DAI and typically show multifocal ovoid and linear hypointensities. DWI may show restricted diffusion, particularly within the corpus callosum.

Differential Diagnosis

Cortical contusions often coexist with DAI in moderate to severe TBI. Cortical contusions are typically superficial lesions, usually located along gyral crests.

Multifocal hemorrhages with "blooming" on T2* (GRE, SWI) scans can be seen in numerous pathologies, including DAI. **Diffuse vascular injury** appears as multifocal parenchymal "black dots." Pneumocephalus may cause multifocal "blooming" lesions in the subarachnoid spaces. Parenchymal lesions are rare.

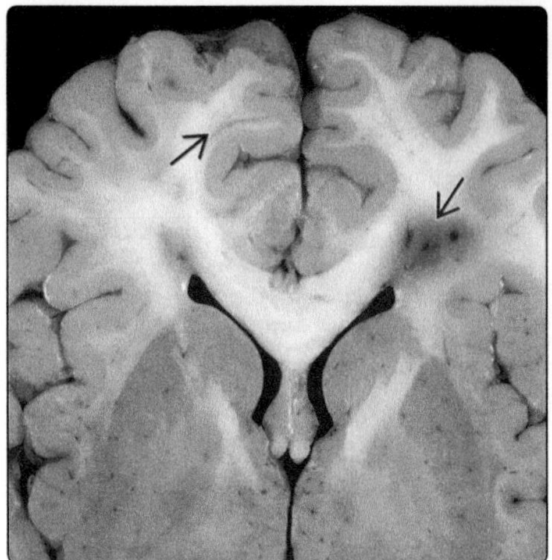

(2-65) Diffuse axonal injury includes linear subcortical, deep periventricular WM hemorrhages ⇒. (Courtesy R. Hewlett, MD.)

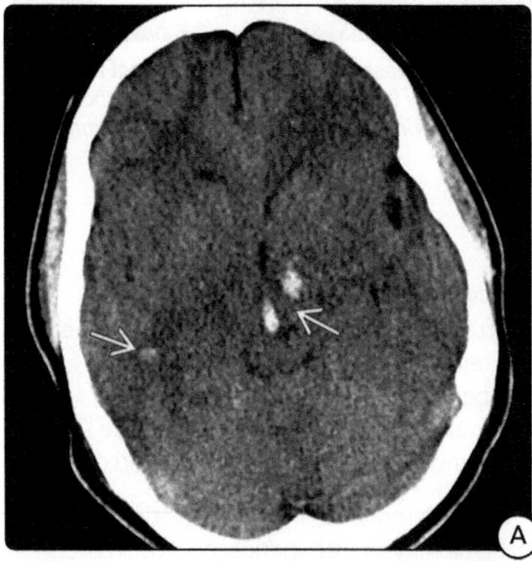

(2-66A) NECT in a patient with severe CHI shows punctate and linear hemorrhagic foci in the subcortical WM, midbrain, and left thalamus ⇒.

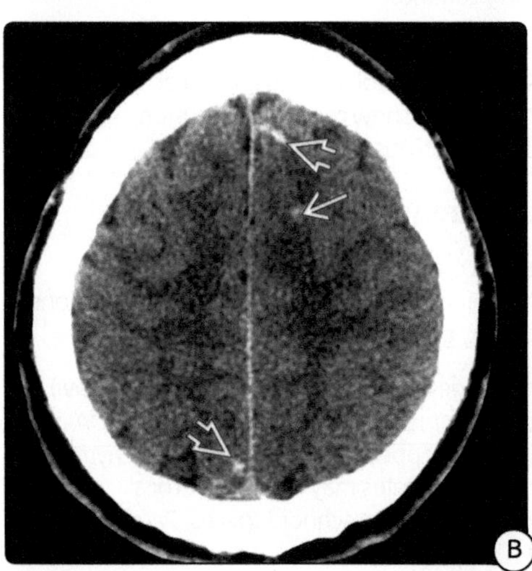

(2-66B) More cephalad scan in the same patient shows additional hemorrhagic foci in the corona radiata ⇒ and subcortical WM ⇒.

Diffuse Vascular Injury

Terminology

Diffuse vascular injury (DVI) probably represents the extreme end of the DAI continuum.

Etiology

DVI is caused by the extreme acceleration/rotational forces that are incurred in high-velocity MVCs. The brain microvasculature, particularly long penetrating subcortical and deep perforating vessels, is disrupted by high tensile forces. The result is numerous small punctate and linear parenchymal hemorrhages.

Pathology

Gross Pathology. Autopsied brains of patients with DVI show numerous small hemorrhages in the subcortical and deep white matter as well as in the deep gray nuclei. Blood is identified along periarterial, perivenous, and pericapillary spaces with focal hemorrhages in the adjacent parenchyma.

Clinical Issues

Epidemiology. Autopsy series suggest that DVI is present in 1-2% of fatal MVC victims and 15% of cases with diffuse brain injury. Although DVI can occur at any age, most occur in adults.

Presentation. Immediate coma from the moment of impact is typical. A very low GCS, often < 6-8, is typical in patients who survive the initial impact.

Imaging

CT Findings. NECT scans may show only diffuse brain swelling with effaced superficial sulci and small ventricles. A few small foci of hemorrhage in the white matter and basal ganglia can sometimes be identified.

MR Findings. T1WI shows only mild brain swelling. T2WI and FLAIR scans may demonstrate a few foci of hyperintensity in the white matter **(2-67A)**. Occasionally, scattered hypointensities can be identified within the hyperintensities, suggesting the presence of hemorrhage.

T2* (GRE/SWI) sequences are striking. Punctate and linear "blooming" hypointensities are seen oriented perpendicularly to the ventricles, predominantly in the subcortical and deep white matter, especially the corpus callosum **(2-67B)**. Additional lesions in the basal ganglia, thalami, brainstem, and cerebellum are often present.

DWI may demonstrate a few foci of restricted diffusion consistent with ischemia caused by the vascular injuries **(2-67C)**.

Differential Diagnosis

The major differential diagnosis is **DAI**. DVI is characterized by innumerable petechial hemorrhages on T2* imaging. It is the number, severity, and extent of the hemorrhages that distinguishes DVI from DAI.

Subcortical (Deep Brain) Injury

Terminology

Subcortical injuries (SCIs) are traumatic lesions of deep brain structures, such as the brainstem, basal ganglia, thalami, and ventricles. Most represent severe shear-strain injuries that disrupt axons, tear penetrating blood vessels, and damage the choroid plexus of the lateral ventricles.

Pathology

Gross Pathology. Manifestations of SCI include deep hemorrhagic contusions, nonhemorrhagic lacerations, intraventricular bleeds, and tSAH **(2-68)**. SCIs usually occur with other traumatic lesions, such as cortical contusions and DAI.

Clinical Issues

Epidemiology. Between 5% and 10% of patients with moderate to severe brain trauma sustain SCIs. SCIs are the third most common parenchymal brain injury after cortical contusions and DAI. As with most traumatic brain injuries, SCIs are most common in male patients between the ages of 15 and 24 years.

Natural History. Prognosis is poor in these severely injured patients. Many do not survive; those who do typically have profound neurologic impairment with severe long-term disability.

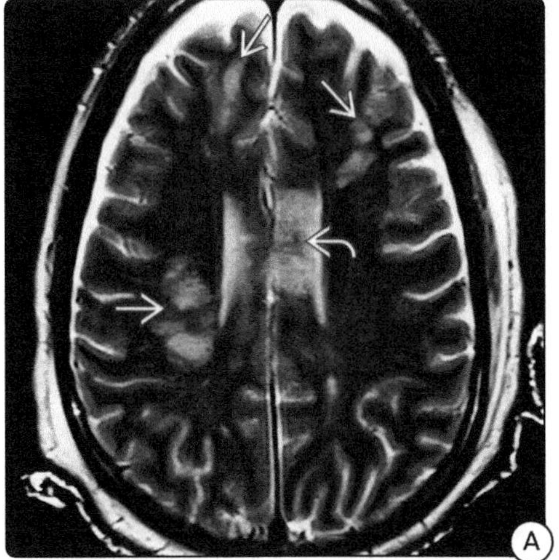

(2-67A) MR 2 days after a normal initial NECT shows hyperintensities in subcortical/deep WM ➡ and corpus callosum ➡.

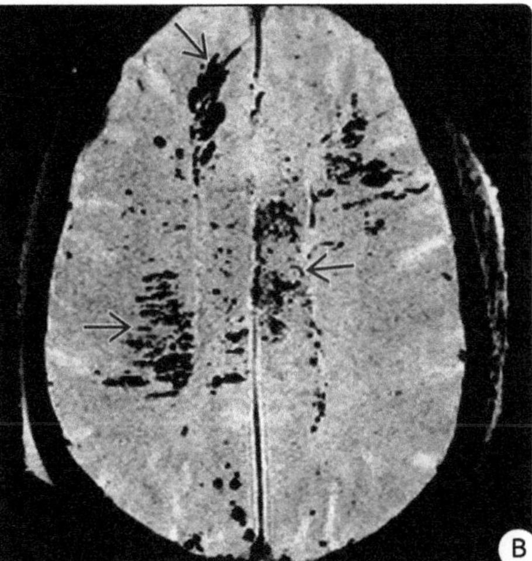

(2-67B) SWI MIP in the same case shows innumerable punctate and linear "blooming" hypointensities ➡, consistent with DVI.

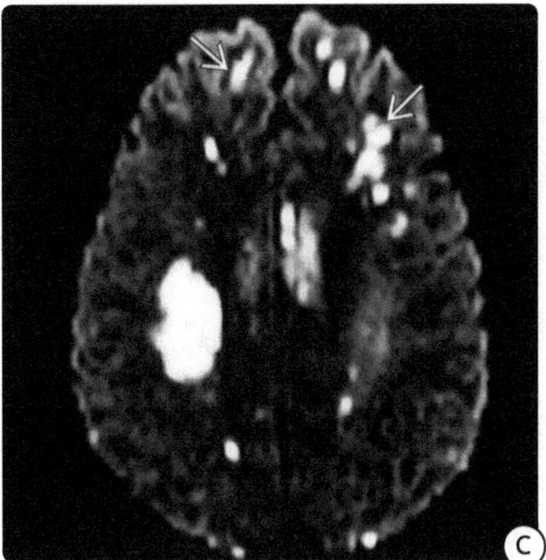

(2-67C) DWI in the same case shows multiple foci of restricted diffusion ➡.

PARENCHYMAL BRAIN INJURIES

Cerebral Contusions
- Most common intraaxial injury
  - Brain impacts skull &/or dura
  - Causes "brain bruises" in gyral crests
  - Usually multiple, often bilateral
  - Anteroinferior frontal, temporal lobes most common sites
- Imaging
  - Superficial petechial, focal hemorrhage
  - Edema, hemorrhage more apparent with time
  - T2* (GRE, SWI) most sensitive imaging

Diffuse Axonal Injury (DAI)
- 2nd most common intraaxial injury
  - Spares cortex, involves subcortical/deep white matter
- Imaging
  - GCS low; initial imaging often minimally abnormal
  - Subcortical, deep petechial hemorrhages ("tip of the iceberg")
  - T2* (GRE, SWI) most sensitive technique

Diffuse Vascular Injury
- Rare, usually fatal
- High-speed, high-impact MVCs
- May represent extreme end of DAI spectrum
- Imaging
  - CT shows diffuse brain swelling
  - T2 and FLAIR show a few scattered hyperintensities
  - SWI shows innumerable linear hypointensities

Subcortical Injury
- "The deeper the injury, the worse it is"
- Basal ganglia, thalami, midbrain, pons
  - Hemorrhages, axonal injury, brain tears

Imaging

General Features. Minimal abnormalities may be present on initial imaging but show dramatic increase on follow-up scans.

SCI typically exists with numerous comorbid injuries. Lesions ranging from subtle tSAH to gross parenchymal hemorrhage are common **(2-69)**. Mass

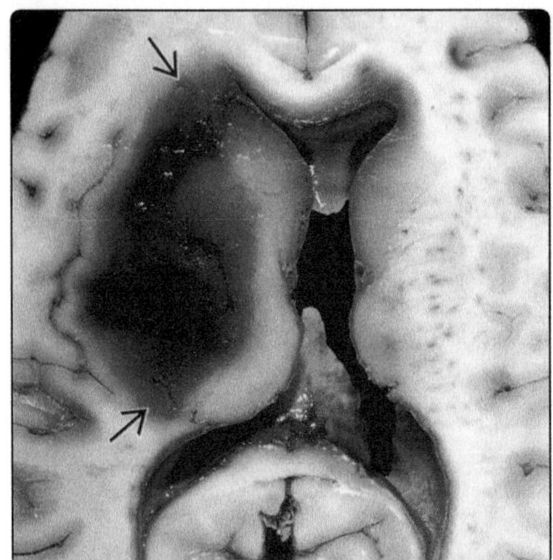

(2-68) High-speed MVC shows a large hemorrhage ⇨ characteristic of severe subcortical injury. (Courtesy R. Hewlett, MD.)

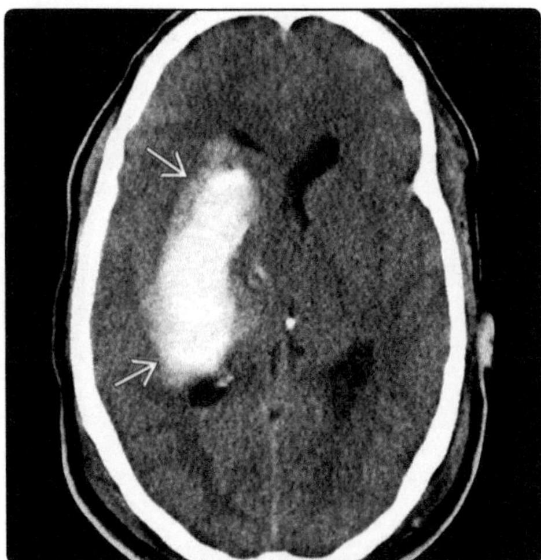

(2-69) NECT in a 38-year-old man in a severe MVA shows a large expanding basal ganglia hematoma ➡. He expired 2 days later.

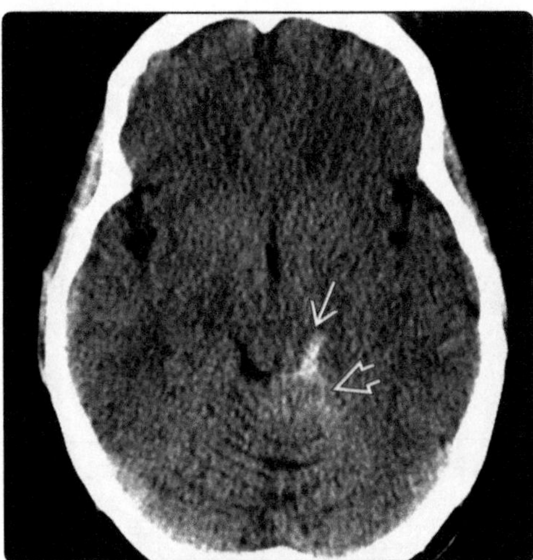

(2-70) NECT of midbrain contusion shows hyperdensity in the left posterolateral midbrain ➡ associated with focal tSAH ➡.

effect with cerebral herniation and gross disturbances in regional blood flow may develop.

CT Findings. NECT scans often show diffuse brain swelling with punctate &/or gross hemorrhage in the deep gray nuclei and midbrain **(2-70)**. Intraventricular and choroid plexus hemorrhages are common and may form a "cast" of the lateral ventricles. Blood-fluid levels are common.

MR Findings. MR is much more sensitive than CT, even though acute hemorrhage is isointense with brain on T1 scans. FLAIR and T2* are the most sensitive sequences. DWI may show foci of restricted diffusion. DTI mapping delineates the pattern of white matter tract disruption.

Differential Diagnosis

Secondary midbrain ("Duret") hemorrhage may occur with severe descending transtentorial herniation. These hemorrhages are typically centrally located within the midbrain, whereas contusional SCIs are dorsolateral.

Miscellaneous Injuries

Pneumocephalus

Differential Diagnosis

Air is air and should not be mistaken for anything else. If wide windows are not used, a ruptured dermoid cyst with fat droplets in the CSF cisterns can mimic subarachnoid air.

Terminology

Intracranial air does not exist under normal conditions. In **pneumocephalus**, air can be found anywhere within the cranium, including blood vessels, and within any compartment. While intracranial air is never normal, it can be an expected and therefore routine finding (e.g., after surgery).

Tension pneumocephalus is a collection of intracranial air under pressure that causes mass effect on the brain and results in neurologic deterioration. Intracerebral **pneumatocele** or "aerocele" is a less commonly used term and refers specifically to a focal gas collection within the brain parenchyma.

Clinical Issues

Epidemiology. Pneumocephalus is present in 3% of all patients with skull fractures and 8% of those with paranasal sinus fractures. Virtually all patients who have supratentorial surgery have some degree of pneumocephalus on imaging studies obtained within the first 24-28 hours.

Natural History and Treatment Options. Unless it is under tension, most intracranial air resolves spontaneously within a few days after trauma or surgery. Occasionally, air collections increase and may require evacuation with duraplasty.

Imaging

General Features. Intracranial air can exist in any compartment (epidural, subdural, subarachnoid, intraventricular, or intraparenchymal) and conforms to the shape of that compartment or potential compartment. The subdural space is the most frequent, and the most common site is frontal.

Epidural air is typically solitary, biconvex in configuration, may cross midline, and does not move with changes in head position **(2-71)**.

Subdural air is confluent, crescentic, and often bilateral, frequently contains air-fluid levels, moves with changes in head position, and surrounds cortical veins that cross the subdural space **(2-72)**.

Subarachnoid air is typically seen as multifocal small "dots" or "droplets" of air within and around cerebral sulci **(2-73)**. **Intraventricular air** forms air-fluid levels, most often in the frontal horns of the lateral ventricles. Intraparenchymal air is uncommon, and such a collection is termed a **pneumatocele (2-74)**. **Intravascular air** conforms to the vascular structure(s) within which it resides.

CT Findings. Air is extremely hypodense on CT, measuring approximately -1,000 HU. The "Mount Fuji" sign of **tension pneumocephalus** is seen as bilateral subdural air collections that separate and compress the frontal lobes, widening the interhemispheric fissure **(2-75)**. The frontal lobes are displaced posteriorly by air under pressure and are typically pointed where they are tethered to the dura-arachnoid by cortical veins, mimicking the silhouette of Mount Fuji.

Distinguishing air from fat on CT is extremely important. With typical narrow soft tissue windows, both appear similarly hypodense. Increasing window width or simply looking at bone CT algorithms (on which air is clearly distinct from the less hypodense fat) helps differentiate fat from air.

MR Findings. Air is seen as areas of completely absent signal intensity on all sequences **(2-76A)**. On T2* GRE, intracranial air "blooms" and appears as multifocal "black dots" **(2-76B)**.

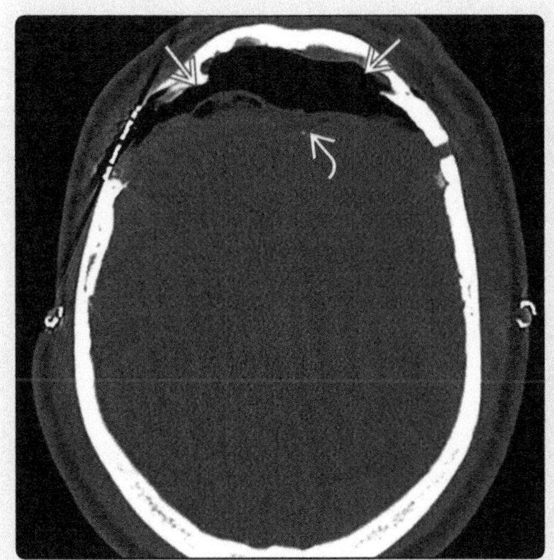

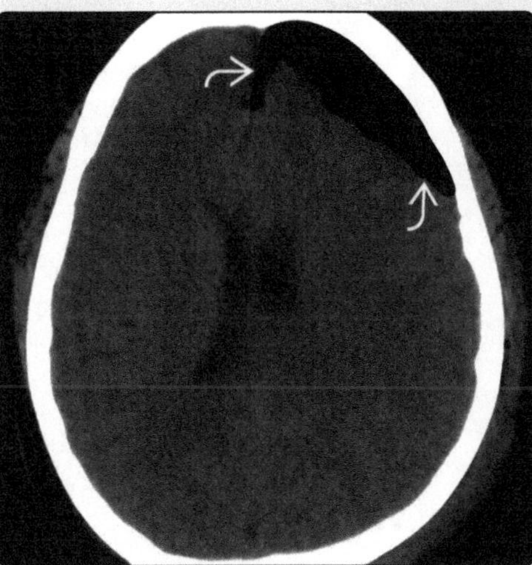

(2-71) *Epidural air is seen in this immediate postoperative NECT following bifrontal craniotomy. The air collection ➡ is continuous across the midline, and the fat packing and dura ➡ are displaced posteriorly, confirming epidural location of air.* ***(2-72)*** *Unilateral subdural air is an expected finding after supratentorial craniotomies. Subdural air ➡ forms a crescent-shaped collection over the hemisphere and does not cross the midline.*

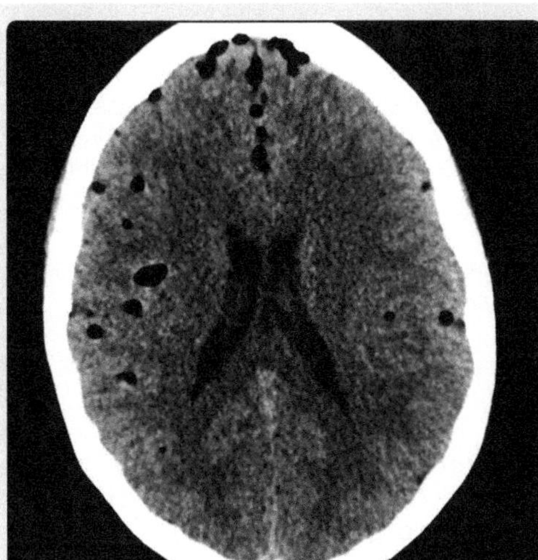

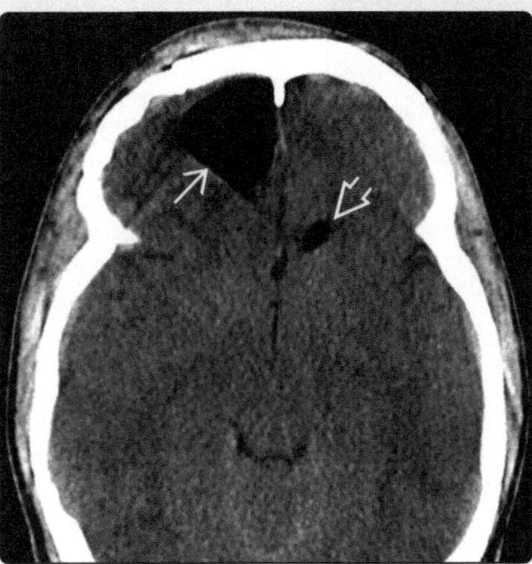

(2-73) *Subarachnoid air appears as scattered, separate "spots" and dots" that collect in the sulci and cisterns.* ***(2-74)*** *NECT scan shows a focal pneumatocele in the right frontal lobe ➡. Some air is also present in the frontal horn of the left lateral ventricle ➡.*

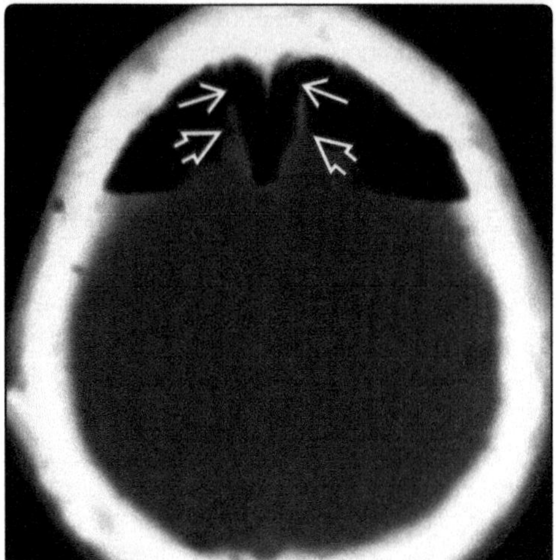

***(2-75)** NECT shows tension pneumocephalus, "Mount Fuji" sign caused by cortical veins ➡ tethering frontal lobes ➡.*

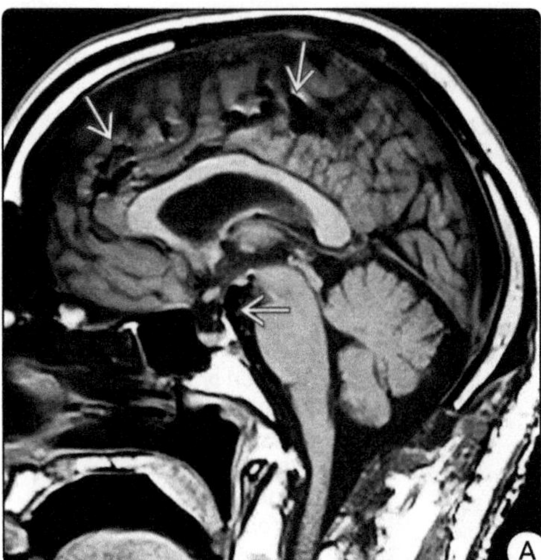

***(2-76A)** Sagittal T1WI shows postoperative pneumocephalus with "spots" and "dots" of air ➡ in the subarachnoid spaces.*

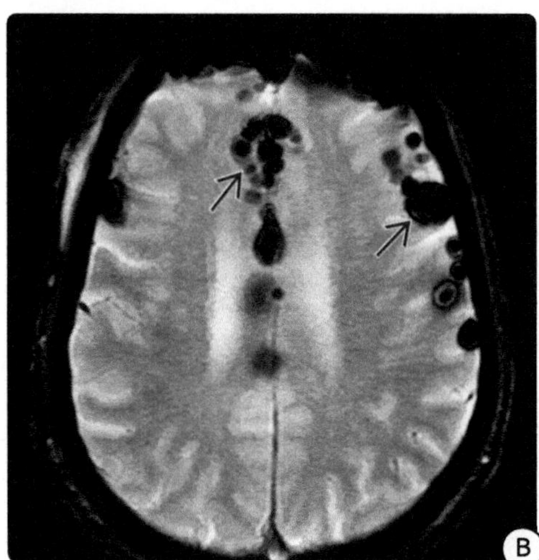

***(2-76B)** T2* GRE scan in the same case shows multifocal "blooming" black dots ➡ representing air in the subarachnoid spaces.*

PNEUMOCEPHALUS

Terminology

- Gross intraventricular hemorrhage common
- Air in intracranial compartment
  - Always abnormal
  - Not always clinically significant
- Tension pneumocephalus
  - Air under pressure → neurologic deterioration

Etiology

- Surgery (most common)
  - Expected after craniotomy
- Trauma (8-10% of cases)
- "Spontaneous" (defect in temporal bone, sinus)

Location

- Epidural
  - Unilateral, biconvex
  - May cross midline
  - Does not move with change in position
- Subdural
  - Confluent, crescentic
  - Often bilateral ± air-fluid level
  - Shows crossing cortical veins
  - Changes with head position
  - Does not cross midline
- Subarachnoid
  - Discrete "spots" and "dots" in sulci, cisterns
- Intraventricular
  - Usually air-fluid levels, frontal horns
- Intraparenchymal
  - Confluent, well delineated

General Imaging Features

- CT
  - Extremely hypodense (-1,000 HU)
  - Fat vs. air? Use wide windows!
- MR
  - Signal void
  - Prominent "blooming" on GRE
  - Alternating dark "holes" ± concentric bright rings
  - Chemical shift artifact in phase-encoding direction

Abusive Head Trauma (Child Abuse)

Radiologists play a key role in the diagnosis of suspected child abuse. Imaging must be performed with care, interpreted with rigor, and precisely described. The final diagnosis of child abuse is typically made by a child abuse pediatrician, who leads a multidisciplinary team (in which the radiologist plays an important role). There is no rush to judgment. Detailed consideration of imaging and medicolegal issues in abusive head trauma is beyond the scope of *Essentials of Osborn's Brain*.

Terminology

The term "nonaccidental trauma" (NAT), a.k.a. nonaccidental injury (NAI) or shaken-baby syndrome (SBS), refers to intentionally inflicted injury. The American Academy of Pediatrics endorses the term **abusive head trauma (AHT)**, which encompasses a spectrum of potential mechanisms of intracranial injury acting independently or in concert, including shaking with or without impact, impact alone, strangulation/suffocation, and hypoxic-ischemic insult.

Etiology

Direct injuries are inflicted by blows to the head, impact of the cranium on an object, such as a wall, or the brain impacting a rigid internal structure, such as the pterion, rough floors of the anterior or middle cranial fossa, falx cerebri, or tentorium cerebelli. Direct impact may result in skull fractures, acute subdural hemorrhage (aSDH), subarachnoid hemorrhage (SAH), contusions in the subjacent brain, parenchymal brain lacerations (PBLs) of the subcortical white matter in the young infant, and "contre-coup" injuries. **Importantly, victims of AHT commonly exhibit no skin, scalp, or calvarial evidence of trauma**, thus supporting shaking alone as the underpinning of intracranial hemorrhage and brain injury in AHT.

AHT may involve linear translational forces with shaking and impact (impactive forces) or complex angular forces without impact (impulsive forces); AHT impulsive forces are commonly commotio forces with acceleration and deceleration often without impact. Resultant subdural and subarachnoid hemorrhages, cerebral edema, infarction, and brainstem or cervical cord injury may predispose the patient to respiratory arrest. Irreversible hypoxic-ischemic injury may result. Death may follow.

Indirect injuries of AHT lead to death and significant neurologic morbidity. The head of an infant or young child is relatively large compared with its body, cervical musculature is comparatively weak, and the incompletely myelinated cerebral white matter relatively fragile. Commotio motion alone (shaking) and potential for whiplash injury of the brainstem and upper cervical cord may lead to death. The most common result of shaking is diffusely distributed aSDH. SAH is a common accompaniment of aSDH. These extraaxial hemorrhages often represent proxies for underlying cerebral edema, early herniation, infarction, parenchymal contusions, subcortical laceration, and axonal shear injuries.

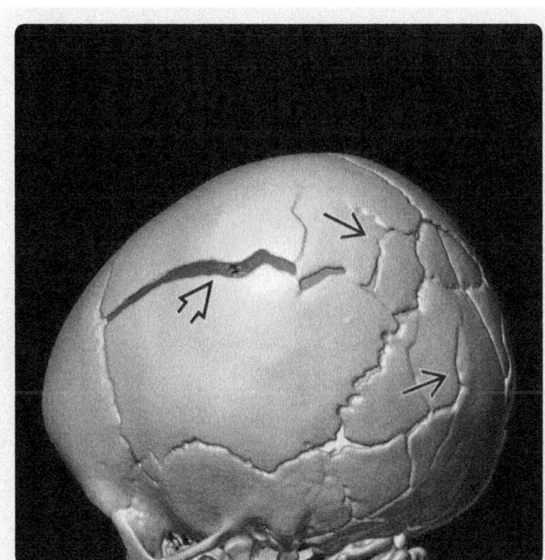

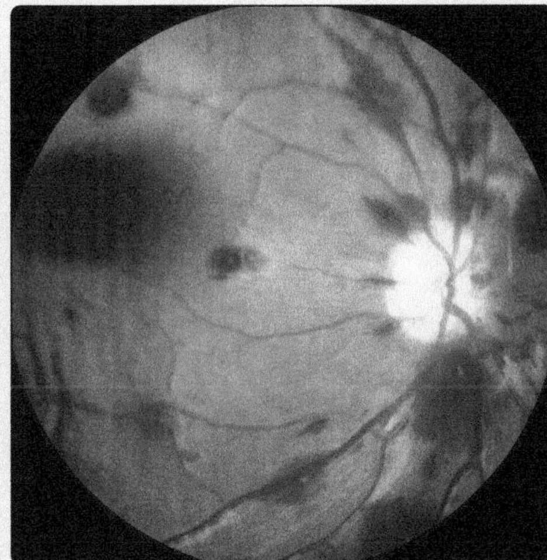

(2-77) 3D NECT in a 6-month-old boy with scalp swelling is shown. There was no history of prior head trauma. Note the diastatic right parietal fracture ⇨ and innumerable occipital and parietal fractures ⇨. Skull fractures are often absent in the setting of abusive head trauma (AHT). ***(2-78)*** *Funduscopic exam in an infant victim of AHT (shaking) shows multiple retinal hemorrhages (RHs). RHs often accompany SDHs. (Courtesy K. Digre, MD.)*

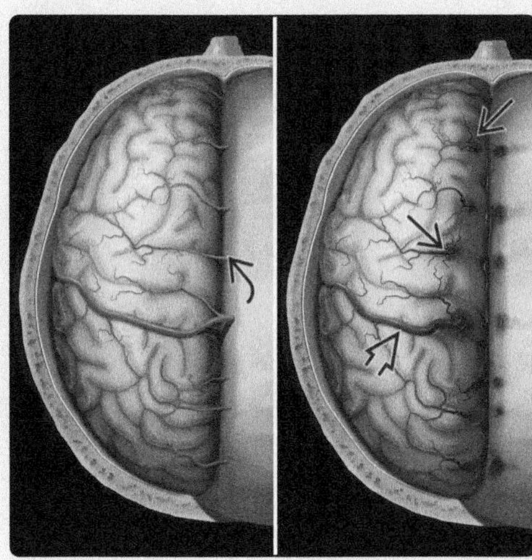

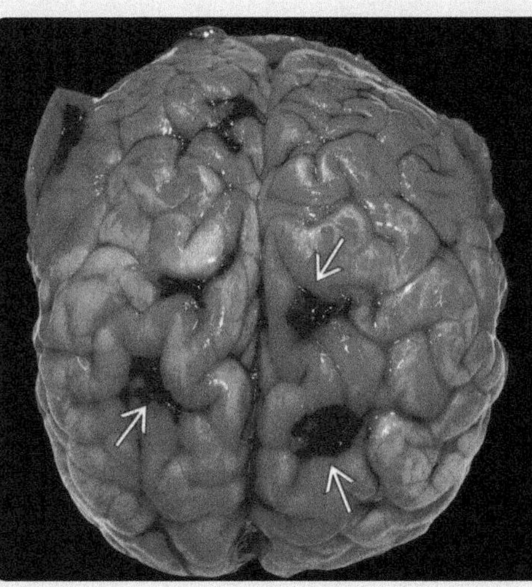

(2-79) (L) Cortical veins bridge subarachnoid space, enter dura ⇨. In AHT (R), numerous torn bridging veins ⇨ are present with thrombosis of the vein of Trolard ⇨. Bridging veins tear at the dural cuff where the veins penetrate the dura of the superior sagittal sinus. ***(2-80)*** *Autopsy photograph in an infant victim of fatal AHT shows numerous traumatically torn and thrombosed convexity bridging veins ➡. (Courtesy C. Rambaud, MD.)*

Pathology

SDH and subdural hygroma (SDHy) (CSF, CT attenuation, and MR signal intensity) detected in a child < 2 years of age are strongly associated with trauma. SDH in a preambulatory infant (< 1 year of age) or young child is highly suspicious for AHT. SDHs of differing ages support multiple traumatic insults and are common in AHT. SDH is the most common intracranial imaging finding in confirmed cases of AHT **(2-81A)**.

Imaging

General Features. Initial imaging in cases of suspected child abuse should include a complete skeletal survey and NECT of the brain in the neurologically symptomatic infant or young child. MR is recommended for children 2 years old or younger. Brain MR obtained 3-5 days after admission helps to optimize the full appraisal of intracranial injury, including estimation of SDH age. Serial imaging (NECT and MR) plays an important role in dating AHT, extraaxial hemorrhage, and characterizing injury patterns.

Radiologists must resist strong dating language when reporting initial NECT findings in AHT. More precision in estimating hemorrhage age and magnitude of injury comes from serial imaging (NECT and MR). Experts emphasize that, although dating of both brain and skeletal injuries is imprecise, the more important goal is determining whether the pattern is that of "differing age" lesions regardless of location.

SDH discovered in the setting of Benign Expansion of the Subarachnoid Spaces (BESS) (a benign transient communicating form of hydrocephalus) in normally developing infants and young children are rare and warrant a thoughtful investigation by the child protective services team.

CT Findings. Identification and characterization of intracranial hemorrhage and detecting cerebral edema and herniation are critical. SDHs are shown in nearly 80% of all AHT cases **(2-**

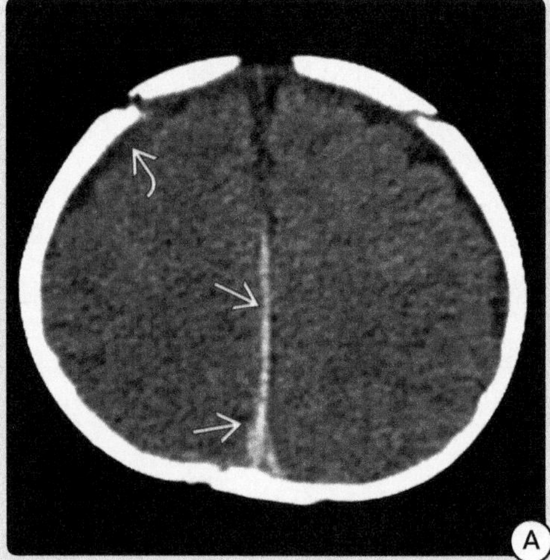

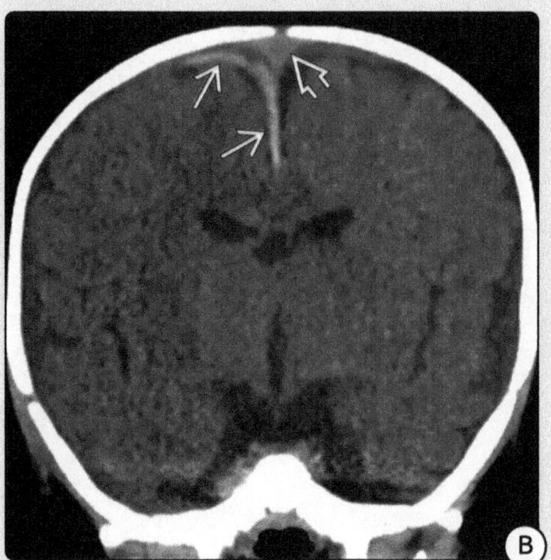

***(2-81A)** Axial NECT in a 3-month-old boy shows acute parafalcine SDH ➡. There was no evidence of scalp or skull injury. Note the hypoattenuating right frontal subdural collection ➡ that MR characterized as a chronic SDH. **(2-81B)** Coronal NECT, MPR shows an acute parafalcine and convexity SDH ➡. Note the triangular shape of the normal superior sagittal dural venous sinus ➡. The falx cerebri limits the medial migration of the SDH.*

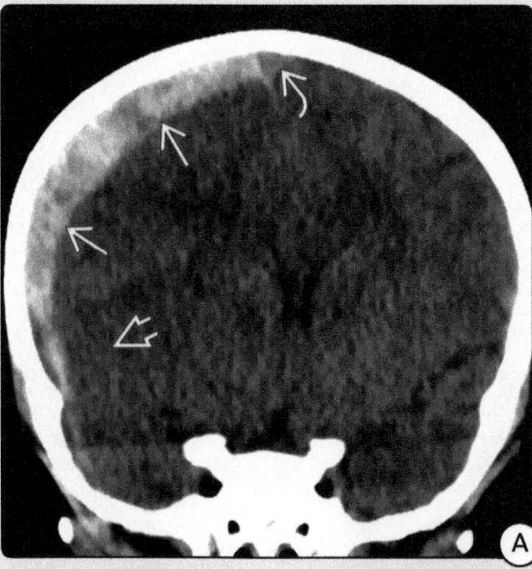

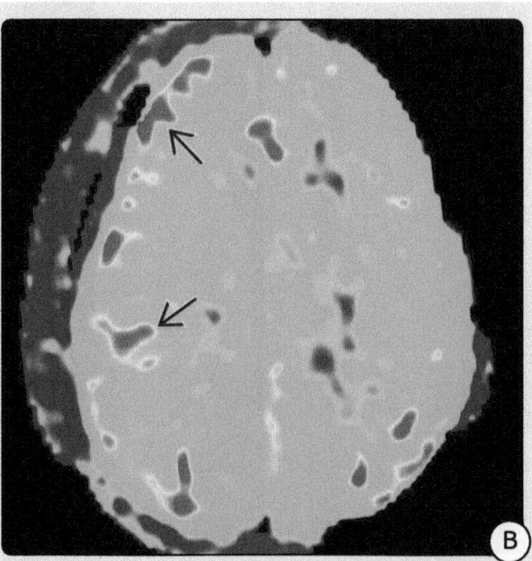

***(2-82A)** Coronal NECT in AHT shows mixed-attenuation SDH ➡ and subfalcine herniation ➡. An acute hematoma was evacuated. Note the loss of GM-WM differentiation ➡ representing cerebral edema. Extensive right hemispheric encephalomalacia followed. **(2-82B)** Arterial spin labeling (ASL) MR after SDH evacuation shows ↑ right cerebral hemispheric blood flow ➡ reflecting disordered autoregulation.*

81A). These are often thin, parafalcine, and convexal in location. SAH frequently accompanies SDH.

Mixed-attenuation SDH is common in the acutely symptomatic AHT patient **(2-82A)**. Dependent SDH (hematohygroma and hematocrit effect) typically reflects a single event, not multiple bleeds **(2-85)**. SDHy (CSF-like on NECT) in children < 2 years should be considered of traumatic etiology **(2-86)**. SDHy can enlarge rapidly. Epidural hematoma is rare in AHT. The presence of SDH and retinal hemorrhages increases the specificity of SDH as a proxy for AHT.

Causes of mixed-attenuation SDHs include the following: (1) aSDH, (2) hyperacute + acute hemorrhage, (3) hematohygroma (SDH + CSF), and (4) old and new SDH. When there is associated underlying cerebral edema and herniation, invariably at the time of surgical drainage, the subdural collection is one of the first three considerations. Innocent rebleeding into a cSDH rarely leads to shift and cerebral edema.

The common origin of SDH and SAH in AHT are torn bridging veins (BVs) **(2-79)**. On NECT, these appear as tubular or comma-shaped high-attenuation extraaxial collections over the parafalcine cerebral convexities. MR shows similarly shaped hypointensities on T2WI, GRE, and SWI. Underlying cerebral ischemia may be detected. These torn and thrombosed BVs represent a sign of trauma **(2-80)**.

MR Findings. SDHs of differing age on T1- and T2-weighted images showing mixed hyper-, hypo-, and isointense components are highly suggestive of AHT. FLAIR is helpful in compartmentalizing extraaxial collections and detecting small extraaxial collections (SDH, SDHy, and SAH) and white matter injury. SDH MR signal heterogeneity confounds estimates of blood dating. Use NECT and MR in conjunction for dating **(2-85)**.

Traumatic SDHy follows CSF on all MR pulse sequences **(2-86)**. Variance from this should invoke the radiologist to consider cSDH vs. hematohygroma **(2-85)** in the differential diagnosis.

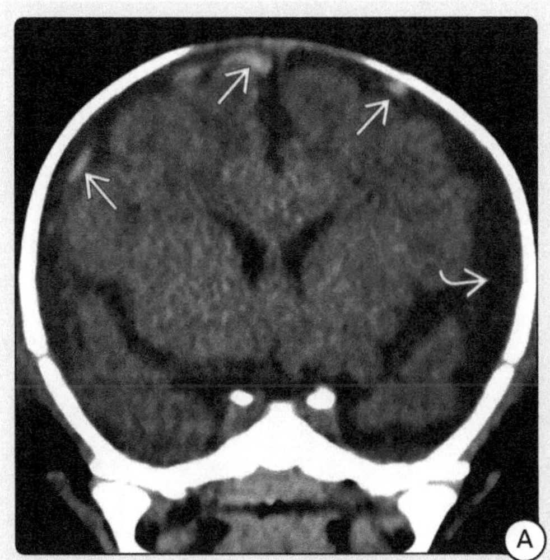

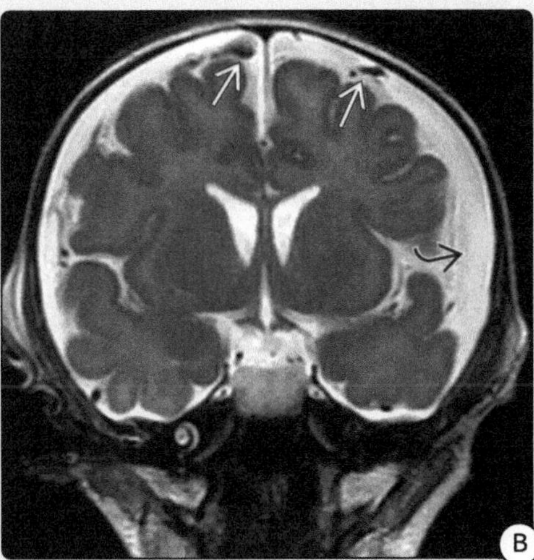

***(2-83A)** Coronal NECT in AHT shows confirmed infant shaking victim showing tubular and comma-shaped convexity hyperattenuating (torn & thrombosed) bridging veins ➡. Note CSF-like subdural collection ➡. MR showed features of hygroma (SDHy). **(2-83B)** Tubular hyperattenuating injured bridging veins from prior coronal NECT show corresponding T2 hypointensities ➡ with associated SDHy ➡ on T2 MR.*

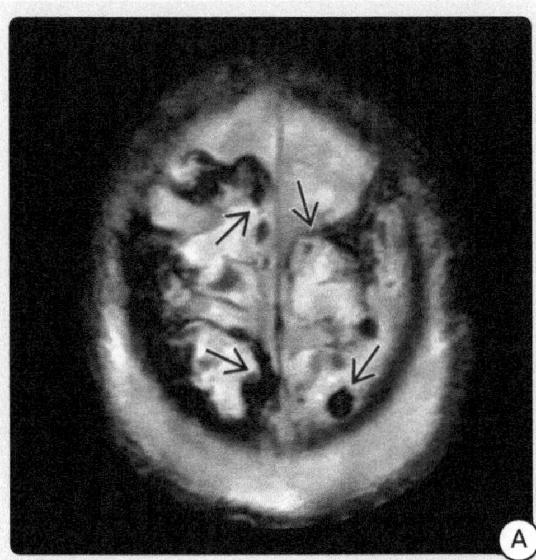

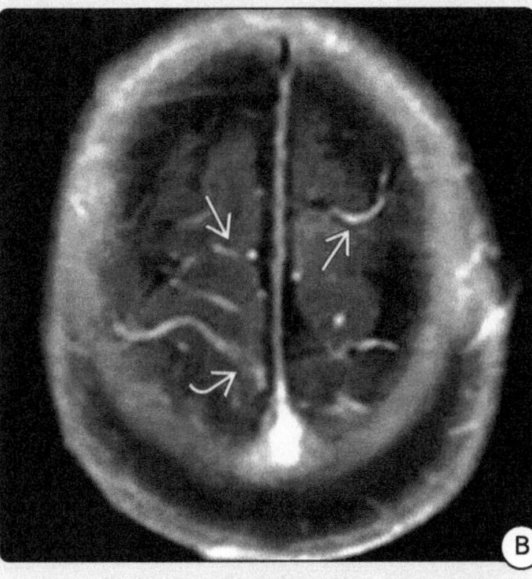

***(2-84A)** Axial SWI shows injured bridging veins in an infant AHT victim with chaotic convexal tubular and rounded hypointensities ➡ that, at autopsy, revealed torn and thrombosed bridging veins. Normal bridging veins converge and enter SSS. **(2-84B)** Axial T1 C+ MR shows the absence of normal bridging veins (normally 12-15/hemisphere). Thrombus is noted in a parietal bridging vein ➡. Note small cortical veins ➡.*

Trauma, both accidental and inflicted, represents the most common causes of SDHy in a child < 2 years of age.

T2* (GRE, SWI) scans are useful techniques for detecting blood products, particularly acute and subacute extraaxial and intraaxial hemorrhage, subtle petechial cortical contusions, PBLs, torn BVs **(2-84A)**, and hemorrhagic axonal injuries. Chronic convexity SDHs often lack susceptibility effect on T2* imaging (appearing deceptively as "simple fluid"); therefore, the radiologist must look for the presence of internal membrane structure within the SDH. DWI and ADC maps are essential for evaluating foci of ischemic injury.

FLAIR, FSE T2, T2*, and post-IV contrast 3D T1-weighted imaging can detect membrane architecture within the SDH. This is the best predictor of cSDH. Macroscopic subdural membrane formation within the SDH requires ~ 4-6 weeks to form. 3D post-IV contrast T1 imaging may display the traumatic disruption of BVs and the presence of traumatic cerebral sinovenous thrombosis **(2-84B)**.

DWI, ADC maps, DTI, FLAIR, and SWI provide insights into parenchymal injuries in AHT. Arterial spin labeling (ASL) pre- and postoperatively reflects alterations in cerebral blood flow following trauma **(2-82B)**. Altered cerebral vascular regulation is a pathophysiologic underpinning of the potentially catastrophic **second impact syndrome**.

Spine and spinal cord injuries are common in infants and children with shaking injuries. MR is the procedure of choice, as significant injuries can occur in the absence of fractures or subluxations. MR of the cervical and thoracic spine is also often performed in conjunction with brain MR in the setting of suspected AHT.

Differential Diagnosis

Accidental TBI is the most common differential diagnosis. Accidents are typically witnessed and more common after the child begins to ambulate. Household falls less than 3 feet do not result in imaging findings that mimic AHT. Accidental head

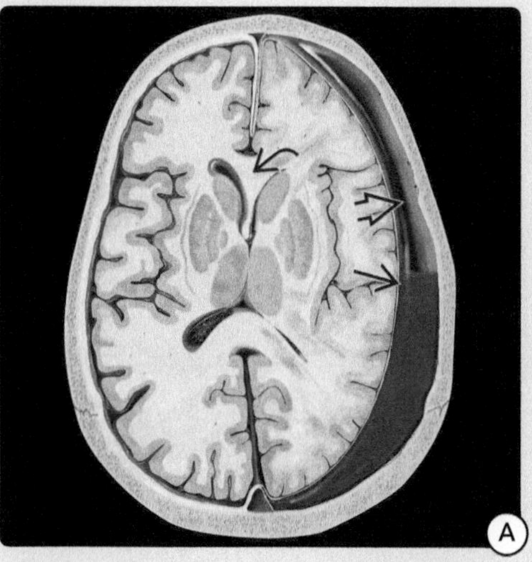

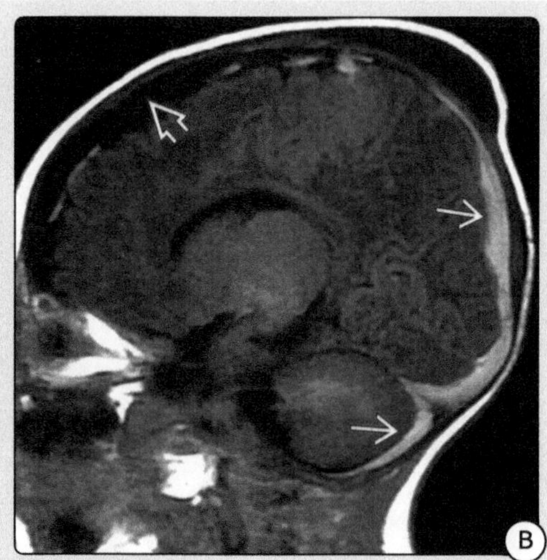

***(2-85A)** Graphic demonstrates hematohygroma and subfalcine shift. Dependent blood forms an interface with serum and CSF. To estimate hemorrhage age, assess the sediment! **(2-85B)** Parasagittal T1WI shows hematohygroma in a 4m victim of shaking. Dependent hyperintense acute hemorrhage (sediment) and CSF-like supernate are shown. Detection of hematohygroma in a child < 2y is a proxy for trauma.*

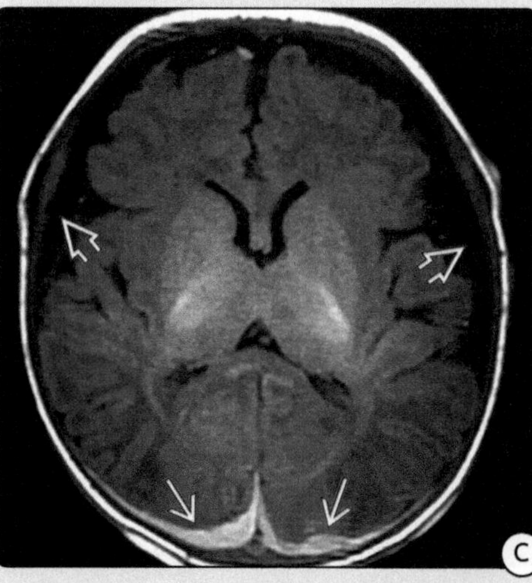

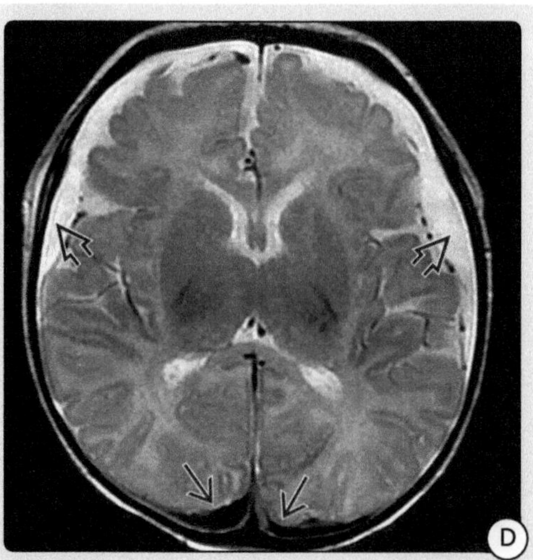

***(2-85C)** Axial T1WI is shown. Dating hematohygroma focuses on the sediment. Note the bilateral hygromas (supernate). Cortical veins hug the lateral cerebral fissures, confirming subdural location of hygroma. **(2-85D)** Axial T2WI shows hypointense acute SDH. This hematohygroma was assessed to reflect a single AHT event. Avoid defaulting to the diagnosis of new and old SDH in the setting of hematohygroma. Also note SDHy.*

trauma is more commonly impactive as opposed to the more common impulsive forces of AHT.

Other uncommon diagnoses, such as **inborn error of metabolism** (e.g., glutaric aciduria and Menkes kinky hair syndrome), can cause retinal hemorrhages and bilateral SDHs.

Selected References: The complete reference list is available on the Expert Consult™ eBook version included with purchase.

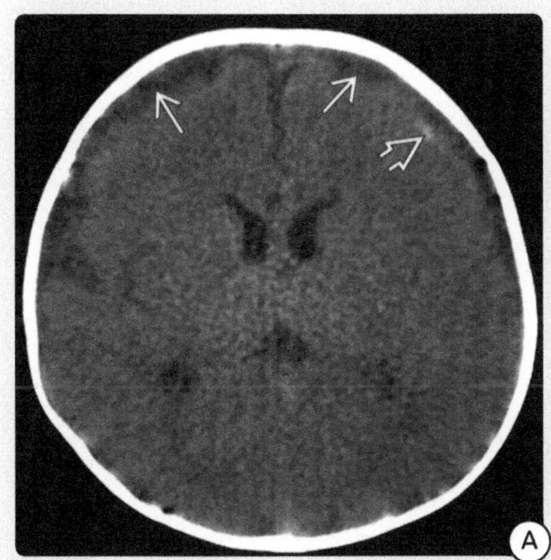

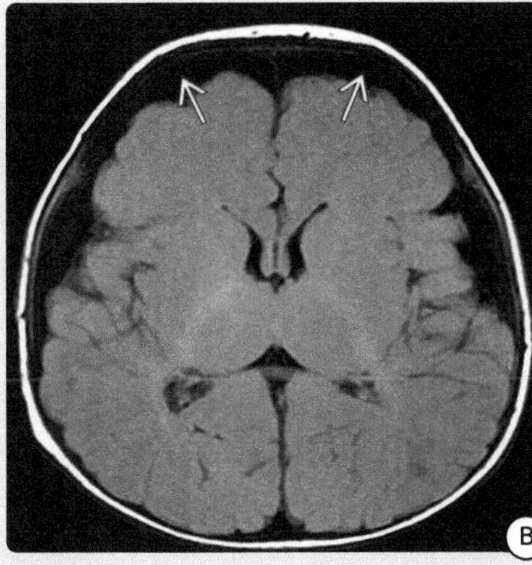

***(2-86A)** Axial NECT in a 2-month-old unresponsive boy shows SAH ➡ and thin, anterior, intermediate-attenuation subdural collections ➡ (DDx = chronic SDH vs. hematohygroma). Thin parafalcine convexal high-attenuation (acute) SDH was also detected (not shown). **(2-86B)** Axial FLAIR MR performed 12 hours after NECT shows enlarging SDHys ➡. These subdural collections followed CSF on all MR pulse sequences.*

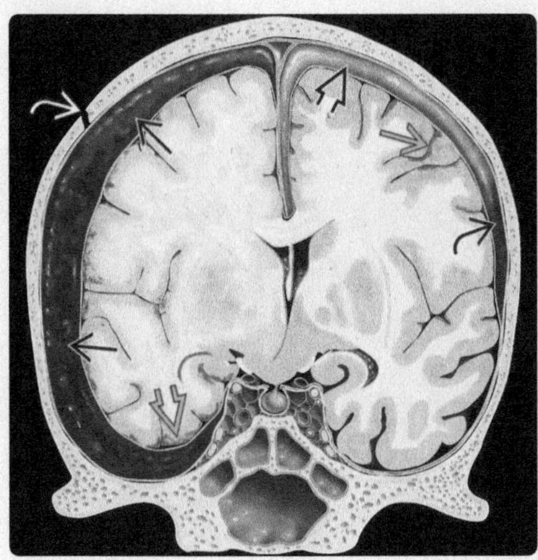

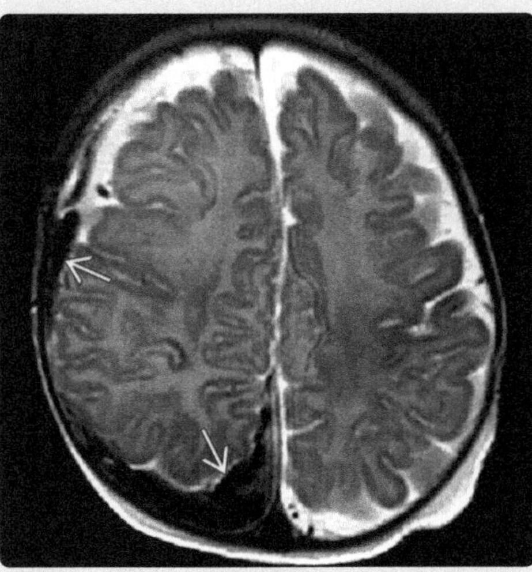

***(2-87)** Graphic shows aSDH ➡, subfalcine herniation, and cSDH ➡ with rebleed ➡. Note SAH ➡, cortical contusions ➡, and fracture ➡. **(2-88)** T2WI in a patient with AHT shows hypointensity in the dependent portion of the right SDH ➡, suggesting a more acute component to the hematoma.*

Secondary Effects and Sequelae of CNS Trauma

Traumatic brain injury (TBI) is not a single "one and done" event. A veritable "cascade" of adverse pathophysiologic events continues to develop after the initial injury. Some—such as progressive hemorrhagic injury—occur within the first 24 hours after trauma. Others (e.g., brain swelling and herniation syndromes) may take a day or two to develop.

Secondary effects of CNS trauma are defined as those that occur after the initial injury. These secondary effects are often more devastating than the initial injury itself and can become life threatening. In this chapter, we consider a broad spectrum of secondary effects that follow brain trauma, beginning with herniation syndromes.

Herniation Syndromes

Brain herniations occur when one or more structures is displaced from its normal or "native" compartment into an adjacent space. They are the most common secondary manifestation of *any* expanding intracranial mass, regardless of etiology.

Relevant Anatomy

Bony ridges and dural folds divide the intracranial cavity into three compartments: Two supratentorial hemicrania (the right and left halves) and the posterior fossa **(3-1)**.

The **falx cerebri** is a broad, sickle-shaped dural fold that attaches superiorly to the inside of the skull on either side of the midline, where it contains the superior sagittal sinus (SSS).

The concave inferior "free" margin of the falx contains the inferior sagittal sinus. As it courses posteriorly, the inferior margin of the falx forms a large open space above the corpus callosum and cingulate gyrus. This open space allows potential displacement of brain and blood vessels from one side toward the other ["subfalcine herniation (SFH)"].

The **tentorium cerebelli** extends inferolaterally from its confluence with the falx, where their two merging dural folds contain the straight sinus. The straight sinus courses posteroinferiorly toward the sinus confluence with the SSS and transverse sinuses.

The tentorium has two concave medial edges that contain a large U-shaped opening called the **tentorial incisura**. "Transtentorial" displacement of brain structures and accompanying blood vessels from the supratentorial

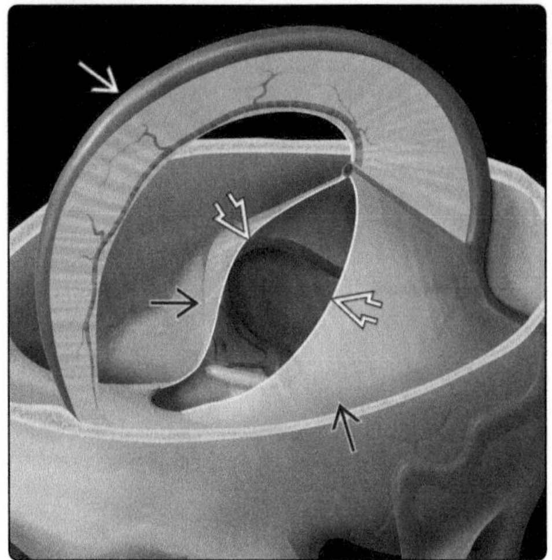

(3-1) Falx ➡ divides supratentorial compartment into 2 halves. Tentorium ➡ forms a U-shaped opening ➡, the tentorial incisura.

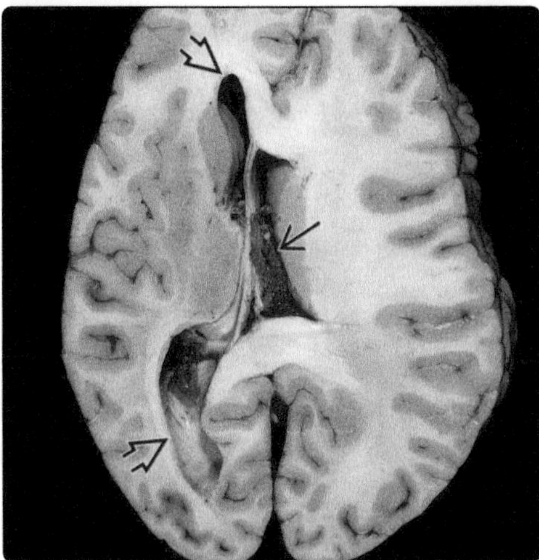

(3-2) L lateral ventricle ➡ is compressed, shifted across midline. Obstructed foramen of Monro causes enlarged R ➡. (R. Hewlett, MD.)

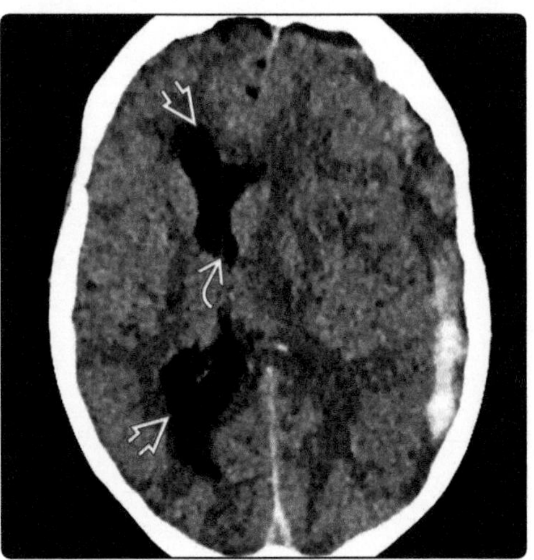

(3-3) SDH with compression, subfalcine herniation of L lateral ventricle ➡ is shown. R lateral ventricle ➡ is enlarged from obstruction.

compartment or posterior fossa can occur in either direction—up or down—through the tentorial incisura.

Relevant Physiology

Once the sutures fuse and the fontanelles close, brain, CSF, and blood all coexist in a rigid, unyielding "bone box." The cerebral blood volume (CBV), perfusion, and CSF volume exist in a delicate balance within this closed box. Under normal conditions, pressures within the brain parenchyma and intracranial CSF spaces are equal.

When extra volume (blood, edema, tumor, etc.) is added to a cranial compartment, CSF in the sulci and subarachnoid cisterns is initially squeezed out. The ipsilateral ventricle becomes compressed and decreases in size. As intracranial volume continues to increase, the mass effect eventually exceeds the brain's compensatory capacity, and intracranial pressure (ICP) begins to rise.

If a mass becomes sufficiently large, brain, CSF spaces, and blood vessels are displaced from one intracranial compartment into an adjacent one, resulting in one or more cerebral herniations.

In turn, cerebral herniations may cause their own cascade of secondary effects. Parenchyma, cranial nerves, &/or blood vessels can become compressed against the adjacent unyielding bone and dura. Secondary ischemic changes, frank brain infarcts, cranial neuropathies, and focal neurologic deficits may develop.

Subfalcine Herniation

Terminology and Etiology

SFH is the most common cerebral herniation and the easiest to understand. In a simple, uncomplicated SFH, an enlarging supratentorial mass in one hemicranium causes the brain to begin shifting toward the opposite side. Herniation occurs as the affected hemisphere pushes across the midline under the inferior "free" margin of the falx, extending into the contralateral hemicranium **(3-2)**.

Imaging

Mass effect displaces the brain from one side toward the other. The ipsilateral ventricle appears compressed and displaced across the midline, while the contralateral ventricle enlarges **(3-3)**. The cingulate gyrus and accompanying anterior cerebral arteries also herniate under the falx.

Complications

Early complications of SFH include unilateral hydrocephalus, seen on axial NECT as enlargement of the contralateral ventricle. As the mass effect increases, the lateral ventricles become progressively more displaced across the midline. This displacement initially just deforms, then kinks, and eventually occludes the foramen of Monro.

If SFH becomes severe, the herniating anterior cerebral artery (ACA) can become pinned against the inferior "free" margin of the falx cerebri and then occluded, causing secondary infarction of the cingulate gyrus.

SUBFALCINE HERNIATION

Etiology and Pathology
- Unilateral hemispheric mass effect
- Brain shifts across midline under falx cerebri

Epidemiology
- Most common cerebral herniation

Imaging
- Cingulate gyrus, ACA, internal cerebral veins displaced across midline
- Foramen of Monro kinked, obstructed
- Ipsilateral ventricle small, contralateral enlarged

Complications
- Obstructive hydrocephalus
- Secondary ACA infarction (severe cases)

Descending Transtentorial Herniation

Transtentorial herniations are brain displacements that occur through the tentorial incisura. Although these displacements can occur in both directions (from top down or bottom up), descending herniations from supratentorial masses are far more common than ascending herniations.

Terminology and Etiology

Descending transtentorial herniation (DTH) is the second most common type of intracranial herniation syndrome. DTH is caused by a hemispheric mass that initially produces side-to-side brain displacement (i.e., SFH). As the mass effect increases, the uncus of the temporal lobe is pushed medially and begins to encroach on the suprasellar cistern. With progressively increasing mass effect, both the uncus and hippocampus herniate inferiorly through the tentorial incisura.

DTH can be unilateral or bilateral. **Unilateral DTH** occurs when a hemispheric mass effect pushes the uncus and hippocampus of the ipsilateral temporal lobe over the edge of the tentorial incisura **(3-4)**. In **bilateral DTH**, both temporal lobes are displaced medially.

"Complete" or **"central" descending herniation** occurs when the supratentorial mass effect becomes so severe that the hypothalamus and optic chiasm are flattened against the skull base, *both* temporal lobes are herniated, and the whole tentorial incisura is completely plugged with displaced tissue **(3-4)**.

Imaging

Axial CT scans in early **unilateral DTH** show that the uncus is displaced medially and the ipsilateral aspect of the suprasellar cistern is effaced **(3-5)**. As DTH increases, the hippocampus also herniates medially over the edge of the tentorium, compressing the quadrigeminal cistern and pushing the midbrain toward the opposite side of the incisura. In severe cases, the temporal horn can even be displaced almost into the midline **(3-6)**.

With **bilateral DTH**, both temporal lobes herniate medially into the tentorial hiatus. With **central descending herniation**, both hemispheres are so swollen that the whole central brain is flattened against the skull base. All the basal cisterns are obliterated as the hypothalamus and optic chiasm are crushed against the sella turcica, and the suprasellar and quadrigeminal cisterns are completely effaced **(3-7)**.

In complete (central) bilateral DTH, the midbrain is compressed and squeezed medially from both sides. Sagittal images show that the midbrain

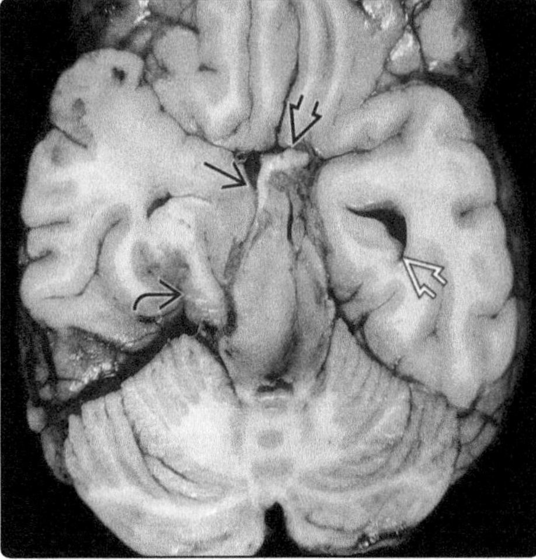

***(3-4)** DTH with uncal ➡, hippocampal ➡ herniation. Suprasellar cistern ➡ is effaced, contralateral ventricle enlarged ➡. (R. Hewlett.)*

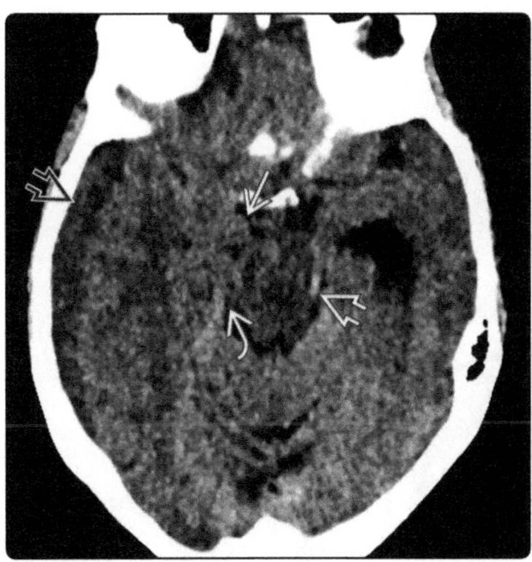

***(3-5)** Subacute SDH ➡, descending transtentorial herniation of uncus ➡, and hippocampus ➡, Kernohan notch ➡ are shown.*

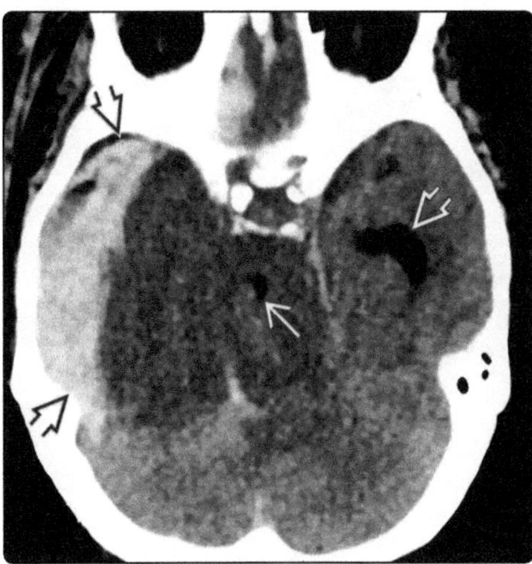

***(3-6)** Large aSDH ➡ displaces the R temporal horn over the tentorial incisura into the midline ➡. L lateral ventricle is enlarged ➡.*

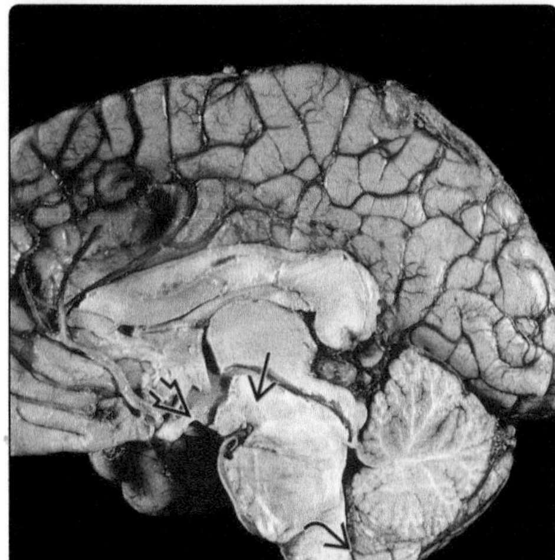

***(3-7)** DTH shows midbrain is kinked inferiorly ➙, hypothalamus is smashed over dorsum sellae ➙, and tonsil is herniated ➙. (R. Hewlett, MD.)*

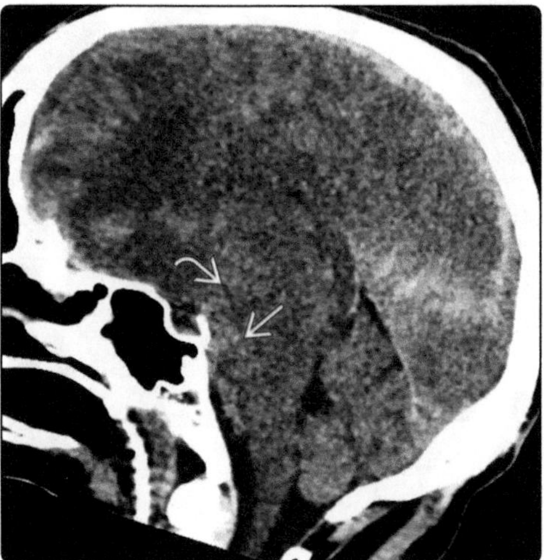

***(3-8)** Sagittal NECT shows traumatic brain swelling with midbrain displaced inferiorly ➙, and the midbrain-pons angle ➙ is obliterated.*

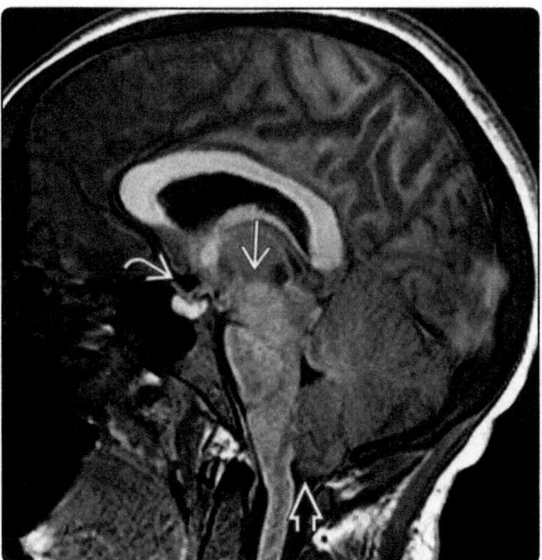

***(3-9)** MP-RAGE shows complete DTH with obliterated suprasellar cistern ➙, downwardly displaced midbrain ➙, & tonsillar herniation ➙.*

is also pushed inferiorly through the tentorial incisura, displacing the pons downward. The angle between the midbrain and pons is progressively reduced from nearly 90° to almost 0° **(3-8)**. In terminal central herniation, the pons eventually pushes the cerebellar tonsils inferiorly through the foramen magnum **(3-9)**.

Complications

Even mild DTH can compress the third cranial (oculomotor) nerve as it exits from the interpeduncular fossa and courses anterolaterally toward the cavernous sinus. This may produce a **pupil-involving third nerve palsy (3-21)**.

Other, more severe complications may occur with DTH. As the temporal lobe is displaced inferomedially, it pushes the posterior cerebral artery (PCA) below the tentorial incisura. The PCA can become kinked and eventually even occluded as it passes back up over the medial edge of the tentorium **(3-22)**, causing a **secondary PCA (occipital) infarct (3-23)**.

Severe uni- or bilateral DTH may cause pressure necrosis of the uncus and hippocampus, causing a secondary hemorrhagic midbrain infarct known as a **Duret hemorrhage (3-4)**.

With complete bilateral DTH, perforating arteries that arise from the circle of Willis are compressed against the central skull base and also occlude, causing **hypothalamic and basal ganglia infarcts (3-25)**.

In a vicious cycle, the hemispheres become more edematous, and ICP soars. If the rising pressure exceeds intraarterial pressure, perfusion is drastically reduced and eventually ceases, causing **brain death (BD)**.

DESCENDING TRANSTENTORIAL HERNIATION

Terminology and Pathology

- Unilateral DTH
  - Temporal lobe (uncus, hippocampus) pushed over tentorial incisura
- Severe bilateral DTH = "complete" or "central" herniation
  - Hypothalamus, chiasm flattened against sella

Epidemiology

- 2nd most common cerebral herniation

Imaging

- Unilateral DTH
  - Suprasellar cistern initially encroached
  - Progressive effacement as herniation worsens
  - Herniating temporal lobe pushes midbrain to opposite side (may cause Kernohan "notch")
- Bilateral DTH
  - Basal cisterns completely effaced
  - Midbrain pushed down behind clivus, compressed on both sides
  - Midbrain-pons angle becomes more acute

Complications

- CNIII compression
  - May cause pupil-involving 3rd nerve palsy
- PCA occlusion
  - Becomes kinked against edge of tentorium
  - Secondary occipital (PCA) infarct may ensue
- Complete "central" DTH
  - If severe ± hypothalamus, basal infarcts
- Compression of contralateral cerebral peduncle ("Kernohan notch")
- Midbrain ("Duret") hemorrhage

Tonsillar Herniation

Two types of herniations occur with posterior fossa masses: Tonsillar herniation and ascending transtentorial herniation (ATH). Tonsillar herniation is the more common of these two herniations.

Terminology and Etiology

In tonsillar herniation, the cerebellar tonsils are displaced inferiorly and become impacted into the foramen magnum **(3-10)**. Tonsillar herniation can be congenital (e.g., Chiari 1 malformation) or acquired.

Acquired tonsillar herniation occurs in two different circumstances. The most common cause is an expanding posterior fossa mass *pushing* the tonsils downward into the foramen magnum.

Inferior tonsillar displacement also occurs with intracranial hypotension. Here, the tonsils are *pulled* downward by abnormally low intraspinal CSF pressure (Chapter 34).

Imaging

Diagnosing tonsillar herniation on NECT scans may be problematic. The foramen magnum usually contains CSF that surrounds the medulla and cerebellar tonsils. Herniation of one or both tonsils into the foramen magnum obliterates most or all of the CSF in the cisterna magna **(3-11A)**.

Tonsillar herniation is much more easily diagnosed on MR. In the sagittal plane, the normally horizontal tonsillar folia become vertically oriented, and the inferior aspect of the tonsils becomes pointed. Tonsils > 5 mm below the foramen magnum are generally abnormal, especially if they are peg-like or pointed (rather than rounded).

In the axial plane, T2 scans show that the tonsils are impacted into the foramen magnum, obliterating CSF in the cisterna magna and displacing the medulla anteriorly **(3-11B)**.

Complications

Complications of tonsillar herniation include obstructive hydrocephalus and tonsillar necrosis.

TONSILLAR HERNIATION

Etiology and Pathology
- Most common posterior fossa herniation
- Can be congenital (Chiari 1) or acquired
- Acquired
  - Most common = secondary to posterior fossa mass effect
  - Less common = intracranial hypotension
  - Rare = severe central DTH, BD

Imaging Findings
- 1 or both tonsils > 5 mm below foramen magnum
- CSF in foramen magnum effaced
- Foramen magnum appears tissue filled on axial NECT, T2WI
- Inferior "pointing" or peg-like configuration of tonsils on sagittal T1WI

Complications
- Obstructive hydrocephalus
- Tonsillar necrosis

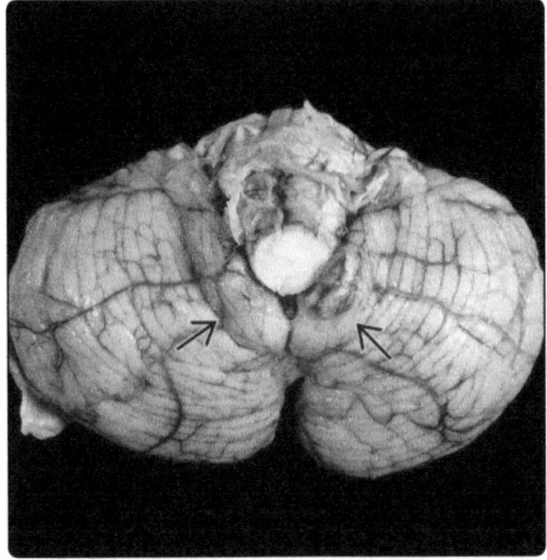

***(3-10)** Herniation shows tonsils displaced inferiorly, "grooved" ⇒ by bony margins of foramen magnum. (Courtesy R. Hewlett, MD.)*

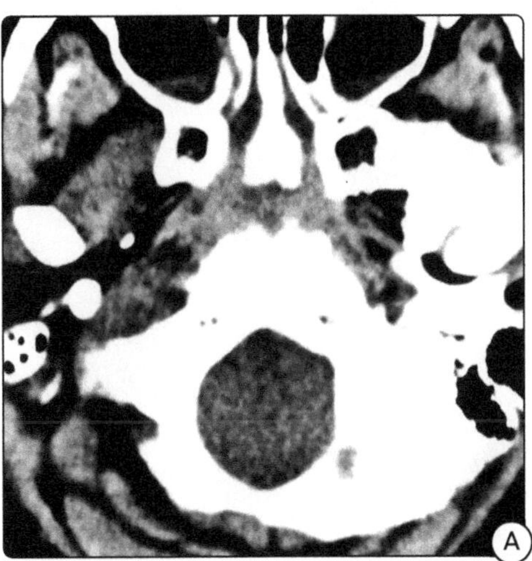

***(3-11A)** NECT in a patient with tonsillar herniation shows only effacement of CSF within the foramen magnum.*

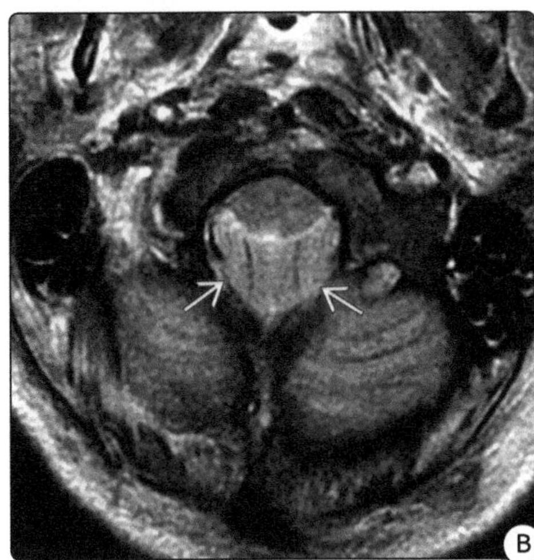

***(3-11B)** T2WI in the same patient shows tonsils ⇒ filling the foramen magnum, displacing the medulla anteriorly.*

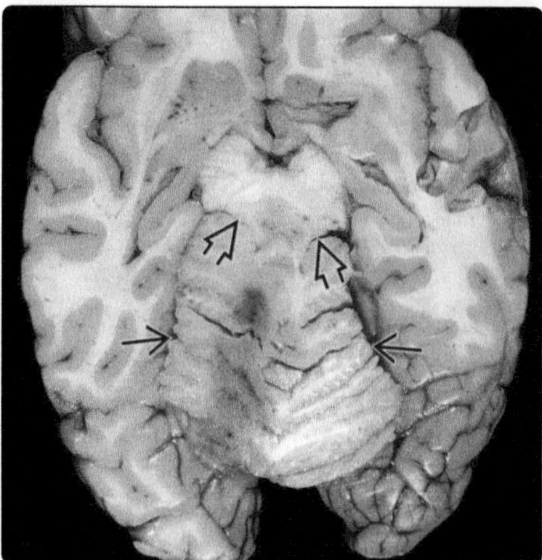

(3-12) Vermis, cerebellum ⇨ push upward to tentorial incisura & compress midbrain/tectum ⇨; ATH. (Courtesy E. T. Hedley-Whyte, MD.)

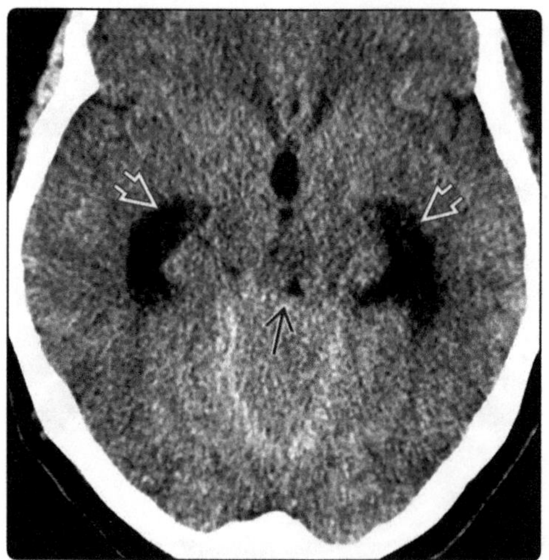

(3-13) NECT shows ATH with obliterated quadrigeminal cistern, compressed tectum ⇨. Note severe obstructive hydrocephalus ⇨.

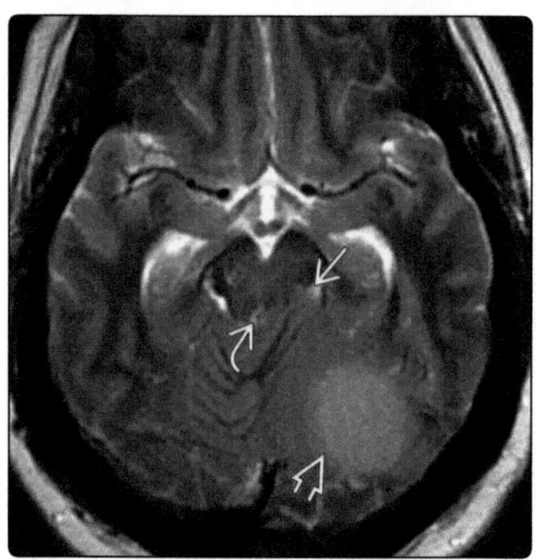

(3-14) T2WI shows unilateral ATH ⇨ from a mass ⇨ pushing the cerebellum up through the tentorial incisura, compressing the aqueduct ⇨.

Ascending Transtentorial Herniation

Terminology and Etiology

In ATH, the cerebellar vermis and hemispheres are pushed upward ("ascend") through the tentorial incisura into the supratentorial compartment. The superiorly herniating cerebellum first flattens and displaces, then effaces the quadrigeminal cistern and compresses the midbrain **(3-12)**.

Imaging

Axial NECT scans show that CSF in the superior vermian cistern and cerebellar sulci is effaced **(3-13)**. The quadrigeminal cistern is first compressed and then obliterated by the upwardly herniating cerebellum **(3-14)**. As the herniation progresses, the tectal plate becomes compressed and flattened **(3-13)**. In severe cases, the dorsal midbrain may actually appear concave instead of convex **(3-12)**. The most common complication of ATH is acute intraventricular obstructive hydrocephalus caused by compression of the cerebral aqueduct **(3-14)**.

ASCENDING TRANSTENTORIAL HERNIATION

Relatively Rare

- Caused by expanding posterior fossa mass
- Neoplasm > trauma
- Cerebellum pushed upward through incisura
- Compresses, deforms midbrain

Imaging Findings

- Incisura filled with tissue, CSF spaces obliterated
- Quadrigeminal cistern, tectal plate compressed/flattened
  - Eventually appear obliterated

Complications

- Hydrocephalus (secondary to aqueduct obstruction)

Other Herniations

The vast majority of cerebral herniations are subfalcine, descending/ascending transtentorial, and tonsillar herniations. Other, less common herniation syndromes are transalar and transdural/transcranial herniations.

Transalar Herniation

Transalar herniation occurs when the brain herniates across the greater sphenoid wing (GSW) or "ala" and can be either ascending (the most common) or descending.

Ascending transalar herniation is caused by a large *middle cranial fossa mass* **(3-15)**. The middle cerebral artery (MCA) branches and sylvian fissure are elevated, and the superior temporal gyrus is pushed above the GSW **(3-16)**.

Descending transalar herniation is caused by a large *anterior cranial fossa mass*. Here, the gyrus rectus is forced posteroinferiorly over the GSW, displacing the sylvian fissure and shifting the MCA backward **(3-17)**.

Transdural/Transcranial Herniation

This rare type of cerebral herniation, sometimes called a "brain fungus" by neurosurgeons, can be life threatening. For transdural/transcranial herniation to occur, the dura must be lacerated, a skull defect (fracture or craniotomy) must be present, and ICP must be elevated.

Traumatic transdural/transcranial herniations typically occur in infants or young children with a comminuted skull fracture that deforms inward with impact, lacerating the dura-arachnoid. When ICP increases, the brain can herniate through the torn dura and across the skull fracture into the subgaleal space.

OTHER HERNIATIONS

Ascending Transalar Herniation
- Most common transalar herniation
- Caused by middle fossa mass
- Sagittal imaging (best appreciated on off-midline images)
  - Sylvian fissure, MCA displaced up/over greater sphenoid ala
- Axial imaging
  - Sylvian fissure/MCA bowed forward
  - Temporal lobe bulges into anterior fossa

Descending Transalar Herniation
- Caused by anterior fossa mass
- Sagittal imaging
  - Sylvian fissure, MCA displaced posteroinferiorly
  - Frontal lobe pushed backward over greater sphenoid ala
- Axial imaging
  - Gyrus rectus pushed posteriorly
  - MCA curved backward

Transcranial/Transdural Herniation
- ↑ ICP + skull defect + dura-arachnoid tear
- Caused by
  - Comminuted, often depressed skull fracture
  - Craniectomy
- Brain extruded through skull, under scalp aponeurosis
- Best appreciated on axial T2WI

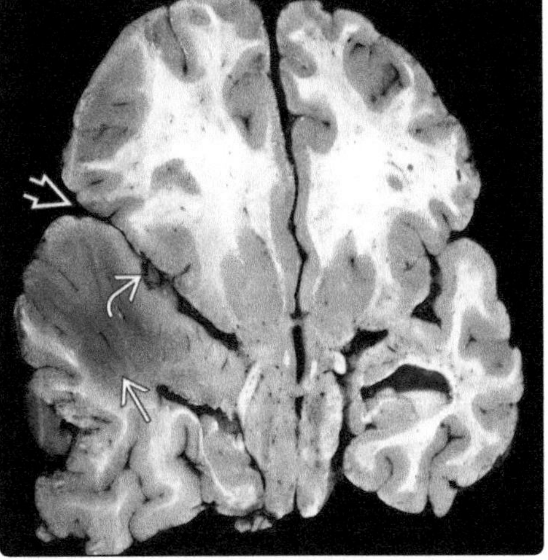

***(3-15)** Temporal lobe mass ➡ pushes sylvian fissure and MCA ➡ up/over the site of greater sphenoid wing ➡. (E. T. Hedley-Whyte, MD.)*

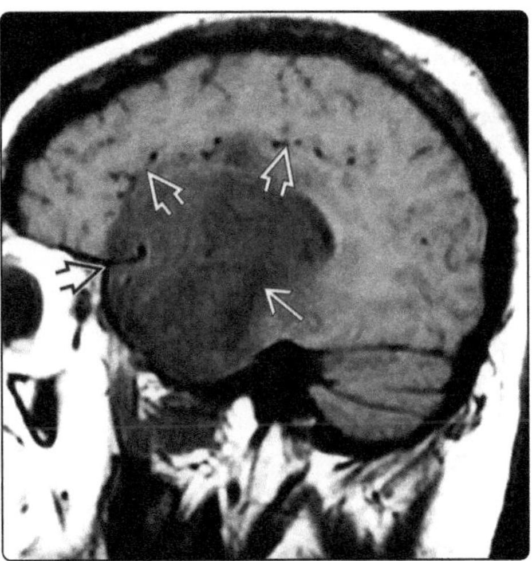

***(3-16)** Ascending transalar herniation shows mass ➡ elevates sylvian fissure, MCA ➡, pushing temporal lobe up/over sphenoid wing ➡.*

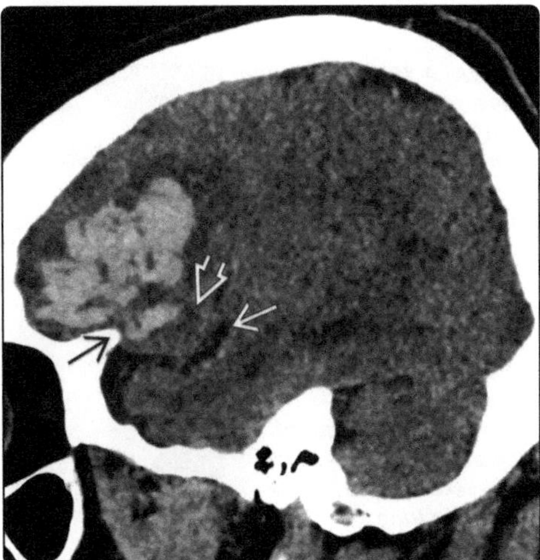

***(3-17)** Descending transalar herniation shows frontal lobe ➡ is pushed over the sphenoid wing ➡, displacing sylvian fissure ➡ posteroinferiorly.*

Edema, Ischemia, and Vascular Injury

TBI can unleash a cascade of physiologic responses that may adversely affect the brain more than the initial trauma. These responses include diffuse brain swelling, excitotoxic responses elicited by glutamatergic pathway activation, perfusion alterations, and a variety of ischemic events, including territorial infarcts.

Posttraumatic Brain Swelling

Cerebral edema is a major contributor to TBI morbidity. Massive brain swelling with severe intracranial hypertension is among the most serious of all secondary traumatic lesions. Mortality approaches 50%, so early recognition and aggressive treatment of this complication are imperative.

Etiology and Epidemiology

Focal, regional, or diffuse brain swelling develops in 10-20% of patients with TBI **(3-18)**. Whether this is caused by increased tissue fluid (cerebral edema) or elevated blood volume (cerebral hyperemia) secondary to vascular dysautoregulation is unclear. In some cases, the trigeminal system may mediate brain swelling associated with subdural bleeding, providing the link between small-volume, thin subdural bleeds and swelling of the underlying brain.

Clinical Issues

Children, young adults, and individuals with repetitive concussive or subconcussive injuries are especially prone to developing posttraumatic brain swelling and are almost twice as likely as older adults to develop this complication. Although gross enlargement of one or both hemispheres occasionally develops rapidly after the initial event, delayed onset is more typical. Severe cerebral edema generally takes between 24 and 48 hours to develop.

In some cases, aggressive measures for control of ICP fail to restore cerebral metabolism and improve neurologic outcome. Decompressive craniectomy as a last resort is often performed, but evidence for reduced risk of death or dependence in severe TBI is lacking.

Imaging

The appearance of posttraumatic brain swelling evolves over time. Initially, mild hemispheric mass effect with sulcal/cisternal compression is seen on NECT scans **(3-19)**.

During the early stages of brain swelling, gray matter-white matter differentiation appears relatively preserved. Although the ipsilateral ventricle may be slightly compressed, subfalcine displacement is generally minimal. However, **if the mass effect is disproportionately greater (≥ 3 mm) than the maximum width of an extraaxial collection, such as a subdural hematoma (SDH), early and potentially catastrophic swelling of the underlying brain parenchyma should be suspected and treated proactively (3-20)**.

MR shows swollen gyri that are hypointense on T1WI and hyperintense on T2WI. Diffusion-weighted scans show restricted diffusion with low apparent diffusion coefficient (ADC) values.

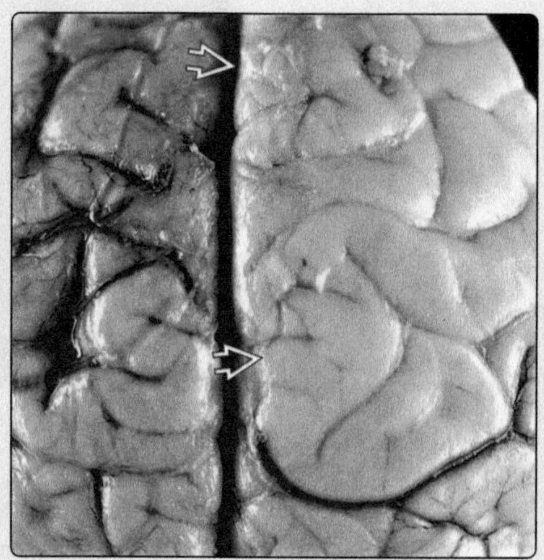

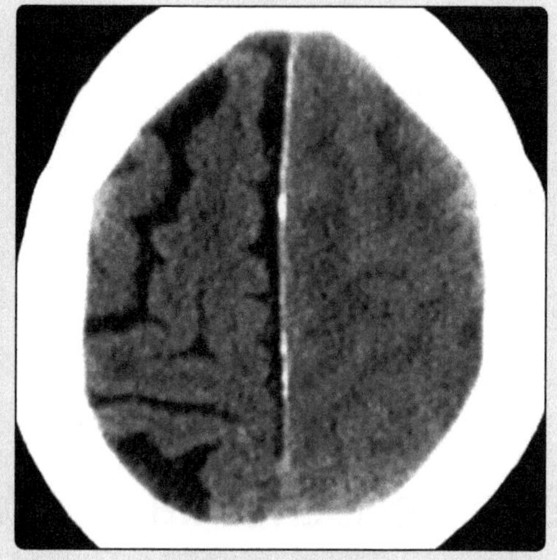

***(3-18)** Autopsy specimen shows unilateral hemispheric swelling ➲ that expands the gyri and compresses and obliterates the sulci. (Courtesy E. T. Hedley-Whyte, MD.) **(3-19)** Axial NECT scan shows normal right sulci and obliterated ("disappearing") convexity sulci over the swollen left hemisphere.*

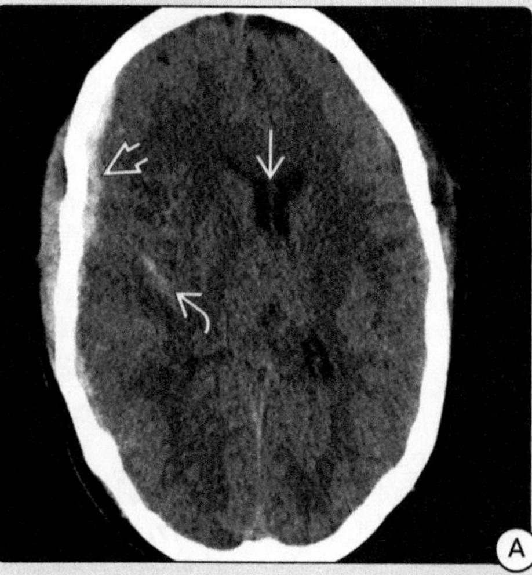

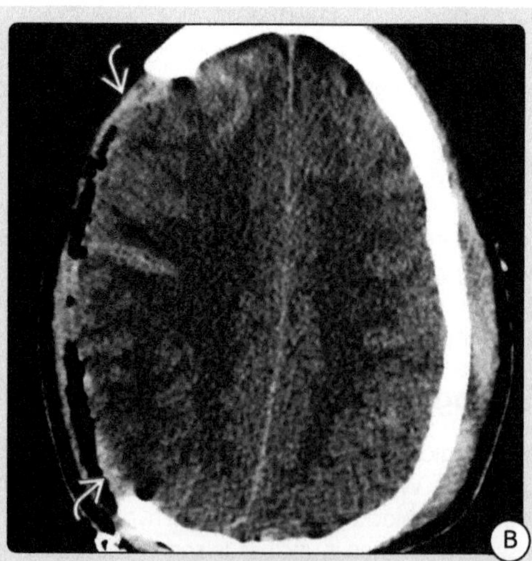

***(3-20A)** A 35-year-old man has a small right aSDH ➲ that measures only 6 mm in max diameter. SFH across the midline measured 15 mm ➲. Note the small amount of tSAH ➲, preserved GM-WM interface. **(3-20B)** Alerted to impending brain swelling, the neurosurgeons immediately evacuated the small aSDH. Because of severe intraoperative brain swelling, an emergency decompressive craniectomy ➲ had to be performed.*

As brain swelling progresses, the demarcation between the cortex and underlying white matter becomes indistinct and eventually disappears. The lateral ventricles appear smaller than normal, and the superficial sulci are no longer visible **(3-29A)**.

POSTTRAUMATIC BRAIN SWELLING

Epidemiology

- 10-20% of TBI
- Can be focal, regional, or diffuse
- Most common in children, young adults
- Potentially catastrophic

Imaging

- Earliest sign
  - SFH ≥ 3 mm than width of epidural or SDH
- Next
  - Sulcal effacement
- Later
  - Indistinct gray-white interfaces
- End stage
  - One or both hemispheres uniformly low density
  - All sulci, cisterns obliterated
  - Small ventricles

Traumatic Cerebral Ischemia, Infarction, and Perfusion Abnormalities

Traumatic ischemia and infarction are uncommon but important complications of TBI. They have a variety of causes, including direct vascular compression, systemic hypoperfusion, vascular injury, vasospasm, and venous congestion. The most common cause of posttraumatic cerebral ischemia is mechanical vascular compression secondary to a brain herniation syndrome.

Posttraumatic Infarcts

The most common brain herniation that causes secondary cerebral infarction is DTH. Severe unilateral DTH displaces the temporal lobe and accompanying PCA inferiorly into the tentorial incisura. As the herniating PCA passes posterior to the midbrain, it courses superiorly and is forced against the hard, knife-like edge of the tentorial incisura. The P3 PCA segment occludes, resulting in occipital lobe infarction **(3-23)** **(3-24)**.

Less commonly, SFH presses the callosomarginal branch of the ACA against the undersurface of the falx cerebri and causes cingulate gyrus infarction **(3-26)**.

With complete bilateral ("central") DTH, penetrating arteries that arise from the circle of Willis are crushed against the skull base, resulting in multiple scattered basal ganglia and hypothalamus infarcts **(3-25)**. Pressure necrosis of the uncus and hippocampus can also occur as the herniated temporal lobes impact the free edge of the tentorial incisura.

Traumatic Cerebral Ischemia

Focal, regional, and generalized perfusion alterations also occur with TBI. Extraaxial hematomas that exert significant focal mass effect on the underlying brain may cause reduced arterial perfusion and cortical ischemia. They may also compress the underlying cortical veins, causing venous ischemia.

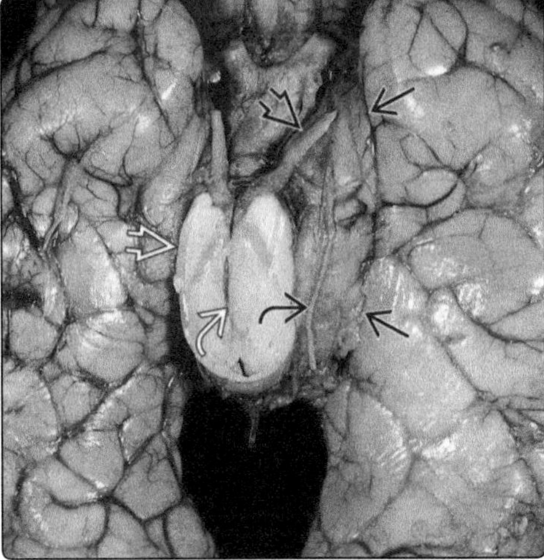

***(3-21)** Temporal lobe herniation by tentorium ➔ compresses CNIII ➔, IV ➔, causes midbrain Kernohan notch ➔ and Duret hemorrhage ➔.*

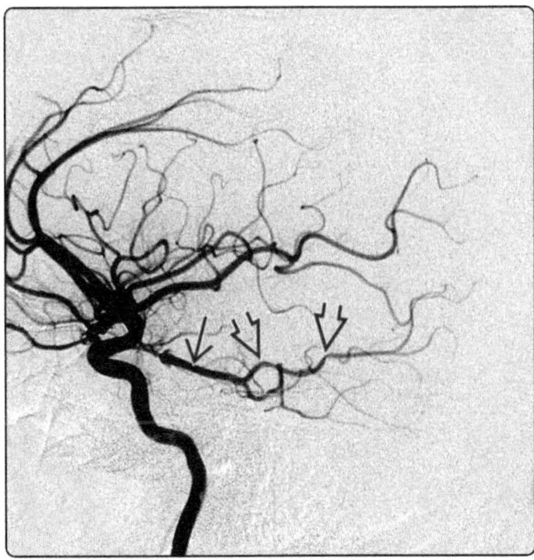

***(3-22)** In DTH, proximal PCA ➔ is displaced inferiorly through incisura, "kinked" ➔, & passes over tentorium edge. (Courtesy R. Hewlett, MD.)*

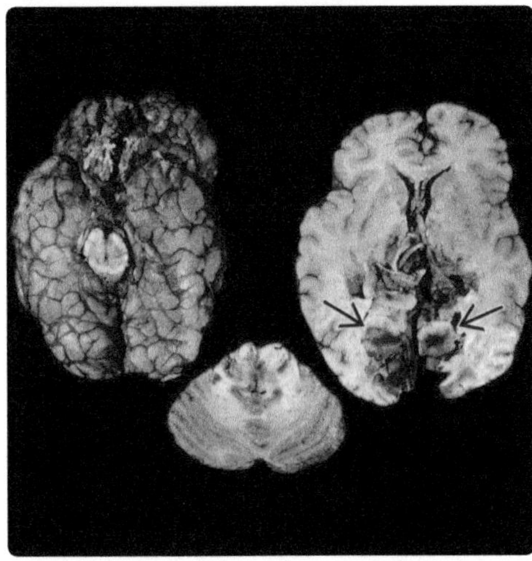

***(3-23)** Autopsy shows bilateral central DTH causing secondary PCA infarcts ➔. (Courtesy R. Hewlett, MD.)*

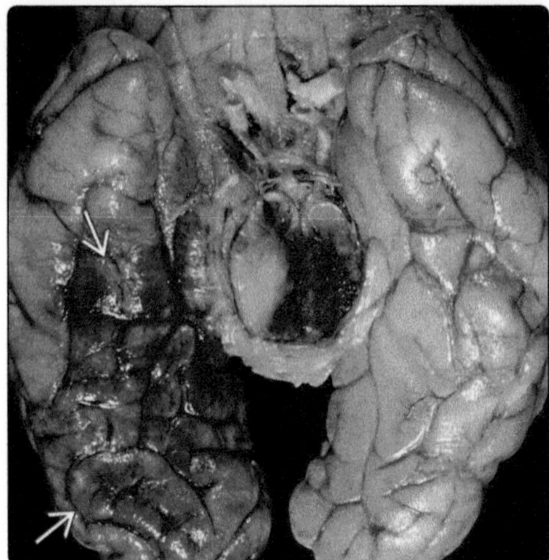

***(3-24)** DTH can occlude the PCA against the tentorial incisura and cause secondary territorial infarction ➡. (Courtesy R. Hewlett, MD.)*

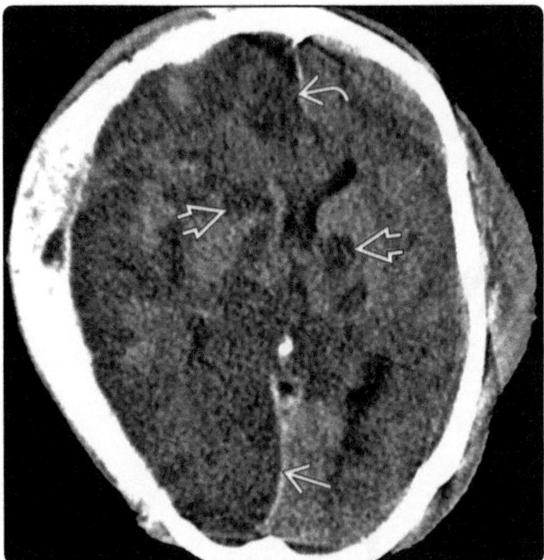

***(3-25)** NECT 5 days after initial trauma shows PCA ➡, anterior cerebral artery ➡, and multiple perforating artery ➡ posttraumatic infarcts.*

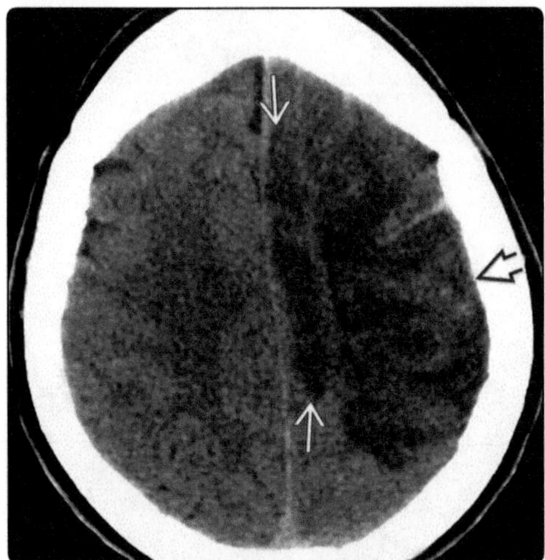

***(3-26)** NECT 5 days after a "malignant" MCA infarct ➡ shows secondary ACA infarction of the left cingulate gyrus ➡.*

Global or generalized **cerebral ischemia** may result from hypoperfusion, hypoxia, membrane depolarization, or loss of cellular membrane integrity and ion homeostasis. Cellular energy failure may induce glutamate-mediated **acute excitotoxic brain injury.**

NECT scans show hypodensity with loss of gray-white differentiation in the affected parenchyma. CT perfusion (CTP) may show decreased cerebral blood flow (CBF) with prolonged time to drain. In cases of excitotoxic brain injury, MR shows swollen, hyperintense gyri on T2/FLAIR that do not correspond to defined vascular territories.

Traumatic Cerebral Perfusion Alterations

In patients with acute SDHs, raised ICP typically leads to reduced cerebral perfusion pressure and impaired CBF. In contrast, patients with mixed or chronic SDHs may have significantly upregulated CBV and CBF in the cortex underlying the chronic SDH **(3-27)**. Mean transit times (MTTs) are often elevated.

Brain Death

Terminology

BD is defined pathophysiologically as complete, irreversible cessation of brain function **(3-28)**. Some investigators distinguish between "whole BD" (all intracranial structures above the foramen magnum), "cerebral death" (all supratentorial structures), and "higher BD" (cortical structures).

The legal definition of BD varies from country to country (e.g., the USA and the United Kingdom) and from state to state. Since the adoption of the Uniform Determination of Death Act, all court rulings in the United States have upheld the medical practice of death determination using neurologic criteria according to state law.

Clinical Issues

BD is primarily a clinical diagnosis. Three clinical findings are necessary to confirm irreversible cessation of all functions of the entire brain, *including the brainstem*: (1) Coma (with a known cause), (2) absence of brainstem reflexes, and (3) apnea.

Complex spontaneous motor movements and false-positive ventilator triggering may occur in patients who are brain dead, so expert assessment is crucial. Once reversible causes of coma (e.g., drug overdose, status epilepticus) are excluded, the clinical diagnosis of BD is highly reliable *if* the determination is made by experienced examiners using established, accepted criteria.

There are no published reports of recovery of neurologic function in adults after a diagnosis of BD using the updated 1995 American Academy of Neurology (AAN) practice parameters.

Imaging

Imaging studies may be helpful in confirming BD but neither replace nor substitute for clinical diagnosis.

CT Findings. NECT scans in BD show diffuse, severe cerebral edema. The superficial sulci, sylvian fissures, and basilar cisterns of both hemispheres are completely effaced **(3-29)**. The normal attenuation relationship between gray and white matter is inverted with gray matter becoming iso- or even hypodense relative to the adjacent white matter (the **"reversal" sign**). The severely edematous, abnormally low-density brain accentuates the prominence of the cerebral vessels and may mimic subarachnoid hemorrhage **(3-29B)**.

In striking contrast to the hypodense hemispheres, density of the cerebellum appears relatively normal (the **"white cerebellum" sign**). Density of the deep gray nuclei and brainstem may be initially maintained; however, all supratentorial structures eventually assume a featureless, uniform hypodensity.

MR Findings. Sagittal T1WI shows complete descending central brain herniation with the optic chiasm and hypothalamus compressed against the skull base and the midbrain "buckled" inferiorly through the tentorial incisura **(3-9)**. The hemispheres appear swollen and hypointense with indistinct gray matter-white matter differentiation.

T2 scans show swollen gyri with hyperintense cortex. DWI in patients with BD typically shows restricted diffusion with decreased ADC in both the cerebral cortex and white matter.

Angiography. Conventional digital subtraction angiography (DSA) shows severe, prolonged contrast stasis in the internal carotid artery. Although most BD patients show no intracranial flow, almost 30% have some proximal opacification of intracranial arteries. The deep venous drainage remains unopacified throughout the examination.

CT angiography (CTA) is emerging as an acceptable, noninvasive alternative to DSA in many jurisdictions. Demonstrating lack of opacification in the MCA cortical segments and internal veins in CTA is an efficient and reliable method for confirming BD.

Nuclear Medicine. Tc-99m scintigraphy shows scalp uptake but absent brain activity ("light bulb" sign). With increased extracranial activity ("hot nose" sign), these findings are both highly sensitive and specific for BD.

Differential Diagnosis

Potentially reversible causes of BD, such as deep coma due to **drug overdose** or **status epilepticus**, must be excluded clinically.

Technical difficulties with imaging studies that may mimic BD include a "missed bolus" on either CTA or nuclear medicine flow studies. Vascular lesions, such as arterial dissection and vasospasm, may also delay or even prevent opacification of intracranial vessels.

Massive cerebral infarction (especially "malignant MCA infarction") with severe edema can mimic BD but is typically territorial and does not involve the entire brain.

BD can also mimic other disorders. **End-stage brain swelling** from severe trauma or profound hypoxic encephalopathy (e.g., following cardiopulmonary arrest) makes the cranial arteries, dura, and dural venous sinuses all seem relatively hyperdense compared with the diffusely edematous low-density brain.

With very low-density brain, comparatively high-density areas are seen along the basal cisterns, sylvian fissures, tentorium cerebelli, and sometimes even within the cortical sulci. This appearance is sometimes termed **pseudosubarachnoid hemorrhage** (pseudo-SAH) **(3-29B)**. Pseudo-SAH should not be mistaken for "real" SAH. The density of pseudo-SAH is significantly lower (between 30 HU and 40 HU) than the attenuation of "real" SAH (between 50 HU and 60 HU).

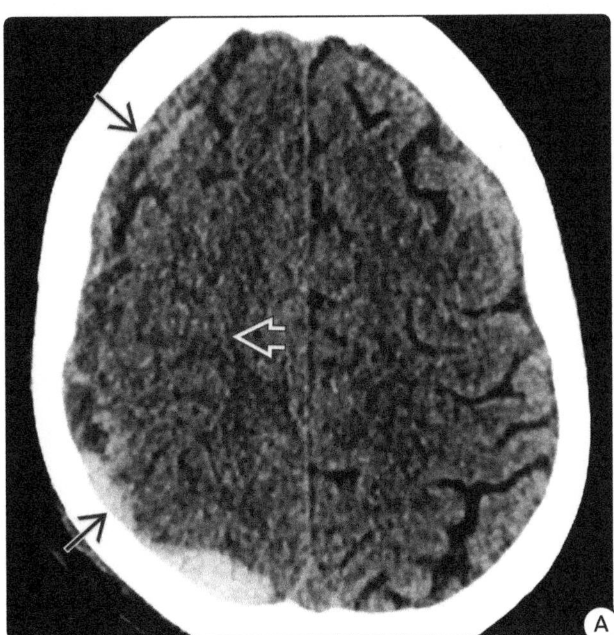

***(3-27A)** NECT in a patient with left hemiparesis shows a mixed-age right SDH ⇨ and cortical swelling ➡ under the SDH.*

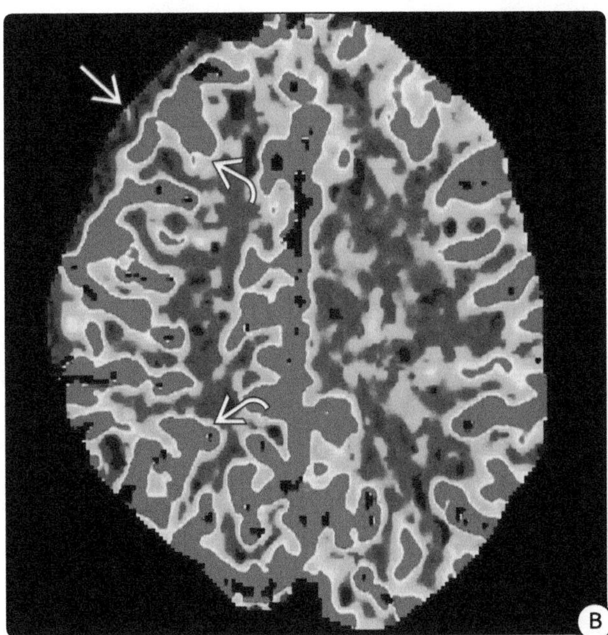

***(3-27B)** CT perfusion shows increased cerebral blood flow ➡ in the cortex under the SDH ➡. (Courtesy C. Hsu, MD.)*

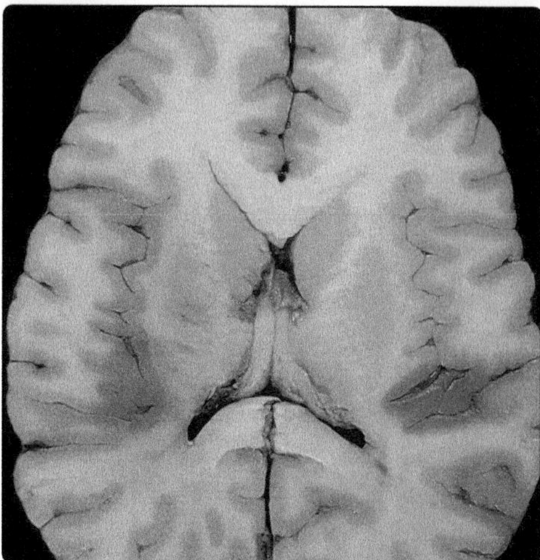

(3-28) Brain death shows diffuse swelling, poor GM-WM discrimination, small ventricles, and effaced surface sulci. (Courtesy R. Hewlett, MD.)

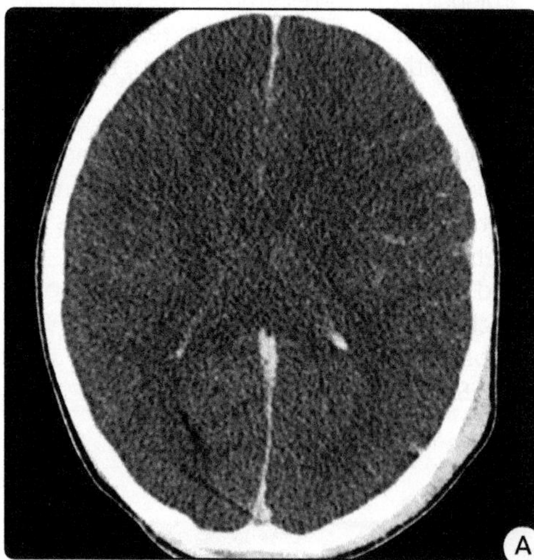

(3-29A) CECT obtained after a near drowning shows diffuse brain swelling with absent GM-WM interface. Lateral ventricles are almost invisible.

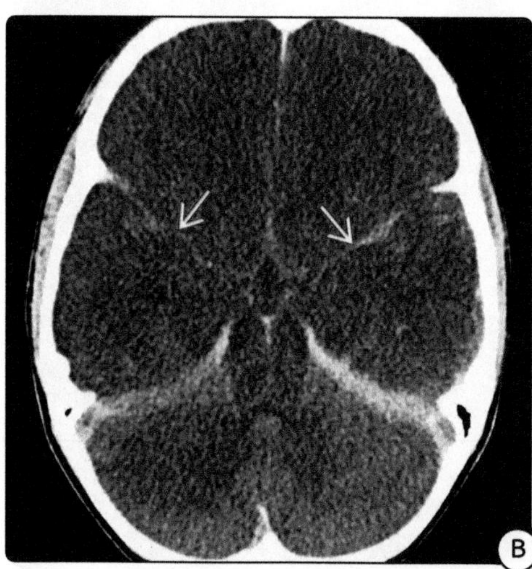

(3-29B) CECT in the same case shows severely attenuated MCAs ➔ and diffuse low-density brain. The patient expired shortly after the study.

BRAIN DEATH

Terminology and Definition

- BD = irreversible cessation of brain function
- Legal definition(s) vary with country, jurisdictions

Clinical Issues

- AAN 2010 checklist (BD in adults)
  - Coma (irreversible, known cause)
  - Neuroimaging explains coma
  - Neurologic examination, apnea testing performed

Ancillary Testing

- Only 1 needs to be performed
- Only if
  - Clinical examination cannot be fully performed, **or**
  - Apnea testing inconclusive/aborted
- Options
  - Cerebral angiogram (many jurisdictions accept DSA)
  - HMPAO SPECT
  - EEG
  - TCD

Imaging Findings

- DSA
  - Severe, prolonged contrast stasis in ICA
  - Most show no intracranial flow
  - 30% have some proximal opacification of intracranial arteries
- CTA, CTP
  - **No** opacification of cortical MCAs and internal cerebral veins on CTA
  - Stasis filling on CTP
- HMPAO SPECT
  - No intracranial opacification of flow studies
  - Scalp uptake but no brain activity ("light bulb" sign)
  - Extracranial uptake ("hot nose" sign)

Differential Diagnosis

- Reversible causes of coma (clinical, laboratory)
  - Drug overdose
  - Status epilepticus
  - Severe hypoglycemia
- Technical issues
  - "Missed" contrast bolus
- Severe brain swelling (other causes)
  - "Malignant" MCA infarct
  - Metabolic (e.g., hyperammonemia)
  - Hypoxic-ischemic encephalopathy

Selected References: The complete reference list is available on the Expert Consult™ eBook version included with purchase.

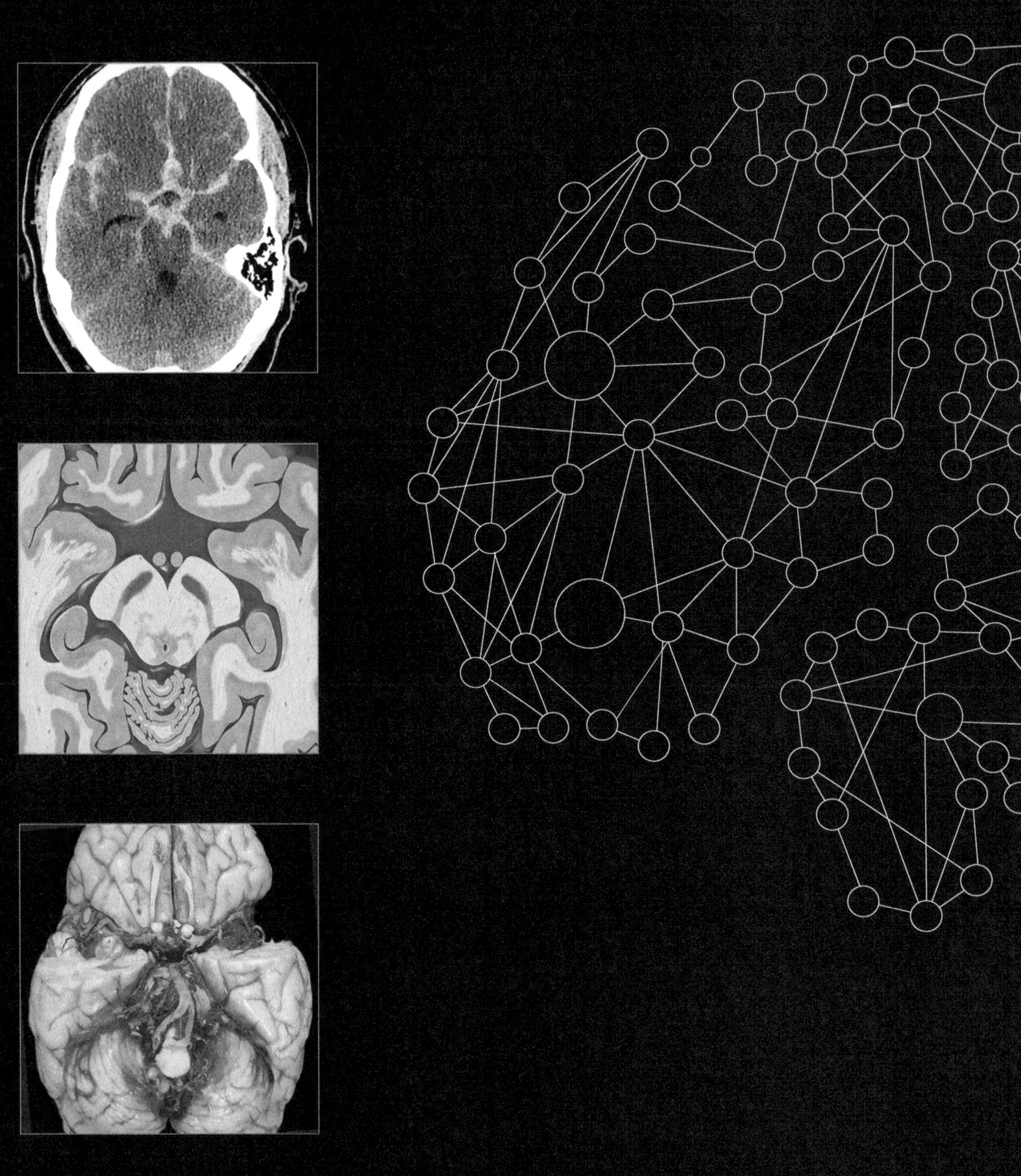

Section 2

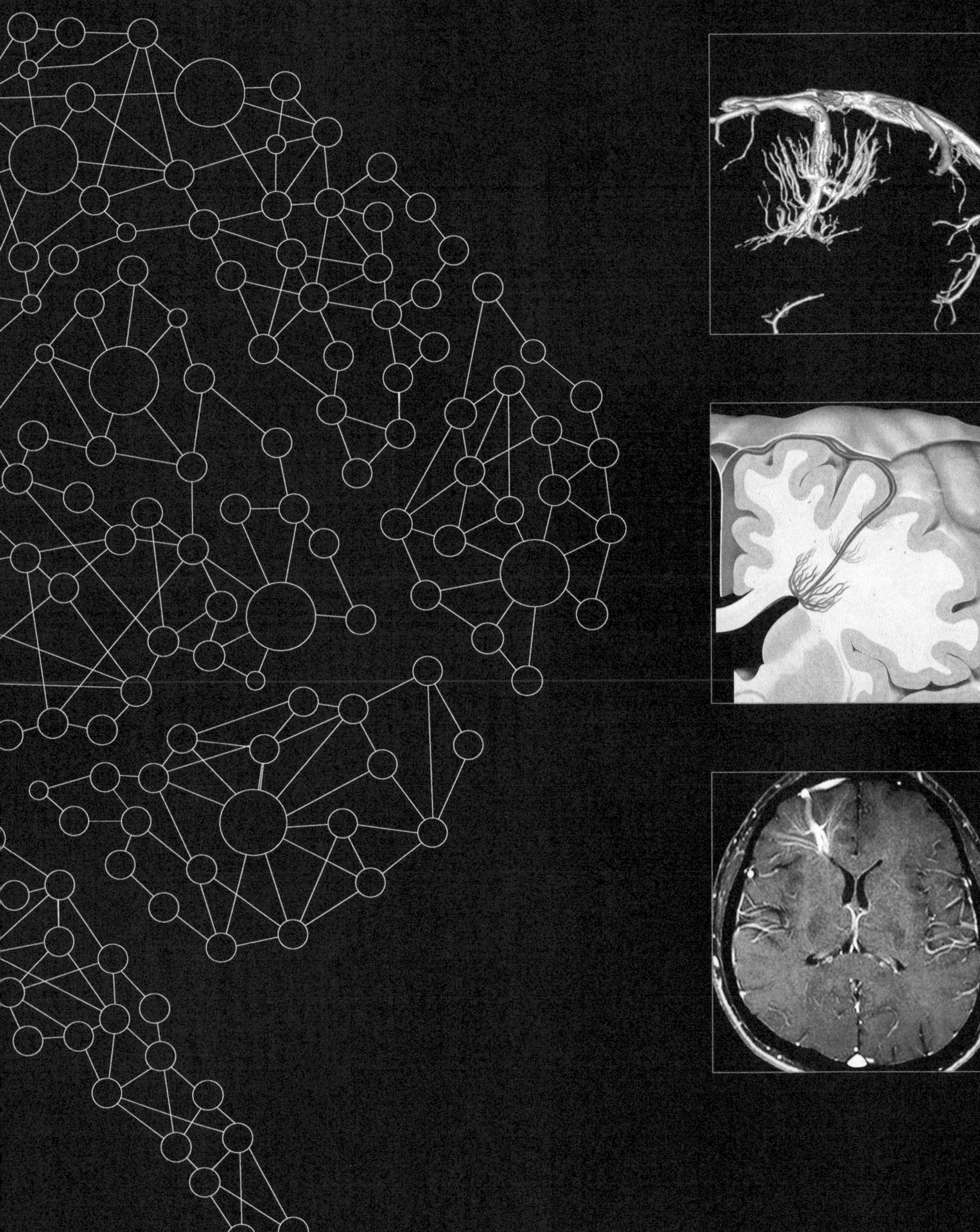

Section 2

Nontraumatic Hemorrhage and Vascular Lesions

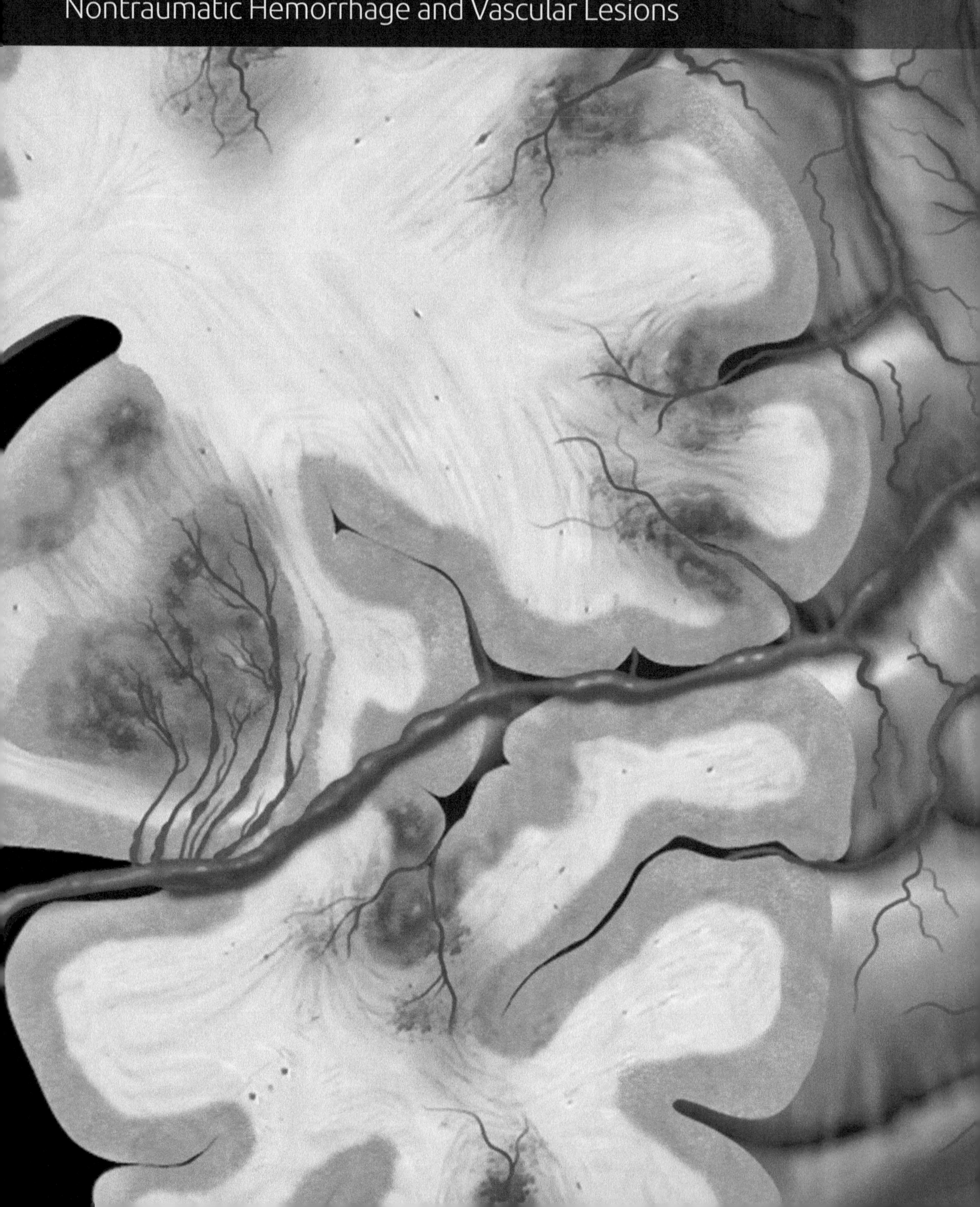

Approach to Nontraumatic Hemorrhage and Vascular Lesions

This part devoted to "spontaneous" (i.e., nontraumatic) hemorrhage and vascular lesions begins with a general discussion of brain bleeds. Subsequent chapters delineate a broad spectrum of vascular pathologies, ranging from aneurysms/subarachnoid hemorrhage (SAH) and vascular malformations to cerebral vasculopathy and strokes. Where appropriate, anatomic considerations and the pathophysiology of specific disorders are included.

Spontaneous (i.e., nontraumatic) intracranial hemorrhage (sICH) and vascular brain disorders are second only to trauma as neurologic causes of death and disability. Stroke or "brain attack"—defined as sudden onset of a neurologic event—is the third leading *overall* cause of death in industrialized countries. Imaging plays a crucial role in the management of stroke patients, both in establishing the diagnosis and stratifying patients for subsequent treatment.

We start this chapter with a brief overview of nontraumatic ICH and vascular diseases of the CNS, beginning with a short discussion of who, why, when, and how to image these patients. We then develop an anatomy-based approach to evaluating nontraumatic ICH. We close the discussion with a pathology-based introduction to the broad spectrum of congenital and acquired vascular lesions that affect the brain.

Imaging Hemorrhage and Vascular Lesions

Who and Why To Image?

Because of its widespread availability and speed, an emergent NECT scan is generally the first-line imaging procedure of choice in patients with sudden onset of an unexplained neurologic deficit.

If the initial NECT scan is negative and no neurologic deficit is apparent, further imaging is often unnecessary. However, if the history and clinical findings suggest a thromboembolic stroke or transient ischemic attack (TIA), additional imaging is indicated.

Emergent NECT imaging is also often obtained in patients with headache to screen for suspected SAH, hydrocephalus, intracranial mass, or other unspecified abnormalities. The updated American College of Radiology (ACR) Appropriateness Criteria indicate that most patients with uncomplicated nontraumatic primary headache do not require imaging.

ACR APPROPRIATENESS CRITERIA: CHRONIC HEADACHE

Chronic Headache (HA), No New Features, Normal Neurologic Examination
- NECT (3), CTA (2): Usually not appropriate
- MR (4): May be (minimally) appropriate

Chronic HA, New Feature or Neurologic Deficit
- Major concerns = mass lesion, brain bleed
- NECT (7), CTA (4): May be appropriate
- MR without/with contrast (8): Usually appropriate

Positional HA
- Major clinical concern = intracranial hypotension
- MR without/with contrast (8): Usually appropriate
- MR spine + MR myelography (7)

ACR APPROPRIATENESS CRITERIA: NEW HEADACHE

Sudden Severe HA ("Worst," "Thunderclap")
- Major concern = ICH
- NECT (9), CTA (8): Highly appropriate
- MR (7), MRA (7): Usually appropriate

New HA in Pregnant Woman
- MR without contrast (8): Usually appropriate
- NECT (7): Usually appropriate

New HA, Suspected Meningitis
- MR without/with contrast (8): Usually appropriate

New HA, Immunosuppressed or Cancer
- MR without/with contrast (9): Highly appropriate

New HA, Focal Neurologic Deficit or Papilledema
- MR without/with contrast (8): Usually appropriate
- MR without contrast (7), NECT (7): Usually appropriate

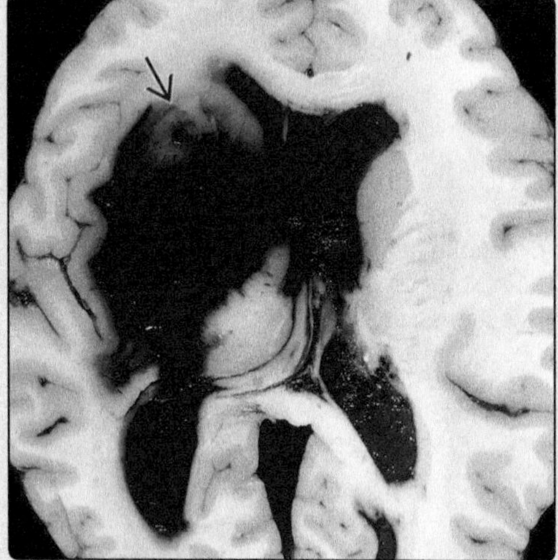

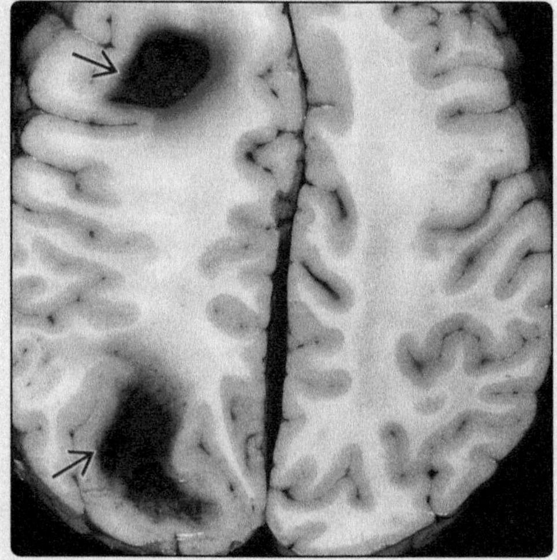

***(4-1)** Autopsy from an elderly adult shows a parenchymal hematoma ➙ centered in the striatocapsular region. External capsule/putamen location is classic for hypertensive hemorrhage. (Courtesy R. Hewlett, MD.) **(4-2)** Autopsy from a middle-aged patient with metastatic renal cell carcinoma shows 2 hemorrhagic metastases ➙ at GM-WM interface, a typical location. (Courtesy R. Hewlett, MD.)*

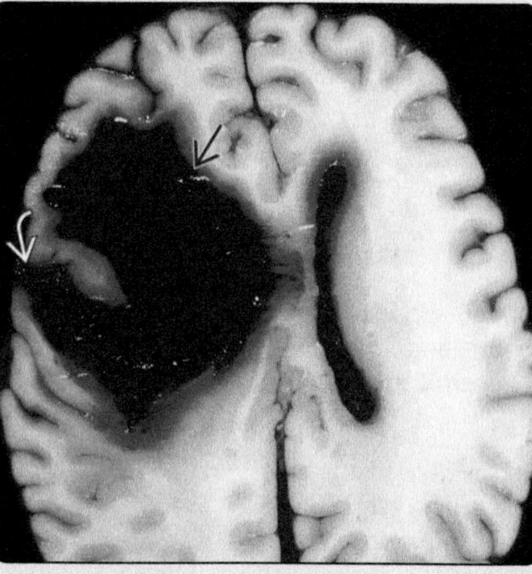

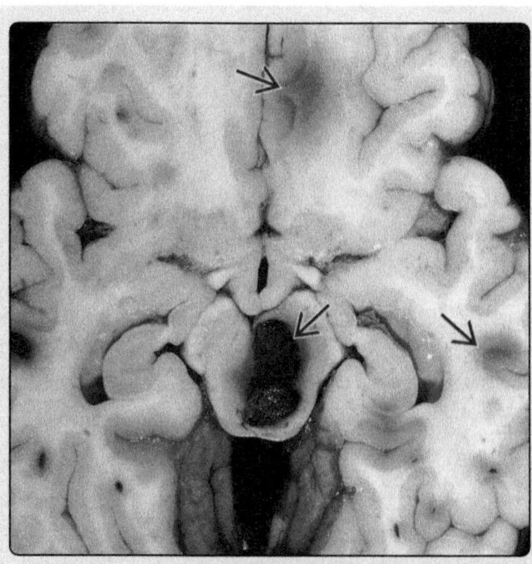

***(4-3)** Autopsy case is from a young patient with a large hematoma ➙ centered in the hemispheric WM with focal extension ➙ through the cortex. Underlying arteriovenous malformation (AVM) was the cause of this fatal intracranial hemorrhage (ICH). (Courtesy R. Hewlett, MD.) **(4-4)** Autopsy case is from a child with multifocal parenchymal hemorrhages ➙ caused by leukemia. (Courtesy R. Hewlett, MD.)*

When and How To Image?

Some of the most challenging questions arise when screening NECT discloses parenchymal hemorrhage. What are the potential causes? Should further emergent imaging be performed?

Many parenchymal "brain bleeds" carry high mortality and morbidity. Early deterioration secondary to rapid hematoma expansion and growth is common in the first few hours after onset. Imaging is crucial in further evaluating and managing these patients.

CTA is indicated in patients with sudden clinical deterioration and a mixed-density hematoma (indicating rapid bleeding or coagulopathy). A "spot" sign with active contrast extravasation caused by rupture of a lenticulostriate microaneurysm (Charcot-Bouchard aneurysm) can sometimes be identified. Contrast extravasation in sICH predicts hematoma expansion and poor clinical outcome.

CTA is also an appropriate next step in children and young/middle-aged adults with spontaneous (nontraumatic) ICH detected on screening NECT. In contrast to elderly patients—in whom hypertensive hemorrhage and amyloid angiopathy are the two most common etiologies of unexplained sICH—vascular malformation is the most common underlying etiology in younger age groups.

Emergency MR is rarely necessary if CTA is negative. However, follow-up MR without and with contrast enhancement can be very useful in patients with unexplained ICH. In addition to the standard sequences (i.e., T1WI, T2WI, FLAIR, DWI, and T1 C+), a T2* sequence—either (or both) GRE or susceptibility-weighted imaging (SWI)—should be obtained.

MR evidence for prior hemorrhage(s) and cerebral "microbleeds" can be very helpful in narrowing the differential diagnosis. Benign ICH typically follows an orderly, predictable evolution on MR scans. MR evidence of disordered or bizarre-looking hemorrhage should raise the possibility of neoplasm,

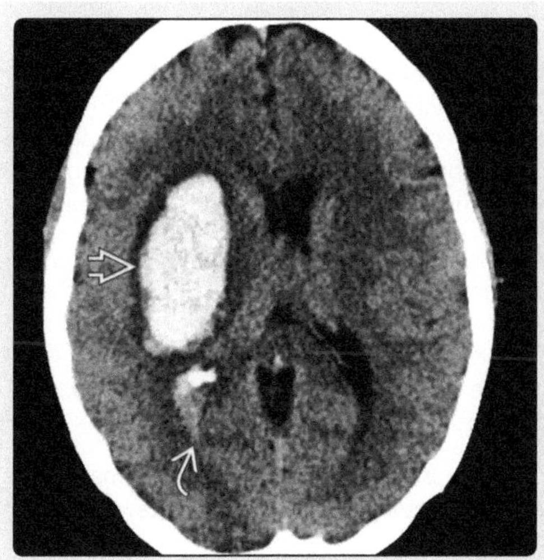

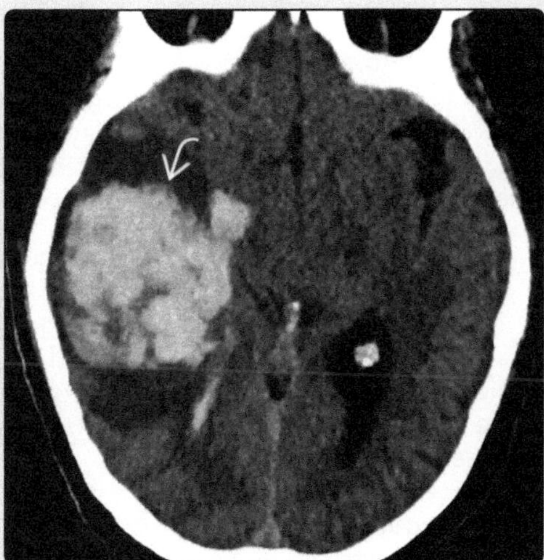

***(4-5)** NECT in a 60y woman with uncontrolled hypertension, sudden-onset, left-sided weakness shows classic putamen-external capsule hypertensive hemorrhage. Note small amount of blood in the right occipital horn. **(4-6)** NECT in a 59y normotensive man with headache, left-sided weakness, lethargy, and vomiting shows a right temporal lobar hemorrhage. CTA was negative. Surgery disclosed glioblastoma.*

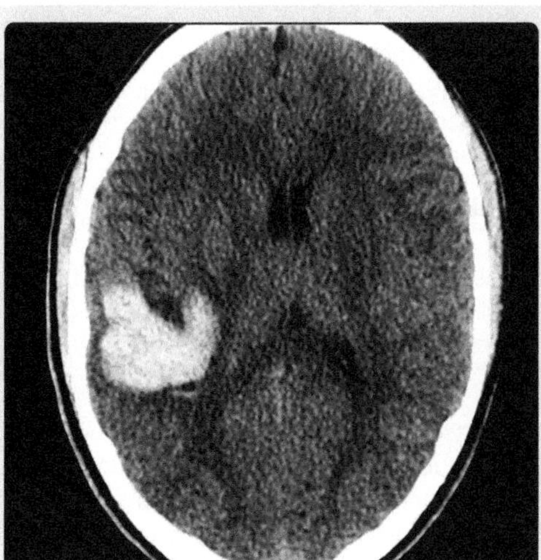

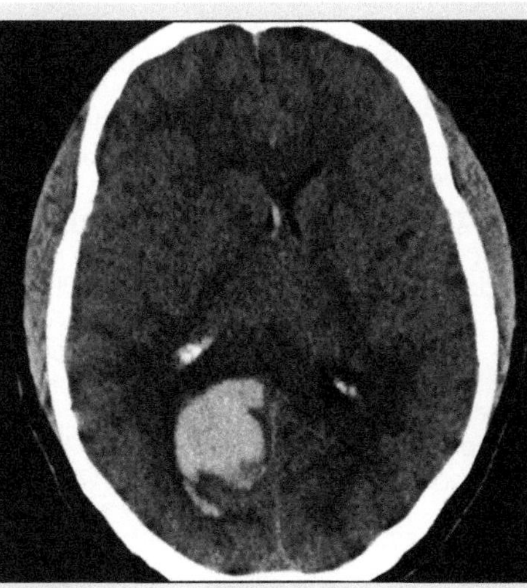

***(4-7)** NECT in a 15-year-old boy with headache, mild left-sided weakness shows a right posterior temporal hematoma. DSA (not shown) disclosed a partially thrombosed AVM. **(4-8)** NECT in a 43-year-old, mildly hypertensive man who presented with a severe occipital headache shows a right occipital lobar hematoma. CTA and DSA (not shown) disclosed straight sinus thrombosis.*

underlying arteriovenous malformation (AVM), or coagulopathy.

If MR demonstrates multiple parenchymal hemorrhages of different ages, the underlying etiology varies with patient age. Multiple microbleeds in elderly patients are typically associated with chronic hypertension or amyloid angiopathy. Cavernous malformations or hematologic disorders are the most common causes in children and young adults.

Approach to Nontraumatic Hemorrhage

Hematoma location, age, and number (solitary or multiple) should be noted.

Intraaxial Hemorrhage

Clinical Issues

Parenchymal hemorrhage is the most devastating type of stroke. Although recent advances have improved the treatment of ischemic strokes, few evidence-based treatments exist for ICH. Strategies are largely supportive, aimed at limiting further injury and preventing associated complications, such as hematoma expansion, elevated intracranial pressure, and intraventricular rupture with hydrocephalus.

Imaging

Parenchymal hematomas are easily recognized on NECT scans by their hyperdensity or, in the case of rapid bleeding or coagulopathy, mixed iso-/hyperdense appearance. Expansion of a parenchymal hematoma into the ventricular system is commonly encountered on initial imaging in patients with sICH and is associated with poor long-term outcome.

Hematomas typically expand the brain, displacing the cortex outward and producing mass effect on underlying structures, such as the cerebral ventricles. The sulci are often compressed, and the overlying gyri appear expanded and flattened. The surrounding brain may appear grossly edematous.

Hematoma signal intensity on standard MR varies with clot age and imaging sequence. T2* (GRE, SWI) scans are especially important in evaluating patients with brain hemorrhage. Susceptibility-weighted imaging is particularly useful in identifying the presence and location of cerebral microbleeds.

Differential Diagnosis

Sublocation of an intraparenchymal clot is very important in establishing putative etiology. The differential diagnosis of sICH varies widely with anatomic location.

If a classic **striatocapsular** or **thalamic** hematoma is found in a middle-aged or elderly patient, hypertensive hemorrhage is by far the most common etiology **(4-1)** **(4-7)**. Drug abuse should be suspected in a young adult with a similar-appearing lesion. Ruptured aneurysms rarely cause lateral basal ganglionic hemorrhage, and neoplasms with hemorrhagic necrosis are far less common than hypertensive bleeds in this location.

Lobar hemorrhages present a different challenge, as the differential diagnosis is much broader. In older patients, amyloid angiopathy, hypertension, and underlying neoplasm (primary or metastatic) are the most common causes **(4-2)** **(4-6)**. Vascular malformations **(4-3)** **(4-7)** and hematologic malignancies **(4-4)** are more common in younger patients. Dural sinus &/or cortical vein thrombosis are uncommon but occur in patients of all ages **(4-8)**.

Hemorrhages at the **gray matter-white matter interface** are typical of metastases **(4-2)**, septic emboli, and fungal infection.

Multifocal hemorrhages confined to the white matter are rare. **"Critical illness-associated" brain microbleeds** have recently been reported, especially in intubated patients with acute respiratory distress syndrome (ARDS) or ECMO. These may be hypoxia related, similar to the microbleeds seen in high-altitude cerebral edema.

When microbleeds are identified in a patient with a history of a febrile illness followed by sudden neurologic deterioration, they are most likely secondary to a hemorrhagic form of acute disseminated encephalomyelitis called acute hemorrhagic leukoencephalopathy (**AHLE, a.k.a. Weston-Hurst disease**).

Clot age can likewise be helpful in suggesting the etiology of an ICH. A hemosiderin-laden encephalomalacic cavity in the basal ganglia or thalamus of an older patient is typically due to an old hypertensive hemorrhage. Cortical/subcortical microbleeds can be seen in cerebral amyloid angiopathy, particularly if siderosis is present.

The most common cause of a hyperacute parenchymal clot in a child is an underlying AVM or (less commonly) cavernous malformation.

Extraaxial Hemorrhage

Spontaneous extraaxial hemorrhages can occur in any of the three major anatomic compartments, i.e., the epidural space, subdural space, and the subarachnoid space. By far, the most common are SAHs **(4-9)** **(4-10)**. In contrast to traumatic hemorrhages, spontaneous bleeding into the epi- and subdural spaces is rare.

Subarachnoid Hemorrhage

Clinical Issues. Patients with nontraumatic SAH (ntSAH) usually present with sudden onset of severe headache ("worst headache of my life"). A "thunderclap" headache is very common.

Imaging. ntSAH is easily distinguished from a parenchymal hematoma by its location and configuration. Blood in the subarachnoid spaces has a feathery, curvilinear, or serpentine appearance as it fills the cisterns and surface sulci **(4-12)**. It follows brain surfaces and rarely causes a focal mass effect.

SAH is hyperdense on NECT scans. Bloody sulcal-cisternal CSF appears dirty on T1WI, hyperintense on FLAIR, and "blooms" on T2* sequences.

Differential Diagnosis. As with parenchymal bleeds, ntSAH sublocation is helpful in establishing an appropriate differential diagnosis. By far, the most common cause of ntSAH is **aneurysmal SAH** (aSAH). As most intracranial aneurysms arise from the circle of Willis and the middle cerebral bifurcation, aSAH tends to spread throughout the basal cisterns and extend into the sylvian fissures **(4-10)**.

Two special, easily recognizable subtypes of SAH are *not* associated with ruptured intracranial aneurysm. Blood localized to the subarachnoid spaces around the midbrain and anterior to the pons is called **perimesencephalic nonaneurysmal SAH** (pnSAH) **(4-11)**. This type of SAH is self-limited, rarely results in vasospasm, and is probably secondary to venous hemorrhage. CTA is a reliable technique to rule out a basilar tip aneurysm. DSA and noninvasive follow-up imaging have had no demonstrable increased diagnostic yield in such cases.

Blood in one or more sulci over the upper cerebral hemispheres is called **convexal SAH (4-12)**. This special subtype of SAH is associated with a number of diverse etiologies, including cortical vein thrombosis and amyloid angiopathy in older patients, as well as reversible cerebral vasoconstriction syndrome in younger individuals.

Despite extensive imaging evaluation, the origin of spontaneous ntSAH remains unidentified in 10-20% of patients. Hydrocephalus and delayed cerebral ischemia in these patients are infrequent, and long-term neurologic outcomes are generally good.

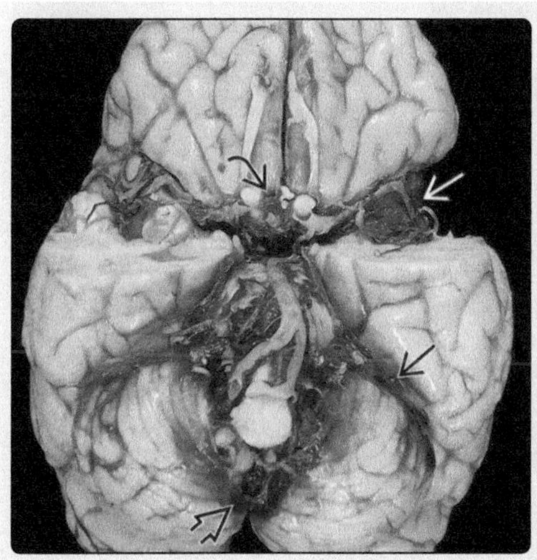

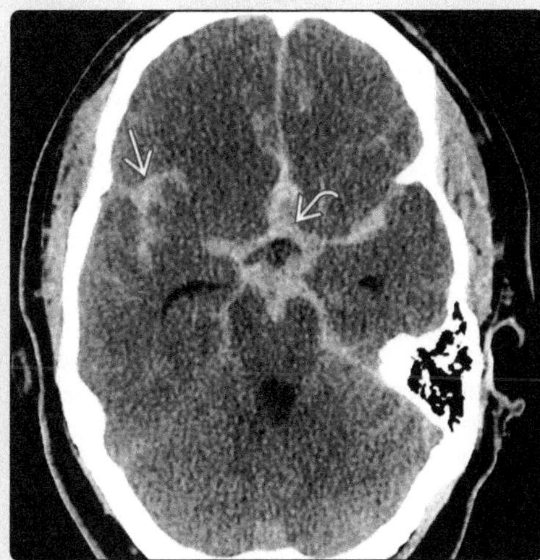

***(4-9)** Autopsy case demonstrates diffuse acute subarachnoid hemorrhage (SAH) in the basal cisterns. Blood fills the sylvian fissures ➔, suprasellar cistern ↷, and cisterna magna ⇨. Hemorrhage coats the surface of the pons and extends laterally into the cerebellopontine angle cisterns ⇨. **(4-10)** NECT scan shows a patient with aneurysmal SAH. Diffuse hemorrhage fills the suprasellar cistern ↷ and sylvian fissures ➔.*

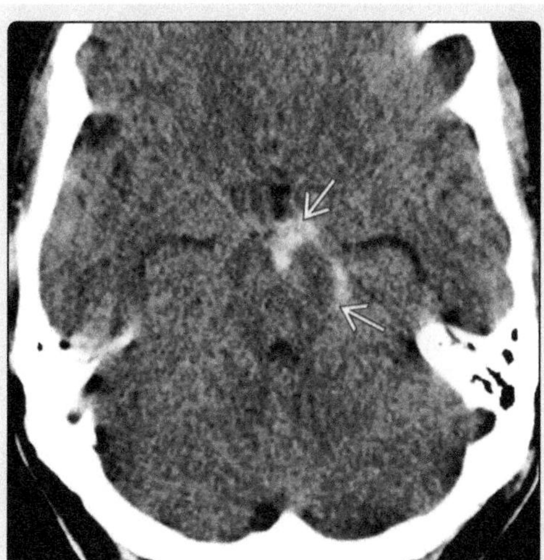

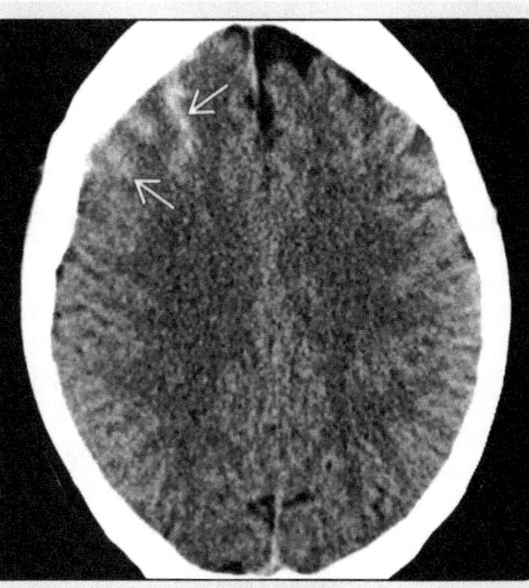

***(4-11)** NECT shows classic perimesencephalic nonaneurysmal SAH ➔ with subarachnoid blood localized around the midbrain, in the interpeduncular fossa, and in the ambient cistern. CTA was negative. **(4-12)** NECT in a young woman with severe headache shows focal subarachnoid blood in right frontal convexity sulci ➔. Basal cisterns (not shown) were normal. This is proven reversible cerebral vasoconstriction syndrome.*

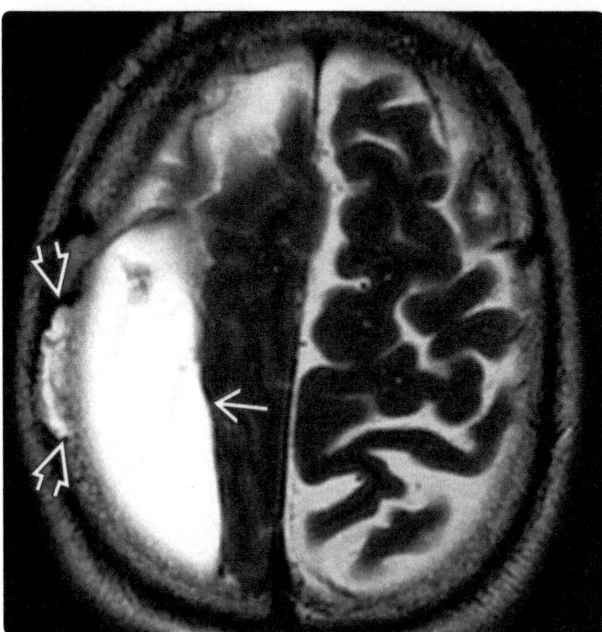

***(4-13)** T2WI shows a chronic epidural hematoma ➡ associated with a well-demarcated hyperintense lesion in the calvarium ➡. Hemangioma was found at surgery.*

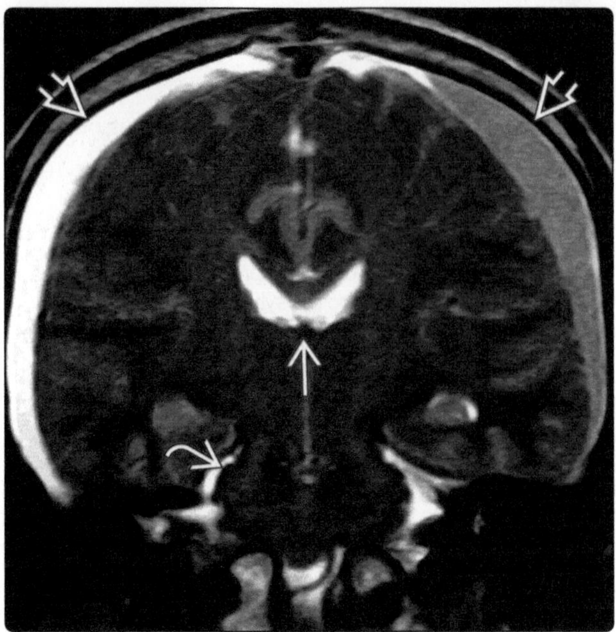

***(4-14)** Coronal T2WI in a patient with severe headaches and intracranial hypotension shows "fat pons" ➡ and lateral ventricles pulled inferiorly ➡ by brain sagging. Bilateral subdural hematomas of different ages are present ➡.*

Epidural Hemorrhage

The pathogenesis of extradural hematomas is almost always traumatic and arises from lacerated meningeal arteries, fractures, or torn dural venous sinuses.

Most spontaneous epidural bleeds are found in the spinal—not the cranial—epidural space and are an emergent condition that may result in paraplegia, quadriplegia, and even death. Elderly anticoagulated patients are most at risk.

Intracranial spontaneous epidural hemorrhages are very rare. Most reported cases are associated with bleeding disorders, craniofacial infection (usually mastoiditis or sphenoid sinusitis), dural sinus thrombosis, bone infarction (e.g., in patients with sickle cell disease), or a vascular lesion of the calvarium (e.g., hemangioma, metastasis, or intradiploic epidermoid cyst) **(4-13)**.

Subdural Hemorrhage

Trauma also causes the vast majority of subdural hematomas (SDHs). Nontraumatic SDHs represent < 5% of all cases.

Many nontraumatic SDHs occur with CSF volume depletion, i.e., dehydration or CSF hypovolemia. Both can become life threatening if sufficiently severe.

Intracranial hypotension can be traumatic, iatrogenic, or spontaneous (see Chapter 34). Most cases of traumatic intracranial hypotension are secondary to CSF leak associated with spinal or dural injury. Iatrogenic intracranial hypotension occurs with dural tear following lumbar puncture, myelography, spinal anesthesia, or cranial surgery. Regardless of etiology, SDH is a common (but not invariable) association **(4-14)**.

Nontraumatic SDHs have been reported in association with a number of other conditions, including hyponatremic dehydration, inherited or acquired coagulation disorders, dural venous sinus thrombosis, and meningitis.

A few cases of spontaneous SDH occur directly adjacent to a lobar peripheral hemorrhage and are associated with an underlying vasculopathy (such as cerebral amyloid disease with pseudoaneurysm formation) or vascular malformation. Others occur without an identifiable antecedent or predisposing condition.

Occasionally, a ruptured cortical artery or saccular aneurysm may result in a nontraumatic intracranial SDH. Dural hemangiomas have also been reported as causes of acute nontraumatic SDH. Elderly patients with intrinsic or iatrogenic coagulopathy can present with an SDH and either minor or no definite evidence for head trauma.

Approach to Vascular Disorders of CNS

Here, we discuss a general approach to vascular disorders in the brain, briefly introducing the major chapters in this part. Details regarding pathoetiology, clinical features, imaging findings, and differential diagnosis are delineated in each individual chapter.

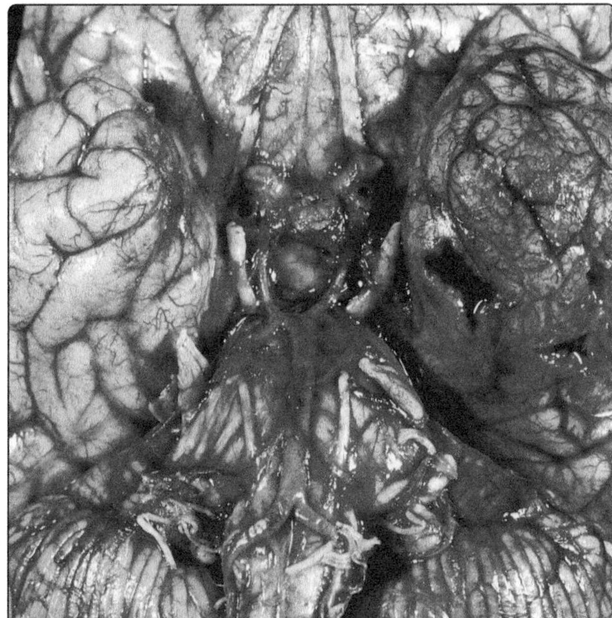

(4-15) Autopsied case shows extensive basilar SAH and vasospasm from a ruptured saccular aneurysm. (Courtesy R. Hewlett, MD.)

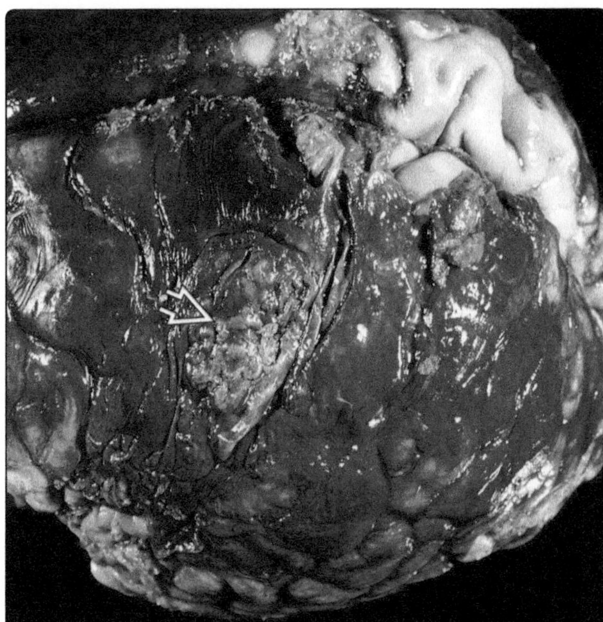

(4-16) Autopsy case shows an AVM causing massive ICH. Note prominent draining veins ➡ over the surface of the hemisphere. (Courtesy R. Hewlett, MD.)

Subarachnoid Hemorrhage and Aneurysms

Trauma is—by far—the most common cause of SAH. Traumatic SAH (tSAH) is found in 100% of patients with fatal severe head injuries and is common in those with moderate to severe nonfatal closed head trauma.

Chapter 6 focuses on *nontraumatic* "spontaneous" SAH, which causes 3-5% of all acute strokes. Of these, nearly 80% are caused by rupture of a saccular aneurysm **(4-15)**. aSAH can generally be distinguished from nonaneurysmal SAH by its distribution on NECT scans.

Classic saccular ("berry") aneurysms, as well as the less common dissecting aneurysms, pseudoaneurysms, fusiform aneurysms, and blood blister-like aneurysms, are discussed in this chapter.

Vascular Malformations

Cerebrovascular malformations (CVMs) are a fascinating, remarkably heterogeneous group of disorders with unique pathophysiology and imaging features. Chapter 7 discusses the four major types of vascular malformations, grouping them according to whether they shunt blood directly from the arterial to the venous side of the circulation without passing through a capillary bed.

CVMs that display arteriovenous (AV) shunting include AVMs **(4-16)** and fistulas. Included in this discussion is the newly described entity called cerebral proliferative angiopathy. Cerebral proliferative angiopathy can mimic AVM on imaging studies but has unique features that may influence treatment decisions.

With few exceptions, most CVMs that lack AV shunting—i.e., developmental venous anomalies (venous "angiomas") along with cavernous malformations and capillary telangiectasias—rarely hemorrhage and are "leave me alone" lesions that are identified on imaging studies but generally do not require treatment.

Lastly, note that the topic of "occult" vascular malformation is not discussed. This is an outdated concept that originated in an era when angiography was the only available technique to diagnose brain vascular malformations prior to surgical exploration. Some vascular malformations, such as cavernous angiomas and capillary telangiectasias, are invisible (and therefore "occult") at angiography but are easily identified on MR.

Arterial Anatomy and Strokes

Chapter 8 begins with a discussion of normal intracranial arterial anatomy and vascular distributions, an essential foundation for understanding the imaging appearance of cerebral ischemia/infarction.

The major focus of the chapter is thromboembolic infarcts in major arterial territories, as they are, by far, the most common cause of acute strokes **(4-17)** **(4-18)**. Subacute and chronic infarcts are briefly discussed. Although typically not amenable to intravascular treatment, they are nevertheless seen on imaging studies and should be recognized as residua from a prior infarct **(4-19)** **(4-20)**.

The discussion of embolic infarcts includes cardiac and atheromatous emboli, as well as lacunar infarcts and the distinct syndrome of fat emboli. The importance of recognizing calcified cerebral emboli on NECT scans is emphasized, as the risk of repeated stroke in these patients is very high.

The pathophysiology and imaging of watershed ("border zone") infarcts and global hypoxic-ischemic brain injury is also included. Miscellaneous strokes, such as cerebral hyperperfusion syndrome, are discussed.

The chapter concludes by illustrating strokes in unusual vascular distributions, including artery of Percheron and "top of the basilar" infarcts.

Venous Anatomy and Occlusions

The venous side of the cerebral circulation is—quite literally—"terra incognita" (an unknown land) to many physicians who deal with brain disorders. Although many could sketch the major arterial territories with relative ease, few could diagram the intracranial venous drainage territories.

The brain veins and sinuses are unlike those of the body. Systemic veins typically travel parallel to arteries and mirror their vascular territories; not so in the brain. Systemic veins have valves, and flow is generally in one direction.

The cerebral veins and dural sinuses lack valves and may thus exhibit bidirectional flow. Systemic veins have numerous collateral pathways that can develop in the case of occlusion. Few such collaterals exist inside the calvarium.

Chapter 9 begins with a brief discussion of normal venous anatomy and drainage patterns before we consider the various manifestations of venous occlusion. Venous thrombosis causes just 1% of all strokes, and its clinical presentation is much less distinctive than that of major arterial occlusion. It is perhaps the type of stroke most frequently missed on imaging studies. Venous stroke can also mimic other disease (e.g., neoplasm), and, in turn, a number of disorders can mimic venous thrombosis.

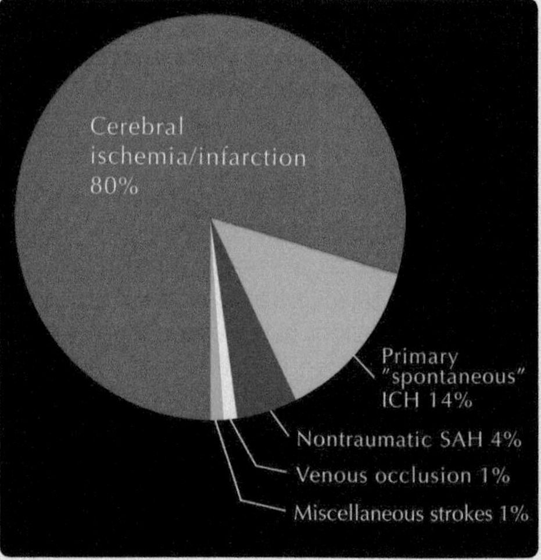

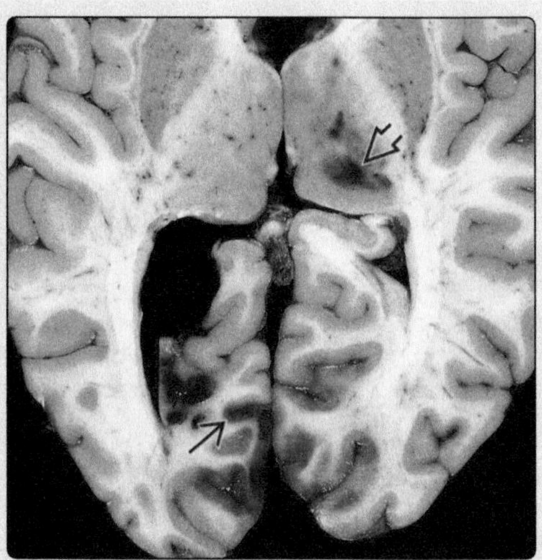

***(4-17)** Diagram shows that cerebral ischemia-infarction represents a vast majority of strokes. The 2nd most common is primary ICH followed by nontraumatic SAH. **(4-18)** Autopsy shows subacute cerebral infarct, hemorrhagic transformation in occipital cortex ⇨, and contralateral thalamus ⇨. Anatomic distribution is of posterior (vertebrobasilar) territorial infarct. (Courtesy R. Hewlett, MD.)*

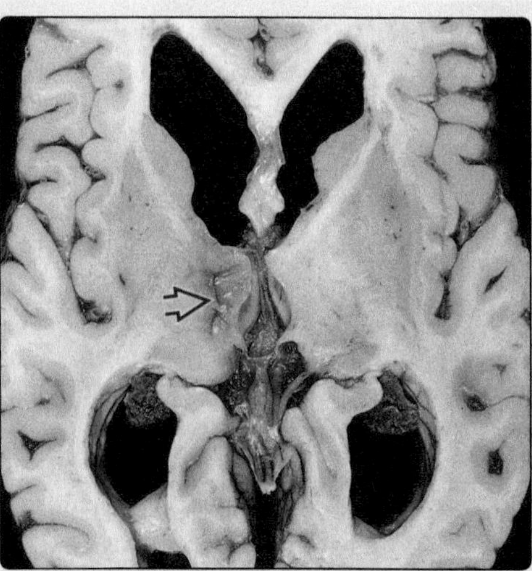

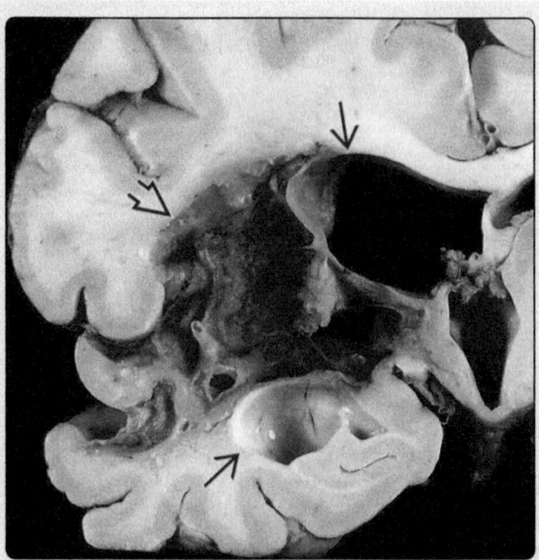

***(4-19)** Autopsied brain shows a chronic healed thalamic infarct ⇨. (Courtesy R. Hewlett, MD.) **(4-20)** Coronal autopsied brain shows encephalomalacic changes of an old middle cerebral artery (MCA) infarct ⇨. Note the enlargement of the adjacent lateral ventricle ⇨. (From DP: Hospital Autopsy.)*

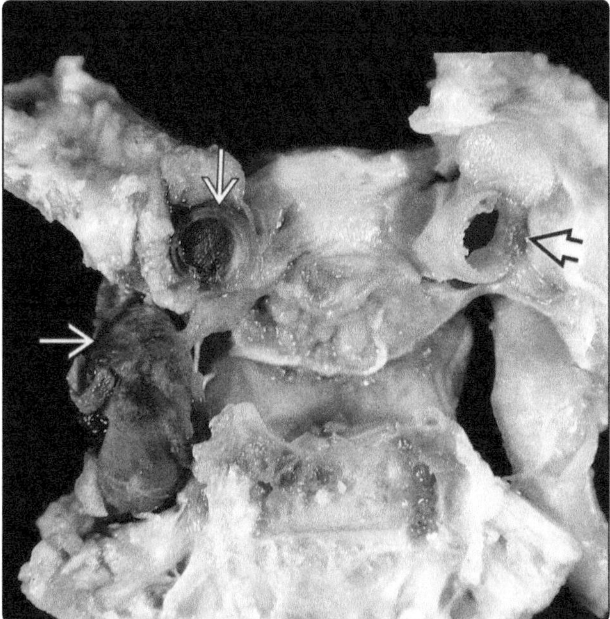

(4-21) Autopsy case shows thrombosis of 1 cavernous/supraclinoid internal carotid artery (ICA) ➡ and atherosclerosis ➡ in the other ICA.

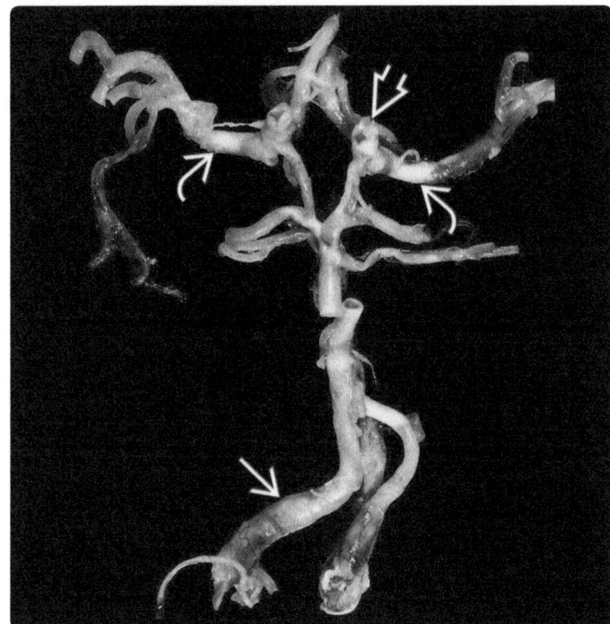

(4-22) Yellowish discoloration and ectasia from atherosclerotic vascular disease is most prominent in the posterior circulation ➡, but the ICAs ➡ and proximal MCAs ➡ are also affected.

Vasculopathy

Chapter 10, the final chapter in this part, is devoted to cerebral vasculopathy. This chapter begins with a review of normal extracranial arterial anatomy with special focus on the carotid arteries and their variants.

The bulk of the chapter is devoted to cerebral vasculopathy and is organized into two parts: Atherosclerosis **(4-21)** and nonatherosclerotic disease. The concept of the "vulnerable" or "at-risk" atherosclerotic plaque is underscored. Indeed, although measuring the percentage of internal carotid artery stenosis has been emphasized since the 1990s as a major predictor of stroke risk and the basis for treatment-related decisions, identifying a rupture-prone plaque is at least as important as determining stenosis.

The relatively new but extremely important topic of high-resolution vessel wall imaging is introduced, and its role in distinguishing between different types of vasculopathy is emphasized.

The much-neglected but important topic of *intracranial* atherosclerosis is also discussed. Whereas major vessel and cardiac thromboemboli cause most arterial strokes, between 5-10% can be attributed to intracranial stenoocclusive disease **(4-21)** **(4-22)**. The topic of arteriolosclerosis (i.e., small vessel vascular disease) is also considered here and again in the subsequent section on metabolic disease.

Nonatheromatous diseases of the cerebral vasculature are much less common than atherosclerosis and its sequelae. However, a number of vasculopathies can have serious consequences and should be recognized on imaging studies. This heterogeneous group of disorders includes fibromuscular dysplasia, dissection, vasospasm, the unusual but important cerebral vasoconstriction syndromes, and the often-confusing topic of vasculitis.

The vasculopathy chapter concludes with the intriguing topic of nonatheromatous microvascular diseases, such as systemic lupus erythematosus, antiphospholipid syndrome, and amyloid angiopathy.

Selected References: The complete reference list is available on the Expert Consult™ eBook version included with purchase.

Spontaneous Parenchymal Hemorrhage

In the absence of trauma, abrupt onset of focal neurological symptoms is presumed to be vascular in origin until proven otherwise. Rapid neuroimaging to distinguish ischemic stroke from intracranial hemorrhage (ICH) is crucial to patient management.

Primary (Spontaneous) Intracranial Hemorrhage

Epidemiology

Cerebral ischemia/infarction is responsible for almost 80% of all "strokes." Spontaneous (nontraumatic) primary ICH (pICH) causes 10-15% of first-time strokes and is a devastating subtype with unusually high mortality and morbidity. Death or dependent state is the outcome in > 70% of all patients.

Natural History

Early deterioration with pICH is common. More than 20% of patients experience a decrease in a Glasgow Coma Scale (GCS) score of two or more points between initial assessment by paramedics and presentation in the ED.

Active bleeding with hematoma expansion (HE) occurs in 25-40% of patients. Patients with large hematomas, history of anticoagulation, or hypertension (HTN) are at particular risk for HE, which may occur several hours after symptom onset. HE is predictive of clinical deterioration and carries significantly increased morbidity and mortality. Therefore, swift diagnosis is needed to direct treatment.

The prognosis is grave, even with prompt intervention. 20-30% of all patients die within 48 hours after the initial hemorrhage. The one-year mortality rate approaches 60%. Only 20% of patients who survive regain functional independence and recover without significant residual neurologic deficits.

Imaging Recommendations

The most recent American Heart Association/American Stroke Association (AHA/ASA) guidelines recommend emergent CT as the initial screening procedure to distinguish ischemic stroke from ICH.

If a parenchymal hematoma is identified, determining its size and etiology becomes critically important in patient triage. CTA is easily obtained at the time of initial imaging and is now included in many institutions as an integral part of acute stroke protocols. If contrast or extravasation within the clot (spot sign) is present, these patients are at risk of HE.

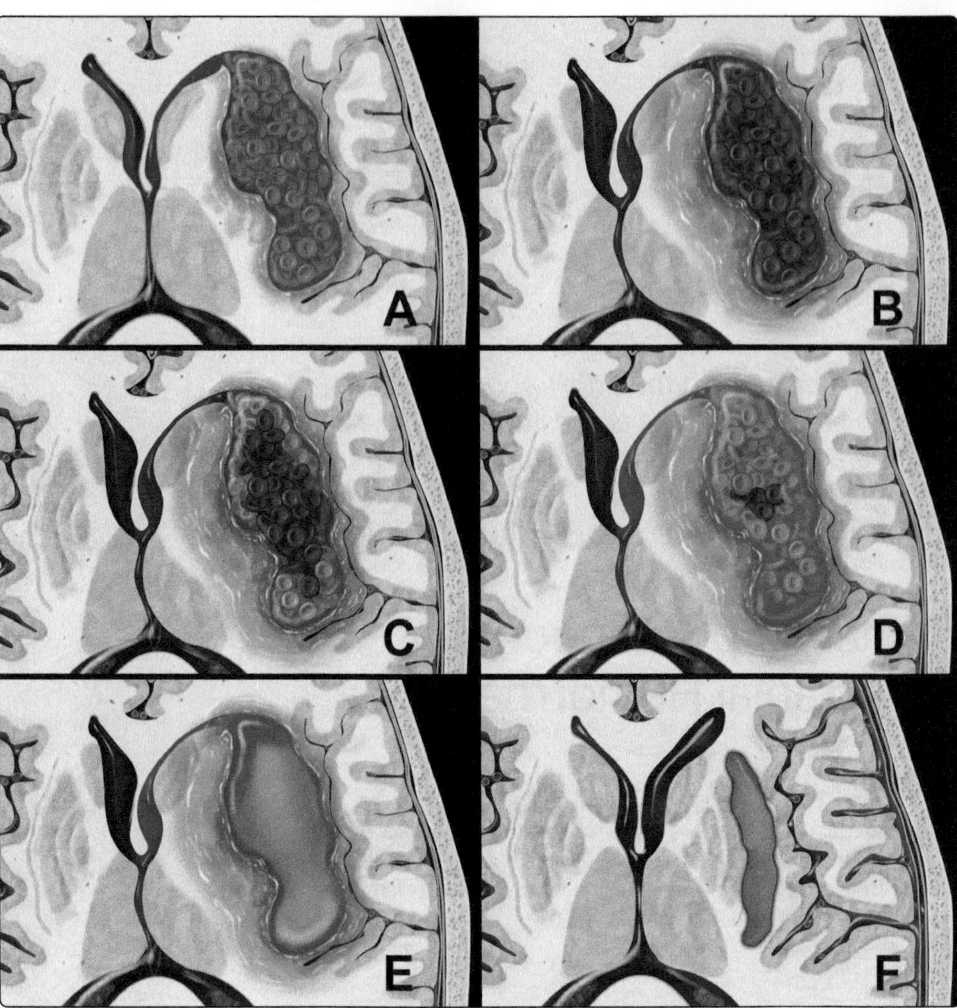

***(5-1)** Brain parenchymal hematomas have a fairly wide range of appearance depending on age of the clot, size of the hematoma, and oxygen tension in the environment. (A) Hyperacute hemorrhage is defined as less than 24 hours old. It consists of a water-rich clot that is 95-98% intracellular oxygenated hemoglobin (oxy-Hgb) [indicated by the intact red blood cells (RBCs) colored red]. (B) Acute clots are between 1 and 3 days old. Here, the hematoma consists mostly of RBCs (blue) containing intracellular deoxy-Hgb, with the conversion first appearing in the intensely hypoxic clot center. Early subacute clots between 3 (C) and 7 days (D) contain mostly RBCs with intracellular met-Hgb (yellow). (E) Late subacute clots (between 1 and 2 weeks) consist primarily of lysed RBCs with a liquid pool of extracellular met-Hgb. The mostly liquidized clot gradually shrinks with time until only a thin, slit-like yellowish residual fluid collection of extracellular met-Hgb surrounded by a hemosiderin rim remains (F).*

The management of unexplained brain bleeds also varies with patient age. If the patient is older than 45 years and has preexisting systemic HTN, a putaminal, thalamic, or posterior fossa ICH is almost always hypertensive in origin. Vascular imaging may or may not be requested.

In contrast, lobar or deep brain bleeds in younger patients or normotensive adults—regardless of age—almost always require further investigation. Contrast-enhanced CT/MR with angiography &/or venography may be helpful in detecting underlying abnormalities, such as arteriovenous malformation, neoplasm, and cerebral sinovenous thrombosis.

In older patients with pICH, MR with T2* (GRE, SWI) is also helpful in detecting the presence of "surrogate markers" of small vessel disease, such as brain microbleeds, white matter hyperintensities, and lacunar infarcts.

Overview

We begin this chapter with a discussion of the pathophysiology of ICH. This provides the basis for considering how pICH looks on imaging studies and why its appearance changes over time. We then consider some major causes of spontaneous ICH, such as HTN and amyloid angiopathy.

"UNEXPLAINED" ICH: WHAT YOU NEED TO KNOW AND DO

Key Clinical Information

- History (any predisposing conditions, e.g., HTN)
- Medications, drugs (prescription, street)

Initial Imaging Survey = NECT ± CTA

Report

- Hematoma size
  - ABC/2 (width x length x height/2)
- Location
- Is there IVH, hydrocephalus?
- Edema, mass effect (herniations, etc.)

Solitary lesions comprise the vast majority of pICHs. The presence of more than one simultaneous *macroscopic* brain bleed is actually quite uncommon, accounting for just 2-3% of all pICHs. Multifocal brain *microbleeds* are much more common. We therefore conclude this chapter with a discussion of multifocal brain microbleeds, their etiology, pathology, imaging appearance, and differential diagnosis.

Evolution of Intracranial Hemorrhage

Pathophysiology of Intracranial Hemorrhage

Clot Formation

Clot formation is a complex physiologic event that involves both cellular (mainly platelet) and soluble protein components. Platelets are activated by vascular injury and aggregate at the injured site. Soluble proteins are activated by both intrinsic and extrinsic arms that merge into a common coagulation pathway, resulting in a fibrin clot.

Hemoglobin Degradation

Hemoglobin (Hgb) is composed of four protein (globin) subunits. Each subunit contains a heme molecule with an iron atom surrounded by a porphyrin ring.

Hgb within red blood cells (RBCs) that are extravasating into a pICH rapidly desaturates. Fully oxygenated Hgb (oxy-Hgb) contains nonparamagnetic ferrous iron. In a hematoma, oxy-Hgb is initially converted to deoxyhemoglobin (deoxy-Hgb).

With time, deoxy-Hgb is metabolized to methemoglobin (met-Hgb), which contains ferric iron. As RBCs lyse, met-Hgb is released and eventually degraded and resorbed. Macrophages convert the ferric iron into hemosiderin and ferritin.

Ferritin is the major source of nonheme iron deposition in the human brain. Although iron is essential for normal brain function, iron overload may have devastating effects. Lipid peroxidation and free radical formation promote oxidative brain injury after ICH that may continue for weeks or months.

Stages of Intraparenchymal Hemorrhage

Five general stages in temporal evolution of hematomas are recognized: Hyperacute, acute, early subacute, late subacute, and chronic. Each has its own features that depend on three key factors: (1) Clot structure, (2) RBC integrity, and (3) Hgb oxygenation status. In turn, imaging findings depend on hematoma stage **(5-1)**.

Hematomas consist of two distinct regions: A central core and a peripheral rim or boundary. In general, Hgb degradation begins in the clot periphery and progresses centrally toward the core.

Hyperacute Hemorrhage. Hyperacute hemorrhage is minutes (or even seconds) to under 24 hours old. Most imaged hyperacute hemorrhages are generally between four and six, but < 24, hours old. Initially, a loose fibrin clot that contains plasma, platelets, and intact RBCs is formed. At this stage, diamagnetic intracellular oxyhemoglobin predominates in the hematoma.

In early clots, intact erythrocytes interdigitate with surrounding brain at the hematoma-tissue interface. Edema forms around the hematoma within hours after onset and is associated with mass effect, elevated intracranial pressure, and secondary brain injury.

Acute Hemorrhage. Acute ICH is defined as between one and three days old. Profound hypoxia within the center of the clot induces the transformation of oxy-Hgb to deoxy-Hgb. Iron in deoxy-Hgb is paramagnetic because it has four unpaired electrons.

Deoxyhemoglobin is paramagnetic, but, as long as it remains within intact red cells, it is shielded from direct dipole-dipole interactions with water protons in the extracellular plasma. At this stage, magnetic susceptibility is induced primarily because of differences between the microenvironments inside and outside of the RBCs.

Early Subacute Hemorrhage. Early subacute hemorrhage is defined as a clot that is from three days to one week old. Hgb remains contained within intact RBCs. Hgb at the hypoxic center of the clot persists as deoxy-Hgb. The periphery of the clot ages more rapidly and therefore contains intracellular met-Hgb. Intracellular met-Hgb is highly paramagnetic, but the intact RBC membrane prevents direct dipole-dipole interactions.

Imaging the Stages of Intraparenchymal Hemorrhage

Stage	Time (Range)	Blood Products	CT	T1	T2	T2*	DWI	ADC
Hyperacute	< 24 hours	Oxy-Hgb	Hyperdense	Isointense	Bright	Rim "blooms"	Bright	Dark
Acute	1-3 days	Deoxy-Hgb	Hyperdense	Isointense	Dark	↑ "blooming"	Dark	Dark
Early subacute	> 3 days to 1 week	Intracellular met-Hgb	Isodense	Bright	Dark	Very dark	Dark	Dark
Late subacute	1 week to months	Extracellular met-Hgb	Hypodense	Bright	Bright	Dark rim, variable center	Bright	Dark
Chronic	> 14 days (≥ months)	Hemosiderin	Hypodense	Dark	Dark	Dark	Dark	Dark

(Table 5-1) *Deoxy-Hgb = deoxyhemoglobin; met-Hgb = methemoglobin; oxy-Hgb = oxygenated hemoglobin.*

A cellular perihematomal inflammatory response develops. Microglial activation occurs as immune cells infiltrate the parenchyma surrounding the clot.

Late Subacute Hemorrhage. Late subacute hemorrhage lasts from one to several weeks. As RBCs lyse, met-Hgb becomes extracellular. Met-Hgb is now exposed directly to plasma water, reducing T1 relaxation time and prolonging the T2 relaxation time.

Chronic Hemorrhage. Parenchymal hemorrhagic residua persist for months to years. Heme proteins are phagocytized and stored as ferritin in macrophages. If the capacity to store ferritin is exceeded, excess iron is stored as hemosiderin. Intracellular ferritin and hemosiderin induce strong magnetic susceptibility.

Chronic hemorrhage in the subarachnoid space typically coats the pial surface of the brain, a condition termed "superficial siderosis" (see Chapter 6). Superficial siderosis is sometimes seen adjacent to intraparenchymal hematomas, especially those associated with amyloid angiopathy (see Chapter 10).

Imaging of Intracranial Parenchymal Hemorrhage

The role of imaging in spontaneous ICH (sICH) is first to identify the presence and location of a clot (the easy part), to "age" the clot (harder), and then to detect other findings that may be clues to its etiology (the more difficult, demanding part).

The appearance of pICH on CT depends on just one factor, electron density. In turn, the electron density of a clot depends almost entirely on its protein concentration, primarily the globin moiety of Hgb. Iron and other metals contribute < 0.5% to total clot attenuation and so have no visible effect on hematoma density.

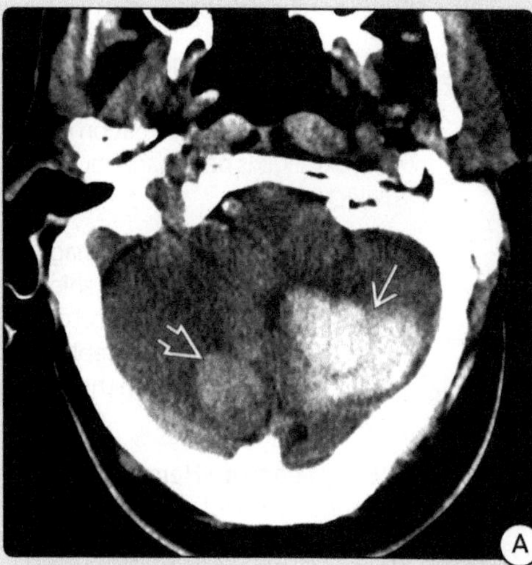

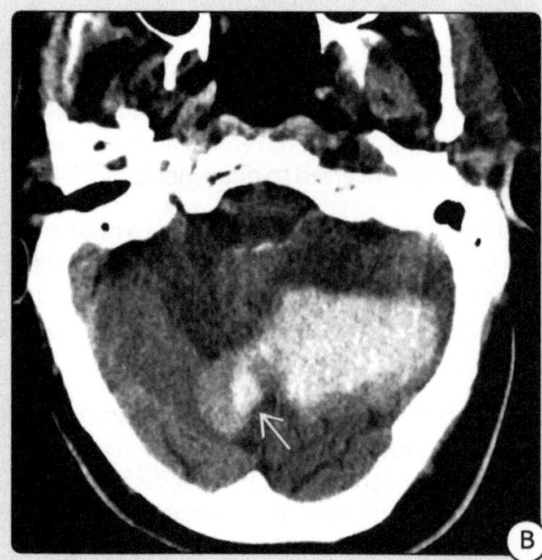

***(5-2A)** NECT in a hypertensive patient shows a large heterogeneous hematoma in the left cerebellar hemisphere ➔ and a smaller, much less hyperdense clot in the right cerebellum ➔. Findings are consistent with a hyperacute (loose, largely unretracted) clot. **(5-2B)** The patient suddenly deteriorated while still in the scanner. Repeat NECT scan now shows additional hemorrhage ➔. The patient died shortly after this scan was performed.*

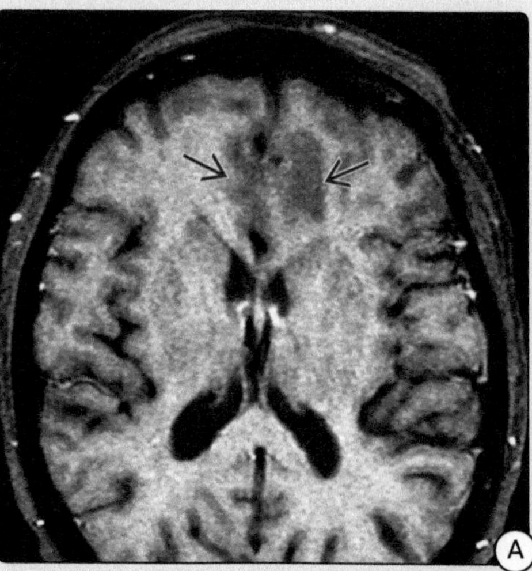

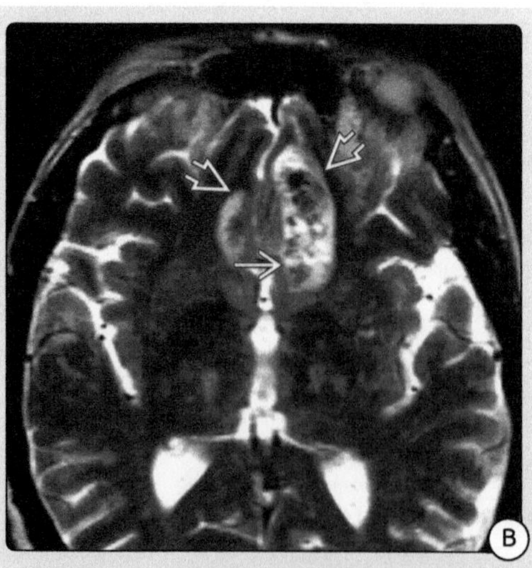

***(5-3A)** Patient is shown with acute myelogenous leukemia, acute visual symptoms. Emergent NECT scan showed no abnormalities. Sudden deterioration prompted MR. T1WI obtained within minutes shows an ill-defined bifrontal mass ➔ that appears isointense with gray matter. **(5-3B)** T2WI obtained 5 minutes later shows a mixed-signal mass ➔ with fluid-fluid levels ➔. This is rapid hyperacute hemorrhage. (Courtesy M. Brant-Zawadzki, MD.)*

In contrast, the imaging appearance of ICH on MR is more complex and depends on a number of factors. Both intrinsic and extrinsic factors contribute to imaging appearance.

Intrinsic biologic factors that influence hematoma signal intensity are primarily related to macroscopic clot structure, RBC integrity, and Hgb oxygenation status. RBC concentration, tissue pH, arterial vs. venous source of the bleed, intracellular protein concentration, and the presence and integrity of the blood-brain barrier also contribute to the imaging appearance of an ICH.

Extrinsic factors include pulse sequence, sequence parameters, receiver bandwidth, and field strength of the magnet. Of these, pulse sequence and field strength are the most important determinants. T1- and T2-weighted images are the most helpful in estimating lesion age. T2* (GRE, SWI) is the most sensitive sequence in detecting parenchymal hemorrhages (especially microhemorrhages).

Field strength also affects imaging appearance of ICH. The MR findings delineated below and in the table **(Table 5-1)** are calculated for 1.5T scanners. At 3.0T, all parts of acute and early subacute clots have significantly increased hypointensity on FLAIR and T2WI.

Hyperacute Hemorrhage

CT. If ICH is imaged within a few minutes of the ictus, the clot is loose, poorly organized, and largely unretracted **(5-2)**. Water content is still high, so a hyperacute hematoma may appear isodense or occasionally even hypodense relative to adjacent brain. If active hemorrhage is present, the presence of both clotted and unclotted blood results in a mixed-density hematoma with hypodense and mildly hyperdense components. Rapid bleeding and coagulopathy may result in fluid-fluid levels.

MR. Oxy-Hgb has no unpaired electrons and is diamagnetic. Therefore, signal intensity of a hyperacute clot depends

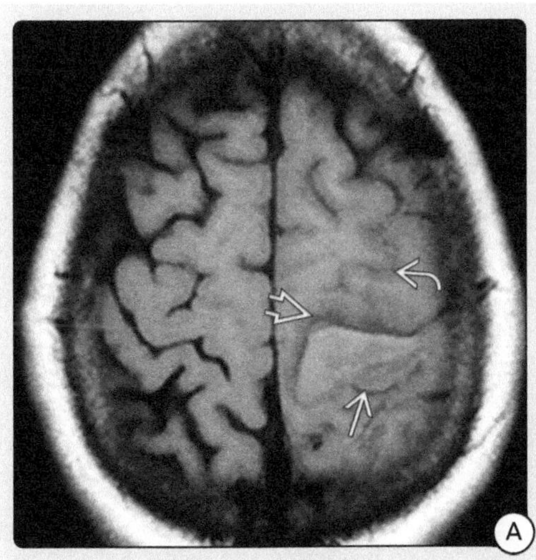

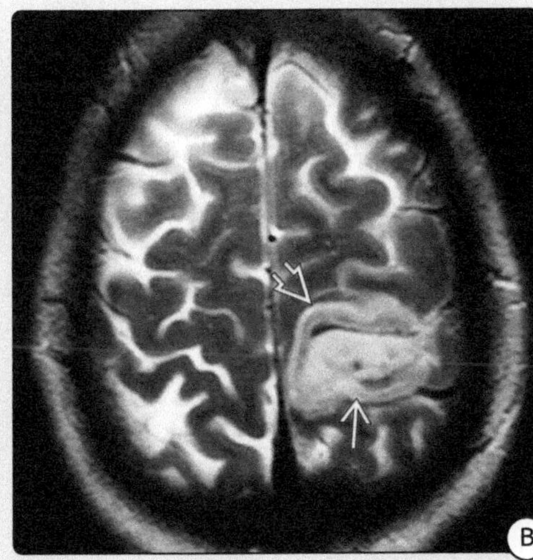

***(5-4A)** MR in a normotensive patient with acute spontaneous intracranial hemorrhage (sICH) on NECT is shown. T1WI shows acute hematoma is intermediate in SI ➡, surrounded by a rim of hypointense vasogenic edema ➡. Adjacent sulcal effacement ➡ may be from subarachnoid hemorrhage (SAH). **(5-4B)** Clot is heterogeneously hyperintense on T2WI ➡. Note vasogenic edema ➡. "Dirty" CSF probably represents SAH.*

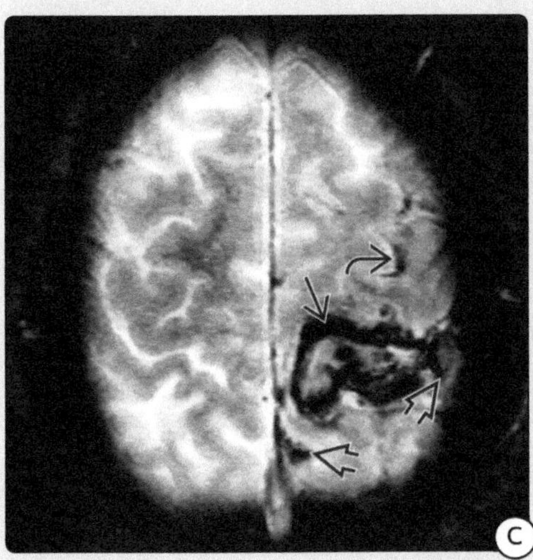

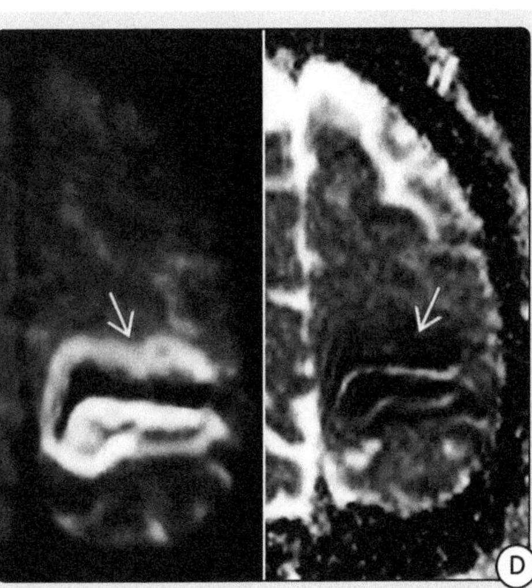

***(5-4C)** T2* GRE scan shows "blooming" around the periphery of the clot ➡ and in the sulci ➡. Tubular hypointensity in adjacent cortical veins ➡ suggests venous thrombosis. **(5-4D)** DWI (L) and ADC map (R) in the same case show restricted diffusion in the layered, heterogeneous acute hematoma ➡.*

mostly on its water content. Hyperacute clots are isointense to slightly hypointense to gray matter on T1WI **(5-3A)**. A hyperacute clot is generally hyperintense on T2 scans, although they can appear quite heterogeneous **(5-3B)**.

Because the macroscopic structure of a hyperacute clot is so inhomogeneous, spin dephasing results in heterogeneous hypointensity ("blooming") on T2* sequences.

Acute Hemorrhage

CT. The hematocrit of a retracted clot approaches 90%. Therefore, an acute hematoma is usually hyperdense on NECT, typically measuring 60-80 HU. Exceptions to this general rule are found if hemorrhage occurs in extremely anemic patients with very low hematocrits or in patients with coagulopathies.

MR. Acute hematomas are low/intermediate signal intensity on T1WI **(5-4A)**. Significant vasogenic edema develops around the clot and is T1 hypointense and T2/FLAIR hyperintense **(5-4B)**. As the clot retracts, water content diminishes. Intracellular deoxyhemoglobin predominates. Deoxyhemoglobin is paramagnetic with four unpaired electrons, and the hematoma becomes more profoundly hypointense on T2WI. Acute hematomas "bloom" on T2* (GRE, SWI) **(5-4C)**. Diffusion restriction is present on DWI and ADC, although the presence of T2 and susceptibility effects can combine to produce a complex appearance in and around acute hematomas **(5-4D)**.

Early Subacute Hemorrhage

CT. Hematoma density gradually decreases with time, beginning with the periphery of the clot. Clot attenuation diminishes by an average of 1.5 HU per day **(5-6)**. At around 7-10 days, the outside of a pICH becomes isodense with the adjacent brain **(5-7B)**. The hyperdense center gradually shrinks, becoming less and less dense until the entire clot

(5-5A) Axial T1 (L) and T2 (R) MR scans in a patient with a 3-day-old left basal ganglionic hematoma are shown. The clot is largely isointense with brain on T1WI ➡ and profoundly hypointense on T2WI ➡. Some T1 shortening ➡ is beginning to appear in this late acute/early subacute hematoma. (5-5B) DTI DWI (L) and ADC (R) in the same case show "T2 blackout" ➡, which is surrounded by a hyperintense rim of "T2 shine-through" ➡.

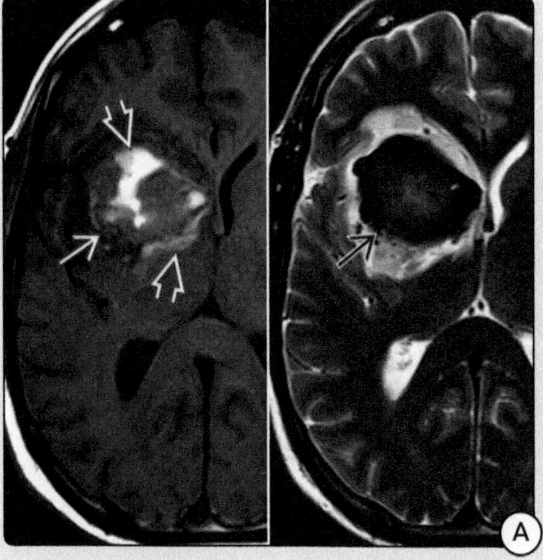

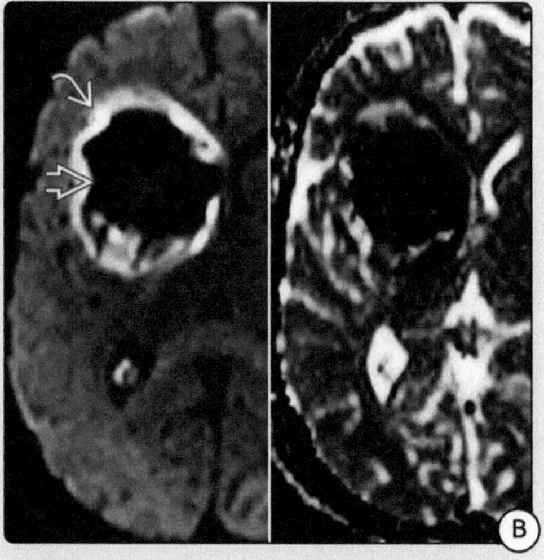

(5-5C) Axial T1 (L) and T2 (R) 3 months later in the same case shows the hematoma is composed mostly of "bright" extracellular dilute-free met-Hgb. Note hypointense rim (hemosiderin/ferritin) ➡ and some isointense clot ➡ remaining in the center of the hematoma. (5-5D) DWI (L), ADC map (R) show that the T2 effect dominates in the DWI, while the ADC is dark, indicating true diffusion restriction in the chronic hematoma.

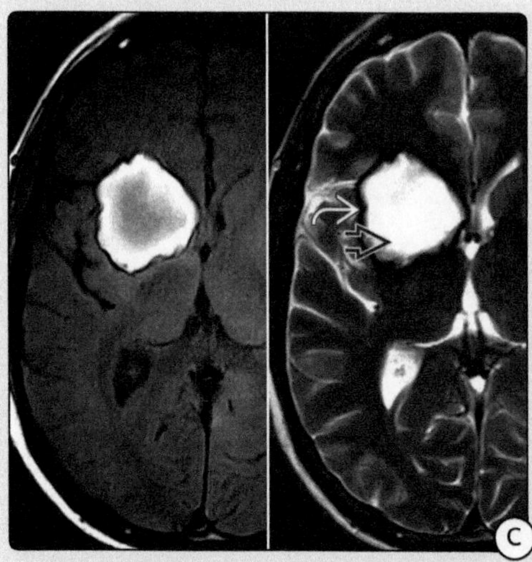

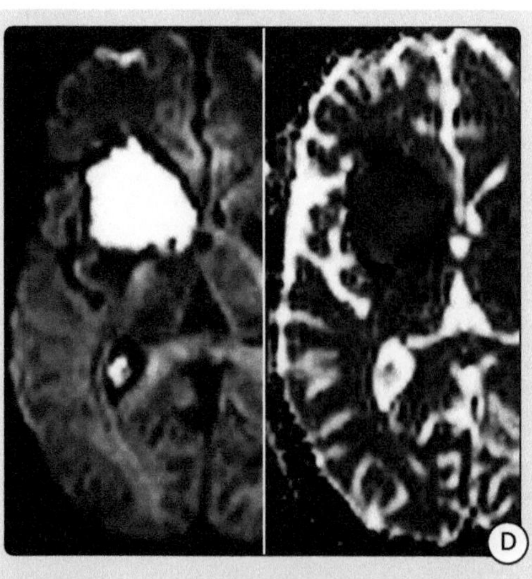

becomes hypodense. A subacute hematoma shows ring enhancement on CECT.

MR. Intracellular methemoglobin predominates around the clot periphery, whereas deoxyhemoglobin persists within the hematoma core. A rim of T1 shortening (hyperintensity) surrounding an isointense to slightly hypointense core is the typical appearance on T1WI **(5-7C)**. Paramagnetic methemoglobin is not very mobile and causes pronounced T2 shortening so early subacute clots are hypointense on T2WI. Profound hypointensity on T2* persists.

Clot appearance on diffusion-weighted imaging (DWI) varies. For many forms of hemorrhage, the T2/T2* effect comprises the dominant contribution to signal intensity and therefore appears markedly hypointense (T2 "blackout effect"). In acute and subacute hemorrhage, true restricted diffusion occurs with the intrinsically long T2 of these hematomas **(5-5D)**. The diffusion signal of hemorrhage at each stage of evolution is summarized in the table **(Table 5-1)**.

Late Subacute Hemorrhage

CT. With progressive aging, a pICH gradually becomes hypodense relative to adjacent brain on NECT scans. Ring enhancement may persist for weeks or up to two or three months.

MR. Once cell lysis occurs, mobile free dilute extracellular methemoglobin predominates in determining signal intensity. Clots develop hyperintensity around their rim on both T1WI and T2WI **(5-5C)**. Eventually, the clot appears very hyperintense on both sequences. A rim of T2* blooming generally persists. With the exception of minor susceptibility artifacts, late subacute clots appear similar on both 1.5T and 3.0T.

Chronic Hemorrhage

CT. A few very small healed hemorrhages may become invisible on NECT scan. From 35-40% of chronic hematomas

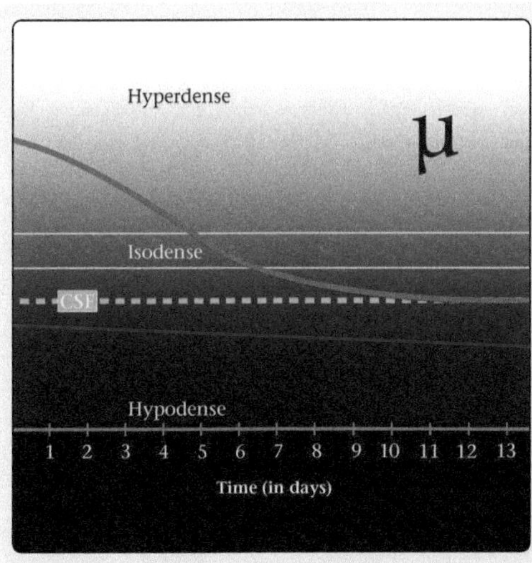

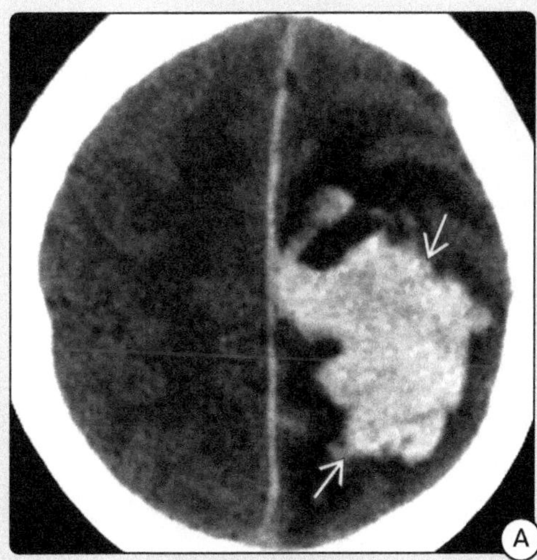

***(5-6)** Graphic depicts time-related progressive decrease in density of brain hematoma relative to parenchyma. Clots are initially hyperdense, become isodense between a few days to a week or so, and then are hypodense. Eventually, a resolving clot becomes nearly isodense with CSF. **(5-7A)** Axial NECT scan in a patient with an acute lobar hypertensive hemorrhage shows relatively uniform hyperdense clot in the left parietal lobe ➡.*

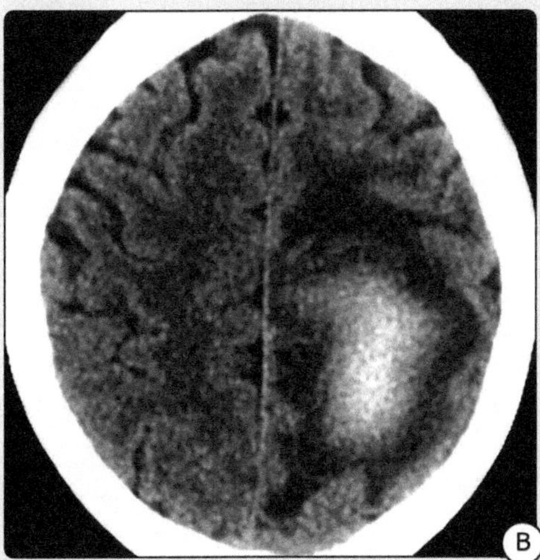

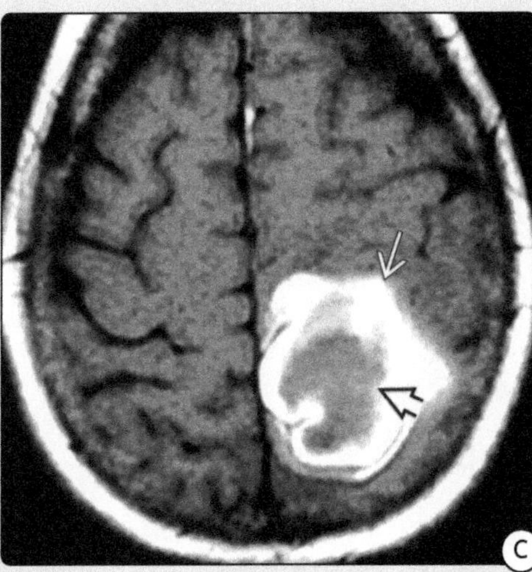

***(5-7B)** Follow-up NECT scan was obtained 1 week later. Clot density has decreased with a gradation from hyperdense in the center to isodense to hypodense at the periphery. **(5-7C)** MR scan was obtained immediately after the follow-up CT scan. T1WI shows that the subacute hematoma is hyperintense around the rim ➡ and nearly isointense in the center ⇨.*

appear as a round or ovoid hypodense focus. Another 25% of patients develop slit-like hypodensities. Between 10-15% of healed hematomas calcify.

MR. Intracellular ferritin and hemosiderin are hypointense on both T1WI and T2WI. A hyperintense cavity surrounded by a "blooming" rim on T2* may persist for months or even years **(5-9)**. Eventually, only a slit-like scar remains as evidence of a prior parenchymal hemorrhage **(5-8)**.

Etiology of Nontraumatic Parenchymal Hemorrhages

There are many causes of nontraumatic ("spontaneous") or unexplained ICH. The role of imaging in such cases is to localize the hematoma, estimate its age from its imaging features, and attempt to identify possible underlying causes.

The effect of age on the pathoetiology of sICH is profound. Knowing the patient's age is extremely important in establishing an appropriately narrowed differential diagnosis.

It can be difficult to discern enhancement within an already hyperdense acute hematoma on CECT scans. Dual-energy CT (DECT) can display the presence of contrast enhancement, potentially helping distinguish between tumor bleeding and nonneoplastic ("pure") hemorrhage. DECT can also help differentiate ICH from extravasated contrast material staining.

MR imaging with standard sequences as well as fat-saturated contrast-enhanced scans can be very helpful. A T2* sequence (GRE &/or SWI) should always be included, as the identification of other prior "silent" microhemorrhages affects both diagnosis and treatment decisions.

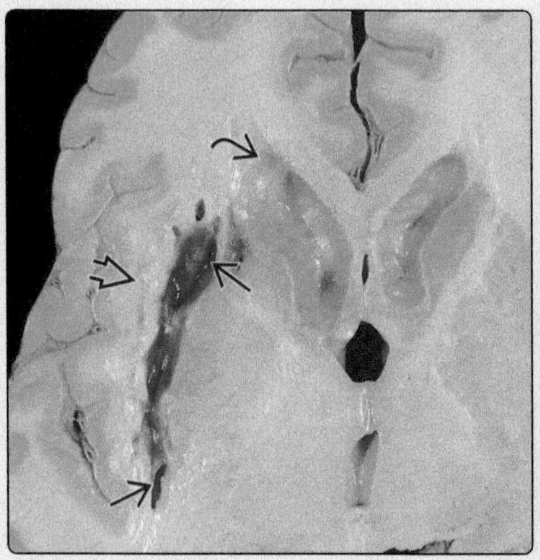

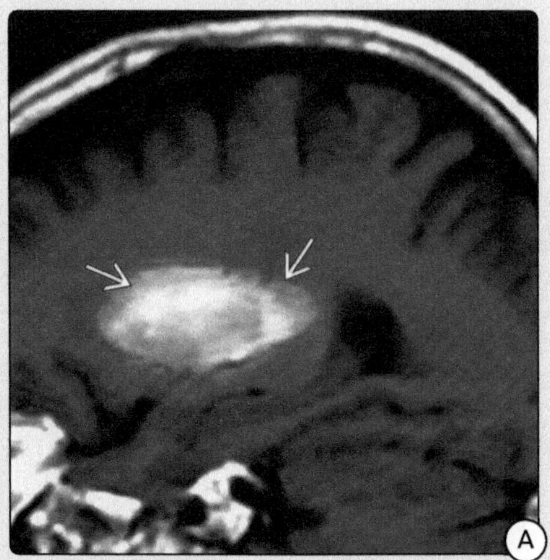

***(5-8)** Gross autopsy case shows residua of remote striatocapsular hemorrhage. A slit-like cavity with a small amount of yellowish fluid is surrounded by dark hemosiderin staining →. Note volume loss with enlarged right frontal horn →, gliotic brain → surrounding old hematoma. (Courtesy R. Hewlett, MD.) **(5-9A)** Sagittal T1WI in a patient 2 years following hypertensive hemorrhage shows ovoid hyperintense cavity →.*

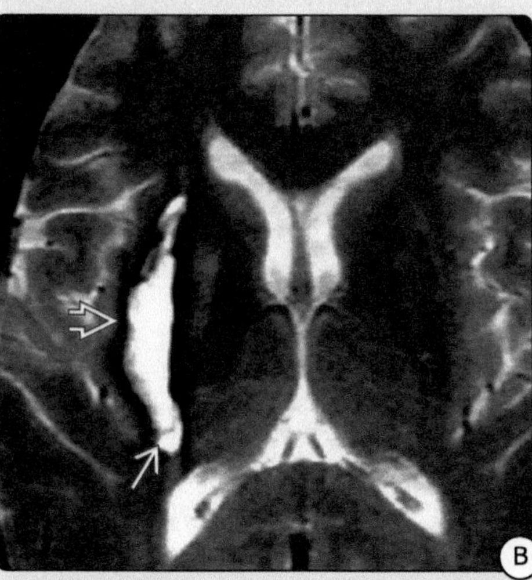

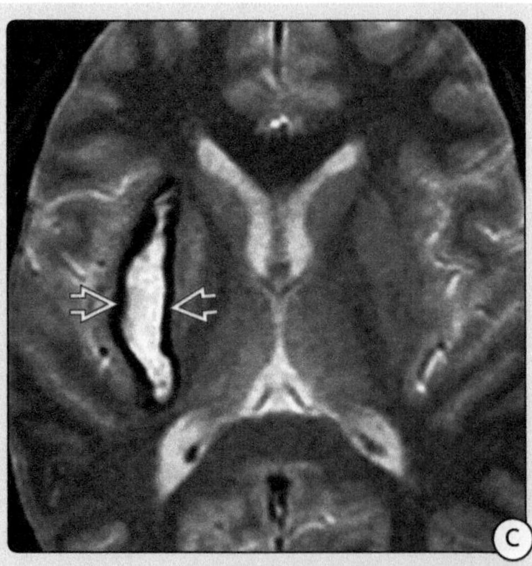

***(5-9B)** Axial standard (not FSE) T2WI shows that the cavity → contains hyperintense fluid (dilute-free extracellular met-Hgb) and is surrounded by a hypointense rim of hemosiderin/ferritin →. **(5-9C)** T2* GRE shows "blooming" → around the rim of the residual cavity. Findings are classic for chronic parenchymal hematoma.*

Newborns and Infants With sICH

ICH in the term newborn is most frequently associated with prolonged or precipitous delivery, traumatic instrumented delivery (e.g., forceps assistance or vacuum extraction), and primiparity. The most common cause of ICH in infants < 34 gestational weeks is **germinal matrix hemorrhage** **(5-10)** **(5-11)**.

The germinal matrix is a highly vascular, developmentally dynamic structure in the brain subventricular zone. The germinal matrix contains multiple cell types, including premigratory/migratory neurons, glia, and neural stem cells. Rupture of the relatively fragile germinal matrix capillaries may occur in response to altered cerebral blood flow, increased venous pressure (e.g., with delivery), coagulopathy, or hypoxic-ischemic injury. Germinal matrix hemorrhage is discussed in greater detail later (Chapter 8).

Isolated choroid plexus and **isolated intraventricular hemorrhage (IVH)** do not involve the germinal matrix. **White matter injury of prematurity** generally does not show evidence of hemorrhage ("blooming") on T2* imaging.

The most common nontraumatic cause of spontaneous IVH in *neonates beyond 34 gestational weeks* is **dural venous sinus thrombosis** (DVST) **(5-12)**. In contrast to older children and adults in whom the transverse sinus is most commonly affected, the straight sinus (85%) and superior sagittal sinus (65%) are the most frequent locations in infants. Multisinus involvement is seen in 80% of cases. Thalamic and punctate white matter lesions are common in infants with DVST.

Children With sICH

The most common cause of sICH in children ages 1-18 years is an underlying **vascular malformation**. Vascular malformations are responsible for nearly 1/2 of spontaneous parenchymal hemorrhages in this age group **(5-13)**.

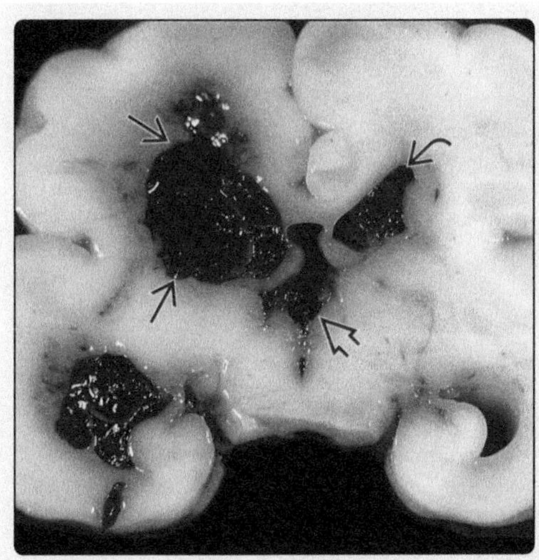

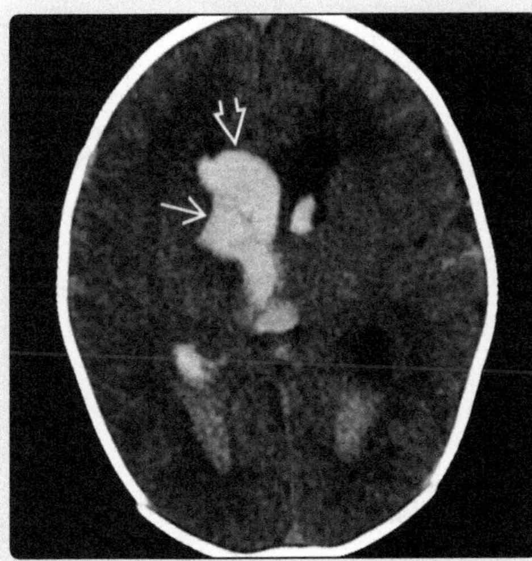

***(5-10)** Autopsied brain of a premature infant shows hemorrhage into the germinal matrix and the adjacent deep periventricular white matter (WM) ➙. Blood is also present in both lateral ➙ and 3rd ➙ ventricles. **(5-11)** NECT in a premature infant shows typical germinal matrix hemorrhage ➙ with dissection into the adjacent ventricles ➙.*

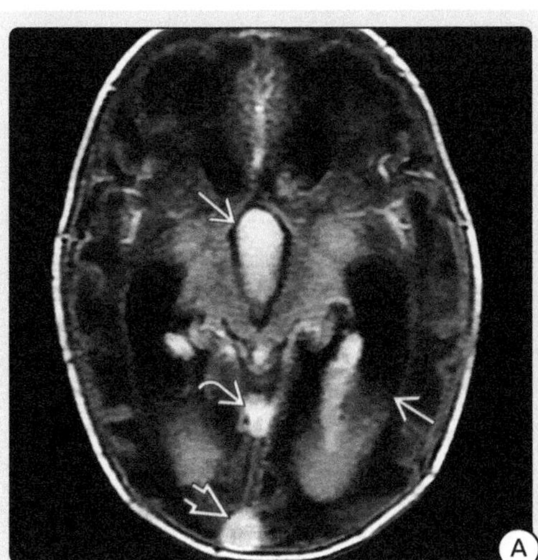

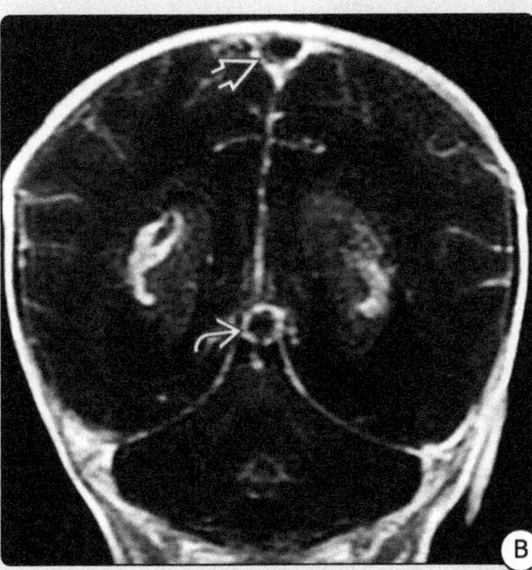

***(5-12A)** T1WI in a septic newborn infant shows blood in the 3rd/lateral ventricles ➙, thrombus in straight sinus ➙, and torcular ➙. **(5-12B)** Coronal T1 C+ MR in the same case shows thrombosis of superior sagittal ➙, straight sinuses ➙ seen here as enhancing dura around nonenhancing clot (empty delta sign).*

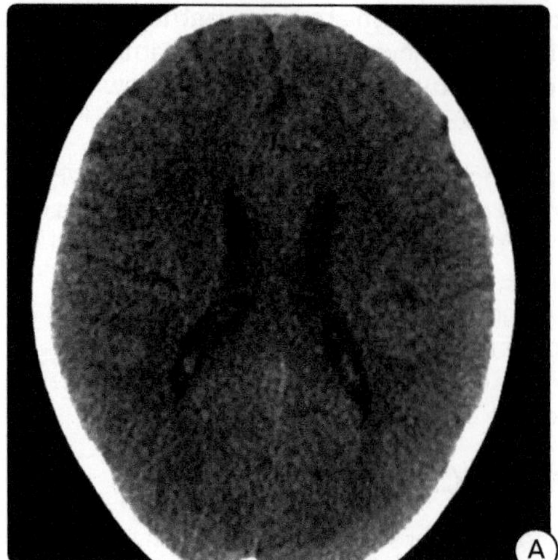

(5-13A) NECT in a child with headaches, family history of multiple cavernous malformations shows no abnormalities.

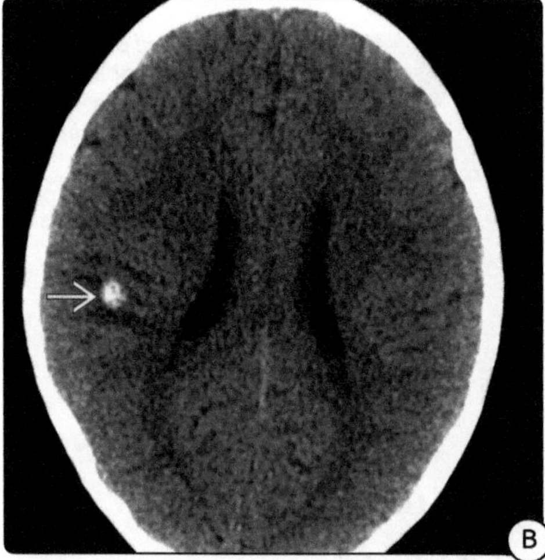

(5-13B) Follow-up scan 1 year later shows a small, solitary, calcified lesion in the right cerebral hemisphere ➡.

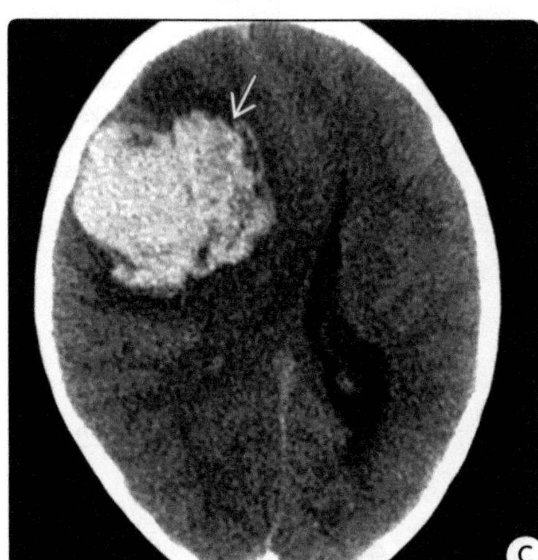

(5-13C) Several weeks later, the child had a severe headache, left-sided weakness, and bleeding into the cavernous malformation ➡.

At least 25% of all arteriovenous malformations hemorrhage by the age of 15 years. Cavernous malformations, especially familial cavernous malformations ("cavernomas"), are a less common but important cause of sICH in children.

Other less common but important causes of pediatric sICH include **hematologic disorders** and **malignancies**, **vasculopathy**, and **venous occlusion/infarction**.

Primary neoplasms are a relatively rare cause of sICH in children **(5-14)**. Infratentorial tumors are more common than supratentorial neoplasms.

Posterior fossa neoplasms that frequently hemorrhage include ependymoma and rosette-forming glioneuronal tumor. Patchy or petechial hemorrhage is more common than large intratumoral bleeds.

Supratentorial tumors with a propensity to bleed include ependymoma and the spectrum of primitive neuroectodermal tumors. Malignant astrocytomas with hemorrhage occur but are rare. In contrast to middle-aged and older adults, hemorrhagic metastases from extracranial primary cancers are *very* rare in children.

sICH IN INFANTS AND CHILDREN

Newborns and Infants
- Common
  - Germinal matrix hemorrhage (< 34 gestational weeks)
  - DVST (≥ 34 gestational weeks)
- Rare
  - Congenital prothrombotic disorder
  - Thrombocytopenia
  - Hemophilia
  - Vitamin K deficiency bleeding
  - Neoplasm

Children
- Common
  - Vascular malformation: ~ 50%
- Less common
  - Hematologic disorder
  - Vasculopathy
  - Dural venous sinus or cortical vein thrombosis
- Rare but important
  - Neoplasm (primary)
  - Drug abuse

Young Adults With sICH

An underlying **vascular malformation** is the most common cause of sICH in young adults as well **(5-15)**. **Drug abuse** is the second most common cause of unexplained hemorrhage **(5-16)**. Cocaine and methamphetamine may induce extreme systemic HTN, resulting in a putaminal-external capsule bleed that looks identical to those seen in older hypertensive adults.

Vasculitis and **reversible cerebral vasoconstriction syndrome** (RCVS) occasionally cause pICH in young adults **(5-17)**.

Venous occlusion/infarction with or without **dural sinus occlusion** is also relatively common in this age group, especially in young women taking oral contraceptives. Severe **eclampsia/preeclampsia** with posterior reversible encephalopathy syndrome (PRES) may cause multifocal posterior cortical and subcortical hemorrhages **(5-19)**. Hemorrhagic neoplasms (both primary and metastatic) are rare.

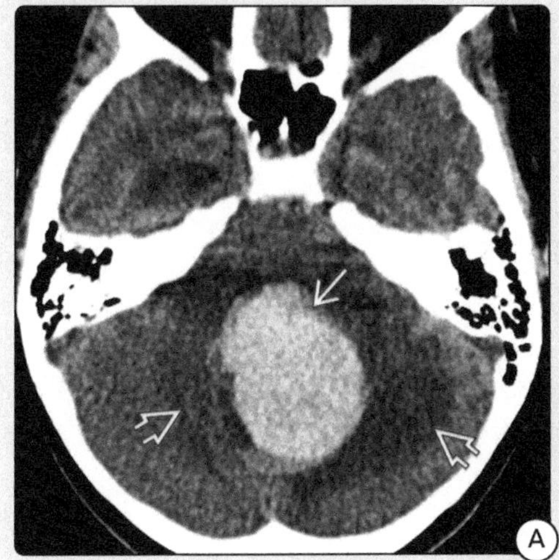

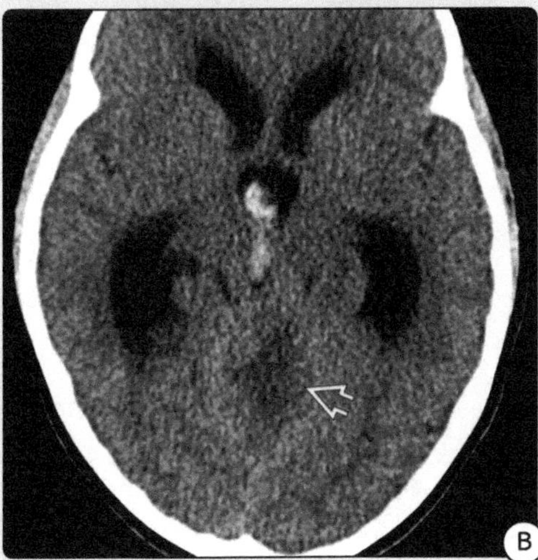

***(5-14A)** Axial NECT in a 10-year-old child with morning nausea and vomiting and sudden onset of severe headache shows a large posterior fossa midline hemorrhage ➡ that involves the 4th ventricle/vermis. Edema is seen in both cerebellar hemispheres ➡. **(5-14B)** More cephalad scan shows upward herniation of the edematous cerebellum ➡ and acute obstructive hydrocephalus. Hemorrhagic pilocytic astrocytoma was found at surgery.*

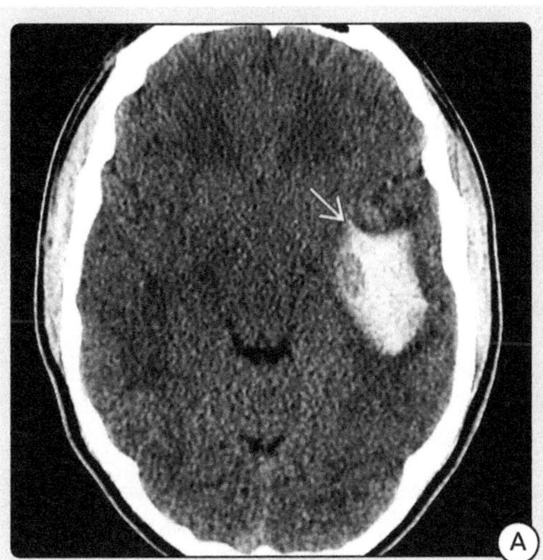

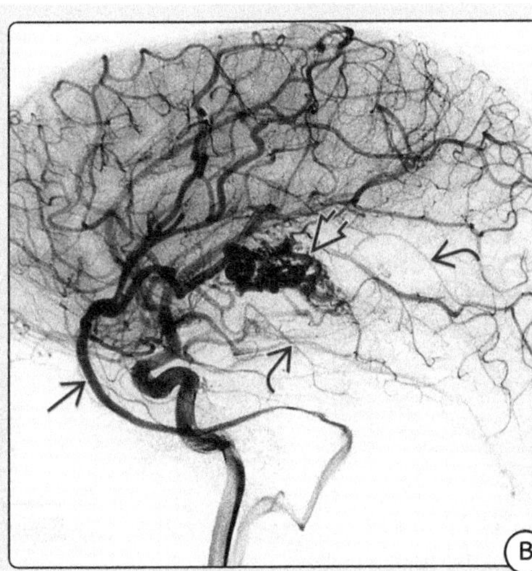

***(5-15A)** NECT in a 15-year-old boy with sudden-onset severe headache and right-sided weakness shows an acute left anterior temporal hematoma ➡. **(5-15B)** Lateral view of the internal carotid angiogram in the same case shows a partially thrombosed arteriovenous malformation ➡ with early draining superficial middle cerebral vein ➡. Most of the avascular mass effect ➡ is from the hematoma.*

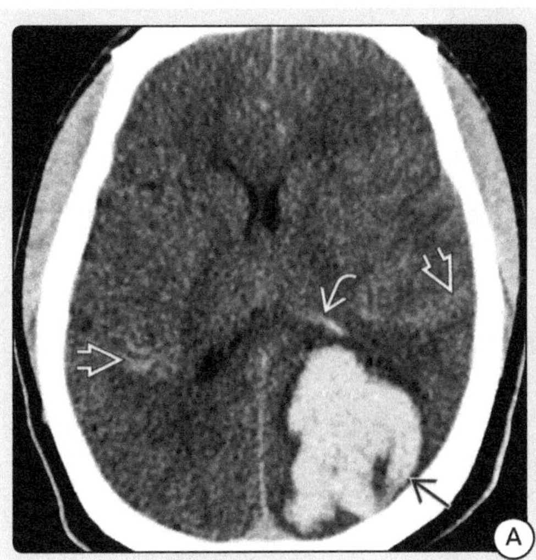

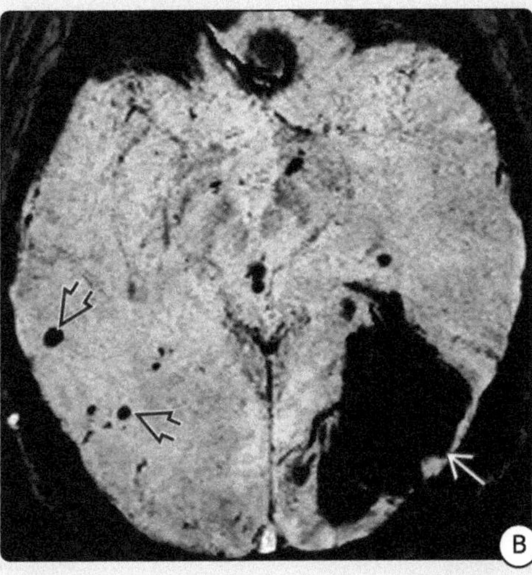

***(5-16A)** NECT in a 33-year-old man with methamphetamine abuse shows a spontaneous left occipital lobe hemorrhage ➡. Note the small amount of intraventricular ➡, subarachnoid ➡ hemorrhage. **(5-16B)** T2* SWI MIP shows the lobar hemorrhage ➡ as well as several small microbleeds ➡. Multiple cavernous malformations were "unmasked" by the drug abuse.*

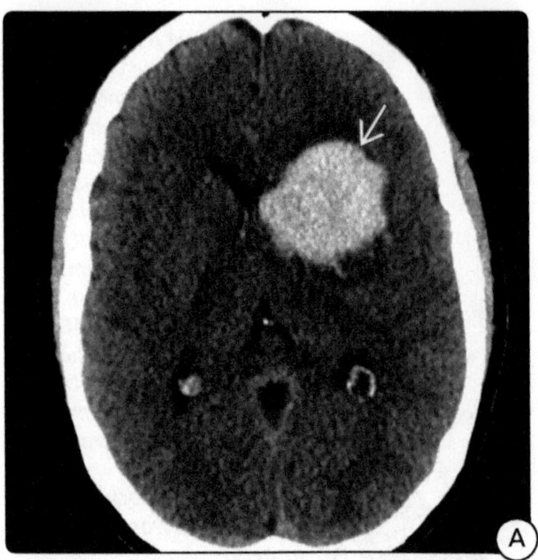

***(5-17A)** NECT in a 37y normotensive man with R-sided weakness shows a left basal ganglionic hemorrhage ➡. Drug screen was negative.*

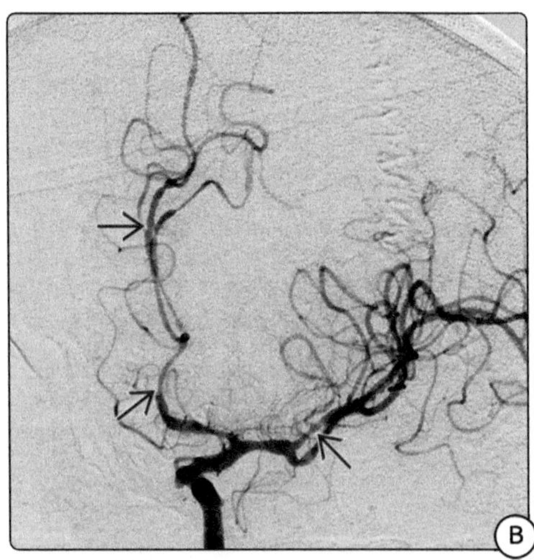

***(5-17B)** Oblique coronal DSA shows multiple areas of arterial dilatations, constrictions in the left ACA, MCA ➡. Initial diagnosis was vasculitis.*

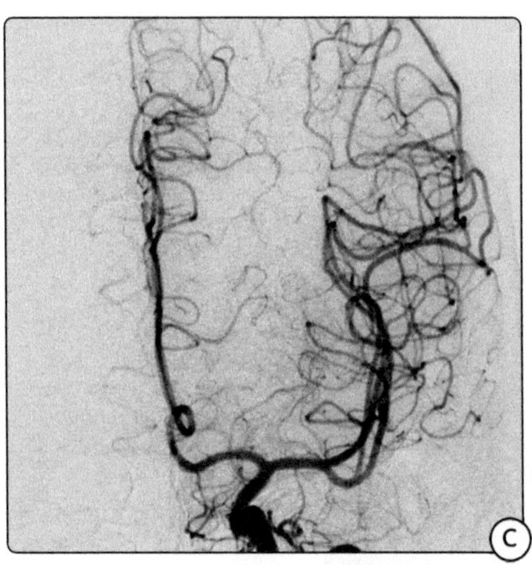

***(5-17C)** Repeat DSA 3 months later is normal. Final diagnosis was reversible cerebral vasoconstriction syndrome (RCVS).*

sICH IN YOUNG AND MIDDLE-AGED ADULTS

Young Adults

- Common
  - Vascular malformation
  - Drug abuse
- Less common
  - Venous occlusion
  - PRES
- Rare but important
  - Vasculitis
  - RCVS
  - Neoplasm

Middle-Aged Adults

- Common
  - HTN
  - Neoplasm (primary or metastatic)
- Less common
  - Dural sinus or cortical vein occlusion
  - Drug abuse
- Rare but important
  - Vascular malformation
  - Vasculitis
  - RCVS
  - Acute hemorrhagic leukoencephalopathy

Middle-Aged and Elderly Adults With sICH

The two most common causes of sICH in middle-aged and elderly patients are HTN and **amyloid angiopathy**, both of which are discussed in detail below. Approximately 10% of spontaneous parenchymal hemorrhages are caused by bleeding into a brain **neoplasm**, generally either a high-grade primary tumor, such as glioblastoma multiforme, or hemorrhagic metastasis from an extracranial primary, such as renal cell carcinoma **(5-20)**.

A less common but important cause of sICH in this age group is **venous infarct**. Venous infarcts are caused by cortical vein thrombosis with or without dural sinus occlusion. Iatrogenic **coagulopathy** is also common in elderly patients, as many take maintenance doses of warfarin for atrial fibrillation.

Occasionally, a ruptured **saccular aneurysm** presents with a focal lobar hemorrhage rather than a subarachnoid hemorrhage. The most common source is an anterior communicating artery aneurysm that projects superolaterally and ruptures into the frontal lobe.

Underlying **vascular malformation** is a relatively rare cause of sICH in older patients. With a 2-4% per year cumulative rupture risk, a first-time arteriovenous malformation bleed at this age can occur but is unusual (so is hemorrhage from a cavernous malformation). However, **dural arteriovenous fistulas (dAVFs)** *do* occur in middle-aged and elderly patients. Although dAVFs rarely hemorrhage unless they have cortical venous (not just dural sinus) drainage, spontaneous thrombosis of the outlet veins may result in sudden ICH.

Rare but important causes of sICH in this age group include **vasculitis** (more common in younger patients) and **acute hemorrhagic leukoencephalopathy**.

sICH IN OLDER ADULTS

Older Adults

- Common
  - HTN
  - Amyloid angiopathy
  - Neoplasm (primary or metastatic)
- Less common
  - Dural sinus or cortical vein occlusion
  - Coagulopathy
- Rare but important
  - Vascular malformation (usually dAVF)

Multiple sICHs

Solitary spontaneous parenchymal hemorrhages are much more common than multifocal bleeds. Etiology varies with patient age.

Multifocal brain bleeds that occur at all ages include venous thrombosis, PRES **(5-19)**, vasculitis (especially fungal), septic emboli, thrombotic microangiopathy, and acute hemorrhagic leukoencephalopathy.

Multiple *nontraumatic* brain bleeds in children and young adults are most often caused by multiple cavernous malformations and hematologic disorders (e.g., leukemia, thrombocytopenia).

The most common causes of multiple ICHs in middle-aged and older adults are HTN, amyloid angiopathy, hemorrhagic metastases **(5-20)**, and impaired coagulation (either coagulopathy or anticoagulation).

MULTIPLE SPONTANEOUS ICHs

Children and Young Adults

- Multiple cavernous malformations
- Hematologic disorder/malignancy

Middle-Aged and Older Adults

- Common
  - Chronic HTN
  - Amyloid angiopathy
- Less common
  - Hemorrhagic metastases
  - Coagulopathy, anticoagulation

All Ages

- Common
  - Dural sinus thrombosis
  - Cortical vein occlusion
- Less common
  - PRES
  - Vasculitis
  - Septic emboli
- Rare but important
  - Thrombotic microangiopathy
  - Acute hemorrhagic leukoencephalopathy

Macrohemorrhages

The top two causes of spontaneous (nontraumatic) intraparenchymal hemorrhage in middle-aged and elderly adults are HTN and amyloid angiopathy; they account for 78-88% of all nontraumatic ICHs. Although

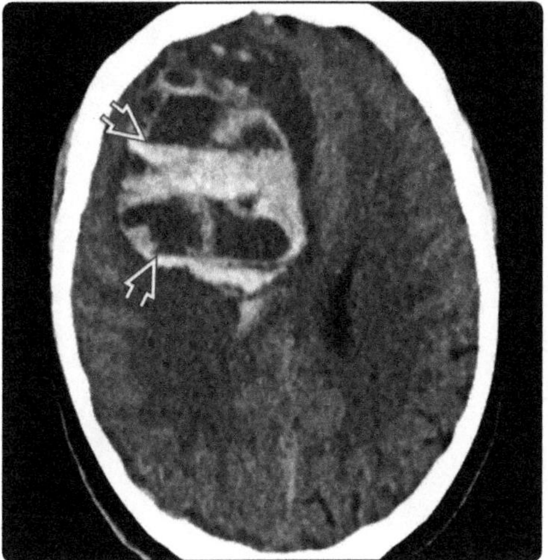

***(5-18)** NECT in an anticoagulated 72-year-old woman shows sICH with multiple blood-fluid levels ➡.*

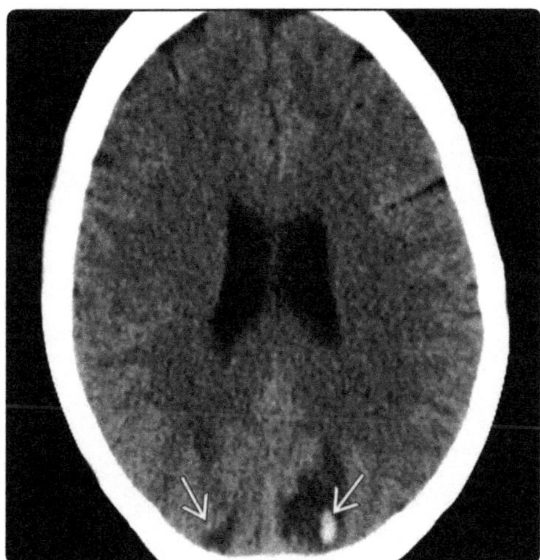

***(5-19)** A 22y eclamptic woman has occipital lesions ➡ with edema, hemorrhage; posterior reversible encephalopathy syndrome (PRES).*

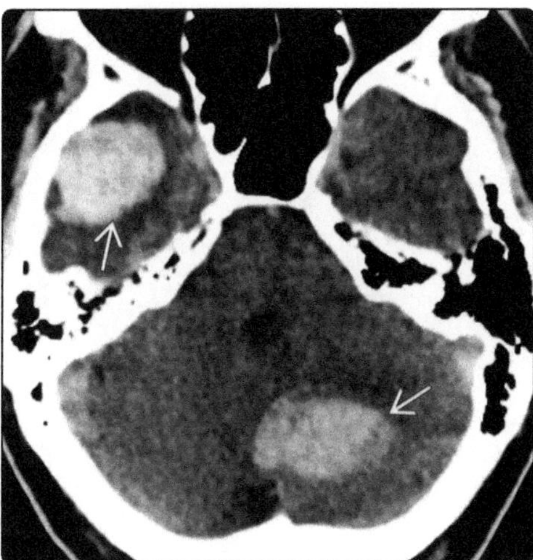

***(5-20)** Axial NECT scan in an elderly patient with known renal cell carcinoma shows multiple hemorrhagic metastases ➡.*

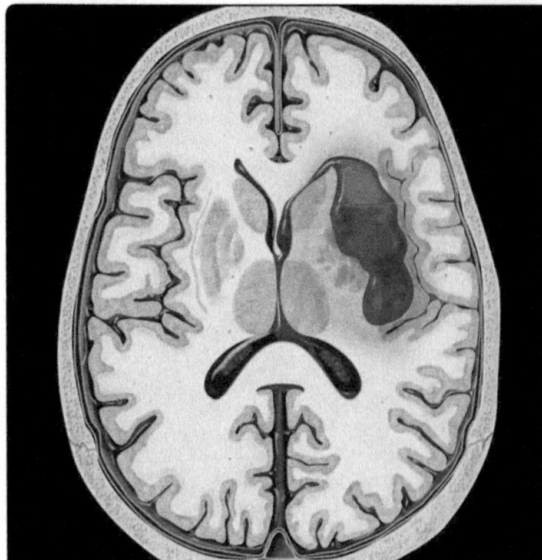

***(5-21)** Graphic depicts acute hypertensive striatocapsular hemorrhage with edema, dissection into the lateral and 3rd ventricles.*

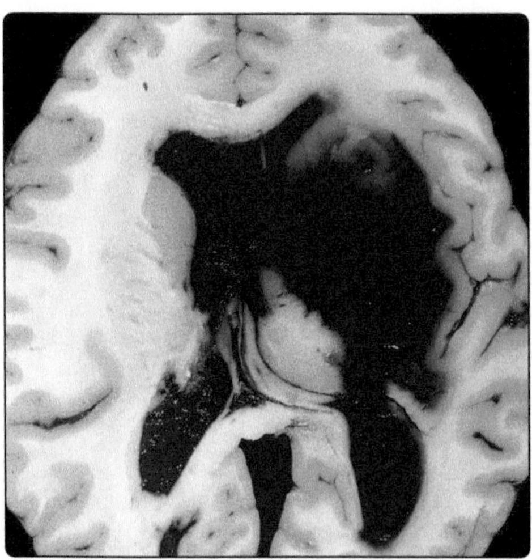

***(5-22)** Autopsy shows acute hypertensive ganglionic hemorrhage with intraventricular hemorrhage. (Courtesy R. Hewlett, MD.)*

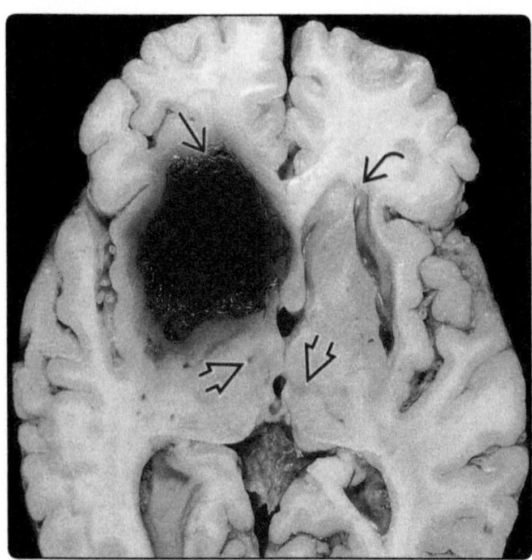

***(5-23)** Autopsy shows acute ➔ and chronic ➔ hICH, small remote thalamic microhemorrhages ➔. (Courtesy R. Hewlett, MD.)*

both can cause extensive nonhemorrhagic "microvascular" disease, their most common manifestations are gross lobar and multifocal microbleeds. We therefore discuss them here.

Hypertensive Intracranial Hemorrhage

Terminology

Hypertensive ICH (hICH) is the *acute* manifestation of nontraumatic ICH secondary to systemic HTN. *Chronic* hypertensive encephalopathy refers to the effects of longstanding HTN on the brain parenchyma and is mostly seen as subcortical white matter disease &/or multifocal microbleeds.

Etiology

HTN accelerates atherosclerosis with lipohyalinosis and fibrinoid necrosis. Penetrating branches of the proximal middle and anterior cerebral arteries, primarily the lenticulostriate arteries (LSAs), are most severely affected, possibly because of their branching angle from the parent vessels.

Progressive weakening and accelerated degeneration of the LSA wall permit formation of small pseudoaneurysms ("Charcot-Bouchard aneurysms" or "bleeding globes"). Ruptured LSA pseudoaneurysm is thought to be the genesis of most striatocapsular hypertensive hemorrhages.

Pathology

Location. The putamen/external capsule is the most common location **(5-21) (5-22)**. These so-called striatocapsular hemorrhages account for nearly 2/3 of all hICHs. The thalamus is the next most common site, responsible for 15-25% **(5-23)**. The pons and cerebellum are the third most common location and cause 10% of all hICHs. Lobar hemorrhages account for another 5-10%.

Multiple microbleeds are common in patients with chronic HTN. HTN-related microbleeds tend to cluster in the basal ganglia and cerebellum with fewer lesions in the cortex and subcortical white matter.

Size and Number. Size varies from tiny submillimeter microbleeds to large macroscopic lesions that measure several centimeters in diameter **(5-23)**. When T2* sequences are used, the majority of patients with hICH have multiple lesions.

Gross Pathology. The most common gross finding in hICH is a large ganglionic hematoma that often extends medially into the ventricles **(5-22)**. Hydrocephalus and mass effect with subfalcine herniation are common complications.

Microscopic Features. Generalized arteriosclerosis with lipohyalinosis and fibrinoid necrosis is common in patients with hICH. In some cases, small fibrosed pseudoaneurysms in the basal ganglia can be identified.

Clinical Issues

Epidemiology. Although the prevalence of hICH has declined significantly, HTN still accounts for 40-50% of spontaneous "primary" intraparenchymal hemorrhages in middle-aged and older adults. hICH is 5-10x less common than cerebral ischemia-infarction, accounting for ~ 10-15% of all strokes.

Demographics. The overall risk of cardiovascular disease—including hICH—is significantly increased with systolic-diastolic HTN, isolated diastolic HTN, and isolated systolic HTN. HTN increases the risk of ICH four times compared with normotensive patients.

Elderly male patients are the demographic group most at risk for hICH with peak prevalence between 45 and 70 years. African Americans are the most commonly affected ethnic group in North America.

Presentation. Large hICHs present with sensorimotor deficits and impaired consciousness. Patients may—or may not—have a history of longstanding untreated systemic HTN.

Natural History. Neurologic deterioration after hICH is common. HE is frequent in the first few hours and is highly predictive of neurologic deterioration, poor functional outcome, and mortality. For each 10% increase in ICH size, there is a 5% increase in mortality and an additional 15% chance of poorer functional outcome.

Mortality rate approaches 80% in patients with large hemorrhages. Of hICH survivors, between 1/3 and 1/2 are moderately or severely disabled.

Treatment Options. Control of intracranial pressure and hydrocephalus are standard. Hematoma evacuation (whether open or stereotactic guided) and craniectomy for brain swelling are controversial.

Imaging

CT Findings. NECT scans typically show a round or ovoid hyperdense mass centered in the lateral putamen/external capsule or thalamus **(5-24A)**. In the presence of active bleeding or coagulopathy, the hemorrhage may appear inhomogeneously hyperdense with lower density areas and even fluid-fluid levels. Intraventricular extension is common. Acute hICH does not enhance on CECT.

MR Findings. Signal intensity on MR changes with clot age and varies from a large acute hematoma to a slit-like hemosiderin "scar." White matter hyperintensities on T2/FLAIR are common findings in patients with hICH. T2*

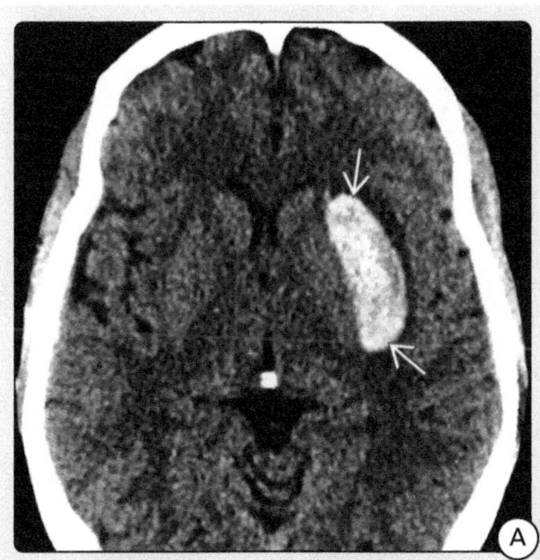

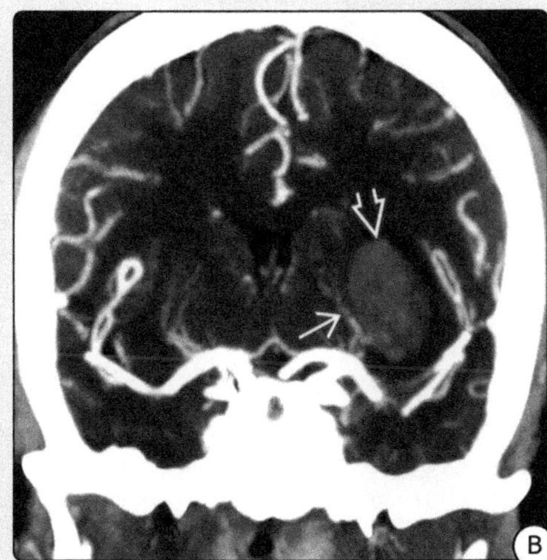

***(5-24A)** Axial NECT scan in a 57-year-old hypertensive woman shows classic left striatocapsular hemorrhage ➡. **(5-24B)** Coronal MIP CTA shows that the left lenticulostriate arteries ➡ are displaced by the hematoma ➡, but there is no evidence of contrast extravasation or "bleeding globe" to suggest increased risk of hematoma expansion.*

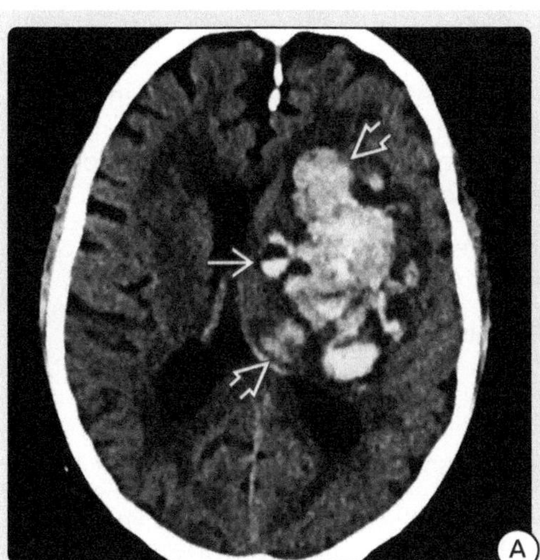

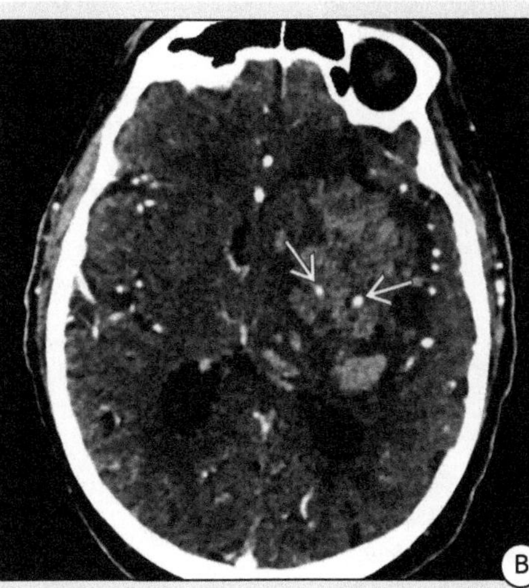

***(5-25A)** NECT in a 73-year-old hypertensive man "found down" shows an acute left basal ganglionic hemorrhage ➡ with mixed hyper-, hypodense foci, fluid-fluid levels ➡, suggesting rapid hemorrhage. **(5-25B)** CTA in the same case shows 2 spot signs with contrast extravasation ➡, indicating active bleeding into the expanding hematoma.*

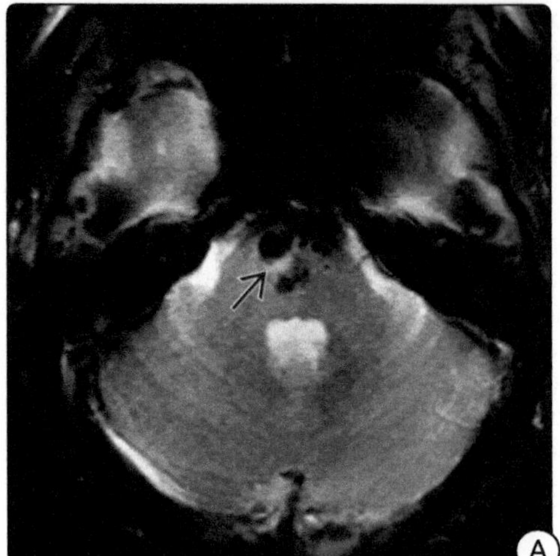

(5-26A) *T2* GRE in a patient with chronic hypertension shows multiple blooming "microbleeds" in the pons ⇒.*

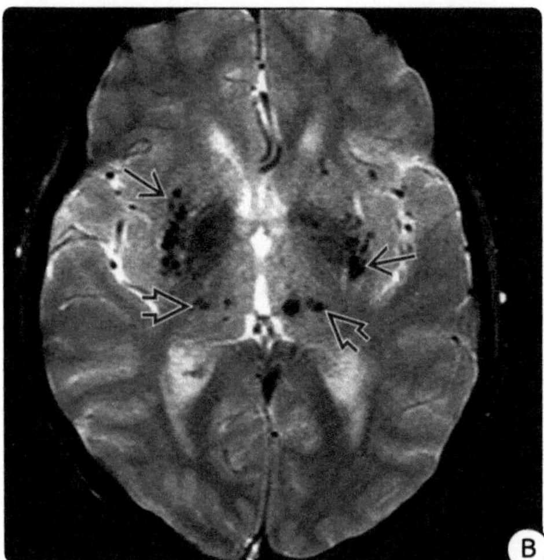

(5-26B) *More cephalad T2* GRE shows multiple microbleeds in the putamina ⇒ and both thalami ⇒.*

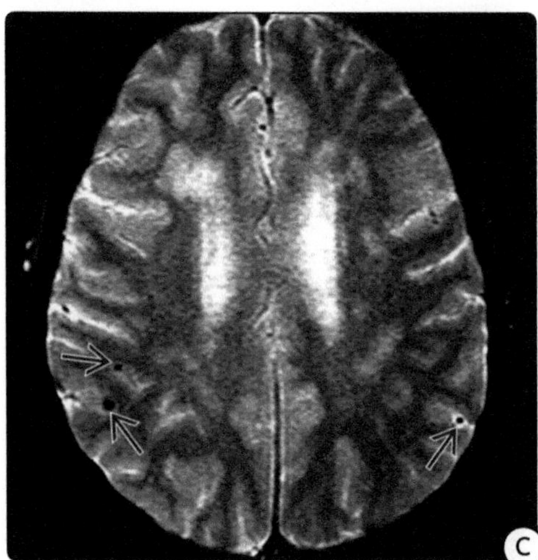

(5-26C) *T2* GRE in the same case shows a few scattered cortical "blooming black dots" ⇒. This is chronic hypertension with microbleeds.*

sequences (GRE, SWI) frequently demonstrate multifocal "blooming black dots," especially in the basal ganglia and cerebellum **(5-26)**.

Angiography. Most hICHs are avascular on CTA **(5-24B)**. However, an enhancing spot sign with contrast extravasation can sometimes be identified in actively bleeding lesions **(5-25)**.

DSA in stroke patients with a classic striatocapsular hemorrhage and a history of HTN is rarely required and usually does not contribute to patient management.

HYPERTENSIVE INTRACRANIAL HEMORRHAGE (hICH)

Location

- Putamen/basal ganglia (60-65%)
- Thalamus (15-25%)
- Pons/cerebellum (10%)
- Lobar hemispheric (5-10%)

Clinical Issues

- 10-15% of all "strokes"
- 40-50% of spontaneous hemorrhages in older adults
- Age, hematoma volume early predictors of death/disability

Imaging

- Classic = hyperdense clot in putamen/external capsule
- Look for old hemosiderin "scar," microbleeds on T2*

Differential Diagnosis

- Cerebral amyloid angiopathy
- Hemorrhagic neoplasm
- Internal cerebral vein thrombosis
- Drug abuse (e.g., cocaine use)

Differential Diagnosis

The major differential diagnosis for hICH is **cerebral amyloid angiopathy** (CAA). Patients with CAA are usually normotensive and have moderately impaired cognition. Although there is some overlap with hICH, the distribution of hemorrhages in CAA is typically lobar and peripheral more often than striatocapsular and central. Cerebellar hemorrhages are common in hICH but rare in CAA.

Hemorrhagic neoplasms (e.g., glioblastoma multiforme or metastasis) are more common in the white matter or gray matter-white matter junction and less common in the basal ganglia and cerebellum.

With the exception of dAVF, first-time hemorrhage from an underlying **vascular malformation** is unusual in middle-aged and elderly patients. **Coagulopathy** can cause or exacerbate spontaneous ICH. Coagulation-related hemorrhages are typically lobar, not striatocapsular.

In younger patients, **drug abuse** (e.g., cocaine use) with extreme HTN can cause putamen/external capsule hemorrhage.

Internal cerebral venous thrombosis can occur at all ages. These hemorrhages tend to be bilateral, thalamic, and more medially located than the striatocapsular bleeds of hICH.

Cerebral Amyloid Angiopathy

CAA is one of three morphologic varieties of cerebral amyloid deposition disease. Because CAA—a.k.a. congophilic angiopathy—is a common cause of spontaneous lobar hemorrhage in elderly patients, we discuss it briefly here.

The full spectrum of cerebral amyloid disease is discussed in greater detail in the chapter on vasculopathy (Chapter 10).

CAA causes ~ 1% of all strokes and 15-20% of primary intracranial bleeds in patients over the age of 60 years. Mean age at onset is 73 years. Patients with CAA are usually normotensive and moderately demented.

NECT may show one or more lobar hematomas, often in different ages of evolution. Some patients with CAA—especially those with "thunderclap" headache—may demonstrate vertex ("convexal") subarachnoid hemorrhage.

MR is the most sensitive study to detect CAA. Multifocal and confluent areas of white matter hyperintensity on T2/FLAIR scans are common. At least 1/3 have petechial microhemorrhages, seen as multifocal "blooming black dots" on T2* (GRE, SWI) sequences. Cortical superficial siderosis is also common and predictive of future lobar hemorrhages.

Remote Cerebellar Hemorrhage

Terminology and Etiology

Remote cerebellar hemorrhage (RCH) is a less well-recognized and often misdiagnosed cause of spontaneous posterior fossa parenchymal hemorrhage in postoperative patients. Most reported cases occur a few hours following supratentorial craniotomy. RCH also occurs as a rare complication of foramen magnum decompression or spinal surgery.

The etiology of RCH is most likely CSF hypovolemia with inferior displacement or "sagging" of the cerebellar hemispheres. Tearing or occlusion of bridging tentorial veins is thought to result in superficial cerebellar hemorrhage with or without hemorrhagic necrosis.

Clinical Issues

RCH is relatively rare, occurring in 0.1-0.6% of patients with supratentorial craniotomies, most often for aneurysm clipping, temporal lobe epilepsy, or tumor resection. There is a slight male predominance. Median age is 51 years.

Many—if not most—cases of RCH are asymptomatic and discovered incidentally at postoperative imaging. The most common symptoms are delayed awakening from anesthesia, decreasing consciousness, and seizures.

Prognosis is generally excellent. Treatment is generally conservative, as hematoma removal is rarely indicated.

Imaging

NECT demonstrates stripes of hyperdense blood layered over the cerebellar folia, the zebra sign. Hemorrhage can be uni- or bilateral, ipsi- or contralateral to the surgical site **(5-30)**.

MR findings are variable, depending on the age/stage of hematoma evolution. "Blooming" black stripes are seen on T2* (GRE, SWI) **(5-31)**.

Microhemorrhages

Cerebral microbleeds (CMBs) represent perivascular collections of hemosiderin-containing macrophages. CMBs are almost always multiple and have many etiologies, ranging from trauma and infection to vasculopathy and metastases. Each is discussed in detail in the respective chapters that deal with the specific pathologic groupings.

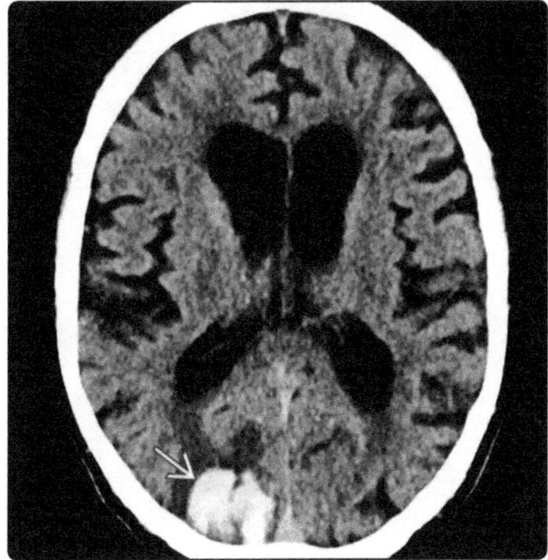

***(5-27)** NECT in an 82y normotensive man with sudden onset of left homonymous hemianopsia shows right occipital lobar hemorrhage ➡.*

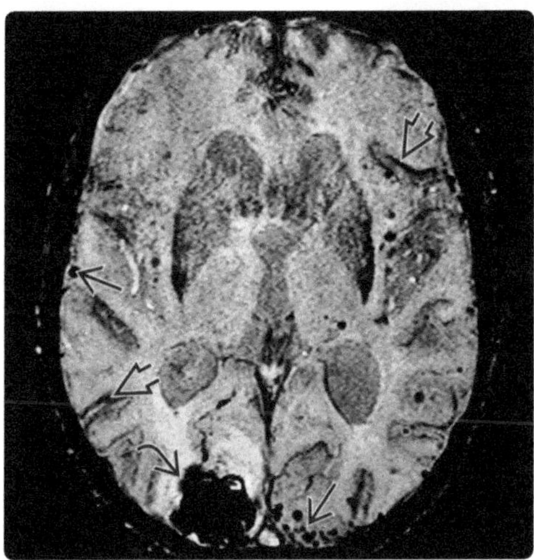

***(5-28)** T2* SWI MIP shows hematoma ⮫, multiple cortical microbleeds ➡, and superficial siderosis ➡. No basal ganglionic lesions are seen.*

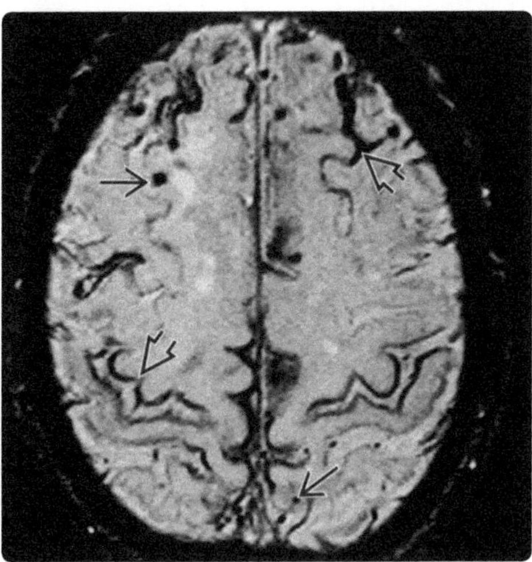

***(5-29)** More cephalad T2* SWI shows more microbleeds ➡ and extensive cortical superficial siderosis ➡. This is amyloid angiopathy.*

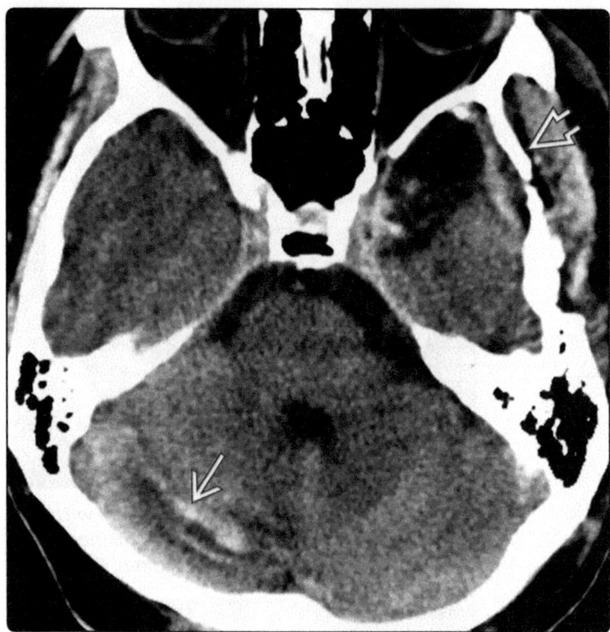

(5-30) NECT scan after supratentorial craniotomy ➡ shows linear "zebra stripes" ➡ of alternating hyperdensity (blood) and low density (edema) in the right cerebellum, consistent with remote cerebellar hemorrhage.

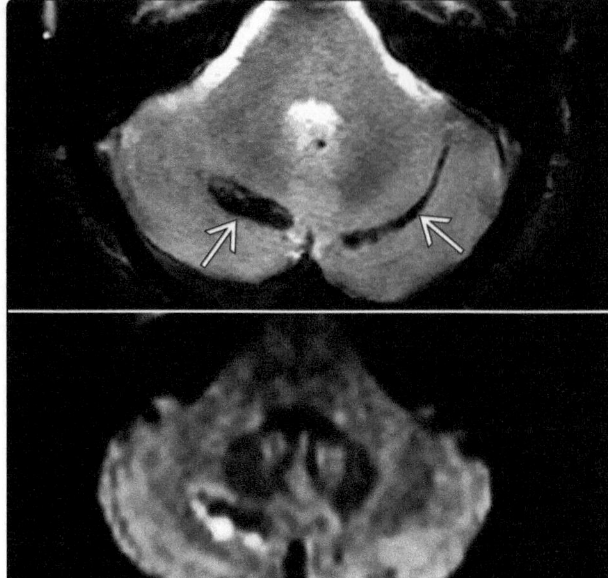

(5-31) Bilateral remote cerebellar hemorrhage followed resection of a supratentorial neoplasm. (Top) T2* GRE shows bilateral "blooming" lesions ➡. (Bottom) DWI shows some restriction in the right acute hemorrhage.

In this section, we briefly summarize two distinct but related differential diagnoses: (1) Entities that cause diffuse brain microbleeds and (2) the differential diagnosis of "black spots" or "blooming black dots" on T2* MR that are *not* caused by microhemorrhages.

Multifocal Brain Microbleeds

A number of entities can cause diffuse brain microhemorrhages. CMBs are best identified on T2* SWI and are often faint or invisible on standard GRE sequences.

Trauma with hemorrhagic vascular or axonal injury is the most common cause of CMBs in children and young adults. **"Critical illness-associated microbleeds"** have recently been described in middle-aged patients with acute respiratory failure who are on mechanical ventilation or extracorporeal membrane oxygenation (ECMO) **(5-33)**.

DIC, **sepsis**, **acute hemorrhagic leukoencephalopathy**, and **high-altitude cerebral edema** are other reported causes of CMBs. Reversible cytotoxic and vasogenic white matter edema with confluent T2/FLAIR hyperintensity may be present along with the CMBs, most likely secondary to capillary failure/leakage.

Chronic HTN and amyloid angiopathy are the two most common pathologies responsible for multiple CMBs in older adults.

"Blooming Black Dots"

Many nonhemorrhagic entities cause multifocal "black dots" on T2* imaging. Calcifications are hypointense on T2* and appear as "blooming black dots" on GRE as well as SWI magnitude images.

Pneumocephalus is common following neurosurgical procedures. Air has very low magnetic susceptibility, and small amounts of intracranial air can be difficult to detect on FSE T2WI. Air causes signal loss on T2* (GRE, SWI) sequences and makes the "blooming black dots" easy to identify (see Fig. 2-76B).

Selected References: The complete reference list is available on the Expert Consult™ eBook version included with purchase.

NONHEMORRHAGIC CAUSES OF "BLOOMING BLACK DOTS" ON T2*

Common
- Pneumocephalus

Less Common
- Multiple parenchymal calcifications
  - Neurocysticercosis
  - Tuberculomas

Rare but Important
- Extracorporeal membrane circulation
- Devices, complications
  - Metallic emboli (heart valves, etc.)

BRAIN MICROBLEEDS: ETIOLOGY, COMMON

Common
- Diffuse axonal/vascular injury
- Cerebral amyloid angiopathy
- Chronic hypertensive encephalopathy
- Hemorrhagic metastases

Less Common
- Multiple cavernous malformations
- Septicemia
- Critical illness associated
  - Hypoxemia, acute respiratory distress syndrome
- Fat emboli
- Vasculitis
  - Fungal
  - Sickle cell
- Coagulopathy

BRAIN MICROBLEEDS: ETIOLOGY, RARE

Rare but Important
- Acute hemorrhagic leukoencephalopathy
- Intravascular lymphoma
- Leukemia
- Radiation/chemotherapy
  - Radiation-induced telangiectasias
  - Mineralizing microangiopathy
  - SMART syndrome (**s**troke-like **m**igraine **a**fter **r**adiation **t**herapy)
- Thrombotic microangiopathy
  - Malignant HTN
  - Disseminated intravascular coagulopathy
  - Hemolytic uremic syndrome (HUS), atypical HUS
  - Thrombotic thrombocytopenic purpura
- High-altitude cerebral edema
- Cerebral malaria

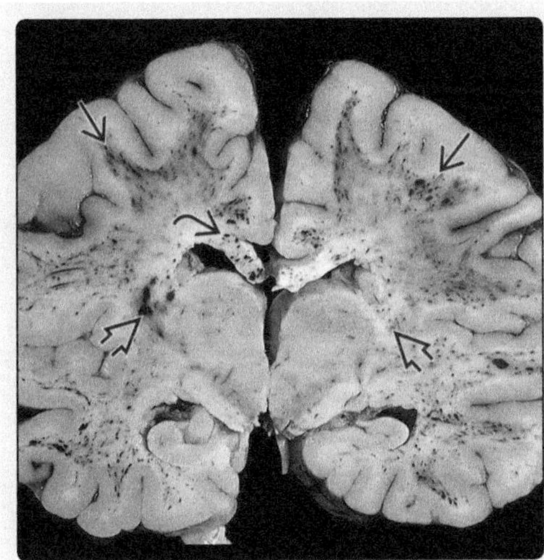

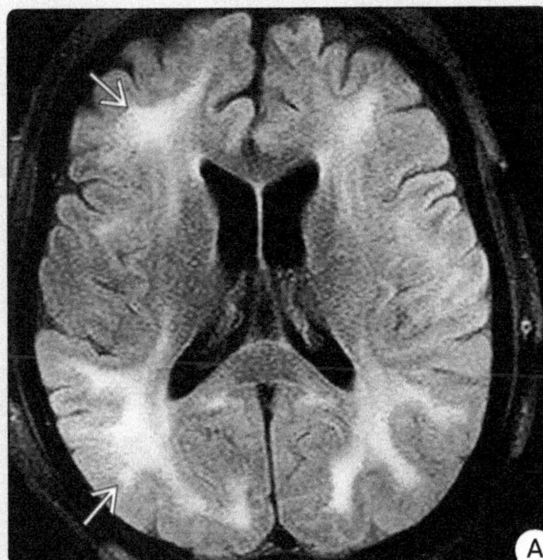

***(5-32)** Coronal autopsy shows innumerable tiny microhemorrhages in the subcortical ➙, deep ➙ white matter in a patient with respiratory failure and sepsis. Corpus callosum ➙ is severely affected. (Courtesy R. Hewlett, MD.) **(5-33A)** FLAIR MR in a 55-year-old intubated man with acute respiratory distress syndrome shows diffuse confluent symmetric hyperintensity ➙ in the subcortical, deep white matter that spares the cortex.*

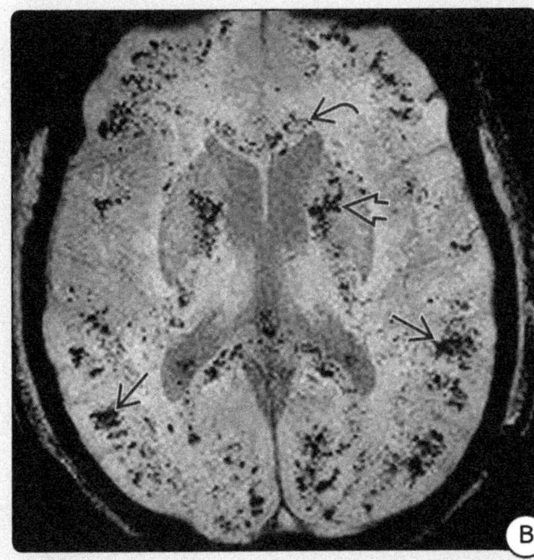

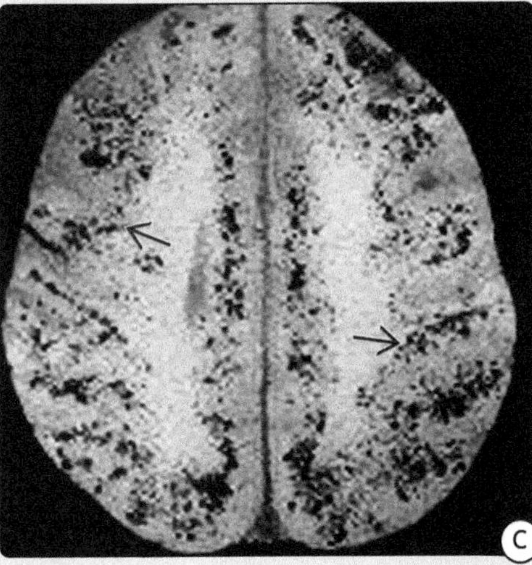

***(5-33B)** T2* SWI MR shows innumerable microbleeds in the subcortical, deep white matter ➙, including the corpus callosum ➙ and internal capsules ➙. **(5-33C)** More cephalad SWI MR shows the diffuse subcortical microbleeds ➙ with striking sparing of the overlying cortex. This is a striking case of critical illness-associated cerebral microbleeds. (Courtesy M. Jhaveri, MD.)*

Subarachnoid Hemorrhage and Aneurysms

Trauma is—by far—the most common cause of intracranial subarachnoid hemorrhage (SAH). Traumatic SAH occurs when blood from contused brain or lacerated vessels extends into adjacent sulci; it was discussed in connection with craniocerebral trauma (Chapter 2). This chapter focuses on nontraumatic SAH and aneurysms.

Subarachnoid Hemorrhage

Spontaneous (i.e., nontraumatic) SAH accounts for 3-5% of all acute "strokes." Approximately 80% of these are caused by a ruptured intracranial saccular aneurysm (SA). Other identifiable causes of nontraumatic SAH (ntSAH) include a variety of entities, such as dissections, venous hemorrhage or thrombosis, vasculitis, amyloid angiopathy, and reversible cerebral vasoconstriction syndrome (RCVS). No identifiable origin is found in 10-12% of patients presenting with ntSAH.

We begin this discussion with **aneurysmal SAH** (aSAH) and its most devastating complications, vasospasm and secondary cerebral ischemia. We then review two special types of nontraumatic, nonaneurysmal SAH: **Perimesencephalic SAH** and an unusual pattern of SAH called convexity or **convexal SAH (cSAH)**. Lastly, we discuss chronic repeated SAH and its rare but important manifestation, **superficial siderosis (SS)**.

Aneurysmal Subarachnoid Hemorrhage

Terminology

aSAH is an extravasation of blood into the space between the arachnoid and pia. The typical location of aSAH (basal cisterns and sylvian and inferior interhemispheric fissures) usually helps distinguish it from other causes of ntSAH (see shaded box, p. 100).

Etiology

aSAH is most often caused by rupture of a saccular ("berry") or (rarely) a blood blister-like aneurysm (BBA). Other less common causes of aSAH include intracranial dissections and dissecting aneurysms.

Pathology

Location. Because most SAs arise from the circle of Willis or middle cerebral artery (MCA) bifurcation, the most common locations for aSAH are the suprasellar cistern and sylvian fissures **(6-1)**.

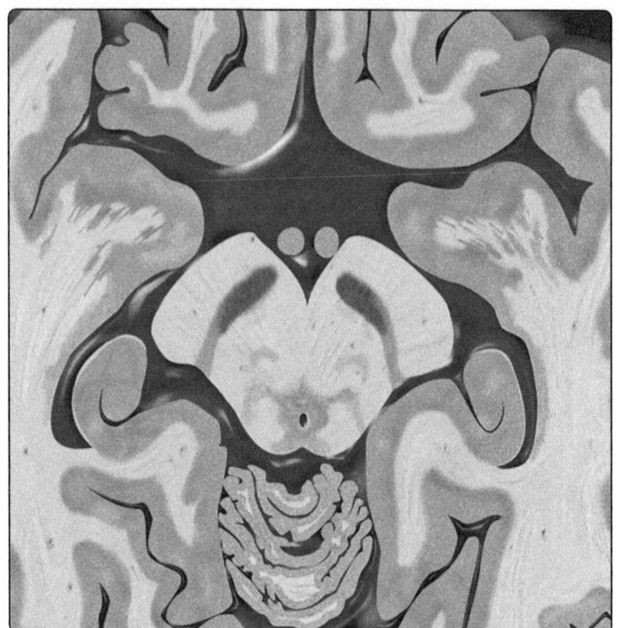

***(6-1)** Axial graphic through the midbrain shows subarachnoid hemorrhage (SAH) in red throughout the basal cisterns. With diffuse distribution of SAH without focal hematoma, statistically the most likely location of the ruptured aneurysm is the ACoA.*

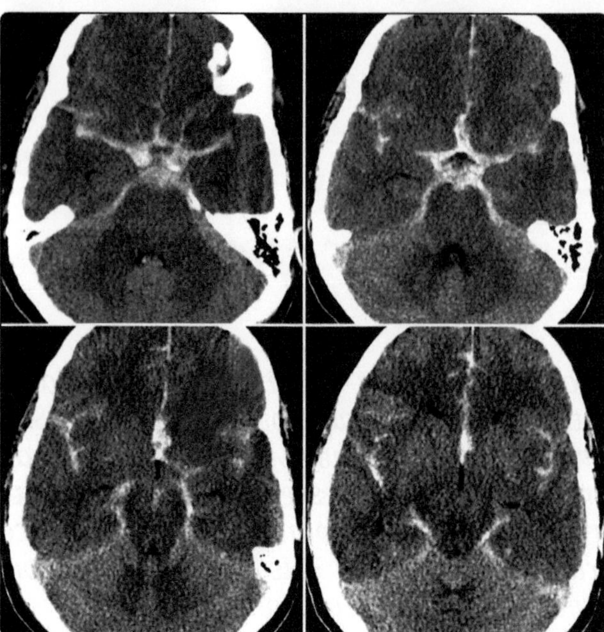

***(6-2)** Series of axial NECT scans shows the typical appearance of aneurysmal SAH. Hyperdensity in the basilar cisterns and sylvian fissures is typical.*

Occasionally, an aneurysm ruptures directly into the brain parenchyma rather than the subarachnoid space. This occurs most frequently when the apex of an anterior communicating artery (ACoA) aneurysm points upward and bursts into the frontal lobe **(6-3)**.

Gross Pathology. The gross appearance of aSAH is typically characterized by blood-filled basal cisterns **(6-13)**. SAH may extend into the superficial sulci and ventricles.

Clinical Issues

Demographics. The overall incidence of aSAH increases with age and peaks between 40 and 60 years old. M:F = 1:2.

aSAH is rare in children. Regardless of their relative rarity, however, cerebral aneurysms cause the majority of spontaneous (nontraumatic) SAHs in children and account for ~ 10% of all childhood hemorrhagic "strokes."

Presentation. At least 75% of patients with aSAH present with sudden onset of the "worst headache of my life." The most severe form is a "thunderclap" headache, an extremely intense headache that comes on "like a boom of thunder" and typically peaks within minutes or even seconds. There are many causes of "thunderclap" headache. The most serious and life threatening is aSAH, although it accounts for just 4-12% of these severe headaches.

1/3 of patients with aSAH complain of neck pain and 1/3 report vomiting. 10-25% experience a "sentinel headache" days or up to two weeks before the onset of overt SAH. These "sentinel headaches" are sudden, intense, persistent, and may represent minor bleeding prior to aneurysm rupture.

SCREENING FOR SUSPECTED ANEURYSMAL SAH

Clinical Issues
- Causes 3-5% of "strokes"
- "Thunderclap" headache (aSAH: 4-12%)
- Peak age = 40-60 years; M:F = 1:2

NECT
- Sensitivity: ~ 100% if performed in first 6 hours
- Lumbar puncture unnecessary *if*
  - CT negative
  - Neurologic examination normal

CTA
- If NECT shows aSAH

Natural History. Although aSAH causes just 3-5% of all "strokes," nearly 1/3 of all stroke-related years of potential life lost before age 65 are attributable to aSAH. The mean age at death in patients with aSAH is significantly lower than in patients with other types of strokes.

aSAH is fatal or disabling in more than 2/3 of patients. Massive SAH can cause coma and death within minutes. Approximately 1/3 of patients with aSAH die within 72 hours; another 1/3 survive but with disabling neurologic deficits.

Treatment Options. The goals of aSAH treatment in patients who survive their initial bleed are (1) to obliterate the aneurysm (preventing potentially catastrophic rebleeding) and (2) to prevent or treat vasospasm.

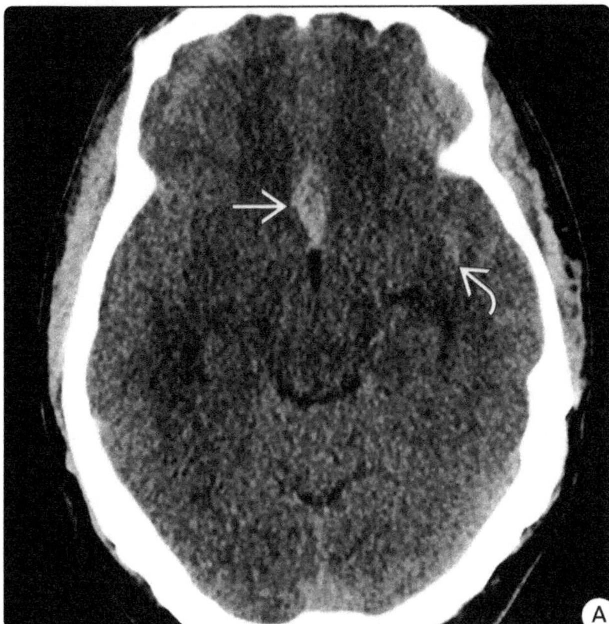

(6-3A) NECT in a 42-year-old man with "thunderclap" headache shows a focal hematoma in the interhemispheric fissure ➡. A small amount of SAH is present in the left sylvian fissure ⮫.

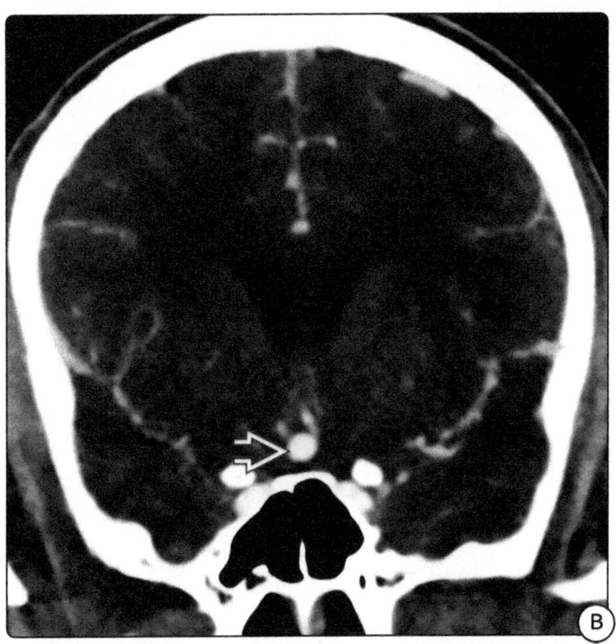

(6-3B) Coronal CTA in the same case demonstrates an 8-mm saccular aneurysm (SA) arising from the ACoA ➡. The aneurysm was successfully treated with endovascular coiling.

Imaging

General Features. NECT is an excellent screening examination for patients with "thunderclap" headache and suspected aSAH. In the first six hours after ictus, the sensitivity of modern CT scanners (16-slice or greater) for detecting aSAH approaches 100%. Lumbar puncture is now considered unnecessary if the NECT is negative and the neurologic examination is normal.

The best imaging clue to aSAH is hyperdense cisterns and sulci on NECT.

CT Findings. The basal cisterns—especially the suprasellar cistern—are generally filled with hyperdense blood **(6-2)**. Although SAH distribution generally depends on location of the "culprit" aneurysm, it is also somewhat variable and not absolutely predictive of aneurysm location.

ACoA aneurysms often rupture superiorly into the interhemispheric fissure **(6-3)**. MCA bifurcation aneurysms usually rupture into the sylvian fissure. Internal carotid-posterior communicating artery (ICA-PCoA) aneurysms generally rupture into the suprasellar cistern. Vertebrobasilar aneurysms often fill the fourth ventricle, prepontine cistern, and foramen magnum with blood.

Intraventricular hemorrhage (IVH) is present in nearly 1/2 of all patients with aSAH. Focal parenchymal hemorrhage is uncommon but, if present, is generally predictive of aneurysm rupture site.

MR Findings. Acute aSAH is isointense with brain on T1WI **(6-4C)**. The CSF cisterns may appear smudged or "dirty" **(6-4D)**. Hyperacute aSAH is isointense with CSF and may be difficult to identify. With time, subarachnoid blood may actually become hypointense **(6-4E)**.

FLAIR is the best sequence to depict acute aSAH. Hyperintensity in the sulci and cisterns is present **(6-4F)** but nonspecific. Other causes of "bright" CSF on FLAIR include hyperoxygenation, meningitis, neoplasm, and artifact.

Angiography. CTA is positive in 95% of aSAH cases if the "culprit" aneurysm is 2 mm or larger **(6-3B)**. Many patients with aSAH and positive CTA undergo surgical clipping without DSA. DSA identifies vascular pathology in 13% of patients with CTA-negative SAH, so such patients should be considered candidates for DSA.

So-called angiogram-negative SAH is found in ~ 15% of cases **(6-4)**. With the addition of 3D rotational angiography and 3D shaded surface displays, the rate of "angiogram-negative" SAH decreases to 4-5% of cases.

IMAGING OF ANEURYSMAL SAH

NECT
- Hyperdense basal cisterns, sulci
- Hydrocephalus common, onset often early

MR
- "Dirty" CSF on T1WI
- Hyperintense cisterns, sulci on FLAIR

Angiography
- CTA positive in 95% if aneurysm ≥ 2 mm
- DSA reserved for complex aneurysm, CTA negative
- "Angiogram-negative" SAH (15%; 5% if 3D used)
- Repeat "2nd look" DSA positive (5%)

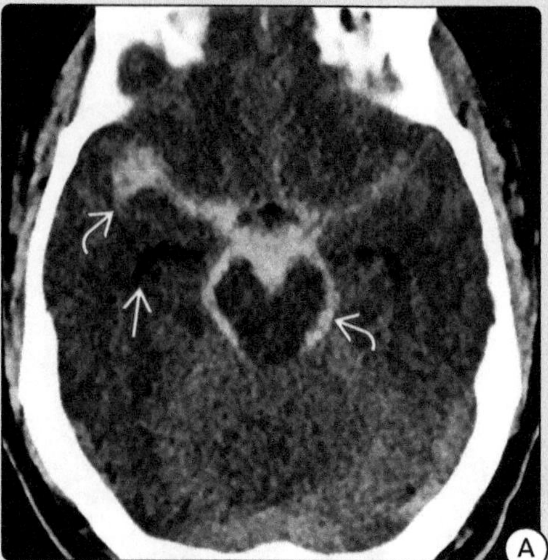

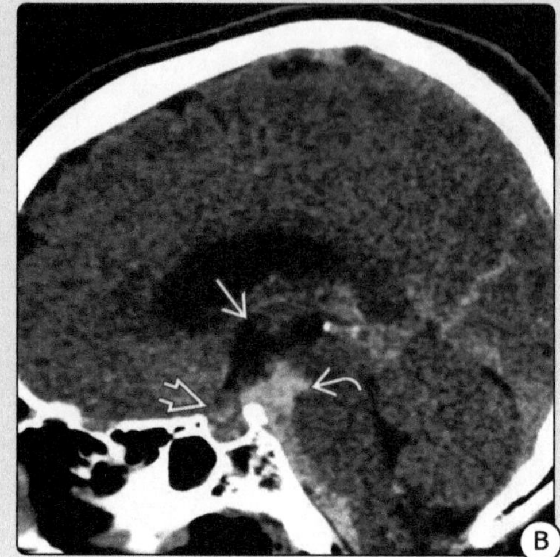

***(6-4A)** NECT in a 58-year-old man with "thunderclap" headache shows typical pattern of aneurysmal (aSAH) filling the basal cisterns, sylvian fissures. Early obstructive hydrocephalus is present. **(6-4B)** Sagittal reformatted NECT shows iso- and hyperdense blood filling the suprasellar, interpeduncular, and prepontine cisterns. Note contrast with normal low-density CSF in the 3rd ventricle.*

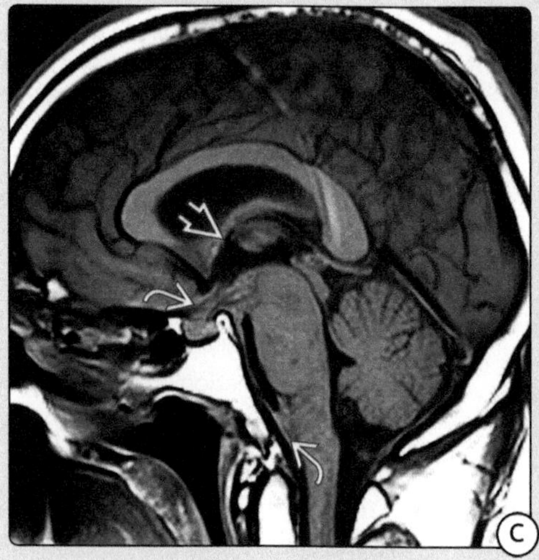

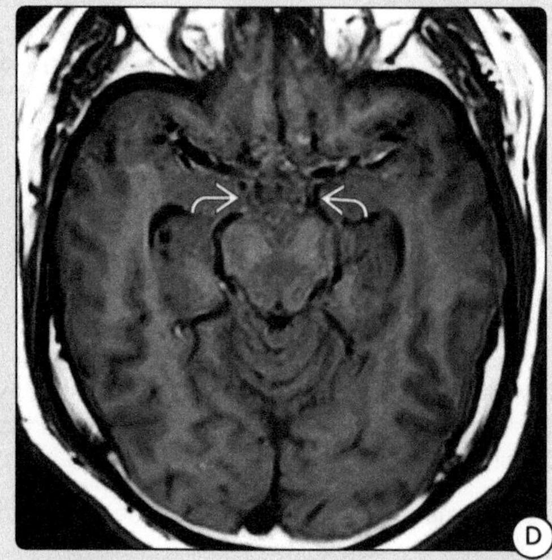

***(6-4C)** Because CTA and DSA were negative, MR was obtained several hours later. Sagittal T1WI shows that "dirty" CSF surrounds basilar artery "flow void" and is nearly isointense with adjacent brain. Note contrast with normal hypointense CSF in the 3rd ventricle. **(6-4D)** Axial T1WI MR shows that the suprasellar cistern is filled with "dirty" CSF that is nearly isointense with the surrounding brain.*

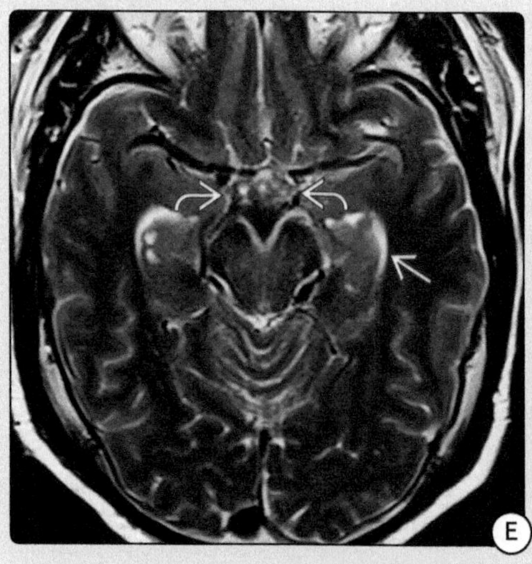

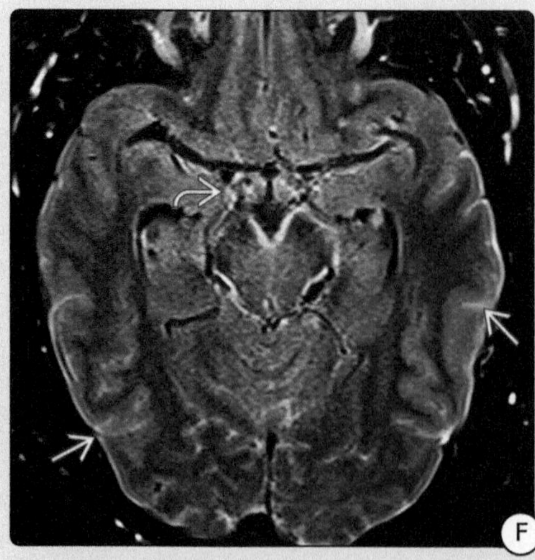

***(6-4E)** T2WI MR shows that CSF in the suprasellar cistern is hypointense as it is mixed with acute hemorrhage. Note contrast with normal hyperintense CSF in the temporal horns of the lateral ventricles. **(6-4F)** CSF in the suprasellar cistern exhibits incomplete suppression on FLAIR. Note hyperintense, nonsuppressing fluid in the superficial sulci from the subarachnoid hemorrhage.*

Differential Diagnosis

The major differential diagnosis of aSAH is **traumatic SAH (tSAH)**. aSAH is generally much more widespread, often filling the basal cisterns. tSAH typically occurs adjacent to cortical contusions or lacerations and is therefore most common in the superficial sulci.

Perimesencephalic nonaneurysmal SAH (pnSAH) is much more limited than aSAH and is localized to the interpeduncular, ambient, and prepontine cisterns. Occasionally, pnSAH spreads into the posterior aspect of the suprasellar cistern. It rarely extends into the sylvian fissures.

Convexal SAH (cSAH) is, as the name implies, localized to superficial sulci over the cerebral convexities. Often, only a single sulcus is affected. Causes of cSAH are numerous and include cortical vein occlusion, amyloid angiopathy, vasculitis, and RCVS.

Pseudo-SAH is caused by severe cerebral edema. The hypodensity of the brain makes blood in the cerebral arteries and veins appear dense, mimicking the appearance of SAH.

Sulcal-cisternal FLAIR hyperintensity on MR is a nonspecific imaging finding. It occurs with hemorrhage, meningitis, carcinomatosis, hyperoxygenation, stroke, and gadolinium contrast (blood-brain barrier leakage or chronic renal failure). FLAIR "bright" CSF can also result from flow disturbances and technical artifacts (e.g., incomplete CSF nulling).

Pyogenic meningitis, meningeal carcinomatosis, and high inspired oxygen concentration may also cause CSF hyperintensity on FLAIR. Prior administration of gadolinium chelates (with or without decreased renal clearance) can result in diffuse delayed CSF enhancement.

Other etiologies of sulcal-cisternal FLAIR hyperintensity include hyperintense vessels with slow flow (e.g., acute arterial strokes, pial collaterals developing after cerebral ischemia-infarction, Sturge-Weber syndrome, moyamoya, and RCVS).

Post-aSAH Cerebral Ischemia and Vasospasm

Cerebral ischemia is the major cause of morbidity and death in patients who survive their initial SAH. Cerebral vasospasm (CVS) is the most common cause of cerebral ischemia and typically occurs 4-10 days after aSAH.

Imaging Post-aSAH Complications

Noninvasive methods to detect early-stage post-aSAH complications include transcranial Doppler ultrasound, CTA, and MR/MRA. Multiple segments of vascular constriction and irregularly narrowed vessels are typical findings on CTA and DSA **(6-5)**. MR with DWI and pMR is most sensitive for detecting early ischemic changes following aSAH.

DSA is typically performed if endovascular treatment or intraarterial administration of antispasmolytic agents, such as nicardipine, is anticipated.

Differential Diagnosis

The differential diagnosis of vasospasm within the context of existing SAH is limited. If the patient has a known aneurysm with recent SAH, the findings of multisegmental vascular narrowing indicate CVS. However, if the SAH is convexal, the differential diagnosis includes **RCVS** and **vasculitis**.

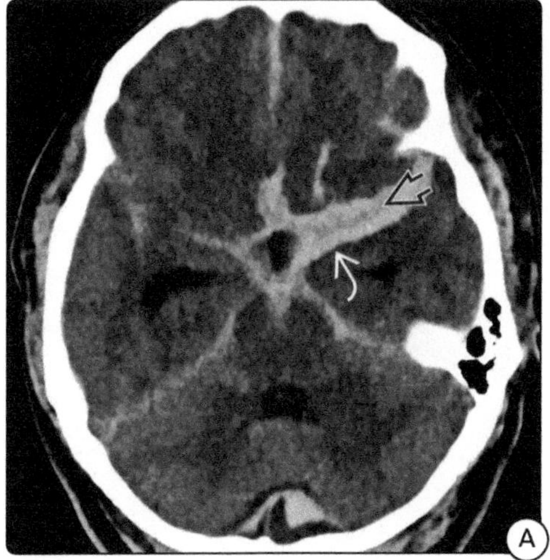

***(6-5A)** NECT in a 43-year-old man with sudden, severe headache shows SAH filling the basal cisterns ➡. Left MCA ➡ is outlined by the SAH.*

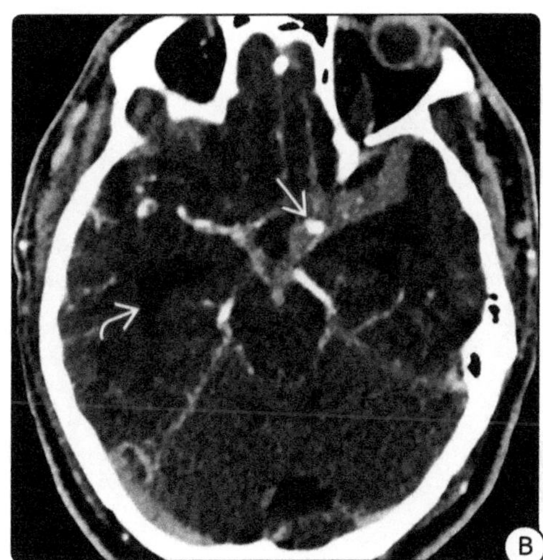

***(6-5B)** CTA shows an 8-mm bilobed aneurysm ➡ at the left internal carotid artery (ICA) bifurcation. Note obstructive hydrocephalus ➡.*

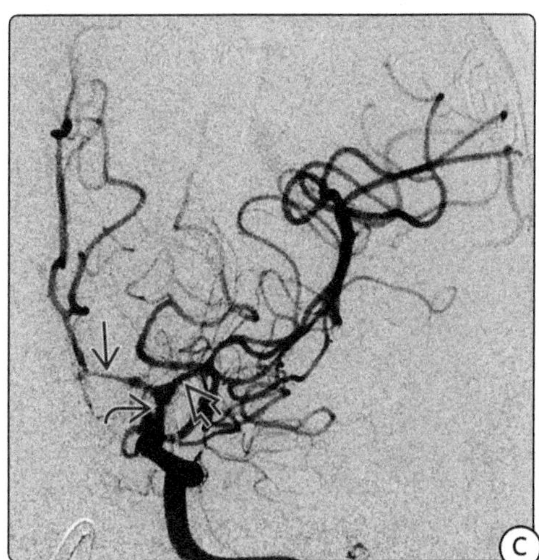

***(6-5C)** DSA 4 days after clipping shows moderate vasospasm involving the distal ICA ➡, proximal A1 ➡, and M1 ➡ segments.*

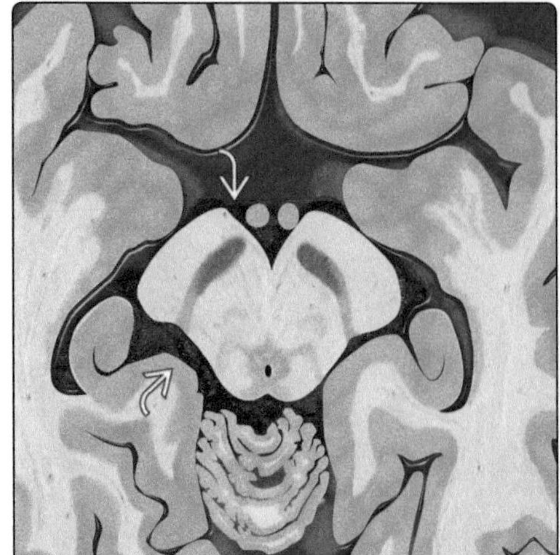

(6-6) In pnSAH, hemorrhage is confined to the interpeduncular fossa and ambient (perimesencephalic) cisterns ➡.

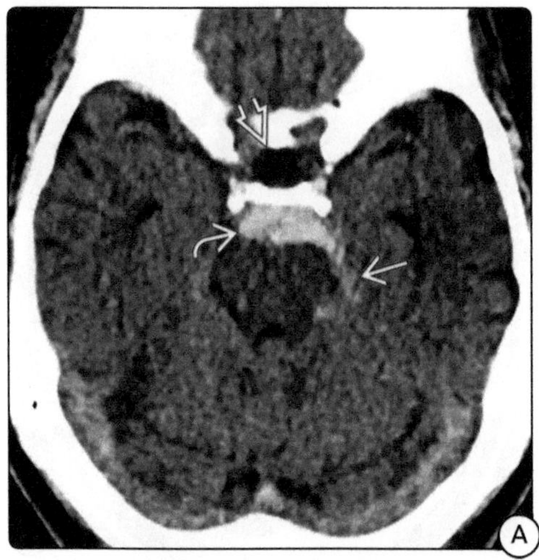

(6-7A) Axial NECT shows pnSAH with blood in the prepontine ➡, left lateral mesencephalic ➡ cisterns. Suprasellar ➡ cistern is normal.

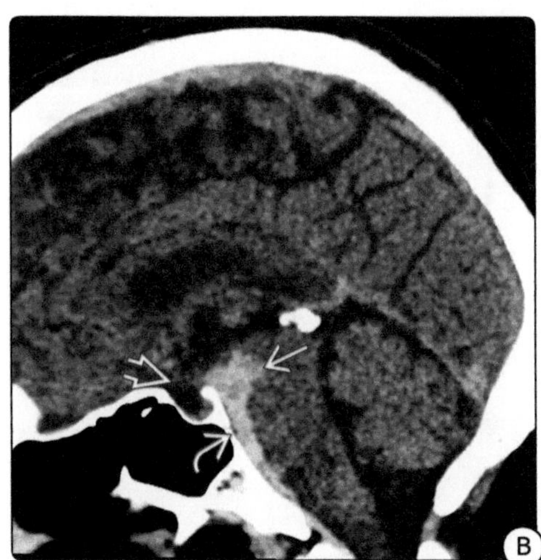

(6-7B) Sagittal reformatted NECT shows prepontine ➡, interpeduncular ➡ blood. The anterior suprasellar cistern is clear ➡. pnSAH.

Other Complications of aSAH

Obstructive hydrocephalus commonly develops in patients with aSAH, sometimes within hours of the ictus, and may be exacerbated by the presence of IVH. Imaging studies show increased periventricular extracellular fluid with "blurred" lateral ventricle margins **(6-5B)**.

Perimesencephalic Nonaneurysmal SAH

Terminology

pnSAH is also known as benign perimesencephalic SAH. pnSAH is a clinically benign SAH subtype that is anatomically confined to the perimesencephalic and prepontine cisterns **(6-6)**.

Etiology

The precise etiology of pnSAH is unknown, and the bleeding source in pnSAH is usually undetermined. Yet most investigators implicate venous—not aneurysmal—rupture as the most likely cause.

Clinical Issues

pnSAH is the most common cause of nontraumatic, nonaneurysmal SAH. The typical presentation is mild to moderate headache with Hunt and Hess grades 1-2. Occasionally, patients experience severe "thunderclap" headache with meningismus.

The peak age of presentation in patients with pnSAH is between 40 and 60 years—identical to that of aSAH. There is no sex predilection.

Most cases of pnSAH follow a clinically benign and uneventful course, although MR demonstrates acute—and usually asymptomatic—ischemic lesions in nearly 1/2 of all cases. Rebleeding is uncommon (< 1%). In contrast to aSAH, vasospasm and delayed cerebral ischemia are rare.

Imaging

pnSAH has well-defined imaging features. NECT scans show focal accumulation of subarachnoid blood around the midbrain (in the interpeduncular and perimesencephalic cisterns) **(6-7)** and in front of the pons. High-resolution CTA is used to rule out underlying aneurysm or dissection. If the initial CTA is negative, there is no significant additional diagnostic yield from DSA.

Differential Diagnosis

The major differential diagnosis of pnSAH is **aSAH**. aSAH is significantly more extensive, spreading throughout the basal cisterns and often extending into the interhemispheric and sylvian fissures.

tSAH would be suggested both by history and imaging appearance. tSAH occurs adjacent to contused brain. It is usually more peripheral, lying primarily within the sylvian fissure and over the cerebral convexities. During closed head injury, the midbrain may be suddenly and forcibly impacted against the tentorial incisura. In such cases, the presence of perimesencephalic blood can mimic pnSAH. In contrast to pnSAH, interpeduncular and prepontine hemorrhage is usually absent.

cSAH is found over the cerebral convexities, not in the perimesencephalic cisterns. Blood within a single sulcus or immediately adjacent sulci is common.

Convexal SAH

Terminology

Isolated spontaneous ntSAH that involves the sulci over the brain vertex is called *convexal* or *convexity SAH* (cSAH). cSAH is a unique type of SAH with a very different imaging appearance from either aSAH or pnSAH: cSAH is restricted to the hemispheric convexities, sparing the basal and perimesencephalic cisterns **(6-8)**.

Etiology

A broad spectrum of vascular and even nonvascular pathologies can cause cSAH. These include dural sinus and cortical vein thrombosis (CoVT), arteriovenous malformations, dural arteriovenous fistulas, arterial dissection/stenosis/occlusion, mycotic aneurysm, vasculitides, amyloid angiopathy, coagulopathies, RCVS, and posterior reversible encephalopathy syndrome.

Clinical Issues

Although cSAH can occur at virtually any age, most patients are between the fourth and eighth decades. Peak age is 70 years.

The clinical presentation of cSAH varies with etiology but is quite different from that of aSAH. Most patients with cSAH have nonspecific headache without nuchal rigidity. Some present with focal or generalized seizures or neurologic deficits.

Patients with cSAH secondary to RCVS may present with a "thunderclap" headache. The vast majority are middle-aged women. cSAH caused by venous thrombosis or vasculitis may have milder symptoms with more insidious onset. Mean age of CoVT accompanied by cSAH is 33 years.

ETIOLOGY OF NONTRAUMATIC CONVEXAL SAH

Common
- Reversible cerebral vasoconstriction syndrome (RCVS)
  - Mean age ≈ 50 years
  - Typical presentation = "thunderclap" headache
- Cerebral amyloid angiopathy (CAA)
  - Mean age ≈ 70 years
  - Symptoms = confusion, dementia, sensorimotor dysfunction

Less Common
- Endocarditis
- CoVT ± dural sinus occlusion

Rare
- Vasculitis

Cerebral amyloid angiopathy (CAA) is the major cause of cSAH in elderly patients. Worsening dementia and headache are the common presentations. cSAH in this age cohort is associated with cognitive impairment and CAA as well as APOE-ε4 overrepresentation compared with age-matched health controls. Between 40-45% experience recurrent cSAH and subsequent lobar hemorrhage (see Chapter 10).

The outcome of cSAH *itself* is generally benign and depends primarily on underlying etiology. Vasospasm and DCI are rare.

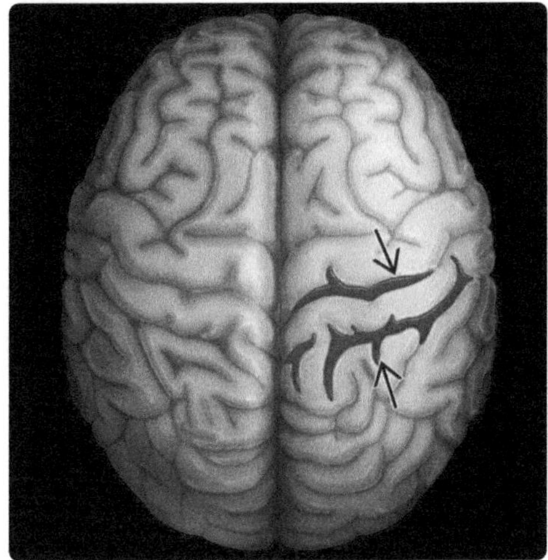

***(6-8)** Graphic depicts convexal SAH (cSAH) with focal subarachnoid blood ➲ in adjacent sulci along the vertex of the left hemisphere.*

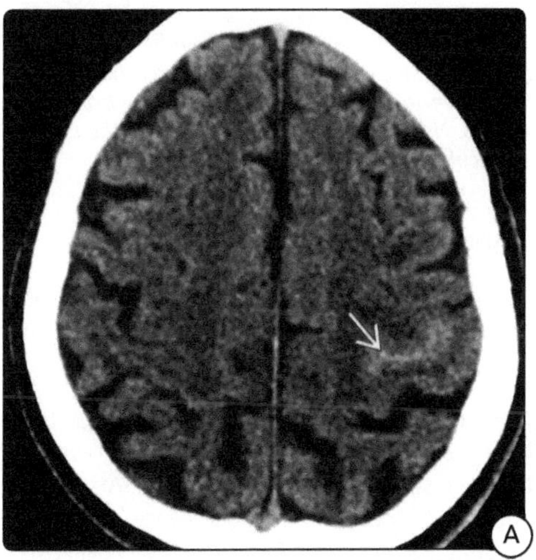

***(6-9A)** NECT in a 78-year-old man with headaches shows subarachnoid blood in a convexity sulcus ➲.*

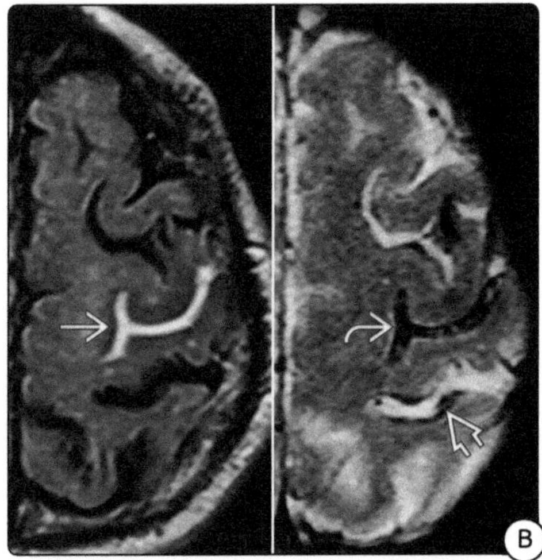

***(6-9B)** FLAIR (L) shows hyperintensity in the convexity sulcus ➲. T2* (R) shows "blooming" of the hemorrhage ➲ & pial siderosis (CAA) ➲.*

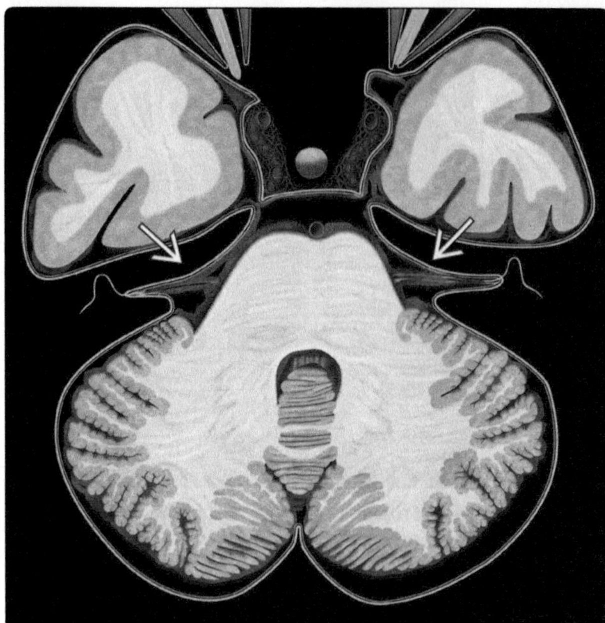

(6-10) Graphic of superficial siderosis shows darker brown hemosiderin staining on surfaces of the brain, meninges, cranial nerves. Notice that CNVII and CNVIII in the CPA-IAC ➡ are particularly affected.

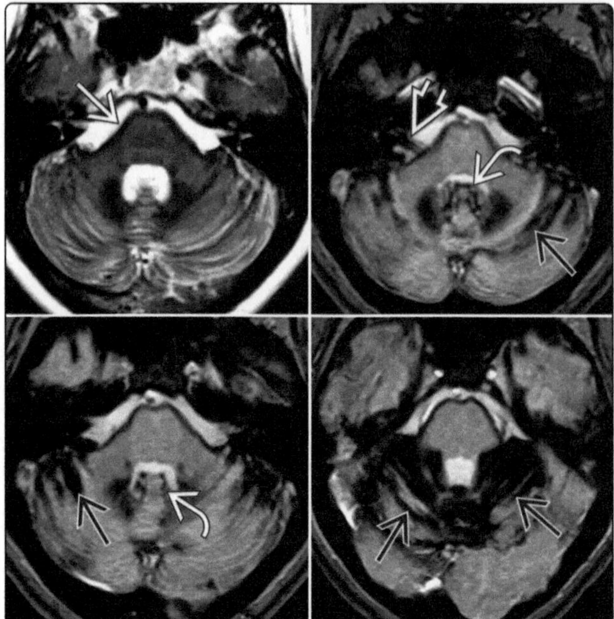

(6-11) FSE T2 shows hypointensity around pons, cerebellum ➡. T2 shows "blooming" along pons, cerebellar hemispheres ➡. Note siderosis along CNVII, CNVIII ➡, hemosiderin deposition in the choroid plexus of the 4th ventricle ➡. cSS.*

Imaging

CT Findings. Most cases of cSAH are unilateral, involving one **(6-9A)** or several dorsolateral convexity sulci. The basal cisterns are typically spared.

MR Findings. Focal sulcal hyperintensity on FLAIR is typical in cSAH **(6-9B)** **(6-12A)**. T2* (GRE, SWI) shows "blooming" in the affected sulci. If the etiology of the cSAH is dural sinus or cortical vein occlusion, a hypointense "cord" sign may be present. Patients with CAA have multifocal cortical and pial microbleeds ("blooming black dots") on T2* **(6-9B)**. They may also show evidence of siderosis and prior lobar hemorrhages of differing ages.

NONTRAUMATIC SAH: ANEURYSMAL vs. NONANEURYSMAL

Aneurysmal SAH
- Widespread; basal cisterns
- Arterial origin
- Complications (vasospasm, ischemia) common

Perimesencephalic Nonaneurysmal SAH
- Focal; perimesencephalic, prepontine cisterns
- Probably venous origin
- Clinically benign; complications, recurrence rare

Convexal SAH
- Superficial (convexity) sulci
- ≥ 60 years? Think CAA!
- ≤ 60 years? Think RCVS!
- All ages: Venous occlusions, vasculitis

Superficial Siderosis

Terminology

Hemosiderin deposition along brain surfaces, cranial nerves, &/or the spinal cord defines the condition known as **superficial siderosis (SS)** **(6-10)**. There are two types of siderosis, which differ in underlying pathologies and clinical presentation. **"Classic" SS** of the CNS primarily affects the infratentorial regions and spinal cord.

The term **"cortical" SS** (cSS) describes a distinct pattern of iron-bearing blood-breakdown product deposition limited to cortical sulci over the convexities of the cerebral hemispheres. In cortical SS, the brainstem, cerebellum, and spinal cord are spared.

Etiology

SS is a consequence of chronic intermittent or continuous minor hemorrhage into the subarachnoid space. Trauma and surgery are the most common causes of classic SS. Other reported etiologies include hemorrhagic neoplasm, vascular malformations, and venous obstruction(s). SS due to repeated aSAH is relatively uncommon.

Cortical SS has many potential causes, but in older individuals, cortical SS is most often associated with CAA.

Pathology

Location. Although it can occur anywhere in the CNS, *classic* SS has a predilection for the posterior fossa (cerebellar folia and vermis, CNVIII) and brainstem.

Cortical SS is seen in 60% of patients with CAA but is rare in non-CAA forms of intracerebral hemorrhages.

Gross Pathology. Brownish yellow and blackish gray encrustations cover the affected structures, layering along the sulci and encasing cranial nerves.

Clinical Issues

Patients with classic SS often present with slowly progressive gait ataxia, dysarthria, and bilateral sensorineural hearing loss. Some patients present with progressive myelopathy. Often, decades pass between the putative event that causes SS and the development of overt symptoms.

As cortical SS most commonly occurs in the setting of CAA, progressive dementia and cognitive decline are common

Imaging

CT is usually normal in patients with SS.

SS on MR is best identified on T2* (GRE, SWI) imaging and is seen as a hypointense rim that follows along brain surfaces and coats the cranial nerves &/or spinal cord **(6-11)**. A characteristic bilinear track-like appearance is common with cortical SS **(6-12B)**.

Despite extensive neuroimaging, the source of the SS often remains occult. In 50% of classic SS, a hemorrhage source is never identified despite extensive investigation of the entire neuraxis.

Differential Diagnosis

The major imaging mimic of classic SS is **"bounce point" artifact**, which makes the posterior fossa surfaces appear artifactually dark.

Most cortical SS mimics contain deoxygenated blood or blood products. **Cerebral veins** appear markedly hypointense on SWI but do not run parallel to the convexity sulci. Slow flow in sulcal arteries (pial collaterals in stroke or moyamoya) can appear hypointense on SWI as well.

In Sturge-Weber syndrome, hypointensity due to gyriform calcifications may be linear and cortical but can be easily identified on NECT and T1 C+ MR. Rare causes of cortical SS include **hemorrhagic subarachnoid metastases**, **neurocutaneous melanosis** (hyperintense on T1WI) and **meningioangiomatosis** (thickened enhancing, sometimes calcified and infiltrating proliferations of meningeal cells and blood vessels).

SUPERFICIAL SIDEROSIS (SS)

Classic SS
- Posterior fossa > > supratentorial
- Brain (typically cerebellum), cranial nerves coated with hemosiderin
- Chronic repeated SAH
- Cause undetermined in ≈ 50%
- Sensorineural hearing loss

Cortical SS
- Cortex over hemisphere convexities
- Most common etiology = CAA
- Transient focal neurologic episodes
- Parallel "track-like" hypointensities on T2*
- High risk of future intracerebral hemorrhage
- Lobar hemorrhages, microbleeds

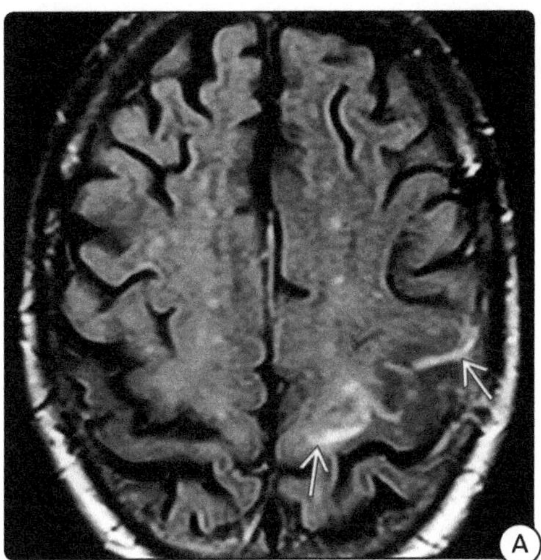

***(6-12A)** FLAIR in an 84-year-old woman with confusion, repeated falls shows left sulcal hyperintensity ➡, suggesting convexal SAH.*

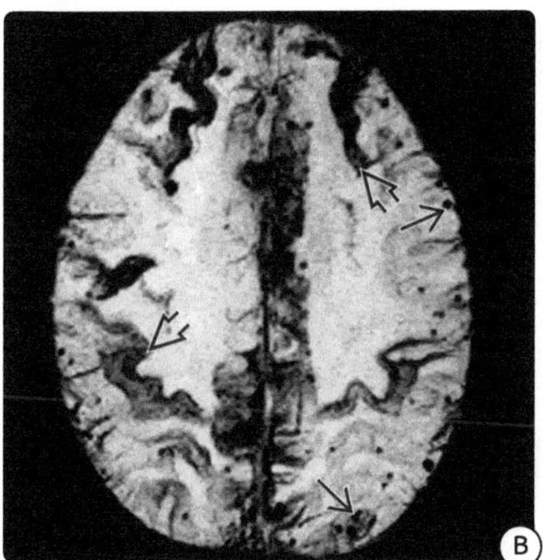

***(6-12B)** T2* SWI several years later shows multiple cortical microbleeds ➡, extensive bilateral cortical SS ➡.*

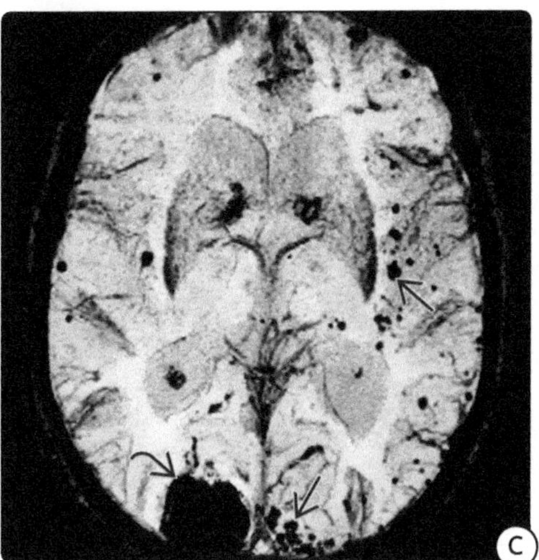

***(6-12C)** More inferior T2* SWI shows more cortical microbleeds ➡, acute R occipital lobar hematoma ➡. Cerebral amyloid angiopathy.*

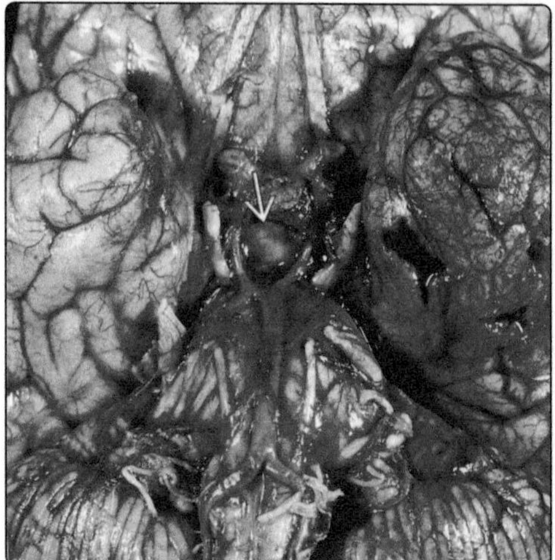

(6-13) Ruptured basilar bifurcation aneurysm ➡ has massive SAH extending throughout all the basilar cisterns. (Courtesy R. Hewlett, MD.)

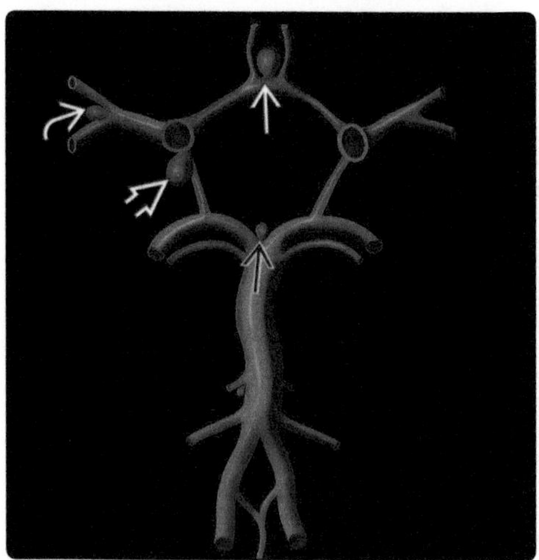

(6-14) Common SA sites are ACoA ➡ and the ICA-PCoA junction ➡. Other locations include the MCA bifurcation ➡ and the basilar tip ➡.

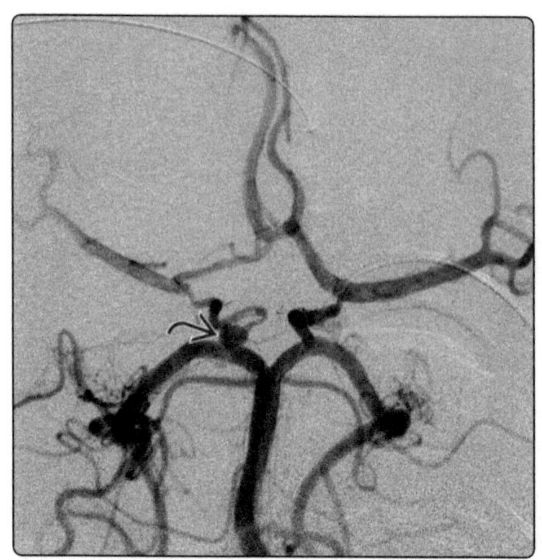

(6-15) Submentovertex DSA shows entire circle of Willis. A small SA ➡ arises from the junction of the right PCoA and the P1 PCA segment.

Aneurysms

Overview

Intracranial aneurysms are classified by their gross phenotypic appearance. The most common intracranial aneurysms are called **saccular** or **"berry" aneurysms** because of their striking sac- or berry-like configuration . Saccular aneurysms (SAs) are acquired lesions that arise from branch points of major cerebral arteries in which hemodynamic stresses are maximal. SAs lack some of the arterial layers (usually the internal elastic lamina and media) found in normal vessels. More than 90% of SAs occur on the "anterior" (carotid) circulation.

Pseudoaneurysms (also sometimes called "false" aneurysms) are focal arterial dilatations that are not contained by any layers of the normal arterial wall. They are often irregularly shaped and typically consist of a paravascular, noncontained blood clot that cavitates and communicates with the parent vessel lumen. Extracranial pseudoaneurysms are more common than intracranial lesions. Intracranial pseudoaneurysms usually arise from mid-sized arteries distal to the circle of Willis. Trauma, drug abuse, infection, and tumor are the usual etiologies.

Blood blister-like aneurysms (BBAs) are a special type of aneurysm recently recognized in the neurosurgical literature. BBAs are eccentric hemispherical arterial outpouchings that are covered by only a thin layer of adventitia. These dangerous lesions are both difficult to detect and difficult to treat. They have a tendency to rupture at a much smaller size and relatively younger age compared with SAs. Although BBAs can be found anywhere, they have a distinct propensity to occur along the supraclinoid internal carotid artery (ICA).

Fusiform aneurysms (FAs) are *focal* dilatations that involve the entire circumference of a vessel and extend for relatively short distances. FAs are more common on the vertebrobasilar ("posterior") circulation. FAs can be atherosclerotic (more common) or nonatherosclerotic in origin. Nonatherosclerotic FAs are often associated with collagen-vascular disorders, such as Marfan or Ehlers-Danlos type IV.

Saccular Aneurysm

Terminology

Saccular ("berry") aneurysms (SAs) are sometimes called "true" aneurysms (to contrast them with pseudoaneurysms).

An SA is a pathologic outward bulge that affects only part of the parent artery circumference. Most SAs lack two important structural components of normal intracranial arteries—the internal elastic lamina and the muscular layer ("media")—and often have a focally thinned wall that is prone to rupture.

Etiology

General Concepts. SAs are *acquired* lesions that develop from abnormal extracellular matrix (ECM) maintenance and excessive hemodynamic stress. SA formation begins with endothelial dysfunction followed by inflammatory cascades, pathologic remodeling, and degenerative changes in vessel walls.

Genetics. Very few SAs are congenital (i.e., present at birth). However, genome-wide association studies have found that several single nucleotide polymorphisms are expressed in SA patients.

Inherited connective tissue disorders, anomalous blood vessels, familial predisposition, and "high-flow" states (i.e., vessels supplying an arteriovenous malformation) all increase the risk of SA development.

Systemic hypertension, smoking, and heavy alcohol consumption contribute significantly to the risk of developing SAs and may augment any underlying genetic propensities.

Anomalous Blood Vessels. Bicuspid aortic valves, aortic coarctation, persistent trigeminal artery, and congenital anomalies of the anterior cerebral artery (ACA) (i.e., A1 asymmetries or infraoptic course of the A1 segment) all carry an increased risk of SA.

Inherited Vasculopathies and Syndromic Aneurysms. Some heritable connective tissue disorders (such as **Marfan** and **Ehlers-Danlos II and IV** syndromes or **fibromuscular dysplasia**) are associated with increased risk of intracranial aneurysms. Arteriopathy—not necessarily with aneurysm formation—is common in patients with **neurofibromatosis type 1** (NF1). **Autosomal dominant polycystic kidney disease (ADPCKD)** carries an increased lifetime risk (4-23%) of developing an SA.

SACCULAR ANEURYSM: ETIOLOGY

General Concepts
- Acquired, not congenital!
- Abnormal hemodynamics, shear stresses → weakened artery wall
- Underlying genetic alterations common

Increased Risk of Saccular Aneurysm
- Anomalous vessels
  - Persistent trigeminal artery
  - Fenestrated ACoA
- Vasculopathies, syndromes
  - Abnormal collagen (Marfan, Ehlers-Danlos)
  - Fibromuscular dysplasia
  - Autosomal dominant polycystic kidney disease
- Familial intracranial aneurysm
  - 4-10x ↑ risk if 1st-order family member with aSAH

Familial Intracranial Aneurysms. A positive family history represents the strongest known risk factor for aSAH (4-10x general population). Up to 20% of patients with SAs have a family history of intracranial aneurysms. SAs in "clusters" of related individuals without any known heritable connective tissue disorder are termed **familial intracranial aneurysms** (FIAs).

Pathology

Location. Most intracranial SAs occur at points of maximal hemodynamic stress. The vast majority arise from major blood vessel bifurcations or branches **(6-13)**. The circle of Willis plus the MCA bifurcations are the most common sites **(6-14)** **(6-15)**. Aneurysms beyond the circle of Willis are uncommon. Many peripheral aneurysms are actually pseudoaneurysms secondary to trauma, infection, or tumor.

Anterior Circulation Aneurysms. 90% of SAs occur on the "anterior" circulation **(6-14)**. The anterior circulation consists of the ICA and its terminal branches, the ACA, and MCA. Approximately 1/3 of SAs occur on the ACoA with another 1/3 arising at the junction of the ICA and the PCoA. Approximately 20% of SAs occur at the MCA bi- or trifurcation.

Posterior Circulation Aneurysms. 10% of SAs are located on the vertebrobasilar ("posterior") circulation. The basilar artery bifurcation is the

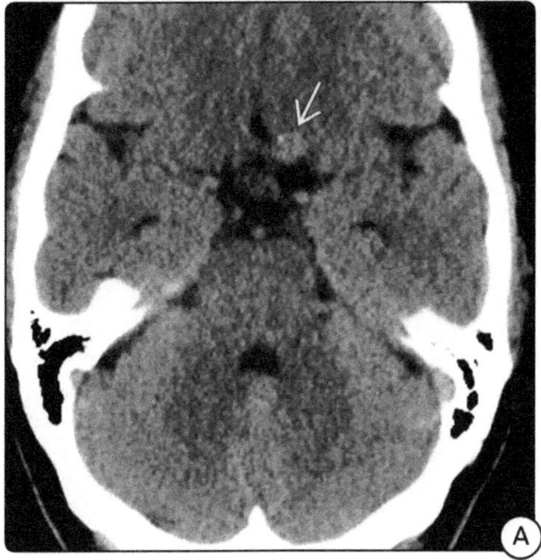

***(6-16A)** NECT in 49y woman with headaches shows rounded hyperdense mass ➡ adjacent to the suprasellar cistern with no evidence for SAH.*

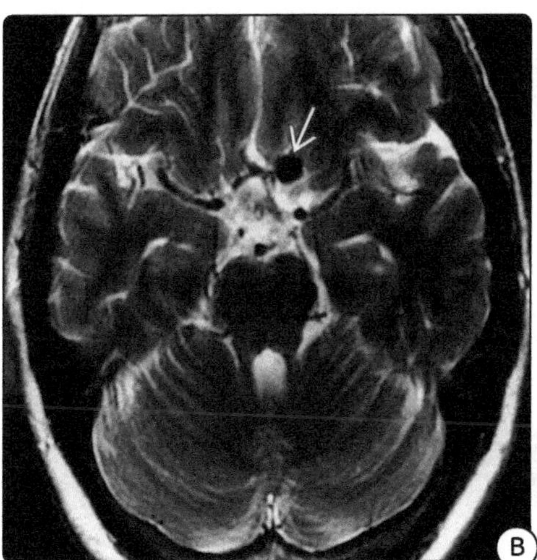

***(6-16B)** T2WI MR in the same case shows a very well-delineated "flow void" ➡ that appears to arise from the circle of Willis.*

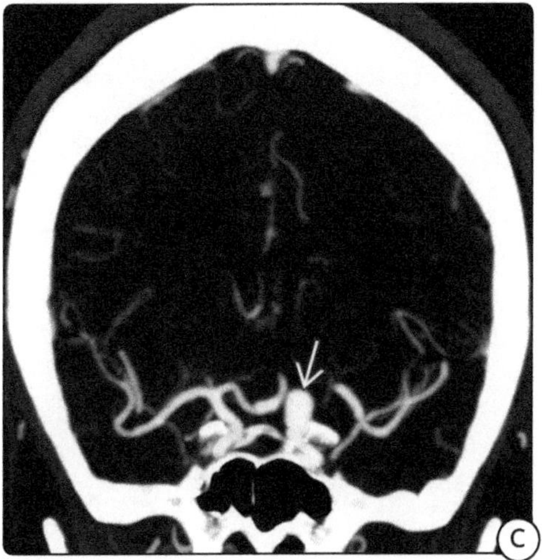

***(6-16C)** Coronal MIP of CTA in the same case shows that a lobulated SA ➡ arises from the distal ICA bifurcation.*

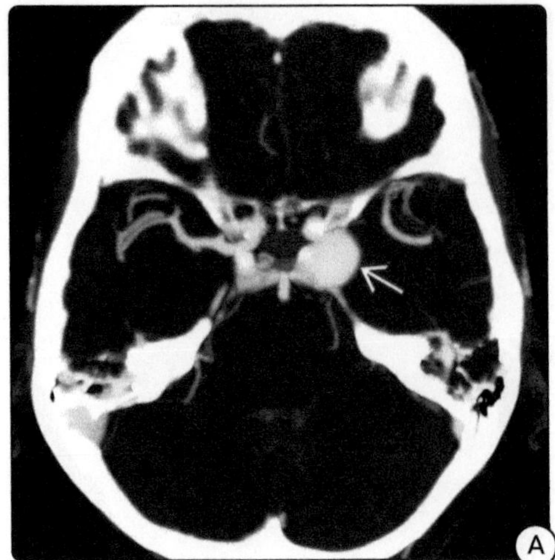

***(6-17A)** MIP of CTA in an 82-year-old woman with diplopia shows a well-delineated, intensely enhancing mass ➡ in the left cavernous sinus.*

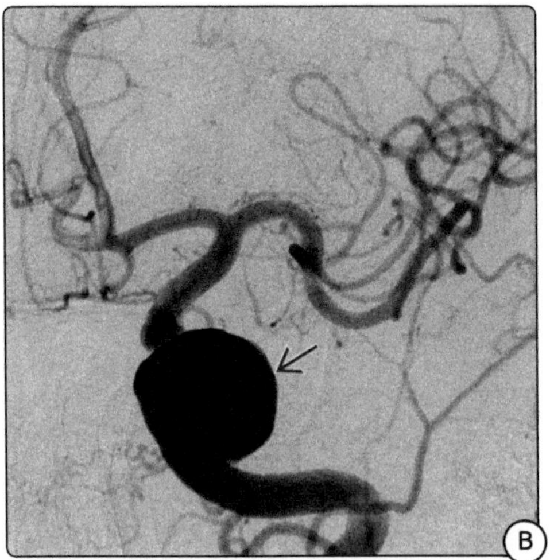

***(6-17B)** Oblique DSA of the left carotid angiogram shows a cavernous ICA aneurysm ➡, but details are difficult to appreciate.*

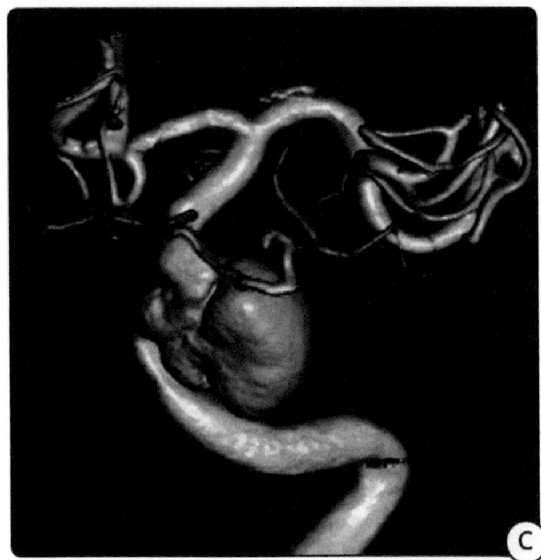

***(6-17C)** 3D rotational DSA with shaded surface display allowed full delineation of the aneurysm and its relationship to the parent vessel.*

most common site, accounting for ~ 5% of all SAs **(6-13)**. The posterior inferior cerebellar artery is the second most common location.

Size and Number. SAs vary in size from tiny (2-3 mm) to large lesions > 1 cm **(6-17)**. SAs that are ≥ 2.5 cm are called "giant" aneurysms. Between 15-20% of aneurysms are multiple and significantly more common in women.

Gross Pathology. The gross configuration of an SA changes with time as the arterial wall is remodeled in response to hemodynamic stresses. As it becomes progressively weakened, the wall begins to bulge outward, forming an SA. The opening (ostium) of an SA can be narrow or broad based. One or more lobules or an apical "tit" may develop. These outpouchings are the most vulnerable rupture site.

Microscopic Features. SAs demonstrate a disrupted or absent internal elastic lamina. The smooth muscle cell layer (media) is generally absent. The wall of an SA is usually quite fragile, consisting of intima and adventitia in a degraded ECM. Variable amounts of thrombus and atherosclerotic changes may also be present, especially in larger "giant" SAs. Inflammatory cell infiltration is a histologic hallmark of SAs.

SACCULAR ANEURYSM: PATHOLOGY

Location
- 90% anterior circulation
  - Circle of Willis, MCA bifurcation
  - ACoA, ICA/PCoA junction most common
- 10% posterior circulation (basilar bifurcation)

Size, Number
- Tiny (1-2 mm) to giant (≥ 2 cm)
- 15-20% multiple (> 2 F:M = 10:1)

Gross, Microscopic Features of SA Walls
- SAs lack internal elastic lamina, media
- Variable thrombus
- Inflammatory changes common

Clinical Issues

Epidemiology. Unruptured intracranial aneurysms (UIAs) are found in 3% of the adult population and are increasingly detected due to more frequent cranial imaging. Asymptomatic unruptured SAs are at least 10x more prevalent than ruptured SAs.

Demographics. Peak presentation is between 40 and 60 years of age. There is a definite female predominance, especially with multiple SAs. SAs are rare in children, accounting for < 2% of all cases. Childhood aneurysms lack female predominance and are more often associated with trauma or infection.

Presentation. Between 80-90% of all ntSAHs are caused by ruptured SAs. The most common presentation is sudden onset of severe, excruciating headache ("thunderclap" or "worst headache of my life").

Cranial neuropathy is a relatively uncommon presentation of SA. Of these, a pupil-involving CNIII palsy from a PCoA aneurysm is the most common. Occasionally, patients with partially or completely thrombosed aneurysms present with a transient ischemic attack (TIA) or stroke.

Natural History. The overall annual rupture rate of all SAs is 1-2%. However, the rupture risk varies according to size, location, and shape of the aneurysm.

Size and Rupture Risk. Aneurysms that are ≥ 5 mm are associated with a significantly increased risk of rupture compared with 2- to 4-mm aneurysms. Demonstrable growth on surveillance imaging is also associated with an increased rupture risk.

Shape/Configuration and Rupture Risk. In addition to size, shape and configuration also matter. Nonsaccular (nonspherical) shape increases rupture risk. The presence of a "daughter" sac (irregular wall protrusion) and increased aspect ratio (length compared with width) are independent predictors of rupture risk.

Location and Rupture Risk. Vertebrobasilar artery aneurysms have a significantly higher rupture risk, as do ICA-PCoA aneurysms. MCA and ACA aneurysms are associated with modest risk. Bifurcation aneurysms are more prone to growth than sidewall aneurysms.

Treatment Options. aSAH is a catastrophic event with high mortality and significant morbidity. Approximately 1/3 of patients die and 1/3 survive with significant residual neurologic deficits. Only 1/4 to 1/3 of patients with aSAH recover with good functional outcome.

Ruptured SAs. Virtually all *ruptured* SAs are treated. Neuroendovascular options, such as coiling (with or without balloon/stent assistance) and flow diversion are increasingly more common. The percentage of patients with cerebral aneurysms treated with craniotomy and clip ligation is decreasing.

Unruptured SAs. The management of *unruptured* SAs (UIAs) is controversial because of their unpredictable natural history. Initial size and multiplicity are significant factors related to aneurysm growth. Recent studies have shown that the growth rate for 7-mm UIAs is significantly faster than that for < 3-mm UIAs.

CLINICAL FEATURES OF SACCULAR ANEURYSMS

Epidemiology
- 3% of population; F > M
- Peak age of presentation: 40-60 years (rare in children)

Presentation
- Most common = SAH
  - Sudden, severe "thunderclap" headache
  - Mass effect (CN palsy) less common

Natural History
- Most SAs don't rupture!
- Incidental finding of SA on imaging increasingly common

What Increases Risk of Rupture?
- Size matters!
  - Rupture risk increases with size
  - ≥ 5 mm greater risk than 2-4 mm
- Shape, configuration matter!
  - Nonround (nonsaccular shape) = ↑ rupture risk!
  - "Daughter" sac or "tit" = ↑ rupture risk!
- Location affects rupture risk!
  - Vertebrobasilar, ICA-PCoA location highest rupture risk
  - MCA, ACA moderate risk; non-PCoA-ICA aneurysms lowest
- **Type**
  - BBAs rupture at smaller size

Imaging

General Features. SAs are round or lobulated arterial outpouchings that are most commonly found along the circle of Willis and at the MCA bifurcation.

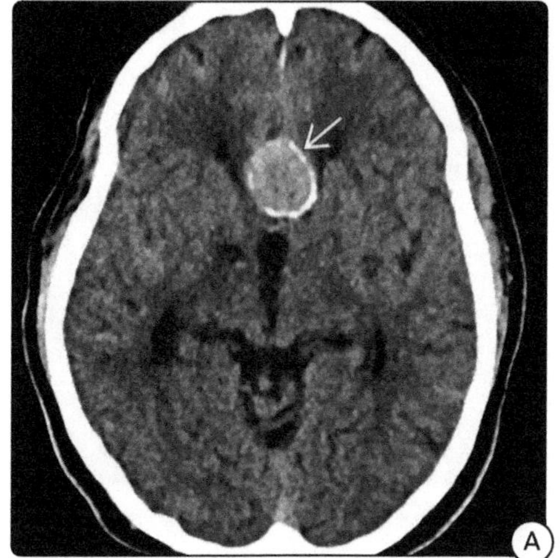

(6-18A) *NECT shows a well-delineated hyperdense midline mass ➡ with peripheral calcification. The lesion is 2.5 cm in diameter.*

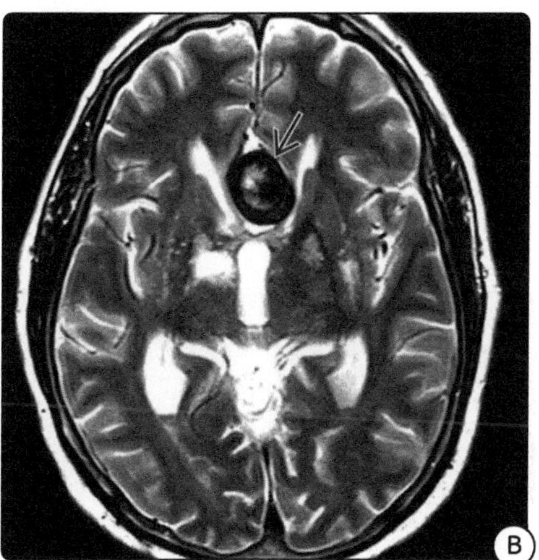

(6-18B) *T2WI MR in the same case shows concentric hypointense layers of thrombus ⇨ surrounding a mixed signal intensity core.*

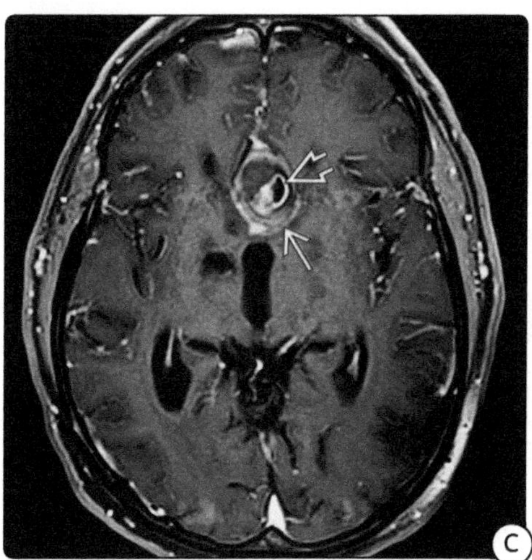

(6-18C) *T1 C+ FS MR shows enhancement ➡ around the thrombosed aneurysm wall and around the residual lumen ➡.*

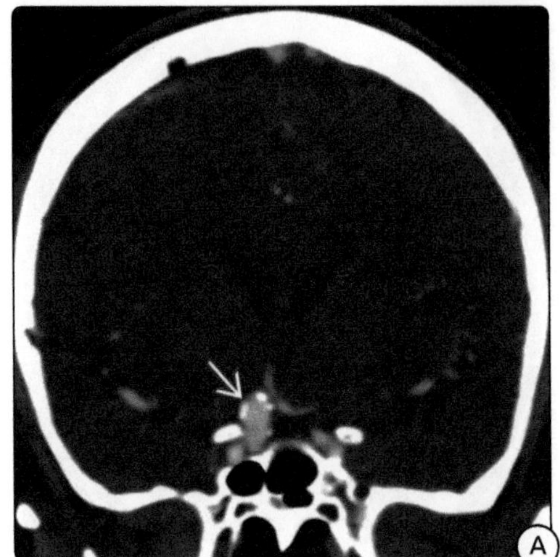

***(6-19A)** Coronal CTA in a 70-year-old woman with headaches shows a partially calcified aneurysm of the distal right ICA ➔.*

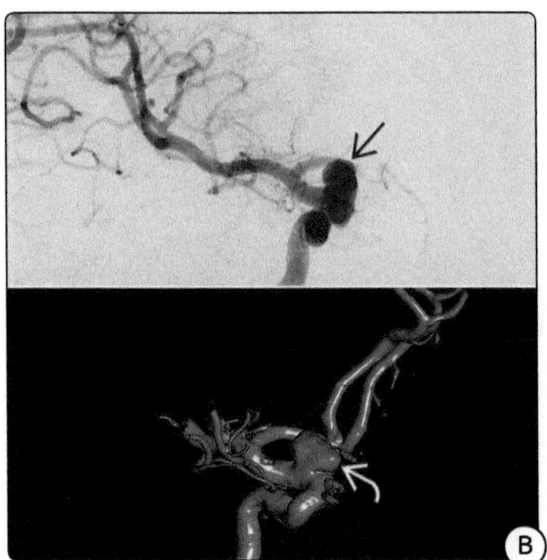

***(6-19B)** (Top) AP DSA in same case shows the aneurysm ➔. (Bottom) 3D SSA shows its detailed complex, multilobulated configuration ➔.*

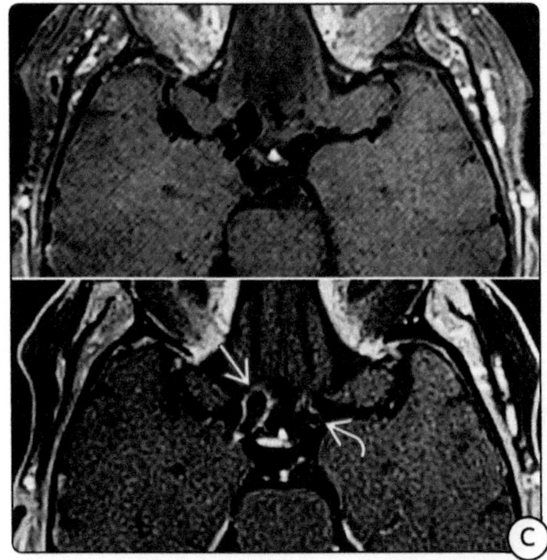

***(6-19C)** T1 C+ FS MR shows strong enhancement of the aneurysm wall ➔ & normal enhancement of left distal ICA ➔. (Courtesy S. McNally, MD.)*

Imaging features depend on whether the aneurysm is unruptured or ruptured (with aSAH) and whether the aneurysm sac is patent or partially or completely thrombosed.

CT Findings. Very small unruptured SAs may be invisible on standard NECT scans. Larger lesions appear as well-delineated masses that are slightly hyperdense to brain **(6-16A)**. Rim **(6-18A)** or mural calcification **(6-19A)** may be present.

Acutely ruptured SAs present with aSAH, which is often the dominant imaging feature and frequently obscures the "culprit" aneurysm. Occasionally, an SA appears as a well-delineated, relatively hypodense filling defect within a pool of hyperdense subarachnoid blood.

A partially or completely thrombosed SA is typically hyperdense compared with the adjacent brain on NECT scans.

Patent SAs show strong, uniform enhancement of the aneurysm lumen. A partially thrombosed SA shows enhancement of the residual lumen. Completely thrombosed SAs do not enhance, although longstanding lesions may demonstrate rim enhancement secondary to reactive inflammatory changes.

MR Findings. MR findings vary with pulse sequence, flow dynamics, and the presence as well as the age of associated hemorrhage (either in the subarachnoid cisterns or within the aneurysm itself).

About 1/2 of all patent SAs demonstrate "flow voids" on T1WI and T2WI **(6-16B)**. The other 1/2 exhibit heterogeneous signal intensity secondary to slow or turbulent flow, saturation effects, and phase dispersion. Propagation of pulsation artifacts in the phase-encoding direction is common. FLAIR scans may show hyperintensity in the subarachnoid cisterns secondary to aSAH.

If the aneurysm is partially or completely thrombosed, laminated clot with differing signal intensities is often present **(6-18)**. "Blooming" on susceptibility-weighted images (GRE, SWI) is common. Contrast-enhanced scans may show T1 shortening in intraaneurysmal slow-flow areas. High-resolution contrast-enhanced MR may demonstrate inflammatory changes in the aneurysm wall **(6-19C)** and adjacent brain **(6-18C)**.

DWI sequences may show ischemic areas secondary to vasospasm or embolized thrombus.

Angiography. High-resolution CTA is a common screening procedure in patients with suspected aSAH. The sensitivity of CTA is > 95% for aneurysms > 2 mm in diameter **(6-16C)**.

Although many patients with aSAH and an SA that has been demonstrated on either CTA or MRA go directly to surgery, conventional DSA is still considered the gold standard for detecting intracranial SAs—especially if endovascular treatment is considered.

Multiple intracranial aneurysms are shown in 15-20% of cases. When more than one aneurysm is identified in aSAH patients, determining which aneurysm ruptured is essential for presurgical planning. Angiographic features suggesting rupture include lobulation or presence of an apical "tit," size (the largest aneurysm is generally, though not always, the one that ruptured), and presence of focal perianeurysmal clot on CT or MR.

Differential Diagnosis

The major differential diagnosis of intracranial SA is a **vessel loop**. Intracranial arteries curve and branch extensively. CTA/DSA with multiple projections, MIP views, and 3D shaded surface displays are helpful in sorting out overlapping or looping vessels from SA.

SACCULAR ANEURYSM: IMAGING AND DDx

Imaging
- Round/lobulated arterial outpouching
- CTA 95% sensitive if aneurysm > 2 mm
- DSA with 3D SSD best delineates architecture

Differential Diagnosis
- Vessel loop
- Arterial infundibulum
  - Conical
  - ≤ 2 mm
  - ICA-PCoA junction
- Blood blister-like aneurysm
  - Hemispherical bulge
  - Along superior surface of supraclinoid ICA
- Pseudoaneurysm
  - Usually distal to circle of Willis, MCA bifurcation
  - History of trauma, drugs, infection, neoplasm

The second most common differential diagnosis is an **arterial infundibulum**. An infundibulum is a focal, symmetric, conical dilatation at the origin of a blood vessel that can easily be mistaken for a small SA. An infundibulum is small, typically < 3 mm in diameter. The distal vessel typically arises from the apex—not the side—of the infundibulum. The PCoA is the most common location for an infundibulum.

A **pseudoaneurysm** may be difficult to distinguish from an SA. Pseudoaneurysms are more common on vessels distal to the circle of Willis and are often fusiform or irregular in shape. Focal parenchymal hematomas often surround intracranial pseudoaneurysms.

A **blood blister-like aneurysm** (BBA) may also be difficult to distinguish from a small, wide-necked SA. Although they can be found in virtually any part of the intracranial circulation, BBAs typically arise along the greater curvature of the supraclinoid ICA, not at its terminal bifurcation or PCoA origin.

Pseudoaneurysm

Pseudoaneurysm is a rare but important underdiagnosed cause of intracranial hemorrhage, accounting for just 1-6% of all intracranial aneurysms. Delayed onset and continued deterioration of neurologic symptoms are common.

Terminology

Pseudoaneurysm—also sometimes called a "false" aneurysm to distinguish it from a "true" SA—is an arterial dilatation with complete disruption of the arterial wall.

Etiology

Pseudoaneurysms are usually caused by a specific inciting event—e.g., trauma, infection, drug abuse, neoplasm, or surgery—that initially weakens and then disrupts the normal arterial wall. Pseudoaneurysms are contained only by relatively fragile, friable cavitated clot and variable amounts of fibrous tissue.

Pathology

Location. Approximately 80% of pseudoaneurysms affecting the carotid and vertebral arteries are extracranial, whereas 20% involve their intracranial segments. Patients with traumatic cavernous/paraclinoid ICA

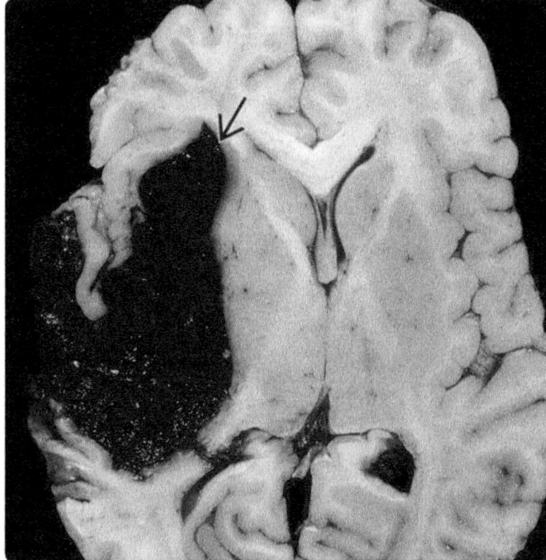

***(6-20)** Large focal right temporal lobe hematoma ⇒ was caused by a ruptured mycotic pseudoaneurysm of the MCA (not shown).*

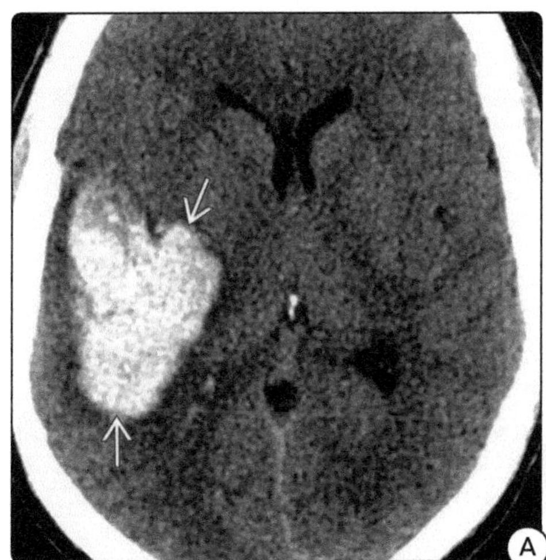

***(6-21A)** NECT shows sICH ➡ in a patient with bacterial endocarditis. History suggests mycotic pseudoaneurysm as possible underlying etiology.*

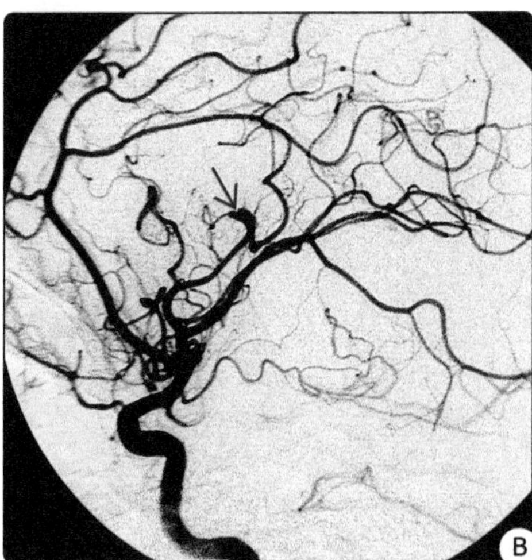

***(6-21B)** DSA demonstrates an irregular fusiform dilatation of an M2 MCA branch ⇒. Mycotic pseudoaneurysm was confirmed at surgery.*

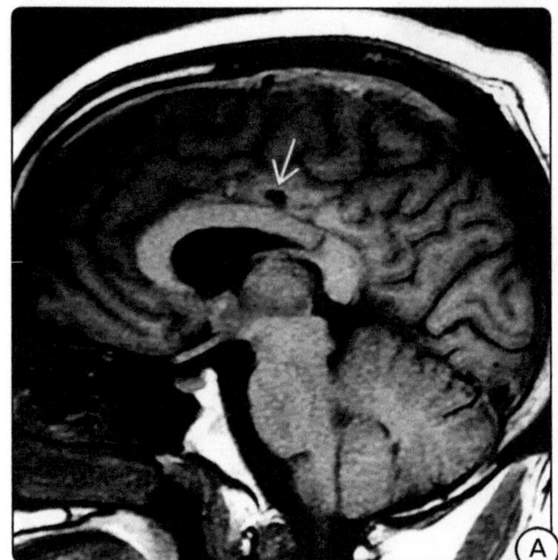

(6-22A) Sagittal T1WI in a 23-year-old man with headaches, remote history of head trauma shows a "flow void" ➡ above the corpus callosum.

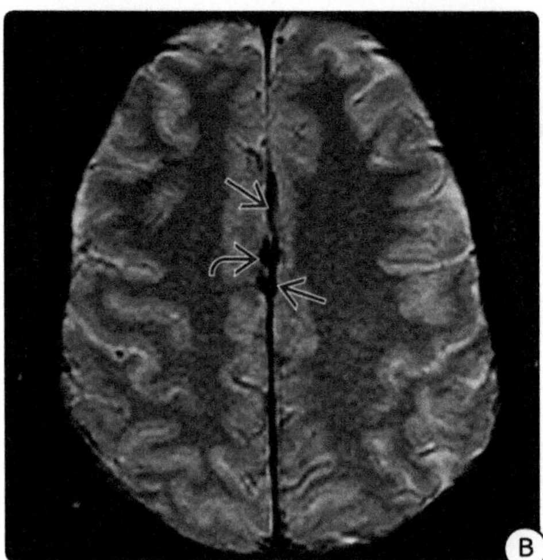

(6-22B) T2 GRE shows some hemosiderin staining along the falx cerebri ➡ adjacent to the flow void ➡.*

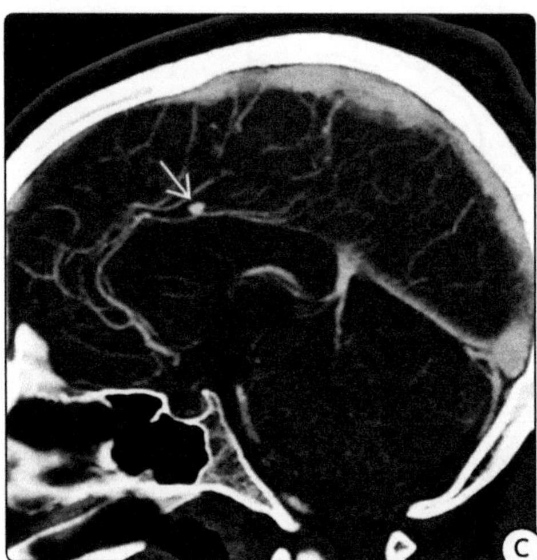

(6-22C) Sagittal CTA shows a pericallosal artery pseudoaneurysm ➡. The ACA was impacted against the falx during closed head injury.

pseudoaneurysms often have skull base fractures. Pseudoaneurysms distal to the circle of Willis are usually infectious (mycotic), drug related, neoplastic (oncotic), or traumatic in origin.

Gross Pathology. Pseudoaneurysms are purplish masses typically contained only by thinned, discontinuous adventitia and organized hematoma. Hematomas associated with pseudoaneurysms are often large and may contain clots of varying ages.

Clinical Issues

As they lack normal vessel wall components, pseudoaneurysms are especially prone to hemorrhage. The interval between the initial injury and neurologic deterioration varies from a few days up to several months.

Imaging

CT Findings. A paravascular parenchymal hematoma is common **(6-21)**. CTA sometimes shows a "spot" sign (focus of contrast enhancement) within a rapidly expanding hematoma.

MR Findings. Hematoma signal varies with clot age and sequence. A "flow void" representing the residual lumen may be present within the hematoma. Intravascular enhancement represents the slow, delayed filling and emptying often seen with pseudoaneurysms.

Angiography. Digital subtraction angiography shows a globular, fusiform, or irregularly shaped "neckless" aneurysm with delayed filling and emptying of contrast agent **(6-21B)**. Endovascular occlusion with a flow-diverting stent is now the method of choice to treat most intracranial pseudoaneurysms.

Differential Diagnosis

The major differential diagnosis of pseudoaneurysm is a "true" aneurysm or **saccular aneurysm**. Location is a helpful feature, as SAs typically occur along the circle of Willis and at the MCA bifurcation.

PSEUDOANEURYSM: IMAGING AND DDx

Imaging Features
- Irregularly shaped outpouching
  - "Neck" usually absent
  - ± surrounding avascular mass effect (cavitated hematoma)
- CTA
  - May show "spot" sign
  - Pseudoaneurysms often small, easily overlooked
  - DSA may be required if CTA is negative
- MR: Look for distal emboli

Differential Diagnosis
- Blood blister-like aneurysm
  - May be form of pseudoaneurysm
- Saccular aneurysm
- Dissecting aneurysm
- Fusiform aneurysm

Blood Blister-Like Aneurysm

Blood blister-like aneurysm (BBA), a.k.a. blister or "dorsal variant blister" aneurysm, is an uncommon but potentially lethal subtype of intracranial pseudoaneurysm. BBAs can be difficult to diagnose and treacherous to treat. They represent ~ 1% of all intracranial aneurysms and 0.5-2.0% of all ruptured aneurysms.

BBAs are small, broad-based hemispheric bulges that typically arise at nonbranching sites of intracranial arteries (most commonly the supraclinoid ICA) **(6-23)**. BBAs have different clinical features and pose special diagnostic and treatment challenges compared with those of typical SAs. Preoperative recognition of a BBA is essential for proper management.

Pathology

Hemodynamic stress and atherosclerosis seem to be the most important factors in formation of a BBA. BBAs are often covered with only a thin fragile fibrin layer or a friable cap of fibrous tissue **(6-24)**. Although BBAs can arise anywhere in the intracranial circulation, the anterosuperior (dorsal) wall of the supraclinoid ICA is the most common site.

Clinical Issues

BBAs exhibit more aggressive behavior compared with SAs. They tend to rupture at an earlier patient age and at a significantly smaller size compared with typical SAs. They are also extremely fragile lesions that lack a definable neck and easily tear during surgical clipping. Intraprocedural rupture is common, occurring in nearly 50% of cases.

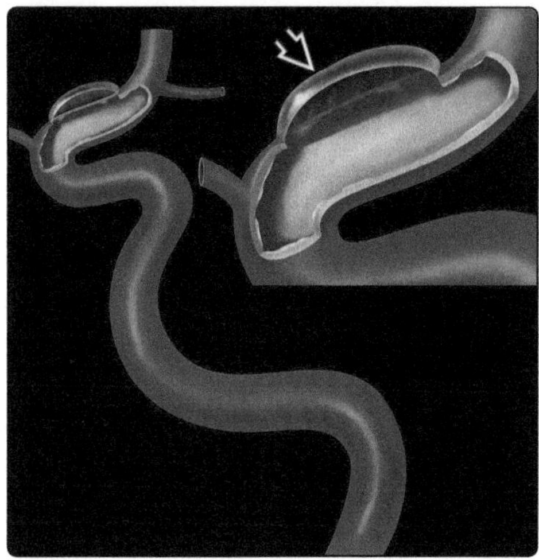

***(6-23)** Blood blister-like aneurysm is seen here as a broad-based hemispheric bulge covered with a tissue-paper-thin layer of adventitia ➡.*

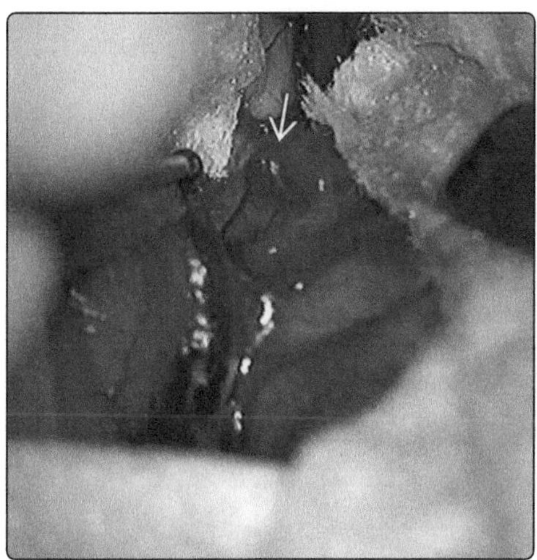

***(6-24)** Intraoperative photograph shows a blood blister-like aneurysm ➡ with blood under the thin, nearly transparent aneurysm wall.*

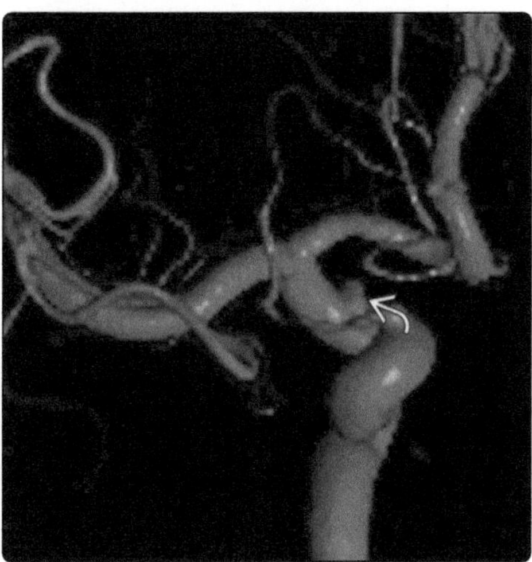

***(6-25)** DSA with SSD in a patient with SAH shows a tiny blood blister-like aneurysm ➡.*

BLOOD BLISTER-LIKE ANEURYSM

Pathology
- Broad-based "blister" covered by thin friable tissue cap
- Usually solitary
- Can occur almost anywhere
- Dorsal wall of supraclinoid ICA most common site

Clinical Issues
- Easily rupture, may cause catastrophic aSAH
- Compared with SAs
  - Rupture at earlier age
  - Rupture at smaller size

Imaging
- Small, easy to miss on CTA
- DSA with 3D shaded surface display best

Treatment
- Endovascular > surgical clipping
  - Flow-diverting stent
  - Stent-assisted coil embolization

Imaging

BBAs are small, often subtle lesions that are easily overlooked. A slight irregularity or small focal hemispherical bulge of the arterial wall may be the only finding **(6-25)**. 3D DSA with shaded surface display has been helpful in identifying these difficult, dangerous lesions.

Fusiform Aneurysm

FAs can be atherosclerotic (common) or nonatherosclerotic (rare). In contrast to SAs, FAs usually involve long, nonbranching vessel segments and are seen as focal circumferential outpouchings from a generally ectatic, elongated vessel.

Atherosclerotic FAs are typically seen in older adults. Nonatherosclerotic FAs can be seen at any age but are most common in children and younger adults.

(6-26A) MIP CTA shows a fusiform aneurysm of the basilar artery as well as dolichoectasia of both supraclinoid ICAs.

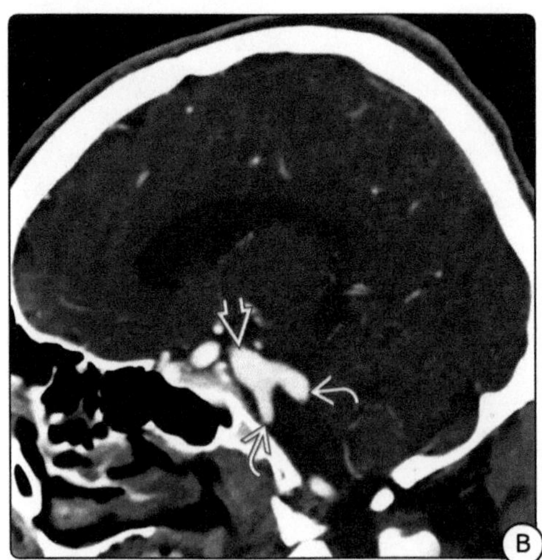

(6-26B) Sagittal CTA in the same case shows the fusiform dilatation of the basilar artery and enlarged ectatic distal vertebral arteries.

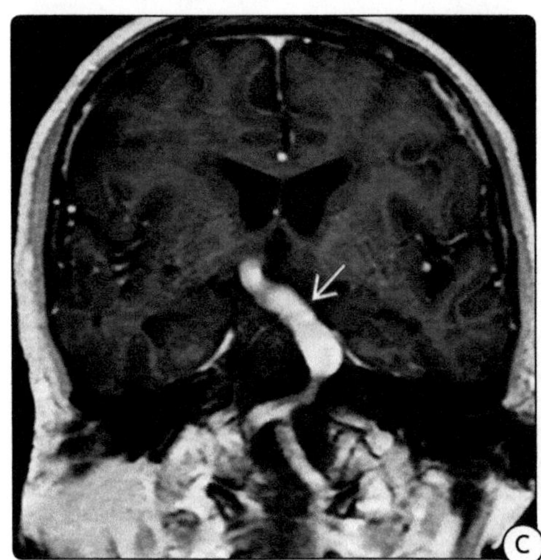

(6-26C) Coronal T1 C+ MR shows the fusiform ASVD basilar aneurysm. Flow is very slow, so the entire vertebrobasilar system is opacified.

Atherosclerotic Fusiform Aneurysm

Terminology

Atherosclerotic FAs (ASVD FAs) are also called aneurysmal dolichoectasias, distinguishing them from the more generalized nonfocal vessel elongations seen as a common manifestation of intracranial atherosclerosis.

Pathology

Arteriectasis is common with advanced atherosclerosis of the cerebral arteries. Fusiform dilatation is a frequent complication. Generalized ASVD with a focally dilated fusiform enlargement is the typical gross manifestation of an ASVD FA.

ASVD FAs are more common in the vertebrobasilar (posterior) circulation and usually affect the basilar artery. Atherosclerotic plaques of foam cells with thickened but irregular intima and extensive loss of elastica and media are present. Layers of organized thrombus surrounding a patent residual lumen are common.

Clinical Issues

Peak age of presentation is the seventh to eighth decade. Posterior circulation TIAs and stroke are the most common presentation. Cranial neuropathy is relatively uncommon.

Imaging

General Features. ASVD FAs are often large (> 2.5 cm in diameter) fusiform or ovoid dilatations that are superimposed on generalized vascular dolichoectasias **(6-26)**.

CT Findings. ASVD FAs are often partially thrombosed and frequently demonstrate mural calcification. Heterogeneously hyperdense clot is often present. The residual lumen enhances intensely following contrast enhancement.

MR Findings. Signal intensity of FAs varies with pulse sequence, degree and direction of flow, and the presence and age of clot within the FA. Slow, turbulent flow in the residual lumen causes complex, sometimes bizarre signal.

FAs are often very heterogeneous on T1WI and strikingly hypointense on T2WI. The residual lumen can be seen as a rounded "flow void" surrounded by complex thrombus that varies from hypointense to hyperintense. Intense enhancement of the residual lumen with prominent phase artifact is common following contrast administration.

Inflammatory changes are common in the walls of ASVD FAs. Vessel wall imaging may show variable enhancement. The enhancement is typically patchy, short segment, and discontinuous.

Angiography. CTA and DSA show generalized enlargement and ectasia of the parent vessel with a focal, round or fusiform, somewhat irregular contour **(6-26)**. In some cases, the residual lumen resides within a larger mass caused by mural thrombus.

Differential Diagnosis

The major differential diagnosis of an ASVD FA is **dolichoectasia**. Dolichoectasias are fusiform elongations of vessels—usually in the posterior circulation—without focal fusiform or saccular dilatations.

Nonatherosclerotic FAs are seen in younger patients who often have an inherited vasculopathy or immune deficiency (see below). Like ASVD FAs, intracranial **dissecting aneurysms** are most common on the vertebrobasilar (posterior) circulation. Findings of generalized ASVD are usually absent.

ATHEROSCLEROTIC FUSIFORM ANEURYSM

Terminology
- ASVD with focally dilated fusiform enlargement
- a.k.a. aneurysmal dolichoectasias

Pathology
- More common in vertebrobasilar artery
- Affects long nonbranching segment
- ASVD with irregular intima
- Extensive loss of elastica, media
- Layers of organized mural, intraluminal thrombus
  - Clot often much larger than residual lumen

Clinical Issues
- Middle-aged, older patients
  - Peak = 60-80 years
  - Most common = posterior circulation TIAs, stroke

Imaging
- CT, CTA
  - Generalized changes of ASVD present
  - Elongated vessel + fusiform or ovoid dilatation
  - Mural Ca^{++}
  - Partial thrombosis common
- MR
  - Layered thrombus in wall, lumen
  - Signal intensity often complex
  - Clot surrounds variably sized residual "flow void"

Differential Diagnosis
- Dolichoectasia
  - Elongated artery
  - No focal fusiform or saccular dilatation
- Dissection, dissecting aneurysm
  - Often younger patients
  - Also posterior circulation
  - ASVD changes minimal/absent
- Nonatherosclerotic fusiform aneurysm
  - Younger patients (including children)
  - Inherited vasculopathy (e.g., Marfan, Ehlers-Danlos type IV)
  - Vascular neurocutaneous syndrome (e.g., NF1)
  - Acquired immune deficiency

Nonatherosclerotic Fusiform Aneurysm

Terminology

Nonatherosclerotic fusiform aneurysms (nASVD FAs) are fusiform elongations that occur in the absence of generalized intracranial ASVD.

Etiology

nASVD FAs occur with collagen vascular disorders (e.g., lupus), inherited vasculopathies (e.g., Marfan, Ehlers-Danlos), and vascular neurocutaneous syndrome (NF1, tuberous sclerosis). Viral infections (varicella, HIV) can also cause nonatherosclerotic vasculopathy.

Pathology

nASVD FAs are focally dilated fusiform arterial ectasias that often involve nonbranching segments of intracranial arteries. Multiple lesions are common. The carotid (anterior) and vertebrobasilar circulations are equally affected.

Clinical Issues

Patients tend to be younger than those with ASVD FAs. nASVD FAs are most common in children and young adults. HIV-associated aneurysmal arteriopathy carries an especially high morbidity.

Imaging

Long segments of tubular, fusiform, or ovoid arterial dilatations are seen in the absence of generalized ASVD. Circumferential involvement of the affected vessels is typical, as is extension into proximal branches.

Differential Diagnosis

Fusiform intracranial dilatations in relatively young patients should suggest the possibility of nASVD vasculopathy and FA with or without accompanying dissection. **Vertebrobasilar dolichoectasia** is seen in older patients with generalized changes of ASVD.

Selected References: The complete reference list is available on the Expert Consult™ eBook version included with purchase.

Vascular Malformations

Brain vascular malformations, a.k.a. cerebrovascular malformations (CVMs), are a heterogeneous group of disorders that exhibit a broad spectrum of biologic behaviors. Some CVMs (e.g., capillary malformations) are almost always clinically silent and found incidentally on imaging studies. Others, such as arteriovenous malformations (AVMs) and cavernous angiomas, may hemorrhage unexpectedly and without warning.

In this chapter, we begin with an overview of CVMs, starting with a discussion of terminology, etiology, and classification. CVMs are grouped according to whether or not they exhibit arteriovenous shunting, and then each type is discussed individually.

Terminology

Two major groups of vascular anomalies are recognized: Vascular *malformations* and vascular *hemangiomas*. All CVMs—the entities considered in this chapter—are malformative lesions and are thus designated as "malformations" or "angiomas." In contrast, vascular "hemangiomas" are true proliferating vasoformative neoplasms. Hemangiomas are classified as nonmeningothelial mesenchymal tumors and discussed in Chapter 22 with meningiomas and other mesenchymal neoplasms.

Classification

CVMs have been traditionally classified by histopathology into four major types: (1) AVMs, (2) venous angiomas (developmental venous anomalies), (3) capillary telangiectasias (sometimes simply termed "telangiectasia" or "telangiectasis"), and (4) cavernous malformations.

Many interventional neuroradiologists and neurosurgeons group CVMs by function, not histopathology. In this functional classification, CVMs are divided into two basic categories: (1) CVMs that display arteriovenous shunting and (2) CVMs without arteriovenous shunting **(Table 7-1)**. The former are potentially amenable to endovascular intervention; the latter are either treated surgically or left alone.

Cerebrovascular Malformations

Type	Etiology	Pathology	Number	Location	Prevalence	Age	Hemorrhage Risk	Best Imaging Clues
CVMs With Arteriovenous Shunts								
AV malformations	Congenital (dysregulated angiogenesis)	Nidus + arterial feeders, draining veins; no capillary bed	Solitary (< 2% multiple)	Parenchyma (85%); supratentorial (15%); posterior fossa	0.04-0.50% of population; 85-90% of CVMs with AV shunting	Peak = 20-40 years (25% by age 15 years)	Very high (2-4% per year, cumulative)	"Bag of worms," "flow voids" on MR
Dural AV fistula	Acquired (trauma; dural sinus thrombosis)	Network of multiple AV microfistulas	Solitary	Skull base; dural sinus wall	10-15% of CVMs with AV shunting	Peak = 40-60 years	Varies with venous draining (increased if cortical veins involved)	Enlarged meningeal arteries with network of tiny vessels in wall of thrombosed dural venous sinus
Vein of Galen malformation	Congenital (fetal arterial fistula to primitive precursor of vein of Galen)	Large venous pouch	Solitary	Behind 3rd ventricle	< 1% of CVMs with AV shunting	Newborn > > infant, older child	Low (but hydrocephalus brain damage common)	Large midline venous varix in neonate with high-output congestive heart failure
CVMs Without Arteriovenous Shunts								
Developmental venous anomaly	Congenital (arrested fetal medullary vein development)	Dilated WM veins; normal brain in between	Solitary (unless BRBNS)	Deep WM, usually near ventricle	Most common CVM (60% of all), between 2-9% of population	Any age	Extremely low unless mixed with cavernous malformation	"Medusa head" of dilated WM veins converging on enlarged collector vein
Sinus pericranii	Congenital	Bluish blood-filled subcutaneous scalp mass	Solitary	Scalp	Rare	Any age (usually childhood)	Extremely low unless direct trauma	Vascular scalp mass connecting through skull defect to intracranial venous circulation
Cavernous malformation	Congenital (CCM, *KRIT1* gene mutations in familial autosomal dominant syndrome; "de novo" lesions continue to form)	Collection of blood-filled "caverns" with no normal brain; complete hemosiderin rim	2/3 solitary (sporadic) ; 1/3 multiple (familial)	Throughout brain		Any age (peak: 40-60 years; younger in familial CCM syndrome)	High (0.25-0.75% per year; 1% per lesion per year in familial)	Varies; most common is solitary "popcorn ball" (locules with blood-fluid levels, hemosiderin rim); multifocal "black dots" in familial
Capillary telangiectasia	Congenital	Dilated capillaries; normal brain in between	Solitary > > multiple	Anywhere but pons; medulla most common	15-20% of all CVMs	Any age (peak: 30-40 years)	Extremely low unless mixed with cavernous malformation	Faint brush-like enhancement, becomes hypointense on T2*

(Table 7-1) *AV = arteriovenous; BRBNS = blue rubber bleb nevus syndrome; CCM = cerebral cavernous malformation; CVM = cerebrovascular malformation; WM = white matter.*

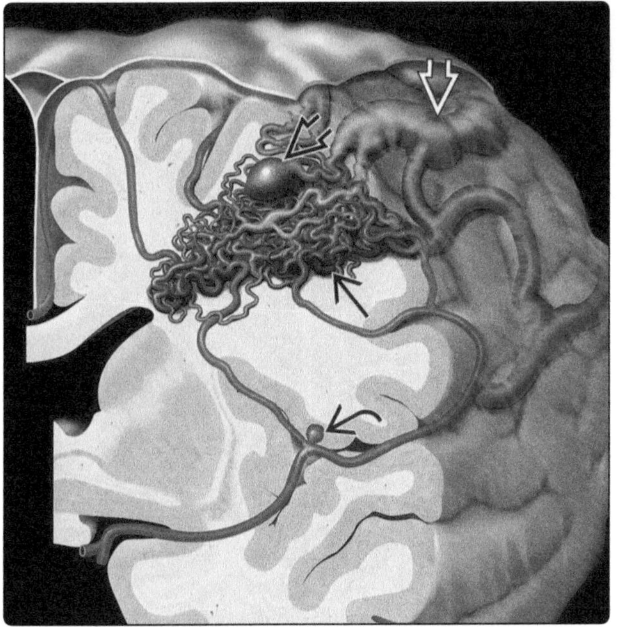

(7-1) Graphic depicts pyramid-shaped arteriovenous malformation (AVM) nidus ➡ with broad base toward cortical surface. Intranidal aneurysm ➡, feeding artery ("pedicle") aneurysm ➡, and enlarged draining veins ➡ are shown.

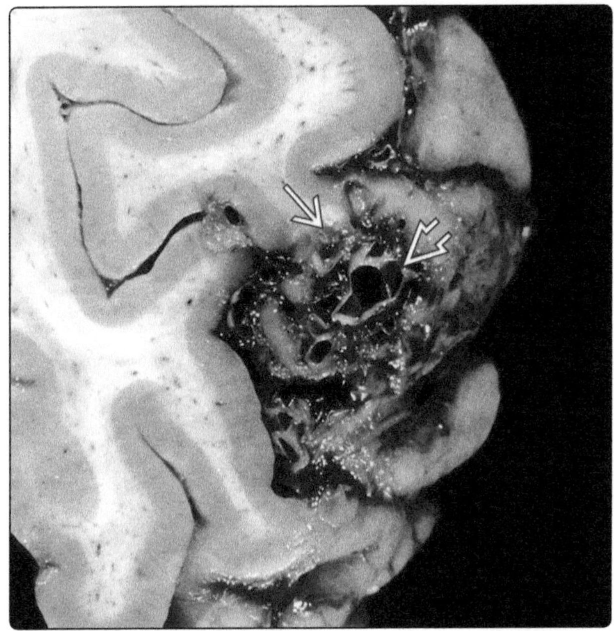

(7-2) Autopsy case demonstrates a classic AVM. The nidus ➡ contains no normal brain. An intranidal aneurysm ➡ is present. (Courtesy R. Hewlett, MD.)

CVMs With Arteriovenous Shunting

Arteriovenous Malformation

Terminology

An arteriovenous malformation (AVM) is a tightly packed "snarl" or "tangle" of serpiginous, thin-walled vessels without an intervening capillary bed. Most brain AVMs (BAVMs) are parenchymal lesions and are also called "pial AVMs," although mixed pial-dural malformations do occur.

Etiology

Genetics. Most AVMs are solitary and nonsyndromic. Somatic *KRAS* mutations activating the MAPK-ERK signaling pathway in brain endothelial cells have recently been identified as playing a key role in BAVM development.

Multiple AVMs are almost always syndromic. The genetic basis for several Mendelian syndromes with BAVM as part of the phenotype have been defined. These include **hereditary hemorrhagic telangiectasia** (HHT, a.k.a. Rendu-Osler-Weber disease), a genetically mediated hereditary disorder characterized by epistaxis, mucocutaneous telangiectases, and visceral AVMs. HHT is discussed in the chapter on neurocutaneous syndromes (Chapter 39).

Pathology

Location. Over 85% of AVMs are supratentorial, located in the cerebral hemispheres **(7-1)**. Only 15% are found in the posterior fossa.

Size. AVMs vary from tiny lesions to giant malformations that can occupy an entire cerebral lobe or hemisphere. Most are intermediate in size with a nidus ranging from 2-6 cm in diameter. Both the feeding arteries and draining veins are usually enlarged.

"Micro"-AVMs have a nidus ≤ 1 cm; feeding arteries and draining veins are usually normal in size. Micro-AVMs are typically associated with HHT.

Number. < 2% of all brain AVMs are multiple. Almost all multiple AVMs are associated with vascular neurocutaneous syndromes.

Gross Pathology. AVMs appear as a compact ovoid or wedge-shaped mass of tangled blood vessels **(7-2)**. Their broadest surface is at or near the cortex with the apex pointing toward the ventricles **(7-1)**. Dilated draining veins are often found on the cortical surface overlying an AVM.

The brain surrounding an AVM often appears abnormal. Hemorrhagic residua, such as gliosis and secondary ischemic changes, are common, as are siderotic changes in the overlying pia.

Microscopic Features. There are no capillaries and no normal brain parenchyma within an AVM nidus. The nidus contains dysplastic, thin-walled vessels with "arterialized" veins, varying amounts of laminated thrombus, dystrophic calcifications, and hemorrhagic residua.

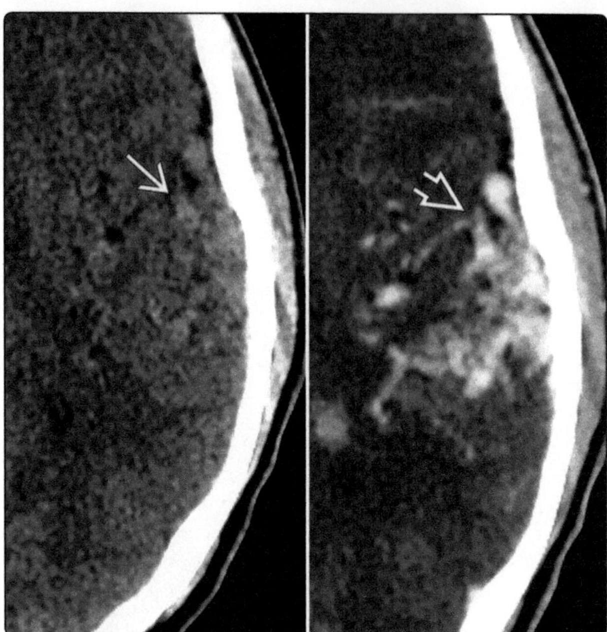

(7-3) *(L) NECT shows serpentine hyperdensities ➡. (R) CECT shows strong uniform enhancement ➡. Wedge-shaped configuration is typical for AVM. Roughly 85% of AVMs are supratentorial.*

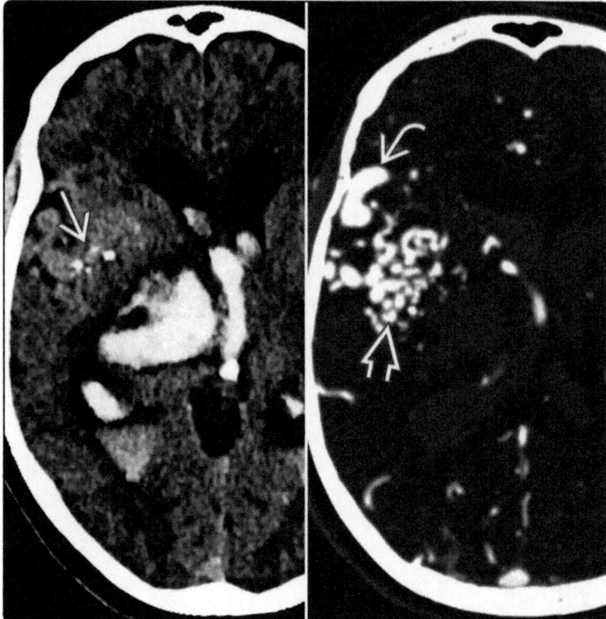

(7-4) *(L) Axial NECT of a 58-year-old woman with "stroke" shows R basal ganglionic spontaneous intracranial hemorrhage (ICH) with intraventricular hemorrhage, Ca^{++} (phleboliths) ➡. (R) CTA shows AVM with nidus ➡, dilated draining veins ➡.*

AVM: ETIOLOGY AND PATHOLOGY

Etiology

- Congenital defect
  - Abnormal vascular development
  - Dysregulated angiogenesis
- **Genetics**
  - Sporadic BAVMs have somatic activating *KRAS* mutations
  - Syndromic BAVMs (e.g., HHT) have known specific mutations

Pathology

- Gross pathology
  - Ovoid or wedge-shaped with broad base toward cortex
  - 3 components: Feeding arteries, nidus (center), draining veins
- Microscopic features
  - Dysplastic thin-walled vessels
  - Ectatic "arterialized" veins
  - Only nonfunctional gliotic brain in nidus

Clinical Issues

Epidemiology. Almost all AVMs are sporadic and solitary. With very rare exceptions ("de novo" AVMs), most are considered congenital lesions. Sporadic (nonsyndromic) AVMs are found in 0.15% of the general population.

Presentation. Peak presentation occurs between 20-40 years of age, although 25% of patients harboring an AVM become symptomatic by age 15. There is no sex predilection.

Headache with parenchymal hemorrhage is the most common presentation, occurring in ~ 1/2 of all patients. Seizure and focal neurologic deficits are the initial symptoms in 25% each. Small micro-AVMs in patients with vascular neurocutaneous syndromes, such as HHT, are often asymptomatic, only discovered when screening imaging studies are performed.

Natural History. The annual hemorrhage risk is ~ 3%, but, depending on the clinical and anatomical features of the AVM, the risk may be as low as 1% per year (in patients whose initial presentation was nonhemorrhagic) or as high as 33% in hemorrhagic lesions with deep brain or brainstem location and exclusively deep venous drainage. Other features associated with bleeding include feeding artery aneurysm and venous outflow restriction.

AVM: CLINICAL ISSUES

Demographics

- Peak age: 20-40 years (mean: 33 years)
- 25% symptomatic by 15 years

Presentation

- Headache with intracranial hemorrhage (ICH) in 50-60%
- Seizure 25%, neurologic deficit 25%

Natural History

- Overall annual ICH risk is 3% but wide variation

Several grading systems have been devised to characterize AVMs and estimate the risks of surgery. The most widely used is the **Spetzler-Martin scale**. Here, AVMs are graded on a scale from 1-5 based on the sum of "scores" calculated from lesion size, location (eloquent vs. noneloquent brain), and venous drainage pattern (superficial vs. deep).

Treatment Options. Embolization, surgery, stereotactic radiosurgery, or a combination of treatments are all current options in treating ruptured (i.e., hemorrhagic) BAVMs.

Imaging

The imaging diagnosis of an uncomplicated AVM is relatively straightforward. However, the presence of hemorrhage or thrombosis can complicate its appearance. Acute hemorrhage may obliterate any typical findings of an AVM. Residua of previous hemorrhagic episodes, such as dystrophic calcification, gliosis, and blood in different stages of degradation, may also complicate its appearance.

General Features. AVMs are complex networks of abnormal vascular channels consisting of three distinct components: (1) feeding arteries, (2) a central nidus, and (3) draining veins **(7-1)**.

CT Findings. AVMs generally resemble a bag of worms formed by a tightly packed tangle of vessels with little or no mass effect on adjacent brain. NECT scans typically show numerous well-delineated, slightly hyperdense serpentine vessels **(7-3)**. Calcification is common **(7-4)**. Enhancement of all three AVM components (feeding arteries, nidus, draining veins) is typically intense and uniform on CECT scans.

CTA is commonly included as part of the initial evaluation in patients who present with nontraumatic "spontaneous" ICH (sICH) and may be helpful in delineating the feeding arteries and draining veins of an underlying AVM **(7-4)**.

MR Findings. The typical appearance of a BAVM is a tightly packed mass or a "honeycomb" of "flow voids" on both T1 and T2 scans **(7-5A)**. Any brain parenchyma within an AVM is typically gliotic and hyperintense on T2WI and FLAIR **(7-5B)**.

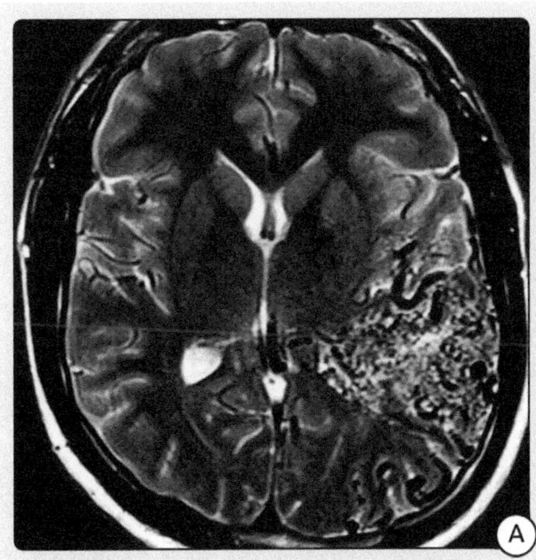

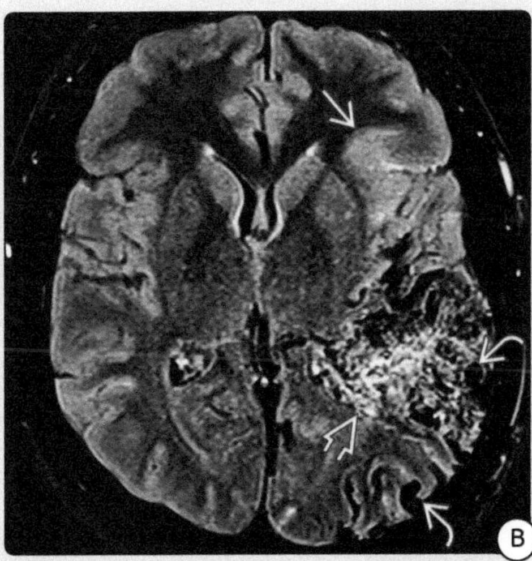

***(7-5A)** T2WI MR in a 29-year-old man with a seizure shows a left parietal AVM with multiple "flow voids." Its "wedge" or pyramidal shape with broad base at the cortical surface is classic. **(7-5B)** FLAIR MR in the same case shows that the nidus contains some hyperintense gliotic brain ➡. Note adjacent gyral swelling of the insula, left temporal lobe ➡ possibly related to vascular steal or postictal state. Dilated cortical veins along the cortex are present ➡.*

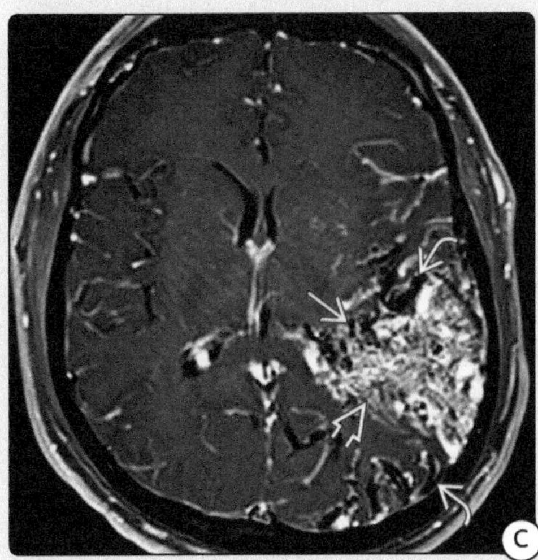

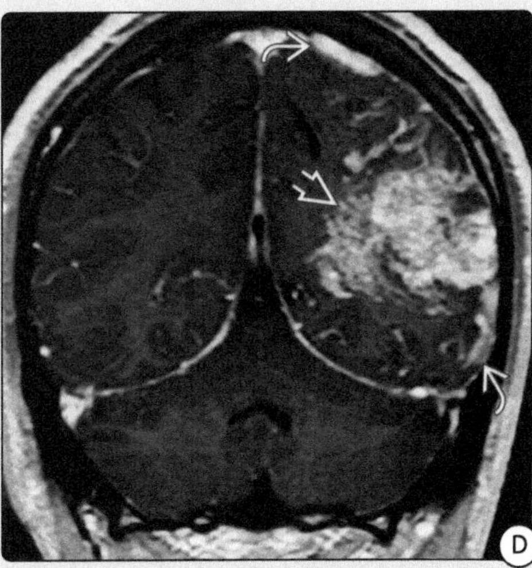

***(7-5C)** T1 C+ FS MR shows that the nidus enhances intensely. "Flow voids" around the nidus ➡ are dilated feeding arteries ➡ and prominent draining veins ➡. **(7-5D)** Coronal T1 C+ MR demonstrates the wedge-shaped configuration of the AVM nidus ➡ especially well. The broad cortical surface of the lesion is apparent, as are enlarged draining cortical veins ➡.*

Contrast enhancement of AVMs is variable, depending on flow rate and direction. Draining veins typically enhance strongly and uniformly **(7-5C)**.

Hemorrhagic residua are common. T2* sequences often show foci of "blooming" both within and around AVMs as well as siderosis in the adjacent pia.

Angiography. All three AVM components (feeding arteries, nidus, venous drainage) must be thoroughly evaluated. The pial **feeding arteries** that supply an AVM are often enlarged and tortuous **(7-6A)**. A flow-induced **"pedicle" aneurysm** is seen in 10-15% of cases.

The **nidus**, the core of the AVM, is a tightly packed tangle of abnormal arteries and veins without an intervening capillary bed **(7-6B)**. Up to 50% contain at least one aneurysmally dilated vessel (**"intranidal aneurysm"**).

As there is no intervening capillary bed between the arterial feeders and draining veins of an AVM, direct arteriovenous shunting within the nidus occurs **(7-6C)**. **Draining veins** typically opacify in the mid to late arterial phase ("early draining" veins) **(7-6B)** **(7-6C)**. Veins draining AVMs are typically enlarged and tortuous and may become so prominent that they form varices and exert local mass effect on the adjacent cortex. Stenosis of one or more "outlet" draining veins may elevate intranidal pressure and contribute to AVM hemorrhage.

Approximately 25% of superficially located, large, or diffuse AVMs have some transdural arterial contributions, so thorough evaluation of the dural vasculature should also be part of the complete angiographic delineation of AVM arterial supply.

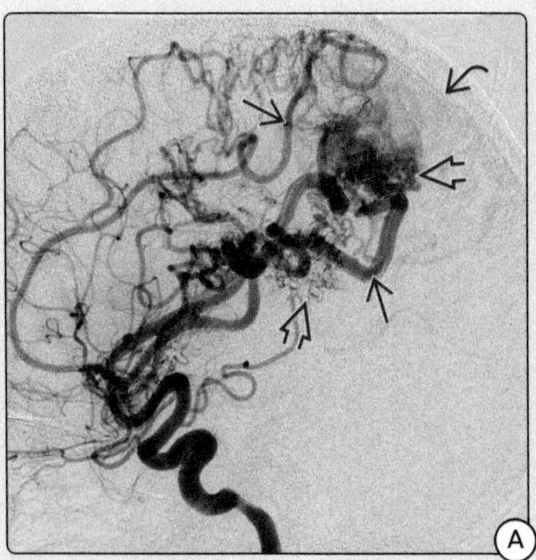

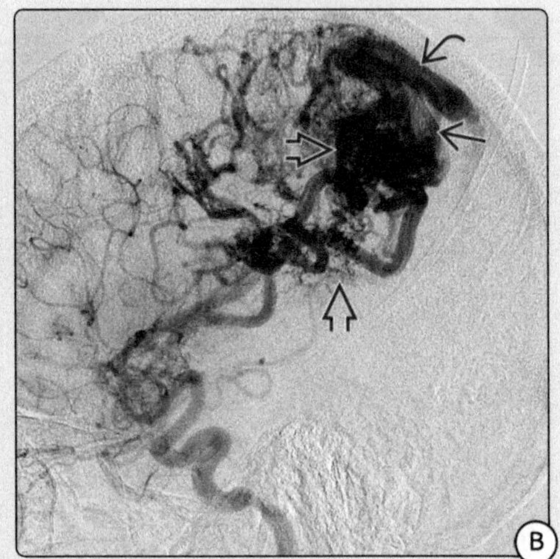

***(7-6A)** Lateral DSA in a 32-year-old man with headache shows enlarged middle cerebral artery (MCA), anterior cerebral artery (ACA) feeding vessels ⇨ with a tangle of smaller vessels in the wedge-shaped nidus ⇨. Faint opacification of the superior sagittal sinus (SSS) ⇨ represents arteriovenous shunting of contrast. **(7-6B)** Late arterial phase of the DSA shows the nidus ⇨ and "early draining" veins ⇨ emptying into the SSS ⇨.*

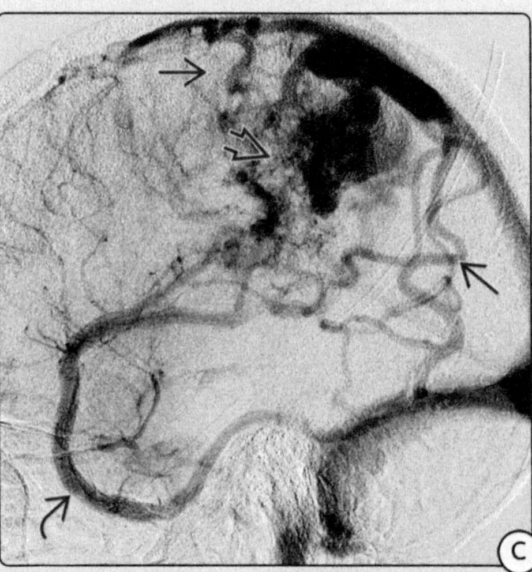

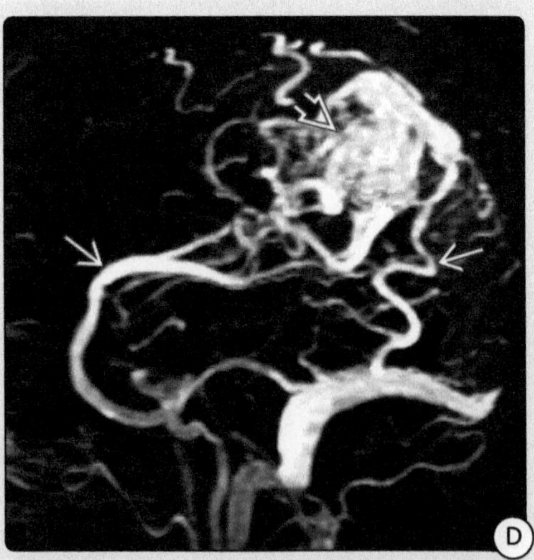

***(7-6C)** Late capillary-early venous phase DSA in the same case shows some residual opacification of the nidus ⇨, multiple enlarged early draining cortical veins ⇨, including a huge superficial middle cerebral vein ⇨. No deep venous drainage was identified; it's Spetzler-Martin grade III AVM. **(7-6D)** 3D MRA in the same case shows the nidus ⇨, multiple draining veins ⇨. Details of the angioarchitecture were best depicted by DSA.*

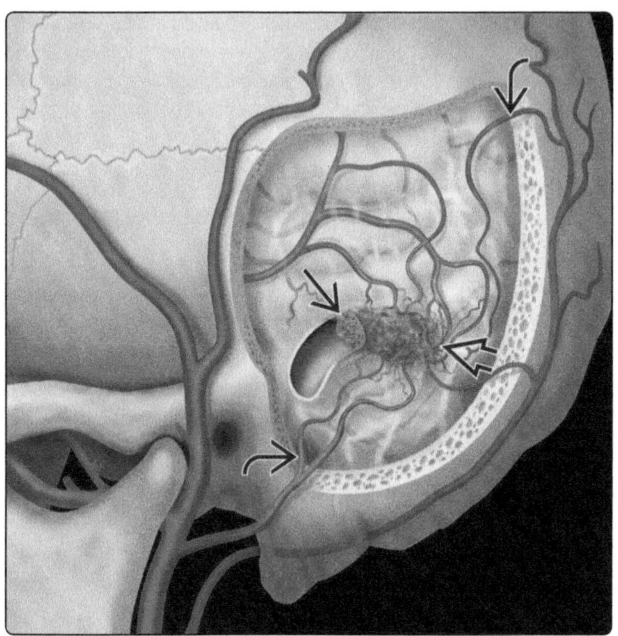

(7-7) Graphic depicts dural arteriovenous fistula (dAVF) with thrombosed transverse sinus with multiple tiny arteriovenous vessels in the dural wall. Lesion is mostly supplied by transosseous feeders from the external carotid artery (ECA).

(7-8) Mass-like surgical specimen from a resected dAVF in the transverse sinus wall shows innumerable crack-like vessels. (Courtesy R. Hewlett, MD.)

Differential Diagnosis

Occasionally, a highly vascular neoplasm, such as **glioblastoma multiforme** (GBM), displays such striking neoangiogenesis that it can mimic an AVM. Most GBMs, even extremely vascular lesions, enhance intensely and contain significant amounts of neoplasm interposed between the enlarged vessels. Sometimes, **densely calcified neoplasms**, such as oligodendroglioma, can mimic the "flow voids" of an AVM.

Cerebral proliferative angiopathy (CPA) is a large, diffuse malformation that has innumerable small feeding vessels, no definable nidus, and *normal brain interposed between the proliferating vascular channels.* CPA is frequently misdiagnosed as a BAVM.

AVM: IMAGING

NECT
- Slightly hyperdense "bag of worms"
- Tightly packed
- Little/no mass effect

CECT
- Strong serpentine enhancement

MR
- "Honeycomb" of "flow voids"
- No normal brain inside

Differential Diagnosis
- Highly vascular neoplasm (e.g., glioblastoma multiforme)
- Cerebral proliferative angiopathy

Dural Arteriovenous Fistula

Dural arteriovenous fistula (dAVF) is the second major type of cerebrovascular malformation that exhibits arteriovenous shunting. Much less common than AVMs, they exhibit a spectrum of biologic behavior that ranges from relatively benign to catastrophic ICH. In this section, we consider typical dAVFs.

A special type of dAVF, carotid-cavernous fistula (CCF), has its own classification schema, distinctive clinical findings, and unique imaging features that differ from dAVFs elsewhere. CCF is discussed separately in this chapter.

Terminology

A dAVF, a.k.a. dural arteriovenous shunt, is a network of tiny, crack-like vessels that shunt blood between meningeal arteries and small venules within the wall of a dural venous sinus.

Etiology

Unlike parenchymal AVMs, adult dAVFs are usually acquired (not congenital). Although the precise etiology is controversial, upregulated angiogenesis in the wall of a thrombosed dural venous sinus is the most commonly cited mechanism.

Pathology

Location. Most dAVFs are found in the posterior fossa and skull base. Between 1/3 and 1/2 occur at the transverse/sigmoid sinus junction. Less common sites are the cavernous sinus (CS) and superior petrosal sinus. dAVFs involving the superior sagittal sinus are rare.

Size and Number. dAVFs account for 10-15% of all intracranial vascular malformations with arteriovenous shunting. Most are solitary. Size varies from tiny single vessel shunts to massive complex lesions with multiple feeders and arteriovenous shunts in the sinus wall.

Gross Pathology. Multiple enlarged dural feeders converge in the wall of a thrombosed dural venous sinus **(7-7)**. A network of innumerable microfistulas connects these vessels directly to arterialized draining veins. These crack-like vessels may form a focal mass within the occluded sinus **(7-8)**.

Clinical Issues

Presentation. Most dAVFs occur in adults. The peak age is 40-60 years, roughly 20 years older than the peak age for AVMs. Clinical presentation varies with location and venous drainage pattern. Uncomplicated dAVFs in the transverse/sigmoid sinus region typically present with either bruit &/or tinnitus. dAVFs in the CS cause pulsatile proptosis, chemosis, retroorbital pain, bruit, and ophthalmoplegia.

"Malignant" dAVFs [lesions with cortical venous drainage (CVD)] may cause focal neurologic deficits, seizures, and progressive dementia.

Natural History. Prognosis depends on location and venous drainage pattern. Most lesions without CVD follow a benign clinical course. Hemorrhage is rare in such cases (~ 1.5% per year). "Malignant" dAVFs often have an aggressive clinical course with high risk for ICH (risk: ~ 7.5% per year).

Treatment Options. Endovascular treatment with embolization of arterial feeders with or without coil embolization of the recipient venous pouch/sinus is most common. Surgical resection of the involved dural sinus wall,

(7-9A) CTA source image in a patient with right-sided tinnitus shows no obvious abnormality, although the right sigmoid sinus ⇨ looks peculiar. (7-9B) Bone CT in the same patient shows multiple enlarged transosseous vascular channels ⇨ in the squama of the right occipital bone.

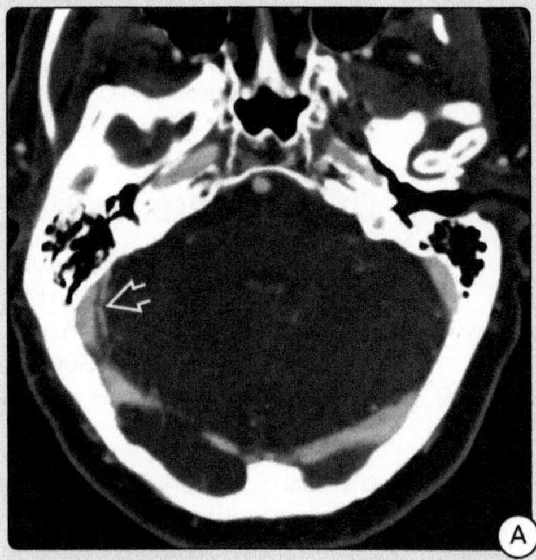

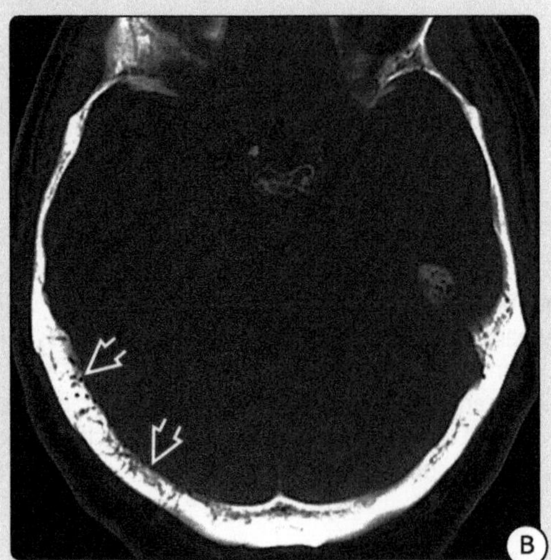

(7-9C) Contrast-enhanced MRA source image shows dural sinus thrombosis ⇨, multiple enhancing vascular channels ⇨ characteristic of posterior fossa dAVF. (7-9D) MRA in the same patient shows innumerable tiny feeding arteries ⇨ supplying a dAVF at the transverse-sigmoid sinus junction. The sinus has partially recanalized ⇨, and the distal sigmoid sinus ⇨ and jugular bulb are partially opacified.

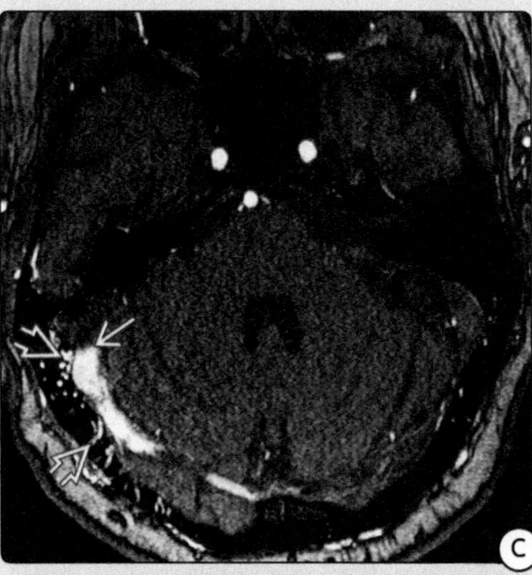

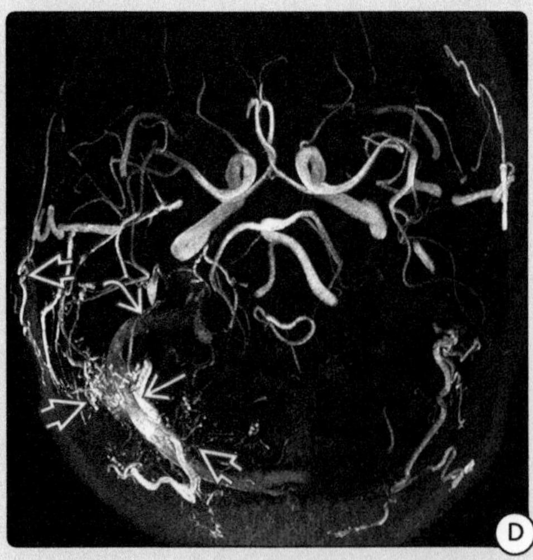

used either alone or in combination with endovascular treatment, is another option.

Imaging

CT Findings. Parenchymal hemorrhage is uncommon in the absence of CVD. An enlarged dural sinus or draining vein can sometimes be identified on NECT scans. Dilated transcalvarial channels from enlarged transosseous feeding arteries can occasionally be seen on bone CT images in patients with pulsatile tinnitus **(7-9A)** **(7-9B)**.

Contrast-enhanced scans may demonstrate enlarged feeding arteries and draining veins. The involved dural venous sinus is often thrombosed or stenotic.

MR Findings. A thrombosed dural venous sinus containing vascular-appearing "flow voids" is the most common finding **(7-9C)** **(7-9D)**. Thrombus is typically isointense with brain on T1 and T2 scans and "blooms" on T2* sequences. Chronically thrombosed, fibrotic sinuses may enhance.

Parenchymal hyperintensity on T2WI and FLAIR indicates venous congestion or ischemia, usually secondary to retrograde CVD.

Angiography. Multiple enlarged dural and transosseous branches arising from the external carotid artery (ECA) are usually present **(7-10A)** **(7-10B)**. Dural branches may also arise from the internal carotid **(7-10C)** and vertebral arteries **(7-10D)**.

Identifying venous drainage is important. dAVFs with normal antegrade venous drainage or minimal reflux into a dural sinus without drainage into cortical veins are considered low-risk lesions. *The presence of CVD puts a dAVF into a higher grade category with increased risk of parenchymal hemorrhage.*

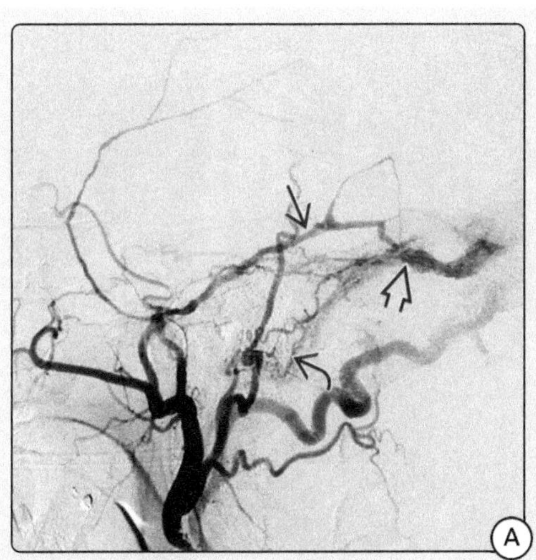

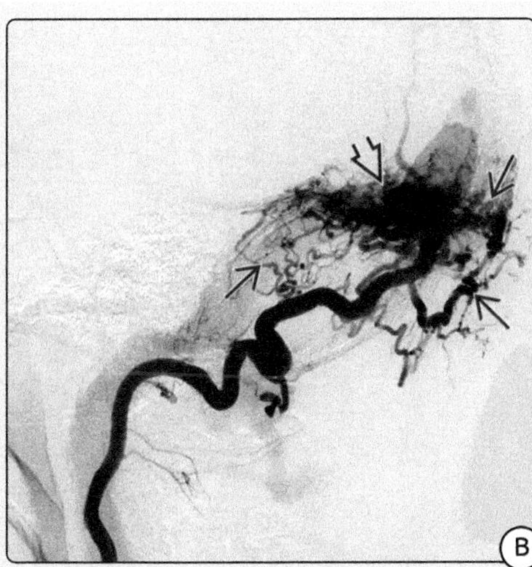

***(7-10A)** Lateral DSA of the ECA in a patient with pulsatile tinnitus shows a dAVF to a partial recanalized transverse sinus. Numerous ECA branches, including the posterior auricular and middle meningeal arteries, supply the fistula. **(7-10B)** Superselective DSA of the occipital artery shows that it is the major contributor to the dAVF in the wall of the transverse sinus through innumerable transosseous perforating branches.*

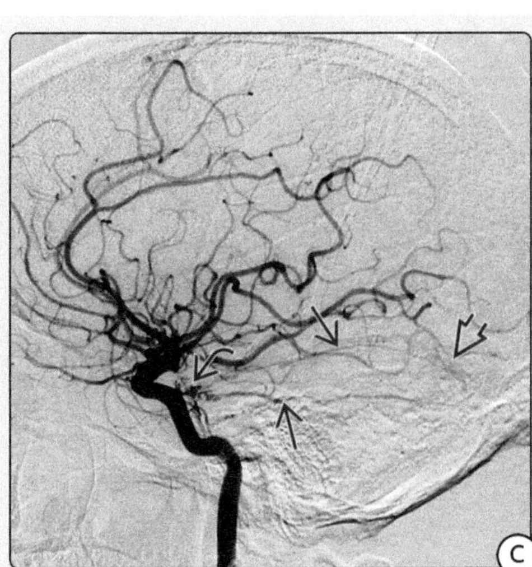

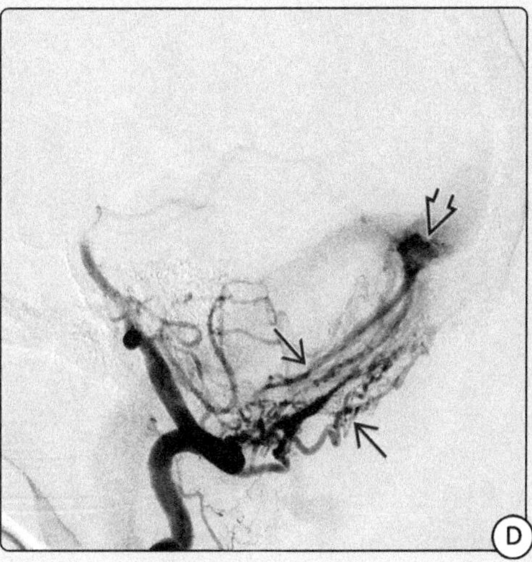

***(7-10C)** Lateral DSA of the left internal carotid artery (ICA) shows a markedly enlarged meningohypophyseal trunk with several marginal tentorial branches supplying the dAVF. **(7-10D)** Lateral DSA of the left vertebral injection shows numerous enlarged posterior meningeal branches that arise from the V3 segment and supply the dAVF.*

Carotid-Cavernous Fistula

Terminology

Carotid-cavernous fistulas (CCFs) are a special type of arteriovenous shunt that develops within the CS **(7-11)**. CCFs are divided into two subgroups, direct and indirect fistulas.

"Direct" CCFs are typically *high-flow* lesions that result from rupture of the cavernous internal carotid artery (ICA) directly into the CS, with or without a preexisting ICA aneurysm. **"Indirect" CCFs** are usually *slow-flow, low-pressure* lesions that represent an AVF between dural branches of the cavernous ICA and the CS.

Etiology

CCFs can be traumatic or nontraumatic. *Direct* CCFs are usually secondary to central skull base fractures. Laceration/transection of the cavernous ICA with direct fistulization into the CS is the typical finding. Spontaneous (i.e., nontraumatic) rupture of a preexisting cavernous ICA aneurysm is a less common etiology. *Indirect* CCFs are nontraumatic lesions and are thought to be degenerative in origin.

Clinical Issues

Epidemiology. An indirect CCF is the second most common intracranial dAVF. Direct high-flow CCFs are much less common.

Demographics. Direct CCFs typically occur with trauma and can occur at any age. Indirect CCFs are most frequent in women 40-60 years of age.

Presentation. Direct CCFs may present within hours to days or even weeks following trauma. Bruit, pulsatile

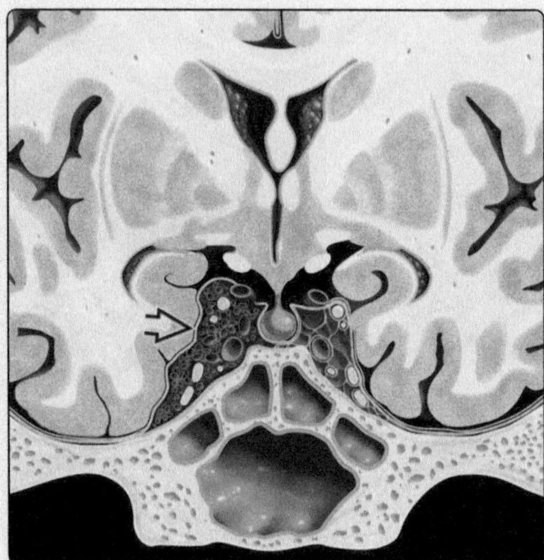

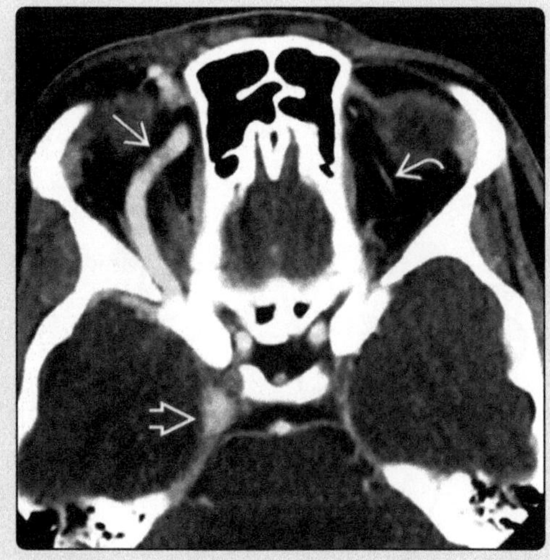

***(7-11)** Coronal graphic depicts a carotid-cavernous fistula (CCF). The right cavernous sinus (CS) ⇒ is enlarged by numerous dilated arterial and venous channels. **(7-12)** CECT scan shows classic findings of CCF. The right CS is enlarged ➡, and the ipsilateral superior ophthalmic vein ➡ is > 4x the size of the left superior ophthalmic vein ➡.*

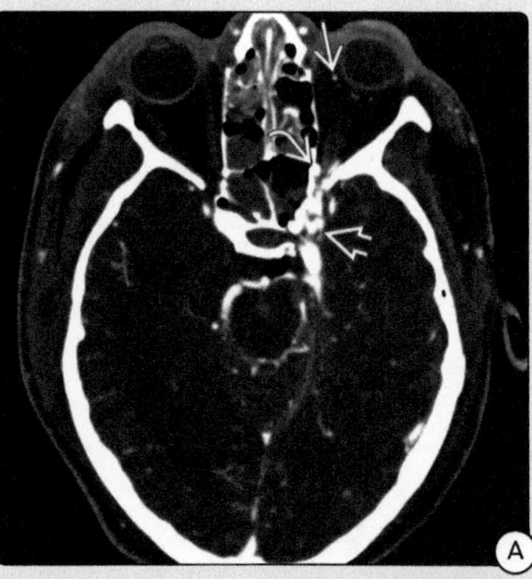

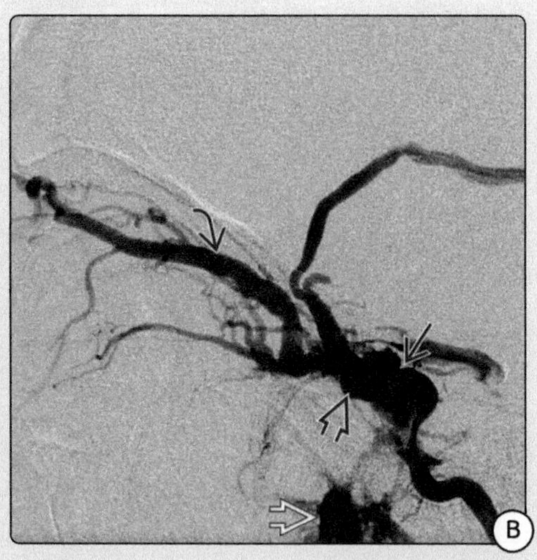

***(7-13A)** A 21-year-old man developed left proptosis following severe trauma with multiple skull base fractures. CTA shows enlarged vessels around the left globe ➡, at the orbital apex ➡, and within the CS ➡. **(7-13B)** DSA shows a direct CCF at the C4-C5 segment ⇒. The enlarged CS ⇒ drains anteriorly into the superior ophthalmic vein ⇒, inferiorly into the pterygoid venous plexus ➡.*

exophthalmos, decreasing vision, and headache are typical. Indirect CCFs cause painless proptosis with variable vision changes.

Treatment Options. Direct CCF fistulae are closed with transarterial-transfistula detachable balloon embolization. Indirect CCFs may be treated conservatively or with superselective embolization.

Imaging

CT Findings. NECT scans may demonstrate a prominent CS with enlarged superior ophthalmic vein (SOV). CECT scans often nicely demonstrate an enlarged SOV and CS **(7-12)**. CTA shows engorgement of the ophthalmic vein and CS **(7-13A)**.

MR Findings. T1WIs may show a prominent "bulging" CS and SOV as well as "dirty" orbital fat. High-flow CCFs may show too many CS "flow voids" on T2WIs. Strong, uniform enhancement of the CS and SOV is typical.

Angiography. *Direct* CCFs typically demonstrate rapid flow with very early CS opacification **(7-13B)**. A single-hole fistula is usually present, typically between the C4 and C5 ICA segments.

Indirect CCFs often have multiple dural feeders from cavernous branches of the ICA (meningohypophyseal and inferolateral trunks) as well as deep branches of the ECA (middle meningeal and distal maxillary branches).

Differential Diagnosis

The major differential diagnosis with CCFs is **cavernous sinus thrombosis** (CST). Both CCF and CST may cause proptosis, intraorbital edema, enlarged extraocular muscles, and the appearance of "dirty" fat. In CST, the CS may appear enlarged, but prominent filling defects are present on T1 C+ MR.

Vein of Galen Aneurysmal Malformation

Different types of vascular malformations share a dilated vein of Galen as a common feature, but only one of these is a true vein of Galen aneurysmal malformation (VGAM). A VGAM is the most common extracardiac cause of high-output cardiac failure in newborns and comprises 30% of pediatric vascular anomalies.

Terminology

VGAM is essentially a direct AVF between deep choroidal arteries and a persistent embryonic precursor of the vein of Galen, the median prosencephalic vein (MPV) of Markowski **(7-14)**.

Etiology

Normally, the developing internal cerebral veins annex drainage of the fetal choroid plexus as the embryonic MPV—the precursor of the vein of Galen—regresses. In a VGAM, a high-flow fistula prevents formation of the definitive vein of Galen. Mutations in Ephrin signaling genes have been identified in nearly 1/3 of VGAMs.

Clinical Issues

Demographics. VGAMs are rare, representing < 1% of all cerebrovascular malformations. Neonatal VGAMs are more common than those presenting in infancy or childhood. There is a definite male predominance (M:F = 2:1).

Presentation. In neonates, high-output congestive heart failure and a loud cranial bruit are typical. Older infants may present with macrocrania and hydrocephalus.

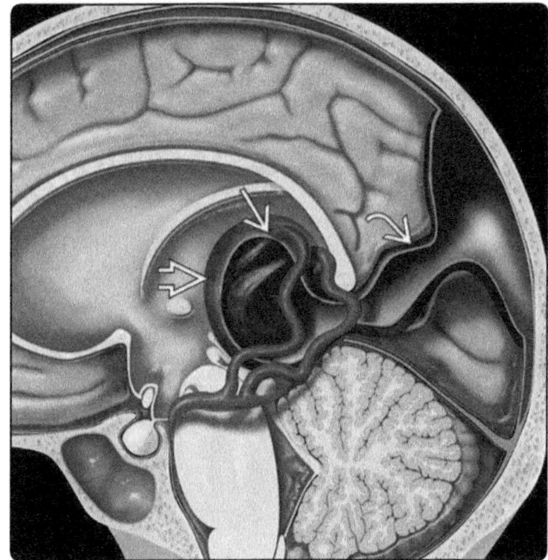

***(7-14)** VGAM with enlarged choroid arteries ➡ draining into venous pouch (dilated median prosencephalic vein) ⬆, falcine sinus ➡.*

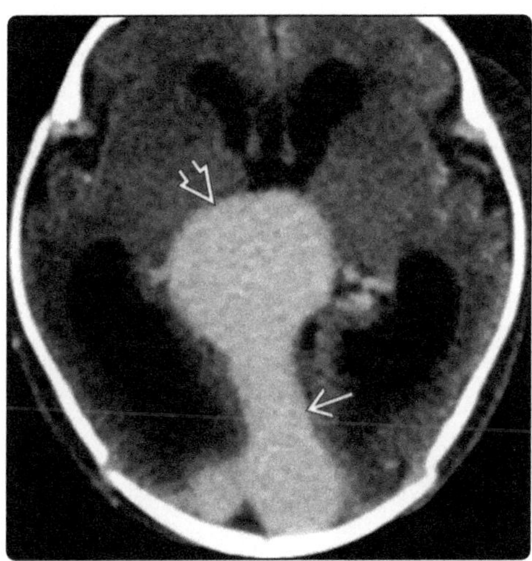

***(7-15)** CECT demonstrates a massive VGAM ⬆ draining into an enlarged falcine sinus ➡, causing obstructive hydrocephalus.*

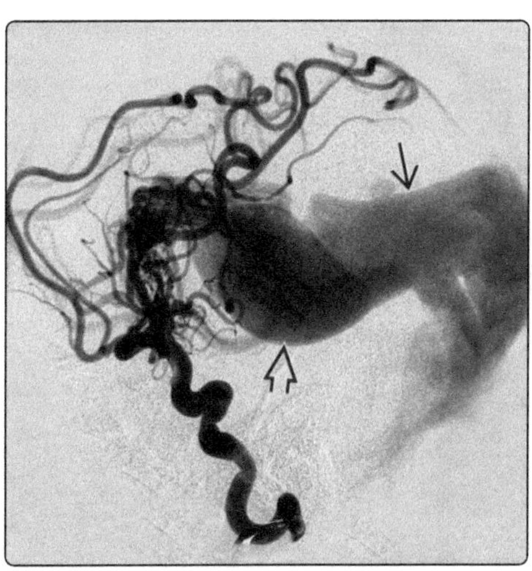

***(7-16)** Lateral DSA shows a VGAM ⬆ draining into a massively enlarged falcine sinus ➡. (Courtesy S. Blaser, MD.)*

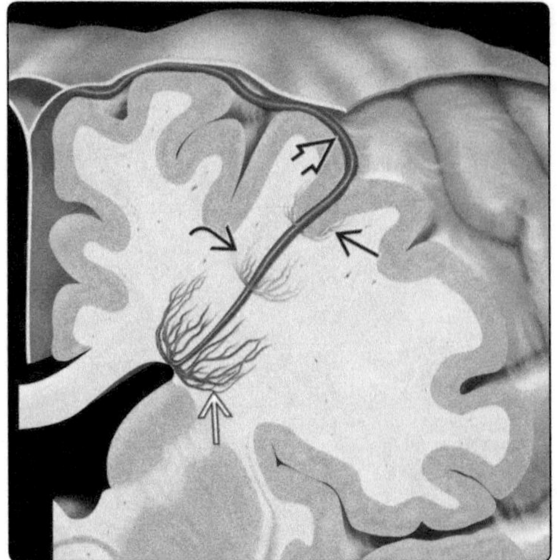

***(7-17)** DVA with enlarged juxtacortical ⇨, subcortical ⇨, periventricular ➡ medullary veins drains into a single transmantle collector vein ⇨.*

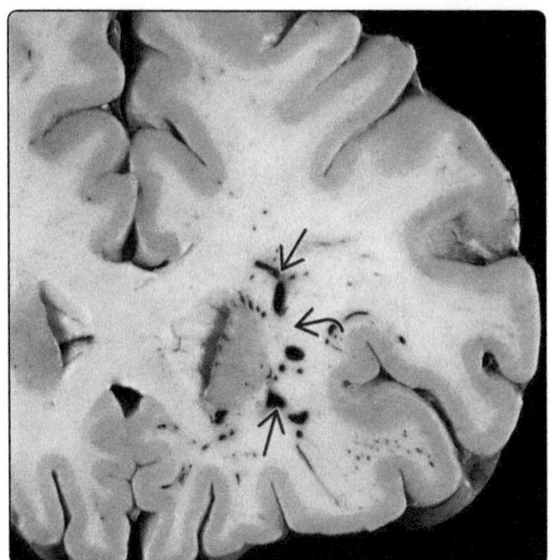

***(7-18)** Coronal autopsy shows a DVA ⇨. Note normal brain ⇨ in between the enlarged medullary veins. (Courtesy P. Burger, MD.)*

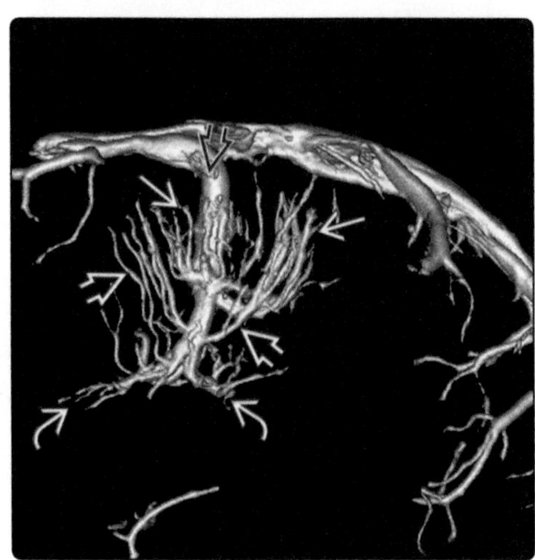

***(7-19)** 3D DSA shows DVA with juxta- ➡ and subcortical ➡, periventricular ➡ medullary veins, collector vein ⇨. (P. Lasjaunias, MD.)*

Natural History. Large VGAMs cause cerebral ischemia and dystrophic changes in the fetal brain. Neonates with untreated VGAMs typically die from progressive brain damage and intractable heart failure. Staged arterial embolization, ideally at 4 or 5 months of age, is the preferred treatment.

Imaging

CT Findings. NECT scans show a well-delineated hyperdense mass at the tentorial apex, usually compressing the third ventricle and causing severe obstructive hydrocephalus. Variable encephalomalacia, hemorrhage, &/or dystrophic calcification in the brain parenchyma are often present. CECT scans show strong uniform enhancement **(7-15)**.

MR Findings. Rapid but turbulent flow in the VGAM causes inhomogeneous signal loss and phase artifact. Enlarged arterial feeders are seen as serpentine "flow voids" adjacent to the lesion.

Angiography. Multiple branches from the pericallosal, choroidal, and thalamoperforating arteries drain directly into an enlarged, aneurysmally dilated midline venous sac **(7-16)**. In > 50% of all VGAMs, the straight sinus is hypoplastic or absent, and venous drainage is into a persistent embryonic **"falcine sinus" (7-14)**.

CVMs Without Arteriovenous Shunting

Developmental Venous Anomaly

Terminology

Developmental venous anomaly (DVA), also called **venous "angioma"** or "venous malformation," is an umbrella-shaped congenital cerebral vascular malformation composed of angiogenically mature venous elements **(7-17)**. Dilated, thin-walled venous channels lie within (and are separated by) normal brain parenchyma.

Etiology

The precise etiology of DVAs is unknown. Most investigators believe it is arrested medullary vein development between 8 and 11 gestational weeks that results in DVAs.

Pathology

Location. Approximately 70% of DVAs are found in the deep white matter, adjacent to the frontal horn of the lateral ventricle. The second most common location is next to the fourth ventricle (15-30%).

DVA depth is defined as where the medullary venous radicles converge into the collector vein. Three depths are recognized: Juxtacortical, subcortical, and periventricular **(7-19)**. Some larger DVAs can have dual or even triple convergence sites.

Size and Number. DVA size varies from tiny, almost imperceptible lesions to giant venous malformations that involve most of the hemispheric white matter.

Between 6-7% of patients with a DVA have two lesions; multiple DVAs occur in 1%. Multiple DVAs have been reported in **blue rubber bleb nevus syndrome** (BRBNS) and other superficial craniofacial venous and venolymphatic malformations.

Gross Pathology. DVAs consist of two elements: A cluster of variably sized prominent medullary (white matter) veins (the so-called "caput medusa") that converges on an enlarged stem or single "collector vein." A DVA is embedded within and drains grossly normal-appearing brain parenchyma, forming its primary or sole venous drainage pathway **(7-18)**.

Hemorrhage and calcification are uncommon unless the DVA is associated with another vascular malformation or the collecting vein becomes thrombosed. The most common "histologically mixed" CVM is a cavernous-venous malformation found in 10-15% of patients with a DVA.

Microscopic Features. Thin-walled, somewhat dilated venous channels are interspersed in normal-appearing white matter. Varying degrees of focal parenchymal atrophy, white matter gliosis, neuronal degeneration, and demyelination may be present within the venous drainage territory of some DVAs.

Clinical Issues

Demographics. DVA is the most common of all intracranial vascular malformations, accounting for 60% of all CVMs. Estimated prevalence on contrast-enhanced MR scans ranges from 2.5-9.0%.

Presentation. DVAs occur in patients of all ages. At least 98% of isolated DVAs are asymptomatic and discovered incidentally. About 2% initially present with hemorrhage or infarct.

DVAs may coexist with a **sinus pericranii**. Sinus pericranii is typically the cutaneous sign of an underlying venous anomaly **(7-22)**. DVAs are also associated with hereditary hemorrhagic telangiectasia (HHT) (4% of cases). Other reported associations include malformations of cortical development.

DEVELOPMENTAL VENOUS ANOMALY

Terminology
- DVA; a.k.a. venous "angioma"

Pathology
- Solitary > > multiple; small > large
- Enlarged white matter veins interspersed with normal brain
- Usually found adjacent to lateral or fourth ventricle

Clinical Issues
- Epidemiology and demographics
    - Most common cerebrovascular malformation (60%)
    - Prevalence on T1 C+ MR = 2-9%
    - All ages, no sex predilection

Natural History
- Usually benign, nonprogressive
- May hemorrhage if mixed with cavernous malformation or collector vein thrombosis

Treatment Options. No treatment is required or recommended for solitary DVAs (they are "leave me alone!" lesions). If a DVA is histologically mixed, treatment is determined by the coexisting lesion. Preoperative identification of such mixed malformations is important, as ligating the collector vein or removing its tributaries may result in venous infarction.

Imaging

General Features. DVAs are composed of radially arranged medullary veins that converge on a transcortical or subependymal large collector vein. The classic appearance is that of a Medusa head or upside-down umbrella **(7-17)**.

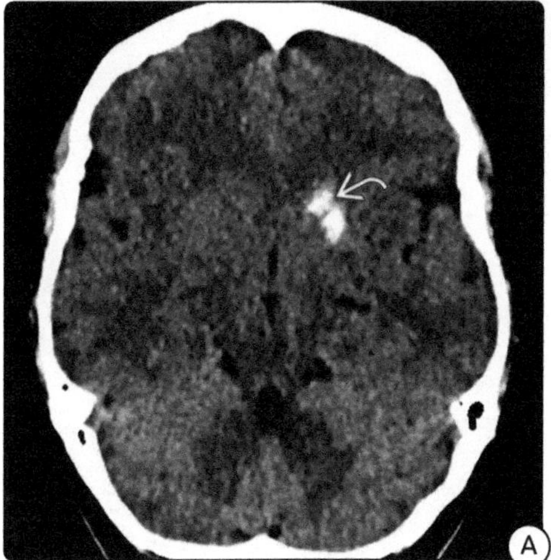

***(7-20A)** NECT in a 34-year-old girl with headaches shows calcification in the left basal ganglia* ➡.

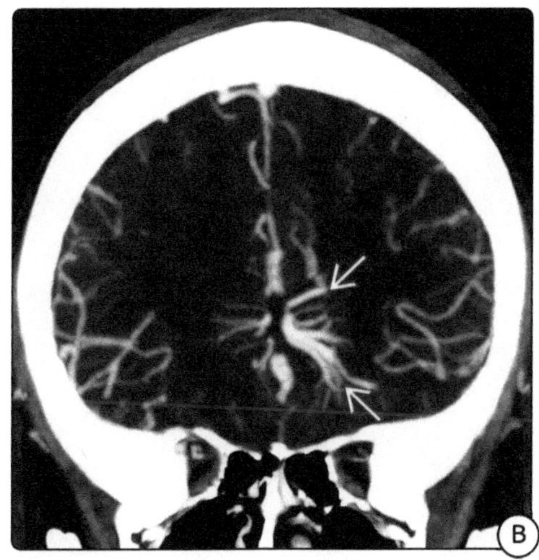

***(7-20B)** Coronal MIP of CT venogram in the same patient shows a large left DVA* ➡.

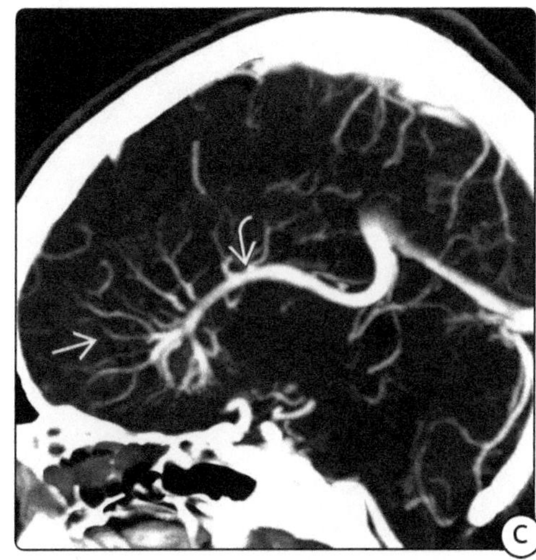

***(7-20C)** Sagittal MIP CTV nicely shows the "Medusa head"* ➡ *of the DVA draining into an enlarged internal cerebral vein* ➡.

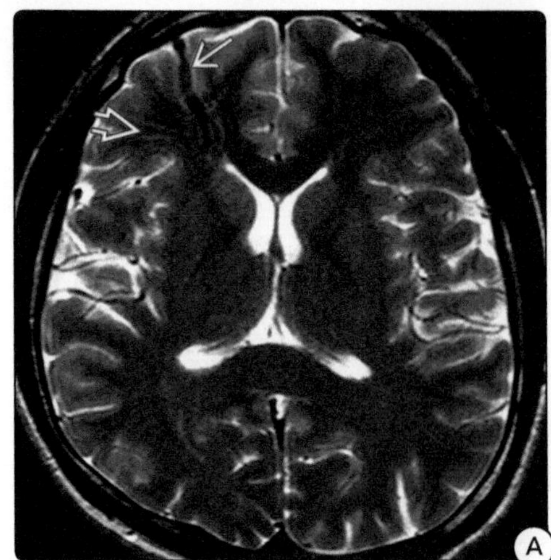

(7-21A) T2 in 32y man with incidental R frontal DVA shows well-defined hypointense draining vein ➡ and hyperintense medullary veins ⇨.

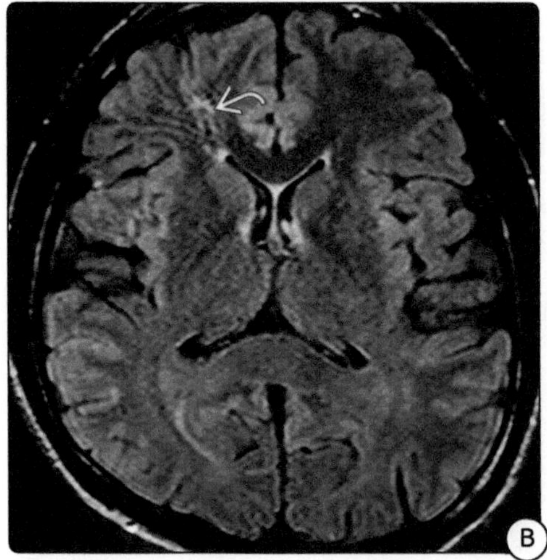

(7-21B) FLAIR shows slight parenchymal hyperintensity ➡ around the DVA.

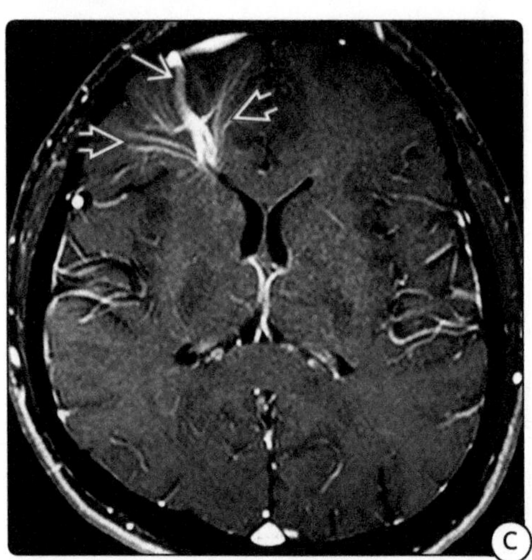

(7-21C) T1 C+ FS MR shows prominent transmantle draining vein ➡, dilated medullary veins forming the classic "Medusa head" ⇨.

CT Findings. NECT scans are usually normal. Unilateral basal ganglia calcification has been reported in the drainage territory of some deep DVAs **(7-20A)**.

CECT scans and CTVs show numerous linear &/or punctate enhancing foci that converge on a well-delineated tubular collector vein **(7-20C)**. In larger DVAs, perfusion CT may show a venous congestion pattern with increased CBV, CBF, and MTT in the adjacent brain parenchyma.

MR Findings. If the DVA is small, it may be undetectable unless contrast-enhanced scans or susceptibility-weighted sequences are obtained.

T2/FLAIR. Large DVAs can exhibit a "flow void" on T2WI **(7-21A)**. Venous radicles of the caput medusa are often hyperintense on T2/FLAIR **(7-21A)**. T2/FLAIR parenchymal abnormalities are present in 10-25% of DVAs **(7-21B)**. The etiology of such associated hyperintensities is unknown but could represent gliosis, venous congestion or ischemia, demyelination, or hypomyelination.

T2* (GRE, SWI). Because flow in the venous radicles of a DVA is typically slow, blood deoxygenates and T2* scans (GRE, SWI) show striking linear hypointensities **(7-25C)**.

If a DVA is mixed with a cavernous malformation, blood products in various stages of degradation may be present and "bloom" on T2* sequences **(7-25)**. Discrete hypointense foci on 3T SWI are seen in the majority of cases, especially in DVAs that are associated with parenchymal hyperintensities on FLAIR. Venous congestion in a DVA may result in microhemorrhages or possibly promote the formation of small cavernous malformations.

T1 C+. T1 C+ sequences show a stellate collection of linear enhancing structures converging on the transparenchymal or subependymal collector vein **(7-21C)**. The collector vein may show variable high-velocity signal loss.

pMR and fMRI. DSC pMR is usually normal in small DVAs. Elevated CBV and CBF with mildly increased MTT are common within larger DVAs. DVAs can strongly resemble neural signal on resting-state fMRI.

Angiography. The arterial phase is normal. The venous phase shows the typical hair-like collection ("Medusa head") of dilated medullary veins within the white matter. A faint, prolonged "blush" or capillary "stain" may be present in some cases.

Nuclear Medicine Studies. More than 3/4 of DVAs are associated with hypometabolism in the adjacent brain parenchyma on FDG PET studies, often in the absence of any other structural abnormalities.

Differential Diagnosis

A histologically mixed vascular malformation in which the DVA provides prominent venous drainage is common. The most common combination is a mixed cavernous-venous malformation **(7-25)**. Unusually large ("giant") **capillary telangiectasias** often have a dominant central collector vein and may therefore resemble a DVA.

DEVELOPMENTAL VENOUS ANOMALY: IMAGING

MR
- T2/FLAIR
  - Collector vein = flow void on T2WI
  - Radicles of "Medusa head" hyperintense on FLAIR
  - 10-25% have T2/FLAIR parenchymal hyperintensities
- T2* (GRE/SWI)
  - Linear hypointensities in radicles, collector vein
  - Blooming foci if mixed with cerebral cavernous malformations
  - 3T SWI may show microbleeds
- T1 C+
  - "Umbrella" of tubular radicles → collector vein
- pMR
  - ↑ CBV/CBF, increased MTT

DSA
- Classic "Medusa head" in venous phase

Sinus Pericranii

Terminology

Sinus pericranii (SP) is a rare benign venous anomaly that consists of an emissary intradiploic vein that connects an intracranial dural venous sinus with an extracranial venous varix **(7-22)**. The dilated venous pouch hugs the external table of the skull.

Pathology

A bluish sac beneath or just above the periosteum of the calvarium is typical. The dilated, blood-filled sac connects with the intracranial circulation through a well-defined bone defect **(7-22)**. The frontal lobe is the most common site, followed by the parietal and occipital lobes. SPs in the middle and posterior cranial fossae are rare.

SP may be associated with single or multiple intracranial DVAs. Other reported associations include craniosynostosis and dural sinus hypoplasia. SP with multiple DVAs is associated with BRBNS.

Imaging

CT Findings. An SP shows strong uniform enhancement after contrast administration **(7-23B)**. The underlying calvarial defect varies in size but is typically well demarcated.

MR Findings. Most SPs are isointense on T1WI and hyperintense to brain on T2WI. "Puddling" of contrast within the SP on T1 C+ is typical unless the lesion is unusually large and flow is rapid. MRV is helpful in delineating both the intra- and extracranial components.

Cerebral Cavernous Malformation

Cerebral cavernous malformations (CCMs) are a distinct type of intracranial vascular malformation characterized by repeated "intralesional" hemorrhages into thin-walled, angiogenically immature, blood-filled locules called caverns. CCMs are discrete, well-marginated lesions that do not contain normal brain parenchyma. Most are surrounded by a complete hemosiderin rim **(7-24)**.

Cavernous malformations exhibit a wide range of dynamic behaviors. They are a relatively common cause of spontaneous nontraumatic ICH in young and middle-aged adults, although they can occur at any age.

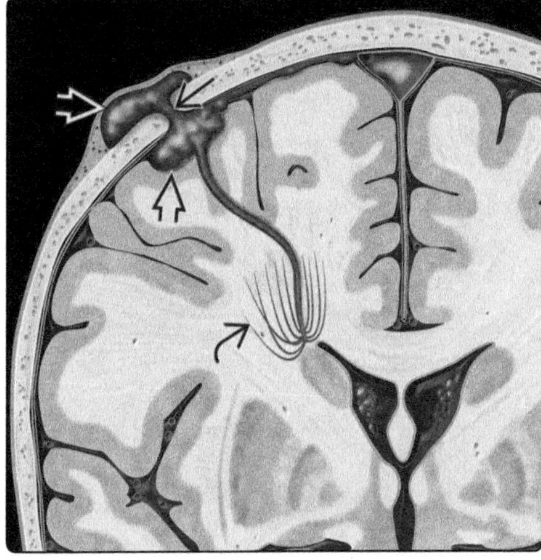

***(7-22)** Sinus pericranii (SP) with extracranial venous pouch ➡, transcalvarial channel ⇨, intracranial pouch ⇨ and associated DVA ↗.*

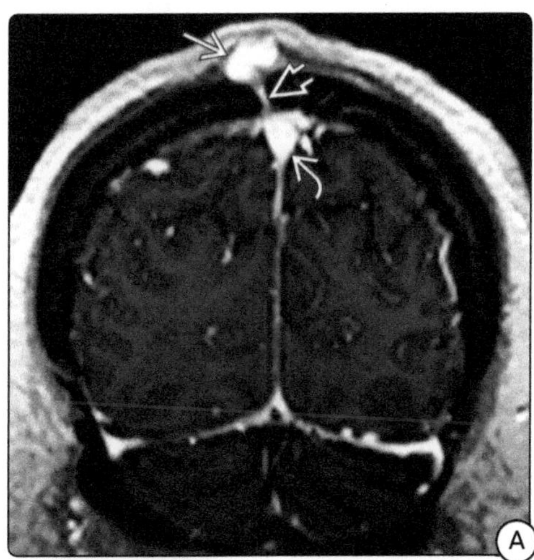

***(7-23A)** Coronal T1 C+ SPGR study shows classic SP. An extracranial venous pouch ➡ connects with the SSS ➡ via a transosseous vein ➡.*

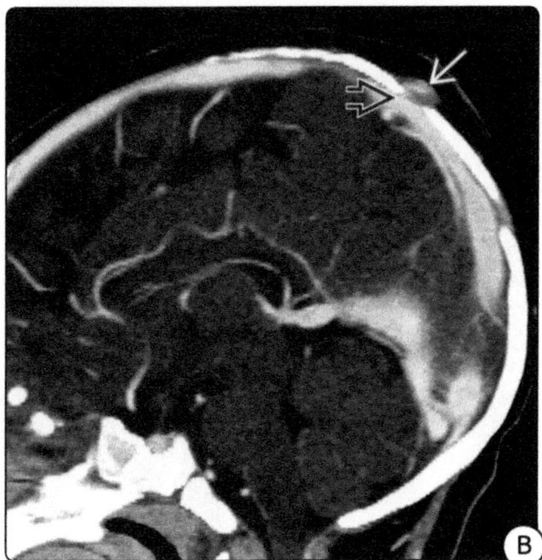

***(7-23B)** Sagittal CTV shows a small SP ➡ connecting to the SSS through an adjacent skull defect ⇨.*

Terminology

CCMs are also known as cavernous "angiomas" or "cavernomas." They are benign malformative vascular hamartomas. CCMs are sometimes erroneously referred to as cavernous hemangiomas. Hemangiomas are benign vascular neoplasms, *not* malformations.

Etiology

General Concepts. CCMs are angiogenically immature lesions with endothelial proliferation and increased neoangiogenesis.

CCMs can be inherited or acquired. Acquired CCMs are rare and usually associated with prior radiation therapy (XRT). Approximately 3.5% of children who have whole-brain XRT develop multiple CCMs with a mean latency interval of ~ 3 years (3-102 months).

Genetics. CCMs can be solitary and sporadic (80% of cases) or multiple and familial (20%). Familial CCMs are inherited as an autosomal dominant disease with variable penetrance and are more common in Hispanic Americans of Mexican descent. Three independent genes have been identified in familial CCMs: *CCM1* (KRIT1), *CCM2* (OSM), and *CCM3* (PDCD10).

Associated Abnormalities. CCMs are the most common component in mixed vascular malformations. Cavernous-venous and cavernous-capillary are the two most frequent combinations.

Pathology

Location and Size. CCMs can occur anywhere in the CNS and range in size from tiny, near-microscopic lesions to giant malformations that can occupy an entire lobe or most of the cerebral hemisphere.

(7-24) Note subacute ⇨, classic "popcorn ball" ⇨ appearances of CCMs. Microhemorrhages are seen as multifocal "blooming black dots" ⇨. (7-25A) Axial NECT in a 30-year-old man with sudden-onset left-sided weakness shows a hyperdense lesion ➡ with a fluid-fluid level ➡ surrounded by peripheral edema ➡.

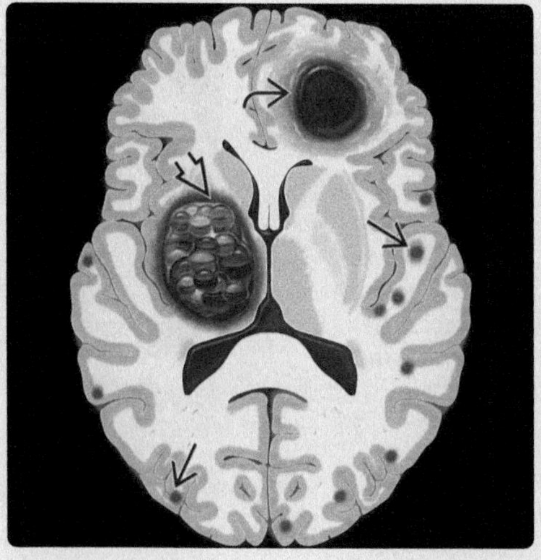

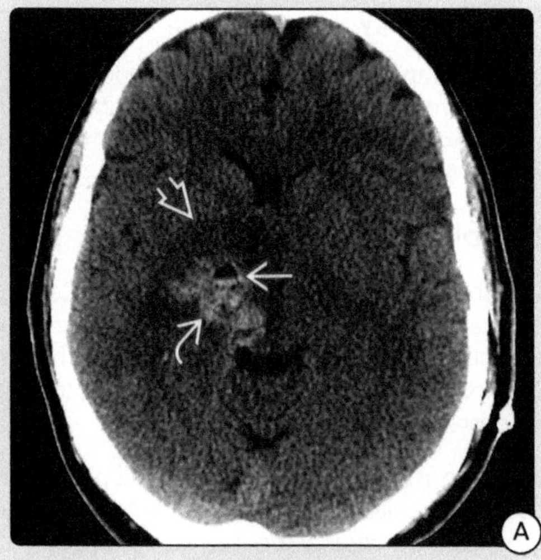

(7-25B) T2 MR shows multiple lesions ➡ with locules containing fluid-fluid levels ➡. (7-25C) T2 SWI MR shows hemorrhagic CCMs ⇨ are mixed with enlarged venous channels containing deoxygenated blood ⇨. This is a mixed vascular malformation, i.e., a cavernous/DVA.*

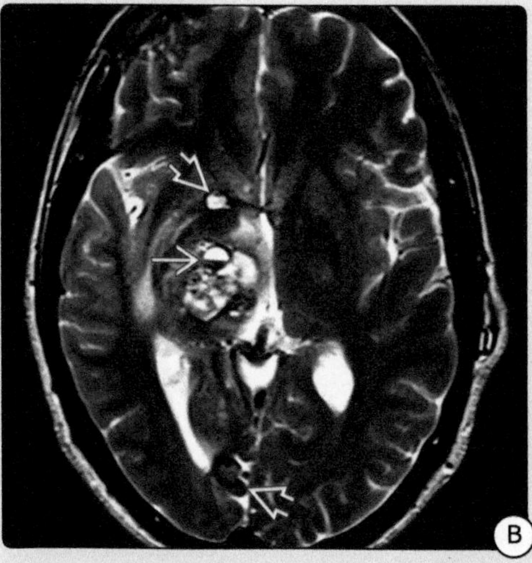

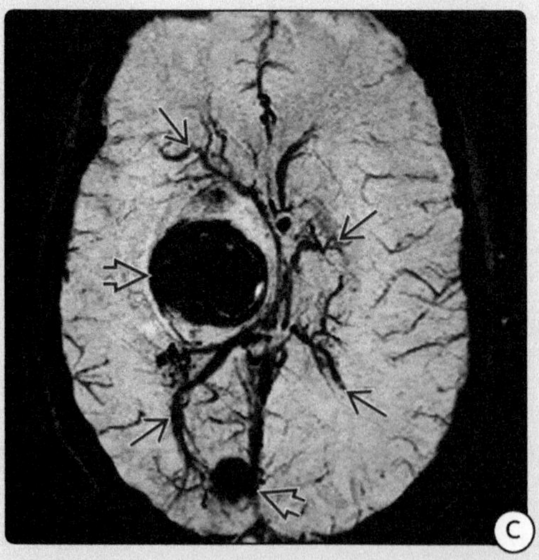

Gross Pathology. A compact, spongy collection of reddish-purple blood-filled "caverns" devoid of intervening neural elements is typical. Most CCMs are surrounded by a rust-colored rim of gliotic, indurated brain.

Staging, Grading, and Classification. The most commonly used classification of CCMs, the Zabramski classification, is based on imaging appearance, not histologic findings (see shaded box on next page).

Clinical Issues

Epidemiology. CCMs are the third most common cerebrovascular malformation (after DVA and capillary telangiectasia) and are found in ~ 0.5% of the population. 2/3 occur as a solitary, sporadic lesion; ~ 1/3 are multiple.

Demographics. CCMs may occur at any age; they cause 10% of spontaneous brain hemorrhages in children. Peak presentation is 40-60 years (younger in the familial multiple cavernous malformation syndrome). There is no sex predilection.

Presentation. 1/2 of all patients with CCMs present with seizures. Headache and focal neurologic deficits are also common. Small lesions, especially microhemorrhages, may be asymptomatic.

Natural History. CCMs have a broad range of dynamic behavior, and the clinical course of individual lesions is both highly variable and unpredictable. Repeated spontaneous intralesional hemorrhages are typical. There is a distinct propensity for lesion growth in all patients. Patients with multiple CCM syndrome typically continue to develop de novo lesions throughout their lives.

Hemorrhage risk with solitary lesions is estimated at 0.25-0.75% per year, cumulative, and greater for women. In the familial multiple CCM form, hemorrhage risk is much higher, approaching 1-5% cumulative risk per lesion per year.

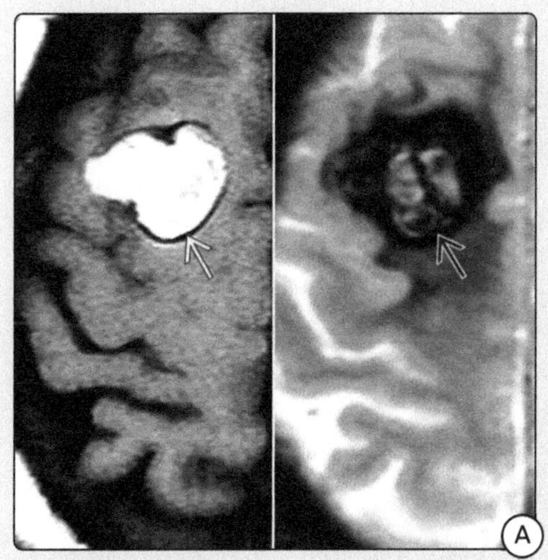

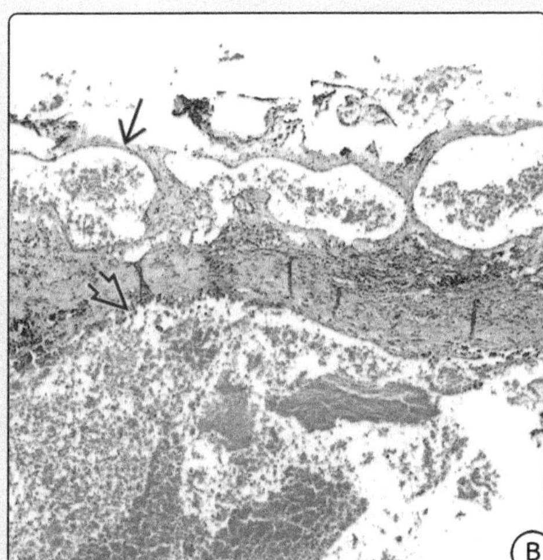

***(7-26A)** Zabramski type I CCM is illustrated. (L) T1 MR shows that the lesion is hyperintense and surrounded by a hypointense hemosiderin rim ➡. (R) T2* GRE scan shows "blooming" hypointensity both around ➡ and within the lesion. **(7-26B)** Microscopic section from the resected specimen in the same case shows a blood-filled cavity ➡ surrounded by thin endothelium-lined vascular channels ➡. (Courtesy R. Hewlett, MD.)*

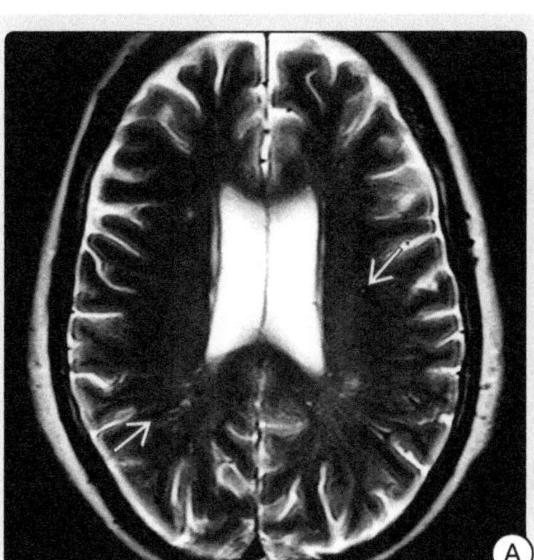

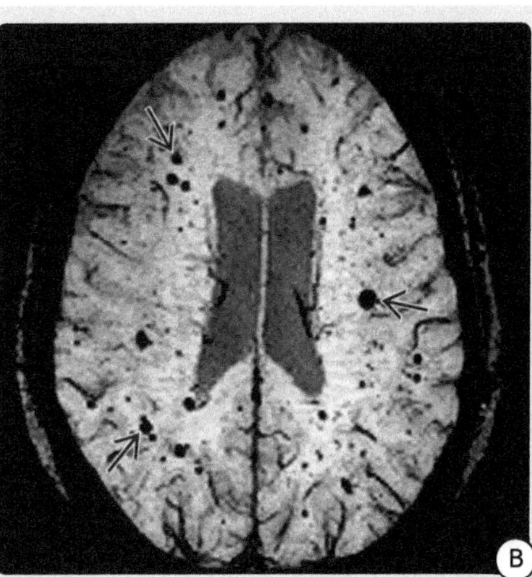

***(7-27A)** Axial FSE T2 MR in a 70-year-old Hispanic woman shows a few scattered faint hypointensities ➡ in the coronal radiata. **(7-27B)** MIP of T2* SWI MR in the same case shows innumerable blooming hypointensities ➡. These are Zabramski type IV CCMs.*

Hemorrhage rates also vary with imaging appearance based on the Zabramski classification (see below). Zabramski type I and II CCMs have a significantly higher hemorrhage rate than types III and IV.

The presence of acute or subacute blood-degradation products on MR (Zabramski I, II) is the strongest indicator for an increased risk of hemorrhage (mean annual hemorrhage rate of 20-25% vs. 3-4% without signs of acute or subacute blood). "Dot-sized" CCMs on T2* (GRE or SWI) that are invisible or barely visible on T1WIs and T2WIs (Zabramski type IV) have the lowest mean annual hemorrhage rate (1%).

CEREBRAL CAVERNOUS MALFORMATIONS

Etiology
- *CCM1*, *CCM2*, or *CCM3* mutations in familial CCM
- Negative inhibition of sprouting angiogenesis lost

Pathology
- Occur throughout CNS
- Solitary (2/3), multiple (1/3, familial)
- Multiple thin-walled blood-filled locules ("caverns")
- No normal brain inside; hemosiderin rim outside

Clinical Issues
- Can present at any age; peak = 40-60 years
- Course variable, unpredictable
  - Repeated intralesional hemorrhages typical
  - Hemorrhage risk = 0.25-0.75% per lesion per year
  - Higher risk, de novo lesions in familial CCM

Imaging

General Features. CCMs occur throughout the CNS. The brain parenchyma is the most common site. A well-circumscribed mixed density/signal intensity mass surrounded by a complete hemosiderin rim ("popcorn ball") is the classic finding. CCMs can vary from microscopic to giant (> 6 cm) lesions. In rare circumstances, a CCM (often mixed with venous malformations) may occupy an entire lobe of the brain.

CT Findings. Large CCMs appear hyperdense **(7-25A)** with or without scattered intralesional calcifications. Most CCMs are well delineated and do not exhibit mass effect unless there is recent hemorrhage.

MR Findings. Findings depend on the stage of evolution and pulse sequence utilized. CCMs have been divided into four types based on imaging appearance (Zabramski classification).

The classic CCM (Zabramski type II) is a discrete reticulated or "popcorn ball" lesion caused by blood products contained within variably sized "caverns" or "locules." Fluid-fluid levels of differing signal intensities are common **(7-25B)**. The mixed signal core is surrounded by a complete hemosiderin rim on T2WI that "blooms" on T2* sequences **(7-25C)**. CCMs with subacute hemorrhage (Zabramski type I) are hyperintense on T1WI and mixed hyper-/hypointense on T2WI **(7-26)**.

T2* scans (GRE, SWI) should always be performed to look for additional lesions. Punctate microhemorrhages are seen as multifocal "blooming black dots" (Zabramski type IV) in many cases with familial CCM **(7-27)**.

Enhancement following contrast administration varies from none (the usual finding) to mild or moderate. If a CCM coexists with a DVA, the venous "angioma" may show strong enhancement.

Angiography. CCMs have no identifiable feeding arteries or draining veins. DSA, CTA, and MRA are usually negative unless the CCM is mixed with another vascular malformation (most commonly a DVA).

Differential Diagnosis

The most common differential diagnosis is a **mixed vascular malformation** in which a CCM is the dominant component. Occasionally, a **hemorrhagic** or **densely calcified neoplasm** (such as a glioblastoma or oligodendroglioma, respectively) can mimic a CCM.

Multifocal "black dots" on T2* scans can be seen in a number of lesions besides type IV CCMs. Chronic hypertensive encephalopathy, amyloid angiopathy, axonal stretch injury, and cortical contusions may have similar appearances.

Hemangiomas are true benign vasoformative neoplasms and should not be mistaken for CCMs. Most are found in the skin and soft tissues of the head and neck. Hemangiomas within the CNS are rare and most commonly found in dural venous sinuses and cranial meninges, not the brain parenchyma.

CEREBRAL CAVERNOUS MALFORMATIONS: IMAGING

CT
- NECT
  - Hyperdense ± scattered Ca^{++}
  - Variable hemorrhage
- DSA

MR (Zabramski Classification)
- Type I: Subacute hemorrhage
  - Hyperintense on T1
  - Hyper-/hypointense on T2
- Type II: Differently aged hemorrhages
  - Mixed signal with hyper/hypointensity on both T1 and T2
  - Classic = "popcorn ball"
  - Look for blood-filled locules with fluid-fluid levels
- Type III: Chronic hemorrhage
- Type IV: Punctate microhemorrhages
  - "Blooming black dots" on T2* (GRE, SWI)

DSA
- Usually negative (unless mixed with DVA)

Capillary Telangiectasia

Terminology

A brain capillary telangiectasia (BCT) is a collection of enlarged, thin-walled vessels resembling capillaries. The vessels are surrounded and separated by normal brain parenchyma.

Etiology

General Concepts. Although their exact pathogenesis is unknown, capillary telangiectasias are probably congenital lesions. BCTs have been reported with hereditary hemorrhagic telangiectasia (HHT).

Cranial irradiation may cause vascular endothelial damage and induce development of multiple cavernous or telangiectatic-like lesions in the brain parenchyma. Patients with radiation-induced capillary telangiectasias typically present with seizures several years after whole-brain XRT. Mean age of onset is 11-12 years, and mean latency period is nearly 9 years.

Genetics. No known genetic mutations have been identified for solitary BCTs. BCTs are the most common vascular malformation in HHT, occurring in 60% of patients. No specific correlation has been observed between genotype and phenotype of brain vascular malformation.

Pathology

Location and Size. BCTs can occur anywhere in the CNS. The pons, cerebellum, and spinal cord are the most common sites **(7-28)**. Solitary lesions are much more common than multiple BCTs. Although "giant" capillary telangiectasias do occur, the vast majority of BCTs are small, typically < 1 cm in diameter.

Gross Pathology. Most BCTs are often invisible to gross inspection. Only 5-10% of BCTs are > 1 cm in diameter. Occasionally, lesions up to 2 cm occur. These can be seen as areas of poorly delineated pink or brownish discoloration in the parenchyma **(7-29)**.

Microscopic Features. A cluster of dilated, somewhat ectatic but otherwise normal-appearing capillaries interspersed within the brain parenchyma is characteristic **(7-31)**. Unless mixed with other malformations (such as cavernous angioma), BCTs do not hemorrhage and do not calcify. Gliosis and hemosiderin deposition are absent.

Clinical Issues

Epidemiology. Capillary telangiectasias are the second most common cerebral vascular malformation, representing between 10-20% of all brain vascular malformations. Skin and mucosal capillary telangiectasias are even more common than brain telangiectasias.

Demographics. BCTs may occur at any age, but peak presentation is between 30-40 years. There is no sex predilection.

Presentation. Most BCTs are asymptomatic and discovered incidentally. A few cases with headache, vertigo, and tinnitus have been reported.

Natural History. Sporadic BCTs are quiescent lesions that do not hemorrhage. BCTs in patients with HHT also have a benign natural history.

Treatment Options. Isolated BCTs do not require treatment. Treatment of mixed lesions is dictated by the associated lesion.

Imaging

General Features. Because normal brain is interspersed between the dilated capillaries of a BCT, no mass effect is present. Unless they are histologically mixed with other CVMs (such as a cavernous malformation), BCTs lack edema, do not incite surrounding gliosis, and neither hemorrhage nor calcify.

CT Findings. Both NECT and CECT scans are usually normal unless the telangiectasia is unusually large **(7-30)**.

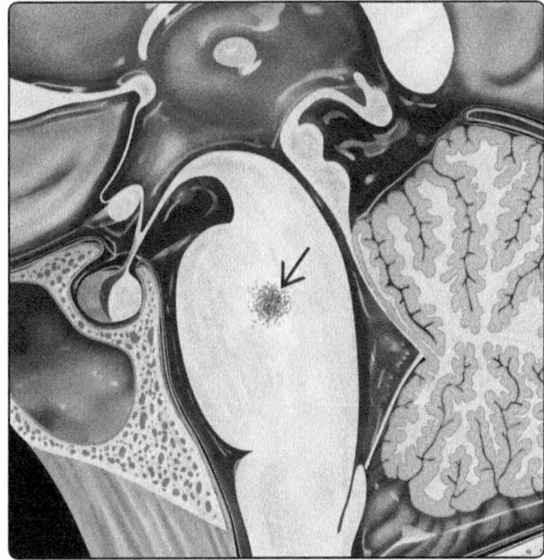

***(7-28)** Graphic depicts pontine capillary telangiectasia ➡ with tiny dilated capillaries interspersed with normal brain.*

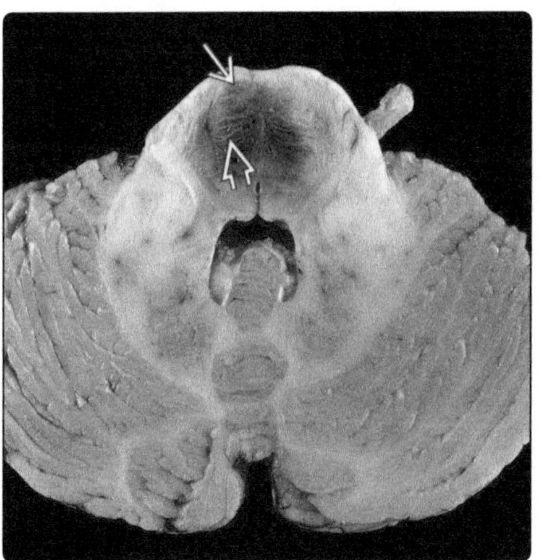

***(7-29)** Autopsy shows large pontine capillary telangiectasia ➡ with pontine fibers ➡ passing through the lesion. (Courtesy B. Horten, MD.)*

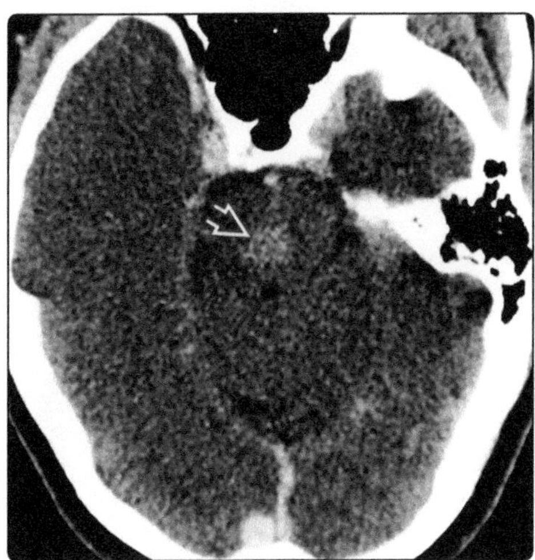

***(7-30)** Axial CECT of the cervical soft tissues shows incidental, asymptomatic large capillary telangiectasia ➡ in the upper pons.*

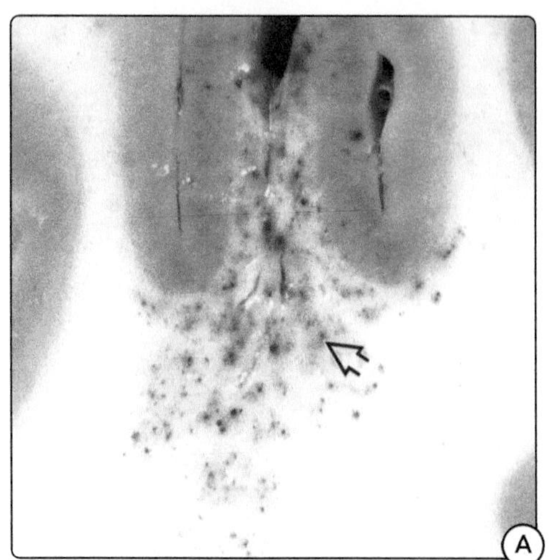

***(7-31A)** Subcortical capillary telangiectasia shows innumerable enlarged pink foci ⇒ in the subcortical WM produced by enlarged capillaries.*

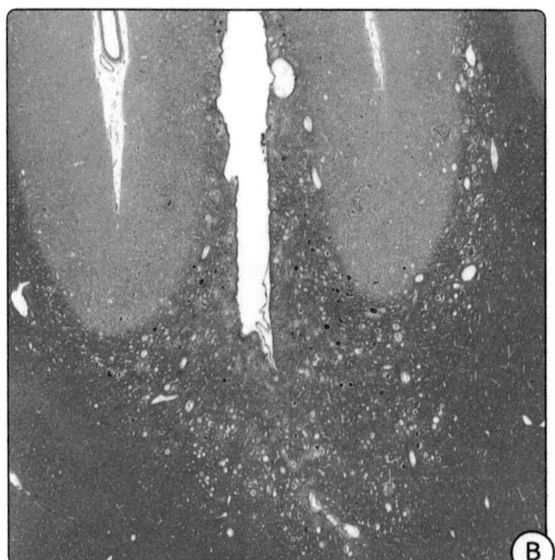

***(7-31B)** Blue myelin stain shows enlarged capillaries in subcortical WM with normal blue-staining WM between the vessels.*

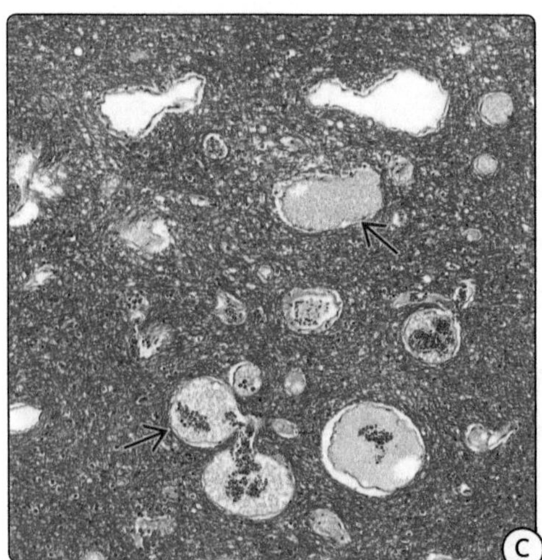

***(7-31C)** Micrograph shows blood-filled, thin-walled enlarged capillaries ⇒, the hallmark of capillary telangiectasia. (Courtesy P. Burger, MD.)*

MR Findings. BCTs are inconspicuous on conventional precontrast MRs **(7-32)**. T1 scans are typically normal. Large BCTs may show faint stippled hyperintensity on T2WI **(7-33A)** or FLAIR, but small lesions are generally invisible.

T2* (GRE, SWI) is the best sequence for demonstrating a BCT **(7-33)**. As blood flow within the dilated capillaries is quite sluggish, oxyhemoglobin is converted to deoxyhemoglobin and is visible as an area of poorly delineated grayish hypointensity.

BCTs typically show faint stippled or poorly delineated brush-like enhancement on T1 C+ **(7-32B)**. Larger lesions may demonstrate a linear focus of strong enhancement within the lesion, representing a draining collector vein **(7-33C)**.

As BCTs are interspersed with normal white matter tracts, DTI shows no displacement or disruption and no alteration of fractional anisotropy.

Differential Diagnosis

Because they show mild enhancement on T1 C+, BCTs are often mistaken for **neoplasms**, yet they do not exhibit mass effect or surrounding edema. Signal intensity loss on T2* and focal brush-like enhancement in a lesion that is otherwise unremarkable on standard sequences easily distinguish BCT from neoplasm.

Radiation-induced vascular malformations are seen as multifocal "blooming black dots" on T2* (GRE, SWI) sequences. Most are cavernous malformations with microhemorrhages, not capillary telangiectasias.

CAPILLARY TELANGIECTASIAS

Pathology

- Cluster of thin-walled, dilated capillaries
  - Normal brain between vascular channels
- Location
  - Pons, cerebellum, spinal cord most common sites
  - **But** can be found anywhere

Clinical Issues

- 10-20% of all cerebrovascular malformations
- All ages
  - Peak: 30-40 years
- Rarely symptomatic
  - Most discovered incidentally at imaging

Imaging

- MR
  - T1/T2 usually normal unless unusually large
  - T2* key sequence (dark gray hypointensity on GRE)
  - May become very hypointense on SWI
  - "Brush-like" enhancement on T1 C+
  - ± prominent central draining vein

Selected References: The complete reference list is available on the Expert Consult™ eBook version included with purchase.

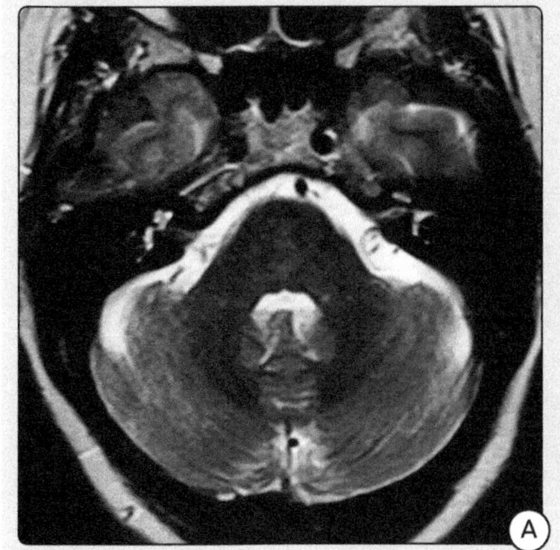

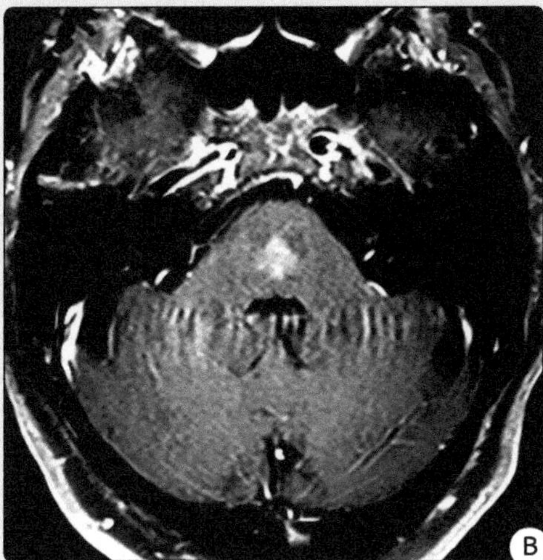

***(7-32A)** Axial T2 MR in a neurologically intact 52y woman is normal. The faint hyperintensities in the cerebellar peduncles are artifactual. **(7-32B)** T1 C+ FS in the same case shows moderate brush-like enhancement in the lesion. The features of normal T2/FLAIR, mild to moderate hypointensity on T2* GRE, and the brush-like enhancement pattern are classic for capillary telangiectasia. The pons is the most common CNS location for capillary telangiectasias.*

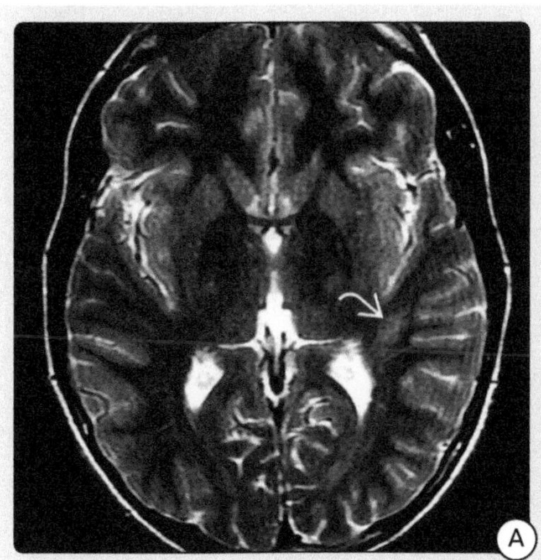

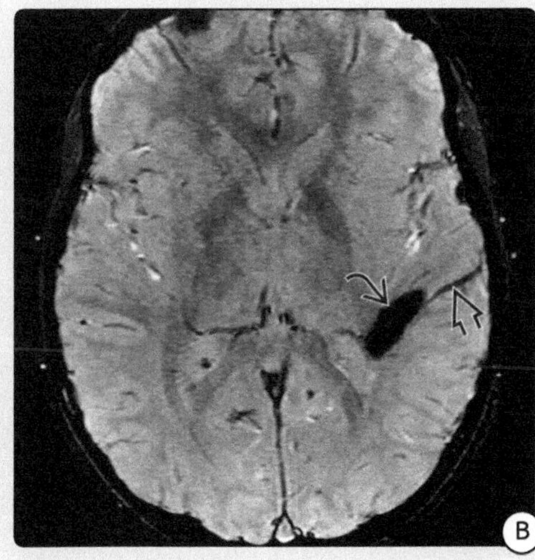

***(7-33A)** Axial T2 MR in a 16-year-old boy with headaches shows a faint, ill-defined hyperintensity in the left parietal white matter. **(7-33B)** T2* SWI MR in the same case shows blooming hypointensity in the lesion and a prominent draining vein.*

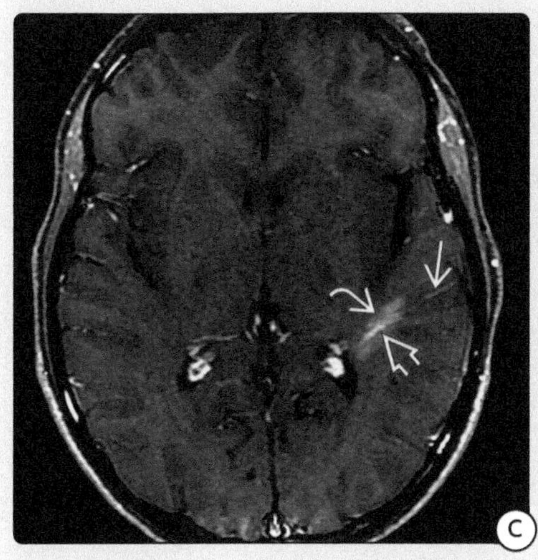

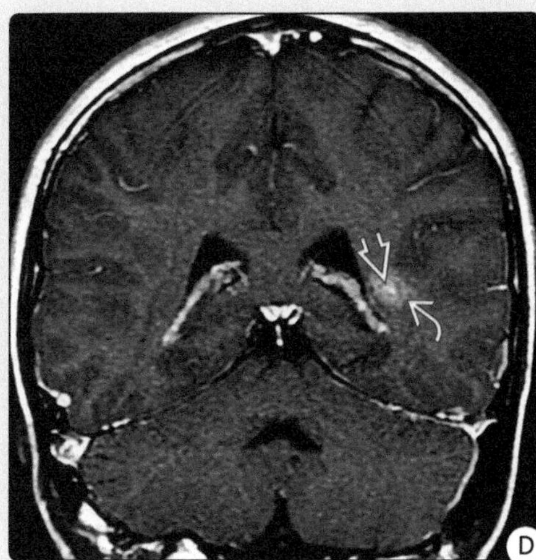

***(7-33C)** T1 C+ FS MR shows brush-like area of enhancement surrounding a prominent central draining vein. A superficial cortical vein also drains the lesion. **(7-33D)** Coronal T1 C+ MR shows the brush-like enhancement of a giant capillary telangiectasia with prominent central draining vein.*

Arterial Anatomy and Strokes

"Stroke" is a generic term that describes a clinical event characterized by sudden onset of a neurologic deficit. However, not all strokes are the same! Stroke syndromes have significant clinical and pathophysiological heterogeneity that is reflected in their underlying gross pathologic and imaging appearances. Arterial ischemia/infarction—the major focus of this chapter—is by far the most common cause of stroke, accounting for 80% of all cases.

The remaining 20% of strokes are mostly hemorrhagic, divided between primary "spontaneous" intracranial hemorrhage (sICH), nontraumatic subarachnoid hemorrhage (SAH), and venous occlusions. Both sICH and SAH were discussed extensively in preceding chapters, and venous occlusions will be discussed in the following chapter.

We begin by briefly reviewing the normal intracranial arteries and their vascular distributions. With this solid anatomic foundation, we then turn our attention to the etiology, pathology, and imaging manifestations of arterial strokes.

Normal Arterial Anatomy and Vascular Distributions

Circle of Willis

Normal Anatomy

The circle of Willis (COW) has 10 components: Two internal carotid arteries (ICAs), two proximal or horizontal (A1) anterior cerebral artery (ACA) segments, the anterior communicating artery (ACoA), two posterior communicating arteries (PCoAs), the basilar artery (BA), and two proximal or horizontal (P1) segments of the posterior cerebral arteries (PCAs) **(8-1) (8-2)**. The middle cerebral artery (MCA) is *not* part of the COW.

Vascular Territory

Important perforating branches arise from all parts of the COW and supply most of the basilar brain structures. COW *variants* are the rule, not the exception. One or more components of the COW is hypoplastic or absent in the majority of cases. A hypoplastic or absent PCoA is the most common COW variant.

Anterior Cerebral Artery

Normal Anatomy

The ACA is the smaller, more medial terminal branch of the supraclinoid ICA. Its first (horizontal) ACA segment is also termed **A1**. Small perforating vessels arise from A1 and supply the medial basal ganglia.

The **A2** or vertical ACA segment extends from the A1-ACoA junction to the corpus callosum rostrum **(8-3)**. The **A3** segment curves anteriorly around the corpus callosum genu then divides into two terminal ACA branches, the pericallosal and callosomarginal arteries.

Vascular Territory

Cortical ACA branches supply the anterior 2/3 of the *medial* hemispheres and corpus callosum, the inferomedial surface of the frontal lobe, and the anterior 2/3 of the cerebral convexity adjacent to the interhemispheric fissure **(8-4)**. Penetrating ACA branches (mainly the medial lenticulostriate arteries) supply the medial basal ganglia, corpus callosum genu, and anterior limb of the internal capsule.

Middle Cerebral Artery

Normal Anatomy

The MCA has four defined segments. The **M1** MCA segment extends laterally from the ICA bifurcation toward the sylvian (lateral cerebral) fissure. Lateral lenticulostriate and anterior temporal arteries arise from M1 **(8-5)**.

M2 (postbifurcation) superior and inferior MCA trunks turn posterosuperiorly in the sylvian fissure, following a gentle curve (the genu or "knee" of the MCA).

MCA branches loop at or near the top of the sylvian fissure, then course laterally under the parts ("opercula") of the

(8-1) Graphic depicts the circle of Willis (COW) with the anterior communicating artery (ACoA) and posterior communicating arteries (PCoAs) connecting the anterior (carotid) circulation to the posterior (vertebrobasilar) circulation. (8-2) Submentovertex 3T MRA shows COW with ACoA and PCoAs. A1s, P1s, and internal carotid arteries (ICAs) are shown.

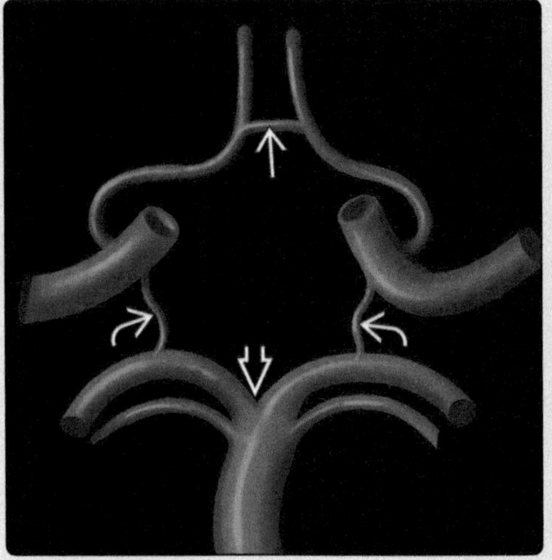

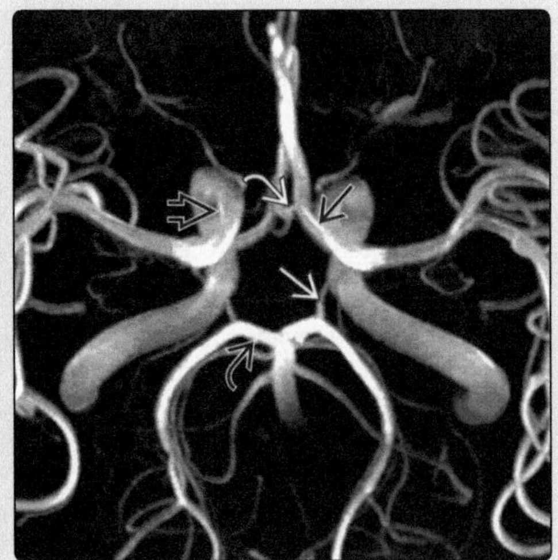

(8-3) Midline graphic shows A2 ascends in front of 3rd ventricle. A3 curves around corpus callosum genu. Pericallosal, callosomarginal arteries are major terminal ACA branches. (8-4) Cortical ACA territory (green) includes the anterior 2/3 of the medial surface of the hemisphere, a thin strip of cortex over the top of the hemisphere vertex, and a small wedge along the inferomedial frontal lobe.

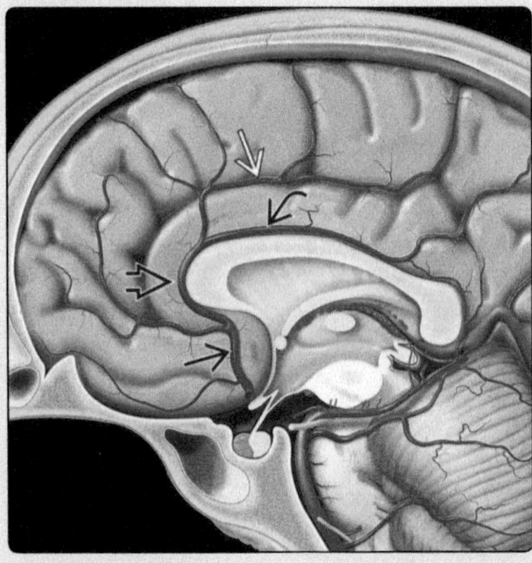

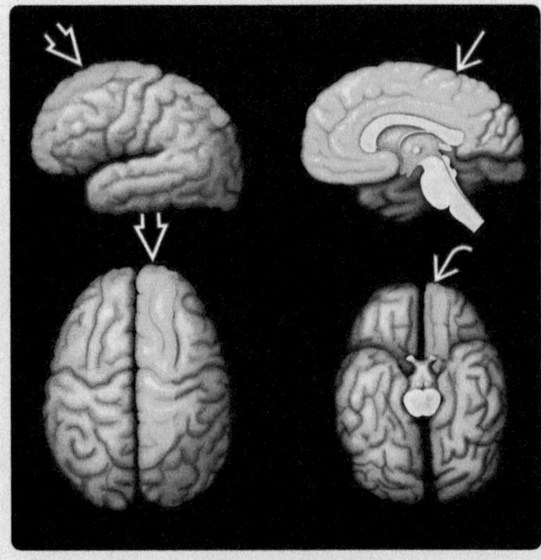

frontal, parietal, and temporal lobes that hang over and enclose the sylvian fissure. These are the **M3** or opercular segments. MCA branches become the **M4** segments when they ramify over the lateral surface of the cerebral hemisphere.

Vascular Territory

The MCA has the largest vascular territory of any of the major cerebral arteries. The MCA supplies most of the *lateral* surface of the cerebral hemisphere with the exception of a thin strip at the vertex (supplied by the ACA) and the occipital and posteroinferior parietal lobes (supplied by the PCA) **(8-6)**. Its penetrating branches supply most of the lateral basal brain structures.

Posterior Cerebral Artery

Normal Anatomy

The two PCAs are the major terminal branches of the distal BA.

The **P1** segment extends laterally from the BA bifurcation to the junction with the PCoA. The P1 segment has perforating branches that course posterosuperiorly in the interpeduncular fossa to enter the undersurface of the midbrain.

The **P2** segment extends from the P1-PCoA junction, running in the ambient (perimesencephalic) cistern as it sweeps posterolaterally around the midbrain **(8-7)**. **P3** (quadrigeminal) is a short segment that lies entirely within the quadrigeminal cistern. It begins behind the midbrain and ends where the PCA enters the calcarine fissure of the occipital lobe. The **P4** segment terminates within the calcarine fissure,

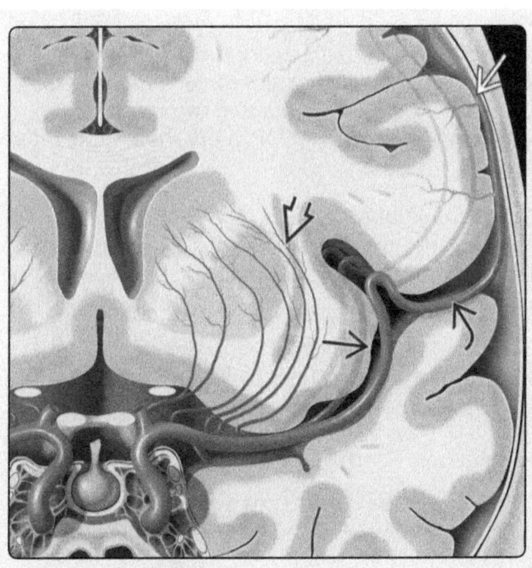

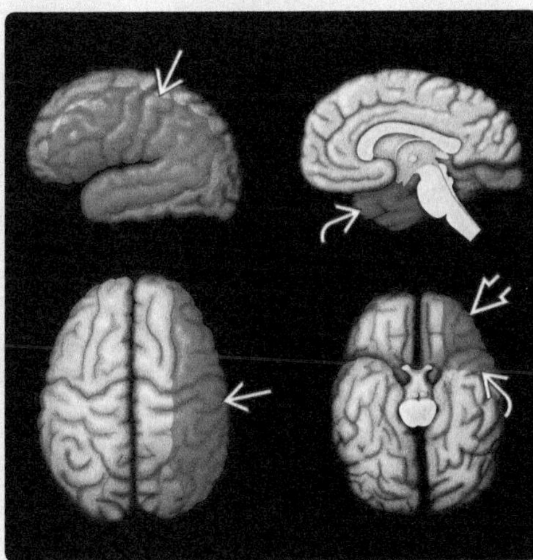

***(8-5)** Coronal graphic shows the lateral lenticulostriate arteries ➡, M2 segments over the insula ➡, M3 segments ➡ running laterally in the sylvian fissure, and M4 (cortical) branches ➡ coursing over the lateral surface of the hemisphere. **(8-6)** Cortical MCA territory (red) supplies most of the lateral surface of the hemisphere ➡, the anterior tip of the temporal lobe ➡, and the inferolateral frontal lobe ➡.*

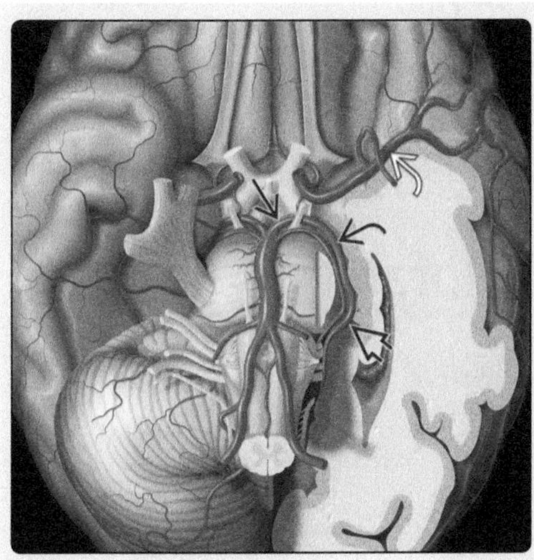

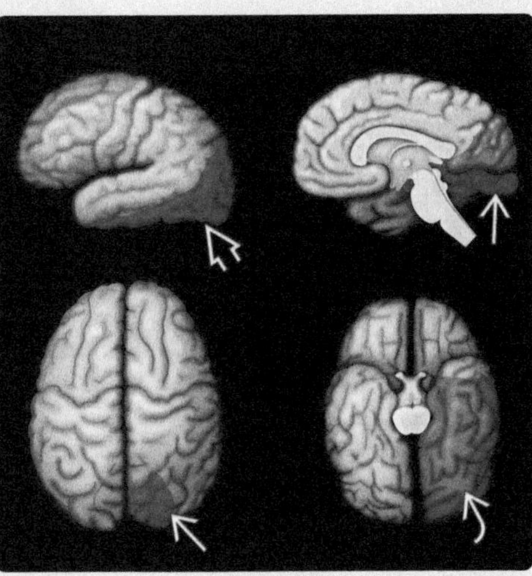

***(8-7)** Submentovertex graphic shows COW, basal brain vessels in relationship to cranial nerves. P1 ➡, P2 ➡, P3 ➡ PCA segments are shown, as is the M1 (horizontal) MCA segment ➡. **(8-8)** Cortical PCA territory (purple) includes the occipital lobe and posterior 1/3 of the medial ➡ and the posterolateral surfaces of the hemisphere ➡, as well as almost the entire inferior surface of the temporal lobe ➡.*

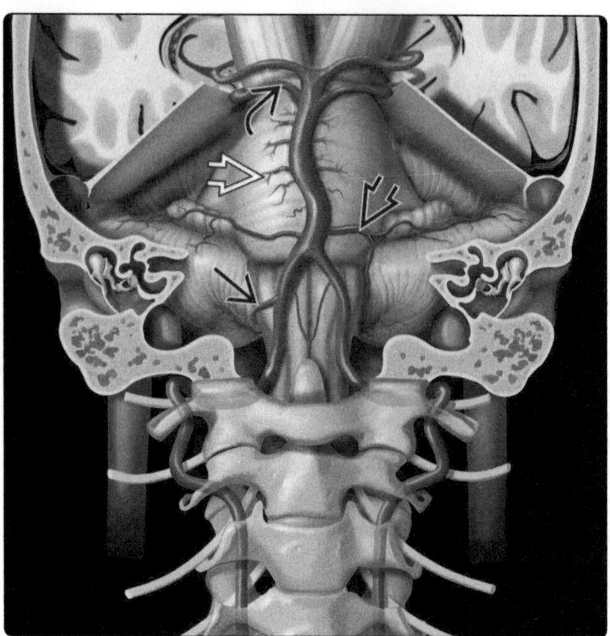

(8-9) Vertebrobasilar system: PICAs ➡ arise from VAs before the basilar junction, curve posteriorly around medulla. AICAs ➡ course laterally to the CPAs. SCAs ➡ arise from the distal BA. Perforating BA branches ➡ supply most of the pons.

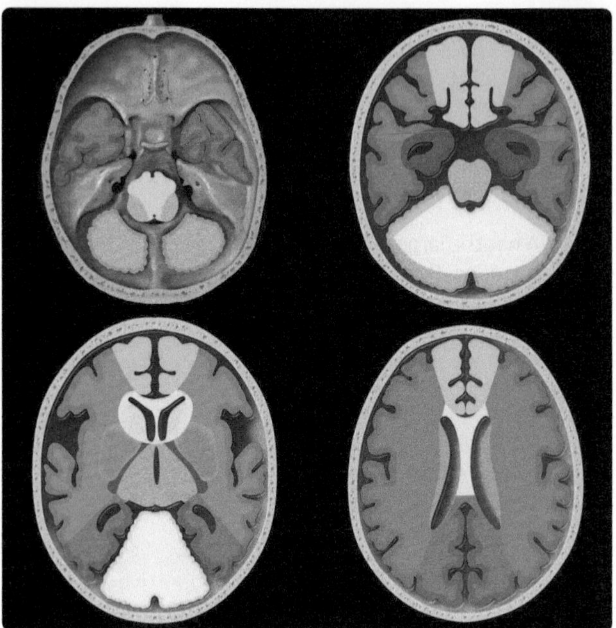

(8-10) Graphics show penetrating artery territories. Medulla (light green) is supplied by VAs, pons and thalami (light purple) from BA, caudate and medial basal ganglia, corpus callosum from ACAs (light green), putamen/globi pallidi from MCAs (blue).

where it divides into the terminal PCA trunks, including the calcarine artery.

Vascular Territory

The PCA supplies most of the *inferior* surface of the cerebral hemisphere with the exception of the temporal tip and frontal lobe. It also supplies the occipital lobe, posterior 1/3 of the medial hemisphere and corpus callosum, and most of the choroid plexus **(8-8)**. Penetrating PCA branches are the major vascular supply to the midbrain and posterior thalami.

Variants and Anomalies

A common normal variant is the **"fetal" origin of the PCA.** Here, the proximal PCA arises from the ICA instead of from the basilar bifurcation. "Fetal" PCA origin is seen in 10-30% of cases. This variant is easily recognized on CT angiography (CTA), MR angiography (MRA), and digital subtraction angiography (DSA).

A rare but important PCA variant is an **artery of Percheron** (AOP). Here, a single dominant thalamoperforating artery arises from the P1 segment and supplies the rostral midbrain and bilateral medial thalami.

Vertebrobasilar System

Normal Anatomy

The vertebrobasilar system consists of the two vertebral arteries (VAs), the BA, and their branches. Four VA segments are identified. Only one—the V4 segment—is intracranial **(8-9)**.

The **V1** (extraosseous segment) arises from the ipsilateral subclavian artery and courses posterosuperiorly to enter the C6 transverse foramen. The **V2** segment courses superiorly through the C6-C3 transverse foramina until it reaches C2, where it first turns superolaterally through the "inverted L" of the transverse foramen and then turns upward to pass through the C1 transverse foramen.

V3 begins after the VA exits the C1 transverse foramen. The **V4** (intracranial) segment extends from the foramen magnum to its junction with the BA. The VAs unite at or near the pontomedullary junction to form the **BA**. After giving off pontine and cerebellar branches, the BA terminates by dividing into the two **PCAs**.

Vascular Territory

The vertebrobasilar system normally supplies all of the posterior fossa structures as well as the midbrain, posterior thalami, occipital lobes, most of the inferior and posterolateral surfaces of the temporal lobe, and upper cervical spinal cord **(8-10)**.

Arterial Infarcts

Acute Cerebral Ischemia-Infarction

Imaging is *the* basis of rapid stroke triage. Because of speed and accessibility, NECT and CTA (with or without CT perfusion) are the most commonly used modalities.

There are four "must know" questions in acute stroke triage that need to be answered rapidly and accurately. (1) Is intracranial hemorrhage or a stroke "mimic" present? (2) Is a large vessel occluded? (3) Is part of the brain irreversibly injured (i.e., is there a core of critically ischemic, irreversibly infarcted tissue)? (4) Is there a *clinically relevant* "penumbra" of ischemic but potentially salvageable tissue?

THE 4 "MUST KNOW" ACUTE STROKE QUESTIONS

- (1) Is there intracranial hemorrhage (or a stroke "mimic")?
- (2) Is a large vessel occluded?
- (3) Is part of the brain irreversibly injured?
- (4) Is an ischemic "penumbra" present?

Terminology

Stroke—a generic term meaning sudden onset of a neurologic event—is also referred to as a cerebrovascular accident (CVA) or "brain attack."

The distinction between cerebral ischemia and cerebral infarction is subtle but important. In cerebral *ischemia*, the affected tissue remains viable, although blood flow is inadequate to sustain normal cellular function. In cerebral *infarction*, frank cell death occurs with loss of neurons, glia, or both.

Timing is important in patient triage. *Hyperacute* stroke designates events within the first 6 hours following symptom onset. In hyperacute stroke, cell death has not yet occurred, so the combined term *acute cerebral ischemia-infarction* is often used. *Acute* strokes are those 6-48 hours from onset.

Etiology

Stroke Subtypes. Atherosclerotic (ASVD) strokes are the most common type of acute arterial ischemia/infarction, representing ~ 40-45% of cases.

Most large artery territorial infarcts are embolic, arising from thrombi that develop at the site of an "at risk" ASVD plaque. The most common site is the carotid bifurcation. The most frequently occluded intracranial vessel is the MCA.

Small vessel disease represents 15-30% of all strokes. Small artery occlusions, also called **lacunar infarcts**, are defined as lesions measuring < 15 mm in diameter. Many are clinically silent, although a strategically located lesion (e.g., in the internal capsule) can cause significant neurologic impairment.

Lacunar infarcts can be embolic, atheromatous, or thrombotic. Most involve penetrating arteries in the basal ganglia/thalami, internal capsule, pons, and deep cerebral white matter.

Cardioembolic disease accounts for another 15-25% of major strokes.

Pathophysiology. An estimated two million neurons are lost each minute when a major vessel, such as the MCA, is suddenly occluded. Cerebral blood flow (CBF) falls precipitously. The center of the affected brain parenchyma—the densely **ischemic core**—typically has a CBF < 6-8 cm^3/100 g/min.

Neuronal death with irreversible loss of function occurs in the core of an acute stroke. A relatively less **ischemic penumbra** surrounding the central core is present in ~ 1/2 of all patients. CBF in the penumbra is significantly reduced, falling from a normal of 60 cm^3/100 g/min to 10-20 cm^3/100 g/min. This ischemic but not-yet-doomed-to-infarct tissue represents physiologically "at risk" but potentially salvageable tissue.

Pathology

Location. The MCA is the most common site of large artery thromboembolic occlusion **(8-11)** followed by the PCA and vertebrobasilar circulation. The ACA is the least commonly occluded major intracranial vessel.

Size and Number. Acute infarcts can be solitary or multiple and vary in size from tiny lacunar to large territorial lesions that can involve much of the cerebral hemisphere.

Gross Pathology. An acutely thrombosed artery is filled with soft purplish clot that may involve the entire vessel or just a short segment.

Gross parenchymal changes are minimal or absent in the first 6-8 hours, after which edema in the affected vascular territory causes the brain to appear pale and swollen. The gray matter-white matter (GM-WM) boundaries become less distinct and more "blurred." As the gyri expand, the adjacent sulci are compressed, and the sulcal-cisternal CSF space is effaced.

Clinical Issues

Epidemiology and Demographics. Stroke is the third leading cause of death in industrialized countries and is the major worldwide cause of adult neurologic disability.

Strokes affect patients of all ages—including newborns and neonates—although most occur in middle-aged or older adults. Children with strokes often have an underlying disorder, such as right-to-left cardiac shunt, sickle cell disease, or inherited hypercoagulable syndrome. Strokes in young adults are often caused by dissection (spontaneous or traumatic) or drug abuse.

Presentation. Sudden onset of a focal neurologic deficit, such as facial droop, slurred speech, paresis, or decreased consciousness, is the most common presentation.

Natural History. Stroke outcome varies widely. Between 20-25% of strokes are considered "major" occlusions and cause 80% of adverse outcomes. Six months after stroke, 20-30% of all patients are dead, and a similar number are severely disabled.

Prognosis in individual patients depends on a number of contributing factors, i.e., which vessel is occluded, the presence or absence of robust collateral blood flow, and whether there is a significant ischemic penumbra.

Uncontrolled brain swelling with herniation and death can result from so-called malignant MCA infarction. In such cases, emergent craniectomy may be the only treatment option.

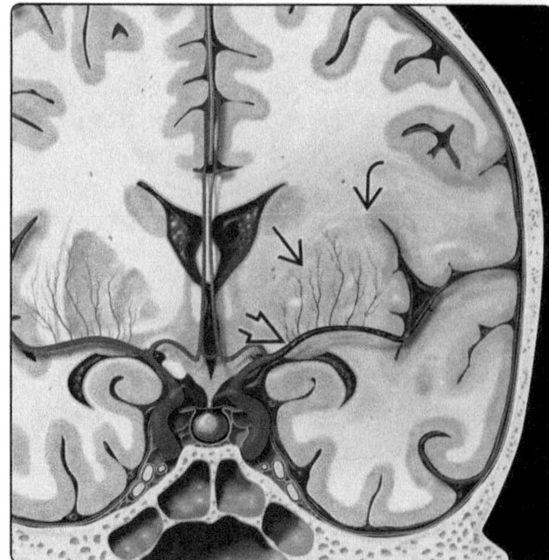

(8-11) *Graphic shows M1 occlusion ➡. Acute ischemia is seen as subtle loss of gray-white interfaces ➡ and "blurred" basal ganglia ➡.*

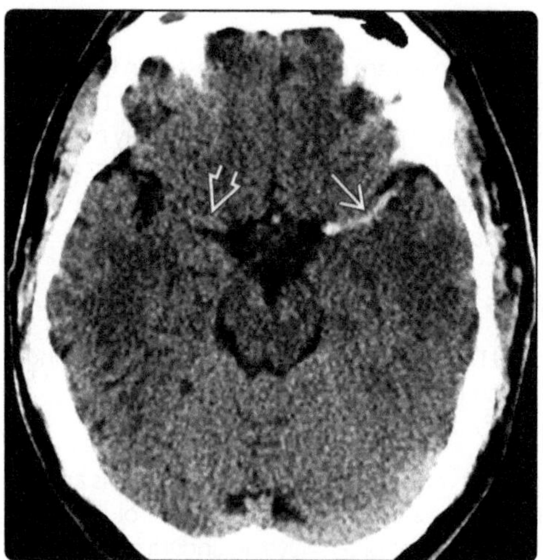

(8-12) *NECT shows "hyperdense MCA" sign ➡ (thrombus in the right MCA) compared to the normal, mild hyperdensity of the left MCA ➡.*

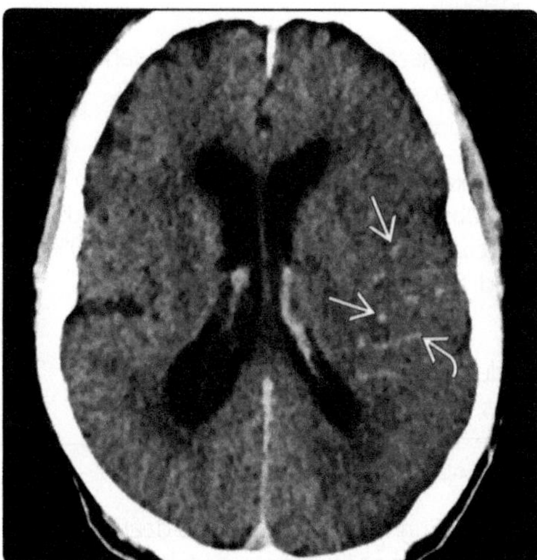

(8-13) *NECT in acute onset of right hemiparesis shows hyperdense thrombus in the left M2 ("dot" sign) ➡ and M3 ➡ MCA branches.*

Treatment Options. Ultrafast stroke triage is essential with the goal of a "door to needle" time (i.e., from arrival in the emergency department to intervention) under 60 minutes.

The single most important factor in successful intervention is patient selection with the two most important considerations being (1) elapsed time from symptom onset and (2) imaging findings.

Once hemorrhage has been excluded by NECT, *intravenous* recombinant tissue plasminogen activator (rTPA) may be administered as patients are transferred to a major stroke center ("drip and ship"), especially if elapsed time is < three hours from ictus (the so-called "golden hours").

Several large studies have shown that the most effective treatment for large vessel clot is mechanical thrombectomy with a stent retriever. Endovascular therapy significantly improves outcomes and reduces long-term disability after ischemic stroke.

Imaging

"Brain Attack" Protocols. The primary goals of emergent stroke imaging are (1) to distinguish "bland" or ischemic stroke from intracranial hemorrhage and (2) to select/triage patients for possible reperfusion therapies.

Most protocols begin with emergent NECT to answer the *first* "must know" question in stroke imaging: Is intracranial hemorrhage or a stroke "mimic" (such as subdural hematoma or neoplasm) present? If a typical hypertensive hemorrhage is identified on the screening NECT and the patient has a history of systemic hypertension, no further imaging is generally required. CTA is sometimes requested to evaluate for active bleeding ("spot" sign).

Once intracranial hemorrhage is excluded, the *second* critical issue is determining whether a major cerebral vessel is occluded. CTA can be obtained immediately following the NECT scan and is the noninvasive procedure of choice for depicting potentially treatable major vessel occlusions. MRA is more susceptible to motion artifact, which is accentuated in uncooperative patients. DSA is typically reserved for patients undergoing intraarterial thrombolysis or mechanical thrombectomy.

The *third* and *fourth* questions can be answered with either CT or MR perfusion (pCT, pMR) studies. Both can depict what part of the brain is irreversibly damaged (i.e., the unsalvageable core infarct) and determine whether there is a clinically relevant ischemic penumbra (potentially salvageable brain).

CT Findings. A complete multimodal acute stroke CT protocol includes nonenhanced head CT, an arch-to-vertex CTA, and dynamic first-pass perfusion CT (pCT). With helical acquisition, the entire protocol can be completed within 15 minutes as a single examination with separate contrast boluses. CTA with CTP improves diagnostic accuracy compared with NECT alone and does not delay IV tPA or endovascular therapy.

NECT. Initial NECT scans—even those obtained in the first 6 hours—are abnormal in 50-60% of acute ischemic strokes if viewed with narrow window width.

The most specific but least sensitive sign is a hyperattenuating vessel filled with acute thrombus. A **"dense MCA" sign** is seen in 30% of cases with documented M1 occlusion **(8-12)**. Less common sites for a hyperdense vessel sign are the intracranial ICA, BA, and MCA branches in the sylvian fissure ("dot" sign) **(8-13)**.

Uncommon but important NECT findings that indicate vascular occlusion include one or more calcified emboli **(8-26)**, most likely from an "at-risk" ulcerated atherosclerotic plaque in the cervical or cavernous ICA. It is critically important to identify calcified cerebral emboli, as they carry a near 50% risk of repeat ischemic stroke.

Blurring and indistinctness of GM-WM interfaces can be seen in 50-70% of cases within the first three hours following occlusion. Loss of the insular cortex (**"insular ribbon" sign**) **(8-15A)** and decreased density of the basal ganglia (**"disappearing basal ganglia" sign**) are the most common findings.

Wedge-shaped parenchymal hypodensity with indistinct GM-WM borders and **cortical sulcal effacement** develops in large territorial occlusions **(8-15B)**. If > 1/3 of the MCA territory is initially involved, the likelihood of a "malignant" MCA infarct with severe brain swelling rises, as does the risk of hemorrhagic transformation with attempted revascularization.

The **A**lberta **S**troke **P**rogram **E**arly **C**omputed **T**omographic **S**core (ASPECTS) is a straightforward, quick, and reproducible measure of early ischemic change **(8-14)**. ASPECTS score is calculated by subtracting one point for each of 10 regions affected. ASPECT score ≤ 7 equates to > 1/3 of the MCA territory and is associated with increased risk of hemorrhage and poor outcome **(8-15)**.

CTA. CTA (with or without CT perfusion) quickly answers the *second* "must know" stroke question **(8-16A)**, i.e., is a major vessel occlusion with a "retrievable" intravascular thrombus present? CTA defines the intravascular thrombus and assesses collateral blood flow.

pCT. The *third* and *fourth* "must know" questions can be answered with whole-brain CT perfusion (pCT). pCT depicts the effect of vessel occlusion on the brain parenchyma itself,

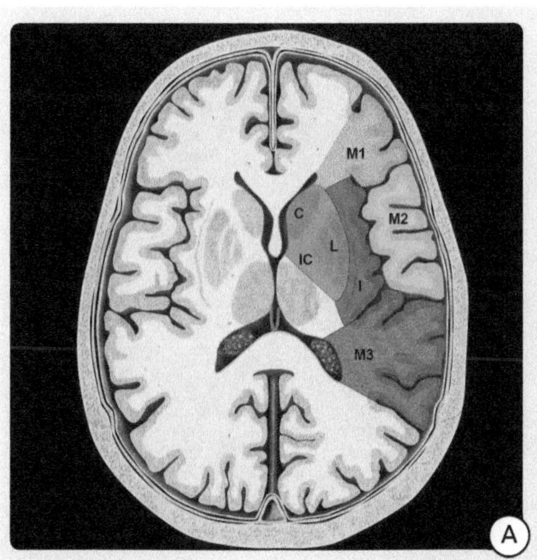

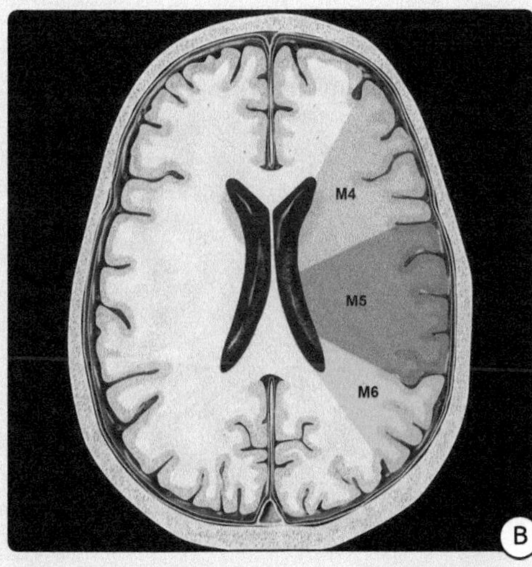

(8-14A) Anatomic regions for calculating ASPECTS score are illustrated. M1-3 represent the MCA cortex with each area allotted 1 point. The insular cortex (I), lentiform nuclei (L), caudate head (C), and internal capsule are scored with 1 point each. (8-14B) More cephalad graphic shows the superior 3 MCA territories. ASPECTS score is calculated by subtracting 1 point for each affected area from 10 (normal total score).

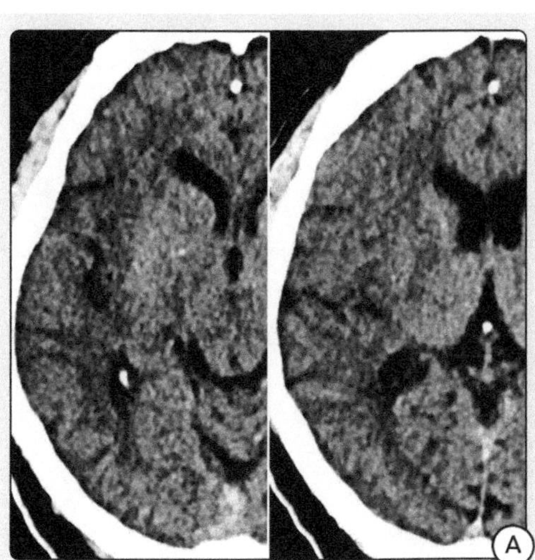

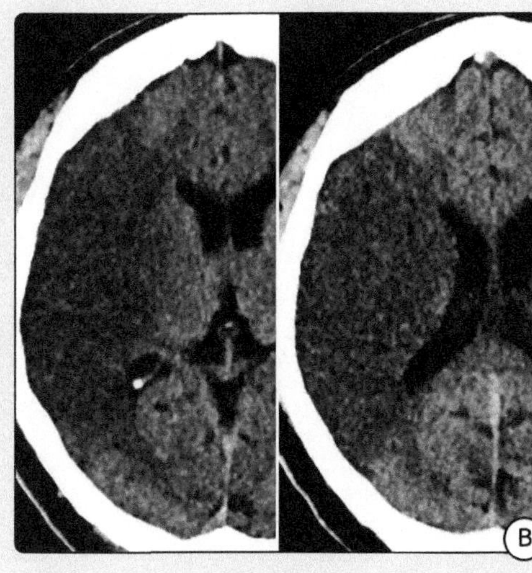

(8-15A) Axial NECTs in a 60-year-old man with acute stroke symptoms show (L) hypodensity in the right insular cortex, M1, M2, and M3 cortical areas. The caudate, lentiform nucleus, and internal capsule are spared. (R) More cephalad NECT shows hypodensity in the M4 to M6 cortical regions. ASPECTS score is 3. (8-15B) At 24 h, the wedge-shaped infarction is sharply delineated. ASPECTS score of 3 has a poor prognosis.

offering a rapid assessment of cerebral hemodynamics and parenchymal viability that is key to acute stroke management **(8-17)**.

pCT has three major parameters: Cerebral blood volume (**CBV**), cerebral blood flow (**CBF**), and mean transit time (**MTT**) or **Tmax**. CBV is the volume of flowing blood in a given volume of brain. CBF is the volume of flowing blood moving through a given volume of brain in a specified amount of time. MTT is the average time it takes blood to transit through a given volume of brain. Automated processing can quickly measure volumes with CBF < 30% and Tmax > 6 seconds as well as calculate mismatch volumes and ratios **(8-17D)**.

All three pCT parameters can also be depicted either visually on a color scale. The standard color scale is graduated from shades of red and yellow to blue and violet. With CBV and CBF, perfusion is portrayed in red/yellow/green (highest) to blue/purple/black (lowest). Well-perfused gray matter (GM) appears red/yellow, white matter (WM) appears blue, and ischemic brain is blue/purple.

The densely ischemic **infarct core**—the irreversibly injured brain—shows matched reduction in *both* CBV and CBF and is seen as a dark blue/purple or black area **(8-17A)**. Prolonged MTT is seen as a red area in contrast to the blue brain, in which transit time is normal **(8-17C)**.

An **ischemic penumbra** with potentially salvageable tissue is seen as a "mismatch" between markedly reduced CBV in the infarcted core and a surrounding area (penumbra) characterized by decreased CBF with normal or even transiently increased CBV. Thus the potentially salvageable brain tissue is equivalent to CBV minus CBF. Between 15-20% of large MCA infarcts cause hypoperfusion with reduced CBF in the *contralateral* cerebellum, a phenomenon called **crossed cerebellar diaschisis**.

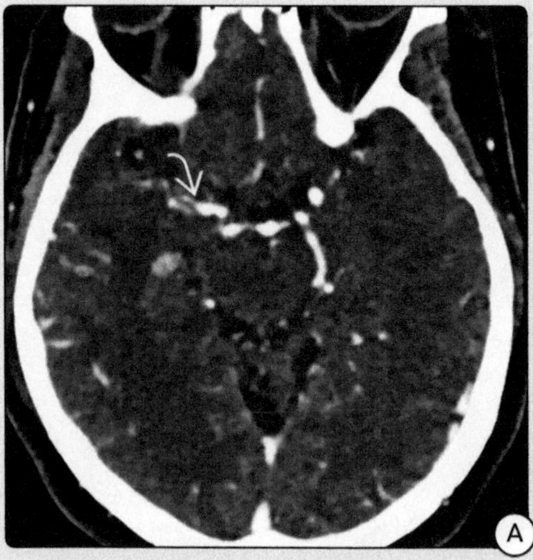

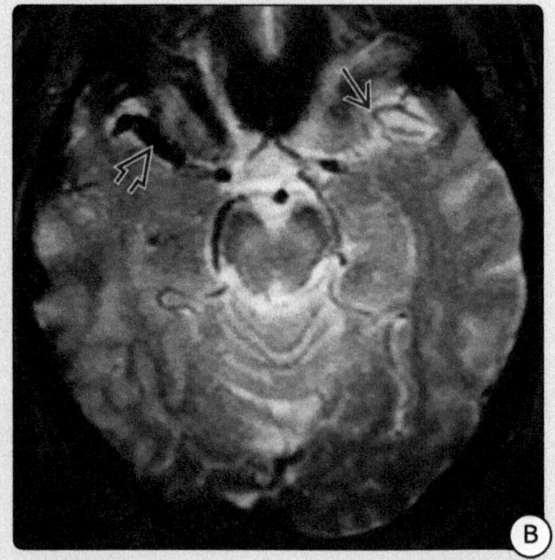

(8-16A) *CT angiogram in a 60-year-old woman in the ER with rapid stroke evaluation shows an abrupt cut-off of the proximal right MCA ➡.* ***(8-16B)*** *T2* GRE shows striking "blooming" of the right M1/proximal M2 MCA thrombus ➡. Compare to normal signal intensity in the left MCA genu ➡.*

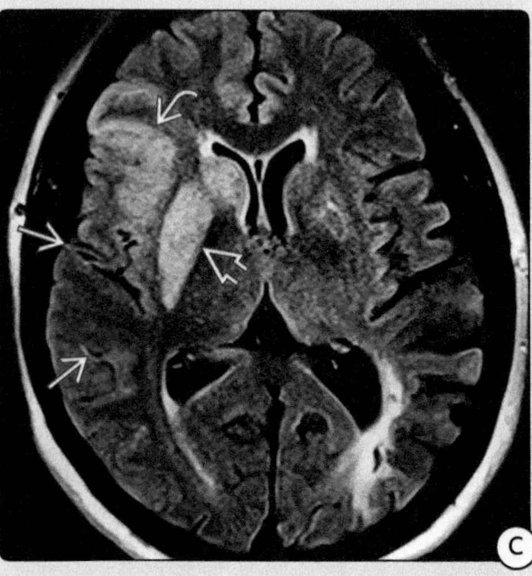

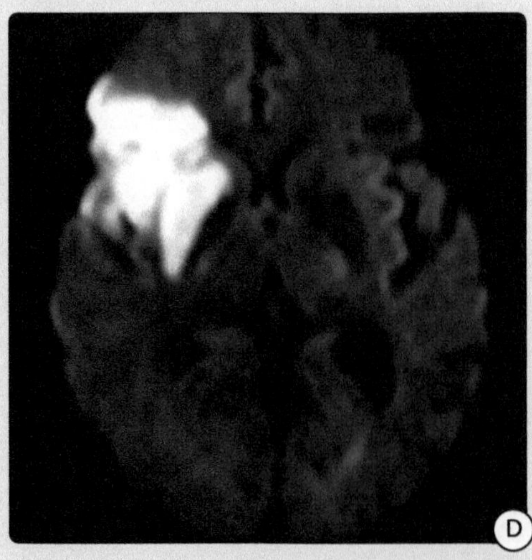

(8-16C) *FLAIR shows hyperintensity in the right basal ganglia ➡ and insular/frontal cortex ➡. Note intravascular signal in the distal cortical branches ➡, indicating slow flow.* ***(8-16D)*** *DWI shows restricted diffusion in the basal ganglia, right frontal lobe. The territory supplied by the posterior division of the right MCA is not affected, indicating that the slow collateral flow seen on FLAIR was sufficient to avoid ischemia.*

MR Findings. Although CT/CTA/pCT is often preferred because of accessibility and speed, "expedited" rapid stroke protocols with only fast FLAIR, T2*, DWI, and pMR can be used. MR is superior to CT in detecting small ischemic and lacunar strokes.

T1WI. T1WI is usually normal within the first 3-6 hours. Subtle gyral swelling and hypointensity begin to develop within 12-24 hours and are seen as blurring of the GM-WM interfaces. With large vessel occlusions, loss of the expected "flow void" in the affected artery can sometimes be identified.

T2/FLAIR. Only 30-50% of acute strokes show cortical swelling and hyperintensity on FLAIR scans within the first 4 hours. Nearly all strokes are FLAIR positive by 7 hours following symptom onset **(8-16C)**. Intraarterial hyperintensity on FLAIR is an early sign of stroke and indicates slow flow, either from delayed antegrade flow or—more commonly—retrograde collateral filling across the cortical watershed **(8-18A)**. FLAIR-DWI "mismatch" (negative FLAIR, positive DWI) has been suggested as a quick indicator of viable ischemic penumbra and eligibility for thrombolysis.

T2* GRE. Intraarterial thrombus can sometimes be detected as "blooming" hypointensity on T2* (GRE, SWI) **(8-16B)**. Large MCA infarcts sometimes exhibit increased hypointensity in deep medullary veins due to prolonged transit time and increased deoxyhemoglobin. Although hemorrhagic transformation may sometimes occur as early as 24-48 hours following ictus, it is more typical of late acute and early subacute infarcts.

T1 C+. Postcontrast T1 scans show intravascular enhancement **(8-18D)**. Parenchymal enhancement is uncommon in acute/hyperacute ischemia.

DWI and DTI. Around 95% of hyperacute infarcts show diffusion restriction on DWI with hyperintensity on DWI **(8-16D)** and corresponding hypointensity on ADC. DTI is even

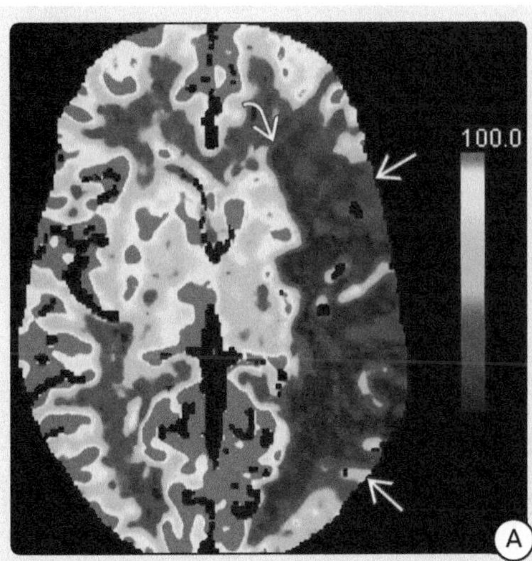

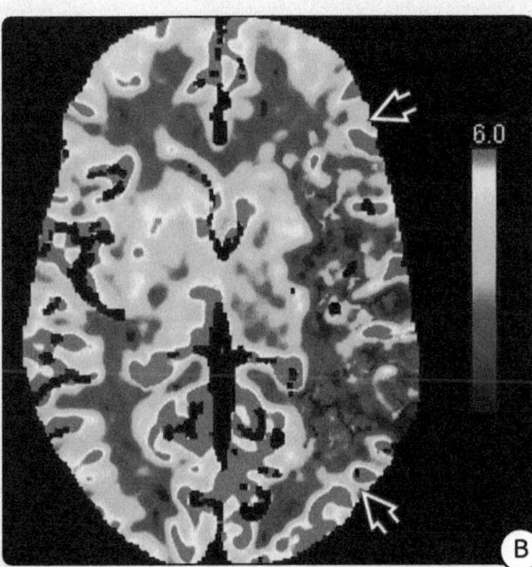

(8-17A) Patient with large left MCA infarct from distal M1 thrombus is shown. pCT shows markedly reduced CBF in the lateral basal ganglia/insula and the entire cortical territory. (8-17B) CBV in the same case shows small areas of preserved blood volume around the margins of the core infarct.

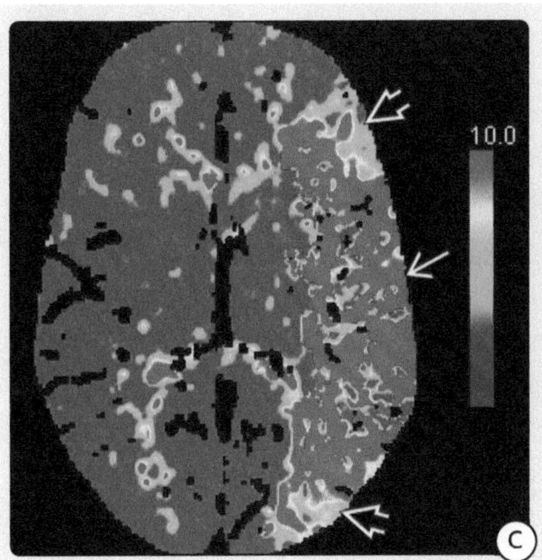

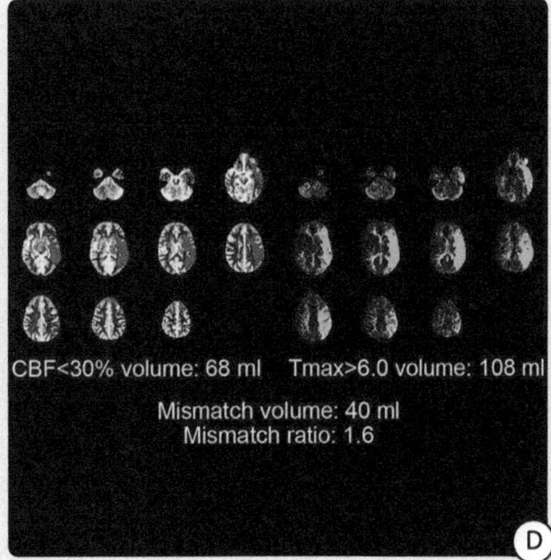

(8-17C) MTT shows severely prolonged transit time in the core infarct. Less severely increased MTT is present at the lesion margins. (8-17D) Automated pCT calculation shows volume with CBF < 30% (pink, representing severely ischemic core infarct) is 68 mL. Volume with Tmax > 6.0 seconds (green) is 108 mL. The mismatch volume is 40 mL and the mismatch ratio is 1.6. Thrombectomy was unsuccessful.

more sensitive than DWI, especially for small pontine and medullary lesions.

pMR. Restriction on DWI generally reflects the densely ischemic core of the infarct, whereas pMR depicts the surrounding "at-risk" penumbra. A **DWI-PWI mismatch** is one of the criteria used in determining suitability for intraarterial thrombolysis.

Angiography. Findings include abrupt vessel "cut-off," a "meniscus" sign, tapered or "rat-tail" narrowing, or tram-track appearance (contrast around intraluminal thrombus). Others are "bare" or "naked" area(s) of nonperfused brain, slow antegrade filling with intraarterial contrast persisting into the capillary or venous phase, and pial collaterals with retrograde filling across the cortical watershed.

Less common signs are hyperemia with a vascular "blush" around the infarcted zone (so-called "luxury perfusion") and "early draining" veins.

Differential Diagnosis

Normal circulating blood is always slightly hyperdense compared with brain on NECT. A "hyperdense vessel" sign can be simulated by **elevated hematocrit** (all the vessels appear dense, not just the arteries), arterial wall **microcalcifications**, and **hypodense brain** parenchyma (e.g., diffuse cerebral edema).

Stroke "mimics" with restricted DWI include **infection, status epilepticus**, and acute **hypoglycemia**. These typically affect cortex in a nonvascular distribution while sparing the underlying subcortical WM.

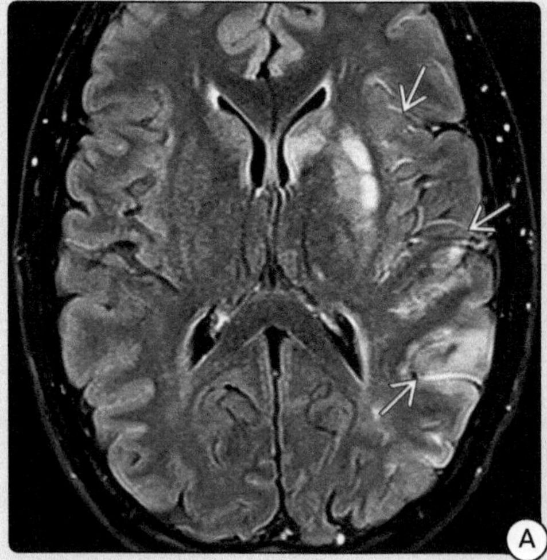

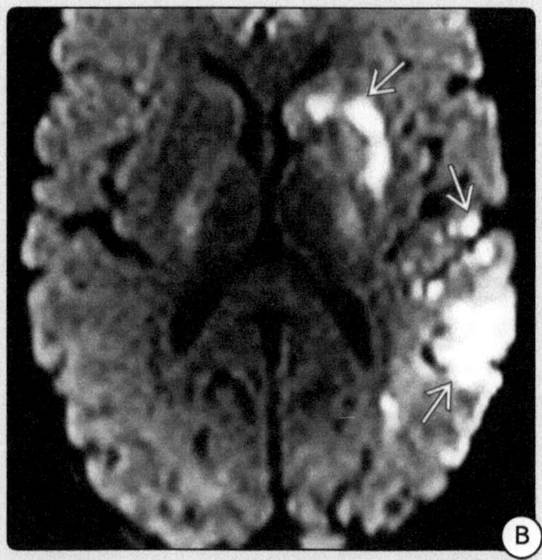

***(8-18A)** Acute stroke in a 47-year-old man shows patchy hyperintensity in the left caudate nucleus, lateral putamen, and parietal cortex. Note multiple linear foci of intravascular hyperintensity ➡, consistent with slow flow in the MCA distribution.* ***(8-18B)** DWI in the same patient shows multiple patchy foci of diffusion restriction ➡, consistent with acute cerebral infarct.*

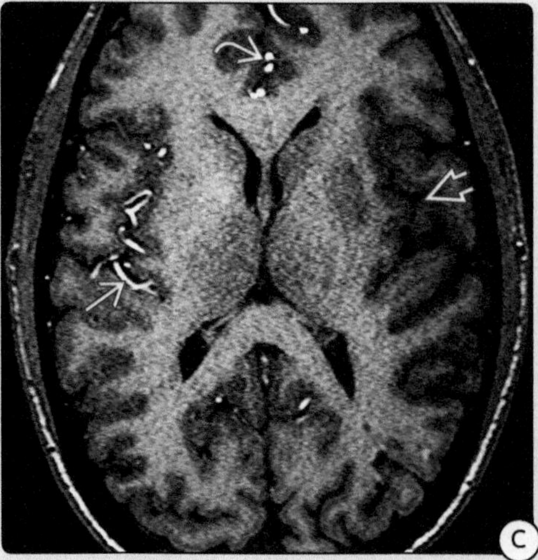

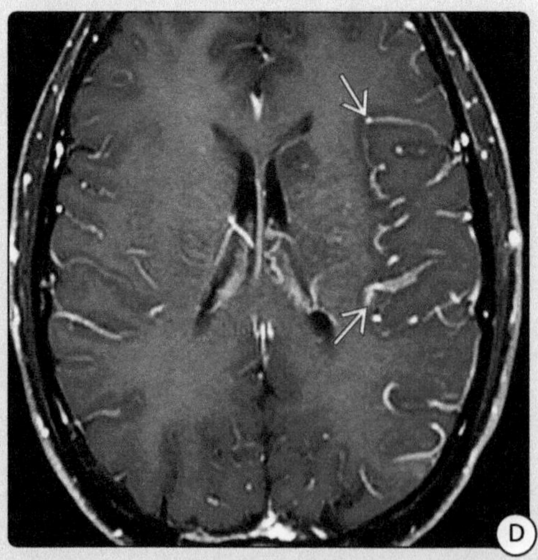

***(8-18C)** Axial source image from 2D TOF MRA shows normal signal intensity in the right MCA ➡ and both ACA branches ➡ but no flow in the left MCA vessels ➡.* ***(8-18D)** Axial T1 C+ FS MR shows striking intravascular enhancement in the left MCA branches ➡, consistent with slow flow in patent (nonthrombosed) vessels.*

ACUTE STROKE IMAGING

NECT
- Hyperdense vessel ± "dot" sign
- "Blurred," effaced GM-WM borders
  - "Insular ribbon" sign
  - "Disappearing" basal ganglia
- Wedge-shaped hypodensity
  - Involves both cortex, WM
- Look for Ca^{++} emboli (≈ 50% risk future stroke)

CECT
- ± enhancing vessels (slow flow, collaterals)

CTA
- Shows site, length of major vessel thrombus
- ASVD
  - Extracranial: Aorta, carotid bifurcation
  - Intracranial: Cavernous ICA, circle of Willis + branches

pCT
- Infarct core (irreversibly damaged brain)
  - Matched perfusion (CBV, CBF both ↓)
  - ↑ MTT
- Ischemic penumbra
  - Perfusion "mismatch" (↓ CBF but normal CBV)

T1WI
- Usually normal in first 4-6 hours
- ± loss of expected "flow void"

T2WI
- Usually normal in first 4-6 hours

FLAIR (use narrow windows)
- 50% positive in first 4-6 hours
  - Cortical swelling, gyral hyperintensity
  - Intraarterial hyperintensity (usually slow flow, not thrombus)

T2* (GRE, SWI)
- Thrombus may "bloom"
- Large infarcts may show prominent hypointense medullary veins
- Microbleeds (chronic hypertension, amyloid)

DWI and DTI
- > 95% restriction within minutes
  - Hyperintense on DWI
  - Hypointense on ADC map
- "Diffusion-negative" acute strokes
  - Small (lacunar) infarcts
  - Brainstem lesions
  - Rapid clot lysis/recanalization
  - Transient/fluctuating hypoperfusion

pMR
- DWI-PWI "mismatch" estimates penumbra
- CBV-CBF, DWI-FLAIR mismatches estimate penumbra

DSA
- Vessel "cut-off," "meniscus" sign, tapered/"rat-tail" narrowing
- "Bare" area of unperfused brain
- Slow antegrade or retrograde filling
- Delayed intraarterial contrast washout
- Luxury perfusion
  - "Blush" around "bare area"
  - "Early draining" veins

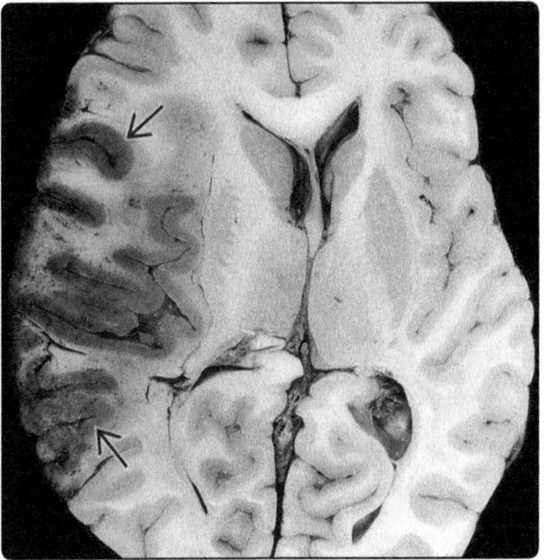

***(8-19)** Late acute/early subacute stroke is shown with mass effect, gyriform hemorrhagic transformation ➡. (Courtesy R. Hewlett, MD.)*

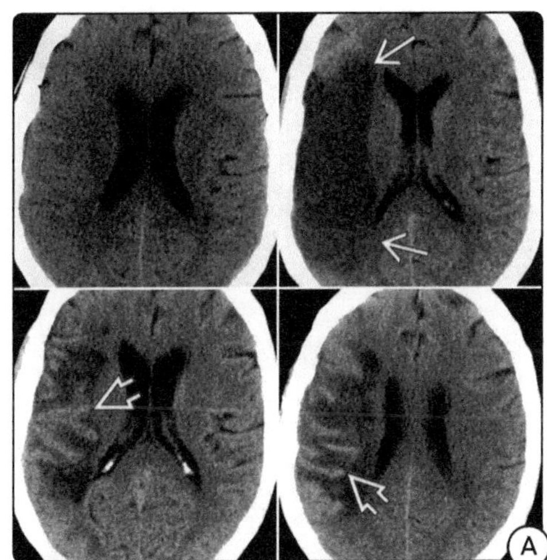

***(8-20A)** (Top) NECT at 2 h shows mild sulcal effacement. At 48 h, wedge-shaped hypodensity ➡ involves GM, WM. (Bottom) HT ➡ at 1 week.*

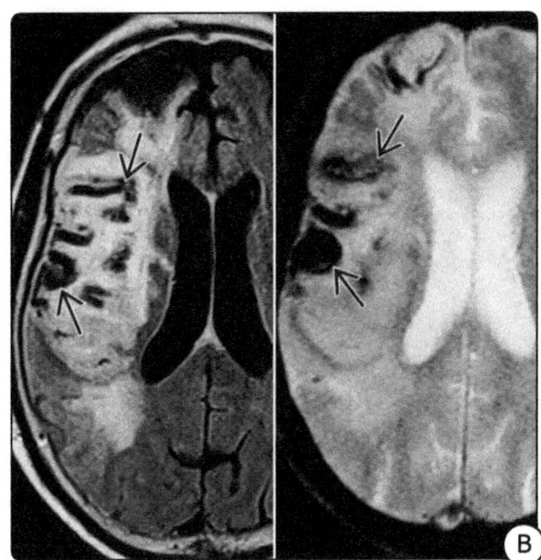

***(8-20B)** FLAIR (L) and GRE (R) in the same case show hemorrhagic transformation ➡ in this example of subacute stroke.*

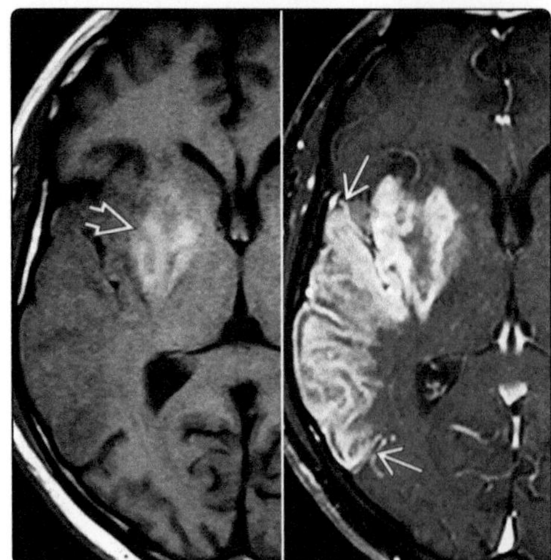

(8-21) MR 2 weeks after right MCA stroke shows HT ➡ (L) and the intense enhancement ➡ characteristic of subacute infarction (R).

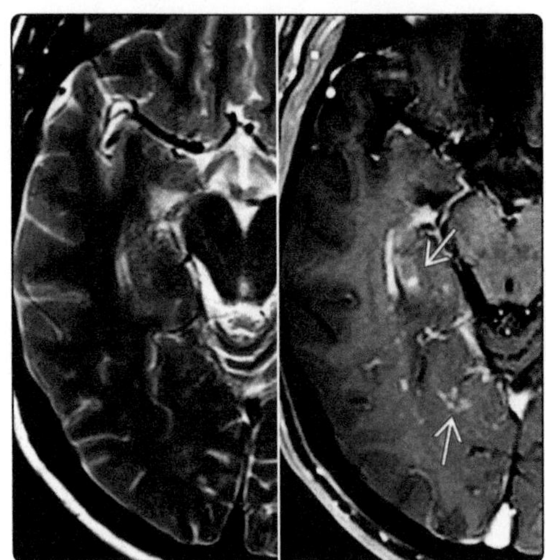

(8-22) T2 "fogging effect" 2 weeks after stroke is shown. (L) T2 appears normal. (R) T1 C+ FS shows patchy enhancement ➡ in PCA infarct.

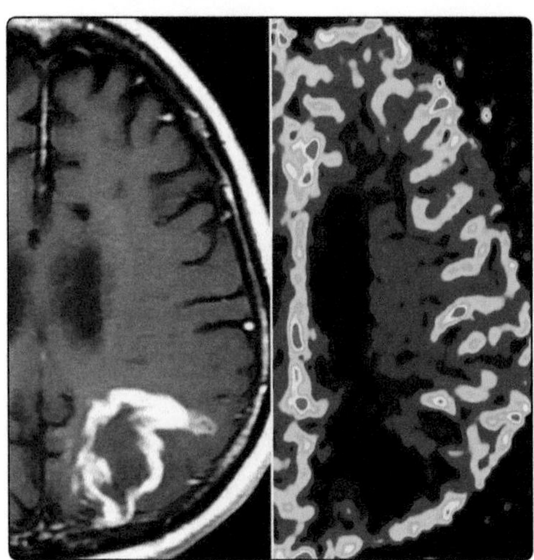

(8-23) (L) Subacute infarct with ring enhancement mimics neoplasm. (R) pMR shows "cold" lesion with profoundly decreased rCBV.

Subacute Cerebral Infarcts

Terminology

Strokes evolve pathophysiologically with corresponding changes reflected on imaging studies. Although there are no firm divisions that demarcate the various stages of stroke evolution, most neurologists designate infarcts as acute, subacute, and chronic.

"Subacute" cerebral ischemia/infarction generally refers to strokes that are between 48 hours and two weeks following the initial ischemic event.

Pathology

Edema and **increasing mass effect** caused by cytotoxic edema become maximal within 3-4 days following stroke onset. Frank tissue necrosis with progressive influx of microglia and macrophages around vessels ensues with reactive astrocytosis around the perimeter of the stroke. Brain softening and then cavitation proceeds over the next two weeks.

Most thromboembolic strokes are initially "bland," i.e., nonhemorrhagic. **Hemorrhagic transformation** (HT) of a previously ischemic infarct occurs in 20-25% of cases between two days and a week after ictus **(8-19)**. Ischemia-damaged vascular endothelium becomes "leaky," and blood-brain barrier permeability increases. When reperfusion is established—either spontaneously or following treatment with tissue plasminogen activator—exudation of red blood cells through the damaged blood vessel walls causes parenchymal hemorrhages. Petechial hemorrhages are more common than lobar bleeds and are most common in the basal ganglia and cortex.

Clinical Issues

HT itself generally does not cause clinical deterioration. HT is actually related to favorable outcome, probably reflecting early vessel recanalization and better tissue reperfusion.

Imaging

General Features. There are significant variations within the subacute time period. Early subacute strokes have significant mass effect and often exhibit HT, whereas edema and mass effect have mostly subsided by the late subacute period.

CT Findings. On NECT, the wedge-shaped area of decreased attenuation seen on initial scans becomes more sharply defined. Mass effect initially increases, then begins to decrease by 7-10 days following stroke onset. HT develops in 15-20% of cases and is seen as gyriform cortical or basal ganglia hyperdensity **(8-20A)**.

CECT follows a "2-2-2" rule. Patchy or gyriform enhancement appears as early as two days after stroke onset, peaks at two weeks, and generally disappears by two months.

MR Findings. Signal intensity in subacute stroke varies depending on (1) time since ictus and (2) the presence or absence of HT.

T1WI. Nonhemorrhagic subacute infarcts are hypointense on T1WI and demonstrate moderate mass effect with sulcal effacement. Strokes with HT are initially isointense with cortex and then become hyperintense **(8-21)**.

T2WI. Subacute infarcts are initially hyperintense compared with nonischemic brain. Signal intensity decreases with time, reaching isointensity at 1-2 weeks (the T2 "fogging effect") **(8-22)**. Early wallerian degeneration can sometimes be identified as a well-delineated hyperintense band that extends inferiorly from the infarcted cortex along the corticospinal tract.

FLAIR. Subacute infarcts are hyperintense on FLAIR **(8-20B)**. By one week after ictus, "final" infarct volume corresponds to the FLAIR-defined abnormality.

T2* (GRE, SWI). Petechial or gyriform "blooming" foci are present if HT has occurred in the infarcted cortex **(8-20B)**. Basal ganglia hemorrhages can be confluent or petechial.

Prominent ipsilateral medullary veins on SWI in MCA territory strokes within 3-7 days of ictus are a significant predictive biomarker of poor clinical outcome. Prominent medullary veins in the contralateral (normal) hemisphere may indirectly reflect increased CBF and are associated with good clinical outcome.

T1 C+. The intravascular enhancement often seen in the first 48 hours following thromboembolic occlusion disappears within three or four days and is replaced by leptomeningeal enhancement caused by persisting pial collateral blood flow. Patchy or gyriform parenchymal enhancement can occur as early as two or three days after infarction **(8-21)** and may persist for 2-3 months, in some cases mimicking neoplasm **(8-23)**.

DWI and pMR. Restricted diffusion with hyperintensity on DWI and hypointensity on ADC persists for the first several days following stroke onset, then gradually reverses to become hypointense on DWI and hyperintense with T2 "shine-through" on ADC. pMR with arterial spin labeling shows crossed cerebellar diaschisis in 50% of patients with subacute ischemic strokes.

SUBACUTE STROKE

Pathology
- Edema, mass effect initially increase
- Vessel damage → HT 25%

CT
- Hypodensity sharply defined
- Gyriform enhancement 2 days to several weeks

MR
- T1WI
  - Iso- to hypointense
  - May see T1 shortening (cortex, basal ganglia)
- T2WI
  - "Fogging effect" (isointensity)
  - ± early wallerian degeneration
- FLAIR
  - Hyperintensity corresponds to final infarct
- T2*
  - "Blooming" HT
  - Prominent medullary veins
- DWI
  - Pseudonormalization
  - T2 "shine-through"
- T1 C+
  - Enhances (gyriform, even ring-like)

Differential Diagnosis
- Neoplasm
- Infection
  - Cerebritis
  - Encephalitis

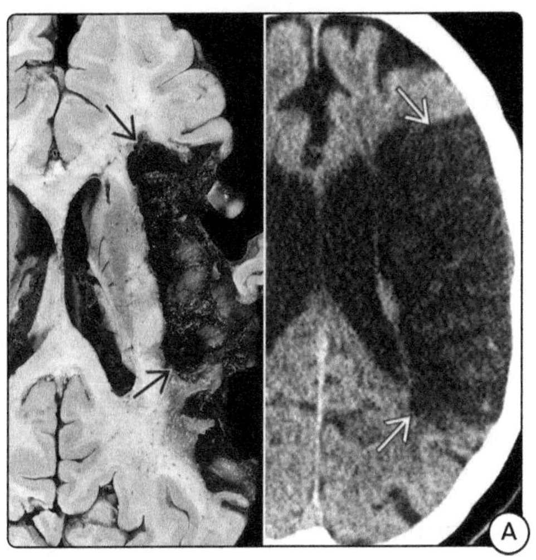

(8-24A) (L) Old MCA infarct with hemorrhagic transformation ⇒. (R. Hewlett, MD.) (R) NECT shows encephalomalacia, old MCA infarct ⇒.

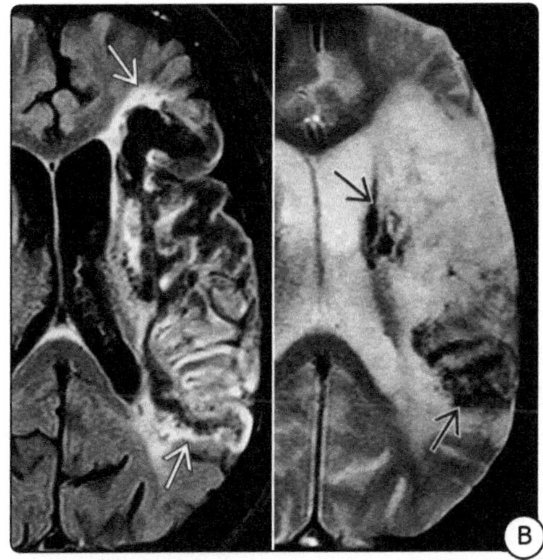

(8-24B) FLAIR (L) shows hyperintensity ⇒ around the cavitated, encephalomalacic area, whereas T2* GRE (R) shows some HT ⇒.

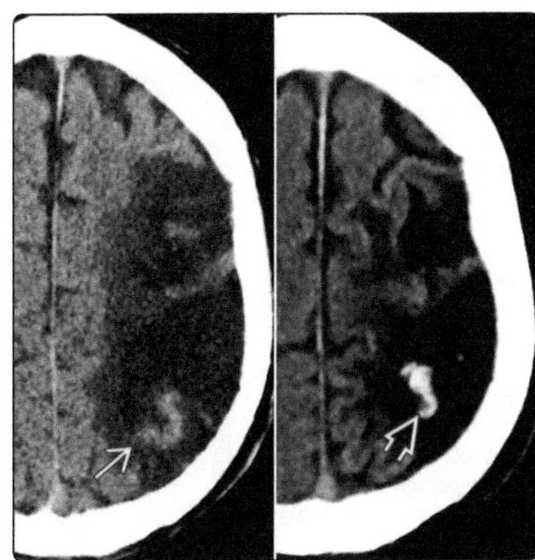

(8-25) (L) NECT of late subacute MCA infarct shows small focus of HT ⇒. (R) Gyriform Ca^{++} ⇒ is present in the same area 3 years later.

Chronic Cerebral Infarcts

Terminology

Chronic cerebral infarcts are the end result of ischemic territorial strokes and are also called postinfarction encephalomalacia.

Pathology

The pathologic hallmark of chronic cerebral infarcts is volume loss with gliosis in an anatomic vascular distribution. A cavitated, encephalomalacic brain with strands of residual glial tissue and traversing blood vessels is the usual gross appearance of an old infarct **(8-24A)**.

Imaging

NECT scans show a sharply delineated wedge-shaped hypodense area that involves both GM and WM and conforms to the vascular territory of a cerebral artery. The adjacent sulci and ipsilateral ventricle enlarge secondary to volume loss in the affected hemisphere **(8-24A)**. Dystrophic calcification occurs but is uncommon **(8-25)**.

Wallerian degeneration with an ipsilateral small, shrunken cerebral peduncle is often present with large MCA infarcts. Look for atrophy of the contralateral cerebellum secondary to crossed cerebellar diaschisis.

Chronic infarcts older than 2-3 months typically do not enhance on CECT.

MR scans show cystic encephalomalacia with CSF-equivalent signal intensity on all sequences. Marginal gliosis or spongiosis around the old cavitated stroke is hyperintense on FLAIR **(8-24B)**. DWI shows increased diffusivity (hyperintense on ADC).

__(8-26A)__ NECT in a 65-year-old man with altered mental status shows a 2-mm, rounded calcification ➔ in the interhemispheric fissure. __(8-26B)__ More cephalad image shows another rounded hyperdensity in the right sylvian fissure ➔.

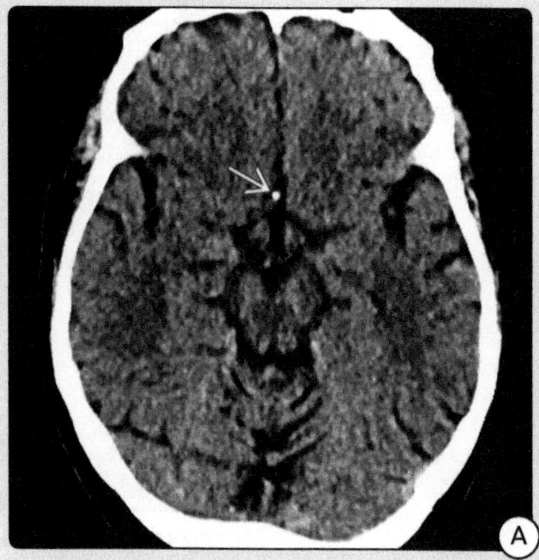

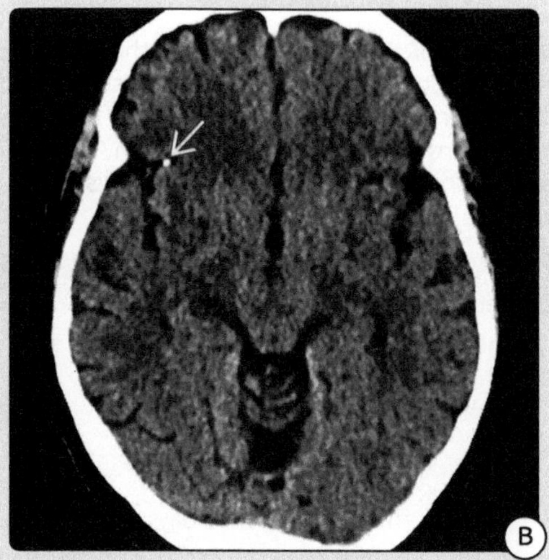

__(8-26C)__ NECT near the vertex shows a 3rd calcification ➔ in a superficial sulcus. __(8-26D)__ Sagittal NECT reformatted from the axial source data shows the calcification lies within a vertex sulcus ➔, not the brain. No parenchymal lesions were present, so these are calcified cerebral emboli in distal arterial branches. These patients are at high risk for recurrent strokes. This patient had a calcified mitral valve.

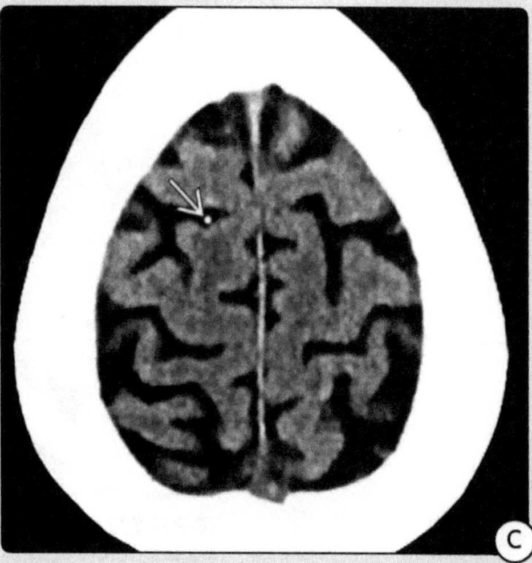

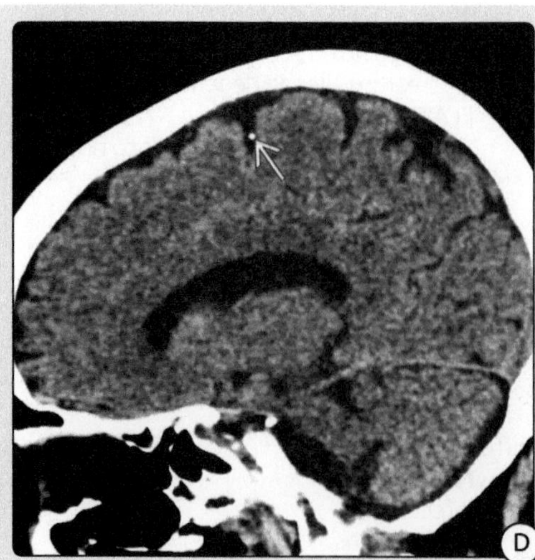

Multiple Embolic Infarcts

Brain emboli are less common but important causes of stroke. Most consist of clots containing fibrin, platelets, and RBCs. Less common emboli include air, fat, calcium, tumor, and foreign bodies (e.g., debris from metallic heart valves).

Cardiac and Atheromatous Emboli

Pathoetiology. Simultaneous small acute infarcts in multiple different vascular distributions are the hallmark of embolic cerebral infarcts **(8-27)**. The heart is the most common source; cardiac emboli can be septic or aseptic. Peripheral signs of emboli, such as splinter hemorrhages, are sometimes present. Echocardiography may demonstrate valvular vegetations, intracardiac filling defect, or atrial or ventricular septal defect.

Ipsilateral hemispheric emboli are most commonly due to atheromatous ICA plaques. Many are clinically silent but convey a high risk for subsequent overt stroke.

Imaging. In contrast to large artery territorial strokes, embolic infarcts tend to involve terminal cortical branches. The GM-WM interface is most commonly affected.

NECT scans show low-attenuation foci, often in a wedge-shaped distribution. Calcified emboli (usually from heart valves or atherosclerotic plaques) are seen as small round or ovoid calcifications within sulci **(8-26)**. These are important to identify as they carry a high risk of recurrent stroke. Septic emboli are often hemorrhagic. CECT scans may demonstrate multiple punctate or ring-enhancing lesions.

MR scans show multifocal peripheral T2/FLAIR hyperintensities. Hemorrhagic emboli cause "blooming" on T2* sequences. The most sensitive sequence is DWI. Small peripheral foci of diffusion restriction in several different

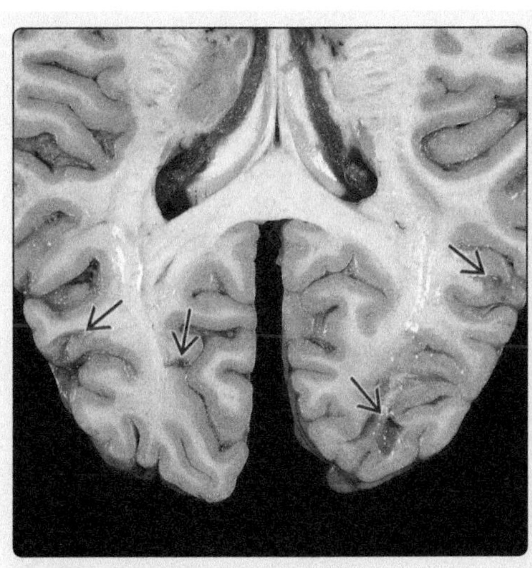

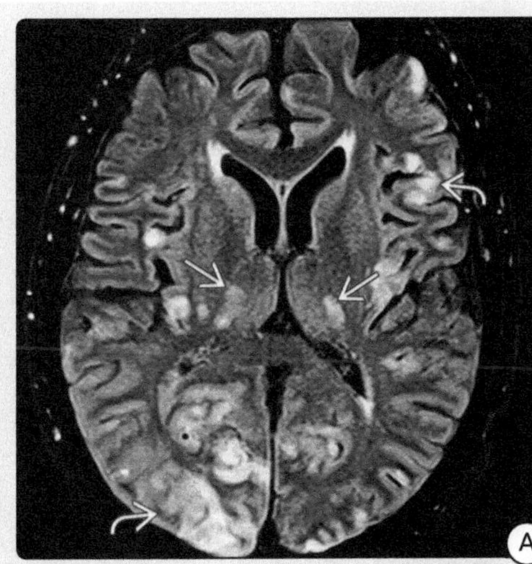

***(8-27)** Autopsy specimen shows multiple old healed infarcts at the gray-white matter (GM-WM) junctions ➡. (Courtesy R. Hewlett, MD.) **(8-28A)** A 70-year-old man with decreasing cognitive function for 1 month became acutely worse. Emergent MR with axial FLAIR shows multifocal bilateral cortical ➡ and basal ganglionic ➡ hyperintensities.*

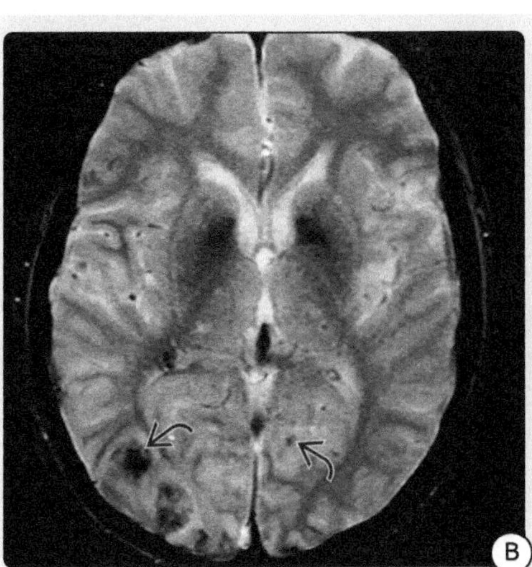

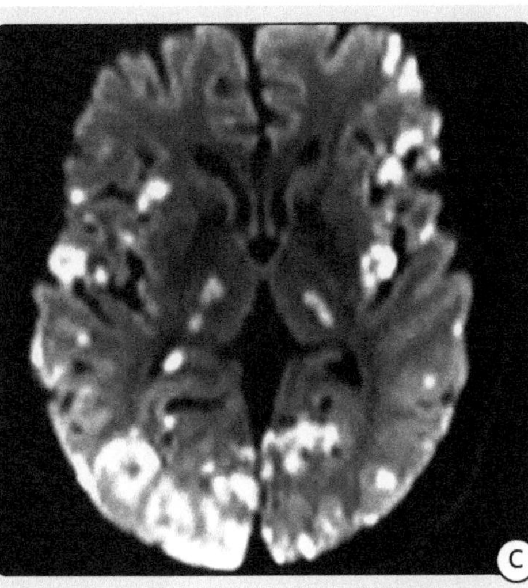

***(8-28B)** T2* GRE shows that some of the cortical lesions ➡ exhibit blooming, consistent with petechial hemorrhages. **(8-28C)** DWI shows restricted diffusion in the lesions. Multiple septic and hemorrhagic embolic infarcts are seen.*

vascular distributions are typical of multiple embolic infarcts **(8-28)**. T1 C+ imaging may show multiple punctate enhancing foci. Septic emboli often demonstrate ring enhancement, resembling microabscesses.

Differential Diagnosis. The major differential diagnosis of multiple embolic infarcts is **hypotensive cerebral infarction**. Hypotensive infarcts are usually caused by hemodynamic compromise and tend to involve the deep internal watershed zones. **Parenchymal metastases** have a predilection for the GM-WM interface, as do embolic infarcts, but generally do not restrict on DWI.

Fat Emboli

Fat embolism syndrome (FES) is an uncommon disorder that presents as hypoxia, neurologic symptoms, &/or a petechial rash in the setting of severely displaced lower extremity long bone fractures. The term "cerebral fat emboli" (CFE) refers to the neurologic manifestations of FES.

Pathoetiology. Two mechanisms have been proposed to explain the effects of FES: (1) Small vessel occlusions from fat particles and (2) inflammatory changes in surrounding tissue initiated by breakdown of fat into free fatty acids and other metabolic byproducts.

The pathologic hallmark of CFE is arteriolar fat emboli with perivascular microhemorrhages **(8-29)**.

Epidemiology and Clinical Issues. The overall incidence of FES in patients with long bone fractures—most commonly the femoral neck—is 1-2%. FES also occurs with pelvic fractures, elective orthopedic procedures (e.g., total hip arthroplasty), anesthesia, and systemic illness (e.g., pancreatitis). FES in patients with bone marrow necrosis secondary to sickle cell crisis has also been reported.

CFE occurs in up to 80% of patients with FES. Signs and symptoms vary in severity and include petechial rash, headache, seizure, drowsiness, altered mental status, and

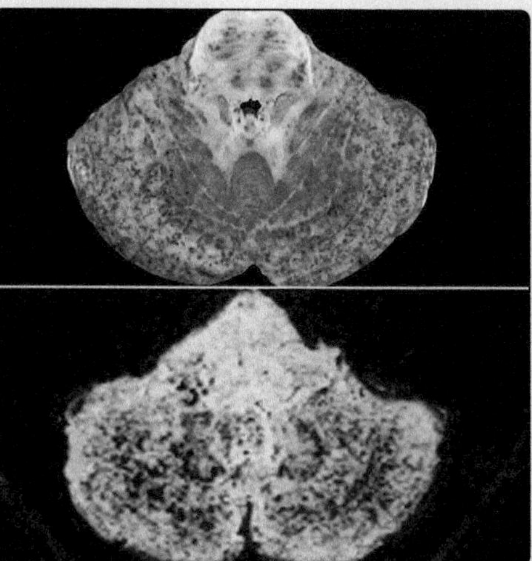

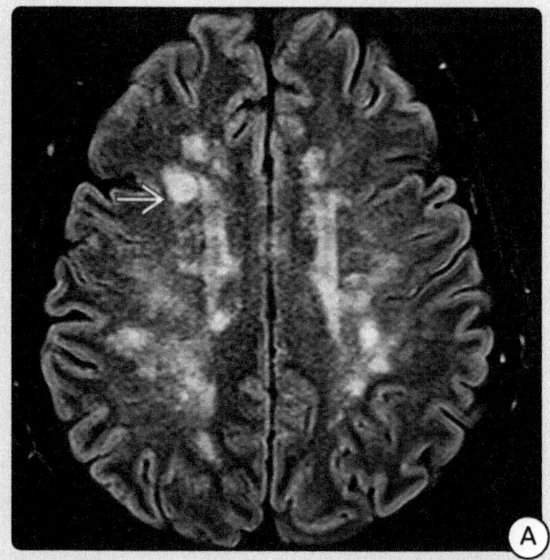

(8-29) (Top) Autopsy case of fat embolism shows innumerable small microbleeds throughout the pons and cerebellum. (Courtesy Klatt, Robbins and Cotran, Atlas of Neuropathology, 2015). (Bottom) MIP SWI in fat embolism shows multiple "blooming black dots." (8-30A) Axial FLAIR MR in a 62-year-old woman with altered mental status following hip surgery shows multiple confluent hyperintense foci ➡ in the deep WM of both hemispheres.

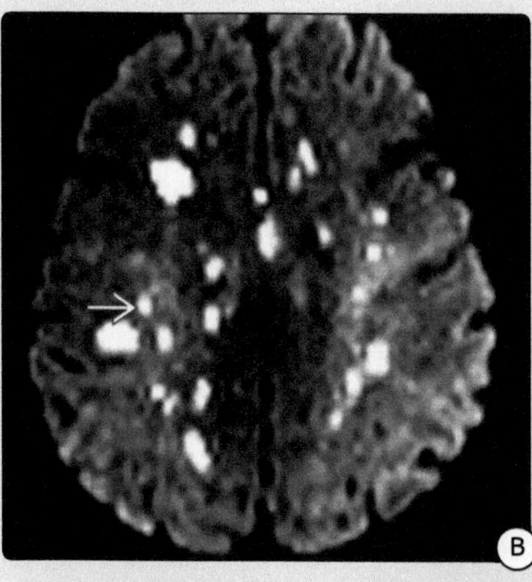

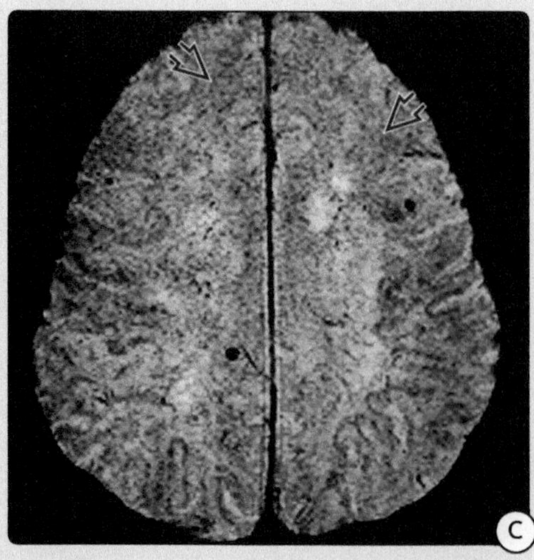

(8-30B) DWI in the same case shows innumerable tiny foci of diffusion restriction in the deep cerebral WM ➡, the so-called star field pattern characteristic of cerebral fat embolism syndrome. (8-30C) T2 SWI in the same case shows literally thousands of tiny blooming hypointense foci throughout the hemispheric WM ⇨ characteristic of microbleeds secondary to cerebral fat embolism syndrome.*

coma. Focal neurologic deficits are less common. Onset is from two hours up to two days after trauma or surgery with a mean of 29 hours.

Imaging. Imaging findings reflect the *effect* of the fat emboli (i.e., multifocal tiny strokes and microhemorrhages) on brain tissue, not the fat itself. NECT scans are therefore usually normal.

MR shows numerous (average = 50) punctate or confluent hyperintensities in the cerebellum, basal ganglia, periventricular WM, and GM-WM junctions on T2/FLAIR **(8-30A)**. DWI shows innumerable tiny punctate foci of diffusion restriction in multiple vascular distributions, the "star field" pattern **(8-30B)**. The deep watershed border zones are commonly involved.

Solitary or multiple small hypointense "blooming" foci can be identified in up to 1/3 of all FES cases on T2* GRE. SWI discloses innumerable (> 200) tiny "black dots" in the majority of patients **(8-30C)**.

Differential Diagnosis. The major differential diagnosis of cerebral FES is **multiple embolic infarcts**. Multiple cardiac or atheromatous embolic infarcts rarely produce the dozens or even hundreds of lesions seen with CFE. Lesions tend to involve the basal ganglia and corticomedullary junctions more than the WM.

Multifocal "blooming" hypointensities on T2* can be seen with severe **diffuse axonal injury (DAI)** or **diffuse vascular injury (DVI)**. As patients with CFE often have polytrauma, the distinction may be difficult on the basis of imaging studies alone. DAI and DVI tend to cause linear as well as punctate microbleeds.

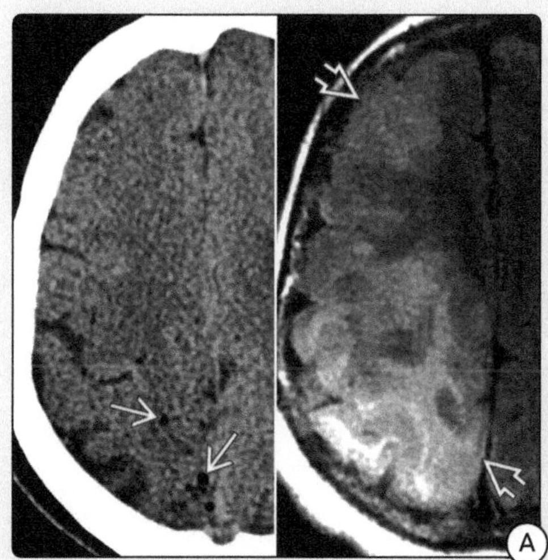

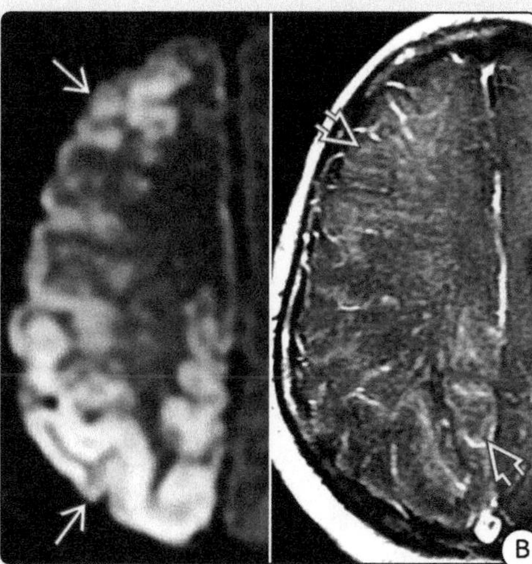

***(8-31A)** 55y woman experienced left hemiparesis after esophageal dilatation. (L) Axial NECT of cerebral gas embolism shows multiple "dots" of air in the brain ➡. (R) FLAIR shows a much more extensive area of diffuse cortical/subcortical WM hyperintensity ➡. **(8-31B)** (L) DWI shows restricted diffusion ➡ in the cortex. (R) T1 C+ shows extensive patchy, linear enhancement ➡ in the cortex and subcortical WM. (Courtesy P. Hildenbrand, MD.)*

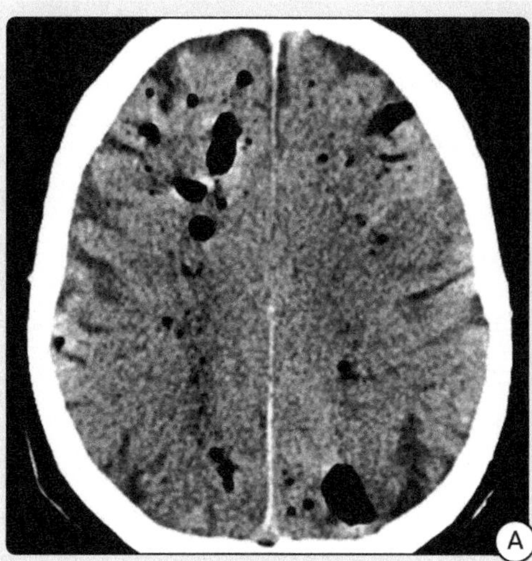

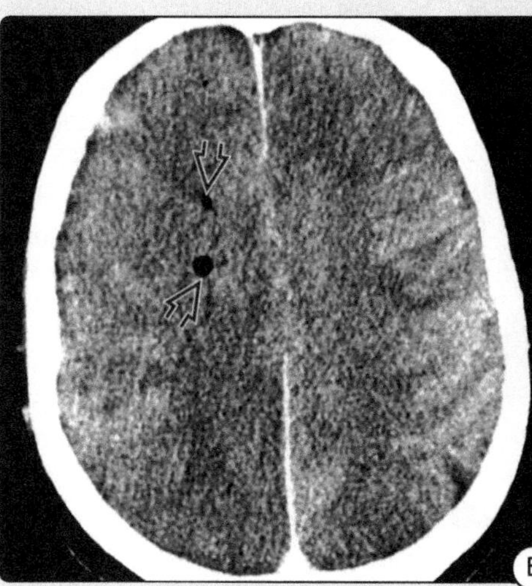

***(8-32A)** Axial NECT scan in a 69-year-old man immediately after cardiac ablation shows massive cerebral gas embolism. **(8-32B)** NECT scan in the same case 1 hour later shows that most of the air has been resorbed with only 2 small parenchymal dots of air ➡ remaining. Severe diffuse cerebral edema is now present.*

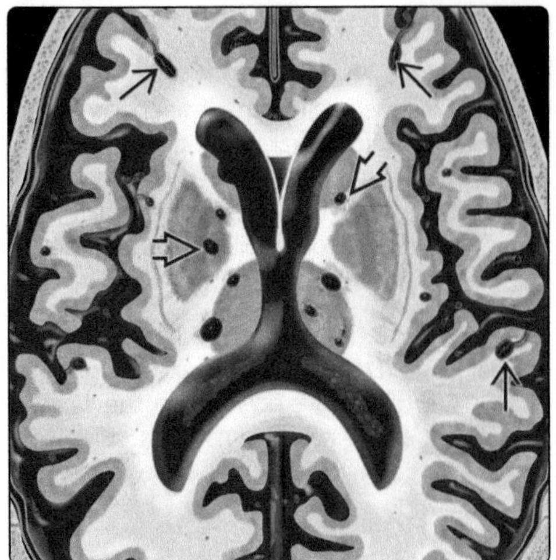

(8-33) Graphic shows lacunar infarctions in thalami, basal ganglia ⇒. Note also prominent perivascular (Virchow-Robin) spaces ⇒.

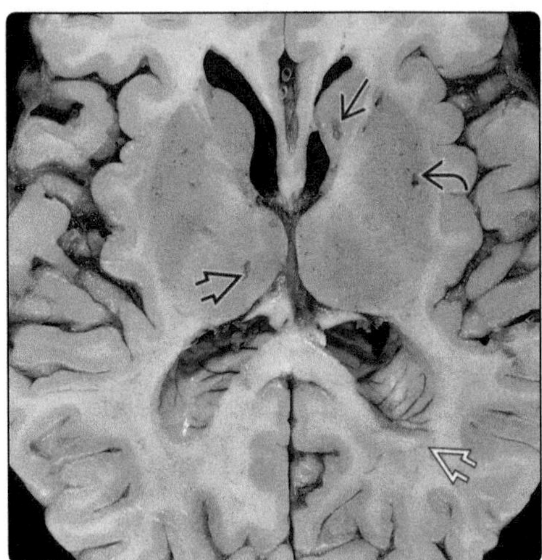

(8-34) Old lacunar infarcts are in the caudate ⇒, putamen ⇒, thalamus ⇒, periatrial WM rarefaction ⇒. (Courtesy R. Hewlett, MD.)

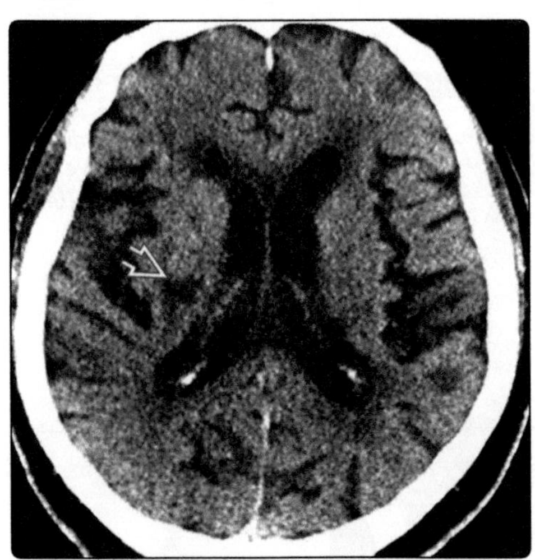

(8-35) NECT shows typical old thalamic lacunar infarct as hypodense, slightly irregular lesion ⇒.

Cerebral Gas Embolism

Pathoetiology. Minor amounts of air in the intracranial venous systems is usually iatrogenic, introduced during intravenous catheter placement.

Massive cerebral gas embolism (CGE) is a potentially catastrophic complication of central venous catheter (CVC) manipulation/disconnection and has been reported with cardiac procedures.

Other etiologies of arterial or venous air embolism include lung biopsy, craniotomy in the sitting position, and angiography. Penetrating trauma, decompression sickness, and hydrogen peroxide ingestion are other causes of gas embolism.

Clinical. Small amounts of CGE may be asymptomatic or mild and transient. In more severe cases, focal neurologic deficit, coma, seizures, and encephalopathy may ensue. Reported mortality of CGE associated with CVCs approaches 20%.

Imaging. Asymptomatic air following intravenous catheter placement is most commonly observed as an incidental finding, typically as dots of air in the cavernous sinus.

Intracranial air bubbles can be identified in 70% of symptomatic CGE cases, appearing on NECT as transient small intravascular rounded or curvilinear hypodensities, typically located at the depths of sulci **(8-31A)**. Intraparenchymal air is less common.

Air is quickly absorbed and can rapidly disappear **(8-32)**. If massive air embolism occurs, cerebral ischemia or diffuse brain swelling typically ensues **(8-32)**.

EMBOLIC INFARCTS

Cardiac and Atheromatous Emboli
- Small, simultaneous, multiple lesions
- Bilateral, multiple vascular distributions
- Typically involve cortex, GM-WM interfaces
- May be Ca^{++}
- ± punctate/ring enhancement
- Usually not hemorrhagic unless septic

Fat Emboli
- 12-72 h after long bone trauma, surgery
- Less commonly from bone marrow necrosis (e.g., sickle cell crisis)
- Arteriolar/capillary fat emboli
- Cause multiple tiny microbleeds
- Multiple foci of restricted diffusion in "star field" pattern (bright spots on dark background)
- Microbleeds best seen on T2* SWI > > GRE
- Deep WM > cortex

Cerebral Gas Embolism
- Usually iatrogenic (procedural) or traumatic
- Can occur with hydrogen peroxide ingestion
- NECT may show transient round or curvilinear air densities in sulcal vessels
- Quickly absorbed, disappear
- If massive, lethal brain swelling ensues rapidly

Lacunar Infarcts

Terminology

The terms "lacuna," "lacunar infarct," and "lacunar stroke" are often used interchangeably. **Lacunae** are 3- to 15-mm CSF-filled cavities or "holes" that most often occur in the basal ganglia or cerebral WM **(8-33)**. They are often observed coincidentally on imaging studies in older patients but are not clearly associated with discrete neurologic symptoms, i.e., they are subclinical strokes. Lacunae are sometimes called "silent" strokes, a misnomer as subtle neuropsychologic impairment is common in these patients.

Lacunar stroke means a clinically evident stroke syndrome attributed to a small subcortical or brainstem lesion that may or may not be evident on brain imaging. The term "état lacunaire" or **lacunar state** designates multiple lacunar infarcts.

Epidemiology and Etiology

Approximately 25% of all ischemic strokes are lacunar-type infarcts. Lacunae are considered macroscopic markers of cerebral small vessel ("microvascular") disease. There are two major vascular pathologies involving small penetrating arteries and arterioles: (1) Thickening of the arterial media by lipohyalinosis, fibrinoid necrosis, and atherosclerosis causing luminal narrowing and (2) obstruction of penetrating arteries at their origin by large intimal plaques in the parent arteries.

The *MTHFR* C677T genotype is correlated with lacunar stroke.

Pathology

Location. Penetrating branches that arise from the circle of Willis and peripheral cortical arteries are small end arteries with few collaterals, so lacunar infarcts are most common in the basal ganglia (putamen, globus pallidus, caudate nucleus), thalami, internal capsule, deep cerebral WM, and pons.

Size and Number. Lacunae are, by definition, 15 mm or less in diameter. Multiple lesions are common. Between 13-15% of patients have multiple simultaneous acute lacunar infarcts.

Gross and Microscopic Appearance. Grossly, lacunae appear as small, pale, irregular but relatively well-delineated cystic cavities **(8-34)**. Brown-staining siderotic discoloration can be seen in old hemorrhagic lacunae. Microscopically, ischemic lacunar infarcts demonstrate tissue rarefaction with neuronal loss, peripheral macrophage infiltration, and gliosis.

Clinical Issues

Independent risk factors for lacunar infarcts include age, hypertension, and diabetes. Other contributing factors include smoking and atrial fibrillation.

Outcome of lacunar stroke is highly variable. Although most lacunae are asymptomatic, "little strokes" can mean "big trouble." A single subclinical stroke—often a lacuna—is associated with increased likelihood of having additional "little strokes" as well as developing overt clinical stroke &/or dementia. Nearly 20% of patients over 65 with WM hyperintensities (WMHs) on T2/FLAIR MR will develop new lacunae within 3 years.

Between 20-30% of patients with lacunar stroke experience neurologic deterioration hours or even days after the initial event. The pathophysiology of "progressive lacunar stroke" is incompletely understood, and no treatment has been proven to prevent or halt progression.

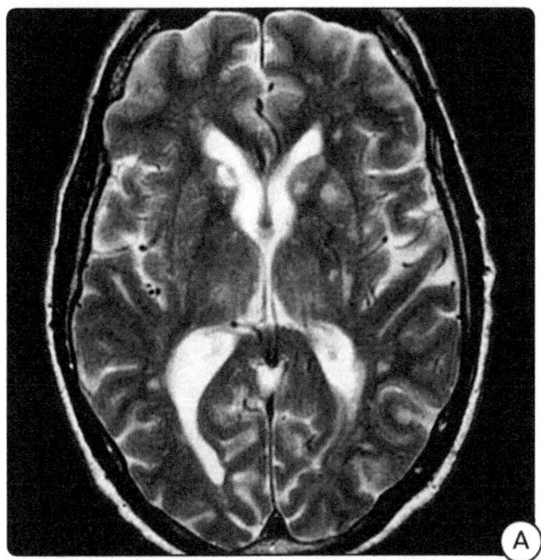

***(8-36A)** Axial T2WI MR shows multiple bilateral rounded and irregular hyperintensities in the basal ganglia and deep cerebral WM.*

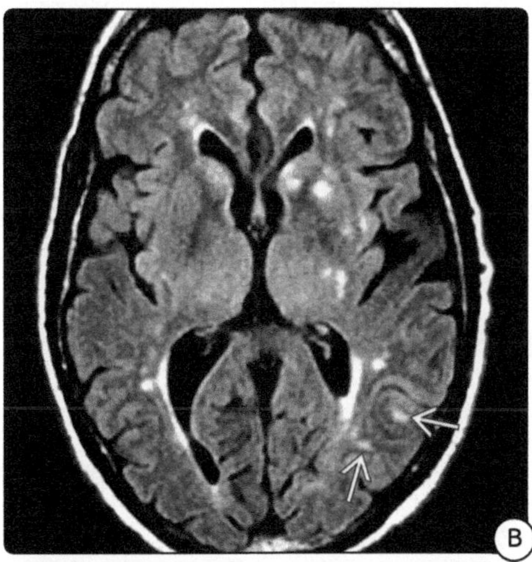

***(8-36B)** FLAIR MR (same case) shows multiple hyperintensities in both hemispheres. Some small subcortical lesions ➡ are also present.*

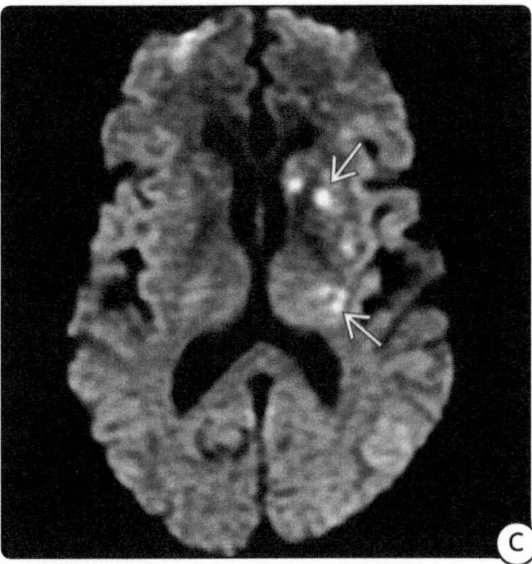

***(8-36C)** Some lesions demonstrate acute restriction ➡. DWI is helpful in distinguishing acute from chronic lacunar infarcts.*

Imaging

Imaging findings vary with whether the lacuna is acute or chronic.

Acute Lacunar Infarcts. Most acute lacunar infarcts are invisible on NECT scans. Acute lacunar infarcts are hyperintense on T2/FLAIR and may be difficult to distinguish from foci of coexisting chronic microvascular disease **(8-36)**. Acute and early subacute lacunae restrict on DWI **(8-36C)** and also usually enhance on T1 C+.

DWI overestimates the eventual size of lacunar infarcts. Cavitation and lesion shrinkage are seen in > 95% of deep symptomatic lacunar infarcts on follow-up imaging.

Chronic Lacunar Infarcts. Old lacunae appear as well-defined but often somewhat irregular CSF-like "holes" in the brain parenchyma on NECT scans **(8-35)**.

Chronic lacunar infarcts are hypointense on T1WI and hyperintense on T2WI. The fluid in the cavity suppresses on FLAIR, whereas the gliotic periphery remains hyperintense. Multifocal WM disease, seen as WMHs, is also common in patients with frank lacunar infarcts.

Most lacunae are nonhemorrhagic and do not "bloom" on T2* sequences. However, parenchymal microbleeds—multifocal "blooming black dots" on T2* (GRE, SWI)—are common comorbidities in patients with lacunar infarcts and chronic hypertension.

Differential Diagnosis

The major differential diagnosis of lacunar infarct is **prominent perivascular spaces** (PVSs). Also known as Virchow-Robin spaces, prominent PVSs are pia-lined, interstitial fluid-filled spaces. Prominent PVSs can be found in virtually all locations and in patients of all ages, although they tend to increase in size and frequency with age. The most common locations for PVSs are the inferior 1/3 of the basal ganglia (clustered around the anterior commissure), subcortical WM (including the external capsule), and the midbrain (see Chapter 28).

PVSs are sharply marginated and ovoid, linear, or round; lacunae tend to be more irregularly shaped. PVSs faithfully follow CSF signal intensity on all MR sequences and suppress completely on FLAIR. The adjacent brain is typically normal, although a thin rim of FLAIR hyperintensity around the PVSs is present in 25% of cases.

Embolic infarcts are typically peripheral (cortical/subcortical) rather than the usual central and deep location of typical lacunae.

Watershed or **"border zone" infarcts** grossly resemble lacunar infarcts on imaging studies. However, "border zone" infarcts occur in specific locations—along the cortical and subcortical WM watershed zones—whereas lacunae are more randomly scattered lesions that primarily affect the basal ganglia, thalami, and deep periventricular WM.

The WMHs associated with **microvascular disease** (primarily lipohyalinosis and arteriolosclerosis) are less well defined and usually more patchy or confluent than the small (< 15 mm) lesions that represent true lacunar infarcts. WMHs tend to cluster around the occipital horns and periventricular WM, not the basal ganglia and thalami.

A few scattered T2/FLAIR hyperintensities are common in the **normal aging brain**. A general guideline is "one white spot per decade" until the age of 50, after which the number and size of WMHs increase at accelerated rates.

LACUNAR INFARCTS

Etiology and Pathology
- Macroscopic markers of "small vessel disease"
- Atherosclerosis, lipohyalinosis
- Along small penetrating arteries (few collaterals)
- Most common in basal ganglia, deep WM

Imaging
- Acute lacunae often invisible on NECT
- T2/FLAIR hyperintense
- Use DWI to distinguish from WMHs of chronic microvascular disease
- Chronic lacunae irregular, CSF-like
- May be surrounded by gliotic rim

Watershed ("Border Zone") Infarcts

Terminology and Epidemiology

Watershed (WS) infarcts, a.k.a. "border zone" infarcts, are ischemic lesions that occur in the junction between two nonanastomosing distal arterial distributions. WS infarcts are more common than generally recognized, constituting 10-12% of all brain infarcts.

Anatomy of Cerebral "Border Zones"

WS zones are defined as the "border" or junction where two or more major arterial territories meet. Two distinct types of vascular border zones are recognized: An external (cortical) WS zone and an internal (deep) WS zone **(8-37)**.

The two major **external WS zones** lie in the frontal cortex (between the ACA and MCA) and parietooccipital cortex (between the MCA and PCA). A strip of paramedian subcortical WM near the vertex of the cerebral hemispheres is also considered part of the external WS.

The **internal WS zones** represent the junctions between penetrating branches (e.g., lenticulostriate arteries, medullary WM perforating arteries, and anterior choroidal branches) and the major cerebral vessels (MCA , ACA, and PCA).

Etiology

Maximal vulnerability to hypoperfusion is greatest where two distal arterial fields meet together. *Hypotension with or without severe arterial stenosis or occlusion can result in hemodynamic compromise.* Flow in the affected WS zone can be critically lowered, resulting in ischemia or frank infarction.

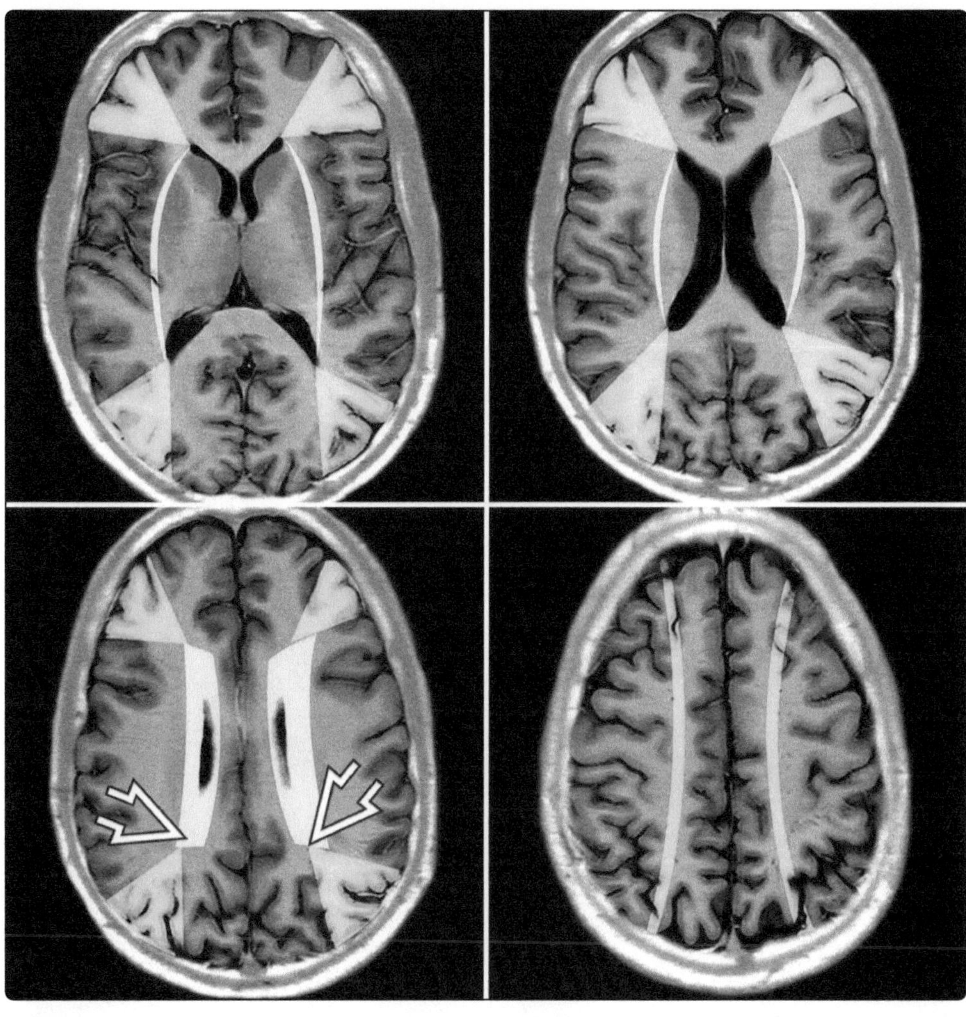

(8-37) *T1-weighted images show 2 vascular watershed (WS) zones with external (cortical) WS zones in turquoise. Wedge-shaped areas between the ACAs, MCAs, and PCAs represent "border zones" between the 3 major terminal vascular distributions. Curved blue lines (lower right) represent subcortical WS. The triple "border zones"* ➡ *represent confluence of all 3 major vessels. Yellow lines indicate the internal (deep WM) WS zone between perforating arteries and major territorial vessels.*

The most susceptible "border zone" is the "triple watershed" where the ACA, MCA, and PCA all converge.

External WS infarcts are the more common type. Most external WS infarcts are *embolic*. Anterior cortical WS embolic infarcts often occur in concert with internal carotid atherosclerosis. External WS infarcts in all three "border zones" are less common and usually reflect *global hypoperfusion*.

Internal WS infarcts are rarely embolic. They represent 35-40% of all WS infarcts and are most often caused by *regional hypoperfusion* secondary to hemodynamic compromise (e.g., ipsilateral carotid stenosis).

Pathology

Location. Internal WS infarcts tend to "line up" in the WM, parallel to and slightly above the lateral ventricles. Cerebellar WS infarcts occur at the borders between the posterior inferior, anterior inferior, and superior cerebellar arteries.

External (cortical) WS infarcts show a bimodal spatial distribution. Anteriorly, they center in the posterior frontal lobe near the junction of the frontal sulcus with the precentral sulcus. Posterior WS infarcts center in the superior parietal lobule posterolateral to the postcentral sulcus. The prevalence of WS infarcts decreases between these two areas. WS infarcts spare the medial cortex.

Size and Number. WS infarcts vary in size from tiny lesions to large wedge-shaped ischemic areas. Multiple lesions are common and can be uni- or bilateral. Bilateral lesions are often related to global reduction in perfusion pressure, usually an acute hypotensive event.

Imaging

Internal WS Infarcts. Internal "border zone" infarcts can be confluent or partial. Confluent infarcts are large, cigar-shaped lesions that lie alongside or just above the lateral ventricles. Partial infarcts are more discrete, rosary-like lesions. They resemble a line of beads extending from front to back in the deep WM **(8-38)**.

Stenosis or occlusion of the ipsilateral ICA or MCA is common with unilateral lesions. The presence and degree of hemodynamic impairment can be determined using a number of methods, including pCT, pMR, SPECT, and PET.

External (Cortical) WS Infarcts. Cortical (external) WS infarcts are wedge- or gyriform-shaped **(8-39)**.

Differential Diagnosis

The major differential diagnosis of WS infarction is **lacunar infarcts**. Lacunar infarcts typically involve the basal ganglia, thalami, and pons and appear randomly scattered. Multiple **embolic infarcts** can also closely resemble WS infarcts. Emboli are often bilateral and multiterritorial but can also occur at vascular "border zones."

Posterior reversible encephalopathy syndrome (PRES) typically occurs in the setting of acute hypertension. The cortex/subcortical WM in the PCA distribution is most commonly affected, although PRES can also involve "border zones" and the basal ganglia. PRES rarely restricts on DWI (vasogenic edema), whereas "border zone" infarcts with cytotoxic edema show acute restriction.

WATERSHED ("BORDER ZONE") INFARCTS

Anatomy and Etiology

- 2 types of vascular "border zones"
  - External (cortical): Between ACA, MCA, PCA
  - Internal (deep WM): Between perforating branches, major arteries
- Etiology
  - Emboli (cortical more common)
  - Regional hypoperfusion (deep WM common)
  - Global hypoperfusion (all 3 cortical WS zones)

Imaging

- External: Wedge or gyriform
- Internal: Rosary-like line of WMHs

Selected References: The complete reference list is available on the Expert Consult™ eBook version included with purchase.

(8-38A) FLAIR MR demonstrates classic findings of internal WS zone ischemia. WM hyperintensities ➡ are not randomly distributed; they lie just above lateral ventricles and line up from front to back. (8-38B) The lesions ➡ restrict on DWI MR. High-grade stenoses were found in both proximal internal carotid arteries.

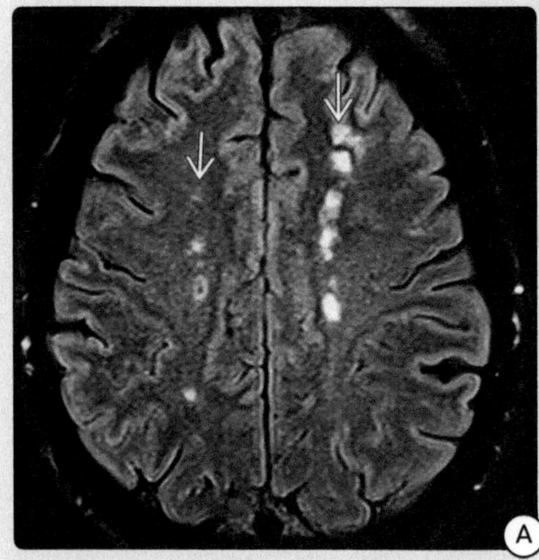

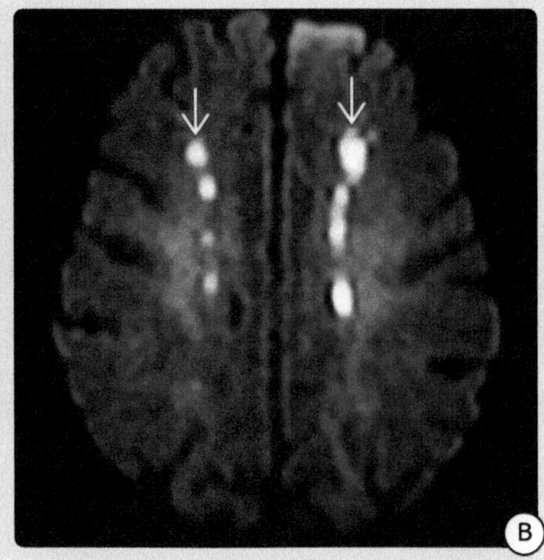

(8-39A) FLAIR MR demonstrates external WS zone ischemia. The WMHs are more peripheral and largely cortical ➡. Some are distinctly gyriform ➡ and lie at the "triple watershed" zone between the ACA, MCA, and PCA cortical distributions. (8-39B) DWI MR shows multiple punctate ➡ and gyriform ➡ foci of restricted diffusion in the cortex. Contrast with internal WS zone infarcts (above).

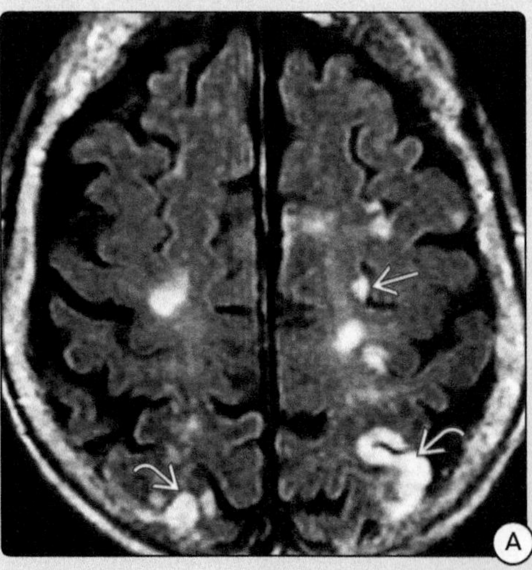

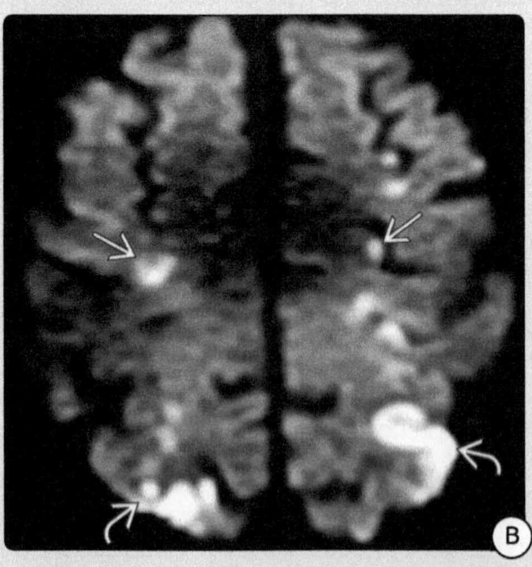

Venous Anatomy and Occlusions

Dural venous sinus and cerebral vein occlusions are relatively rare, accounting for only 1% of all strokes. They are notoriously difficult to diagnose clinically and are frequently overlooked on imaging studies, as attention is focused on the arterial side of the cerebral circulation.

Familiarity with both normal venous anatomy and drainage patterns is essential for understanding the imaging appearance of sinovenous occlusive disease. Therefore, in this chapter, we first briefly review the normal gross and imaging anatomy of the cerebral venous system. Because ~ 1/2 of all venous occlusions result in parenchymal infarcts, we also discuss their drainage territories.

Normal Venous Anatomy and Drainage Patterns

The intracranial venous system has two major components, the **dural venous sinuses** and the **cerebral veins**.

Dural Venous Sinuses

Dural sinuses and venous plexuses are endothelium-lined channels that are contained between the outer (periosteal) and inner (meningeal) dural layers.

Superior Sagittal Sinus (SSS)

The SSS is a large, curvilinear sinus that parallels the inner calvarial vault. It runs posteriorly in the midline at the junction of the falx cerebri with the calvarium **(9-1)**. The SSS increases in diameter as it courses posteriorly, collecting a number of unnamed, small, superficial cortical veins and the larger anastomotic vein of Trolard.

Inferior Sagittal Sinus (ISS)

Compared with the SSS, the ISS is a much smaller and more inconstant curvilinear channel that lies in the bottom of the falx cerebri. It terminates at the falcotentorial junction where it joins the vein of Galen (VofG) and basal veins of Rosenthal to form the straight sinus (SS).

Straight Sinus (SS)

The SS is formed by the junction of the ISS and VofG. It runs posteroinferiorly from its origin at the falcotentorial apex to the venous sinus confluence.

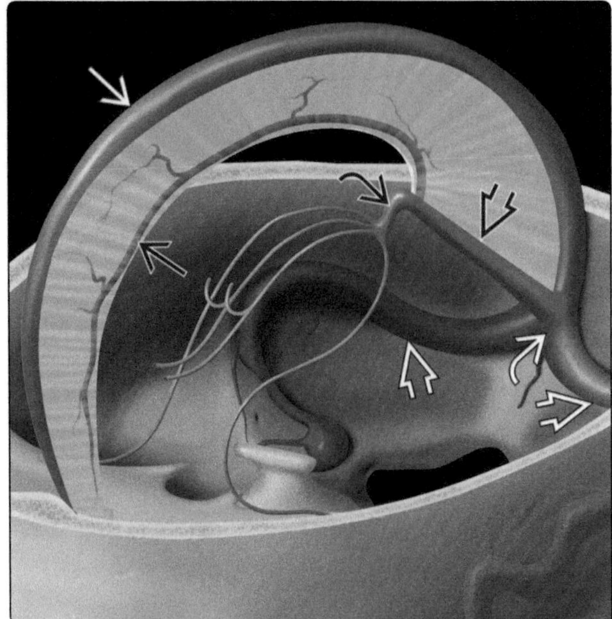

(9-1) *Falx cerebri extends from the crista galli to the falcotentorial junction and holds the SSS ➡ and the ISS ➡. VofG ➡ receives the ICVs and basal vein of Rosenthal. Straight sinus ➡, sinus confluence ➡, transverse sinuses (TSs) ➡ are shown.*

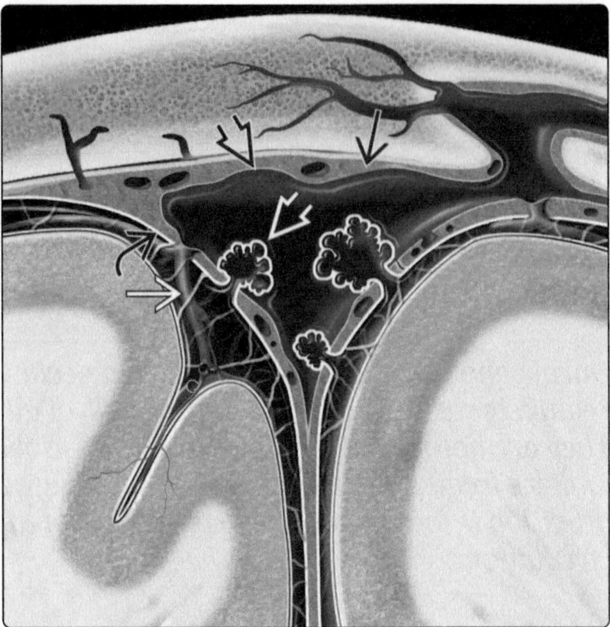

(9-2) *The SSS ➡ is between the outer ➡ and inner ➡ dural layers. CSF-containing projections (arachnoid granulations) ➡ extend from the subarachnoid space (SAS) into the SSS. Cortical veins ➡ also enter the SSS.*

SS variants are relatively uncommon. A **persistent falcine sinus** is an unusual variant that is identified on 2% of normal CTAs. Here, a midline venous structure—the persistent falcine sinus—connects the ISS or VofG directly with the SSS.

Sinus Confluence and Transverse Sinuses (TSs)

The SS terminates by joining the SSS and TSs to form the **venous sinus confluence** (torcular herophili). The TSs are contained between attachments of the tentorium cerebelli to the inner table of the skull. The TSs curve laterally and then turn inferiorly to become the sigmoid sinuses.

The two TSs are frequently asymmetric with the right side typically larger than the left. Hypoplastic or stenotic segments are present in 1/3 of the general population. Filling defects caused by arachnoid granulations and fibrous septa are also common.

Sigmoid Sinuses and Jugular Bulbs

The sigmoid sinuses are the inferior continuations of the TSs. They follow a gentle S-shaped curve, descending behind the petrous temporal bone to terminate by becoming the internal jugular veins (IJVs). Side-to-side asymmetry of the sigmoid sinuses is common and normal.

Cavernous Sinus (CS)

The CSs are irregularly shaped, heavily trabeculated/compartmentalized venous sinuses that lie along the sides of the sella turcica and extend from the superior orbital fissures anteriorly (where they receive the superior ophthalmic veins) to the clivus and petrous apex posteriorly. The two CSs communicate extensively with each other via intercavernous venous plexuses.

The CSs contain the two cavernous internal carotid arteries (ICAs) and abducens (CNVI) nerves. CNIII, CNIV, CNV1, and CNV2 are actually *within* the lateral dural wall, not inside the CS proper.

The size and configuration of the CSs are relatively constant on imaging studies. The lateral walls normally appear straight or concave (not convex), and the venous blood enhances quite uniformly.

Arachnoid Granulations (AGs)

The dural sinuses frequently contain **arachnoid granulations** (AGs), CSF-containing projections that extend from the subarachnoid space (SAS) into dural venous sinuses **(9-2)**. Although AGs can occur in all dural venous sinuses, the most common locations are the TS and SSS.

Cerebral Veins

The cerebral veins are subdivided into three groups: (1) Superficial ("cortical" or "external") veins, (2) deep cerebral ("internal") veins, and (3) brainstem/posterior fossa veins.

Superficial Cortical Veins

Between 8-12 superficial cortical veins course over the cerebral convexities, cross the subarachnoid space, pierce the arachnoid membrane and inner (meningeal) layer of the dura, and drain directly into the SSS **(9-2)**. A dominant anastomotic superficial cortical vein, the **vein of Trolard** (VofT) may be present. The VofT courses upward from the sylvian fissure to join the SSS

The **superficial middle cerebral vein** (SMCV) lies over the sylvian fissure and drains the brain surrounding the lateral cerebral fissure. The **deep middle cerebral vein** (DMCV) collects tributaries from the insula and basal ganglia then anastomoses with the **basal vein of Rosenthal** (BVR), which, in turn, drains into the VofG.

A prominent posterior anastomotic vein, the **vein of Labbé**, courses inferolaterally over the temporal lobe to drain into the TS **(9-4)**.

All three named superficial anastomotic veins—the vein of Trolard, vein of Labbé, and SMCV—vary in size, maintaining a reciprocal relationship with each other. If one or two are dominant, the third anastomotic vein is usually hypoplastic or absent.

Deep Cerebral Veins

Innumerable small **medullary veins** originate between 1 cm and 2 cm below the cortex and course straight through the white matter toward the ventricles where they terminate in subependymal veins. DSA and contrast-enhanced MR may show faint linear stripes of contrast parallel to the ventricles. T2* susceptibility-weighted imaging (SWI) best depicts the medullary veins because the deoxygenated blood is paramagnetic.

The **subependymal veins** course under the ventricular ependyma, collecting blood from the basal ganglia and deep white matter (via the medullary veins). The **thalamostriate veins** receive tributaries from the caudate nuclei and thalami, curving medially to unite with the septal veins near the foramen of Monro to form the paired **internal cerebral veins** (ICVs).

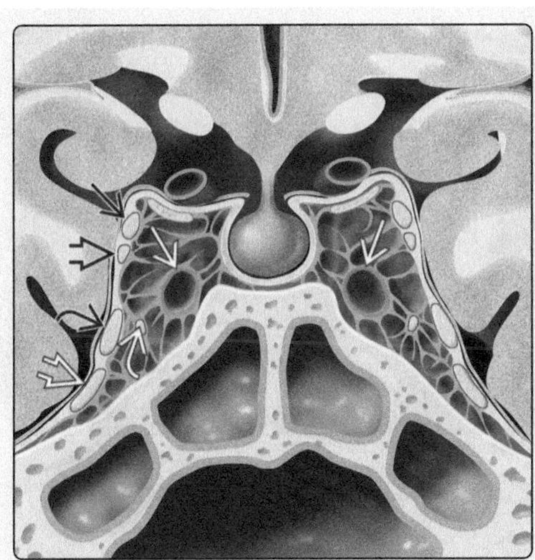

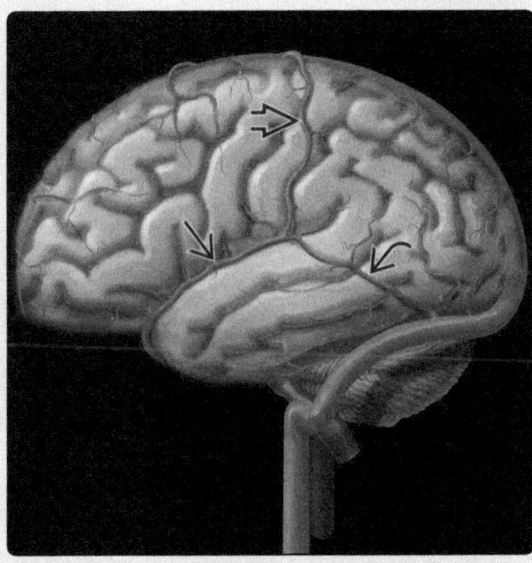

***(9-3)** Coronal graphic shows the trabeculated CSs and their contents. Internal carotid arteries ➡ and CNVI ➡ are inside the CSs. CNIII ➡, CNIV ➡, CNV1 ➡, and CNV2 ➡ lie in the lateral dural wall. **(9-4)** Lateral graphic depicts the superficial cortical veins. The 3 named anastomotic veins—Trolard ➡, Labbé ➡, and the superficial middle cerebral vein ➡ —are depicted. 1 or 2 of the superficial cortical veins are usually dominant.*

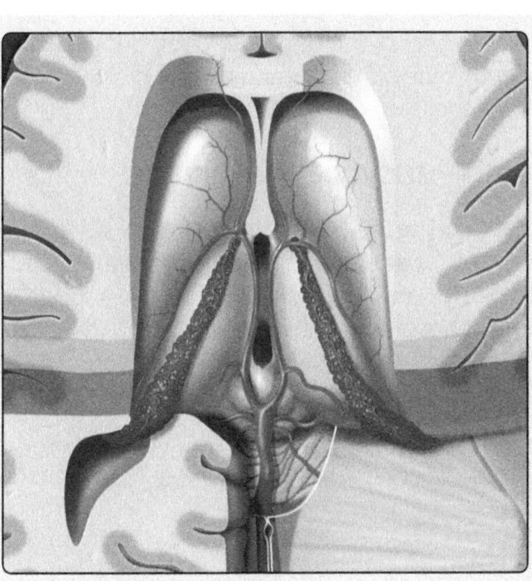

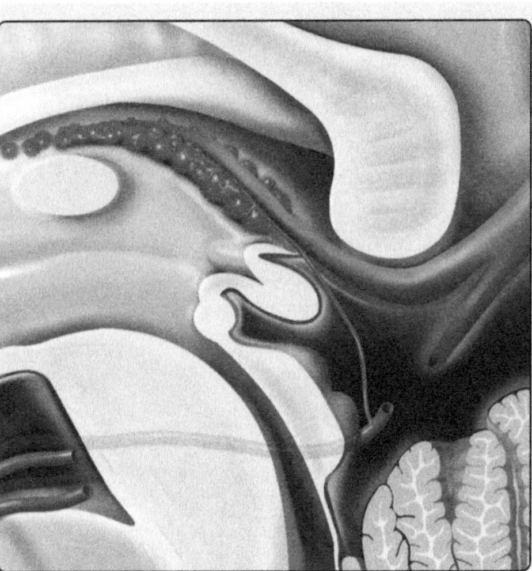

***(9-5)** Deep venous drainage is seen from the top down. Septal, caudate veins converge near the foramen of Monro to form internal cerebral veins. ICVs drain into the vein of Galen and straight sinus. **(9-6)** Lateral graphic shows ICVs coursing posteriorly within velum interpositum, joining with basal veins of Rosenthal to form the vein of Galen.*

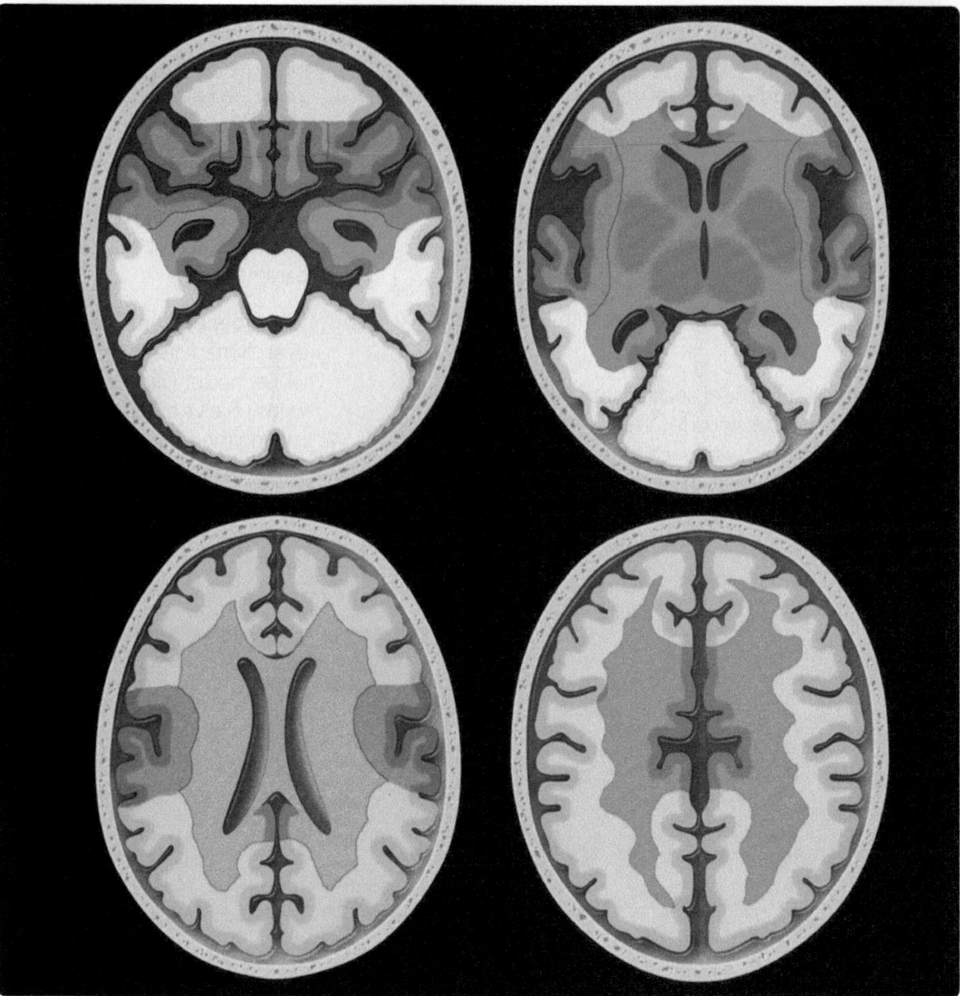

***(9-7)** Color-coded anatomic diagram depicting brain venous drainage territories is shown at 4 representative levels: The base of the brain (upper left), basal ganglia and internal capsules (upper right), middle of the lateral ventricles (lower left), and upper corona radiata above the level of the corpus callosum (lower right). Superficial parts of the brain (cortex, subcortical white matter) are drained by cortical veins (including the vein of Trolard) and superior sagittal sinus (shown in green). Central core brain structures (basal ganglia, thalami, internal capsules, lateral and 3rd ventricles) and most of the corona radiata are drained by the deep venous system (internal cerebral veins, vein of Galen, straight sinus) (red). The veins of Labbé and the transverse sinuses drain the posterior temporal, inferior parietal lobes (yellow). The sphenoparietal and cavernous sinuses drain the area around the sylvian fissures (purple).*

The **ICVs** and **VofG** provide drainage for most of the deep brain structures. The paired ICVs course posteriorly in the cavum velum interpositum and terminate by uniting with each other and the BVR to form the VofG. The VofG (great cerebral vein) curves posterosuperiorly under the corpus callosum splenium, uniting with the ISS to form the SS.

Venous Drainage Territories

The cerebral venous drainage territories are both less familiar and somewhat more variable than the major arterial distributions. Intracranial venous drainage follows four basic patterns: A peripheral (brain surface) pattern, a deep (central) pattern, an inferolateral (perisylvian) pattern, and a posterolateral (temporoparietal) pattern **(9-7)**. Accurately diagnosing and delineating venous occlusions depends on understanding these specific venous drainage territories.

Peripheral (Surface) Brain Drainage

Most of the mid and upper surfaces of the cerebral hemispheres together with their subjacent white matter drain centrifugally (outward) via cortical veins into the SSS.

Deep (Central) Brain Drainage

The basal ganglia, thalami, and most of the hemispheric white matter all drain centripetally (inward) into the deep cerebral veins. The ICVs, VofG, and SS together drain virtually the entire central core of the brain.

The most medial aspects of the temporal lobes, primarily the uncus and the anteromedial hippocampus, also drain into the galenic system via the DMCVs and BVR.

Inferolateral (Perisylvian) Drainage

Parenchyma surrounding the sylvian (lateral cerebral) fissure consists of the frontal, parietal, and temporal opercula plus the insula. This perisylvian part of the brain drains via the SMCV into the sphenoparietal sinus and CS.

Posterolateral (Temporoparietal) Drainage

The posterior temporal lobes and inferolateral aspects of the parietal lobes drain via the SPSs and anastomotic vein of Labbé into the TSs.

Cerebral Venous Thrombosis

Dural venous sinus, superficial (cortical) vein, and deep vein occlusions are collectively termed cerebral venous thrombosis (CVT). CVT is an elusive diagnosis with a great diversity of causes and clinical presentations; it is also easily overlooked on imaging studies.

We begin with the most common intracranial venous occlusion, dural sinus thrombosis. We next discuss superficial vein thrombosis and follow with deep cerebral occlusions. We conclude the discussion with a consideration of cavernous sinus (CS) thrombosis/thrombophlebitis.

Dural Sinus Thrombosis

Terminology

Cerebral dural sinus thrombosis (DST) is defined as thrombotic occlusion of one or more intracranial venous sinuses **(9-8)**. DST can occur either in isolation or in combination with cortical &/or deep venous occlusions.

Etiology

The majority of CVTs are acquired disorders. Oral contraceptive use and pregnancy/puerperium are the most common causes. Others include trauma, infection, inflammation, hypercoagulable states, elevated hemoglobin levels, dehydration, collagen-vascular disorders (such as antiphospholipid syndrome), vasculitis (such as Behçet syndrome), drugs, and Crohn disease. Between 20-35% of all patients with CVT have an inherited prothrombotic condition.

CEREBRAL VENOUS THROMBOSIS: CAUSES

Common
- Oral contraceptives
- Prothrombotic conditions
  - Deficiency of proteins C, S, or antithrombin III
  - Resistance to activated protein C (V Leiden)
  - Prothrombin gene mutations
  - Antiphospholipid, anticardiolipin antibodies
  - Hyperhomocysteinemia
- Puerperium, pregnancy
- Metabolic (dehydration, thyrotoxicosis, etc.)

Less Common
- Infection
  - Mastoiditis, sinusitis
  - Meningitis
- Trauma
- Neoplasm-related causes

Rare but Important
- Collagen-vascular disorders (e.g., antiphospholipid antibody syndrome)
- Hematologic disorders (e.g., polycythemia)
- Inflammatory bowel disease
- Vasculitis (e.g., Behçet disease)

Pathology

When thrombus forms in a dural sinus, venous outflow is restricted. This results in venous congestion, elevated venous pressure, and hydrostatic displacement of fluid from capillaries into the extracellular spaces of the

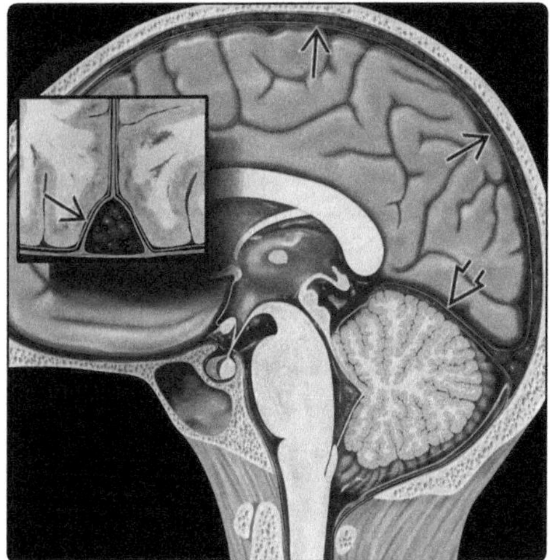

***(9-8)** Sagittal graphic shows SSS ⇒ and straight sinus ⇒ thrombosis. Insert shows pathologic basis of "empty delta" sign.*

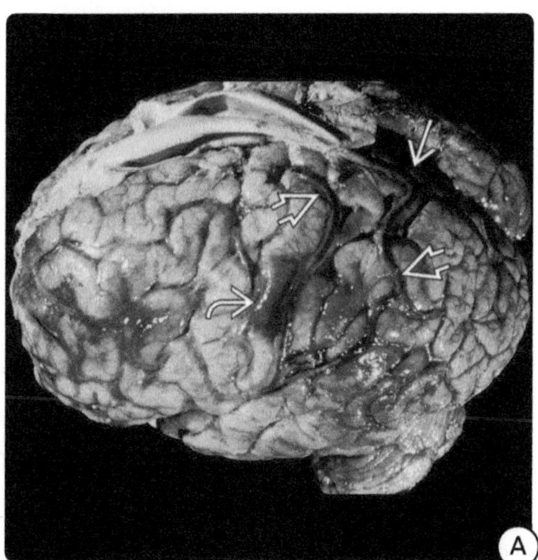

***(9-9A)** Autopsy case demonstrates acute SSS ➡, cortical vein ➡ thrombosis, and venous infarcts ➡.*

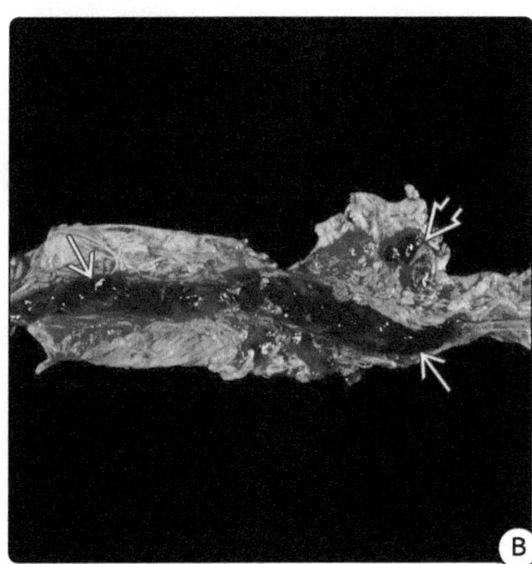

***(9-9B)** Gross photograph from the same case shows "currant jelly" clot in the SSS ➡, cortical veins ➡. (Courtesy E. T. Hedley-Whyte, MD.)*

brain. The result is blood-brain barrier breakdown with vasogenic edema. If a frank venous infarct develops, cytotoxic edema ensues.

Location. The transverse sinus is the most commonly thrombosed dural venous sinus followed by the superior sagittal sinus (SSS).

Gross Pathology. In acute DST, the affected dural sinus appears distended by a soft, purplish clot that can be isolated to the sinus or may extend into adjacent cortical veins **(9-9)**. In chronic DST, firm proliferative fibrous tissue fills the sinus and thickens the dura-arachnoid. Associated brain injury in DST varies from venous congestion to ischemia to petechial hemorrhages and frank hemorrhagic infarcts.

Clinical Issues

Epidemiology. CVTs represent between 1-2% of all acute strokes. Although CVT can occur at any age (from neonates to the elderly), it is most commonly seen in young individuals. Nearly 80% of patients are younger than 50 years of age.

Demographics. CVT predominantly affects women (F:M = 3:1). A sex-specific risk factor (oral contraceptives, pregnancy, puerperium, and hormone replacement therapy) is present in nearly 2/3 of all women with CVT. Mean age at presentation is nearly a decade younger in women compared with men (34 years vs. 42 years).

Presentation. The clinical manifestations of CVT are varied, often nonspecific, and may be subtle—especially in neonates, children, and the elderly.

Nonfocal headache is the most common symptom, occurring in nearly 90% of cases. Headache often slowly increases in severity over several days to weeks. Nearly 25% of patients present without focal neurologic findings.

(9-10A) NECT in a 22-year-old woman with "thunderclap" headache was obtained to evaluate for subarachnoid hemorrhage. Note hyperdensity of straight sinus ➡, torcular (venous confluence) ➘. The left thalamus also appears hypodense ⇨. (9-10B) More cephalad NECT shows hyperdense thrombus filling and expanding the SSS ➡. Note hyperdensity in an adjacent superficial cortical vein ("cord" sign) ➦.

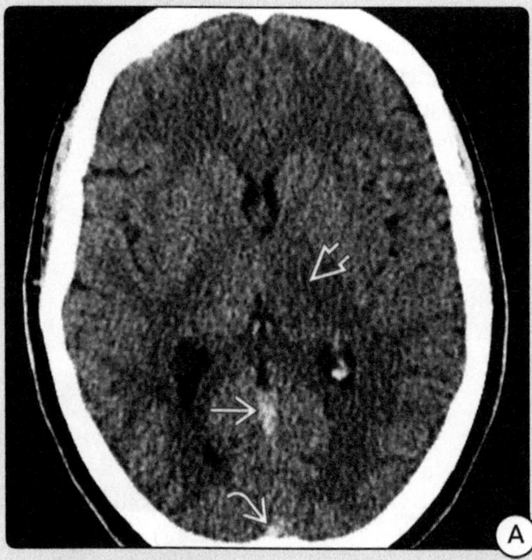

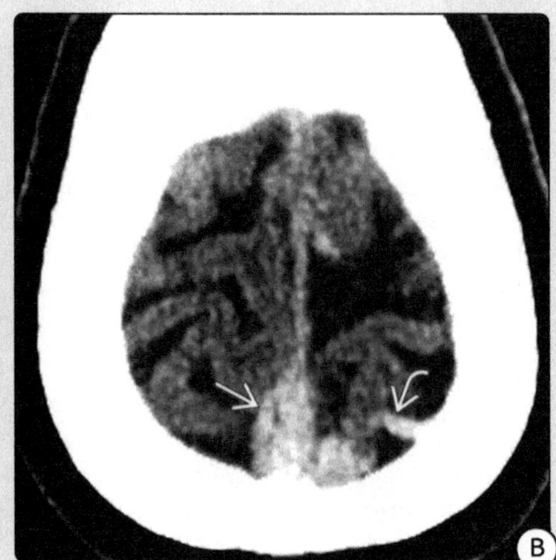

(9-10C) CECT in the same case shows classic "empty delta" sign ➡ formed by enhancing dura around nonenhancing thrombus. (9-10D) Sagittal CTA shows extensive thrombus filling the SSS ➡, straight sinus ⇨, vein of Galen ➦, and torcular (sinus confluence) ⇨.

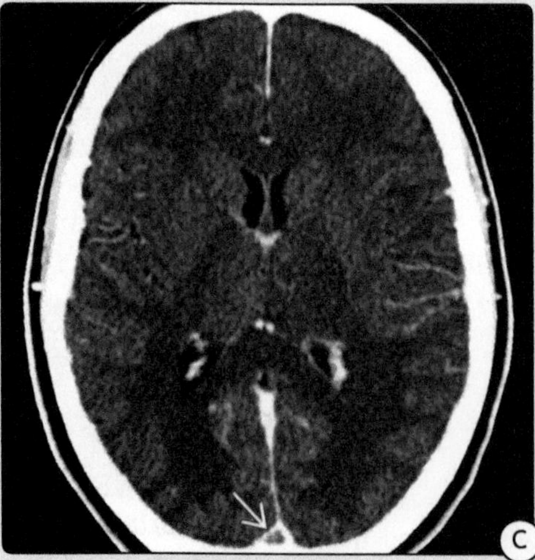

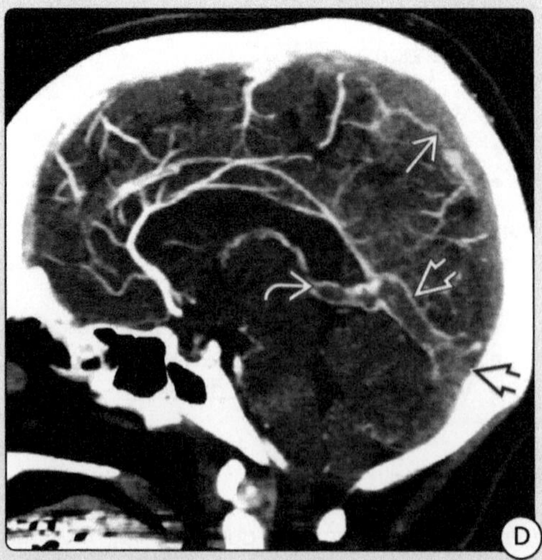

Natural History. Many DSTs recanalize spontaneously without long-term sequelae. In some cases, a thrombosed or partially recanalized venous sinus forms an arteriovenous fistula in the adjacent dural wall.

Prompt recognition of DST has a significant impact on clinical outcome. Diagnostic delay—averaging seven days in large series—is associated with increased death and disability.

Imaging

Keys to the early neuroradiologic diagnosis of DST are (1) a high index of suspicion, (2) careful evaluation of dural sinus density/signal intensity and configuration, and (3) knowledge of normal venous drainage patterns.

CT Findings. *NECT is normal in up to 25-30% of CVT cases, so a normal NECT scan does* **not** *exclude the diagnosis of CVT!* Early signs are often subtle. Slight hyperdensity compared with the carotid arteries is seen in 50-60% of cases and may be the only hint of sinus or venous occlusion. When present, a hyperattenuating vein ("cord" sign) **(9-10B)** or dural venous sinus sign **(9-10A)** **(9-11A)** is both a sensitive and specific sign of cerebral venous occlusive disease. Parenchymal edema with or without petechial hemorrhage in the territory drained by the thrombosed sinus is a helpful but indirect sign of DST.

In 70% of cases, CECT scans show an **"empty delta" sign** caused by enhancing dura surrounding nonenhancing thrombus **(9-10C)**. "Shaggy," enlarged, or irregular veins suggest collateral venous drainage.

MR Findings. Diagnosing CVT on MR can be challenging because thrombus and normal venous flow can have similar signal intensities. The imaging appearance of DST also varies significantly with imaging sequence and clot age.

Acute DST. An acutely thrombosed sinus often appears moderately enlarged ("fat sinus" sign) and displays abnormally convex—not straight or concave—margins **(9-11C)**. The "flow

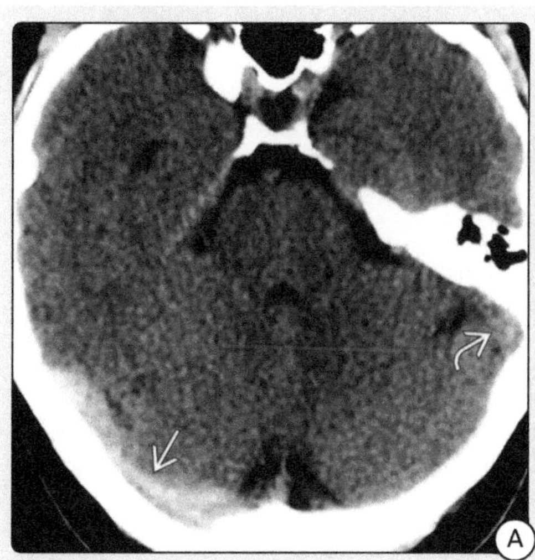

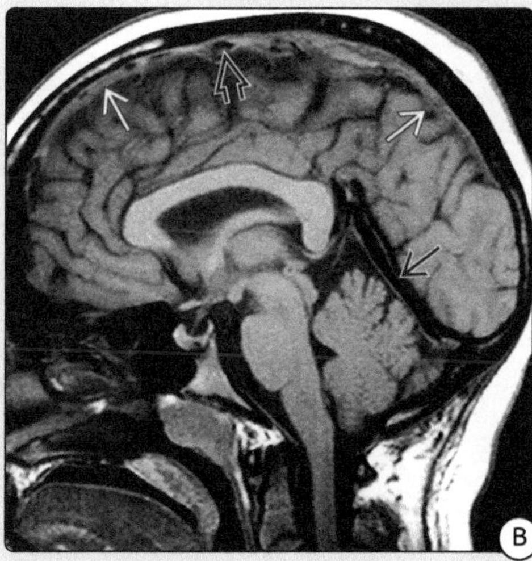

***(9-11A)** Axial NECT scan in a 29-year-old pregnant woman with headaches, papilledema shows hyperdense right TS ➡ compared with the left sigmoid sinus ➡. **(9-11B)** Sagittal T1 MR in the same patient shows a normal "flow void" in the straight sinus ➡. The SSS shows an absent "flow void" and—except for the CSF-filled arachnoid granulations ➡ —appears filled with clot ➡ that is almost isointense with brain.*

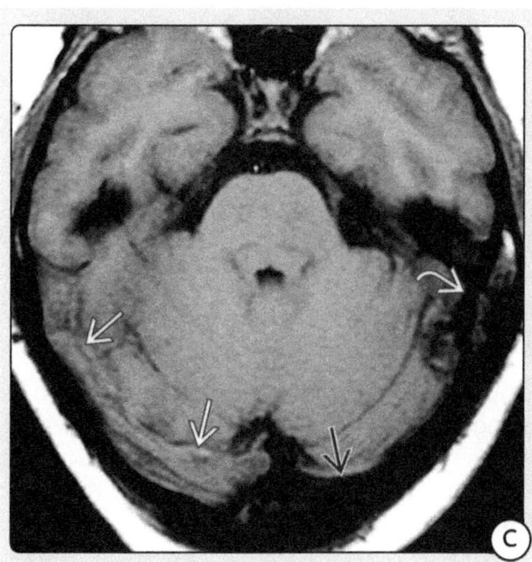

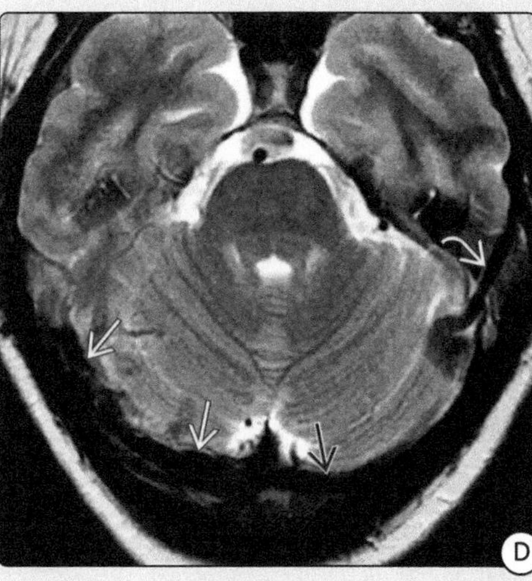

***(9-11C)** Axial T1 MR in the same patient shows an enlarged right TS that appears filled with an isointense clot ➡. Compare with the normal "flow void" in the left vein of Labbé ➡ and TS ➡. **(9-11D)** Axial T2 MR in the same patient shows that the thrombosed right TS ➡ appears very hypointense and mimics the "flow voids" of the patent left TS ➡ and vein of Labbé ➡; this is acute dural sinus thrombosis (DST).*

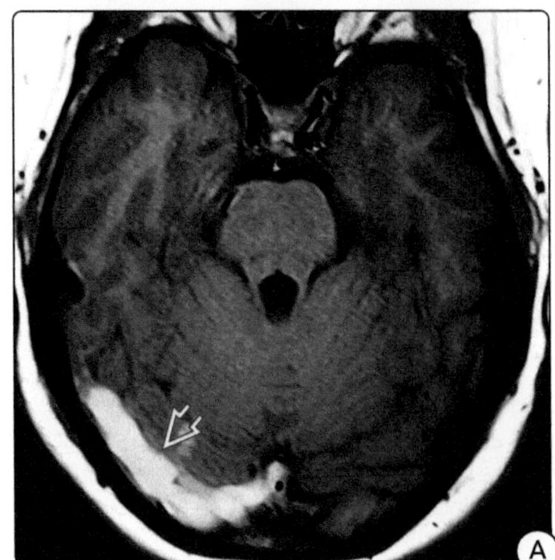

(9-12A) Axial T1 MR shows classic early subacute hyperintense thrombus ➡ in the occluded right TS.

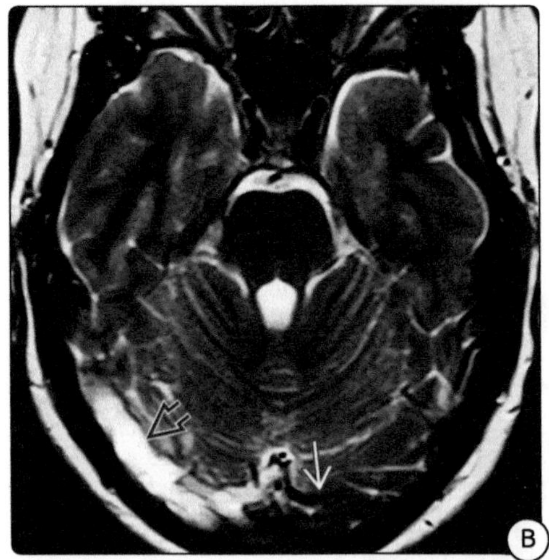

(9-12B) Axial T2 MR shows that subacute thrombus is hyperintense ➡. Contrast with normal "flow void" in the hypoplastic left TS ➡.

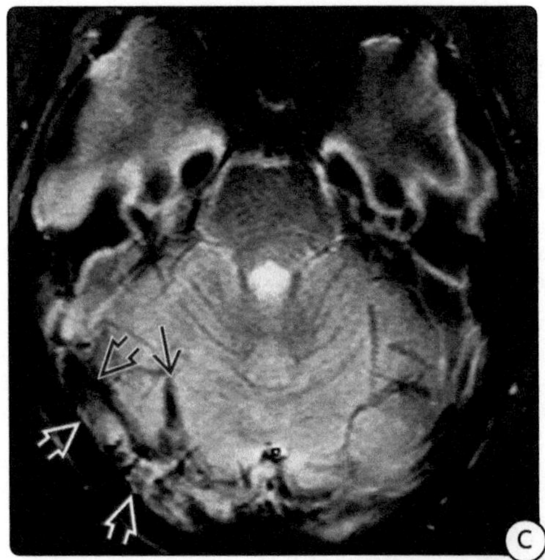

(9-12C) T2* GRE shows that thrombus is mostly hyperintense ➡ with some residual "blooming" in the right TS ➡, tentorial tributary veins ➡.

void" of rapidly moving blood typically seen in large venous sinuses disappears **(9-11B)**. Acute DST appears *isointense* with the underlying cortex on **T1WI (9-11C)**.

As hemoglobin in blood clots rapidly desaturates to deoxyhemoglobin, it becomes very *hypointense* relative to brain on **T2WI (9-11D)**. Therefore, the acute T2 "dark" DST mimics normal intrasinus "flow void." Most acute thrombi are hyperintense on FLAIR. Venous congestion may cause brain swelling with hyperintense parenchymal changes on T2/FLAIR.

Acute venous clots "*bloom*" on **T2* (GRE, SWI)**. SWI shows the profoundly hypointense clot and slow flow with deoxygenated blood in dilated cortical veins. The appearance may nonetheless be confusing, as normal-flowing but deoxygenated venous blood also appears hypointense.

Extensive acute (or longstanding chronic) DST may result in collateral venous drainage through the medullary (white matter) veins into the deep subependymal veins. The medullary veins enlarge and contain desaturated hemoglobin; thus, they are seen on T2* sequences as prominent linear hypointensities entering the subependymal veins at right angles **(9-24C)**.

When seen in cross section, **T1 C+** scans demonstrate an "*empty delta*" sign, similar to the appearance on CECT and CTA/CTV. Intrasinus thrombi usually appear as elongated *cigar-shaped* nonenhancing filling defects on axial T1 C+.

Coronal 2D unenhanced TOF **MRV** may demonstrate *absent flow*, especially if the thrombus is in the SSS. As the transverse sinuses often have hypoplastic segments, a "flow gap" must be interpreted with caution. **Contrast-enhanced MRV** has the highest sensitivity of all MR sequences for visualizing acute DST.

Late Acute DST. As the intrasinus thrombus organizes, the clot begins to exhibit T1 shortening and becomes progressively hyperintense.

With T2 prolongation, a thrombosed sinus progresses from appearing very hypointense to iso- and then hyperintense with brain on both T2WI and FLAIR. T2* can be misleading, as clot signal gradually approaches that of normal sinuses. Late acute DST continues to exhibit an "empty delta" sign on T1 C+.

Subacute DST. Subacute thrombus is hyperintense on all sequences (T1, T2, FLAIR, T2*) **(9-12)**.

Chronic DST. Clot signal in chronic DST is quite variable and depends on the degree of clot organization. Chronic organized, fibrotic thrombus eventually becomes isointense with brain on T1WI and remains isointense to moderately hyperintense on T2WI. As blood has resorbed and largely disappeared, there is little or no T2* "blooming." CTA/CTV readily demonstrates nonenhancing thrombus within the intensely enhancing dura.

Longstanding cerebral venous sinus thrombosis may develop significant collateral drainage through the medullary veins. This is seen as tortuous, corkscrew, or "squiggly" white matter vessels on CTV and intraparenchymal "flow voids" on T2WI that enhance on T1 C+ scans. The enlarged collateral veins sometimes become so prominent that they mimic an arteriovenous malformation on SWI and DSA **(9-13)**.

Dura-arachnoid thickening is also common in longstanding chronic DST. In some cases, the dural thickening becomes so pronounced that it appears very hypointense on T2WI.

Differential Diagnosis

Normal dura and **circulating blood** are mildly hyperdense on NECT scans. If a dural venous sinus appears unusually hyperdense, compare it to density of the ICAs. A dural sinus measuring > 70 Hounsfield units is likely thrombosed.

Asymmetry of the transverse sinuses is common. A **hypoplastic segment** is seen in 1/4 to 1/3 of imaged cases and may mimic DST. A **high-splitting torcular** can mimic an "empty delta" sign on CECT.

Giant arachnoid granulations are focal round or ovoid CSF-like filling defects in the sinuses, whereas clots tend to be elongated, cigar-shaped lesions (see "Venous Occlusion Mimics" section later in the chapter).

DURAL SINUS THROMBOSIS: MR

Acute
- "Fat" sinus with bulging convex walls
- T1 isointense, T2 profoundly hypointense
- T2* "blooms," T1 C+ shows "empty delta"

Late Acute
- T1 mixed isointense, mildly hyperintense
- T2/FLAIR mildly hypointense/isointense
- T2* "blooms"

Subacute
- T1 hyperintense, T2/FLAIR hyperintense
- T2* hyperintense

Chronic
- T1 isointense, T2/FLAIR moderately hyperintense
- T2*, T1 C+ show "squiggly" parenchymal enhancement
- T1 C+ shows thick, enhancing dura

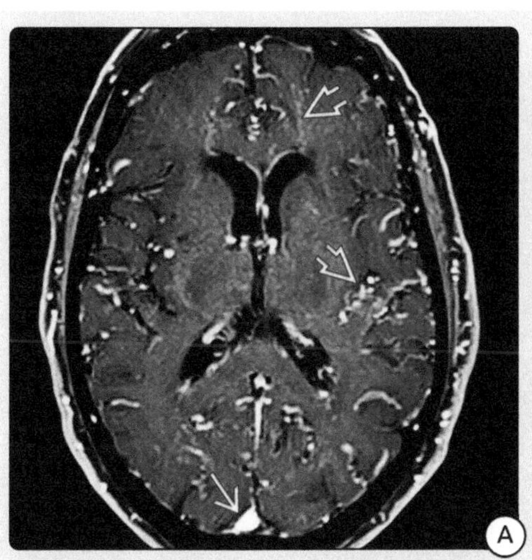

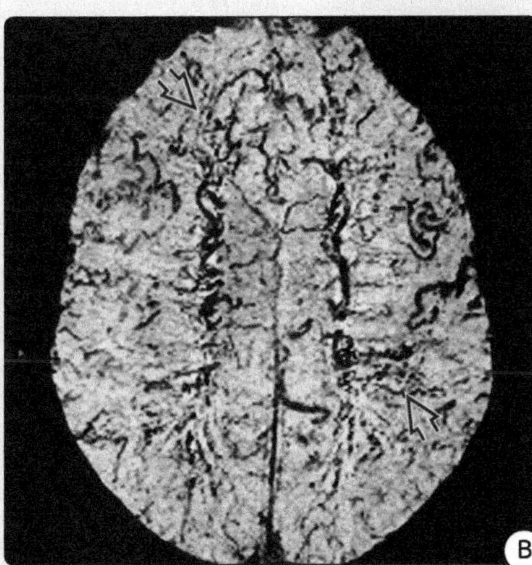

***(9-13A)** Axial T1 C+ FS MR in chronic DST shows thrombosed SSS enhancing intensely ➡. Tortuous, corkscrew vessels in the parenchyma and sulci also enhance intensely ➡. **(9-13B)** Axial T2* SWI shows prominent tortuous, corkscrew "squiggly" medullary veins in both cerebral hemispheres ➡.*

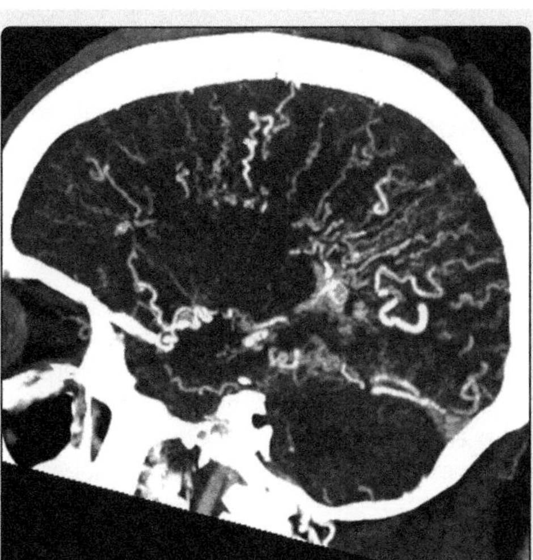

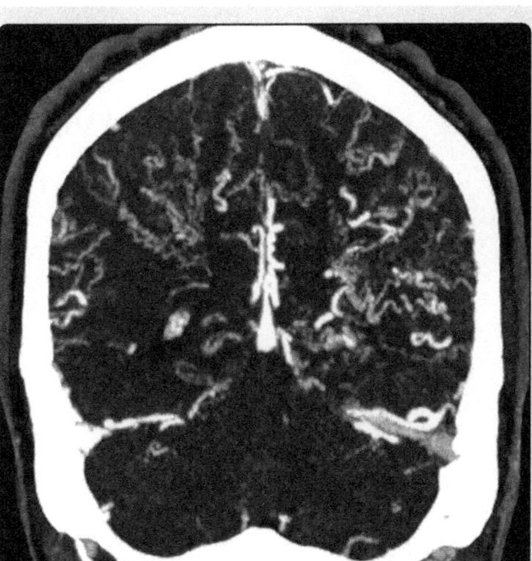

***(9-14)** Sagittal MIP of CT venogram shows innumerable "corkscrew" enlarged, tortuous medullary veins that are providing collateral venous drainage. **(9-15)** Coronal CT venogram shows the absence of a normal SSS and cortical veins. The tortuous "corkscrew" vessels are massively enlarged medullary veins.*

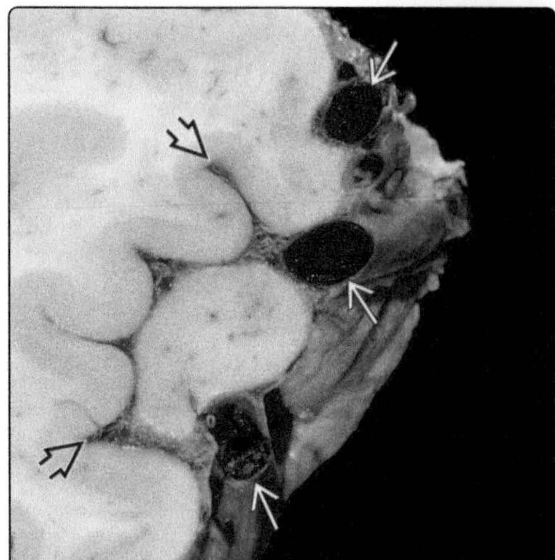

(9-16) Autopsy case shows thrombus in several cortical veins ➡ ("cord" sign) and adjacent convexal subarachnoid hemorrhage ⇨.

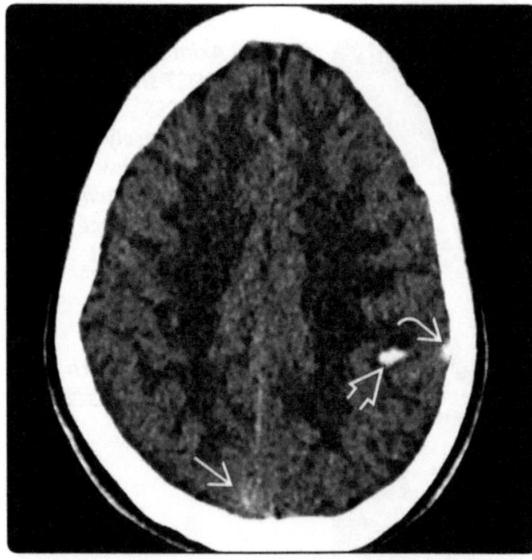

(9-17) NECT shows small parenchymal hemorrhage ⇨ and "cord" sign ↪ of thrombosed cortical vein. SSS ➡ is normal.

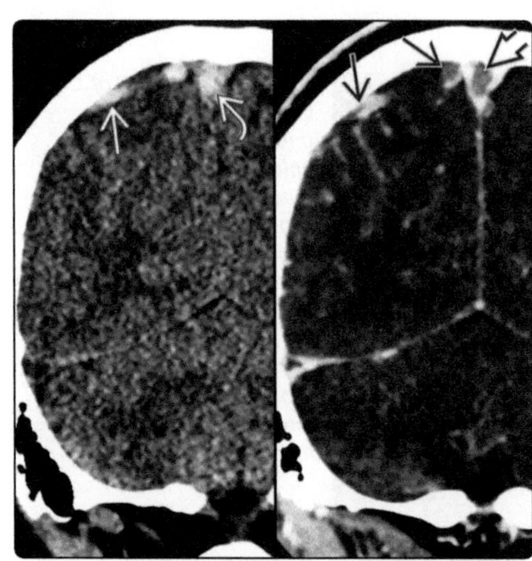

(9-18) (L) Coronal NECT shows hyperdense SSS ↪, thrombosed VofT ➡. (R) CTV shows "empty delta" in SSS ⇨ and filling defects → in VofT.

Superficial Cerebral Vein Thrombosis

Superficial cerebral vein thrombosis (SCVT) can occur without or with DST **(9-16)**. When it occurs without accompanying DST, SCVT is termed isolated cortical vein thrombosis.

Superficial Vein Thrombosis *Without* DST

Isolated SCVT (iSVCT) without DST is rare, representing only 5% of all sinovenous occlusions. The clinical outcome of iSVCT is generally good.

iSCVT usually presents with a nonspecific headache. Approximately 10% of patients report sudden onset of a "thunderclap" headache that clinically mimics aneurysmal subarachnoid hemorrhage.

Symptoms such as focal neurologic deficits, seizures, and impaired consciousness are less common than with dural sinus or deep vein thrombosis.

The imaging diagnosis of iSCVT can be problematic. NECT is usually negative, although some cases may demonstrate focal **convexal subarachnoid hemorrhage** or a **"cord" sign**, representing a hyperdense thrombosed vein **(9-17)**.

CTA/CTV or DSA may show a thin round or tubular layer of contrast surrounding the thrombus.

The MR diagnosis of SCVT—whether with or without dural sinus involvement—is difficult to establish using only standard T1- and T2-weighted sequences. Acute thrombi are isointense with brain on T1WI and hypointense on T2WI, making them difficult to distinguish from normal "flow voids."

FLAIR may demonstrate focal convexal subarachnoid hemorrhage seen as hyperintense sulcal CSF. Cortical-subcortical hyperintensities consistent with vasogenic edema are common associated findings.

Intraluminal thrombus can sometimes be seen as a linear hyperintensity on FLAIR or DWI. Venous ischemia may result in transient diffusion restriction.

T2* (GRE, SWI) sequences are key to the noninvasive diagnosis of SCVT. With a sensitivity of > 95%, they are by far the best imaging sequences for detecting thrombosed cortical veins. A well-delineated tubular hypointensity with "blooming" of hemoglobin degradation products within the clot is observed at all stages of evolution, persisting for weeks. Patchy or petechial hemorrhages in the underlying cortex and subcortical white matter are common, as is associated convexal subarachnoid hemorrhage.

Superficial Vein Thrombosis *With* DST

Two general types of SCVT with DST are recognized: DST that involves one or more small cortical draining veins and DST that affects one of the great anastomotic veins (Trolard or Labbé).

Imaging findings of SCVT with accompanying DST are similar to those of DST alone. In addition to clot in the sinus, thrombus extends into one or more cortical veins **(9-9)**. SSS occlusion with SCVT may affect the superolateral surfaces of the hemispheres with variable amounts of edema and petechial hemorrhage involving the cortex and subcortical white matter **(9-9A)**. If the anastomotic vein of Trolard is dominant, its occlusion may result in lobar hemorrhage.

Transverse sinus occlusion that extends into a dominant vein of Labbé often causes extensive posterior temporal and anterior parietal hemorrhage.

SUPERFICIAL CORTICAL VEIN THROMBOSIS

Superficial Thrombosis With DST
- DST extends into adjacent veins
- Edema, hemorrhage in cortex, adjacent white matter
- Can be extensive if vein of Trolard or Labbé occluded

Superficial Thrombosis Without DST
- Rare (5% of all CVTs)
- May cause convexal subarachnoid hemorrhage
- May see "cord" sign
- Deoxygenated thrombus can mimic normal "flow voids" on T2WI
- T2* (GRE, SWI) key to diagnosis
  - "Blooming" thrombus in vein(s)

Deep Cerebral Venous Thrombosis

Deep cerebral venous thrombosis (DCVT) is a potentially life-threatening disorder with a combined mortality/disability rate of 25%.

Etiology and Pathology

The deep cerebral venous system [the internal cerebral veins (ICVs) and basal vein of Rosenthal, together with their tributaries, the vein of Galen, and straight sinus] is involved in ~ 15% of all patients with cerebral venoocclusive disease **(9-22)**.

DCVT can occur either alone or in combination with other sinovenous occlusions. Isolated DCVT is present in 25-30% of cases. DCVT is almost always bilateral and results in symmetric venous congestion/infarction of the basal ganglia and thalami.

Clinical Issues

Initial symptoms of DCVT are variable and nonspecific, making diagnosis difficult. Most patients present with headache (80%) followed by rapid neurologic deterioration and impaired consciousness (70%). Focal neurologic findings are frequently absent.

Imaging

Early NECT findings may be subtle. Hyperdense ICVs and straight sinuses resemble a contrast-enhanced scan **(9-23)**. Hypodense "fading" or "disappearing" thalami with effacement of the border between the deep gray nuclei and internal capsule are key but nonspecific findings of DCVT.

MR is the imaging modality of choice. Acute thrombus is isointense on T1WI **(9-24A)** and hypointense on T2WI (pseudo-"flow void"). Venous congestion causes hyperintensity with swelling of the thalami and basal ganglia on T2/FLAIR in 70% of cases.

The most sensitive sequence is T2* GRE on which acute clots show distinct "blooming." Venous congestion in the medullary and subependymal veins is also hypointense due to slow flow and hemoglobin deoxygenation **(9-24C)**.

CTA/CTV and DSA show absent opacification in deep venous drainage system, and MRV shows absence of flow.

Differential Diagnosis

Extensive acute DCVT may make the NECT scan resemble a normal **contrast-enhanced CT** **(9-23)**.

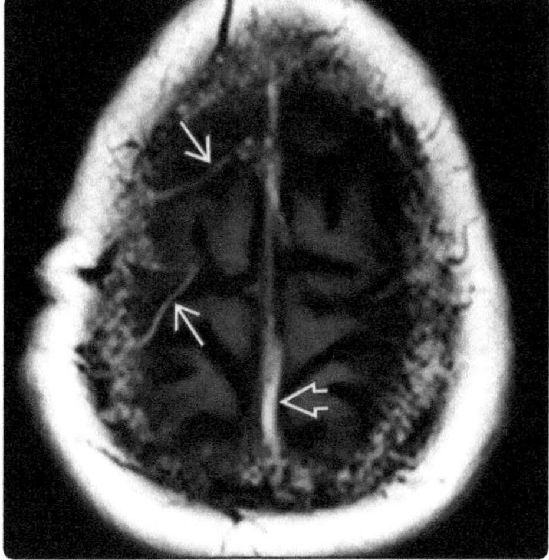

***(9-19)** Axial T1 MR in a patient with headache and normal NECT shows slight T1 shortening in the SSS ➡ and right cortical veins ➡.*

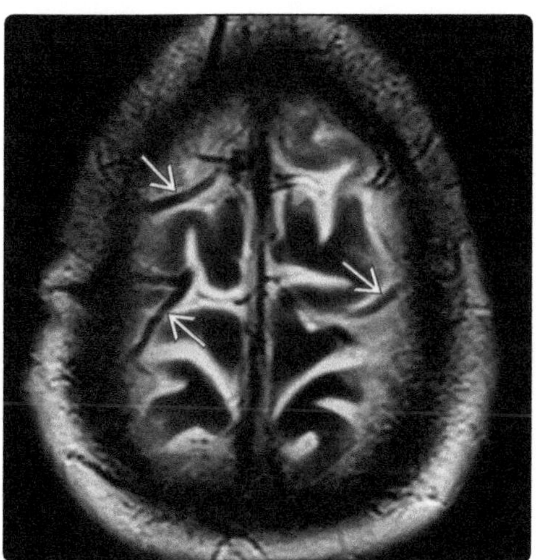

***(9-20)** Axial T2 MR appears superficially normal but acute hypointense thrombus in the cortical veins ➡ mimics normal "flow voids."*

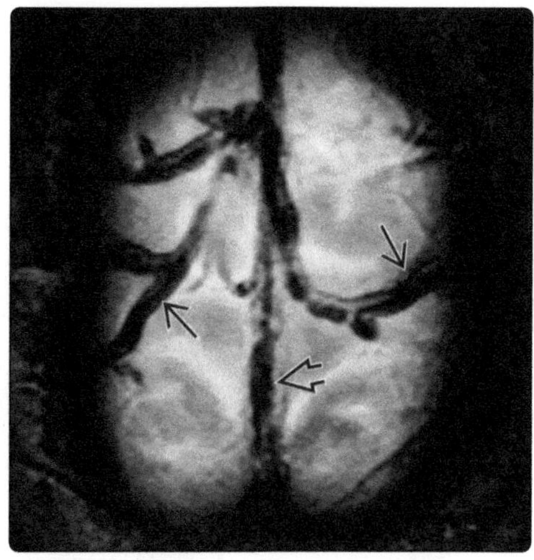

***(9-21)** T2* GRE shows acutely thrombosed cortical veins, seen as curvilinear hypointensities ➡. The adjacent SSS is also occluded ➡.*

(9-22) Thrombosis of both ICVs, VofG, SS are shown. Note thalamic hemorrhages and engorgement of WM medullary veins. (9-23) NECT in deep vein thrombosis shows hyperdense ICVs, straight sinus, and hypodense edematous thalami.

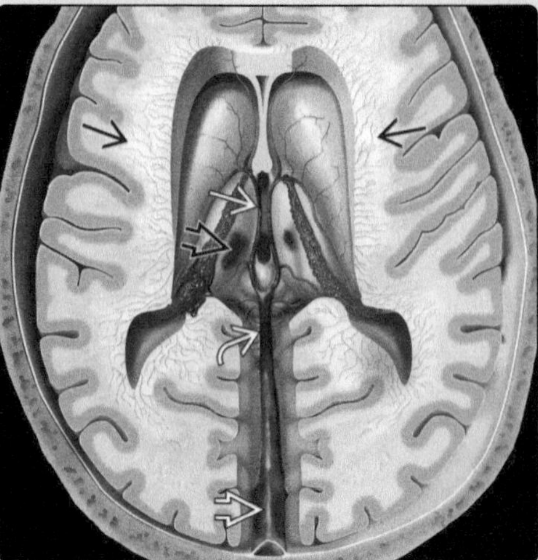

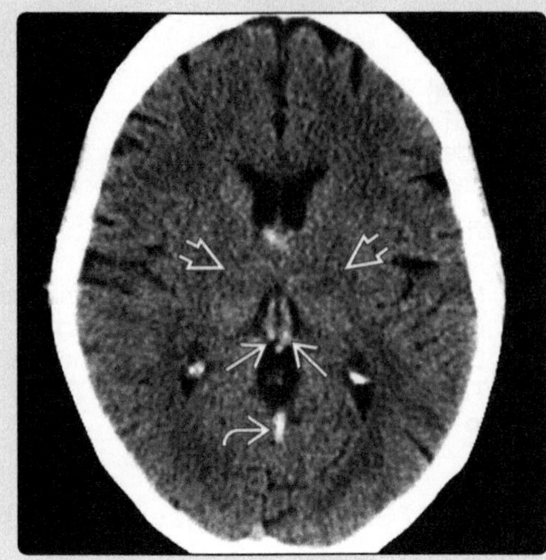

(9-24A) Sagittal T1 MR in deep venous occlusion shows isointense clot in the ICVs, vein of Galen, and straight sinus. (9-24B) Axial T2 GRE in the same case shows "blooming" thrombus in both ICVs and thalamostriate veins with hypointensity from slow flow in deep medullary veins.*

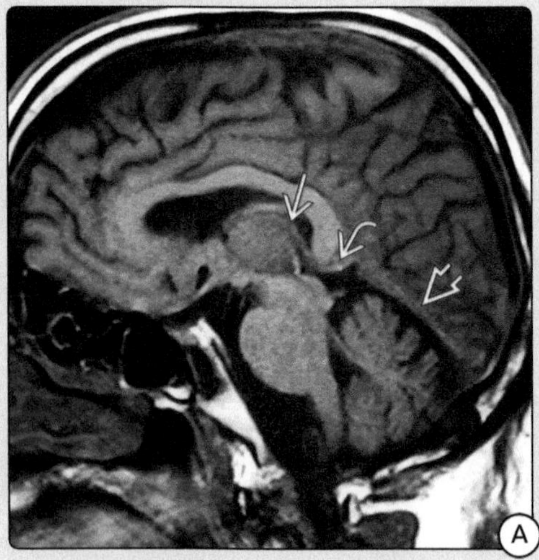

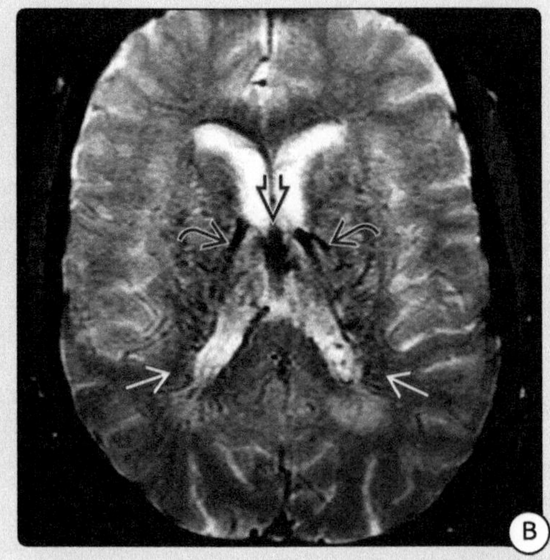

(9-24C) More cephalad T2 shows hypointensity from deoxyhemoglobin in engorged subependymal and deep WM medullary veins. (9-24D) NECT obtained 2 days later shows findings of end-stage deep venous occlusion with thrombus in the ICVs, as well as confluent hypodensity in the entire central brain plus thalamic hemorrhage. The patient expired shortly after this scan.*

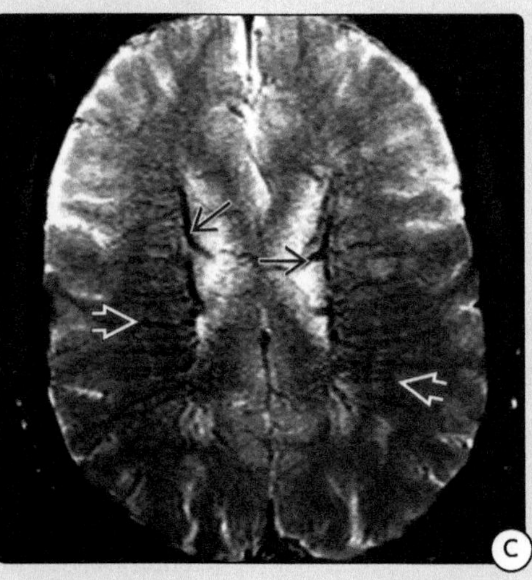

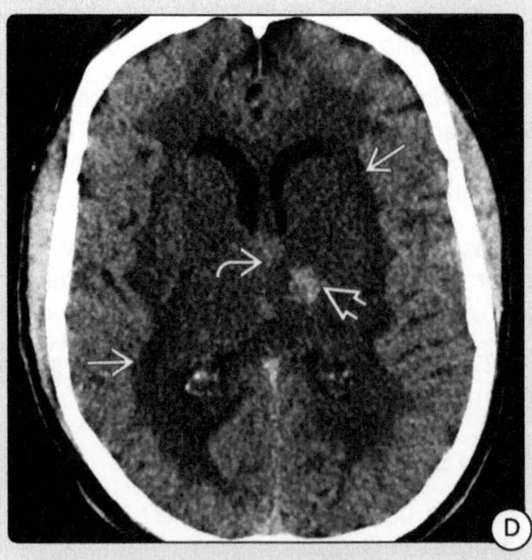

DEEP VENOUS THROMBOSIS

Pathology

- Uncommon (15% of CVTs)
- Usually both ICVs ± VofG, SS involved

Imaging

- Hyperdense ICVs (may look like CECT scan)
- Bithalamic edema common
- Variable hemorrhage
- CTV shows nonopacification of deep (Galenic) veins
- DSA shows absent visualization of ICVs ± VofG, SS
- Differential diagnosis
  - Neoplasm (bithalamic glioma)
  - Top of basilar, artery of Percheron thrombosis
  - Wernicke encephalopathy

Cavernous Sinus Thrombosis/Thrombophlebitis

Cavernous thrombosis/thrombophlebitis is the most common form of septic cerebral venous sinus thrombosis, a rare but potentially lethal condition with significant morbidity and high mortality.

Terminology

Cavernous sinus thrombosis (CST) is a blood clot in the cavernous sinus (CS). If it occurs in conjunction with sinus infection, it is termed cavernous sinus thrombophlebitis **(9-25)**.

Etiology and Pathology

The CS is composed of numerous heavily trabeculated venous spaces that have numerous valveless communications with

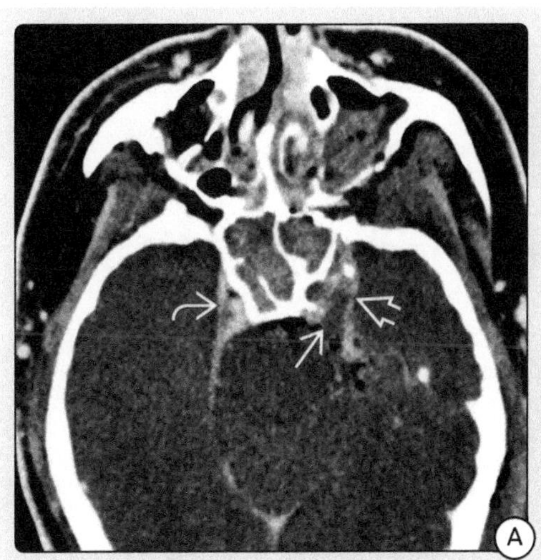
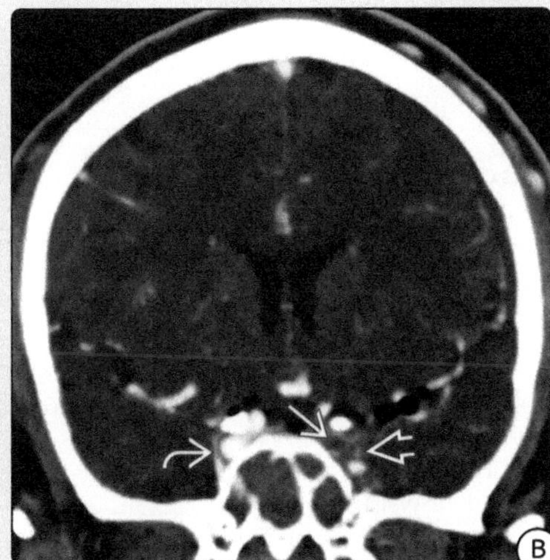

***(9-25A)** CECT source image from CTA in a 28-year-old man with polytrauma shows filling defects in the left CS ➡. The affected CS has a lightly convex lateral margin ➡ compared with the normal right CS ➡. **(9-25B)** Coronal CTA in the same patient shows occlusion of the left cavernous internal carotid artery (ICA) ➡. The left CS remains unopacified because it is filled with thrombus ➡. Compare this to the normal right CS ➡.*

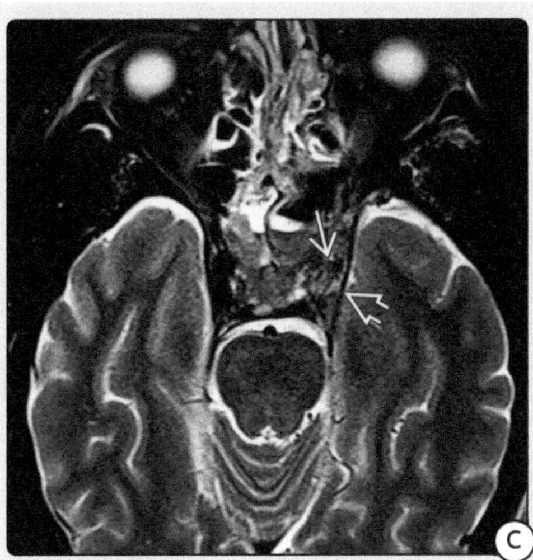
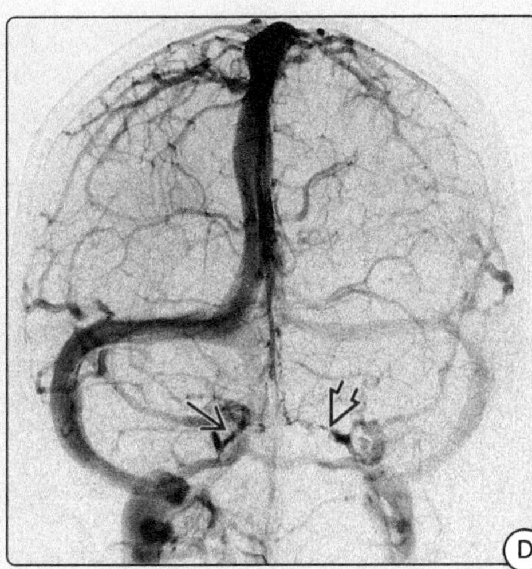

***(9-25C)** Axial T2 MR in the same case shows left ICA occlusion, seen as an absent "flow void" ➡. The left CS is filled with iso-/hypointense clot ➡. **(9-25D)** Venous phase of the right ICA angiogram demonstrates the difficulty in diagnosing CST on DSA. The right CS ➡ is opacified, draining inferiorly into the pterygoid venous plexus. Left CS is not visualized, and subtle thrombus ➡ is present, seen here as a filling defect.*

veins in the orbit, face, and neck. Infection can thus spread easily through these venous conduits into the CS.

CST usually occurs as a complication of sinusitis or other midface infection. *Staphylococcus aureus* is the most frequent pathogen. Other less common agents include anaerobes and angioinvasive fungal infections.

Otomastoiditis, odontogenic disease, trauma, and neoplasm are less frequent causes of CST.

Clinical Issues

Epidemiology. CS thrombosis without trauma, infection, or multiple other dural venous sinus occlusions is extremely rare.

Presentation. Headache, especially in the CNV1 and CNV2 distributions, and fever are usually the earliest symptoms. Orbital pain with edema, chemosis, proptosis, ophthalmoplegia, and visual loss is present in 80-100% of cases.

Natural History. Untreated CST can be fatal. Even with antibiotics, the mortality rate of CS thrombophlebitis is 25-30%.

Imaging

CT Findings. CS thrombophlebitis causes proptosis, "dirty" orbital fat, periorbital edema, sinusitis, and lateral bulging of the CS walls and may demonstrate a thrombosed superior ophthalmic vein (SOV) on NECT. CECT scans demonstrate multiple irregular filling defects in the expanded CS and SOVs **(9-25)**.

MR Findings. MR scans show enlarged CSs with convex lateral margins. Acute thrombus is isointense with brain on T1WI and demonstrates variable hypointensity on T2WI. Nonenhancing filling defects within the enhancing dural walls of the CS and thrombosed orbital veins on T1 C+ are the definitive imaging findings in CST.

Look for the normal intracavernous carotid artery "flow void," as CS thrombophlebitis can lead to thrombosis or pseudoaneurysm formation **(9-25C)**.

Angiography. Nonvisualization of the CS on DSA can be a normal finding and does not indicate the presence of CS thrombosis **(9-25D)**.

Differential Diagnosis

The differential diagnosis of CST includes neoplasm, carotid-cavernous fistula, and inflammatory disorders. **Neoplasms** (e.g., lymphoma, metastases) enhance uniformly. **Carotid-cavernous fistula** causes "flow voids," and **inflammatory disorders** (e.g., sarcoid, inflammatory pseudotumors) enhance strongly and uniformly.

CAVERNOUS SINUS THROMBOSIS/THROMBOPHLEBITIS

Pathoetiology
- Numerous valveless communications between CS, orbit, face
- CS thrombosis secondary to sinusitis, dental disease > trauma, neoplasm
- Spontaneous, isolated CS thrombosis rare

Clinical Issues
- Headache, cranial neuropathy
- Proptosis, chemosis common

Imaging
- NECT may be normal early
  - Look for sinusitis, "dirty" orbit fat
  - Lateral bulging of CS walls
- CECT/CTV
  - Nonenhancing filling defects on CECT
  - Nonopacification on early-phase CTV
- MR
  - T1WI isointense, laterally bulging walls
  - T2 iso-/hypointense
  - Look for cavernous carotid thrombosis (loss of "flow void")
  - T1 C+ shows nonenhancing filling defects

Venous Occlusion Mimics

We conclude this chapter on venous anatomy and occlusions with a brief discussion of conditions that can mimic—or obscure—venous thrombosis.

Sinus Variants

The major differential diagnosis of cerebral venous thrombosis is a **congenital anatomic variation**. The right transverse sinus (TS) is usually the dominant venous sinus and is often significantly larger than the left side. A **hypoplastic TS** segment is present in 1/4 to 1/3 of all imaged cases and is *especially* common in the nondominant sinus (usually the left TS) **(9-26A)**. In such instances, the ipsilateral jugular bulb is typically small. Correlation with bone CT can also be helpful in demonstrating a small bony jugular foramen or sigmoid sinus groove. A hypoplastic TS or sigmoid sinus is also often—but not invariably—associated with alternative venous outflow pathways, such as a persistent occipital sinus or prominent mastoid emissary veins.

Variations in the torcular herophili (sinus confluence) are also common. A **high-splitting**, **segmented**, or **multichanneled sinus confluence** can have a central nonopacified area that mimics dural sinus thrombosis (DST).

The absence of occluded draining veins, enlarged venous collateral channels, or abnormally thick dural enhancement supports the diagnosis of TS sinus hypoplasia or anatomic variant vs. true cerebral venous sinus thrombosis.

Flow Artifacts

A **"flow gap"** on 2D TOF MRV can result from a number of factors, including slow intravascular or in-plane flow or complex blood flow patterns. Flow parallel to the plane of acquisition (in-plane flow) can cause signal loss on MR venography and is most prominent in vertically oriented structures, such as the distal sigmoid sinus. Use of inferior saturation pulses with axial 2D TOF MRV can saturate flow in parts of the curving superior sagittal sinus (SSS) but can be avoided by imaging in the coronal plane.

Arachnoid Granulations and Septations

Another key differential diagnosis of DST is **giant arachnoid granulation** (AG). Giant AGs are round or ovoid short-segment filling defects that exhibit CSF-like attenuation on NECT and do not enhance on CECT scans.

MR appearance of AGs is more problematic than its CT findings. Giant AGs often do not follow CSF signal intensity (SI) on all sequences. CSF-incongruent SI is seen on at least one sequence (usually FLAIR) in 80% of MRs. Even large AGs do not fill the entire sinus, as most thrombi do, and, unlike clots, may show central linear enhancement. Brain tissue may *herniate* into the dural venous sinuses, often part of a complex giant AG.

Septations or **trabeculations** are fibrotic bands looking like linear filling defects in sinuses. One to five septa are in 30% of TSs, most often right TS.

Other Venous Occlusion Mimics

Less common entities can mimic dural sinus or cerebral vein occlusion: Elevated hematocrit, unmyelinated brain, diffuse cerebral edema, and subdural hematoma (SDH).

High Hematocrit

The most common cause of a false-positive diagnosis of DST on NECT scan is an elevated hematocrit (i.e., patients with polycythemia vera or longstanding right-to-left cardiac shunts). This causes the appearance of a hyperdense sinus relative to the brain parenchyma. However, the intracranial arteries in patients with high hematocrits are also similarly hyperdense.

Unmyelinated Brain

Infants and young children often have *higher* hematocrits than adults with relatively *lower* density of their unmyelinated brains. High-attenuation blood vessels *and* low-attenuation brain make all vascular structures (including dural sinuses and cortical veins) seem relatively hyperdense to dural sinus.

Diffuse Cerebral Edema

Diffuse cerebral edema with decreased attenuation of the cerebral hemispheres makes the dura and all the intracranial vessels—both veins *and* arteries—appear relatively hyperdense compared with the low-density brain.

Subdural Hematoma

Acute SDH that layers along the straight sinus and medial tentorium can cause hyperdensity that may mimic DST on NECTs. Dense thrombus surrounds the less dense flowing blood in the SSS and sinus confluence, mimicking an "empty delta" sign, seen *only* on contrast-enhanced scans!

Selected References: The complete reference list is available on the Expert Consult™ eBook version included with purchase.

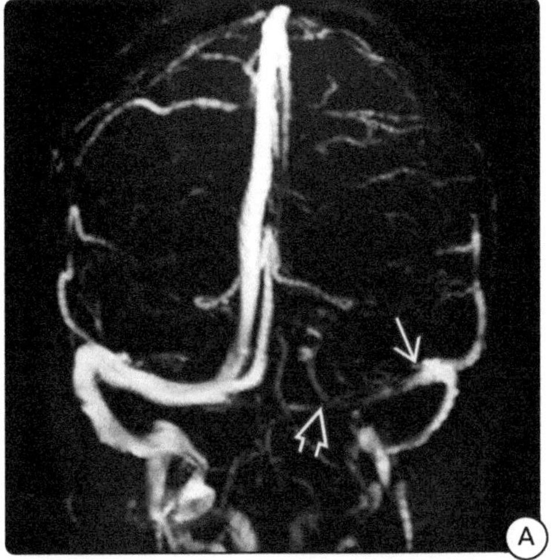

***(9-26A)** MR venogram in a 22-year-old woman shows a dominant right TS. The left TS shows a "missing" segment ➡, possible filling defect ➡.*

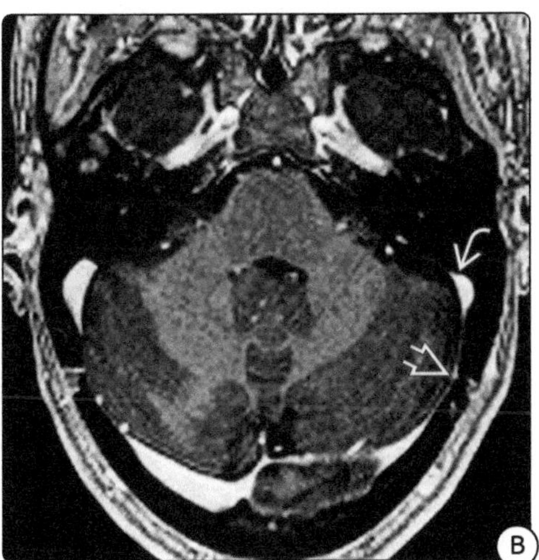

***(9-26B)** Axial MP-RAGE shows hypoplastic but patent left TS ➡ and a small sigmoid sinus ➡.*

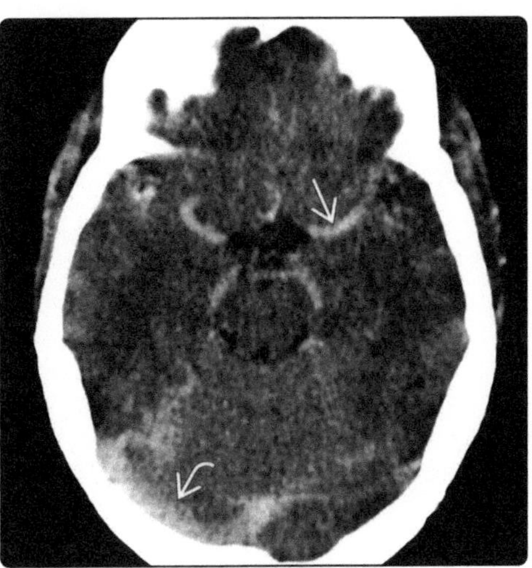

***(9-27)** NECT in polycythemia with elevated hematocrit shows hyperdense right transverse sinus ➡. Arteries ➡ are also hyperdense.*

Vasculopathy

The generic term "vasculopathy" literally means blood vessel pathology—of any kind, in any vessel (artery, capillary, or vein). Evaluating the craniocervical vessels for vasculopathy is one of the major indications for neuroimaging. Large vessel atherosclerotic vascular disease (ASVD) is the single most prevalent vasculopathy in the head and neck, whereas carotid stenosis or embolization from ASVD plaques are the most common causes of ischemic strokes.

We begin this chapter with atherosclerosis, starting with a general discussion of atherogenesis. Extracranial ASVD and carotid stenosis are followed by a brief overview of intracranial large and medium artery ASVD. We conclude the discussion with arteriolosclerosis, the most common brain "microvascular disease."

The broad spectrum of nonatheromatous vasculopathy is then addressed. Finally, we devote the last section of this chapter to non-ASVD diseases of the cerebral macro- and microvasculature. While arteriolosclerosis is by far the most common cause of small vessel vascular disease, nonatherogenic microvasculopathies, such as amyloid angiopathy, can have devastating clinical consequences.

Atherosclerosis

Atherosclerotic vascular disease (ASVD) is by far the most common cause of mortality and severe long-term disability in industrialized countries, so it is difficult to overemphasize its importance. It affects all arteries, of all sizes, in all parts of the body.

The principal cause of cerebral infarction is atherosclerosis and its sequelae. Over 90% of large cerebral infarcts are caused by thromboemboli secondary to ASVD. We begin with extracranial ASVD before concluding with a brief discussion of the clinical and imaging manifestations of intracranial ASVD, including its microvascular manifestations.

Atherogenesis and Atherosclerosis

Terminology

The term "atherosclerosis" was originally coined to describe progressive "hardening" or "sclerosis" of blood vessels. The term "atheroma" (Greek for porridge) designates the material deposited on or within vessel walls.

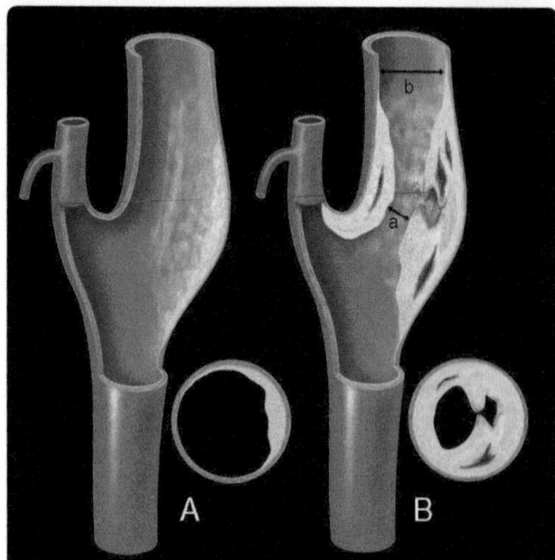

***(10-1)** (A) Mild ASVD with "fatty streaks." (B) Severe ASVD; % stenosis = (b - a)/b x 100; b = normal lumen, a = residual lumen diameter.*

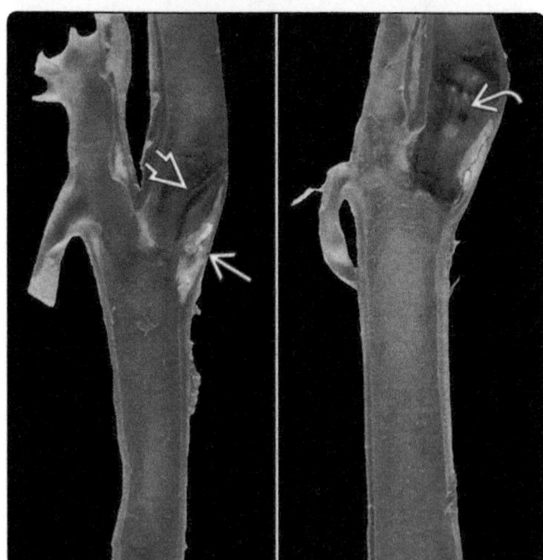

***(10-2)** (L) Stable ASVD shows fatty plaque, intact intima. (R) Initially "at-risk" plaque now shows ulceration, disrupted intima.*

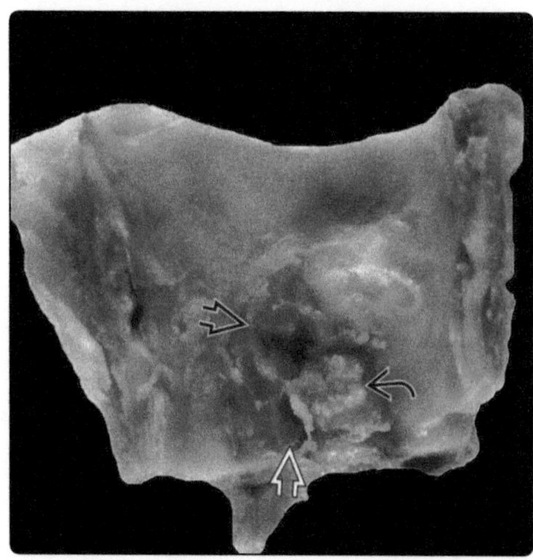

***(10-3)** Carotid endarterectomy shows ulcerated intima, calcification, intraplaque hemorrhage. (Courtesy J. Townsend, MD.)*

"Plaque" is used to describe a focal atheroma together with its epiphenomena, such as ulceration, platelet aggregation, and hemorrhage.

Atherogenesis is the degenerative process that results in atherosclerosis. **Atherosclerosis** is the most common pathologic process affecting large elastic arteries (e.g., the aorta) and medium-sized muscular arteries (e.g., the carotid and vertebral arteries). **Arteriolosclerosis** describes the effects of atherogenesis on smaller arteries (and is treated separately at the end of this section). **ASVD** is the generic term describing atherosclerosis in any artery, of any size, in any area of the body.

Etiology

General Concepts. Plasma lipids, connective tissue fibers, and inflammatory cells accumulate at susceptible sites in arterial walls, forming focal atherosclerotic plaques. Angiogenic factors cause vasa vasorum proliferation, formation of immature vessels, and loss of capillary basement membranes. Neoangiogenesis is closely associated with plaque progression and is likely the primary source of intraplaque hemorrhage.

Pathology

Location. ASVD occurs preferentially at highly predictable locations. In the extracranial vasculature, the most common sites are the proximal internal carotid arteries (ICAs) and common carotid artery (CCA) bifurcations, followed by the aortic arch and great vessel origins.

Size and Number. ASVD plaques vary in size from small, almost microscopic lipid deposits to large, raised, fungating, ulcerating lesions that can extend over several centimeters and dramatically narrow the parent vessel lumen. Multiple lesions in multiple locations are common.

Gross Pathology. ASVD plaques develop in stages **(10-1)**. The first detectable lesion is lipid deposition in the intima, seen as yellowish "fatty streaks." Other than "fatty streaks" and slightly eccentric but smooth intimal thickening, visible changes at this early stage are minimal.

Microscopic Features. ASVD plaques are classified histopathologically as "stable," "vulnerable," or "ulcerated."

Stable Plaques. Uncomplicated **stable plaques**—the basic lesions of atherosclerosis—consist of cellular material, lipid, and an overlying fibrous cap. The intima covering a stable plaque is thickened, but its exterior surface remains intact. No ulceration or intraplaque hemorrhage is present **(10-2)**.

Vulnerable Plaques. As a necrotic core of lipid-laden foam cells, cellular debris, and cholesterol gradually accumulates under the elevated fibrous cap, the cap thins and becomes prone to rupture (**"vulnerable" plaque**) **(10-2)**.

Proliferating small blood vessels also develop around the periphery of the necrotic core. **Neovascularization** can lead to **subintimal hemorrhage**, which enlarges the necrotic core, further weakening the overlying fibrous cap.

Ulcerated Plaques. Plaque **ulceration** occurs when the fibrous cap weakens and ruptures through the intima, releasing necrotic debris **(10-3)**. Plates and fibrin aggregate within the ulcerated denuded endothelium. These aggregates can be pulled into the rapidly flowing main artery slipstream, causing arterioarterial embolization to distal intracranial vessels.

Clinical Issues

Epidemiology and Demographics. Most patients with symptomatic lesions are middle aged or elderly. However, atherosclerosis is increasingly common in younger patients, contributing to the rising prevalence of strokes in patients younger than 45 years.

Presentation. Many ASVD lesions remain asymptomatic until they cause hemodynamically significant stenosis or thromboembolic disease. Transient ischemic attacks (TIAs) and "silent strokes" are common precursors of large territorial infarcts.

Natural History. The natural history of ASVD is also highly variable. ICA occlusion poses an especially high risk for eventual stroke with over 70% of these patients eventually experiencing ischemic cerebral infarction.

Treatment Options. Treatment options include prevention, medical therapy (lipid-lowering regimens), and surgery or endovascular therapy.

Extracranial Atherosclerosis

Extracranial ASVD is the single largest risk factor for stroke. That risk starts with the aortic arch, an underrecognized source of intracranial ischemic strokes. Complete imaging evaluation of patients with thromboembolic infarcts in the brain should include investigation of the aortic arch.

Aortic Arch/Great Vessels

Aortic ASVD is more common in the descending thoracic aorta than in the ascending aorta or arch. However, late diastolic retrograde flow from complex plaques in the proximal descending aorta distal to the left subclavian artery (SCA) origin can reach all supraaortic arteries. Retrograde flow extends to the left SCA orifice in nearly 60% of cases, the left CCA in 25%, and the brachiocephalic trunk in 10-15%.

Aortic emboli involve the left brain in 80% of cases and show a distinct predilection for the vertebrobasilar circulation. This striking geographic distribution is consistent with thromboemboli arising from ulcerated plaques in the descending aorta that are then swept by retrograde flow into left-sided arch vessels.

Carotid Bifurcation/Cervical Internal Carotid Arteries

Between 20-30% of all ischemic infarcts are caused by carotid artery stenosis. Therefore, determining the degree of carotid stenosis on imaging studies is now both routine and required.

Using data from the North American Symptomatic Carotid Endarterectomy Trial (NASCET), carotid stenosis is classified as moderate (50-69%), severe (70-93%), and "preocclusive" or critical (94-99%) **(10-6)**. Patients with critical stenosis are at high risk for embolic stroke as long as the ICA lumen is patent.

In addition to stenosis degree, several recent studies have demonstrated the importance of also assessing the morphologic features of ASVD plaques. Rupture of an "at-risk" plaque with a large necrotic core under a thin fibrous cap is responsible for the majority of acute thrombi. As distal embolization from proximal ASVD-related clots is a common cause of cerebral ischemia/infarction, *identifying rupture-prone "vulnerable" plaques is at least as important as determining stenosis!*

CT Findings. The most common imaging findings in extracranial ASVD are mural calcifications, luminal irregularities, varying degrees of vessel stenosis, occlusion, and thrombosis. Elongation, ectasia, and vessel tortuosity can occur with or without other changes of ASVD.

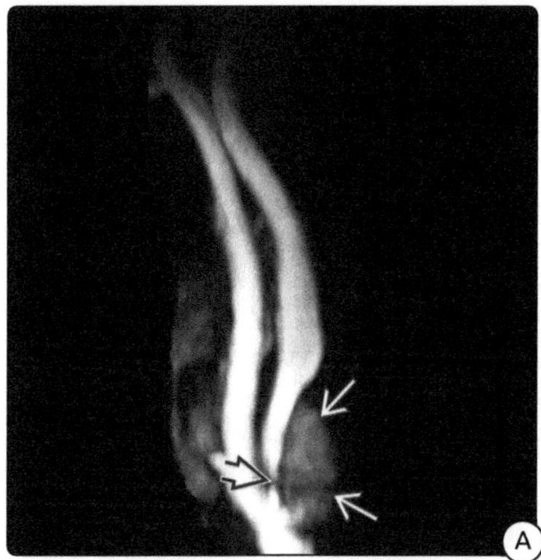

***(10-4A)** Oblique 3T MRA shows very high-grade stenosis of the right carotid artery with a "flow gap" ⇨ caused by a large ASVD plaque ➡.*

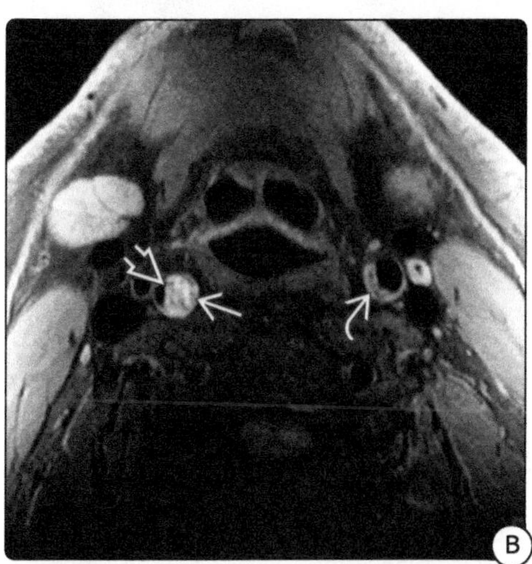

***(10-4B)** MP-RAGE shows intraplaque hemorrhage ➡ with tiny residual lumen ➡ in the R ICA, subintimal hemorrhage ➡ in the L ICA.*

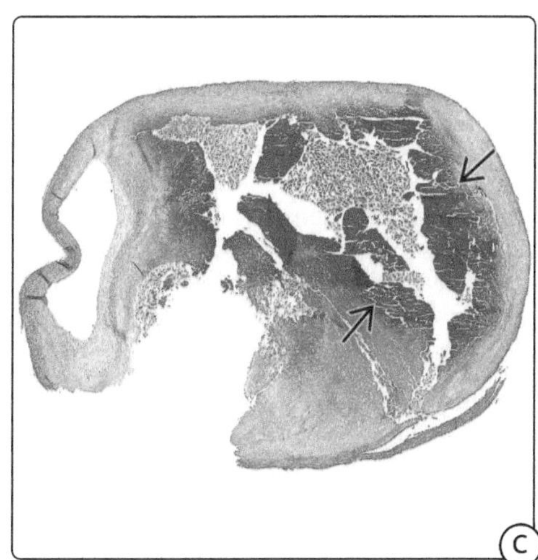

***(10-4C)** Right ICA endarterectomy shows that plaque hyperintensity is due to acute hemorrhage ⇨, not lipid. (Courtesy S. McNally, MD.)*

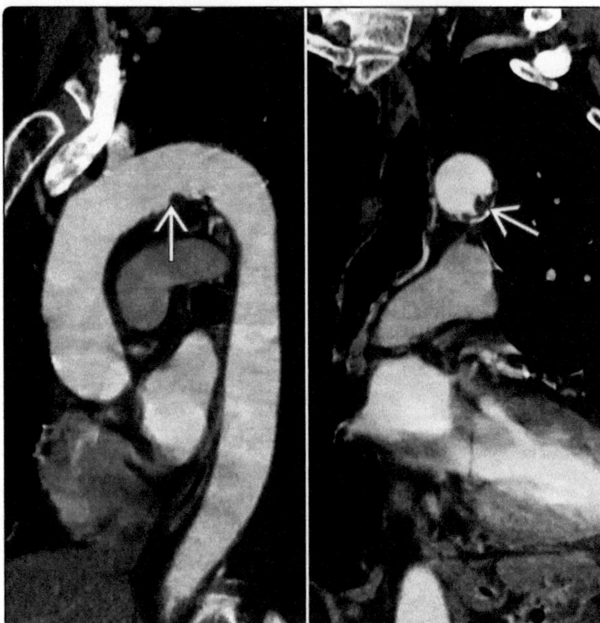

(10-5) (L) "Candy cane" oblique, (R) coronal views show atherosclerotic plaque ➡ along the lesser curvature of the aortic arch. (Courtesy G. Oliveira, MD.)

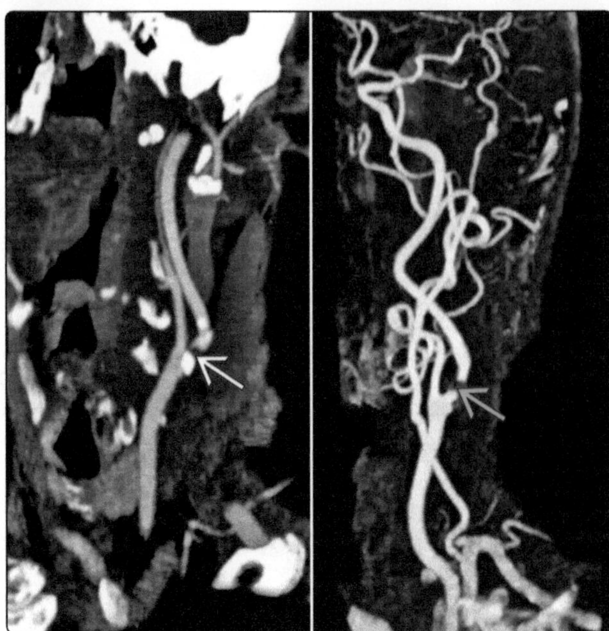

(10-6) (L) DSA ➡ and (R) MRA show critical ICA stenosis with a "flow gap" ➡ characteristic of a high-grade flow-limiting lesion.

NECT scans easily show vessel wall calcifications. Large atherosclerotic plaques may demonstrate one or more subintimal low-density foci. These represent the lipid-rich core of a "soft" plaque. High-density subintimal foci indicate intraplaque hemorrhage. Both findings carry increased risk of plaque rupture and concomitant distal embolization.

CTA source images display the carotid lumen in cross section. Nonstenotic smooth luminal narrowing is the most common finding in ASVD. Ulcerations—seen as irregularly shaped contrast-filled outpouchings from the lumen—are detected with 95% sensitivity and 99% specificity. Intraluminal thrombi are also readily demonstrated ("doughnut" sign). Carotid occlusion is seen as contrast ending blindly in a blunted, rounded, or pointed pouch in the proximal ICA.

In addition to calculating percentage of stenosis **(10-1)**, plaque morphologic characteristics should be described in detail, as stenosis alone does not define complete stroke risk in symptomatic patients. Intraplaque hemorrhage has been identified as an independent risk factor for ischemic stroke at *all* degrees of stenosis, including symptomatic patients with low-grade lesions (< 50%). Therefore, accurate characterization of plaque morphology is important for patient management.

MR Findings. High-resolution MR imaging can be used to characterize carotid plaques, allowing identification of individual plaque components, including lipids, hemorrhage, fibrous tissue, and calcification.

High signal intensity on T1-weighted fat-suppressed scans, MRA source images, or MP-RAGE sequences represents hemorrhage into complicated "vulnerable" atherosclerotic plaques, not lipid accumulation **(10-4)**. Unlike intraparenchymal brain bleeds, plaque hemorrhages may remain hyperintense for up to 18 months. Vulnerable plaques are usually hyperintense on T2WI, whereas stable plaques are isointense on both T1- and T2WI.

T1 C+ FS scans may show enhancement around plaque margins, consistent with neovascularity in a vulnerable "at-risk" plaque.

Contrast-enhanced or unenhanced 2D TOF MRA is 80-85% sensitive and 95% specific for the detection of ICA > 70% ICA stenosis. Signal loss with a "flow gap" occurs if the stenosis is > 95%. Compared with CTA and DSA, MRA tends to overestimate the degree of stenosis.

Vertebral Arteries

ASVD in the extracranial vertebral arteries (VAs) accounts for up to 20% of all posterior circulation ischemic strokes. Although mid- and distal cervical segment lesions occur, extracranial ASVD is most common at or near the VA origin.

A special type of VA pathology is called **subclavian steal**. Here, the SCA or brachiocephalic trunk is severely stenotic or occluded *proximal* to the VA origin. Flow reversal in the affected VA occurs as blood is recruited (i.e., "stolen") from the opposite VA, crosses the basilar artery (BA) junction, and flows in retrograde fashion down the VA into the SCA to supply the shoulder and arm distal to the stenosis/occlusion **(10-7)**.

Noninvasive imaging of subclavian steal can be problematic. Because superior saturation bands are applied in 2D TOF MRA, reversed flow direction in a VA can mimic occlusion. Standard TOF MRA alone may not be adequate to differentiate *reversed* flow from *absent* flow, so confirmation and quantification with additional imaging is usually required.

Differential Diagnosis

The major differential diagnoses of extracranial ASVD include dissection, dissecting aneurysm, vasospasm, and fibromuscular dysplasia (FMD). All usually spare the carotid bulb.

Dissection (either traumatic or spontaneous) is more common in young/middle-aged patients and occurs in the *middle* of extracranial vessels. Extracranial dissections typically terminate at the exocranial opening of the carotid canal. Most are smooth or display minimal irregularities, whereas calcifications and ulcerations—common in carotid plaques—are absent.

Midsegment vessel narrowing with a focal mass-like outpouching of the lumen is typical of **dissecting aneurysm**. **Vasospasm** is more common in the intracranial vessels. When it involves the cervical carotid or vertebral arteries, it also typically spares the proximal segments.

FMD spares the carotid bulb and usually affects the middle or distal aspects of the extracranial carotid and vertebral arteries. A "string of beads" appearance is typical. Long-segment tubular narrowing is less common and may reflect coexisting dissection.

EXTRACRANIAL ATHEROSCLEROSIS

Etiology
- Multifactorial, progressive disease
- Plasma lipids accumulate in susceptible sites
- Lipids incite inflammatory response

Pathology
- Predictable locations
  - Carotid bifurcation, proximal ICA (carotid "bulb")
  - Aortic arch, great vessel origins
- 1st sign = fatty streaks, intimal thickening
- Stable plaque
  - Subintimal smooth muscle cells, macrophages accumulate
  - Fibrous cap formed under intact intima
- "Vulnerable" plaque
  - Necrotic core of cellular debris, cholesterol ± calcifications
  - Plaque thins, becomes prone to rupture
  - Neovascularization, subintimal hemorrhage
- Ulcerated plaque
  - Fibrous cap ruptures through intima
  - Denuded intima → platelet, fibrin aggregates
  - May embolize to intracranial circulation

Clinical Issues
- Identifiable risk factors in patients with ischemic stroke
  - Older age (> 60 years)
  - Diabetes mellitus
  - Elevated LDL
  - Hypertension
  - ± history of heart disease

Intracranial Atherosclerosis

One of the most serious and disabling manifestations of ASVD is stroke. Most acute ischemic strokes are thromboembolic, most often secondary to cardiac sources or plaques in the cervical ICA.

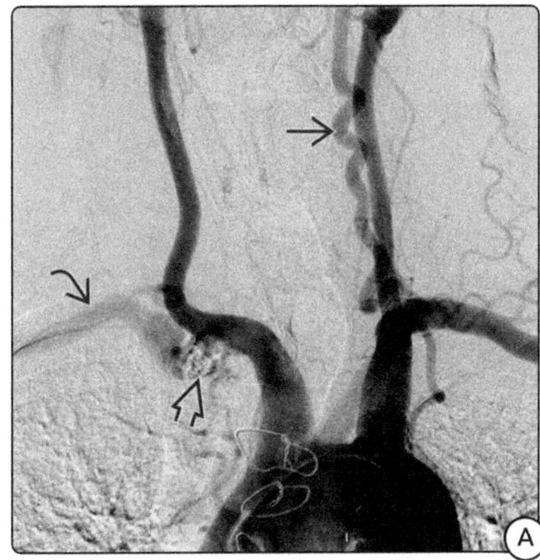

***(10-7A)** DSA shows Ca^{++} ➡, faint contrast in distal SCA ➡. The right VA is unopacified. The left VA is enlarged and tortuous ➡.*

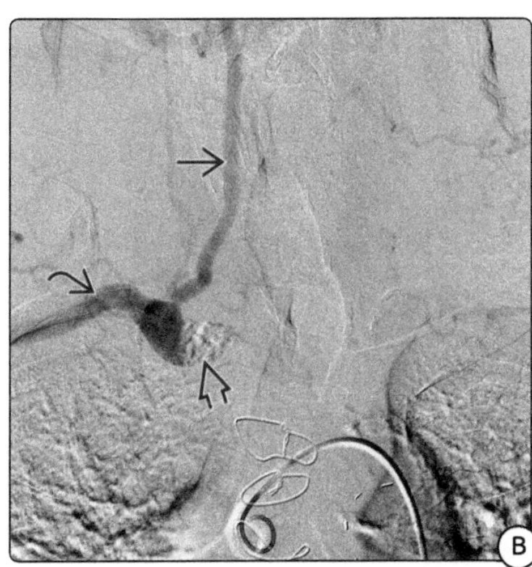

***(10-7B)** Retrograde filling of right VA ➡ and SCA ➡ distal to Ca^{++} ➡ and high-grade stenosis shows classic subclavian steal.*

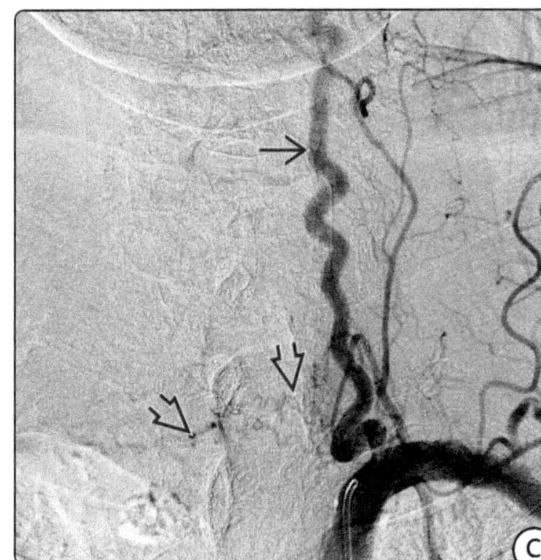

***(10-7C)** Left SCA angiogram shows prominent VA ➡ and muscular branches ➡ collateralizing to the right SCA vascular distribution.*

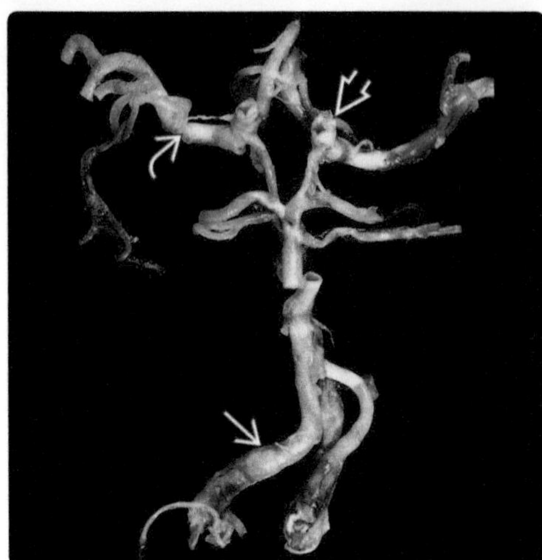

***(10-8)** Intracranial ASVD. Most severe disease is in the vertebrobasilar system, ICAs, and proximal MCAs. (Courtesy R. Hewlett, MD.)*

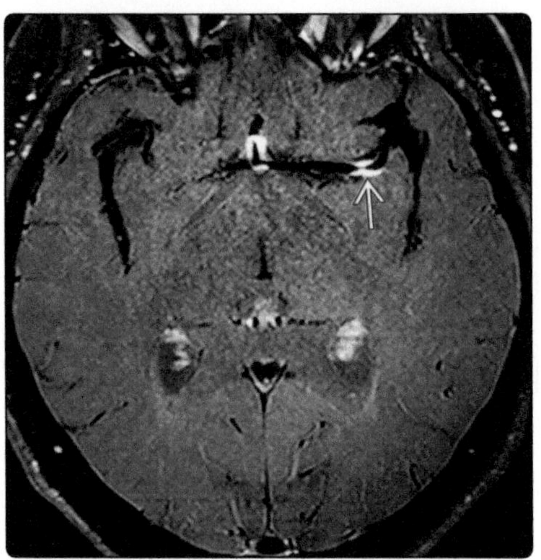

***(10-9)** T1 C+ "black blood" vessel wall imaging in a patient with cryptogenic stroke shows stenosis, enhancement around distal M1 MCA.*

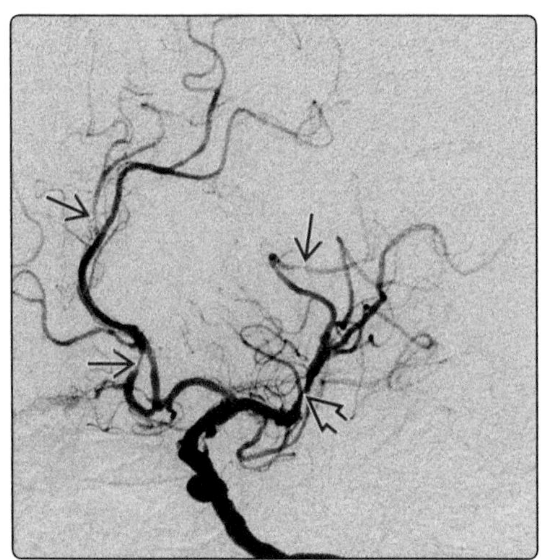

***(10-10)** DSA in a patient with deep watershed infarcts shows severe ASVD. High-grade stenosis of the M2 MCA is present.*

Many clinicians focus on extracranial carotid artery disease, considering intracranial ASVD (IASVD) a relatively infrequent cause of stroke. However, IASVD accounts for 5-10% of all ischemic strokes. Nearly 1/2 of all patients with fatal cerebral infarction have at least one intracranial plaque-associated luminal stenosis at autopsy **(10-8)**.

Ectasia

Generalized nonfocal vessel elongation is called "ectasia," "dolichoectasia," "arteriectasis," or "dilative arteriopathy." Ectasias can involve any part of the intracranial circulation but are most common in the vertebrobasilar arteries ("vertebrobasilar dolichoectasia") and supraclinoid ICA.

Atherosclerotic Fusiform Aneurysm

Atherosclerotic fusiform aneurysms (FAs) are focal arterial enlargements that are usually superimposed on an ectatic artery. ASVD FAs were discussed in detail in Chapter 6. ASVD FAs are most common in the vertebrobasilar circulation. When they occur in the anterior circulation, they can produce a rare but dramatic manifestation called a giant "serpentine" aneurysm.

Intracranial Stenoocclusive Disease

Atherosclerosis that causes large artery intracranial occlusive disease (LAICOD) is now a well-defined yet relatively neglected and poorly understood stroke subtype. Recent studies have shown that the overall prevalence of IASVD in patients with concurrent extracranial disease varies between 20% and 50%, and 12% of patients have diffuse (multifocal) IASVD.

Overall, symptomatic patients with moderate to severe stenosis (i.e., 70-99%) in the intracranial circulation have a 25% 2-year risk for recurrent stroke.

The availability of endovascular techniques, such as intracranial angioplasty, has opened new treatment avenues for LAICOD. A variety of balloon-expandable, drug-eluting, and self-expanding stents are also now available as options.

Imaging. Mural calcifications are common on NECT with patterns varying from scattered stippled foci to thick continuous linear ("railroad track") deposits. CTA or DSA may show solitary or multifocal stenoses alternating with areas of poststenotic dilatation. When ASVD affects distal branches of the major intracranial vessels, the appearance can mimic that of vasculitis (see below).

High-resolution "black blood" vessel wall imaging on MR directly depicts IASVD and is a reliable tool for identifying IASVD and measuring plaque burden. Intramural hemorrhage and irregular, noncircumferential short-segment enhancing foci are common findings.

Differential Diagnosis. The major differential diagnoses of IASVD are vasculitis, vasospasm, and dissection.

Vasculitis occurs at all ages but is more common in middle-aged patients. Vasculitis and ASVD appear virtually identical on angiography (MRA, CTA, or DSA). Remember: The most common cause of a vasculitis-like pattern in an older patient isn't vasculitis; it's ASVD!

Vasospasm spares the cavernous ICA and is usually more diffuse than ASVD. A history of trauma, subarachnoid hemorrhage, or drug abuse (typically with sympathomimetics) is common. **Intracranial dissection**—especially in the anterior circulation—is rare and usually occurs in young patients.

INTRACRANIAL ATHEROSCLEROSIS (ICASVD)

Epidemiology
- Found in 1/3 of patients in population-based imaging studies
  - Causes 8-10% of strokes in USA, Europe
  - > 50% in Asia

Clinical Issues
- Moderate/severe stenosis → 25% 2-year stroke risk

Imaging
- Mural calcifications
- Irregular narrowing ± ulcerations
- Deep watershed ischemia, lacunae
- High-resolution vessel wall imaging
  - Wall hemorrhage
  - Enhancement irregular, short segment, noncircumferential

Arteriolosclerosis

Arteriolosclerosis, also known less specifically as cerebral "microvascular disease," is a microangiopathy that typically affects small arteries (i.e., arterioles), especially in the subcortical and deep cerebral white matter (WM). Aging, chronic hypertension, hypercholesterolemia, and diabetes mellitus are the most common factors that predispose to cerebral microvascular disease.

Pathology

Generalized volume loss, multiple lacunar infarcts, and deep WM spongiosis are typical. Stenosis or occlusion of small vessels by arteriolosclerosis and lipohyalinosis probably results in WM microinfarctions.

Imaging

CT scans show patchy &/or confluent subcortical and deep WM hypodensities. Periventricular lesions have a broad or confluent base with the ventricular surface and are especially prominent around the atria of the lateral ventricles.

MR shows patchy or confluent periventricular and subcortical WM hypointensities on T1WI. The lesions are hyperintense on T2WI and are especially prominent on FLAIR. T2* (GRE, SWI) sequences often demonstrate multifocal "blooming" hypointensities, especially in the presence of chronic hypertension.

Differential Diagnosis

The major differential diagnosis is **age-related hyperintensities** in the periventricular WM. Scattered T2/FLAIR WM hyperintensities are almost universal after age 65. **Enlarged perivascular (Virchow-Robin) spaces** (PVSs) can be seen in patients of all ages and in virtually all locations, although they do increase with age. Unlike arteriolosclerosis, PVSs suppress on FLAIR.

Demyelinating disease typically causes ovoid or triangular periventricular lesions that abut the callososeptal interfaces, which are rarely involved by arteriolosclerosis.

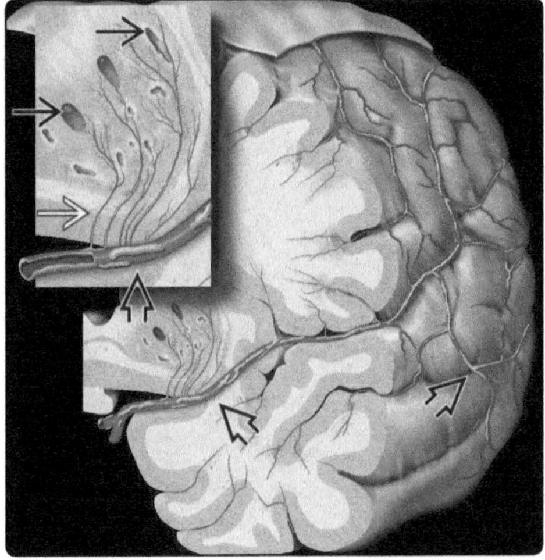

***(10-11)** ASVD involves MCA ➡ and its branches, including penetrating (lenticulostriate) arteries ➡. Note lacunar infarcts ➡.*

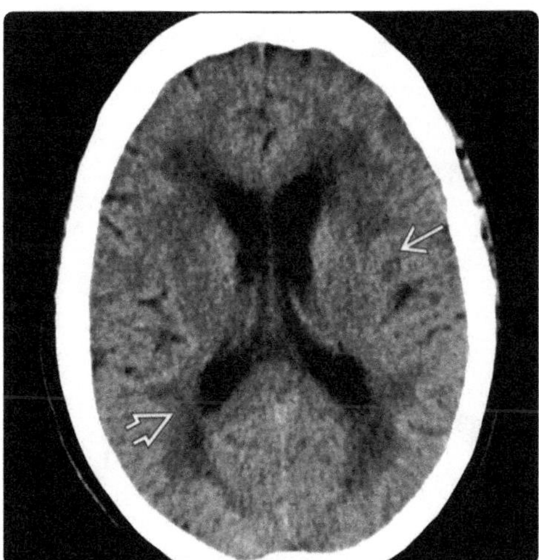

***(10-12)** NECT in chronic hypertension shows patchy ➡ and confluent ➡ hypodensities in the subcortical, deep periventricular WM.*

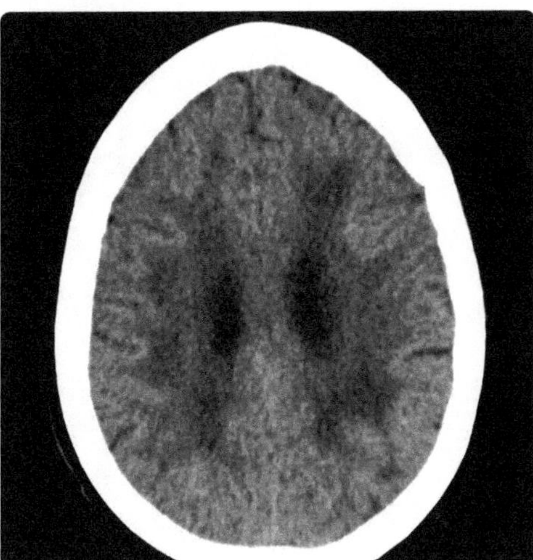

***(10-13)** More cephalad NECT shows cortical sparing, typical of "microvascular disease" (arteriolosclerosis and lipohyalinosis).*

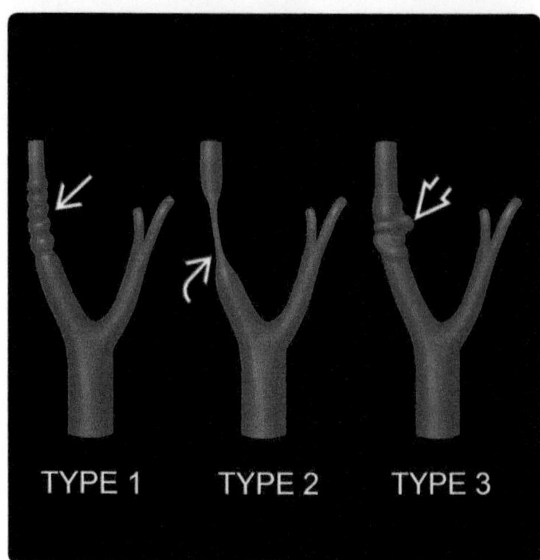

***(10-14)** Type 1 FMD = "string of beads" ➡, type 2 as tubular stenosis ➡, type 3 as focal corrugations ± diverticulum ➡.*

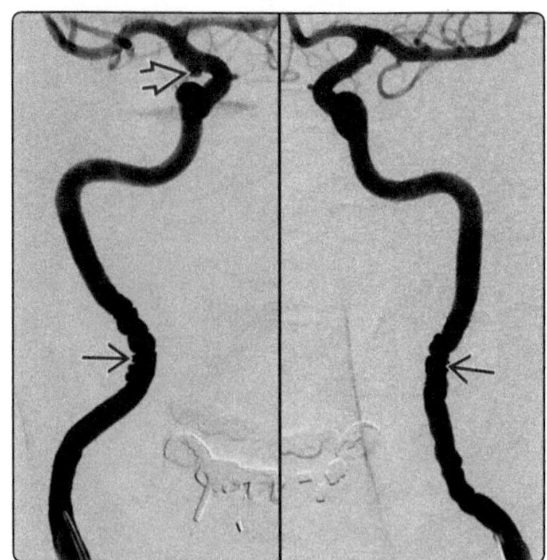

***(10-15)** DSA shows type 1 FMD in midcervical segments ➡ and small unruptured saccular aneurysm ➡ of the right supraclinoid ICA.*

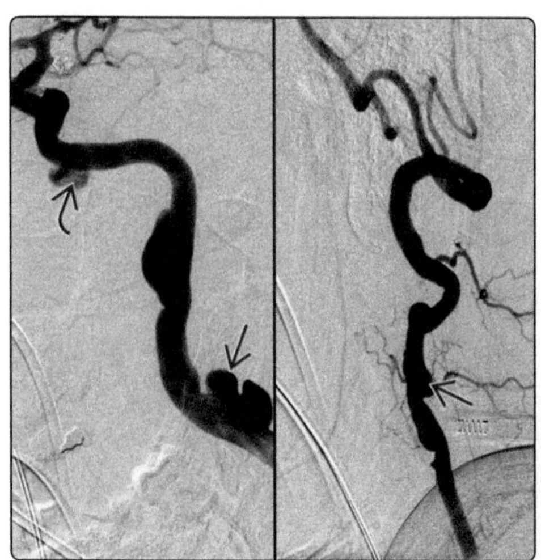

***(10-16)** (L) DSA of internal carotid, (R) vertebral arteries with type 3 FMD show diverticulum-like outpouchings ➡ and saccular aneurysm ➡.*

Nonatheromatous Vascular Diseases

Although atherosclerotic vascular disease (ASVD) is by far the most common disease to affect the craniocervical vasculature, a number of other nonatheromatous disorders can affect the brain, causing stroke or stroke-like symptoms. In this section, we briefly discuss some of the most important entities, including fibromuscular dysplasia (FMD), vasculitis, and non-ASVD noninflammatory vasculopathies, such as cerebral amyloid disease.

Fibromuscular Dysplasia

Terminology

FMD is an uncommon segmental nonatherosclerotic, noninflammatory disease of unknown etiology. FMD is a polyvascular disease that affects medium and large arteries in many areas of the body.

Pathology

Location. Although virtually any artery in any location can be affected, FMD affects some arteries far more than others. The renal arteries are affected in 75% of cases; ~ 35% of these are bilateral. Patients with known renal artery FMD often have cerebrovascular disease (and vice versa).

The cervicocephalic vessels are involved in up to 75% of cases. The internal carotid artery (ICA) is the most common site; FMD typically involves the middle of the ICA and spares the bifurcation. Vertebral artery (VA) FMD is seen in 20% of cases. Approximately 1/2 of all cervicocephalic FMD cases involve more than one artery (usually either both ICAs or one ICA and one VA). Intracranial FMD is very rare.

Multiple arterial systems are involved in 25-30% of cases. When multisystem disease is present, the renal arteries are almost always involved.

FMD carries an increased risk of developing intracranial saccular aneurysms. Intracranial saccular aneurysms are present in ~ 7-10% of patients with cervical FMD.

Staging, Grading, and Classification. FMD is classified histologically into three categories according to which arterial wall layer is affected (media, intima, or adventitia) **(10-14)**.

By far, the most common type (type 1) is **medial fibroplasia**, accounting for ~ 60-85% of all FMD cases. The media has alternating thin and very thick areas formed by concentric rings of extensive fibrous proliferations and smooth muscle hyperplasia.

Intimal fibroplasia (type 2) accounts for < 10% of FMD cases. The intima is markedly thickened, causing smooth, long-segment narrowing.

Adventitial (periarterial) fibroplasia (type 3) is the least common type of FMD, accounting for < 5% of cases. Dense collagen replaces the delicate fibrous tissue of the adventitia and may infiltrate the adjacent periarterial tissues.

Clinical Issues

Epidemiology. Once thought to be a relatively rare vasculopathy, overall prevalence of FMD is estimated between 4-6% in the renal arteries and 0.3-3.0% in the cervicocephalic arteries. FMD is identified in 0.5% of all patients screened with CTA for ischemic neurologic symptoms.

FMD primarily affects individuals between the ages of 20 and 60 years. Sex disparity in FMD is striking with a 9:1 female predominance.

Presentation. Sudden onset of high blood pressure in a young woman is a classic presentation of renal FMD. FMD is found in ~ 1% of hypertensive patients and is the second leading cause of renovascular hypertension (after ASVD).

Cervical FMD can present with headache, pulsatile tinnitus/bruit, dizziness, neck pain, transient ischemia attack, stroke, or dissection (often with Horner syndrome, i.e., ptosis, pupil constriction, and facial anhidrosis). Between 5-6% of patients are asymptomatic at the time of diagnosis.

Natural History. The natural history of FMD is unclear, as many cases are now discovered incidentally on imaging studies. Overall, 1 in 5 patients with FMD will have dissections and 1 in 5 patients will have aneurysms.

Imaging

Technical Considerations. CTA is noninvasive and accurately depicts FMD in the cervicocephalic arteries. Visualization of the intracranial vessels should be included to detect the presence of associated aneurysms. TOF MRA can be problematic, as artifacts caused by patient motion or in-plane flow and susceptibility gradients can mimic the appearance of FMD.

Because multisystem disease is common, patients with newly diagnosed carotid &/or vertebral FMD should also have their renal arteries examined. The prevalence of renal FMD is 40-45% in patients with cephalocervical disease.

Imaging Findings. Type 1 FMD (medial fibroplasia) is seen as an irregular "corrugated" or "string of beads" appearance with alternating areas of constriction and dilatation **(10-15)**. In type 2 (intimal fibroplasia), a smooth, long-segment tubular narrowing is present. In type 3 (adventitial) FMD, asymmetric diverticulum-like outpouchings from one side of the artery are present **(10-16)**.

All three cervical FMD subtypes spare the carotid bifurcations and great vessel origins, involve the middle segments, and are most common at the C1-C2 level. Complications of cervicocephalic FMD include dissection, intracranial aneurysm with or without subarachnoid hemorrhage (SAH) **(10-16)**, and arteriovenous fistulas. Other less common manifestations of FMD include vascular loops and fusiform vascular ectasias.

Differential Diagnosis

The major differential diagnosis of FMD is **atherosclerosis**. FMD is most common in young women, a group that is generally at low risk for ASVD. FMD involves the middle to distal portions of the affected arteries, sparing the carotid bifurcation.

Arterial standing waves are a form of transient vasospasm that can be misinterpreted as type 1 FMD on catheter angiograms. The regular "corrugated" appearance contrasts with the irregular "string of beads" of FMD **(10-21A)**. Standing waves resolve spontaneously on repeat angiography (including CTA or MRA) or after the administration of vasodilators.

The smooth, tapered "tubular" narrowing of type 2 (intimal FMD) can be difficult to distinguish from **spontaneous dissection**, which also occurs as a complication of FMD. The asymmetric, diverticulum-like outpouchings sometimes seen in FMD can mimic **traumatic cervical pseudoaneurysms**.

Other **nonatherosclerotic vasculopathies**, such as Takayasu arteritis and giant cell arteritis, can mimic tubular (i.e., intimal) FMD.

FIBROMUSCULAR DYSPLASIA

Pathology
- Nonatherosclerotic, noninflammatory arteriopathy
- 10% familial
- Commonly affects medium-sized/large arteries
  - Renal: 75%
  - Cervical arteries: 75%
  - ICA: 50%
  - VA: 20-25%
  - Multiple vessels: 50%
  - Intracranial very rare
- Classified by affected arterial wall layer
  - Type 1: Medial fibroplasia
  - Type 2: Intimal fibroplasia
  - Type 3: Adventitial (periarterial) fibroplasia

Clinical Issues
- Any age
  - But 20-60 years most common
- F:M = 9:1
- Presentation
  - Can be asymptomatic, incidental (0.5% of cervical CTAs)
  - Most common = renovascular hypertension
  - Headache, pulsatile tinnitus
  - Neck pain, Horner syndrome
  - Stroke
- Natural history
  - 1 in 5 patients will have dissection
  - 1 in 5 patients will develop saccular aneurysm

Imaging
- Midsegments of cervical ICA, VA affected
- Spares carotid bulbs, artery origins
- Usually terminates before entering skull base
- Appearance
  - "String of beads" (type 1): 60-85%
  - Smooth, long-segment narrowing (type 2): 10%
  - Adventitial (periarterial narrowing): ≤ 5%

Differential Diagnosis
- Atherosclerosis
  - Involves bulb > midsegment
- Arterial "standing waves"
  - Type of vasospasm occurs with catheter angiograms
- Dissection (can occur with FMD)

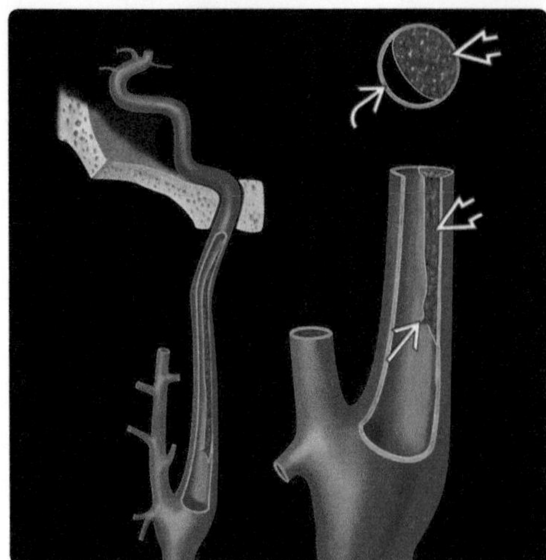

(10-17) Extracranial ICA dissection shows intimal tear ➡ and subintimal thrombus ➡ compressing residual lumen ➡. Bulb is spared.

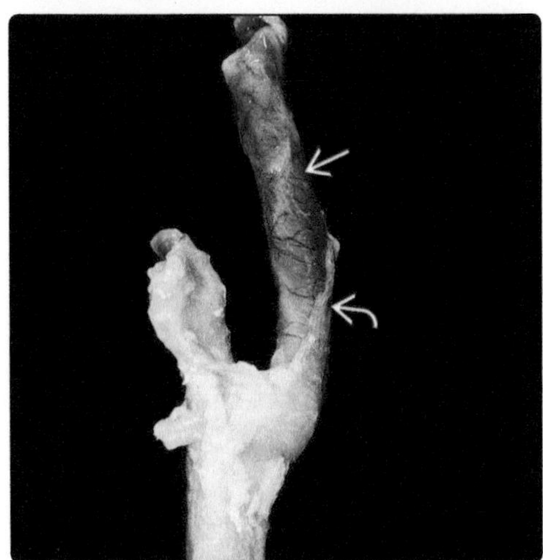

(10-18) Extracranial ICA dissection shows extensive mural thrombus ➡. Dissection begins ➡ distal to the bulb. (Courtesy R. Hewlett, MD.)

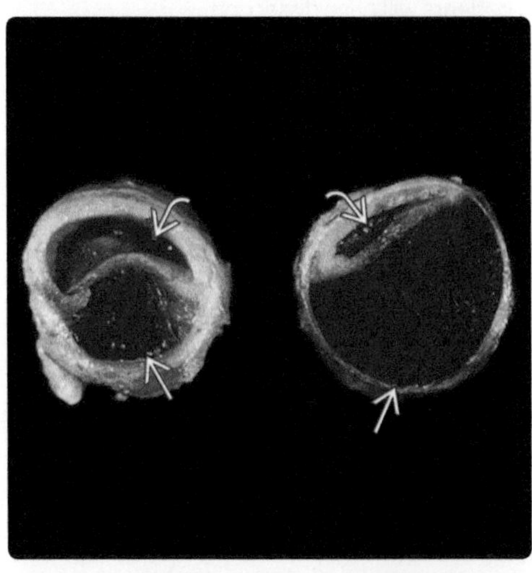

(10-19) Axial sections show carotid dissection with subintimal hematoma ➡, compressed residual lumen ➡. (Courtesy R. Hewlett, MD.)

Dissection

Craniocervical arterial dissection (CAD) is strongly associated with ischemic events, primarily artery-to-artery embolism, so early diagnosis and appropriate treatment are essential.

Terminology

A **dissection** is a tear in at least one layer of the vessel wall that permits blood to penetrate into and delaminate (split apart or "dissect") wall layers **(10-17)**.

A **dissecting aneurysm** is a dissection characterized by an outpouching that extends beyond the vessel wall. Most occur with subadventitial dissections and are more accurately designated as **pseudoaneurysms** (i.e., they lack all normal vessel wall components).

Etiology

Extracranial CAD is more common than intracranial CAD. Almost 60% of *extracranial* dissections are "spontaneous," i.e., nontraumatic. Most have an underlying vasculopathy, such as FMD, Marfan syndrome, or other connective tissue disorder (e.g., Ehlers-Danlos type 4). Less common predisposing conditions include hypertension, migraine headaches, vigorous physical activity, hyperhomocysteinemia, and recent pharyngeal infection.

Traumatic extracranial dissections occur with blunt or penetrating injury, but sports (e.g., wrestling) or chiropractic manipulations have also been implicated.

Intracranial dissections can be either traumatic or spontaneous. Iatrogenic dissections (typically secondary to endovascular procedures) are becoming increasingly common.

Pathology

Location. Extracranial dissections typically occur in the most mobile segment of a vessel, often starting or ending where the vessel transitions from a relatively free position to a position fixed by an encasing bony canal. The extracranial ICA is the most common overall site in the head and neck. Extracranial ICA dissections spare the carotid bulb and often extend up to—but only occasionally into—the skull base **(10-21A)**. Vertebral dissections are most common between the skull base and C1 and between C1 and C2.

The most frequently involved intracranial site is the VA. Dissections in the anterior circulation are even less common. They almost always involve the supraclinoid ICA with or without extension into the proximal middle cerebral artery (MCA).

Size and Number. Dissections can be limited to a focal intimal tear and small subintimal hematoma. Most are solitary, long-segment lesions that extend for several centimeters. Approximately 20% involve two or more vessels. Multiple dissections are more common if an underlying vasculopathy, such as Marfan, Ehlers-Danlos type 4, or FMD, is present.

Gross Pathology. An intimal tear permits dissection of blood into the vessel wall, resulting in a medial or subendothelial hematoma that may narrow or occlude the vessel lumen **(10-19)**. Occasionally, dissections—especially in the VA—extend through the adventitia and present with SAH.

Clinical Issues

Epidemiology and Demographics. Craniocervical arterial dissection (CAD) is the most common cause of ischemic stroke in young and middle-aged adults. Peak age is 40 years.

Presentation. Neck pain and headache are the most common symptoms. One or more lower cranial nerve palsies, including postganglionic Horner syndrome, may occur.

Natural History. The natural history of most *extracranial* CADs is benign. Approximately 90% of stenoses resolve and 60% of all occlusions recanalize. Recurrent dissection is rare. *Intracranial* CAD is much more problematic. Stroke is more common, and spontaneous recanalization is less frequent.

Imaging

General Features. Dissections can present as stenosis, occlusion, or aneurysmal dilatation.

CT Findings. NECT may show crescent-shaped thickening caused by the wall hematoma. Posterior fossa SAH is seen in 20% of intracranial VA dissections.

MR Findings. Fat-saturated T1WI is the best sequence for demonstrating CAD. A hyperintense crescent of subacute blood adjacent to a narrowed "flow void" in the patent lumen is typical **(10-20)**. T2WI may show laminated thrombus that "blooms" on T2*.

At least 1/2 of all patients with cervicocephalic dissections have cerebral or cerebellar infarcts, best depicted on DWI. Multiple ipsilateral foci of diffusion restriction are typical findings.

Angiography. *Extracranial* ICA dissections typically spare the carotid bulb, beginning 2-3 cm distal to the bifurcation and terminating at the exocranial opening of the carotid canal **(10-21A)**. Vertebral dissections are most common around the skull base and upper cervical spine.

CTA and MRA demonstrate an eccentrically narrowed lumen surrounded by a crescent-shaped mural thickening. A dissection flap can sometimes be identified **(10-21B)**. Pseudoaneurysms are common. An opacified double lumen ("true" plus "false" lumen) occurs in < 10% of cases.

The most common finding on DSA is a smooth or slightly irregular, tapered midcervical narrowing **(10-21A)**. CAD with occlusion shows a tapered "rat-tail" termination. Occasionally, a subtle intimal tear or flap, a double lumen, narrowed or occluded true lumen, or pseudoaneurysm can be identified. If the dissection is subadventitial and does not narrow the vessel lumen, DSA can appear entirely normal; the paravascular hematoma must be detected on cross-sectional imaging.

Intracranial dissections are more difficult to diagnose than their extracranial counterparts. They are significantly smaller and findings are often subtle.

Differential Diagnosis

The major differential diagnosis of *extracranial* arterial dissection is type 2 (intimal) **FMD**. A common complication of FMD is dissection, so the two conditions may be indistinguishable.

Atherosclerosis is more common in older patients. ASVD typically involves the great vessel origins and carotid bulb, sites that are almost always spared by dissection. Multiple vessels are usually affected. Dissections are usually solitary unless an underlying vasculopathy is present.

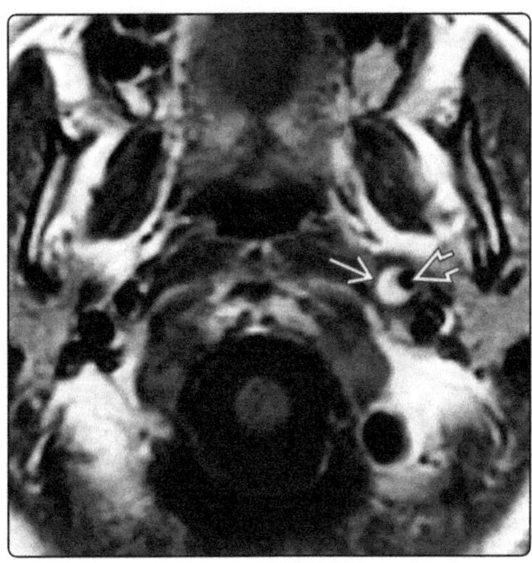

(10-20) Axial T1 MR shows subacute subintimal hematoma, crescent-like hyperintensity ➡ around narrow "flow void" ➡ of midcervical ICA.

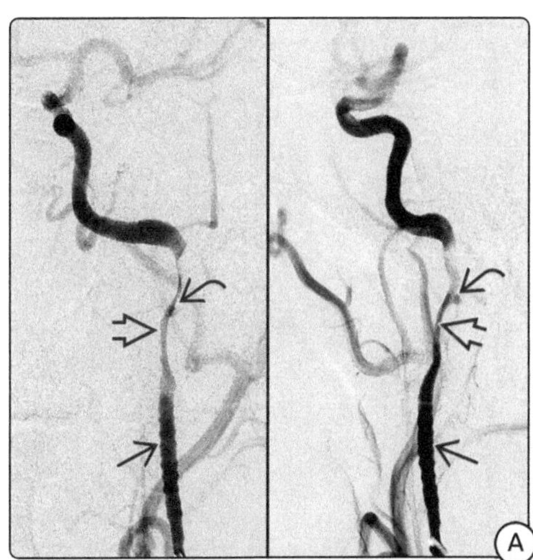

(10-21A) (L) AP, (R) lateral DSA show cervical ICA dissection ➡ to skull base, pseudoaneurysm ➡, arterial "standing waves" ➡.

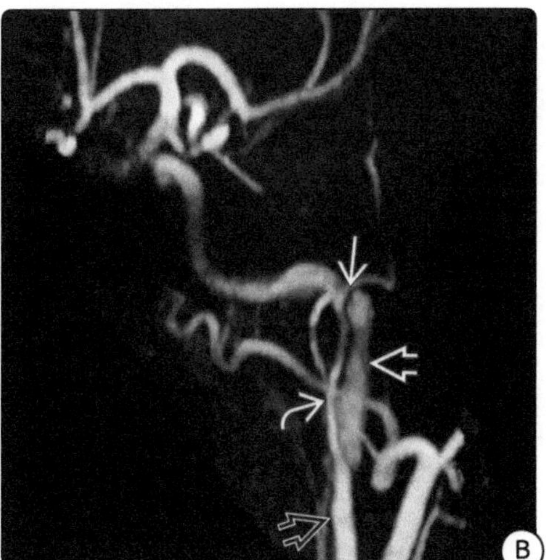

(10-21B) 2D TOF MRA in the same case clearly depicts dissection flap ➡, lumen ➡, subintimal hematoma ➡. Proximal ICA is normal ➡.

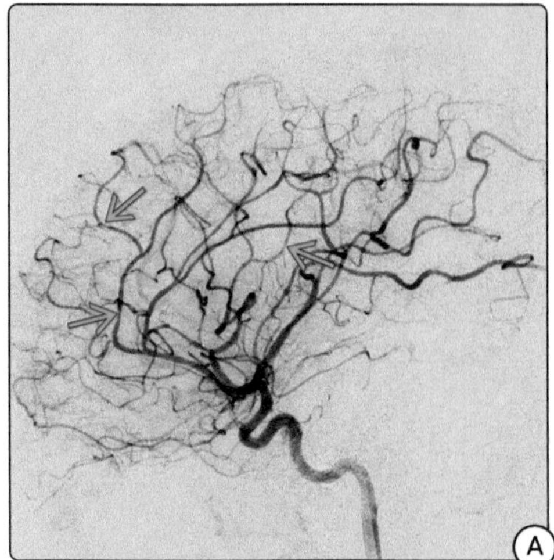

***(10-22A)** DSA in a 35-year-old woman with "thunderclap" headache shows only multifocal "beaded" arterial segments ⇨.*

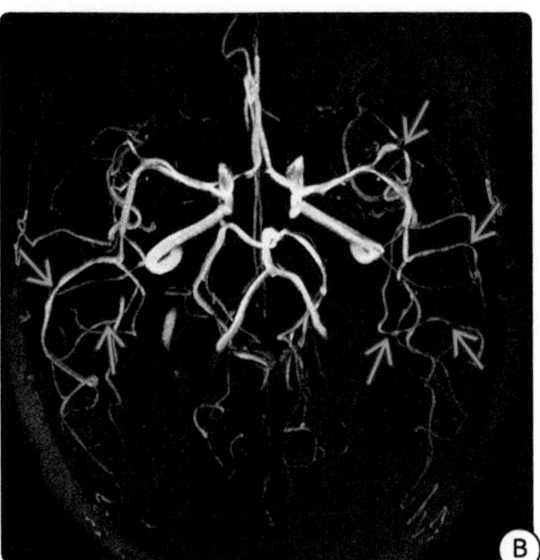

***(10-22B)** DSA 3 days later shows dramatic worsening with multiple bilateral "beaded" 2nd- and 3rd-order MCA branches ⇨.*

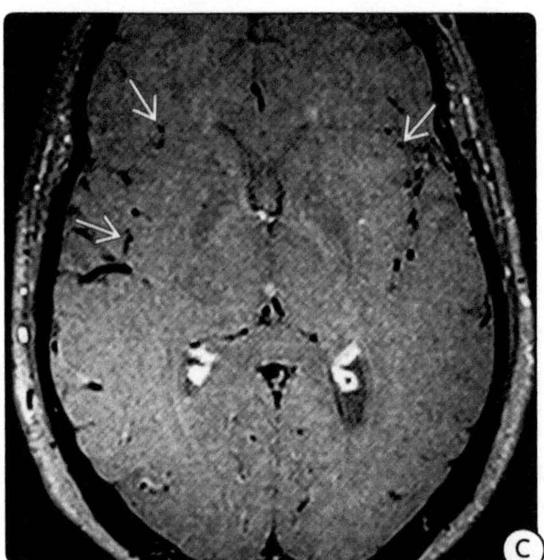

***(10-22C)** High-resolution "black blood" contrast-enhanced vessel wall imaging shows constricted vessels with no wall enhancement ➡; RCVS.*

DISSECTION

Terminology
- Vessel wall tear → blood penetrates into, splits layers apart
  - Intramural hematoma formed
  - With or without pseudoaneurysm

Pathoetiology
- "Spontaneous" (nontraumatic): 60%; traumatic: 40%
  - Underlying vasculopathy (FMD, Marfan, etc.): 40%
- Location
  - Extracranial ICA (spares bulb, usually terminates at skull base)
  - Vertebral artery (skull base-C1, C1-C2 most common)
  - Intracranial = extracranial (vertebral > > carotid)
  - Multiple arteries: 20% (look for underlying vasculopathy)

Clinical Issues
- Most common cause of stroke in young, middle-aged adults
  - Occurs at all ages but peak = 40 years
- Neck pain, headache

Imaging Findings
- Eccentric, crescent-shaped mural hematoma
  - Hyperintense on T1 FS
  - "Blooms" on T2*
  - Look for infarcts on DWI
- Long segment, smooth narrowing of vessel lumen typical
- ± pseudoaneurysm

Vasoconstriction Syndromes

Vasospasm with multifocal foci of arterial constriction and dilation is a common, well-recognized complication of aneurysmal SAH (aSAH) and is the most common cause of severe cerebral vasoconstriction (see Chapter 6). Vasospasm and vasospasm-like arterial constrictions can also occur in the absence of aSAH, trauma, or infection.

Terminology

Reversible cerebral vasoconstriction syndrome (RCVS) now encompasses what was once considered a group of distinct clinical entities, including Call-Fleming syndrome, postpartum angiopathy, drug-induced angiopathy, migrainous vasospasm, and "thunderclap" headache with reversible vasospasm.

The International Headache Society diagnostic criteria for RCVS include severe acute headache, a uniphasic disease course, no evidence for *aneurysmal* SAH (*convexal* SAH is common), normal/near-normal CSF, and imaging demonstration of segmental cerebral artery vasoconstrictions that resolve within 3 months.

Etiology

The exact etiology of RCVS is unknown. Some authors posit that, rather than representing a single specific disease entity, the broad heterogeneity of clinical and imaging manifestations associated with RCVS suggests that it may represent a common end point of numerous diverse disease processes.

RCVS may result from deregulation in vascular tone induced by sympathetic overactivity (including sympathomimetic medications and recreational drugs), endothelial dysfunction, and oxidative stress.

Brain biopsies have demonstrated no histopathologic evidence for vasculitis or inflammatory infiltrates within the constricted, diffusely thickened vessel walls often associated with RCVS.

REVERSIBLE CEREBRAL VASOCONSTRICTION SYNDROME (RCVS)

Terminology
- Vasospasm with multifocal arterial constrictions
- RCVS now encompasses several entities
  - Call-Fleming syndrome
  - Postpartum angiopathy
  - Drug-induced angiopathies
  - Migrainous vasospasm, etc.

Pathoetiology
- Unknown
  - May represent end point of several disease processes
- Dysregulated vascular tone
- No histopathologic evidence for vasculitis, inflammation

Clinical Issues
- International Headache Society criteria for RCVS
  - Severe acute headache ("thunderclap" characteristic, nonspecific)
  - Uniphasic course
  - No evidence for aSAH
  - Normal/near-normal CSF
  - Imaging shows segmental vasoconstrictions; resolve in 3 months
- Demographics
  - 20-50 years most common
  - F:M = 2.5:1.0
- Other: Vasoactive medications, pregnancy, etc.: 25-60%

Imaging Findings
- Multifocal arterial constrictions
  - Multiple vascular territories involved
- "Beaded" appearance
  - Characteristic but nonspecific
- High-resolution vessel wall imaging
  - No/minimal enhancement
  - ± thickened wall, reduced lumen
- Other
  - cSAH
  - Strokes

Differential Diagnosis
- Posterior reversible encephalopathy syndrome (PRES)
  - Overlaps, often coexists with RCVS
- aSAH-related vasospasm
- Vasculitis
  - Concentric, long-segment wall enhancement

Clinical Issues

RCVS most commonly affects patients between the ages of 20-50 years, although cases have also been reported in children and older adults. There is a slight female predominance (2.5:1.0).

Although "thunderclap" headache is characteristic, it is not specific for RCVS. A waxing and waning course with repeated episodes during 1-3 weeks is common.

A history of migraine headaches is elicited in 20-40% of cases. An exogenous "trigger," such as vasoactive medications and postpartum state, is reported in 25-60% of cases.

Imaging

The diagnosis of RCVS requires demonstration of multifocal segmental arterial constrictions in multiple vascular territories on CTA, MRA, or DSA **(10-22)**. A "beaded" appearance with multifocal areas of narrowing interspersed with normal segments is typical. Initial imaging may be unremarkable during the first week after symptom onset, so repeat examination may be necessary.

High-resolution vessel wall imaging typically shows no or minimal enhancement **(10-22)**.

Convexal (cortical) SAH (cSAH) is identified in ~ 1/3 of cases, whereas strokes are seen in 6-39% and concomitant PRES in 9-38%.

Differential Diagnosis

RCVS and posterior reversible encephalopathy syndrome (**PRES**) overlap in both their clinical and imaging features and may occur concurrently. PRES-like reversible cerebral edema is seen in up to 1/3 of RCVS cases, and RCVS-like vasoconstrictions can be identified in the majority of PRES patients.

The other major differential diagnoses of RCVS are **aSAH-related vasospasm** and **CNS vasculitis**. In aSAH, the vasospasm is typically long-segment narrowing of arteries in/around the circle of Willis. In RCVS, the segmental vasoconstrictions preferentially involve the more distal (second- and third-order) branches. Vessel wall imaging can also help distinguish RCVS from vasculitis. Concentric or tram-track wall enhancement is common in vasculitis; it is mild or absent in RCVS.

Vasculitis and Vasculitides

Terminology

The generic terms "vasculitis" and "angiitis" denote inflammation of blood vessels affecting arteries, veins, or both. The plural "vasculitides" is a more generic term that is often used interchangeably. "Arteritis" is more specific and refers solely to inflammatory processes that involve arteries.

Etiology

Vasculitis can be caused by infection, collagen-vascular disease, immune complex deposition, drug abuse, and even neoplasms (e.g., lymphomatoid granulomatosis). The general pathologic features of many vasculitides are quite similar **(10-23)**. As a result, the definitive diagnosis depends primarily on hematologic and immunohistochemical characteristics.

Isolated CNS vasculitis in which thorough clinical and laboratory examination does not identify another disorder causing the vascular inflammation is called **primary arteritis of the CNS (PACNS)**. This contrasts with the many *secondary* causes of CNS vasculitis.

Pathology

Although the vasculitides are a heterogeneous group of CNS disorders, they are characterized histopathologically by two cardinal features: Inflammation and necrosis in blood vessel walls. Infarcts in multiple vascular distributions are common.

Imaging

As imaging in most vasculitides is similar regardless of etiology, this discussion will focus on the general features of vasculitis as it affects the brain.

CT Findings. NECT scans are relatively insensitive and are often normal. Rarely, vasculitis causes convexal SAH.

Multifocal hypodensities in the basal ganglia and subcortical WM with or without patchy enhancement on CECT are common.

MR Findings. Involvement of the cortex/subcortical WM together with the basal ganglia is strongly suggestive of vasculitis. T1 scans can be normal or show multifocal cortical/subcortical and basal ganglia hypointensities. T2/FLAIR scans demonstrate hyperintensities in the same areas. T2* (GRE, SWI) may show parenchymal microhemorrhages &/or SAH in some cases.

Patchy enhancement with punctate and linear lesions is common on T1 C+ scans. Dural and leptomeningeal thickening/enhancement occur in some cases of granulomatosis with polyangiitis. Acute lesions with cerebral

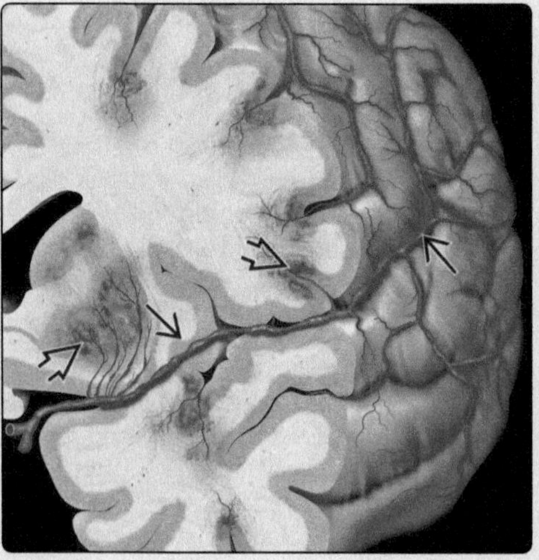

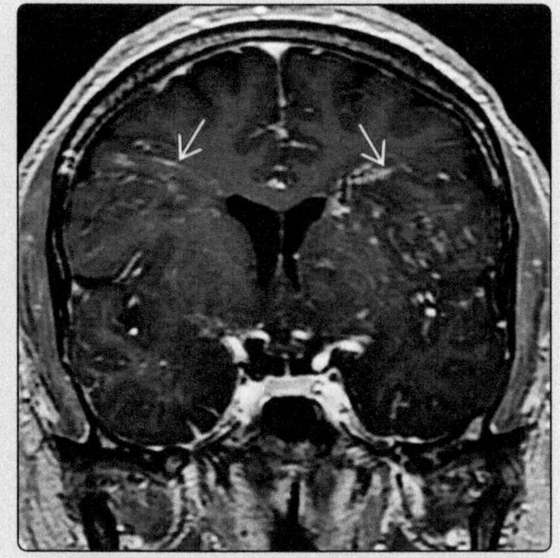

***(10-23)** Graphic shows vasculitis ⇒ with multifocal infarcts, scattered hemorrhages ⇒ in the basal ganglia and at the GM-WM junction. **(10-24)** Coronal T1 C+ MR shows bilateral, prominent linear patterns of enhancement ⇒. This is biopsy-proven primary arteritis of the CNS (PACNS).*

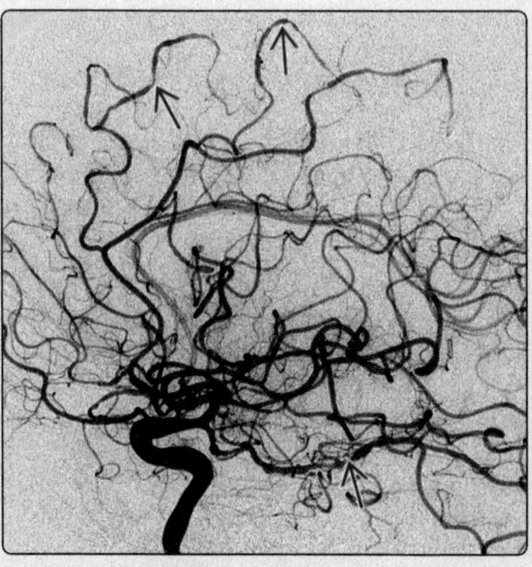

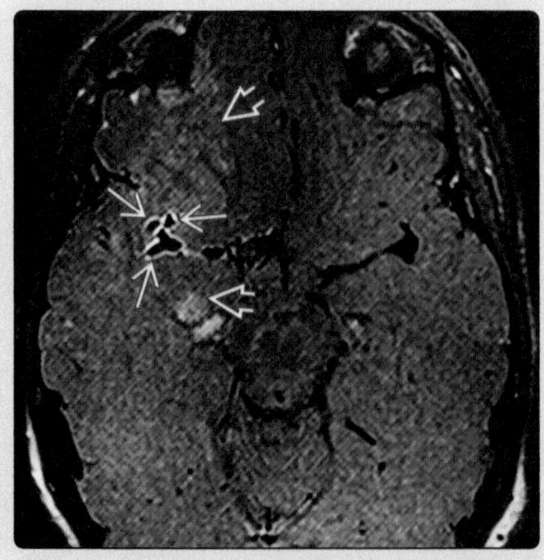

***(10-25)** DSA in a patient with streptococcal meningitis and multiple foci of restricted diffusion on MR shows multifocal segmental "beaded" areas of arterial narrowing and dilatation ⇒, classic findings of vasculitis (in this case, secondary vasculitis). **(10-26)** "Black blood" contrast-enhanced vessel wall imaging in proven autoimmune vasculitis shows circumferential, linear enhancement in the right MCA ⇒, subacute infarct ⇒.*

ischemia show multiple foci of diffusion restriction in the cortex, subcortical WM, and basal ganglia.

High-resolution "black blood" vessel wall imaging shows thickening and multifocal homogeneous smooth, intense, concentric enhancement of the vessel wall.

Angiography. Findings include multifocal irregularities, stenoses, and vascular occlusions **(10-25)**. Pseudoaneurysm formation and branch occlusions occur but are less common than luminal irregularities. Distal branches are more commonly affected than proximal arterial segments.

Differential Diagnosis

The major differential diagnosis of vasculitis is ASVD. **ASVD** typically occurs in older patients and involves larger, more proximal intracranial arteries, although it sometimes affects second- and third-order branches. Vessel wall imaging usually shows mild noncircumferential or no wall enhancement.

Vasospasm can also mimic vasculitis. Vasospasm most commonly affects the major cerebral vessels. A history of trauma or SAH is common but not invariably present. **RCVS** and **postpartum angiopathy** can be indistinguishable from vasculitis.

Other Macro- and Microvasculopathies

A broad spectrum of both inherited and acquired noninflammatory, nonatherosclerotic diseases can involve the intracranial vasculature. We briefly review a few of the more important miscellaneous vasculopathies.

Sickle Cell Disease

Sickle cell disease (SCD) is the most common worldwide cause of childhood stroke. African American and African Brazilian children are the most affected children outside of continental Africa.

Clinical Issues. The most common CNS complication of SCD is stroke. Stroke risk is highest between the ages of 2 and 5 years. Approximately 75% of SCD-related strokes are ischemic, and 25% are hemorrhagic. Hemorrhagic strokes are more common in adult-onset SCD.

Imaging. MR scans often demonstrate subcortical and WM hyperintensities along the deep watershed zone on T2/FLAIR **(10-27B)**. A moyamoya-like pattern with supraclinoid ICA stenosis may develop with especially severe SCD **(10-27C)**. An "ivy" sign with serpentine hyperintensities in the cerebral sulci from leptomeningeal collaterals can sometimes be seen on FLAIR.

Moyamoya Disease

Terminology. Moyamoya disease (MMD) is an idiopathic progressive arteriopathy characterized by stenosis of the distal (supraclinoid) ICAs and formation of an abnormal vascular network at the base of the brain **(10-28)**. Multiple enlarged "telangiectatic" lenticulostriate, thalamo-perforating, leptomeningeal, dural, and pial arteries develop as compensatory circulation. These "moyamoya collaterals" can become so extensive that they resemble the "puff of smoke" from a cigarette, the Japanese term for which the disease is named **(10-29)**.

Clinical Issues. MMD has worldwide distribution but is most prevalent in Japan and Korea. 2/3 of cases occur in children, and at least 1/2 of these occur under the age of 10 years. Between 1/4 and 1/3 present in adults with peak presentation in the fifth decade.

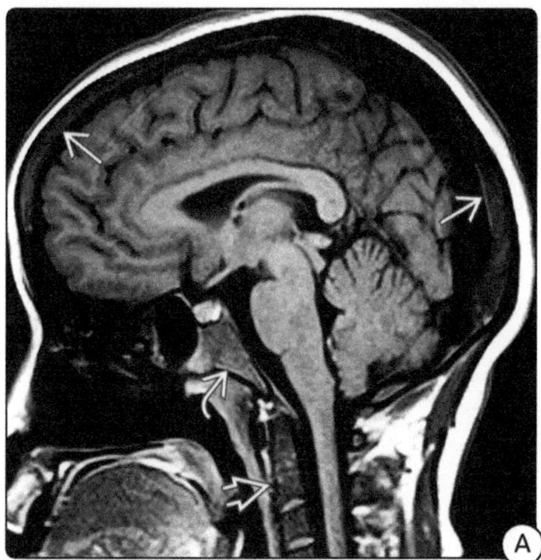

***(10-27A)** T1 MR in 29y woman with SCD shows thick calvarium with hypointense marrow ➡. Clivus ➡, vertebral bodies ➡ are hypointense.*

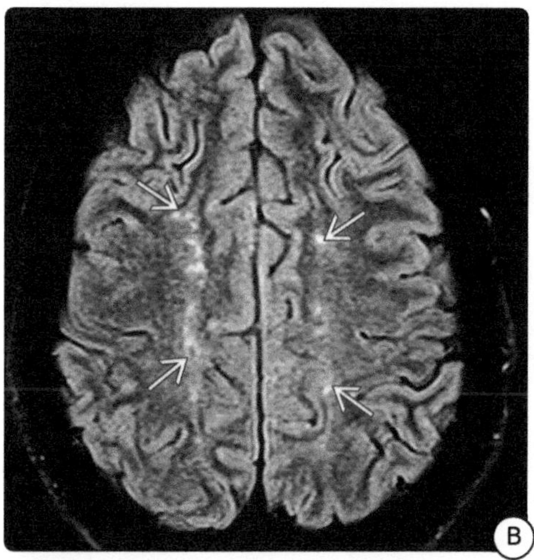

***(10-27B)** FLAIR MR in the same patient shows punctate hyperintensities in both watershed zones ➡, a common finding in SCD.*

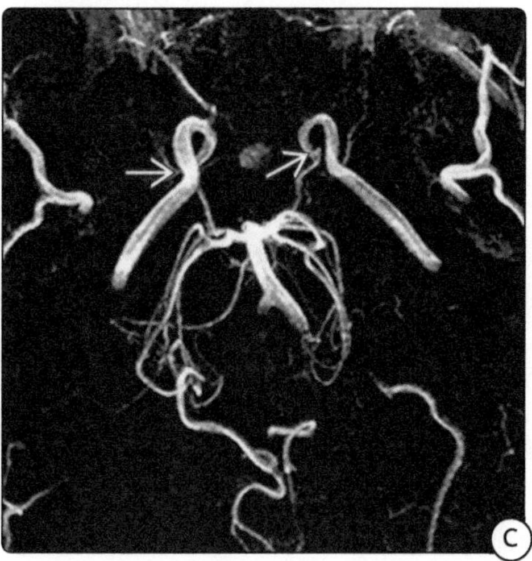

***(10-27C)** Submentovertex MIP of the MRA in the same patient shows occlusion of both supraclinoid ICAs ➡.*

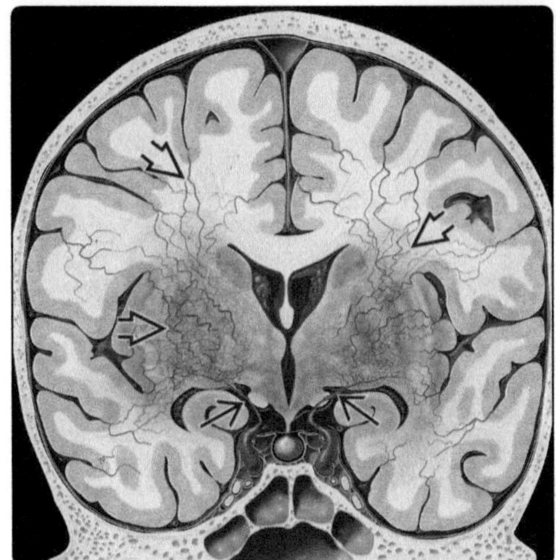

(10-28) MMD shows severely narrowed supraclinoid ICAs ➔, striking "puff of smoke" from extensive basal ganglia, WM collaterals ➔.

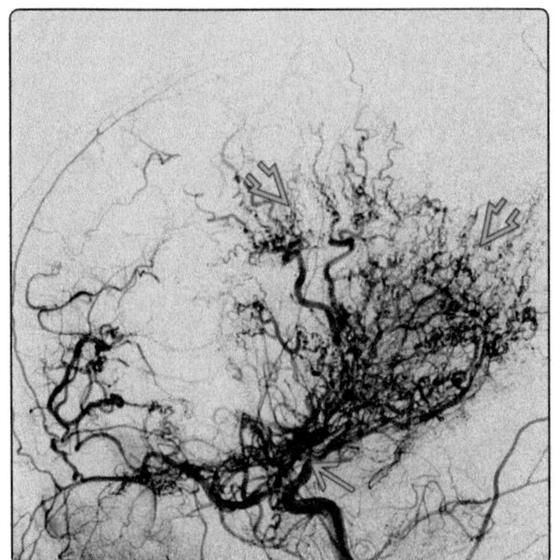

(10-29) MMD in a 3y child shows near-total supraclinoid ICA stenosis ➔ with innumerable tortuous enlarged moyamoya-like collaterals ➔.

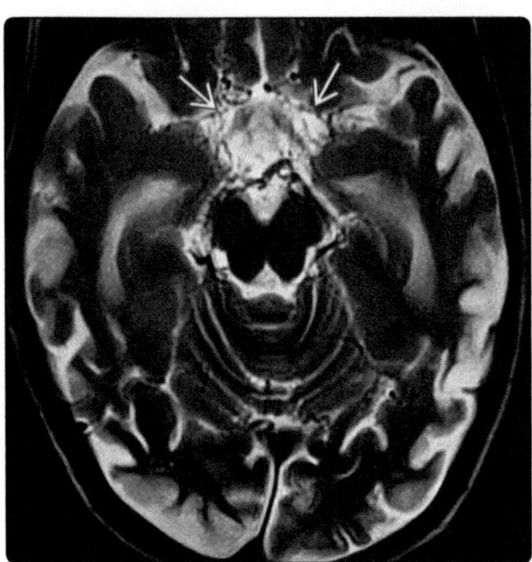

(10-30) T2WI in MMD shows severely narrowed thread-like supraclinoid ICAs, MCAs ➔ with marked cortical atrophy. (Courtesy H. Els, MD.)

When MMD presents in childhood, the initial symptoms are usually ischemic. In adults, ~ 1/2 of all patients develop intracranial hemorrhage from rupture of the fragile moyamoya collateral vessels. The other 50% present with TIAs or cerebral infarcts.

MMD is relentlessly progressive. A recently proposed new system, the Berlin grading system, can be used to stratify clinical severity and predict postoperative morbidity in revascularization surgery.

Imaging. T1 and T2 scans show markedly narrowed supraclinoid ICAs with multiple tortuous, serpentine "flow voids" **(10-30)**. The appearance of multiple tiny collateral vessels in enlarged CSF spaces has been likened to "swimming worms in a bare cistern." T1 C+ scans often show contrast stagnating in slow-flowing collateral vessels, both in the brain parenchyma and over its surface.

An "ivy" sign with sulcal hyperintensity from slow flow in leptomeningeal collaterals is sometimes seen on FLAIR and correlates with decreased vascular reserve in the affected hemisphere. Microbleeds on T2* GRE scans are associated with increased risk of overt cerebral hemorrhage.

DSA, CTA, and MRA show predominantly anterior circulation disease with marked narrowing of both supraclinoid ICAs ("bottle neck" sign). The PCAs are less commonly involved. Prominent lenticulostriate and thalamoperforator collaterals are present, forming the "puff of smoke" appearance characteristic of moyamoya. Numerous transosseous and transdural collaterals from the extracranial to intracranial circulation may develop.

MOYAMOYA DISEASE (MMD)

Terminology
- Moyamoya = "puff of smoke"
- MMD = progressive arteriopathy → stenosis supraclinoid ICAs

Clinical Issues
- Worldwide distribution, most common in Japan
- Children (70%, usually < 10 years)
  - TIAs, stroke
- Adults (30%)
  - Hemorrhage > stroke
- Revascularization (encephalo-duro-arterial-synangiosis, extracranial-intracranial bypass)

Imaging
- Stenosis/occlusion of supraclinoid ICAs
- Innumerable basal collaterals
- Strokes (acute, chronic)
- Hemorrhage

Differential Diagnosis. Other slowly developing occlusive vasculopathies may develop multiple small moyamoya-like collateral vessels. These include **radiation therapy**, **neurofibromatosis type 1**, **trisomy 21**, **sickle cell disease**, and even **atherosclerosis.**

Classic moyamoya typically affects *both* supraclinoid ICAs with relative sparing of the posterior circulation. A unilateral acquired, usually atherosclerotic, **"segmental" high-grade stenosis** or occlusion of the M1 MCA with a network of small vessels bridging the gap between the horizontal and distal segments should be differentiated from MMD.

CADASIL

CADASIL is the acronym for **c**erebral **a**utosomal **d**ominant **a**rteriopathy with **s**ubcortical **i**nfarcts and **l**eukoencephalopathy. CADASIL is an autosomal dominant disease of the cerebral microvasculature that primarily affects smooth muscle cells in penetrating cerebral and leptomeningeal arteries.

Etiology and Pathology. CADASIL is caused by point mutations in the *NOTCH3* gene. Fourteen distinct familial forms of CADASIL have been identified with mutations in different *NOTCH3* exons.

The pathologic hallmark of CADASIL is accumulation of granular osmiophilic material in the basement membranes of small arteries and arterioles that causes severe fibrotic thickening and stenosis.

Clinical Issues. CADASIL is the most common monogenic heritable cause of lacunar stroke and vascular dementia in adults. At initial presentation, only 35% of patients have a first-degree relative with known CADASIL.

The classic clinical presentation involves a young to middle-aged adult without identifiable vascular risk factors ("cryptogenic stroke"). The main manifestations are recurrent ischemic strokes, migraine headache with aura (often the earliest manifestation of the disease), psychiatric disturbances, and progressive cognitive impairment. Symptom onset is generally in the third decade and follows a progressive course, causing disability and dementia in 75% of cases.

Imaging. Characteristic imaging patterns may precede overt symptoms by more than a decade. Typical findings are multiple lacunar infarcts in the basal ganglia and high signal intensity lesions in the subcortical and periventricular WM.

Bilateral, multifocal T2 and FLAIR hyperintensities in the periventricular and deep WM begin to appear by age 20. Involvement of the **anterior temporal lobe** and **external capsule** has high sensitivity and specificity in differentiating CADASIL from common cerebral small vessel disease **(10-31A)**.

Lacunar infarcts in the subcortical WM, basal ganglia, thalamus, internal capsule, and brainstem are found in 75% of patients between 30-40 years of age and increase in both number and prominence with age. Mild to moderate generalized cerebral atrophy is a relatively late finding and is independently associated with the extent of cognitive decline.

Cerebral microbleeds (CMBs) are found on T2* scans in 25% of patients between 40 and 50 years old and are seen in nearly 50% of patients over 50. Cortical superficial siderosis is absent.

Differential Diagnosis. The imaging differential diagnosis of CADASIL includes **ASVD** (usually spares the anterior temporal lobe WM), mitochondrial encephalomyopathy with lactic acidosis and stroke-like episodes (**MELAS**), **vasculitis**, and **antiphospholipid syndromes**.

Other hereditary small vessel diseases that can mimic CADASIL include **CARASIL** (**c**erebral **a**utosomal-**r**ecessive **a**rteriopathy with **s**ubcortical **i**nfarcts and **l**eukoencephalopathy).

Systemic Lupus Erythematosus

Terminology. Systemic lupus erythematosus (SLE or "lupus") is a multisystem complex autoimmune disorder. When overt CNS symptoms are present, the disorder is termed CNS lupus (CNS SLE) or neuropsychiatric systemic lupus erythematosus (NPSLE).

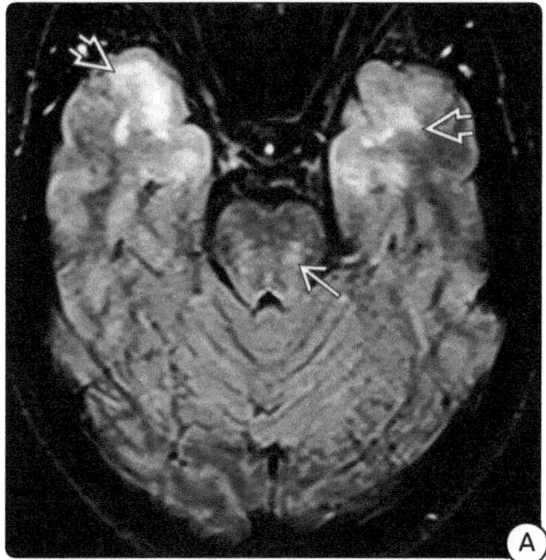

***(10-31A)** FLAIR in 32y woman with repeat strokes shows patchy/confluent WM hyperintensities in anterior temporal lobes ➾ and pons ➾.*

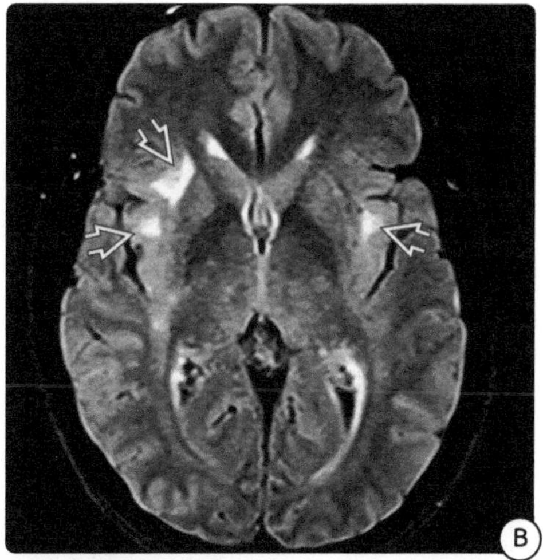

***(10-31B)** More cephalad FLAIR MR in the same case demonstrates lesions in both external capsules ➾.*

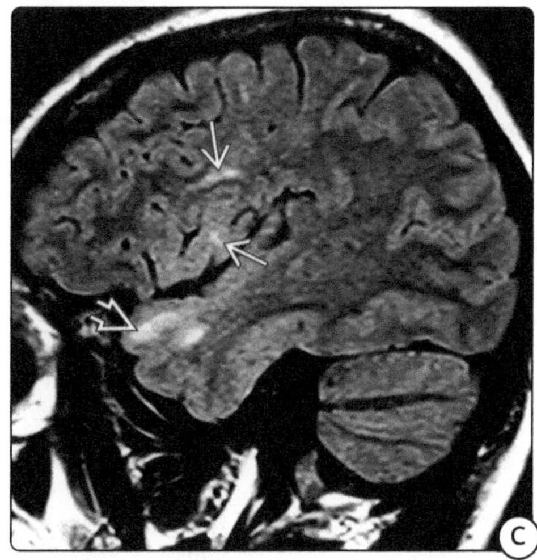

***(10-31C)** Sagittal FLAIR shows anterior temporal subcortical WM ➾, external capsule lesions ➾; proven CADASIL with NOTCH3 mutation.*

Etiology. SLE is an autoimmune disorder characterized by immune complex deposition, vasculitis, and vasculopathy. Circulating autoantibodies may be present years before overt clinical SLE symptoms emerge.

CNS SLE is generally considered an angiopathic disease, although neural autoimmune damage, demyelination, and thromboembolism may be contributing factors. Lupus-related cerebral ischemia/infarction can result from coagulopathy (secondary to antiphospholipid syndrome), accelerated atherosclerosis (often associated with corticosteroid treatment), thromboembolism (secondary to Libman-Sacks endocarditis), or a true primary lupus vasculitis.

Clinical Issues. CNS SLE occurs in 30-40% of lupus cases and can be a serious, potentially life-threatening manifestation of SLE. It occurs at all ages with peak onset between the second and fourth decades. In adults, over 90% of patients are female. In children, the F:M ratio is 2-3:1.

Imaging. Initial NECT scans are often normal or show scattered patchy cortical/subcortical hypodensities. Large territorial infarcts and dural sinus occlusions occur but are less common. Spontaneous intracranial hemorrhages can occur in SLE patients with uremia, thrombocytopenia, and hypertension.

MR findings vary from normal to striking. The most common finding, seen in 25-50% of newly diagnosed NPSLE patients, is that of multiple small subcortical and deep WM hyperintensities on T2/FLAIR **(10-32)**. Large, confluent lesions that resemble acute disseminated encephalomyelitis (ADEM) occur but are generally seen only in patients with CNS symptoms **(10-33)**. Diffuse cortical, basal ganglia, and brainstem lesions—suggestive of vasculopathy or vasculitis—are also common.

Acute lesions demonstrate transient enhancement on T1 C+ studies and restricted diffusion. pMR in patients with NPSLE

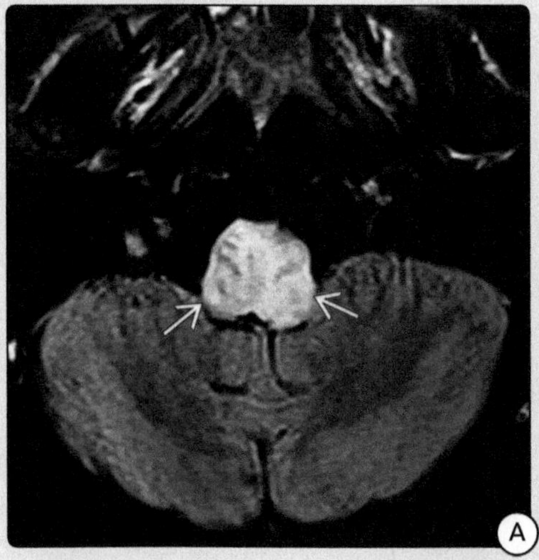

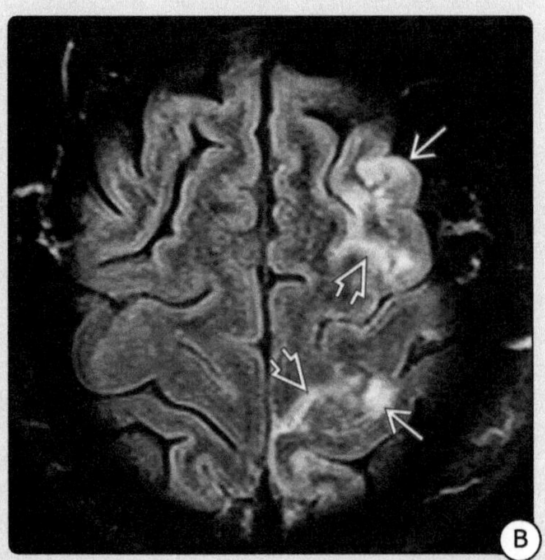

***(10-32A)** Axial FLAIR MR in a 33y woman with acute exacerbation of her CNS lupus shows confluent hyperintensity expanding the medulla ➡. **(10-32B)** FLAIR MR through the vertex in the same patient shows patchy cortical and subcortical hyperintensities in the left frontal and parietal lobes ➡. Mild mass effect with sulcal effacement ➡ is present. The right hemisphere appears normal.*

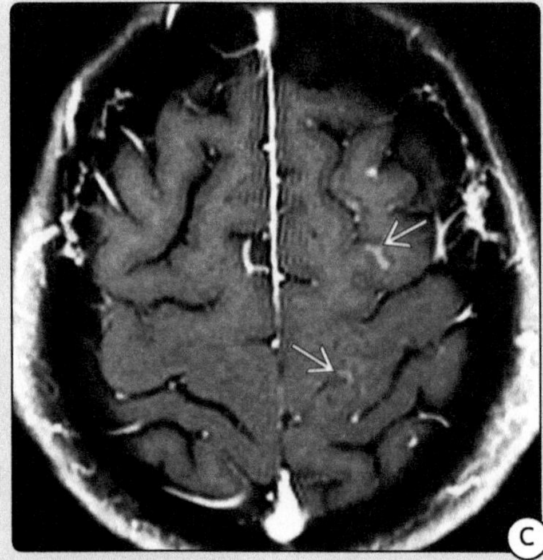

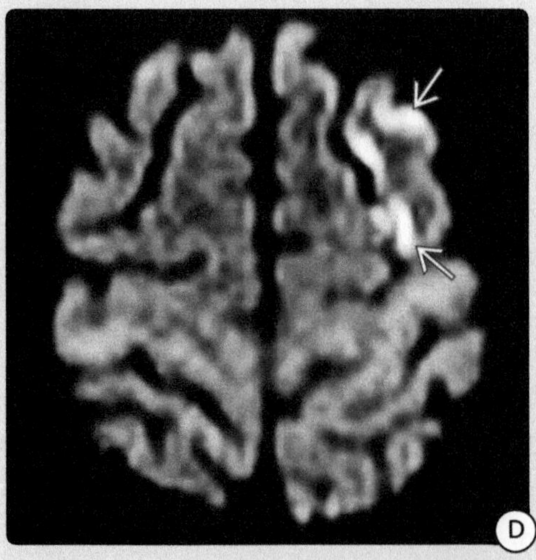

***(10-32C)** T1 C+ FS MR in the same patient shows mild patchy enhancement in the cortex and subcortical WM of the left hemisphere ➡. **(10-32D)** DWI MR shows foci of restricted diffusion in the right frontal cortex ➡.*

shows elevated cerebral blood volume and cerebral blood flow.

Dural venous sinus and cortical/deep venous thrombosis occur in 20-30% of NPSLE cases. Systemic hypertension is common in SLE patients. Posterior reversible encephalopathy syndrome (PRES) is a rare but treatable manifestation of CNS lupus.

Differential Diagnosis. The imaging differential diagnosis of NPSLE is broad and includes **arteriolosclerosis** ("small vessel disease"), **multiple sclerosis (MS), Susac syndrome**, non-lupus **antiphospholipid syndromes, Lyme disease**, and **other vasculitides**, such as primary angiitis of the CNS.

There is a significant overlap of lupus with antiphospholipid syndrome (APS); between 25-40% of SLE patients have APS. While there are no universally accepted diagnostic imaging criteria for NPSLE, the presence of multifocal infarcts and "migratory" edematous areas is suggestive of the disease.

Antiphospholipid Syndrome

Terminology and Etiology. Antiphospholipid syndrome (APS) is a multisystem disorder characterized by arterial or venous thrombosis, early strokes, cognitive dysfunction, and pregnancy loss.

Clinical Issues. The diagnosis of APS requires the presence of at least one clinical criterion (e.g., vascular thrombosis or pregnancy morbidity) and one laboratory finding, i.e., persistently positive lupus anticoagulant, antiphospholipid antibodies (e.g., anticardiolipin antibodies), or anti-β2 glycoprotein 1 antibody.

Mean age of onset is 50 years. There is a 2:1 female predominance (women with APS are often initially diagnosed because of pregnancy loss).

CNS involvement in APS is common. Manifestations of CNS APS include cerebrovascular disease with arterial thrombotic

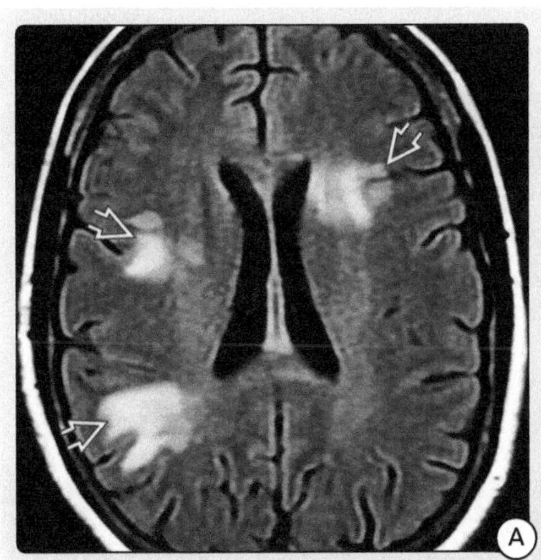

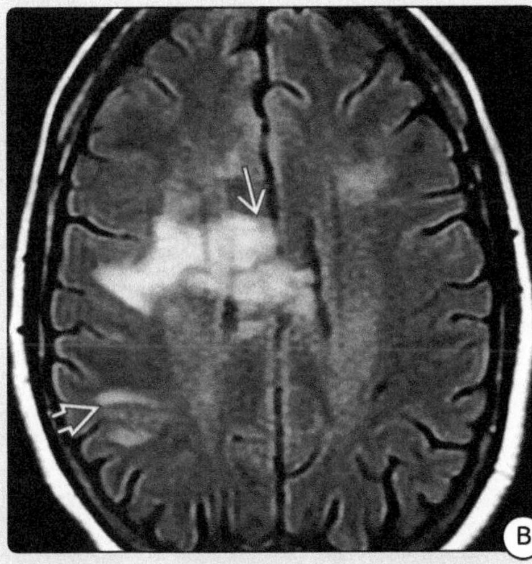

***(10-33A)** Axial FLAIR MR in a 55-year-old woman with unusual neuropsychiatric symptoms shows patchy and confluent hyperintensities in the subcortical and deep periventricular WM ➡. **(10-33B)** Axial FLAIR MR in the same patient shows subcortical WM lesions ➡ in addition to "fluffy" confluent lesions that cross the corpus callosum ➡ and resemble acute disseminated encephalomyelitis.*

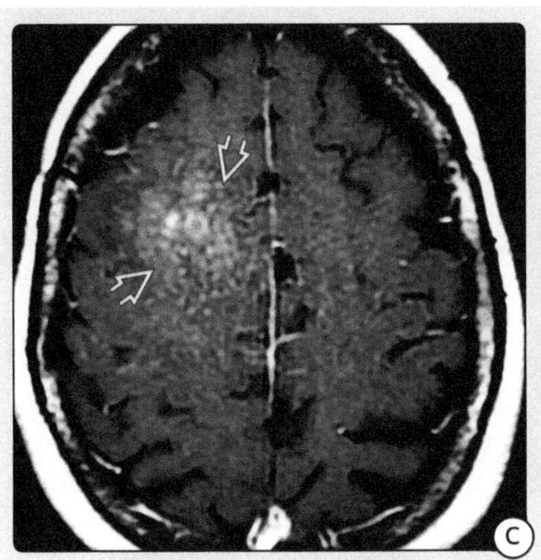

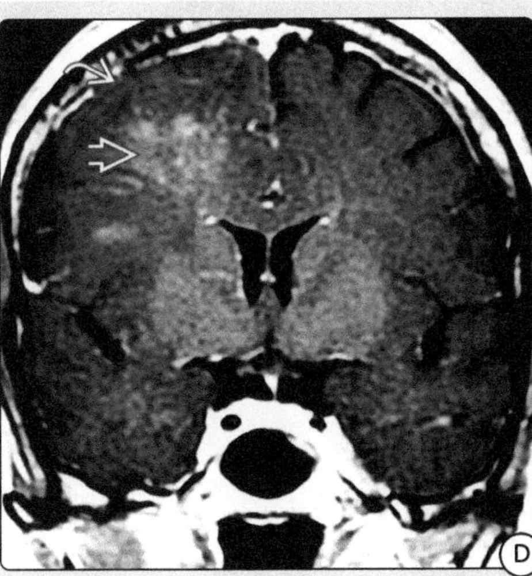

***(10-33C)** Coronal T1 C+ MR in the same patient shows mild punctate and linear foci of enhancement in the subcortical and deep cerebral WM ➡. **(10-33D)** Coronal T1 C+ MR shows patchy and linear enhancing foci in the subcortical WM ➡. Note the burr hole ➡ from biopsy. Histopathologic examination disclosed CNS lupus vasculitis.*

events (early-onset TIA, stroke) or venous occlusions, MS-like syndromes, seizure, headache, and cognitive dysfunction.

Imaging. Mixed-age multifocal cortical/subcortical infarcts, parietal-dominant atrophy with relative sparing of the frontal and temporal lobes, and "too many for age" deep WM hyperintensities on T2/FLAIR scans are typical findings in APS **(10-34)**. Both arterial and venous thromboses are common.

Differential Diagnosis. APS in the CNS can be difficult to distinguish from **multiple sclerosis**. **Multiinfarct ("vascular") dementia** usually lacks the parietal-dominant atrophy of APS. **SLE** commonly occurs with APS and may present with similar clinical and imaging findings.

Cerebral Amyloid Disease

Terminology. Cerebral amyloid disease occurs in several forms. The most common is an age-related microvasculopathy termed **cerebral amyloid angiopathy** (CAA). Rarely, cerebral amyloid disease presents as an **amyloid β-related angiitis** (ABRA) with diffuse inflammatory changes that primarily affect the WM.

Etiology. Imbalance between Aβ production and clearance is considered the key element causing formation of CNS amyloid deposits in small cerebral vessels. Aβ is normally cleared through the brain's "glymphatics." Failure to clear Aβ from the brain has two major consequences: (1) Intracranial hemorrhages associated with rupture of Aβ-laden vessels in CAA and (2) altered neuronal function caused by pathologic accumulation of Aβ and other soluble metabolites in Alzheimer disease (AD). The most frequent vascular abnormality seen in AD is CAA.

Genetics. CAA can be primary or secondary, sporadic or familial. Sporadic CAA is much more common than familial CAA and is strongly associated with presence of the *APOE*E4* allele.

Hereditary forms of CAA are generally familial and occur as an autosomal dominant disorder with several recognized subtypes. Hereditary CAA is generally more severe and earlier in onset compared with the sporadic disease form.

Pathology. Gross pathologic findings include major lobar hemorrhages of different ages, cortical petechial hemorrhages ("microbleeds"), small cerebral infarcts, and WM ischemic lesions **(10-35)**.

On Congo red stains, CAA vessels have a salmon-colored "congophilic" appearance. A characteristic yellow-green color ("birefringence") appears when the affected vessels are viewed using polarized light.

Aβ-related angiitis demonstrates mural and perivascular inflammatory changes with necrosis, variable numbers of multinucleated giant cells, epithelioid histiocytes, eosinophils, and lymphocytes.

Clinical Issues. Advancing age is the strongest known risk factor for developing CAA. Sporadic CAA usually occurs in patients older than 55 years, whereas the hereditary forms present one or two decades earlier.

CAA causes 5-20% of all nontraumatic cerebral hemorrhages and is now recognized as a major cause of spontaneous intracranial hemorrhage and cognitive impairment in the elderly.

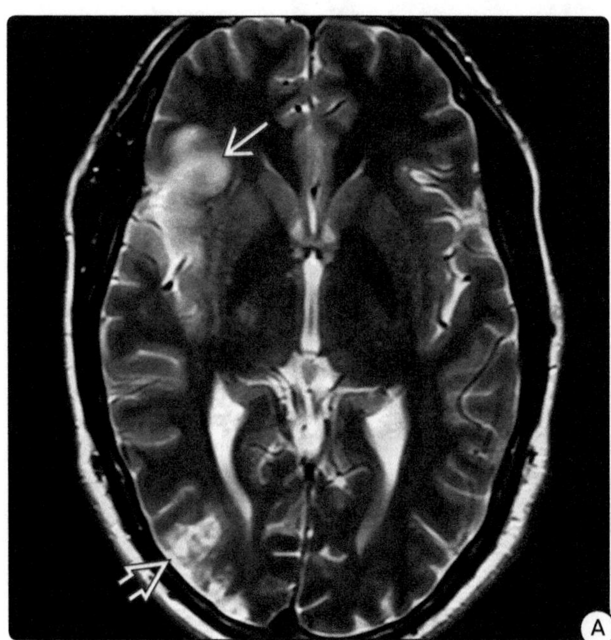

***(10-34A)** Axial T2 MR in a 36-year-old man with documented APS and multiple strokes shows acute gyral edema ➡, parietal encephalomalacia ➡.*

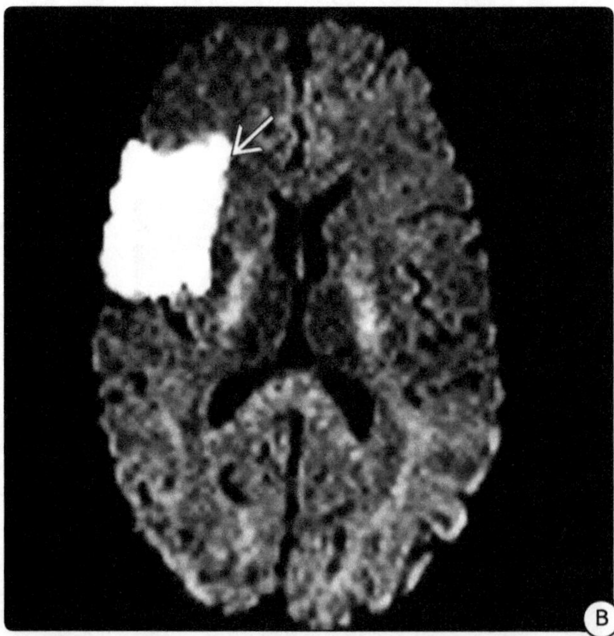

***(10-34B)** DTI trace image in the same patient shows acute restriction in the anterior division of the right MCA ➡.*

The most common clinical manifestations of CAA are focal neurologic deficits (with recurrent lobar hemorrhages) and cognitive impairment (with multiple chronic microbleeds).

Patients with Aβ-related angiitis also tend to be younger than those with sporadic, noninflammatory CAA. The clinical presentation of patients with CAA-related inflammation (e.g., ABRA) differs, usually resembling an autoimmune-mediated vasculitis or a subacute meningoencephalitis.

Imaging

CT. NECT scans in patients with acute manifestations of CAA typically show a hyperdense lobar hematoma with varying peripheral edema. Multiple irregular confluent WM hypointensities together with generalized volume loss are common.

Occasionally, patients with CAA can present with so-called **convexal subarachnoid hemorrhage** (cSAH). In cSAH, one or more adjacent convexity sulci demonstrate curvilinear hyperdensity consistent with blood.

MR. Signal intensity of a CAA-associated lobar hematoma varies with clot age **(10-36)**. Acute hematomas are isointense on T1WI and iso- to hypointense on T2WI.

The vast majority of patients with CAA have focal or patchy confluent WM hyperintensity on T2/FLAIR. Lobar lacunae are present in 25% of cases. Larger, asymmetric areas of confluent WM hyperintensity on T2/FLAIR with or without microhemorrhages are characteristic of ABRA. Mass effect is typically absent unless ABRA or a focal amyloid mass ("amyloidoma") is present.

In addition to residua from lobar hemorrhages **(10-36)**, T2* (GRE, SWI) sequences demonstrate multifocal punctate "blooming black dots" in the leptomeninges, cortex, and subcortical WM **(10-37B)**. The basal ganglia and cerebellum are relatively spared.

Both ABRA and amyloidoma may show such striking enhancement on T1 C+ that they mimic meningitis, encephalitis, or neoplasm **(10-37)**.

Differential Diagnosis. The major differential diagnosis of CAA is **chronic hypertensive encephalopathy** (CHtnE). The microbleeds associated with CHtnE often involve the basal ganglia and cerebellum. Peripheral microbleeds occur but are less common than CAA-related microhemorrhages, which typically affect the cortex and leptomeninges.

Hemorrhagic lacunar infarcts can demonstrate "blooming" hemosiderin deposits. The basal ganglia and deep cerebral WM are the most common sites, helping distinguish these infarcts from the peripheral microbleeds of CAA.

Multiple cavernous angiomas (Zabramski type 4) typically involve the subcortical WM, basal ganglia, and cerebellum. The cortex is a less common site. "Locules" of blood with fluid-fluid levels and hemorrhages at different stages of evolution are often present in addition to multifocal "blooming black dots" on T2*.

Hemorrhagic metastases at the GM-WM junction can resemble CAA. The multifocal microbleeds typical of CAA lack mass effect, peripheral edema, and enhancement.

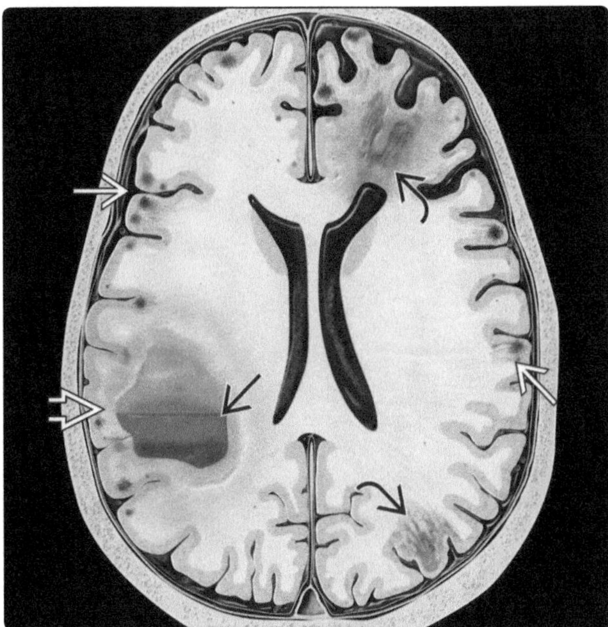

***(10-35)** Acute hematoma ➡ with fluid level ➡ is shown. Microbleeds ➡ and old lobar hemorrhages ➡ are typical findings in cerebral amyloid disease.*

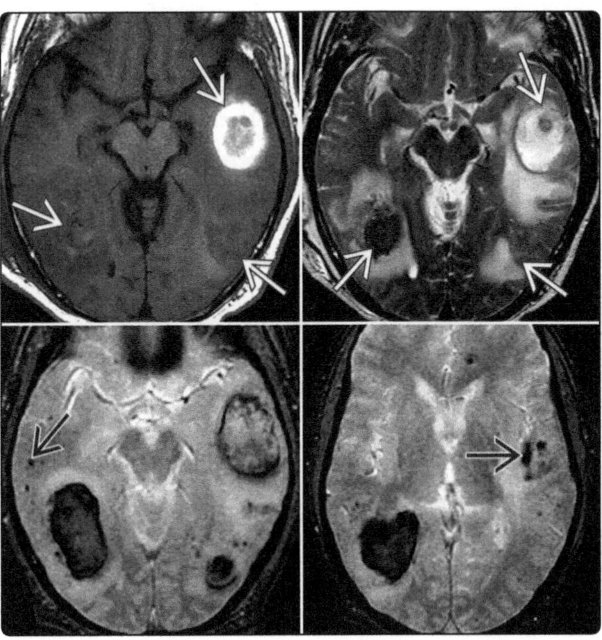

***(10-36)** MR scans demonstrate multiple lobar hemorrhages of different ages ➡, multifocal peripheral "blooming black dots" ➡ that are classic for CAA.*

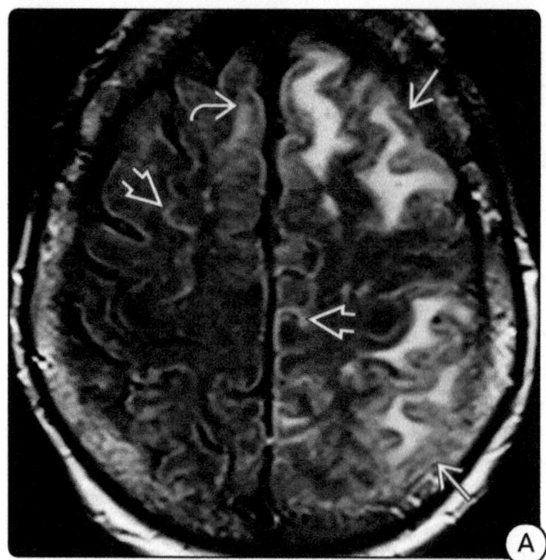

***(10-37A)** FLAIR shows confluent L WM hyperintensity ➡, patchy R cortical, subcortical hyperintensities ➡, and hyperintense sulci ➡.*

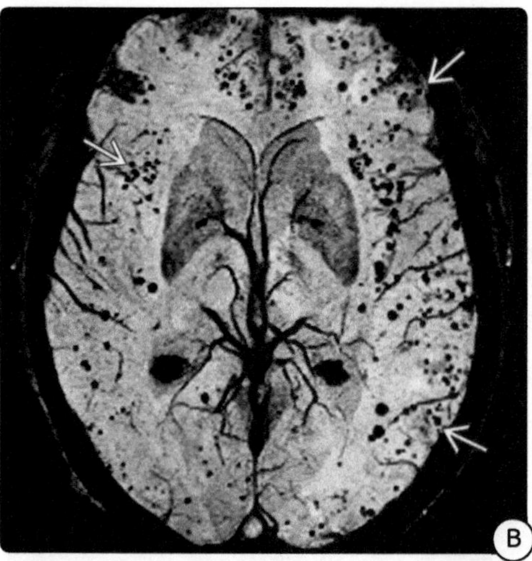

***(10-37B)** T2* SWI shows innumerable peripheral "blooming black dots" in both hemispheres ➡ with sparing of the basal ganglia and thalami.*

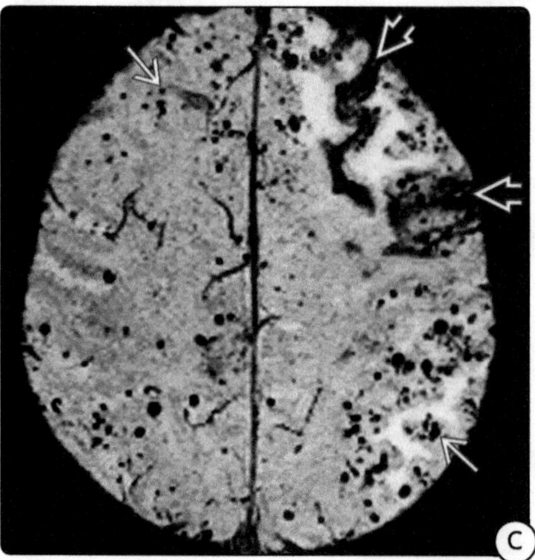

***(10-37C)** Cephalad T2* shows of siderosis ➡ and numerous microhemorrhages ➡. CAA-related inflammation [amyloid β-related angiitis (ABRA)].*

CEREBRAL AMYLOID DISEASE

Pathology
- Aβ40 deposited in meningeal, cortical arterioles
  - "Congophilic" angiopathy
  - Mural, perivascular inflammation common
- Vessel walls thicker but weaker
- Lobar bleeds
- Perivascular microhemorrhages

Clinical Issues
- Causes 5-20% of spontaneous intracranial hemorrhages in elderly patients
  - ↑ age = strongest risk factor
  - Most patients > 55 years old
- Normotensive, demented older adult typical

Imaging
- Classic NECT findings
  - Lobar hemorrhages of different ages
  - Convexal subarachnoid hemorrhage
- MR shows multifocal microbleeds
  - "Blooming" hypointensities on T2*
  - Typically cortical, meningeal (pial)
  - Cerebellum, brainstem, basal ganglia generally spared
  - Cortical superficial siderosis common
- Less common = Aβ-related inflammatory angiitis
  - T2/FLAIR parenchymal hyperintensity
  - Edema, mass effect
  - ± T2* "blooming" microbleeds
  - ± sulcal-cisternal enhancement
- Rare = intracerebral amyloidoma (focal mass)

Selected References: The complete reference list is available on the Expert Consult™ eBook version included with purchase.

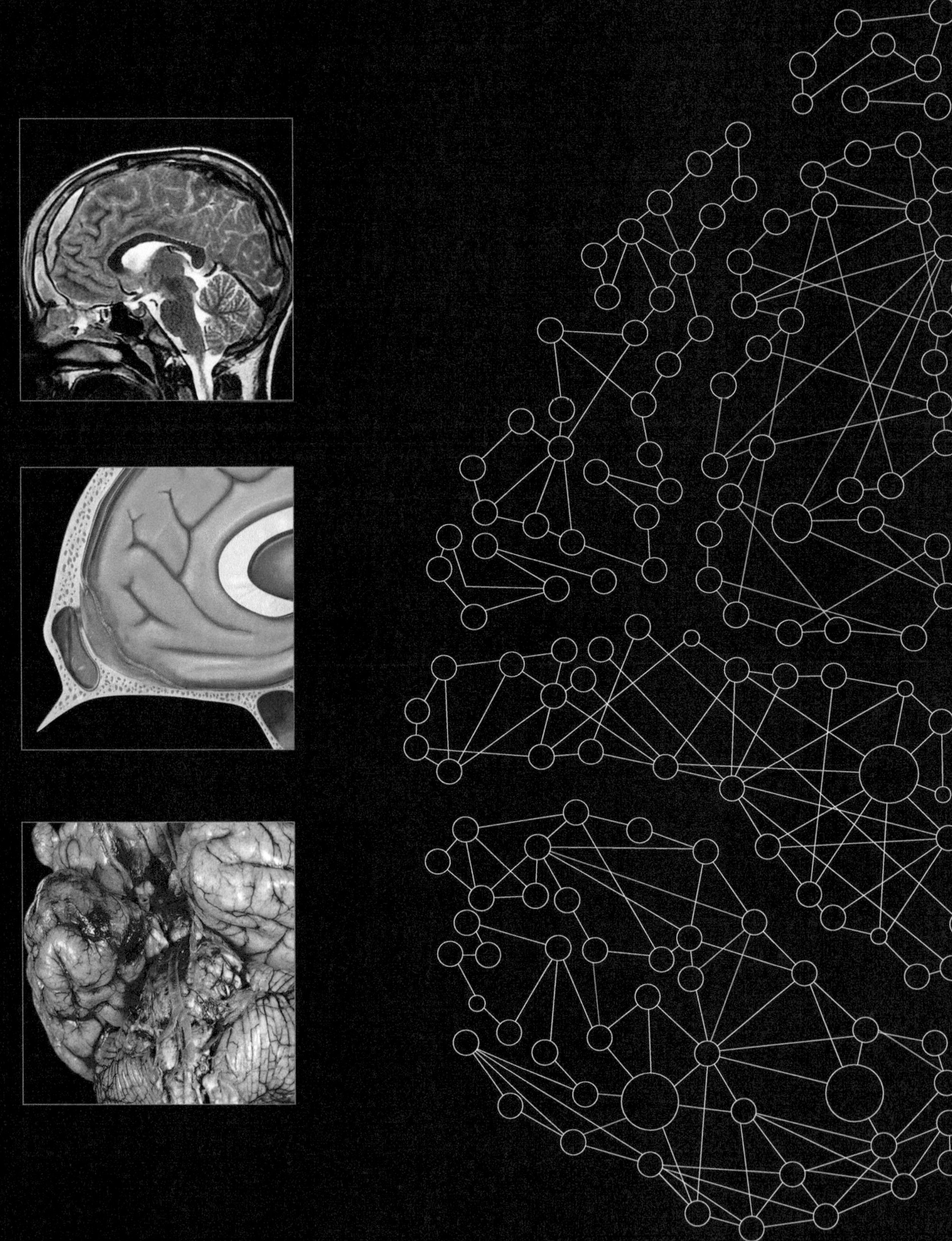

Section 3

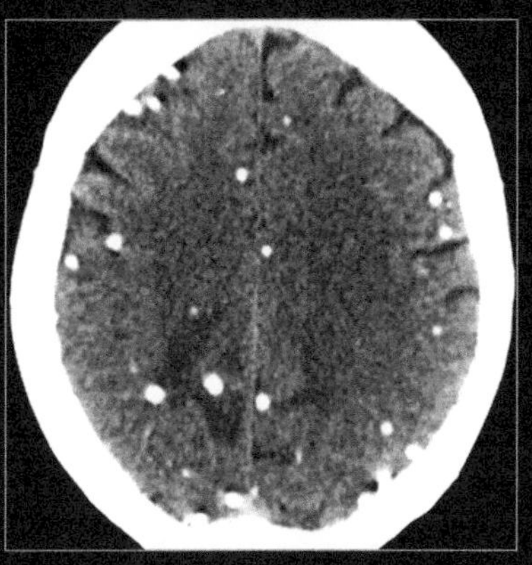

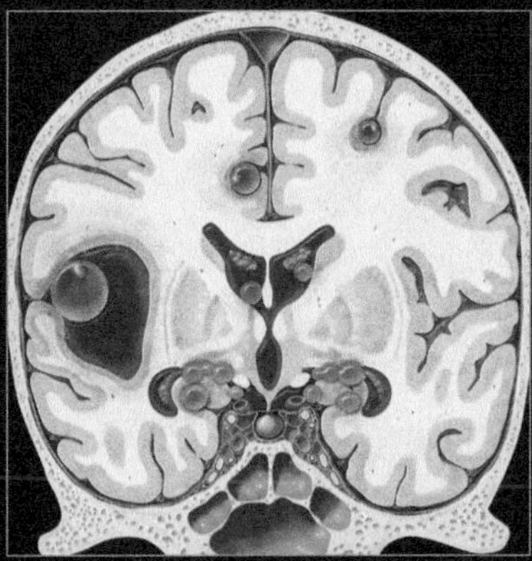

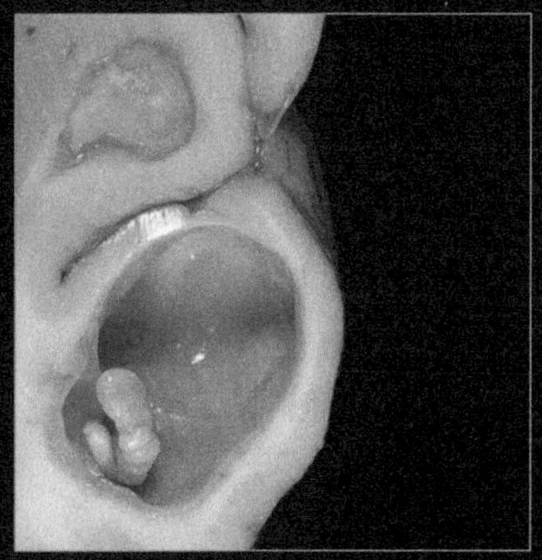

Section 3

Infection, Inflammation, and Demyelinating Diseases

Approach to Infection, Inflammation, and Demyelination

Although any part of the human body can become inflamed or infected, the brain has long been considered an "immunologically protected" site because of the blood-brain barrier (BBB). Although CNS infections are considerably less common than their systemic counterparts, the brain is by no means invulnerable to onslaught from pathogenic organisms.

The role of medical imaging in the emergent evaluation of intracranial infection ideally should be supportive, not primary. But in many health care facilities worldwide, triage of acute CNS disease frequently uses brain imaging as an initial noninvasive "screening procedure." Therefore, the radiologist may be the first—not the last—to recognize the presence of possible CNS infection.

In this part, we devote chapters 12 and 13 to CNS infections. HIV/AIDS is covered in Chapter 14. The last chapter, Chapter 15, considers the surprisingly broad spectrum of noninfectious idiopathic inflammatory and demyelinating disorders that affect the CNS.

CNS Infections

The concept that the brain was an "immune privileged" organ in which the BBB was a relative fortress that restricted pathogen entry and limited inflammation has recently undergone significant revision. Lymphocytes circulate through the normal healthy brain, immune responses can occur without lasting consequence, and cross-talk between the brain and extra-CNS organs is both extensive and robust.

Evidence has also recently emerged that there is extensive CSF and interstitial fluid (ISF) exchange throughout the brain, a process now termed "glymphatics."

A pathway of waste removal from the CNS does exist and is facilitated by CSF entering the brain parenchyma and spinal cord via aquaporin 4 water channels on astrocytes that surround the brain vasculature. This wave of CSF entry drives ISF toward the perivenous space where it collects and drains through lymphatic channels in the dural sinuses through foramina at the skull base to the deep cervical lymph nodes. The process flushes extracellular debris (including β-amyloid) from the parenchyma.

The presence of these drainage systems within the CNS is evidence that there is a constant flow and exchange of proteins within the brain and the blood. CD4(+) central and effector memory T cells are found in healthy CSF. The brain is therefore not a "privileged organ" that is immunologically isolated from the rest of the body but rather is actively monitored by—and accessible to—blood-borne lymphocytes and their mediators.

A surprisingly large number of pathogens, including many neurotropic viruses, can infect the CNS. Well over 200 different organisms have been described as causing CNS infections of one type or another. Routes of entry include transsynaptic spread (e.g., herpesviruses), "hiding" within blood-borne lymphocytes that access the brain (e.g., HIV and JC viruses), and using the choroid plexus as a gateway into the CNS.

In this text, we divide infections into congenital and acquired disorders. Congenital infections are discussed in Chapter 12. Because this is a relatively short discussion, we combine these with acquired pyogenic and viral infections.

Our discussion of pyogenic infections begins with meningitis followed by a consideration of focal brain infections (cerebritis, abscess), ventriculitis **(11-1)**, and pus collections in the extraaxial spaces (subdural/epidural empyemas) **(11-2)**. We close the chapter with CNS manifestations of acquired viral infections.

The pathogenesis and imaging of tuberculosis (TB), fungal infections, and parasitic and protozoal infestations are considered in Chapter 13.

HIV/AIDS

In the more than three decades since AIDS was first identified, the disease has become a worldwide epidemic. With the development of effective combination antiretroviral therapies, HIV/AIDS has evolved from a virtual death sentence to a chronic but manageable disease if the treatment is (1) available and (2) affordable. As treated patients with HIV/AIDS

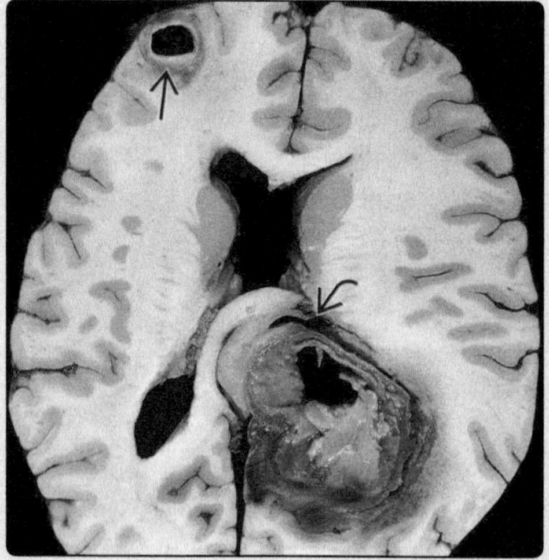

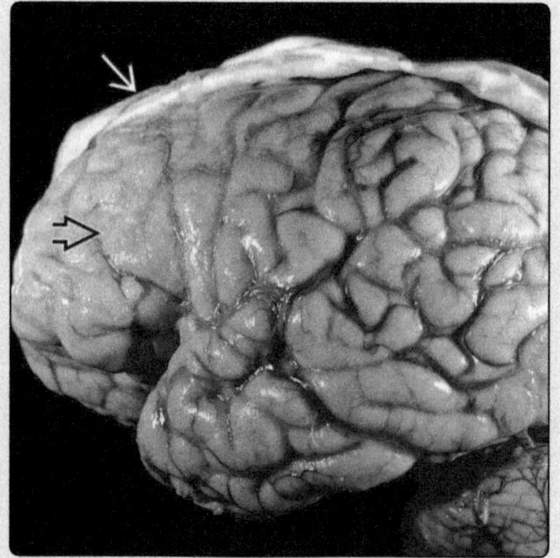

***(11-1)** Note the small, well-encapsulated frontal lobe abscess ➡ has a larger, less well-defined lesion in contralateral hemisphere. Large abscess ruptured into the ventricle ➡, causing pyocephalus and death. (Courtesy R. Hewlett, MD.) **(11-2)** Autopsy shows the dura ➡ reflected up to reveal purulent-appearing collection in the underlying subdural space ➡, typical findings for pyogenic subdural empyema. (Courtesy R. Hewlett, MD.)*

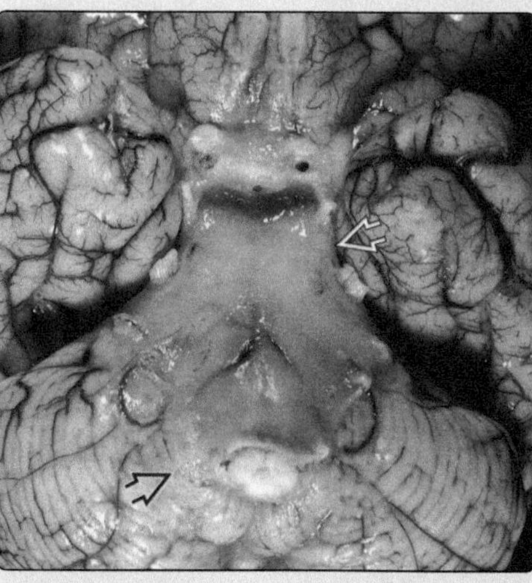

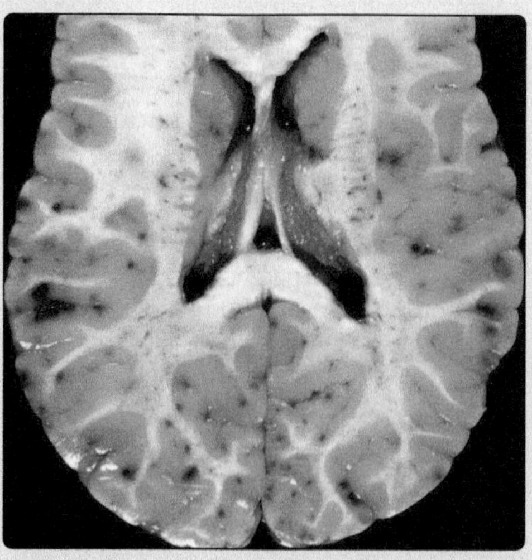

***(11-3)** Autopsy case of tuberculous meningitis shows thick exudate filling the basal cisterns ➡ and covering the pial surfaces of the frontal/temporal lobes and cerebellum ➡. (Courtesy R. Hewlett, MD.) **(11-4)** Axial cut section of an autopsied brain in a patient with septicemia shows multifocal petechial hemorrhages, primarily in the cortex and GM-WM interfaces. (Courtesy R. Hewlett, MD.)*

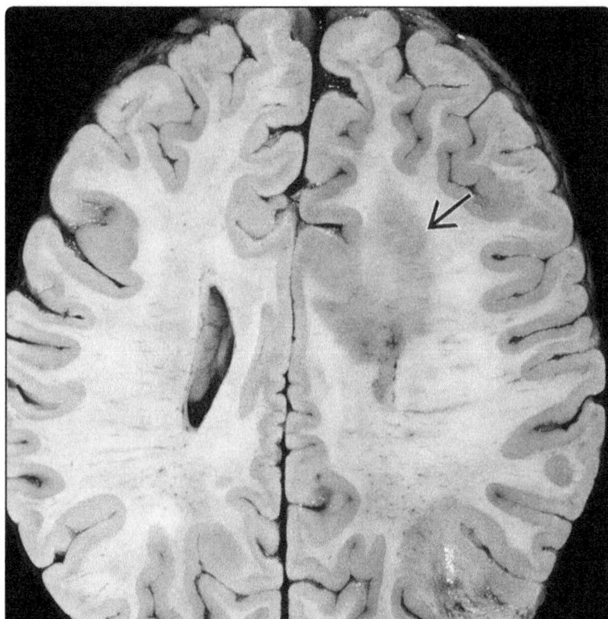

***(11-5)** Axial autopsied brain shows a solitary "horse-shoe" postinfectious tumefactive demyelinating lesion ➡.*

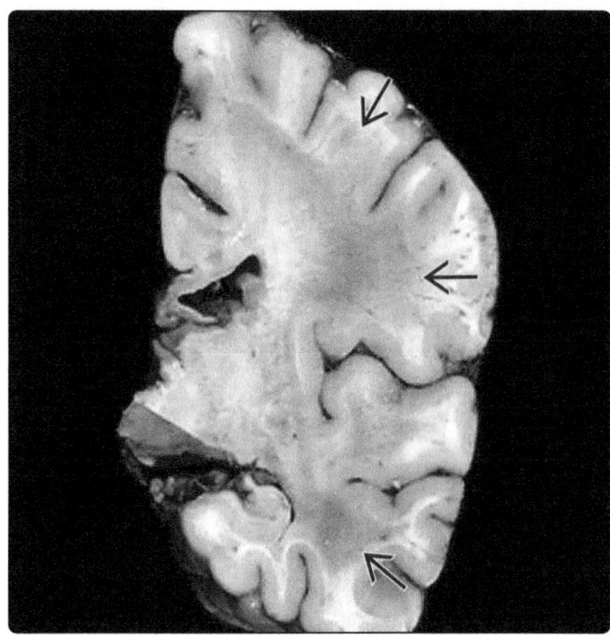

***(11-6)** Coronal gross pathology in a case of severe multiple sclerosis shows confluent demyelination in the subcortical white matter ➡. Note sparing of the subcortical U-fibers.*

now often survive for a decade or longer, the imaging spectrum of HIV/AIDS has also evolved.

Treated HIV/AIDS as a chronic disease looks very different from HIV/AIDS in so-called high-burden regions of the world. In such places, HIV in socioeconomically disadvantaged patients often behaves as an acute, fulminant infection. Comorbid diseases, such as TB, malaria, or overwhelming bacterial sepsis, are common complications and may dominate the imaging presentation.

Complications of HAART treatment have created their own set of recognized disorders, such as immune reconstitution inflammatory syndrome (IRIS). In Chapter 14, we consider the effect of HIV itself on the CNS (HIV encephalitis), as well as opportunistic infections, IRIS, miscellaneous manifestations of HIV/AIDS, and HIV-associated neoplasms.

Demyelinating and Inflammatory Diseases

The final chapter in this part is devoted to demyelinating and noninfectious inflammatory diseases of the CNS **(11-5)**.

Inflammation is not synonymous with infection. Inflammation (from the Latin meaning "to ignite" or "set alight") is the response of tissues to a variety of pathogens (which may or may not be infectious microorganisms). The inflammatory "cascade" is complex and multifactorial. It involves the vascular system, immune system, and cellular responses, such as microglial activation, the primary component of the brain's innate immune response.

The CNS functions as a unique microenvironment that responds differently than the body's other systems to infiltrating immune cells. The brain white matter is especially susceptible to inflammatory disease. Inflammation can be acute or chronic, manageable or life threatening. Therefore, imaging plays a central role in the identification and follow-up of neuroinflammatory disorders.

The bulk of Chapter 15 is devoted to multiple sclerosis (MS) **(11-6)**. Also included is a discussion of MS variants and the surprisingly broad spectrum of idiopathic (noninfectious) inflammatory demyelinating diseases (IIDDs), such as neuromyelitis optica. Susac syndrome is a retinocochleocerebral vasculopathy that is often mistaken for MS on imaging studies, so it too is discussed in the context of IIDDs.

Postinfection, postvaccination, autoimmune-mediated demyelinating disorders are considered next. Acute disseminated encephalomyelitis (ADEM) and its most fulminant variant, acute hemorrhagic leukoencephalitis (AHLE), are delineated in detail.

We close the chapter with a discussion of neurosarcoid and inflammatory pseudotumors, including the rapidly expanding category of IgG4-related disorders.

Selected References: The complete reference list is available on the Expert Consult™ eBook version included with purchase.

Congenital, Acquired Pyogenic, and Acquired Viral Infections

Infectious diseases can be conveniently divided into congenital/neonatal and acquired infections. There are unique infectious agents that affect the developing brain. The stage of fetal development at the time of infection is often more important than the causative organism. The clinical manifestations of fetal and neonatal infection and long-term neurologic consequences compared with infections that affect the more mature or fully developed brain will be emphasized below.

We then delineate the first major category of acquired infections, i.e., pyogenic infections. We start with meningitis, the most common of the pyogenic infections. Abscess, together with its earliest manifestations (cerebritis), is discussed next, followed by considerations of ventriculitis (a rare but potentially fatal complication of deep-seated brain abscesses) and intracranial empyemas.

We close the chapter with a discussion of the pathologic and imaging manifestations of acquired viral infections.

Congenital Infections

Parenchymal calcifications are the hallmark of most congenital infections and have been reported with cytomegalovirus (CMV) **(12-2A)**, toxoplasmosis **(12-3)**, congenital herpes simplex virus (HSV) infection, rubella, congenital varicella-zoster virus (VZV), Zika virus, and lymphocytic choriomeningitis virus (LCMV).

Infections of the fetal brain result in a spectrum of injury and malformation that depends more on the timing of infection than the infectious agent itself. Infections early in fetal development (e.g., during the first trimester) usually result in miscarriage, severe brain destruction, &/or profound malformations, such as anencephaly, agyria, and lissencephaly.

When infections occur later in pregnancy, encephaloclastic manifestations and myelination disturbance (e.g., demyelination, dysmyelination, and hypomyelination) predominate. Microcephaly with frank brain destruction and widespread encephalomalacia are common.

With few exceptions (toxoplasmosis and syphilis), most congenital/perinatal infections are viral and usually secondary to transplacental passage of the infectious agent. Zika virus is a relative newcomer to the list of viruses recognized as a cause of congenital CNS infection and is capable of causing profound brain destruction and resultant microcephaly. Zika virus infection

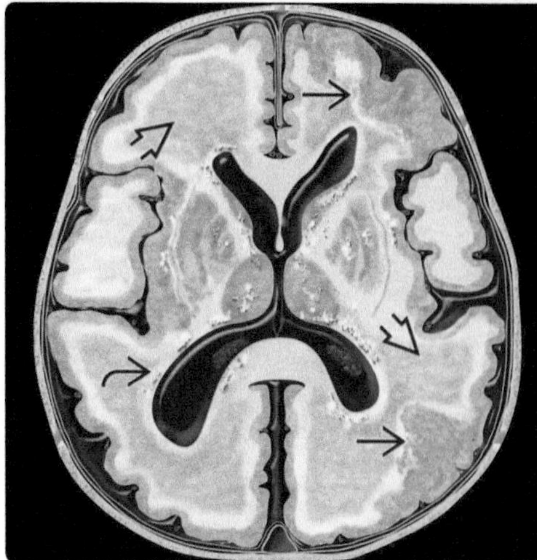

***(12-1)** Congenital CMV is shown with periventricular parenchymal calcifications ⇨, damaged WM ⇨, and dysplastic cortex ⇨.*

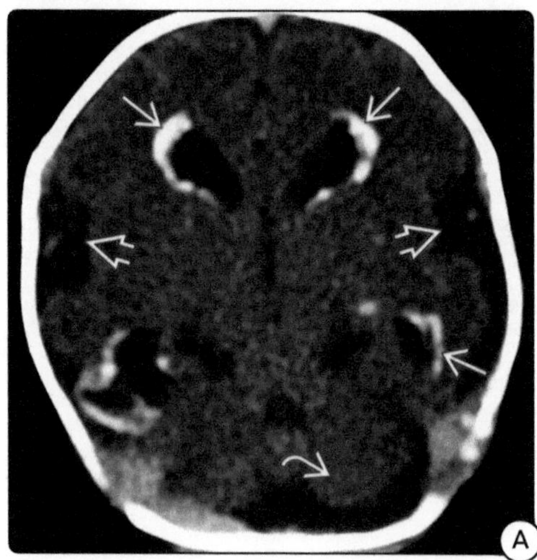

***(12-2A)** NECT in a newborn with CMV shows broad sylvian fissures ⇨, periventricular Ca^{++} ⇨, and cerebellar hypoplasia ⇨.*

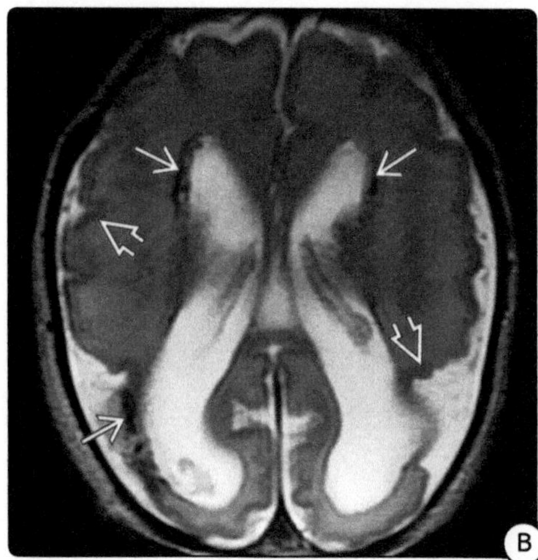

***(12-2B)** T2 MR in the same patient shows ventriculomegaly, periventricular Ca^{++} ⇨, and simplified gyral pattern (polymicrogyria) ⇨.*

represents the first reported congenital CNS infection to be mostly transmitted by mosquitoes.

Six members of the herpesvirus family cause neurologic disease in children: HSV-1, HSV-2, VZV, Epstein-Barr virus (EBV), CMV, and human herpesvirus 6 (HHV-6).

Aside from CMV, HSV-2, Zika virus, and congenital HIV (vertically transmitted), congenital CNS infections have become less common due to immunization programs, prenatal screening, and global infection surveillance.

TORCH Infections

Terminology

Congenital infections are often grouped together and simply called **TORCH** infections—the acronym for **to**xoplasmosis, **r**ubella, **c**ytomegalovirus, and **h**erpes. If congenital **s**yphilis is included, the grouping is called TORCH(S) or (S)TORCH.

Etiology

In addition to the recognized "classic" TORCH(S) infections, a host of new organisms have been identified as causing congenital and perinatal infections. These include Zika virus, LCMV, human parvovirus B19, human parechovirus, hepatitis B, VZV, tuberculosis, HIV, and the parasitic infection toxocariasis.

Imaging

CMV, toxoplasmosis, rubella, Zika virus, VZV, LCMV, and HIV may all cause parenchymal calcifications **(12-1)**. The location and distribution of the calcifications may strongly suggest the specific infectious agent. CMV—the most common congenital infection in developed countries—causes periventricular calcifications **(12-2A)**, cysts, cortical clefts, polymicrogyria (PMG) **(12-2B)**, schizencephaly, and white matter injury.

Early CNS infection with Zika virus leads to severe microcephaly and calcifications at the gray matter-white matter junction. Rubella and HSV cause lobar destruction, cystic encephalomalacia, and nonpatterned calcifications. Congenital syphilis is relatively rare, causing basilar meningitis, arterial strokes, and scattered dystrophic calcifications. Congenital HIV is associated with basal ganglia calcification, atrophy, and aneurysmal arteriopathy.

TORCH(S), Zika virus, and LCMV infections should be considered in newborns and infants with microcephaly, parenchymal calcifications **(12-3)**, chorioretinitis, and intrauterine growth restriction.

The timing of the gestational infection determines the magnitude and appearance of the brain insult. For example, early gestational CMV infection causes germinal zone necrosis with subependymal cysts and dystrophic calcifications **(12-4)**. White matter volume loss occurs at all gestational ages and can be diffuse or multifocal. Malformations of cortical development are very common, with PMG having the greatest prevalence **(12-2B)**.

Herpes Simplex Virus: Congenital and Neonatal Infections

Terminology

CNS involvement in HSV infection is called **congenital** or **neonatal HSV** when it involves neonates. In contradistinction, herpes simplex encephalitis (HSE) (which is also sometimes called herpes simplex virus encephalitis) describes encephalitis in individuals beyond the first postnatal month. In this section, we discuss neonatal HSV. HSE is discussed subsequently with other acquired viral infections.

Etiology

Approximately 2,000 infants in the USA annually are diagnosed with either HSV-1 or HSV-2 neonatal infection. The vast majority (85%) of cases are acquired at parturition while 10% are contracted postnatally. Only 5% of cases are due to **in utero** transmission.

Pathology

Neonatal HSV encephalitis is a diffuse disease without the predilection for the temporal lobes and limbic system seen in older children and adults. Early changes include meningoencephalitis with necrosis and hemorrhage. Atrophy with gross cystic encephalomalacia and parenchymal calcifications is typical of late-stage HSV. Near-total loss of brain substance with hydranencephaly is seen in severe cases.

Imaging

Unlike childhood or adult HSE, neonatal HSV CNS infection is much more diffuse. Both gray and white matter are affected. Radiologists should strongly consider neonatal HSV encephalitis when cranial imaging at 2-3 weeks of neonatal life shows unexplained diffuse cerebral edema, with leptomeningeal enhancement, without or with cerebral parenchymal hemorrhage. Early MR with diffusion is advised.

CT Findings. NECT may be normal early in the disease or show diffuse hypoattenuation involving both cortex and subcortical white matter reflecting cerebral edema. Hemorrhages may present as multifocal punctate, patchy, and curvilinear regions of hyperattenuation in the basal ganglia, white matter, and cortex.

MR Findings. In the acute and subacute stages of neonatal HSV, multifocal lesions (67%), deep gray matter involvement (58%), hemorrhage (66%), "watershed" pattern of injury (40%), and the occasional involvement of the brainstem and cerebellum may occur. T1WI may be normal or show hypointensity in affected areas **(12-6)**. T2WIs show hyperintensity in the cortex, white matter, and basal ganglia. Hemorrhagic foci on T2* sequences are common. Late-stage disease shows severe volume loss with enlarged ventricles and multicystic encephalomalacia **(12-6D)**.

DWI is key for the initial diagnosis of neonatal HSV encephalitis. In 1/2 of all patients, DWI demonstrates bilateral or significantly more extensive disease than seen on conventional MR.

Foci of patchy enhancement, typically a meningeal pattern of enhancement, are common on T1 C+ scans. In later stages, T1 shortening and T2 hypointensity with "blooming" on T2* GRE/SWI secondary to hemorrhagic foci may develop **(12-6C)**.

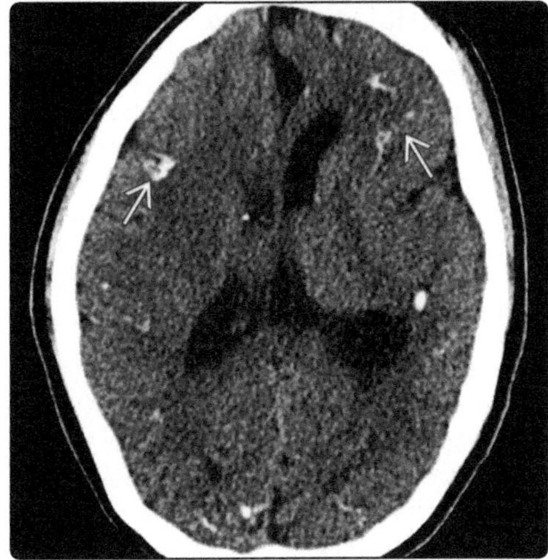

***(12-3)** 12 year old with congenital toxoplasmosis shows Ca^{++} in the cerebral cortex and subcortical WM ➡.*

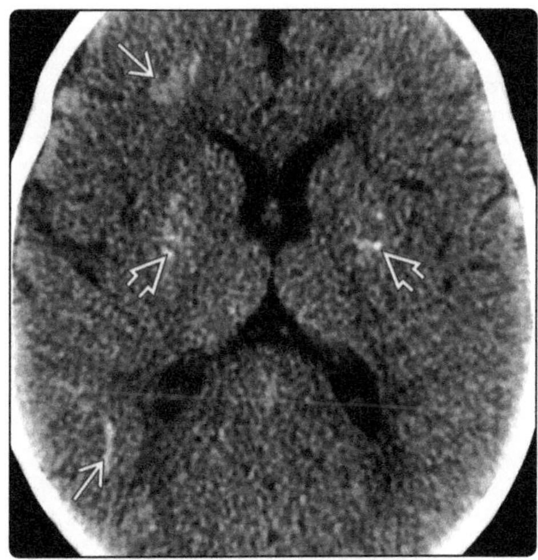

***(12-4)** NECT in an 18-month-old boy with congenital rubella shows subcortical ➡ and basal ganglia ➡ Ca^{++}.*

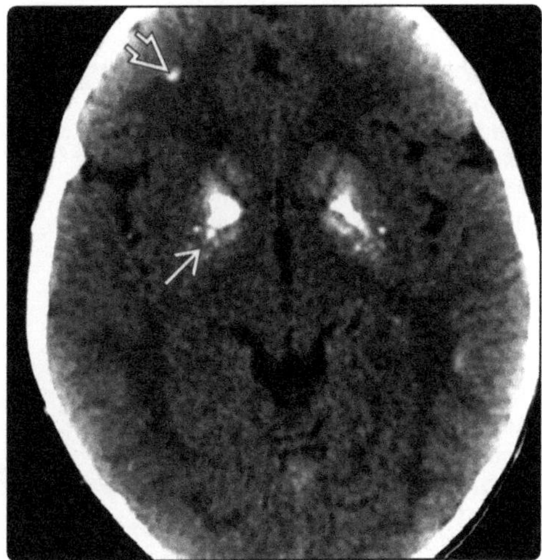

***(12-5)** NECT in a 5-year-old child with congenital HIV shows bilateral basal ganglia ➡ and subcortical ➡ Ca^{++}.*

Differential Diagnosis

The major differential diagnoses for neonatal HSV are **other TORCH and non-TORCH infections**. Because the initial imaging features of acute and subacute HSV encephalitis are often so nonspecific and may manifest with generalized cerebral edema, metabolic, toxic, and hypoxic-ischemic insults must also be considered in the differential diagnosis.

Congenital (Perinatal) HIV

The imaging presentation of congenital HIV infection is quite different from the findings in acquired HIV/AIDS. The most striking and consistent finding is atrophy, particularly in the frontal lobes. Bilaterally symmetric basal ganglia calcifications are common **(12-5)**. Ectasia and fusiform enlargement of intracranial arteries are found in 3-5% of cases.

Differential Diagnosis

The differential diagnosis of congenital HIV is other TORCH infections. **CMV** is characterized by periventricular calcifications, microcephaly, and cortical dysplasia. Other than volume loss, the brain in congenital HIV appears normal. **Toxoplasmosis** is much less common than CMV and causes scattered parenchymal calcifications, not symmetric basal ganglia lesions. **Pseudo-TORCH** calcifications involve cortex and white matter, basal ganglia, brainstem, and cerebellum.

Other Congenital Infections

In congenital **rubella** ("German measles") infection, the timing of infection dictates the magnitude of destructive changes. Reported findings include microcephaly, parenchymal calcifications including cortical calcifications **(12-4)**, delayed myelination, periventricular and basal ganglia cysts, frontal-dominant white matter lesions (NECT hypoattenuating and

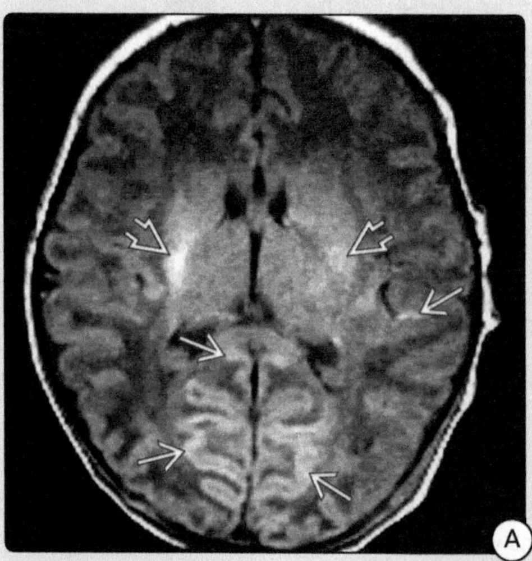

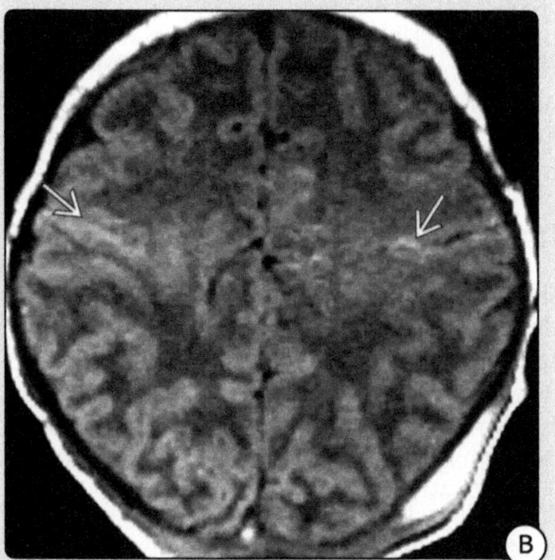

***(12-6A)** A 4-week-old infant born to an HSV-2(+) mother had several days of fever and lethargy. T1 MR shows multiple bilateral cortical ➡ and basal ganglia ⇨ foci of T1 shortening, suggestive of subacute hemorrhage. **(12-6B)** More cephalad scan in the same patient shows additional areas of cortical T1 shortening ➡. Susceptibility-weighted MR with filtered phase maps aids in differentiating hemorrhage from calcification.*

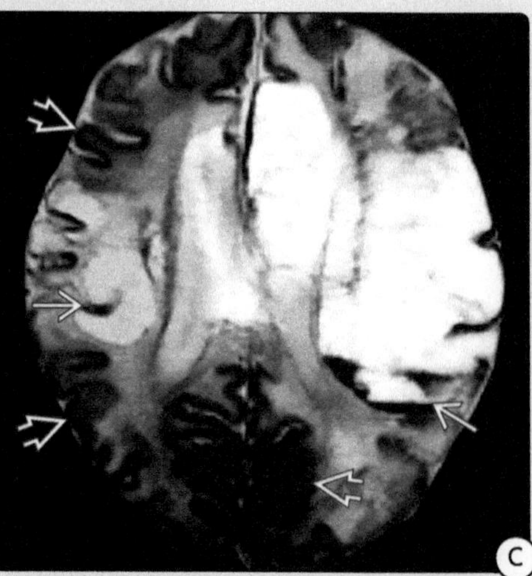

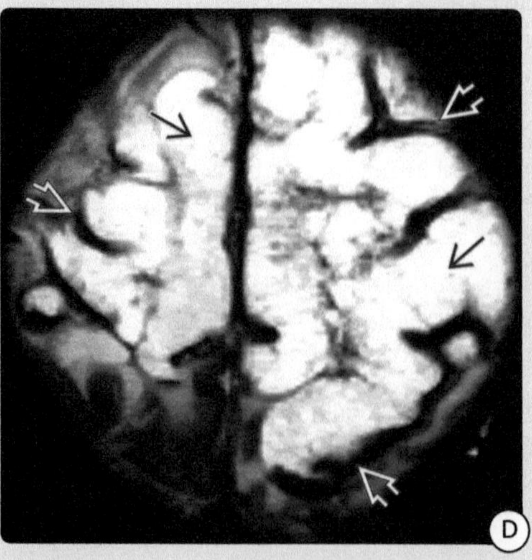

***(12-6C)** T2 MR in the same infant 1 month later shows extensive multicystic encephalomalacia with blood-fluid levels ⇨. Note ribbon-like T2 shortening within the cortex ➡ reflecting hemorrhage &/or Ca^{++}. **(12-6D)** T2 MR through the convexity in the same patient illustrates holohemispheric cystic encephalomalacia ⇨ underlying regions of gyral T2 shortening ➡. This case illustrates early and late changes of congenital HSV.*

MR T2 hyperintense), and atrophy, and, in severe cases, total brain destruction has been described. Imaging findings are nonspecific. Late infection causes generalized brain volume loss, dystrophic calcifications, and regions of demyelination &/or gliosis.

Congenital **varicella-zoster virus** infection ("chickenpox") causes microcephaly, parenchymal calcifications, ventriculomegaly, and polymicrogyria with nonpatterned necrosis of white matter, lobar cortical and subcortical tissues, and deep gray nuclei.

SELECTED CONGENITAL AND PERINATAL INFECTIONS: NEUROIMAGING FINDINGS AND COMMON CAUSES

Cytomegalovirus
- Microcephaly, Ca^{++} at caudostriatal groove, polymicrogyria (PMG), cysts, WM abnormalities, cerebellar hypoplasia, vertical hippocampi

Toxoplasmosis
- Macrocephaly, hydrocephalus, scattered Ca^{++}, lack of cortical malformations

Herpes Simplex Virus
- Early-diffuse cerebral edema, multifocal lesions, DWI abnormalities, hemorrhage, watershed infarctions, leptomeningeal enhancement, late cystic encephalomalacia

Lymphocytic Choriomeningitis Virus
- May precisely mimic features of CMV, negative routine TORCH testing

Zika Virus
- Microcephaly, ventriculomegaly, Ca^{++} at GM-WM junctions, cortical malformations

Rubella Virus
- Microcephaly, Ca^{++} (basal ganglia, periventricular, and cortex) may cause lobar destruction

Varicella-Zoster Virus
- Necrosis of WM, deep GM nuclei, cerebellum ventriculomegaly, cerebellar aplasia, PMG

Syphilis
- Basilar meningitis, stroke, scattered Ca^{++}

HIV
- Atrophy, basal ganglia Ca^{++}, fusiform arteriopathy

Human Parechovirus
- Confluent periventricular WM abnormality mimic of perinatal periventricular leukomalacia

Human Parvovirus B19
- WM, cortical, and basal ganglia injury in setting of severe fetal anemia

Acquired Pyogenic Infections

Meningitis

Meningitis is a worldwide disease that leaves up to 1/2 of all survivors with permanent neurologic sequelae. Despite advances in antimicrobial therapy and vaccine development, bacterial meningitis represents a significant cause of morbidity and mortality. Infants, children, and the elderly or immunocompromised patients are at special risk. In this section, we focus on the etiology, pathology, and imaging findings of this potentially devastating disease.

Terminology

Meningitis is an acute or chronic inflammatory infiltrate of meninges and CSF. **Pachymeningitis** involves the dura-arachnoid; **leptomeningitis** affects the pia and subarachnoid spaces.

Etiology

Many different infectious agents can cause meningitis. Most cases are caused by acute pyogenic (bacterial) infection. Meningitis can also be acute lymphocytic (viral) or chronic (tubercular or granulomatous).

The most common responsible agent varies with age, geography, and immune status. Group B β-hemolytic streptococcal meningitis is the leading cause of newborn meningitis in developed countries, whereas enteric, gram-negative organisms (typically *Escherichia coli*, less commonly *Enterobacter* or *Citrobacter*) cause the majority of cases in developing countries.

Vaccination has significantly decreased the incidence of *Haemophilus influenzae* meningitis, so the most common cause of childhood bacterial meningitis is now *Neisseria meningitidis*.

Adult meningitis is typically caused by *Streptococcus pneumoniae* or *N. meningitidis* (meningococci). The tetravalent meningococcal vaccine used to vaccinate adolescents in the USA does not contain serotype B, the causative organism of 1/3 of all cases of meningococcal disease in industrialized countries.

Listeria monocytogenes, *S. pneumoniae*, gram-negative bacilli, and *N. meningitidis* affect adults over the age of 55 as well as individuals with chronic illnesses.

Tuberculous meningitis is common in developing countries and in immunocompromised patients (e.g., HIV/AIDS patients and solid organ transplant recipients).

Pathology

Cloudy CSF initially fills the subarachnoid spaces followed by development of a variably dense purulent exudate that covers the pial surfaces **(12-7)**. The basal cisterns and subarachnoid spaces are the most commonly involved sites by meningitis

(12-8) followed by the cerebral convexity sulci. Vessels within the exudate may show inflammatory changes and necrosis **(12-9)**.

Clinical Issues

Presentation. Presentation depends on patient age. In adults, fever (≥ 38.5°C) and either headache, nuchal rigidity, or altered mental status are the most common symptoms. Fever, lethargy, poor feeding, and irritability are common among infected infants. Seizures occur in 30% of patients.

Natural History. Despite rapid recognition and effective therapy, meningitis still has significant morbidity and mortality rates. Death rates from 15-25% have been reported in disadvantaged children with poor living conditions.

Complications are both common and numerous. **Extraventricular obstructive hydrocephalus** is one of the earliest and most common complications. The choroid plexus can become infected, causing choroid plexitis and then **ventriculitis**. Infection can also extend from the pia along the perivascular spaces into the brain parenchyma itself, causing **cerebritis** and then **abscess**.

Sub- and epidural **empyemas** or sterile **effusions** may develop. **Cerebrovascular complications** of meningitis include vasculitis, thrombosis, and occlusion of both arteries and veins.

Imaging

General Features. The "gold standard" for the diagnosis of bacterial meningitis is CSF analysis. Remember: **Imaging is neither sensitive nor specific for the detection of meningitis!** Therefore, imaging should be used in conjunction with—and not as a substitute for—appropriate clinical and laboratory evaluation.

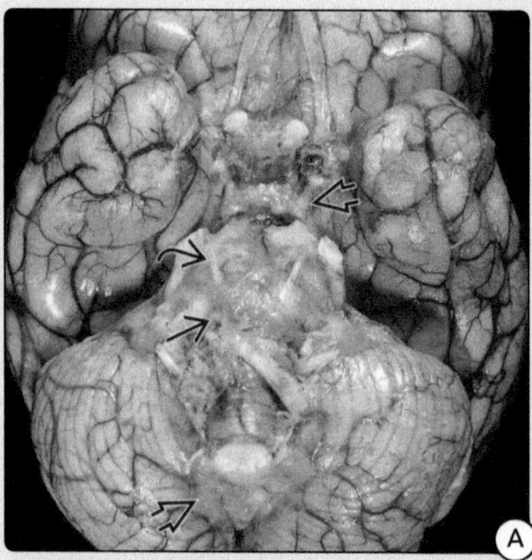

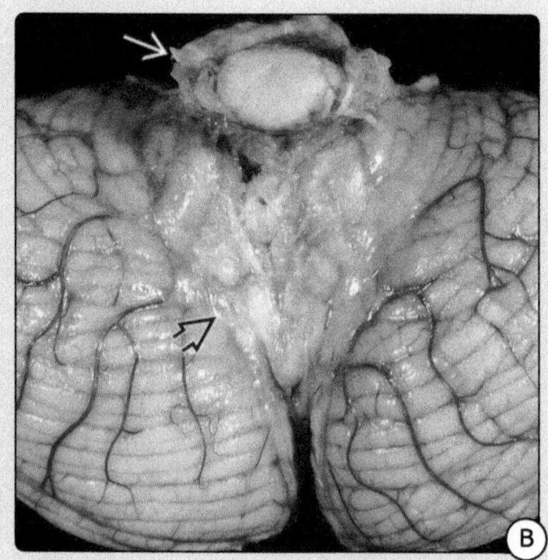

***(12-7A)** Autopsied brain shows typical changes of severe meningitis with dense purulent exudate covering the pons ➡, coating the cranial nerves ➡, and filling the basal cisterns ➡. **(12-7B)** As seen in this autopsy photograph, the exudate coats the medulla ➡ and completely fills the cisterna magna ➡. (Courtesy R. Hewlett, MD.)*

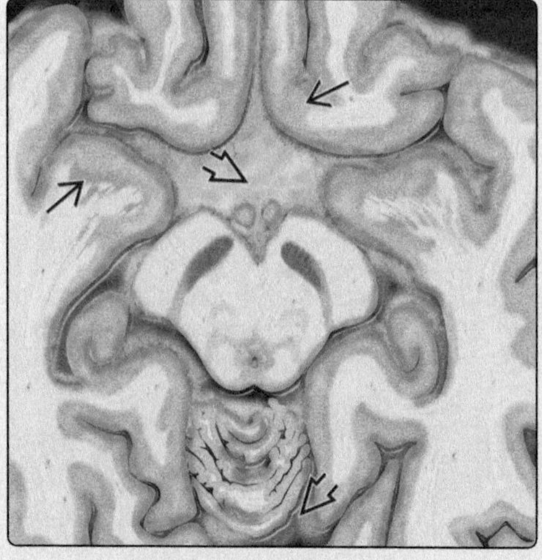

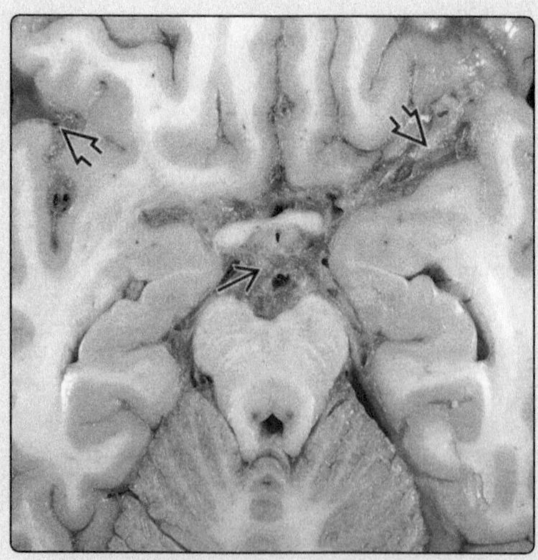

***(12-8)** Graphic of meningitis shows purulent exudate involving the leptomeninges and filling the basal cisterns and sulci ➡. The underlying brain is mildly hyperemic ➡. Venous and arterial spasm/occlusion may result in parenchymal infarction. **(12-9)** Axial autopsy section shows meningitis with exudate completely filling the suprasellar cistern ➡ and sylvian fissures ➡. (Courtesy R. Hewlett, MD.)*

Imaging studies are best used to confirm the diagnosis and assess possible complications. While CT is commonly employed as a screening examination in cases of headache and suspected meningitis, both the primary and acute manifestations of meningitis as well as secondary complications are best depicted on MR.

CT Findings. Initial NECT scans may be normal or show only mild ventricular enlargement **(12-10B)**. "Blurred" ventricular margins indicate acute obstructive hydrocephalus with accumulation of extracellular fluid in the deep white matter. Bone CT should be carefully evaluated for sinusitis and otomastoiditis.

As the cellular inflammatory exudate develops, it replaces the normally clear CSF **(12-11)**. Subtle effacement of surface landmarks may occur as sulcal-cisternal CSF becomes almost isodense with brain **(12-10A)**. In rare cases, subtle hyperattenuation may be present in the basal subarachnoid spaces.

CECT may show intense enhancement of the inflammatory exudate as it covers the brain surfaces, extending into and filling the sulci.

MR Findings. The purulent exudates of acute meningitis are isointense with underlying brain on T1WI, giving the appearance of "dirty" CSF. The exudates are isointense with CSF on T2WI and do not suppress on FLAIR. Hyperintensity in the subarachnoid cisterns and superficial sulci on FLAIR is a typical but nonspecific finding of meningitis **(12-10C)**.

DWI is especially helpful in meningitis, as the purulent subarachnoid space exudates usually show restriction **(12-12B)**. pMR may demonstrate multiple regions of increased cerebral blood flow.

Pia-subarachnoid space enhancement occurs in 50% of patients **(12-10D)**. A curvilinear pattern that follows the gyri and sulci (the "pial-cisternal" pattern) is typical **(12-12A)** and more common than dura-arachnoid enhancement.

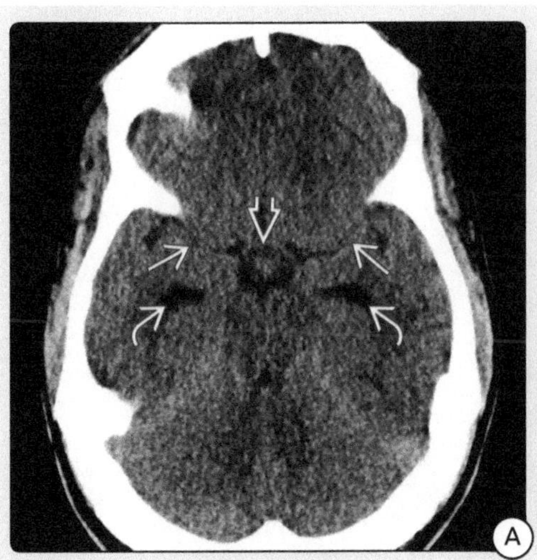

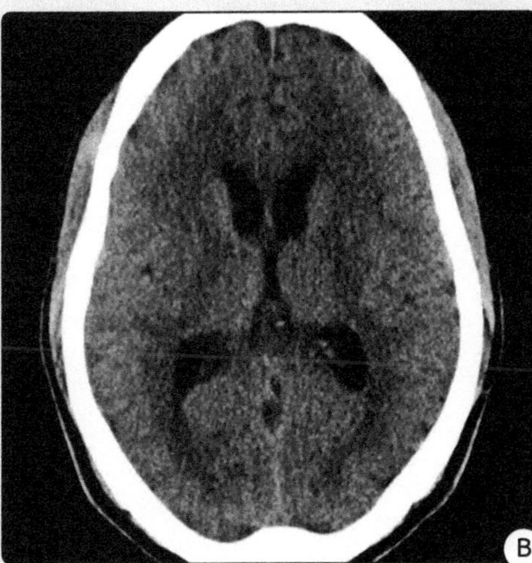

***(12-10A)** NECT in a 25-year-old man w/ headache & fever shows mild enlargement of both temporal horns ➡. CSF in the suprasellar cistern ➡ appears mildly hyperdense ("dirty"), and the sylvian fissures ➡ appear effaced. **(12-10B)** More cephalad NECT shows that the lateral and 3rd ventricles are slightly enlarged. Note poor visualization of the superficial sulci, leading to a somewhat "featureless" appearance. Scan was initially read as normal.*

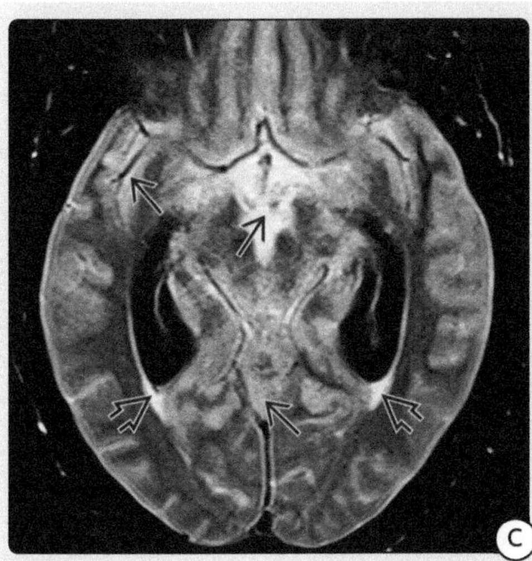

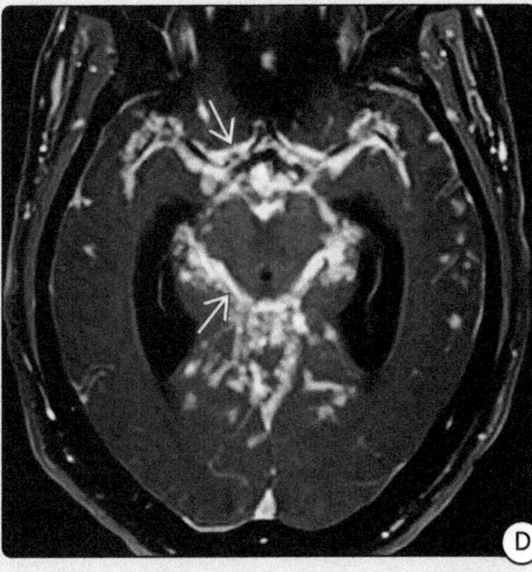

***(12-10C)** The patient returned 3 weeks later with increasing headaches and altered mental status. FLAIR shows the basal cisterns, and sulci are all hyperintense ➡. Progressive hydrocephalus is noted, and transependymal interstitial edema is seen ➡. **(12-10D)** T1 C+ FS MR in the same case shows diffuse linear and nodular sulcal-cisternal enhancement ➡. This is pyogenic meningitis and has led to associated hydrocephalus.*

Postcontrast T2-weighted FLAIR and delayed postcontrast T1-weighted sequences may be helpful additions in detecting subtle cases.

Complications of Meningitis. Other than hydrocephalus **(12-13)**, complications from meningitis are relatively uncommon **(12-14)**. Postmeningitis reactive **effusions**—sterile CSF-like fluid pockets—develop in 5-10% of children treated for acute bacterial meningitis. NECT shows bilateral crescentic extraaxial collections that are iso- to slightly hyperdense compared with normal CSF.

Effusions are iso- to slightly hyperintense to CSF on T1WI and isointense on T2WI. They are often slightly hyperintense relative to CSF on FLAIR. Effusions usually do not enhance on T1 C+ and do not restrict on DWI, differentiating them from subdural empyemas.

Less common complications include pyocephalus (ventriculitis), empyema, cerebritis &/or abscess, venous occlusion, and ischemia. All are discussed separately below.

Differential Diagnosis

The major differential diagnosis of infectious meningitis is noninfectious meningitis. Other causes of meningitis include **noninfectious inflammatory disorders** (e.g., rheumatoid or systemic lupus erythematosus-associated meningitis, IgG4-related disease, drug-related aseptic meningitis, and multiple sclerosis) and neoplastic or **carcinomatous meningitis**. All can appear identical on imaging, so correlation with clinical information and laboratory findings is essential. **Remember**: *Sulcal/cisternal FLAIR hyperintensity is a nonspecific finding and can be seen with a number of different entities (see box on next page).*

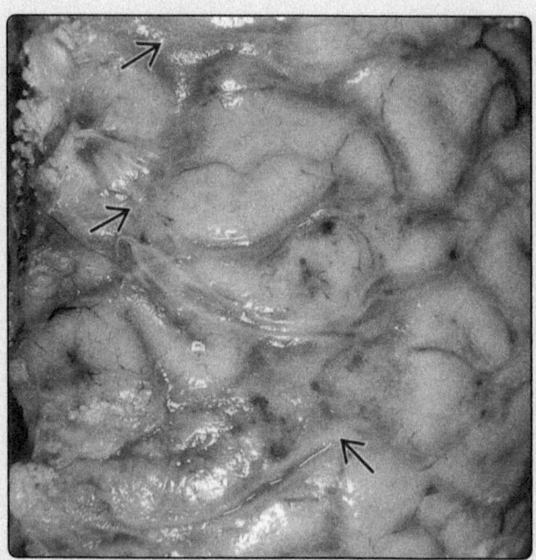

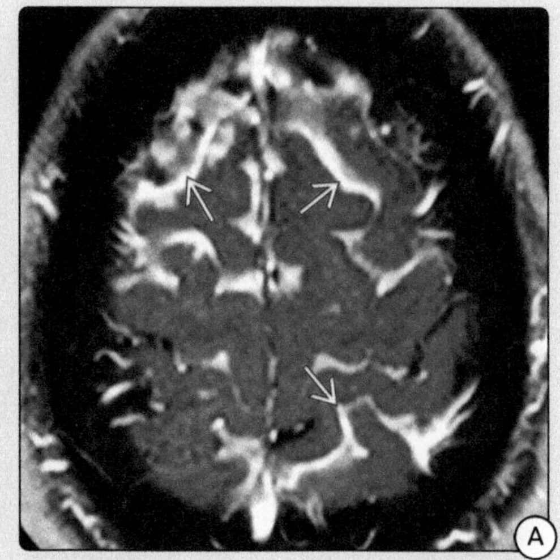

(12-11) Autopsy case with close-up view shows typical changes of pyogenic meningitis. The convexity sulci are filled with purulent exudate ➡. (Courtesy R. Hewlett, MD.) (12-12A) T1 C+ FS MR in a case of acute pyogenic meningitis shows that diffuse, intensely enhancing exudate fills the convexity sulci ➡. FLAIR imaging is also sensitive in detecting SAS pathology.

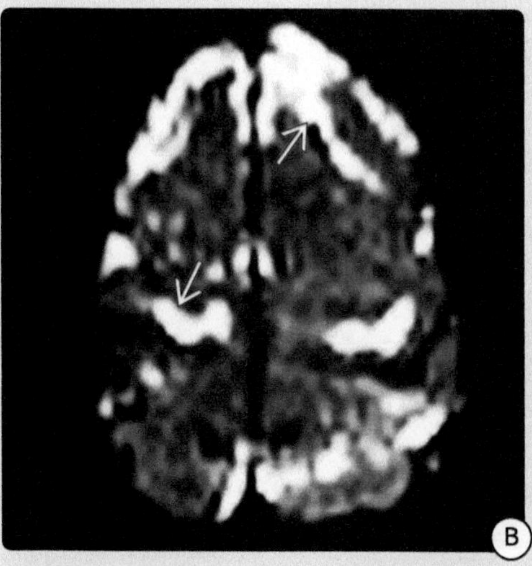

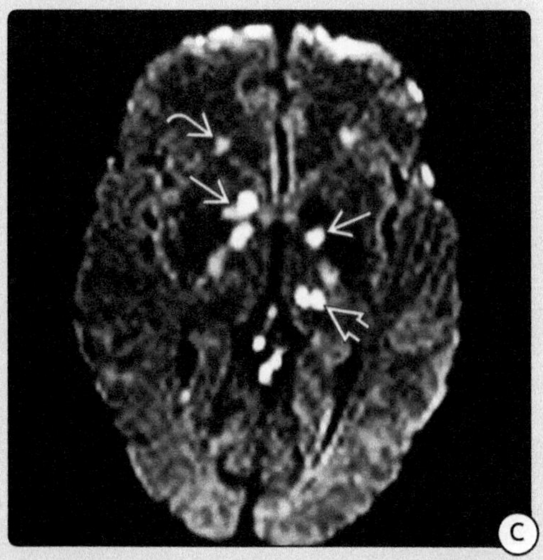

(12-12B) DWI MR in the same patient shows that the viscous pus filling the convexity sulci restricts strongly ➡. This is streptococcal meningitis with secondary vasculitis. (12-12C) DWI MR in the same case shows multifocal acute basal ganglia ➡, thalamic ➡, and deep parenchymal infarcts ➡.

CAUSES OF HYPERINTENSE CSF ON FLAIR

Common

- Blood
  - Subarachnoid hemorrhage
- Infection
  - Meningitis
- Artifact
  - Susceptibility; flow
- Tumor
  - CSF metastases

Less Common

- High inspired oxygen
  - 4-5x signal with 100% O_2
- Prominent vessels
  - Stroke (pial collaterals); "ivy" sign (moyamoya); pial angioma (Sturge-Weber)

Rare but Important

- Fat (ruptured dermoid)
- Gadolinium in CSF
  - Renal failure; blood-brain barrier leakage

Abscess

Terminology

A cerebral abscess is a localized infection of the brain parenchyma.

Etiology

Most abscesses are caused by hematogeneous spread from an extracranial location (e.g., lung or urinary tract infection and endocarditis). Abscesses may also result from penetrating injury or direct geographic extension from sinonasal and otomastoid infection. These typically begin as extraaxial infections, such as empyema or meningitis, and then spread into the brain itself.

Abscesses are most often bacterial, but they can also be fungal, parasitic, or (rarely) granulomatous. Although myriad organisms can cause abscess formation, the most common agents in immunocompetent adults are *Streptococcus* species, *Staphylococcus aureus*, and pneumococci. *Enterobacter* species like *Citrobacter* are a common cause of cerebral abscess in neonates. *Streptococcus intermedius* is emerging as an important cause of cerebral abscess in immunocompetent children and adolescents. In 20-30% of abscesses, cultures are sterile, and no specific organism is identified.

Proinflammatory molecules, such as tumor necrosis factor-α and interleukin-1β, induce various cell adhesion molecules that facilitate extravasation of peripheral immune cells and promote abscess development.

Bacterial abscesses are relatively uncommon in immunocompromised patients. *Klebsiella* is common in diabetics, and fungal infections by *Aspergillus* and *Nocardia* are common in transplant recipients. In patients with HIV/AIDS, toxoplasmosis and tuberculosis are the most common opportunistic infections.

In children, predisposing factors for cerebral abscess formation include meningitis, uncorrected cyanotic heart disease, sepsis, suppurative pulmonary infection, paranasal sinus or otomastoid trauma, or suppurative infections, endocarditis, and immunodeficiency or immunosuppression states.

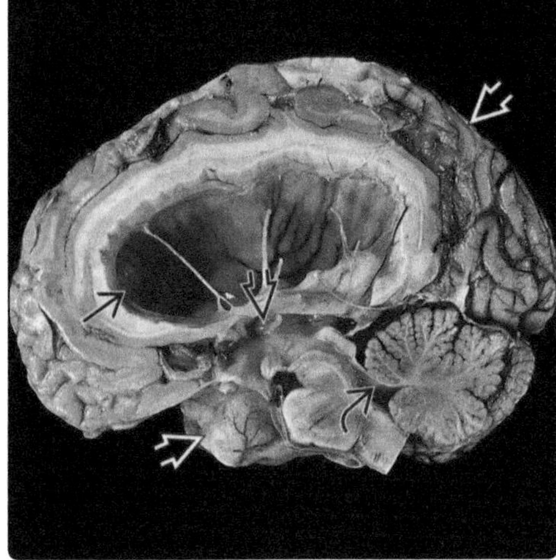

***(12-13)** Autopsy of meningitis ➡ with EVOH shows lateral ➡, 3rd ➡, 4th ventricular ➡ aqueductal dilation. (Ellison, Neuropath, 3e.)*

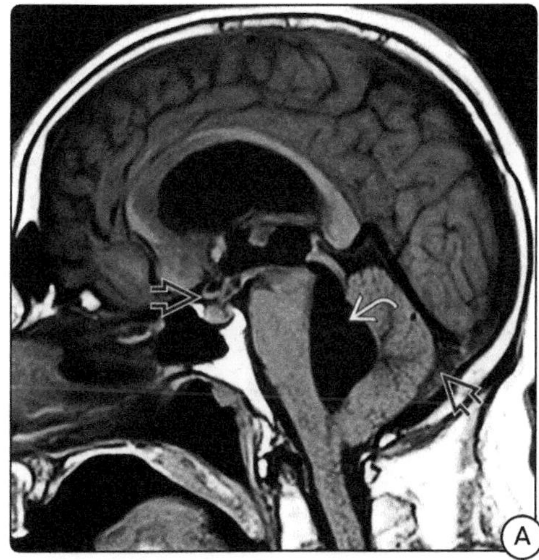

***(12-14A)** Sagittal T1 MR shows basilar meningitis ➡. Lateral, 3rd ventricles are enlarged; 4th ventricle ➡ appears "ballooned" or obstructed.*

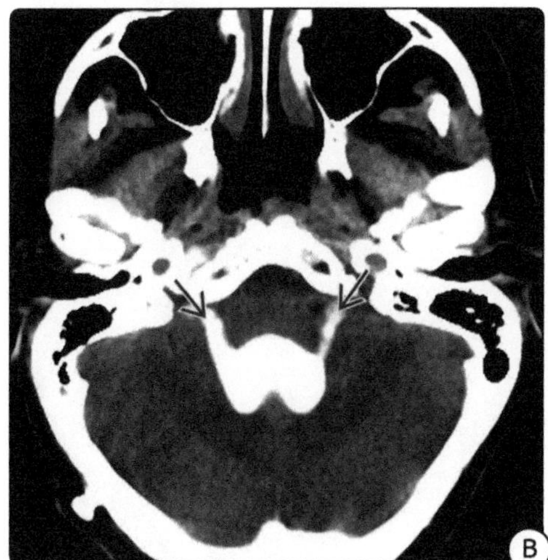

***(12-14B)** CT ventriculogram shows dilated 4th ventricle, obstructed outflow at foramina of Luschka ➡. EVOH is secondary to meningitis.*

(12-15) Graphic of early cerebritis shows focal unencapsulated mass of petechial hemorrhage, inflammatory cells, and edema ➡.

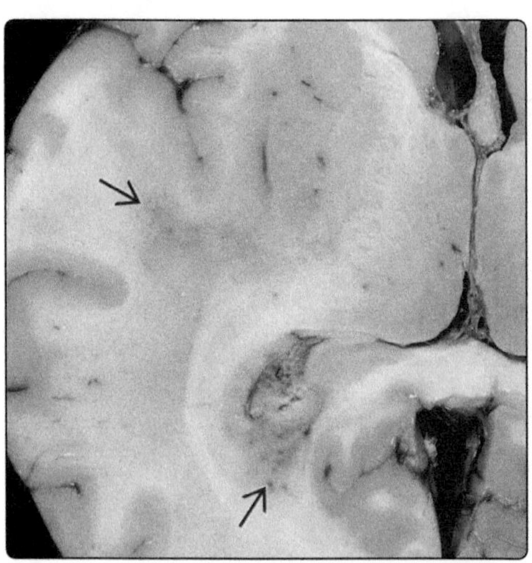

(12-16) Autopsy specimen shows foci of early cerebritis, unencapsulated edema, and petechial hemorrhages ➡. (Courtesy R. Hewlett, MD.)

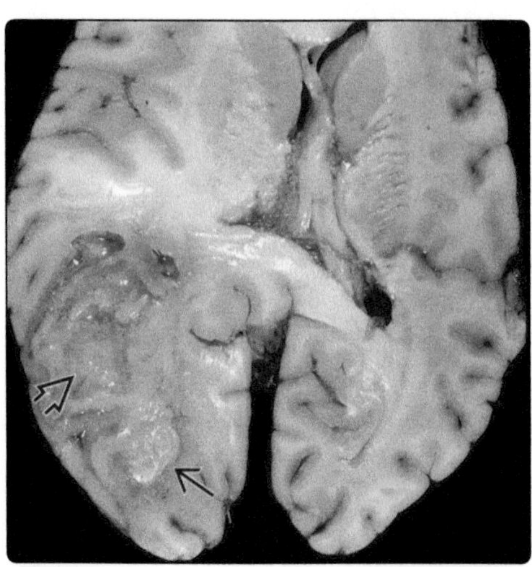

(12-17) Autopsied late cerebritis demonstrates coalescing lesion with some central necrosis ➡, the beginnings of an ill-defined abscess rim ➡.

Pathology

Four general stages are recognized in the evolution of a cerebral abscess: (1) Focal suppurative encephalitis/early cerebritis, (2) focal suppurative encephalitis/late cerebritis, (3) early encapsulation, and (4) late encapsulation. Each has its own distinctive pathologic appearance, which, in turn, determines the imaging findings.

Focal Suppurative Encephalitis. Sometimes also called the **"early cerebritis"** stage of abscess formation, in this earliest stage, suppurative infection is focal but not yet localized **(12-15)**. An unencapsulated, edematous, hyperemic mass of leukocytes and bacteria is present for 1-3 days after the initial infection **(12-16)**.

Focal Suppurative Encephalitis With Confluent Central Necrosis. The next stage of abscess formation is also called **"late cerebritis"** and begins 2-3 days after the initial infection **(12-17)**. This stage typically lasts between a week and 10 days.

Patchy necrotic foci within the suppurative mass form, enlarge, and then coalesce into a confluent necrotic mass. By days 5-7, a necrotic core is surrounded by a poorly organized, irregular rim of granulation tissue consisting of inflammatory cells, macrophages, and fibroblasts. The surrounding brain is edematous and contains swollen reactive astrocytes.

BRAIN ABSCESS: PATHOLOGY AND EVOLUTION

Stages

- Focal suppurative encephalitis (days 1-2)
  - Edematous, suppurative mass
  - No visible necrosis or capsule
- Focal suppurative encephalitis with confluent central necrosis (days 2-7)
  - Necrotic foci form, begin to coalesce
  - Poorly organized irregular rim
- Early encapsulation (days 5-14)
  - Coalescent core
  - Well-defined wall of fibroblasts, collagen
- Late encapsulation (> 2 weeks)
  - Wall thickens, then shrinks
  - Inflammation; edema decreases/disappears

Early Encapsulation. The **"early capsule"** stage starts around 1 week. Proliferating fibroblasts deposit reticulin around the outer rim of the abscess cavity. The abscess wall is now composed of an inner rim of granulation tissue at the edge of the necrotic center **(12-20)** and an outer rim of multiple concentric layers of fibroblasts and collagen **(12-21)**. The necrotic core liquefies completely by 7-10 days, and newly formed capillaries around the mass become prominent.

Late Capsulation. The **"late capsule"** stage begins several weeks following infection and may last for several months.

With treatment, the central cavity gradually involutes and shrinks. Collagen deposition further thickens the wall, and the surrounding vasogenic edema disappears. The wall eventually contains densely packed reticulin and is lined by sparse macrophages. Eventually, only a small gliotic nodule of collagen and fibroblasts remains.

Clinical Issues

Demographics. Brain abscesses are rare. Only 2,500 cases are reported annually in the USA. Brain abscesses occur at all ages but are most common in patients between the third and fourth decades. Almost 25% occur in children under the age of 15 years. The M:F ratio is 2:1 in adults and 3:1 in children.

Presentation and Prognosis. Headache, seizure, and focal neurologic deficits are the typical presenting symptoms. Fever is common but not universal. CSF cultures may be normal early in the infection.

Brain abscesses are potentially fatal but treatable lesions. Rapid diagnosis, stereotactic surgery, and appropriate medical treatment have reduced mortality to 2-4%.

Imaging

General Features. Imaging findings evolve with time and are related to the stage of abscess development. MR is more sensitive than CT and is the procedure of choice.

Early Cerebritis. Very early cerebritis may be invisible on CT. A poorly marginated cortical/subcortical hypodense mass is the most common finding **(12-18A)**. Early cerebritis often shows little or no enhancement on CECT.

Early cerebritis is hypo- to isointense on T1WI and hyperintense on T2/FLAIR. T2* GRE may show punctate "blooming" hemorrhagic foci. Patchy enhancement may or may not be present. DWI shows diffusion restriction **(12-18B)**.

Late Cerebritis. A better-delineated central hypodense mass with surrounding edema is seen on NECT. CECT typically shows irregular rim enhancement **(12-19A)**.

Late cerebritis has a hypointense center and an iso- to mildly hyperintense rim on T1WI. The central core of the cerebritis is hyperintense on T2WI, whereas the rim is relatively hypointense. Intense but somewhat irregular rim enhancement is present on T1 C+ images **(12-19B)**.

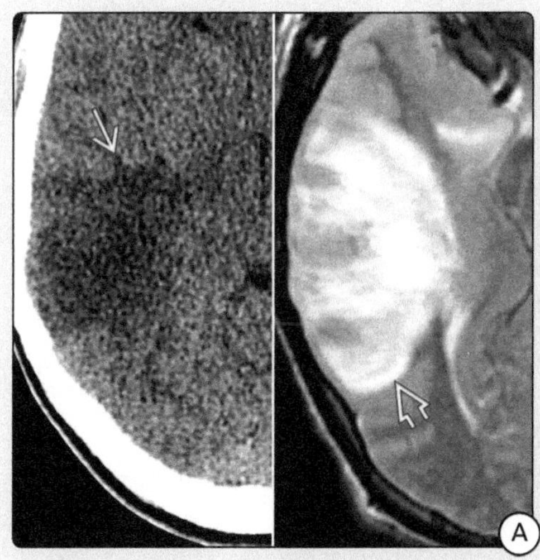

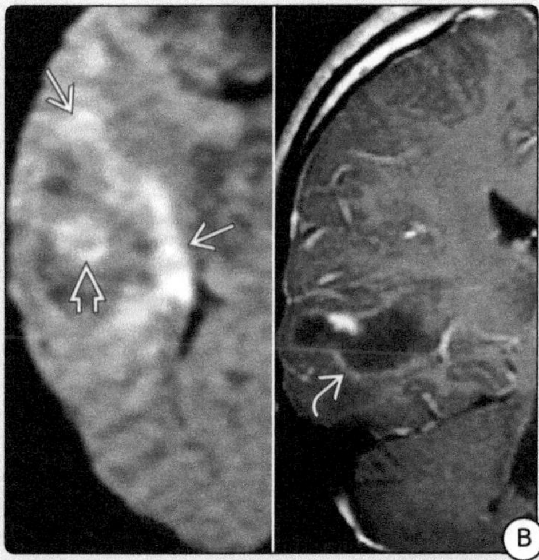

(12-18A) (L) NECT shows ill-defined hypoattenuation ➡ and mass effect within the right temporal lobe. Arterial infarction was suspected. (R) T2 MR shows a hyperintense right temporal lobe mass ➡. (12-18B) (L) DWI MR shows restricted diffusion at the periphery ➡, center ➡ of the lesion. (R) Coronal T1 C+ MR shows a faint rim of peripheral enhancement ➡. This is the early cerebritis stage of abscess formation.

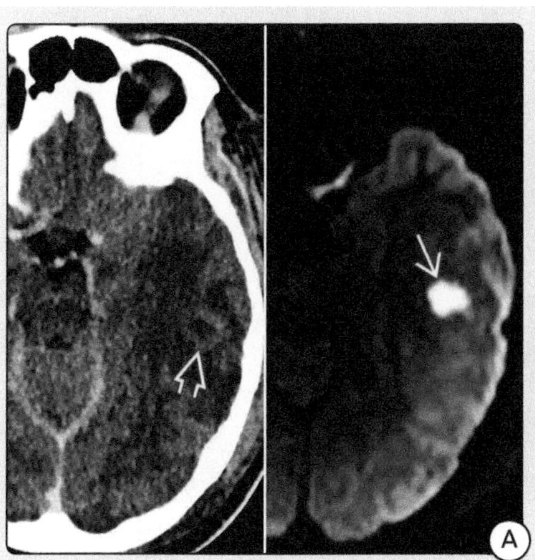

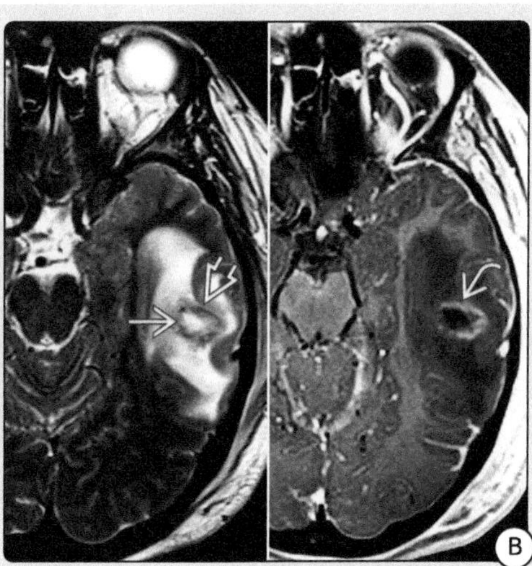

(12-19A) (L) CECT shows faint, ill-defined left temporal lobe ring-enhancing lesion with peripheral edema ➡. (R) DWI MR shows strong diffusion restriction ➡ in the center of the mass. (12-19B) (L) The mass exhibits a hyperintense center ➡, hypointense periphery ➡ on T2WI. (R) Irregular, poorly defined enhancing rim ➡ is seen on T1 C+ FS. This is the late cerebritis stage of abscess formation.

Late cerebritis restricts strongly on DWI **(12-19A)**. MRS shows cytosolic amino acids (0.9 ppm), lactate (1.3 ppm), and acetate (1.9 ppm) in the necrotic core **(12-24)**. The abscess wall demonstrates low rCBV on pMR.

BRAIN ABSCESS IMAGING: CEREBRITIS STAGES

Early Cerebritis
- CT
  - Ill-defined hypodense mass on NECT
  - Usually no enhancement
- MR
  - T2/FLAIR heterogeneously hyperintense
  - T2* ± petechial hemorrhage; DWI+ (often mild)
  - T1 C+ may show patchy enhancement

Late Cerebritis
- CT
  - Round/ovoid hypodense mass on NECT
  - ± thin, irregular ring on CECT
- MR
  - T2-/FLAIR-hyperintense center, hypointense irregular rim
  - T2* GRE-hypointense rim; restricts on DWI
  - Moderate/strong but irregular enhancing rim

Early Capsule. Abscesses are now well-delineated, round or ovoid masses with liquefied, hyperintense *cores* on T2/FLAIR. The *rims* of abscesses are usually thin, complete, smooth, and hypointense on T2WI. A "double rim" sign demonstrating two concentric rims, the outer hypointense and the inner hyperintense relative to cavity contents, is seen in 75% of cases **(12-23A)**.

The necrotic core of encapsulated abscesses restricts strongly on DWI **(12-23C)**. T1 C+ sequences show a strongly enhancing rim **(12-23B)** that is thinnest on its deepest (ventricular) side **(12-25B)** and "blooms" on T2*.

Late Capsule. With treatment, the abscess cavity gradually collapses while the capsule thickens even as the overall mass diminishes in size. The shrinking abscess often assumes a "crenulated" appearance, much like a deflated balloon **(12-25A)**.

Contrast enhancement in the resolving abscess may persist for months, long after clinical symptoms have resolved **(12-25C)**.

BRAIN ABSCESS IMAGING: CAPSULE STAGES

Early Capsule
- Well-defined mass + strongly enhancing rim
- Core: T2/FLAIR hyperintense, restricts on DWI
- Wall: "Double rim" sign (hyperintense inner, hypointense outer)

Late Capsule
- Wall thickens, cavity and edema reduce
- Enhancing focus may persist for months

Differential Diagnosis

The differential diagnosis of abscess varies with its stage of development. Early cerebritis is so poorly defined that it can be difficult to characterize and can mimic many lesions, including **cerebral ischemia** or neoplasm.

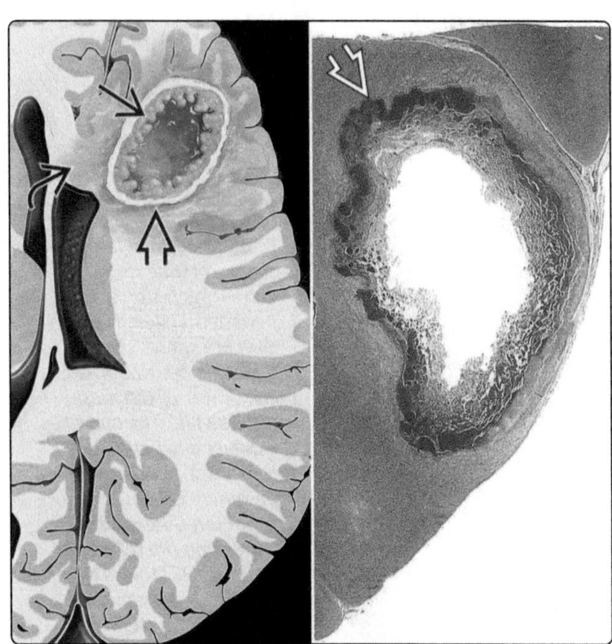

***(12-20)** (L) Graphic shows edema ⇨ surrounding early capsule abscess. Well-defined double-layered wall ⇨ surrounds a central core of necrosis, inflammatory debris ⇨. (R) Micrograph shows double-layered abscess wall ➡. (Ellison, Neuropath, 3e.)*

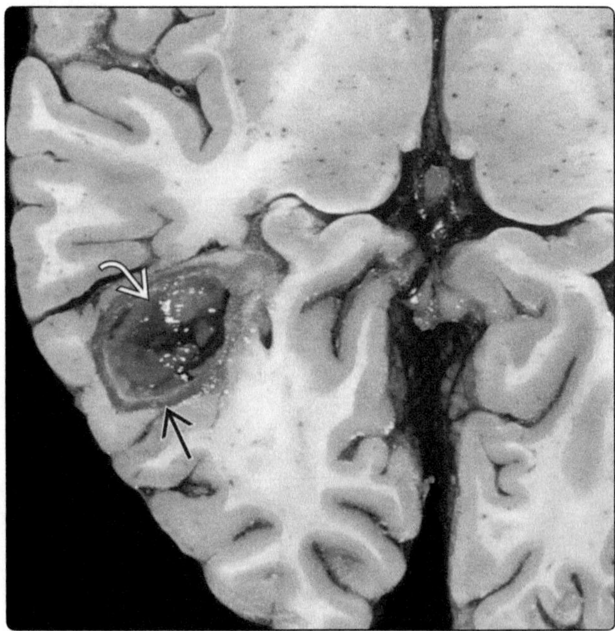

***(12-21)** Abscess at early capsule stage is shown. Necrotic core ➡ is surrounded by a double-layered, well-developed capsule ⇨. (Courtesy R. Hewlett, MD.)*

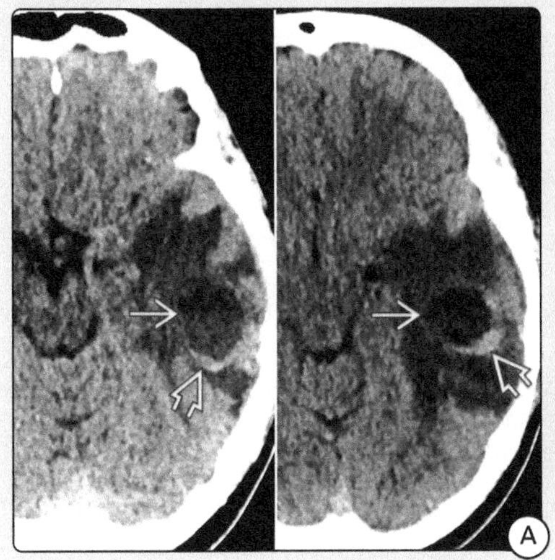

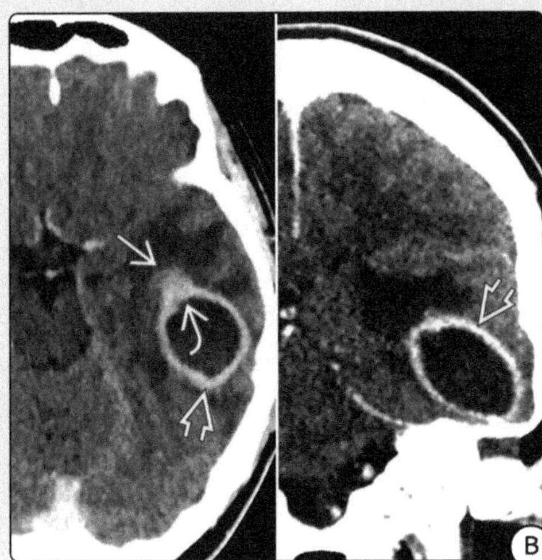

(12-22A) (L and R) NECT scans show large, well-defined lesion with hyperdense rim and a hypodense center. (12-22B) Axial (L), coronal (R) CECT scans show complete, well-delineated rim enhancement. The abscess has progressed from late cerebritis to the early capsule stage. Note the wall defect with the adjacent area of new cerebritis.

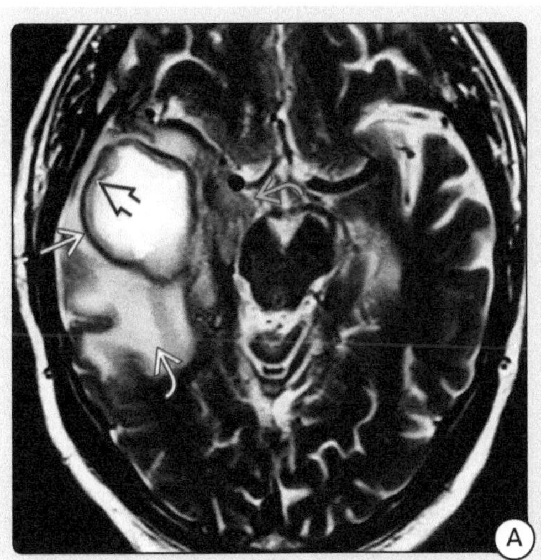

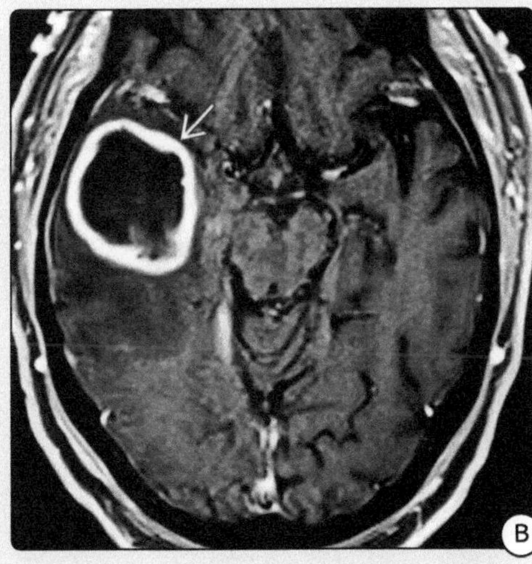

(12-23A) T2 MR in the early capsule stage of abscess development shows the classic "double rim" sign with a hypointense outer rim and a mildly hyperintense inner rim surrounding a very hyperintense necrotic core. Note the peripheral edema and mass effect (uncal herniation). (12-23B) T1 C+ FS MR in the same case shows intense enhancement of the well-developed abscess capsule.

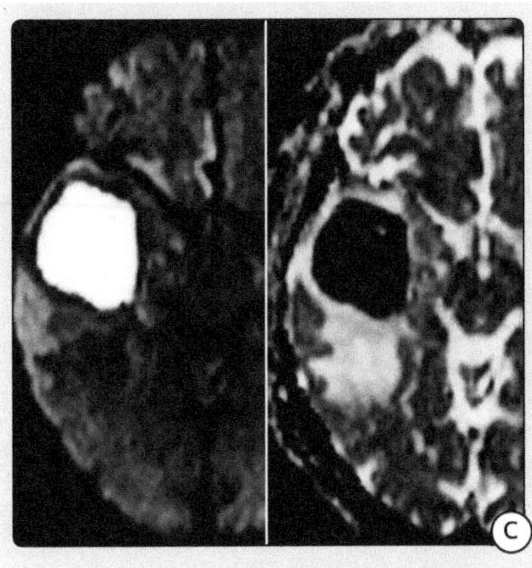

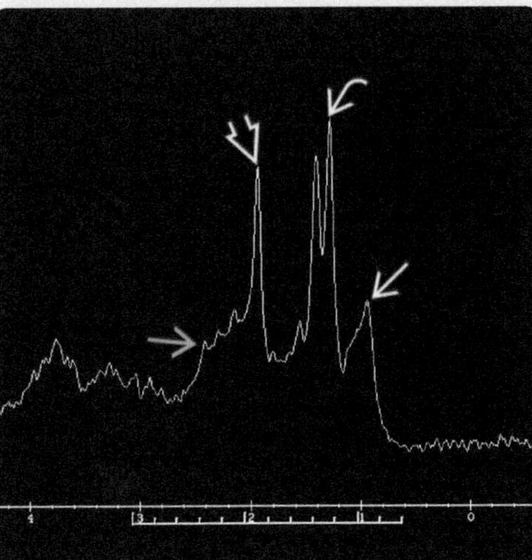

(12-23C) DWI MR (L) and ADC map (R) in the same case show that necrotic contents of the abscess cavity restrict strongly, whereas the wall of the capsule itself does not. (12-24) MRS in another late cerebritis/early capsule abscess with TR 2,000 TE 35 shows amino acids (valine, leucine, isoleucine) at 0.9 ppm, acetate at 1.9 ppm, lactate at 1.3 ppm, and succinate at 2.4 ppm.

Once a ring develops around the necrotic center, the differential diagnosis is basically that of a generic ring-enhancing mass. Although there are many ring-enhancing lesions in the CNS, the most common differential diagnosis is infection vs. **neoplasm (glioblastoma or metastasis)**.

Tumors have increased rCBV in their "rind," usually do not restrict (or if they do, not as strongly as an abscess), and do not demonstrate cytosolic amino acids on MRS.

Less common entities that can appear as a ring-enhancing mass include **demyelinating disease**, in which the ring is usually incomplete and "open" toward the cortex. Resolving hematomas can exhibit a vascular, ring-enhancing pattern.

BRAIN ABSCESS: DIFFERENTIAL DIAGNOSIS

Early Cerebritis

- Encephalitis (may be indistinguishable)
- Stroke
  - Vascular distribution
  - Usually involves both cortex, WM
- Neoplasm (e.g., diffusely infiltrating low-grade astrocytoma)
  - Usually does not enhance or restrict

Late Cerebritis/Early Capsule

- Neoplasm
  - Primary (glioblastoma)
  - Metastasis
- Demyelinating disease
  - Incomplete ("horseshoe") enhancement

(12-25A) Axial T1 C+ FS MR in a 65-year-old man with a history of dental abscess and headaches for 2-3 weeks shows a left posterior frontal thick-walled ring-enhancing mass ➡. Findings are consistent with late capsule stage of abscess development. (12-25B) Coronal T1 C+ FS MR in the same case shows the abscess wall ➡ is thinnest on its deepest side ➡ next to the lateral ventricle. Note edema and mass effect on the ventricle.

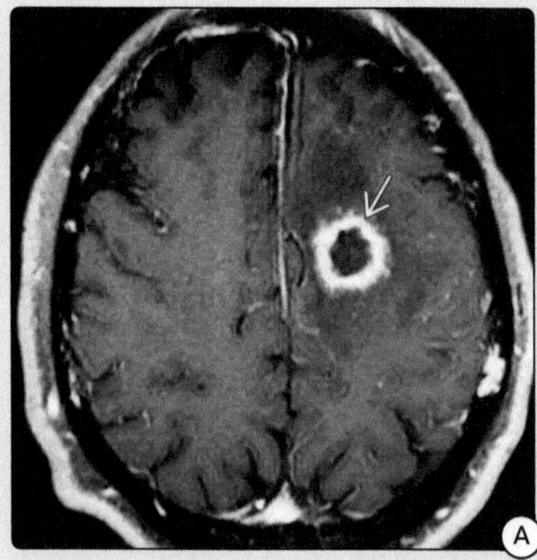

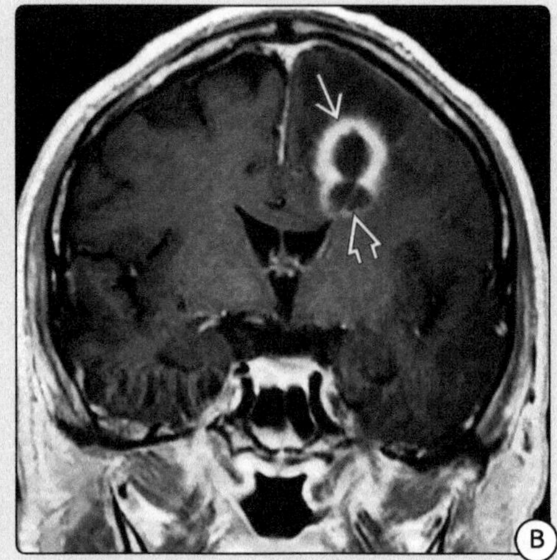

(12-25C) The patient was treated with intravenous antibiotics for 6 weeks. Follow-up scan at the end of treatment shows a small residual enhancing nodule ➡ with almost complete resolution of the surrounding edema. (12-25D) Follow-up T1 C+ FS MR 1 year later shows that only a small hypointense nonenhancing focus remains ➡.

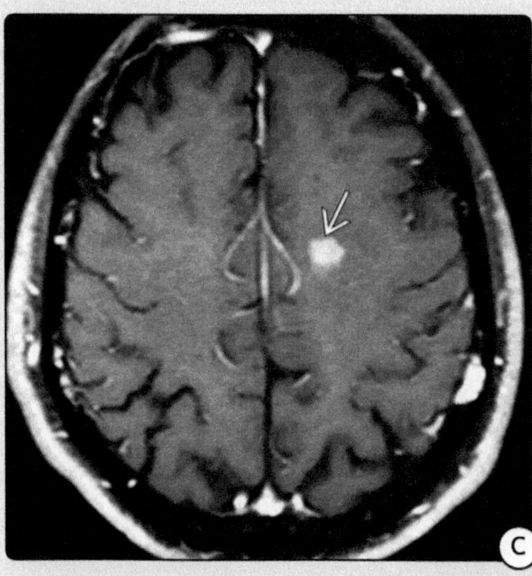

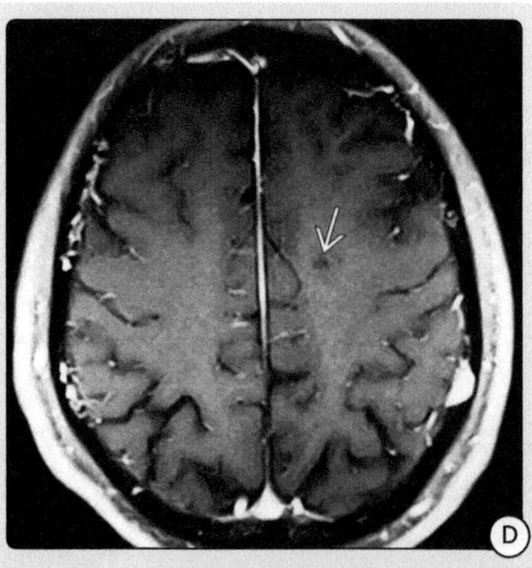

Ventriculitis

Primary intraventricular abscess is rare. A collection of purulent material in the ventricle is more likely due to intraventricular *rupture* of a brain abscess (IVRBA), a catastrophic complication. Ventriculitis also occurs as a complication of meningitis and neurosurgical procedures, such as external ventricular drainage. Recognition and prompt intervention are necessary to treat this highly lethal condition.

Terminology

Ventriculitis is also called **ependymitis, pyocephalus**, and (less commonly) ventricular empyema.

Etiology

Infection of the ventricular ependyma most often occurs when a pyogenic abscess ruptures through its thin, medial capsule into the adjacent ventricle. Risk of IVRBA increases if an abscess is deep seated, multiloculated, &/or close to the ventricular wall. The most common pathogens causing ventriculitis are *Staphylococcus*, *Streptococcus*, and *Enterobacter*. Infections are often multidrug resistant and difficult to treat.

Pathology

Autopsy examination shows that the ependyma, subependymal region, and choroid plexus are congested and covered with pus **(12-26)**. Hemorrhagic ependymitis may be present. Hydrocephalus with pus obstructing the aqueduct is common.

Clinical Issues

Overall mortality is 25-85%. Only 40% of patients survive with good functional outcome.

Imaging

MR should be the first-line imaging modality in cases of suspected ventriculitis. Irregular ventricular debris that appears hyperintense to CSF on T1WI and hypointense on T2WI with layering in the dependent occipital horns is typical.

The most sensitive sequences are FLAIR and DWI. A "halo" of periventricular hyperintensity is usually present on both T2WI and FLAIR scans. DWI shows striking diffusion restriction of the layered debris **(12-27B)**.

Ependymal enhancement is seen in only 60% of cases and varies from minimal to moderate **(12-27A)**. When present, ependymal enhancement tends to be relatively smooth, thin, and linear rather than thick and nodular.

Differential Diagnosis

Thin, linear ependymal enhancement of the periventricular and ependymal veins is normal, especially around the frontal horns and bodies of the lateral ventricles.

Primary neoplasms, such as **glioblastoma**, **primary CNS lymphoma**, and **germinoma**, can spread along the ventricular ependyma. Rarely, **metastases** from an extracranial neoplasm can cause irregular ependymal thickening and enhancement.

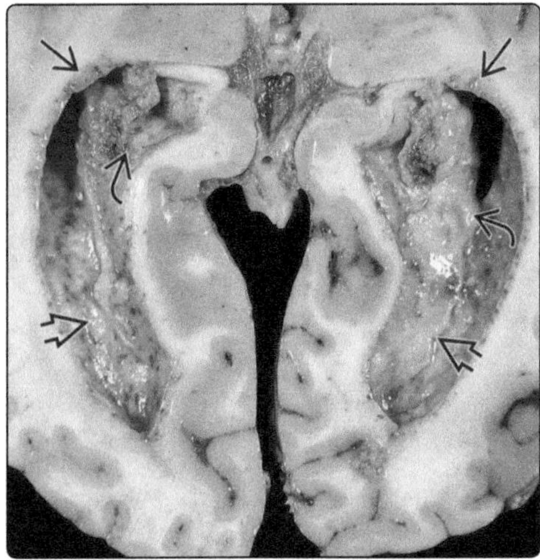

***(12-26)** Autopsy of IVRBA shows ependymal infection ➡, choroid plexitis ➡, pus adhering to ventricular walls ➡. (Courtesy R. Hewlett, MD.)*

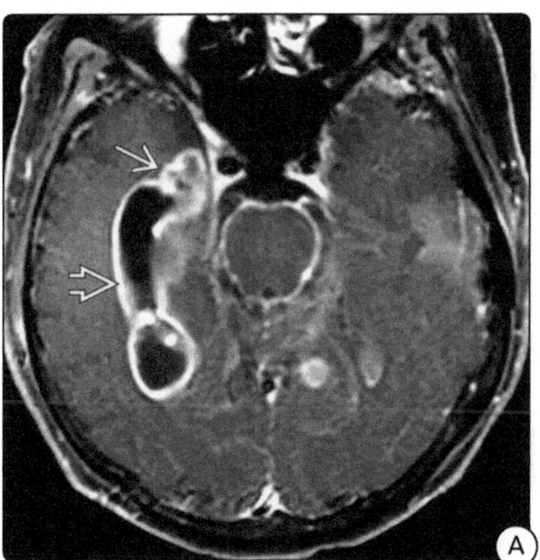

***(12-27A)** Axial T1 C+ FS MR shows meningitis and an abscess ➡ with intraventricular rupture (ventriculitis) ➡.*

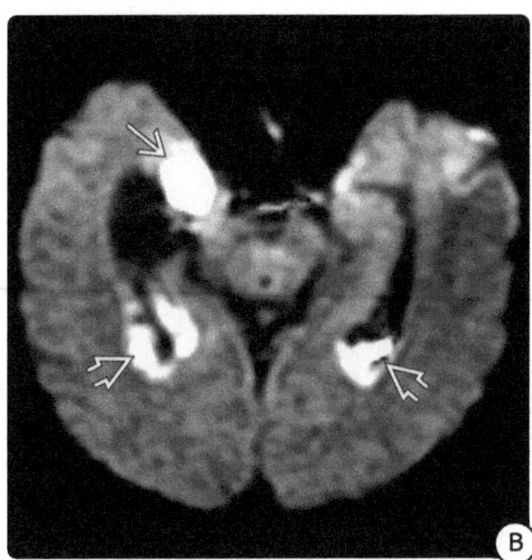

***(12-27B)** DWI MR in the same patient shows that the abscess viscous contents ➡ and ventricular purulent debris ➡ restrict.*

(12-28) Purulent frontal sinusitis ➡ with extension into epidural space causes epidural empyema ⇨ and frontal lobe cerebritis ➡.

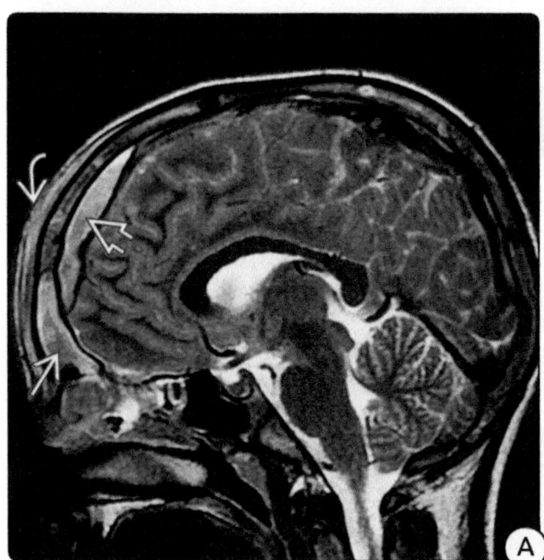

(12-29A) Sagittal T2 MR is from a child with frontal sinusitis ➡ causing scalp cellulitis ➡ and epidural empyema ➡.

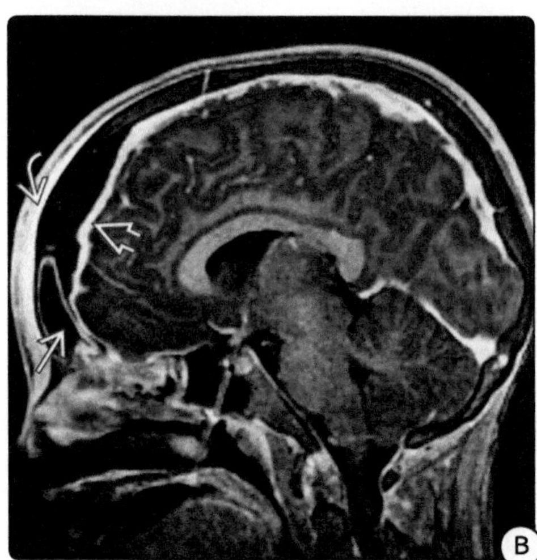

(12-29B) T1 C+ MR shows the frontal sinusitis ➡, cellulitis ➡, and enhancing endosteal dura ➡ displaced by the epidural empyema.

Empyemas

Extraaxial infections of the CNS are rare but potentially life-threatening conditions. Early diagnosis and prompt treatment are essential to maximize neurologic recovery.

Terminology

Empyemas are pus collections that can occur in either the subdural or epidural space.

Etiology

Empyemas in infants and young children are most commonly secondary to bacterial meningitis. In older children and adults, over 2/3 occur as an extension of infection from paranasal sinus disease, while 20% are secondary to otomastoiditis. Rare causes include penetrating head trauma, neurosurgical procedures, or hematogenous spread of pathogens from a distant extracranial site.

Pathology

Empyemas are extraaxial pus collections **(12-28)**. Subdural empyemas (SDEs) are much more common than epidural empyemas (EDEs). Empyemas range from small, focal epidural collections to extensive subdural infections that spread over most of the cerebral hemisphere and extend into the interhemispheric fissure. The most common locations are the frontal and frontoparietal convexities.

Clinical Issues

Presentation. Empyemas can occur at any age. The most common clinical presentation is headache followed by fever. Preceding symptoms of sinusitis or otomastoiditis are common. Meningismus, seizures, and focal motor signs are also frequent.

"Pott puffy tumor"—a fluctuant ("doughy"), tender erythematous swelling of the frontal scalp—is considered a specific sign for frontal bone osteomyelitis with a subperiosteal abscess. Most occur in the setting of untreated frontal sinusitis that breaches the posterior table of the sinus.

Natural History. Untreated empyemas can spread quite rapidly, extending from the extraaxial spaces into the subjacent brain. Besides cerebritis and abscess formation, the other major complication of empyema is cortical vein thrombosis with venous ischemia.

Imaging

Imaging is essential to the early diagnosis of empyema. NECT scans may be normal or show a hypodense extraaxial collection **(12-30A)** that demonstrates peripheral enhancement on CECT. Bone CT should be evaluated for signs of sinusitis and otomastoiditis.

MR is the procedure of choice for evaluating potential empyemas. T1 scans show an extraaxial collection that is mildly hyperintense relative to CSF. SDEs are typically crescentic and lie over the cerebral hemisphere. The extracerebral space is widened, and the underlying sulci are compressed by the collection. SDEs often extend into the interhemispheric fissure but do not cross the midline.

EDEs are biconvex and usually more focal than SDEs. The inwardly displaced dura can sometimes be identified as a thin hypointense line between the epidural collection and the underlying brain **(12-29A)**. In contrast to SDEs, frontal EDEs may cross the midline, confirming their epidural location.

Empyemas are iso- to hyperintense compared with CSF on T2WI and are hyperintense on FLAIR **(12-30B)**. Hyperintensity in the underlying brain parenchyma may be caused by cerebritis or ischemia (either venous or arterial).

SDEs typically demonstrate striking diffusion restriction on DWI **(12-30C)**. EDEs are variable but usually have at least some restricting component.

Empyemas show variable enhancement depending on the amount of granulomatous tissue and inflammation present **(12-29B)**. The encapsulating membranes, especially on the outer margin, enhance moderately strongly **(12-29B)**.

Differential Diagnosis

The major differential diagnosis of extraaxial empyema is a nonpurulent extraaxial collection, such as subdural effusion, subdural hygroma, and chronic subdural hematoma.

A **subdural effusion** is usually postmeningitic, typically bilateral, and does not restrict on DWI. Because of its increased proteinaceous contents, effusions are typically hyperintense to CSF on FLAIR.

A **subdural hygroma** is a sterile, nonenhancing, nonrestricting CSF collection that occurs with a tear in the arachnoid, allowing escape of CSF into the subdural space. Hygromas are usually posttraumatic or postsurgical and behave exactly like CSF on imaging studies.

A **chronic subdural hematoma** (cSDH) is hypodense on NECT. Signal intensity varies with chronicity. Early cSDHs are hyperintense compared with CSF on both T1WI and T2/FLAIR. They may show some residual blood that "blooms" on T2* (GRE, SWI). The encapsulating membranes enhance and may show diffusion restriction. In contrast to SDEs, the cSDH contents themselves typically do not restrict on DWI. Very longstanding cSDHs look similar to CSF and may show little or no residual evidence of prior hemorrhage.

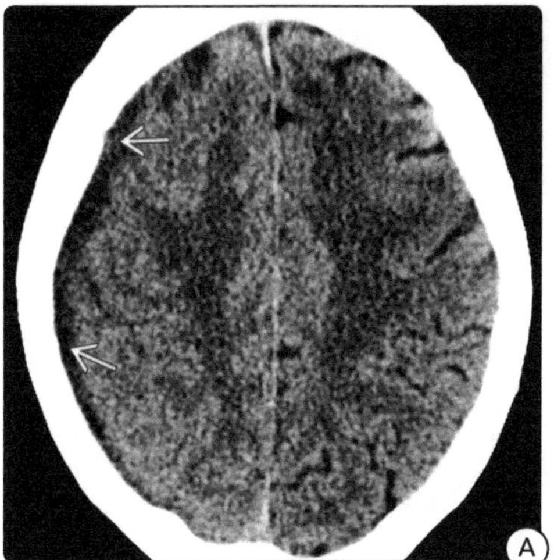

(12-30A) NECT in a patient with sinusitis shows hypodense subdural fluid ➡ that is slightly hyperattenuating compared with sulcal CSF.

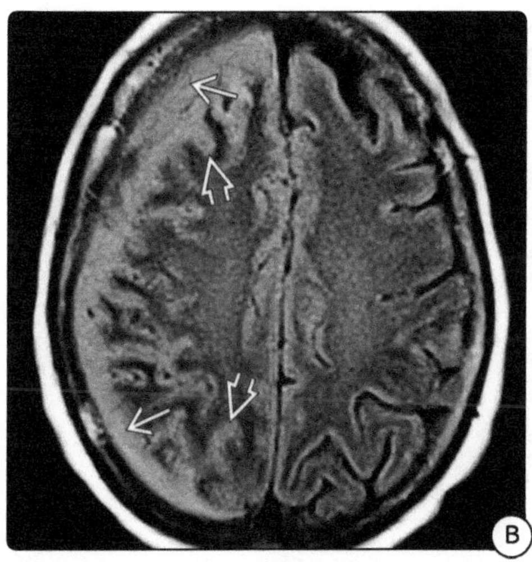

(12-30B) Fluid collection ➡ does not suppress on FLAIR MR. Underlying sulci are hyperintense, suggesting meningitis. Note cortical edema ➡.

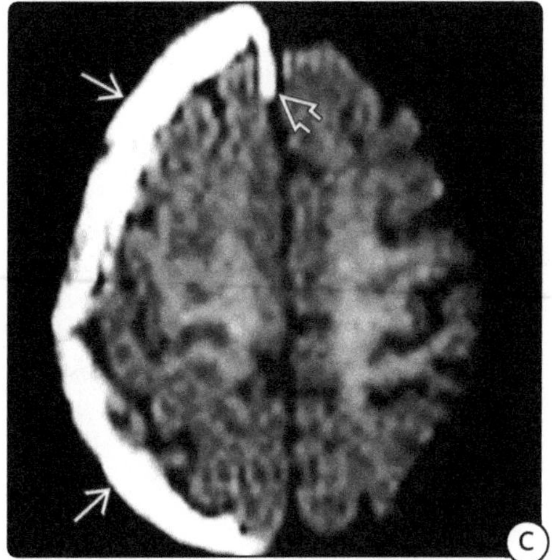

(12-30C) DWI MR shows that SDE ➡ restricts. Interhemispheric extension ➡ does not cross the midline. Streptococcus pneumoniae was cultured.

EMPYEMAS

Pathology
- Subdural empyemas (SDEs) > > epidural empyemas (EDEs)
- EDE focal (usually next to sinus, mastoid)
- SDE spreads diffusely along hemispheres, tentorium/falx

Imaging
- Bone CT: Look for sinus, ear infection
- EDE is focal, biconvex; can cross midline
- SDE is crescentic, covers hemisphere, may extend into interhemispheric fissure
- SDEs restrict strongly on DWI; EDEs variable

Differential Diagnosis
- Chronic SDH, subdural hygroma, effusion

Acquired Viral Infections

A number of both familiar and less well-known but emerging viruses can cause CNS infections. In this section, we focus on neurotropic herpesvirus infections, which can promote acute fulminant CNS disease and become latent with the potential of reactivation that may last for decades.

Eight members of the herpesvirus family are known to cause disease in humans. These are herpes simplex virus 1 (HSV-1) and HSV-2, varicella-zoster

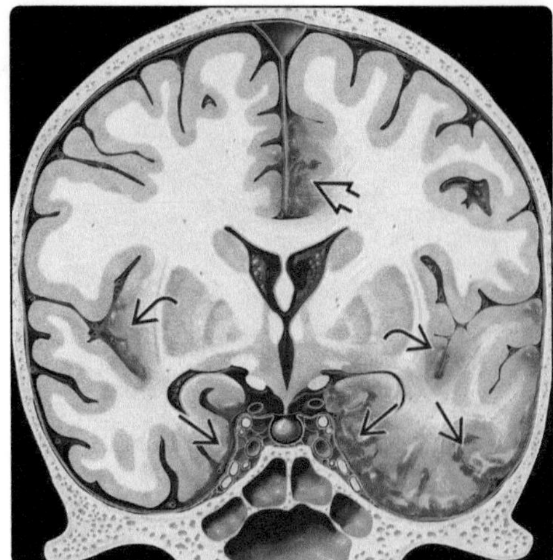

(12-31) Graphic shows herpes encephalitis with bilateral, asymmetric involvement of temporal lobes ➩, cingulate gyri ➩, and insula ➩.

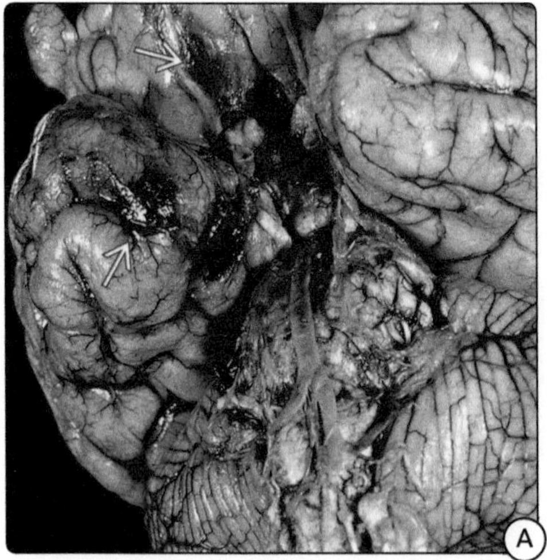

(12-32A) Autopsy of HSE shows hemorrhagic lesions in the basal medial temporal lobes and subfrontal regions ➡. (Courtesy R. Hewlett, MD.)

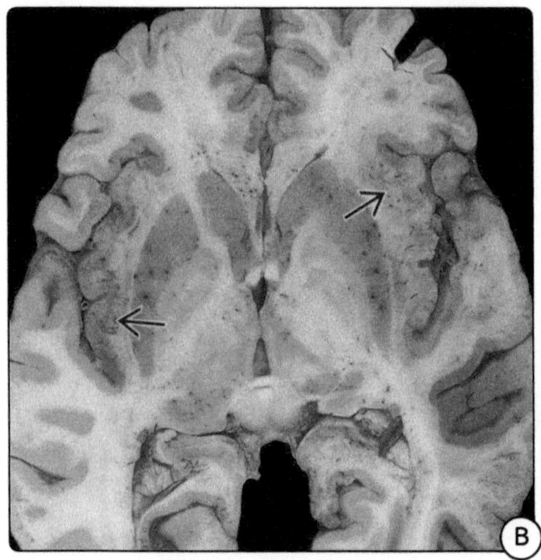

(12-32B) Axial section in the same case shows petechial hemorrhages in insular cortex of both temporal lobes ➩. (Courtesy R. Hewlett, MD.)

virus (VZV), Epstein-Barr virus (EBV), cytomegalovirus (CMV), and human herpesvirus (HHV)-6, HHV-7, and HHV-8. Each has its own disease spectrum, clinical setting, and imaging findings.

Congenital HSV-2 and CMV were both considered earlier, as their manifestations in newborn infants differ from those of acquired herpesvirus infections. HSV-1 and HHV-6 are discussed in this section. VZV and EBV are discussed later in the chapter under "Miscellaneous Acute Viral Encephalitides."

Herpes Simplex Encephalitis

Etiology

After the neonatal period, over 95% of HSE is caused by reactivation of HSV-1, an obligate intracellular pathogen. The virus initially gains entry into cells in the nasopharyngeal mucosa, invades sensory lingual branches of the trigeminal nerve, then passes in retrograde fashion into the trigeminal ganglion. It establishes a lifelong latent infection within sensory neurons of the trigeminal ganglion, where it can remain dormant indefinitely.

Pathology

Location. HSE has a striking affinity for the limbic system **(12-31)**. The anterior and medial temporal lobes, insular cortex, subfrontal area, and cingulate gyri are most frequently affected **(12-32A)**. Bilateral but asymmetric disease is typical **(12-32B)**. Extratemporal, extralimbic involvement occurs but is more common in children compared with adults. When it occurs, extralimbic HSE most often involves the parietal cortex. Brainstem-predominant infection is uncommon. The basal ganglia are usually spared.

Gross Pathology. HSE is a fulminant, hemorrhagic, necrotizing encephalitis. Massive tissue necrosis accompanied by numerous petechial hemorrhages and severe edema is typical. Inflammation and tissue destruction are predominantly cortical but may extend into the subcortical white matter. Advanced cases demonstrate gross temporal lobe rarefaction and cavitation.

Clinical Issues

Epidemiology. HSV-1 is the most common worldwide cause of sporadic (i.e., nonepidemic) viral encephalitis, and HSE may occur at any age. It follows a bimodal age distribution with 1/3 of all cases occurring between the ages of 6 months and 3 years and 1/2 seen in patients older than 50. There is no sex predilection.

Natural History. Typical initial presentation of an HSE is a viral prodrome followed by fever, headache, seizures, and altered mental status. Mortality rates range from 50-70%. Rapid clinical deterioration with coma and death is typical. Nearly 2/3 of survivors have significant neurologic deficits despite antiviral therapy.

HERPES SIMPLEX ENCEPHALITIS (HSE)

Etiology
- > 95% caused by HSV-1

Pathology
- Necrotizing, hemorrhagic encephalitis
- Limbic system
  - Anteromedial temporal lobes, insular cortex
  - Subfrontal region, cingulate gyri

Imaging
- Bilateral > unilateral; asymmetric > symmetric
- FLAIR most sensitive
- DWI shows restriction

Imaging

CT Findings. NECT is often normal early in the disease course. Hypodensity with mild mass effect in one or both temporal lobes and the insula may be present **(12-33A)**. CECT is usually negative, although patchy or gyriform enhancement may develop after 24-48 hours **(12-33C)**.

MR Findings. MR is the imaging procedure of choice. T1 scans show gyral swelling with indistinct gray-white interfaces **(12-34A)**. T2 scans demonstrate cortical/subcortical hyperintensity with relative sparing of the underlying white matter. FLAIR is the most sensitive sequence and may be positive before signal changes are apparent on either T1- or T2WI. Bilateral but asymmetric involvement of the temporal lobes and insula is characteristic of HSE but not always present.

T2* (GRE, SWI) may demonstrate petechial hemorrhages after 24-48 hours. Gyriform T1 shortening, volume loss, and confluent curvilinear "blooming" foci on T2* are seen in the subacute and chronic phases of HSE.

HSE shows restricted diffusion early in the disease course **(12-34B)**, sometimes preceding visible FLAIR abnormalities. Enhancement varies from none (early) to intense gyriform enhancement several days later **(12-34D)**.

Differential Diagnosis

The major differential diagnoses for HSE are neoplasm, acute cerebral ischemia, status epilepticus, other encephalitides (especially HHV-6), and autoimmune/paraneoplastic limbic encephalitis. Primary neoplasms, such as **diffusely infiltrating astrocytoma**, usually involve white matter or white matter plus cortex.

Acute cerebral ischemia-infarction occurs in a typical vascular distribution involving both the cortex and white matter. **Status epilepticus** is usually unilateral and typically involves just the cortex. Postictal edema is transient but generally more widespread, often involving most or all of the hemispheric cortex.

HHV-6 encephalitis usually involves just the medial temporal lobes, but, if extrahippocampal lesions are present, it may be difficult to distinguish from HSE solely on the basis of imaging findings.

Antibody-mediated CNS disorders, such as **limbic encephalitis** and **autoimmune encephalitis**, often have a more protracted, subacute onset and frequently present with altered mental status of unclear etiology. In some cases, imaging findings may be virtually indistinguishable from those of HSE.

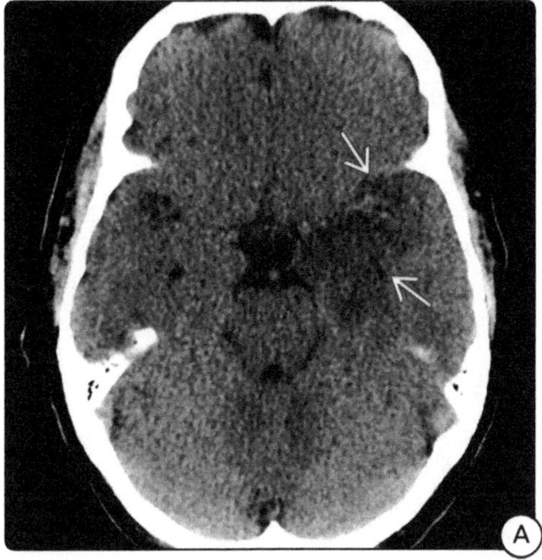

***(12-33A)** NECT in 60-year-old woman w/ altered mental status shows ill-defined, low-attenuation temporal lobe mass ➡, but it was called normal.*

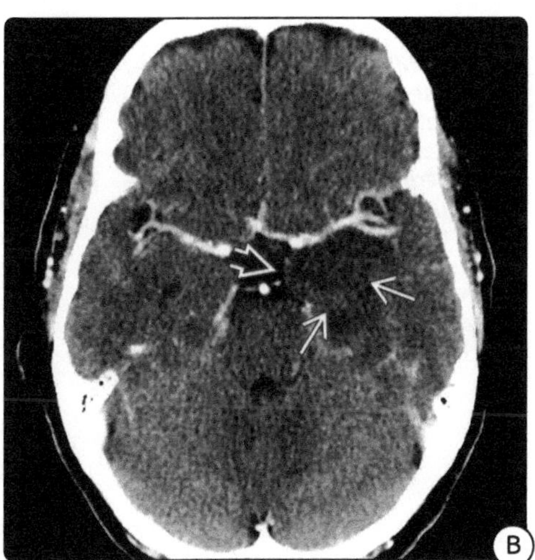

***(12-33B)** CECT in the same case obtained 48 hours later shows a hypoattenuating temporal lobe mass ➡. Note uncal herniation ➡.*

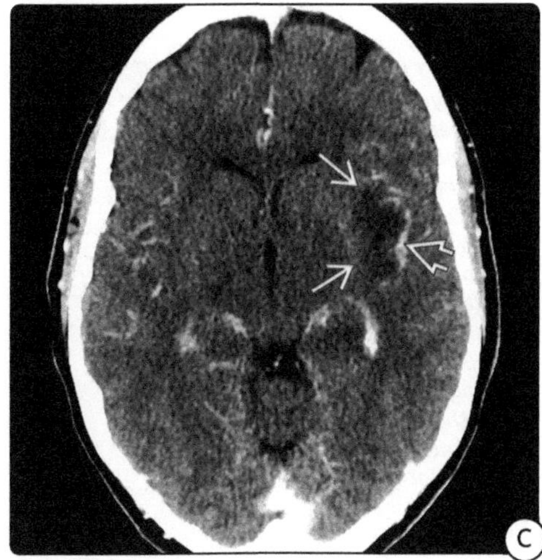

***(12-33C)** More cephalad CECT shows a hypoattenuating insular mass ➡ with superficial gyriform enhancement ➡.*

HHV-6 Encephalopathy

Etiology

More than 90% of the general population is seropositive for HHV-6 by 2 years of age. Most primary infections are asymptomatic, after which the virus remains latent. HHV-6 can become pathogenic in immunocompromised patients, especially those with hematopoietic stem cell or solid organ transplantation.

Imaging

NECT scans are typically normal. MR shows predominant or exclusive involvement of one or both medial temporal lobes (hippocampus and amygdala) **(12-35)**. Extrahippocampal disease is less common than with HSE. Transient hyperintensity of the mesial temporal lobes on T2WI and FLAIR with restriction on DWI is typical. T2* (GRE, SWI) scans show no evidence of hemorrhage.

Differential Diagnosis

The major differential diagnosis is **HSE**. The disease course of HSE is more fulminant. Extratemporal involvement and hemorrhagic necrosis are common in HSE but rare in HHV-6 encephalopathy. In contrast to HSE, in HHV-6, MR abnormalities tend to resolve with time. **Postictal hippocampal hyperemia** is transient, and extrahippocampal involvement is absent.

(12-34A) MR in the same patient shows left temporal lobe hypointensity ⇒ on T1WI (L), hyperintensity ⇒ on FLAIR (R). (12-34B) DWI MR in the same case shows restricted diffusion ⇒ in the anterior temporal lobe cortex (L) and insular cortex (R).

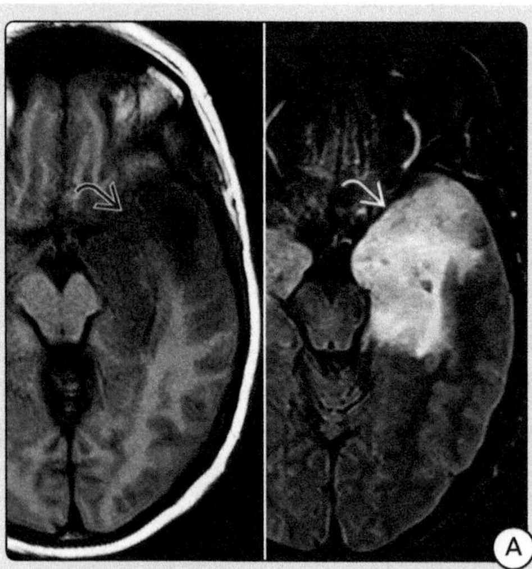

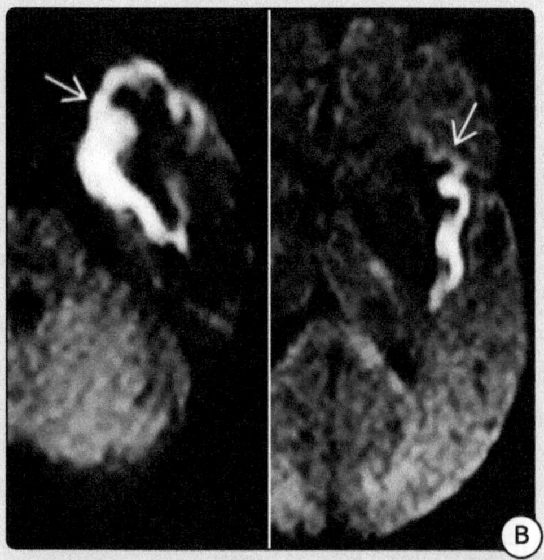

(12-34C) T1 C+ FS MR shows gyriform enhancement in the left insula and low-attenuation edema. (12-34D) Coronal T1 C+ MR shows gyriform cortical enhancement ⇒ but also pial (leptomeningeal) enhancement ⇒. This is PCR-proven HSE meningoencephalitis. Note the ipsilateral ventricular compression and displacement.

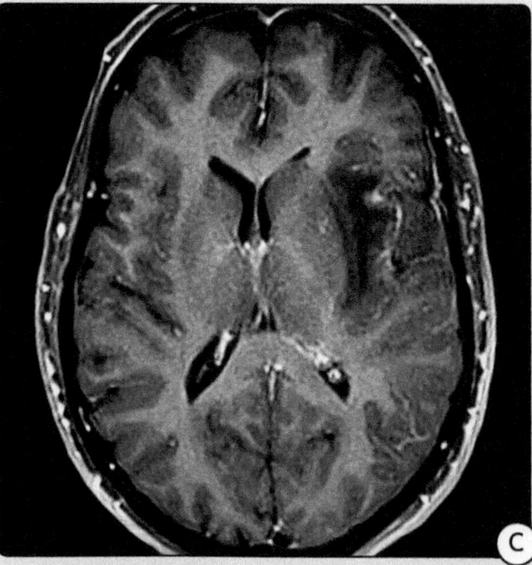

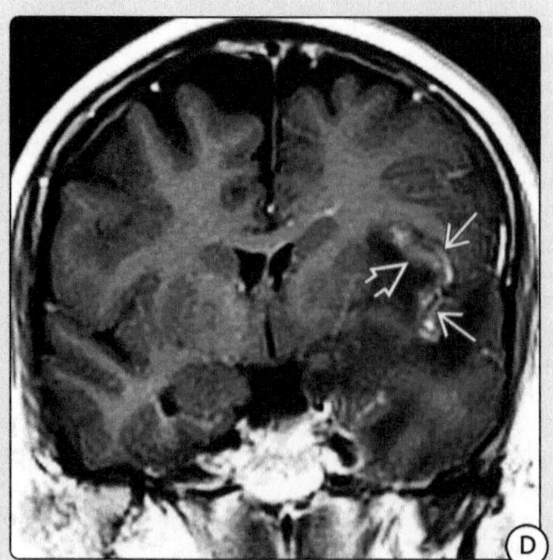

HHV-6 ENCEPHALITIS

Clinical Issues
- Patients often immunocompromised
  - Hematopoietic stem cell, solid organ transplants

Imaging Findings
- Bilateral medial temporal lobes
  - Symmetric > asymmetric involvement
  - Extratemporal lesions less common than in HSE
- T2/FLAIR hyperintense
- Restricts on DWI

Differential Diagnosis
- HSE, limbic encephalitis
- Postictal hyperemia

Miscellaneous Acute Viral Encephalitides

Many viruses can cause encephalitis. Over 100 different viruses in more than a dozen families have been implicated in CNS infection. HSV-1, EBV, mumps, measles, and enteroviruses are responsible for most cases of encephalitis in immunocompetent patients. CSF or serum analysis with pathogen identification by PCR amplification establishes the definitive diagnosis. Nevertheless, imaging is essential to early diagnosis and treatment.

Varicella-Zoster Encephalitis

VZV, which causes chickenpox (varicella) and shingles (zoster), also causes Bell palsy, Ramsay-Hunt syndrome, meningitis, encephalitis, myelitis, Reye syndrome, and postherpetic neuralgia.

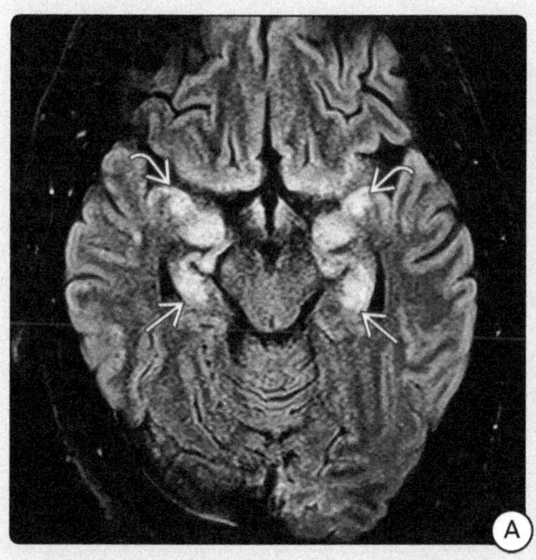

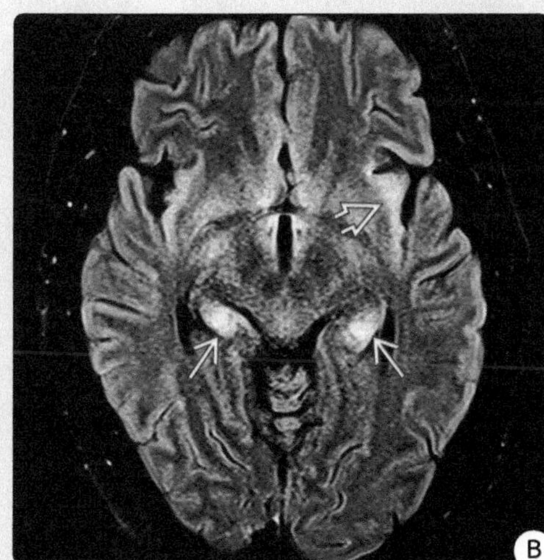

***(12-35A)** Axial FLAIR MR in a 43-year-old man with proven HHV-6 encephalitis shows bilaterally symmetrical hyperintensity in the hippocampi ➡ and anteromedial temporal lobes ➡, including the amygdalae. **(12-35B)** More cephalad FLAIR MR shows involvement of the hippocampal tails ➡ and left insular cortex ➡.*

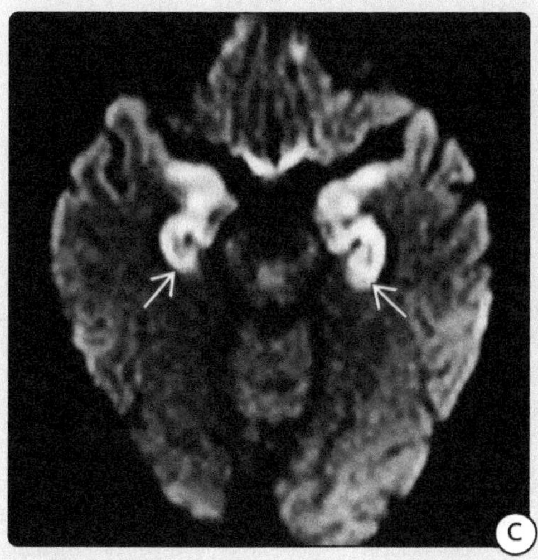

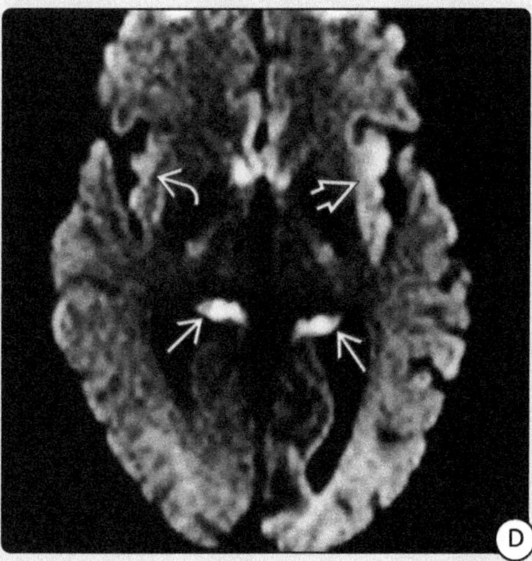

***(12-35C)** DWI MR shows strong, symmetric diffusion restriction ➡ in the hippocampi, medial temporal lobes, and amygdalae. **(12-35D)** DWI MR shows restricted diffusion in the hippocampal tails ➡ and left insular cortex ➡. There is also mild involvement of the right insular cortex ➡. This is variant HHV-6 encephalitis with extrahippocampal involvement.*

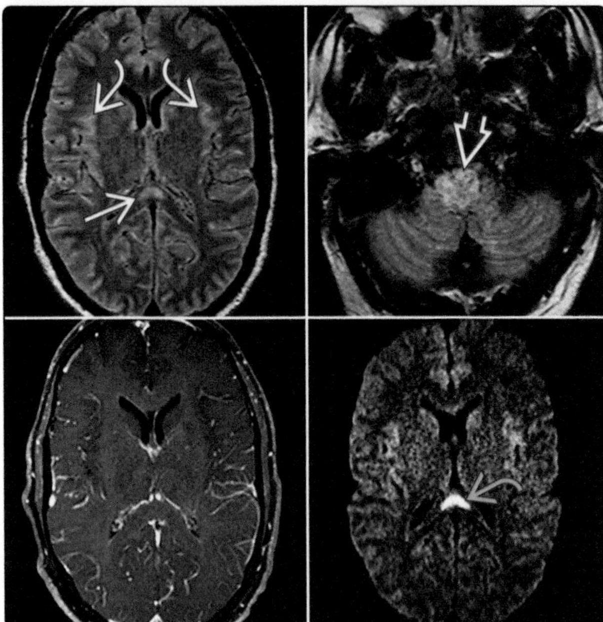

(12-36) FLAIR MR of EBV encephalitis in a 29-year-old man with headache, fever, diplopia, and somnolence shows sulcal hyperintensities ➡, focal lesion in CC splenium ➡, medulla ➡. WM lesions do not enhance; splenium lesion restricts on DWI ➡.

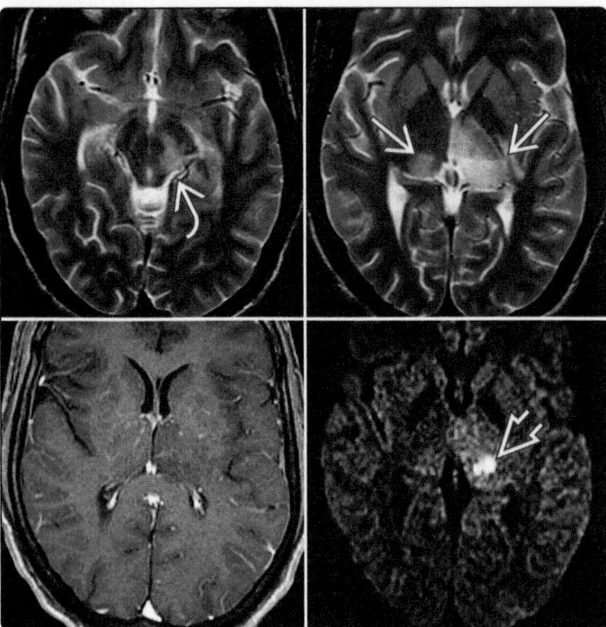

(12-37) Typical findings of West Nile virus (WNV) encephalitis include bilateral but asymmetric nonenhancing lesions in the basal ganglia ➡ and midbrain ➡. DWI may demonstrate restriction ➡.

Meningitis is the most frequent overall manifestation (50% of cases) and the most common clinical presentation in immunocompetent patients (90%). Encephalitis is the second most common CNS presentation (42%) but the most common manifestation in immunodeficient patients (67%). The most common presentation in children is acute cerebellitis with diffuse cerebellar swelling and hyperintensity on T2/FLAIR.

VZV may cause a vasculopathy of both intra- and extracerebral arteries. Ischemic or hemorrhagic strokes, aneurysms, subarachnoid and parenchymal hemorrhages, arterial ectasias, and dissections have all been described.

Epstein-Barr Encephalitis

EBV causes infectious mononucleosis. Neurologic complications occur in < 7% of cases, but occasionally, CNS disease can be the sole manifestation of EBV infection. Bilateral diffuse T2/FLAIR hyperintensities in the basal ganglia and thalami are common. Patchy white matter hyperintensities are seen in some cases. EBV can also cause a transient, reversible lesion of the corpus callosum splenium that demonstrates restricted diffusion **(12-36)**. The differential diagnosis of EBV includes ADEM and other viral infections, especially West Nile virus (WNV).

West Nile Virus Encephalitis

WNV CNS infection can result in meningitis, encephalitis, and acute flaccid paralysis/poliomyelitis. The definitive diagnosis is made by PCR. Bilateral hyperintensities on T2/FLAIR in the basal ganglia, thalami, and brainstem are typical **(12-37)**. WNV may cause a transient corpus callosum splenium lesion. Lesions restrict on DWI but rarely enhance.

Influenza-Associated Encephalopathy

Influenza-associated encephalitis or encephalopathy (IAE) usually affects children younger than 5 years old. Many viruses have been reported as causing IAE, most recently H3N2 and influenza A (H1N1 a.k.a. swine flu). The morbidity and mortality are particularly impressive among patients with trisomy 21.

Imaging studies are abnormal in the majority of cases. Symmetric bilateral thalamic lesions, hemispheric edema, and reversible lesions in the corpus callosum splenium and WM are common. Findings resembling posterior reversible encephalopathy syndrome (PRES) have also been reported.

Miscellaneous Infectious Viral Encephalitides

A host of other viral encephalitides have been identified. While some (such as rotavirus encephalitis) are widespread, others (e.g., Japanese encephalitis, LaCrosse encephalitis, Nipah virus encephalitis) currently have a more restricted geographic distribution.

Arthropod-borne (ticks and mosquitoes) viruses represent an underappreciated cause of encephalitis in older pediatric patients and adults. Most of these viruses are from the Flaviviridae family. MR demonstrates T2-hyperintense lesions of the thalami, substantial nigra, basal ganglia, brainstem, cerebellum, and cerebral cortical and hemispheric WM.

Selected References: The complete reference list is available on the Expert Consult™ eBook version included with purchase.

Tuberculosis and Fungal, Parasitic, and Other Infections

In this chapter, we continue the delineation of acquired infections that we began in Chapter 12 with pyogenic and viral CNS infections.

We first turn our attention to mycobacterial infections, focusing primarily on tuberculosis followed by a brief discussion of fungal and parasitic infections. We close the chapter with a brief consideration of miscellaneous and emerging CNS infections to remind us that the "hot zone" is right outside our windows, no matter where we live!

Mycobacterial Infections

Mycobacteria are small, rod-shaped, acid-fast bacilli that are divided into three main groups, each with a different signature disease: (1) *Mycobacterium tuberculosis* (tuberculosis), (2) nontuberculous mycobacteria ("atypical" mycobacterial spectrum infections), and (3) *Mycobacterium leprae* (leprosy). *M. tuberculosis* causes > 98% of CNS tuberculosis (TB) and is therefore the major focus of our discussion.

Tuberculosis

Etiology

Most TB is caused by *M. tuberculosis*. Human-to-human transmission is typical. Animal-to-human transmission via *Mycobacterium bovis*, a common pathogen in the past, is now rarely encountered. Neurotuberculosis is secondary to hematogeneous spread from extracranial infection, most frequently in the lungs.

Pathology

CNS TB has several distinct pathologic manifestations. Acute/subacute TB **meningitis** (TBM) constitutes 70-80% of cases. An inflammatory reaction ("exudate") with a variable admixture of exudative, proliferative, and necrotizing components in subarachnoid cisterns is typical finding **(13-1)**.

The second most common manifestation of neurotuberculosis is a focal parenchymal infection with central caseating necrosis (TB granuloma or **tuberculoma**). True CNS abscesses are rare. TB **pseudoabscess** is found in 20% of TB patients coinfected with HIV.

Location. TBM has a striking predilection for the basal cisterns, although exudates in superficial convexity sulci do occur. Most tuberculomas occur in cerebral hemispheres, especially frontal and parietal lobes and basal ganglia.

Size and Number. Tuberculomas vary in size. The majority are small (< 2.5 cm), and the "miliary" nodules are often just a few millimeters in diameter. "Giant" tuberculomas can reach 4-6 cm.

Tuberculomas also vary in number, ranging from a solitary lesion to innumerable small "miliary" lesions.

Gross Pathology. TBM is a dense exudate that coats the brain surfaces and cranial nerves **(13-2)**. The suprasellar/chiasmatic region, ambient cisterns, and interpeduncular fossa are most commonly involved **(13-3)**. **Tuberculomas** with "caseating" necrosis have a creamy (cheese-like) necrotic center surrounded by a grayish granulomatous rim **(13-4)**.

Clinical Issues

Demographics. TB is endemic in many developing countries and reemerging in developed countries because of widespread immigration and HIV/AIDS.

CNS TB occurs in both immunocompetent and immunocompromised patients. Among people with latent TB infection, HIV is the strongest known risk factor for progression to active TB. In TB and HIV/AIDS coinfection, each disease also greatly amplifies the lethality of the other.

CNS TB occurs at all ages, but 60-70% of cases occur during the first two decades. There is no sex predilection.

Presentation. The most common manifestation of active CNS TB is meningitis (TBM). Presentation varies from fever and headache with mild meningismus to confusion, lethargy, seizures, and coma. Symptoms of increased intracranial pressure and cranial neuropathies are common.

Focal neurologic deficits may occur; **one of the most common "brain tumors" in endemic countries is tuberculoma, which accounts for 10-30% of all CNS mass lesions.**

Natural History and Treatment. Prognosis depends on the patient's immune status as well as treatment. Untreated TB can be fatal in 4-8 weeks. Even with treatment, 1/3 of patients

(13-1) Coronal graphic shows basilar TB meningitis (TBM) ➾ and tuberculomas ➙, which often coexist. Note the vessel irregularity ➾ and early basal ganglia ischemia related to arteritis. (13-2) Autopsy case shows typical findings of TBM with dense exudates extending throughout the basal cisterns ➙. Gross appearance is indistinguishable from that of pyogenic meningitis. (Courtesy R. Hewlett, MD.)

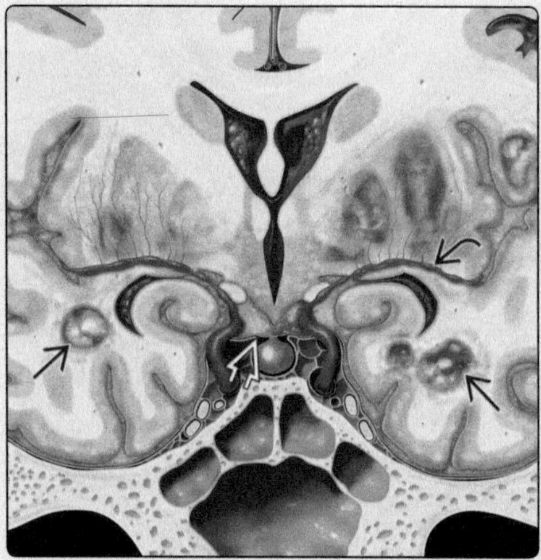

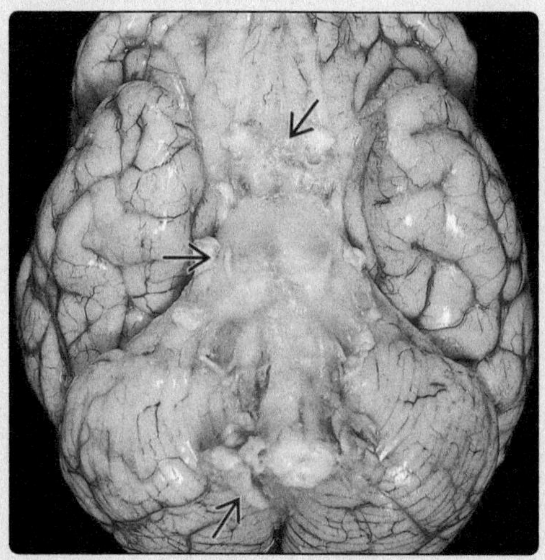

(13-3) Axial section through the suprasellar cistern in another autopsied case of TBM shows thick exudate ➙ filling the suprasellar cistern and coating the pons. Note the extremely small diameter of the supraclinoid internal carotid arteries ➾ due to TB vasculitis. (Courtesy R. Hewlett, MD.) (13-4) Surgically resected TB gumma shows the solid "cheesy" appearance of a caseating granuloma. (Courtesy R. Hewlett, MD.)

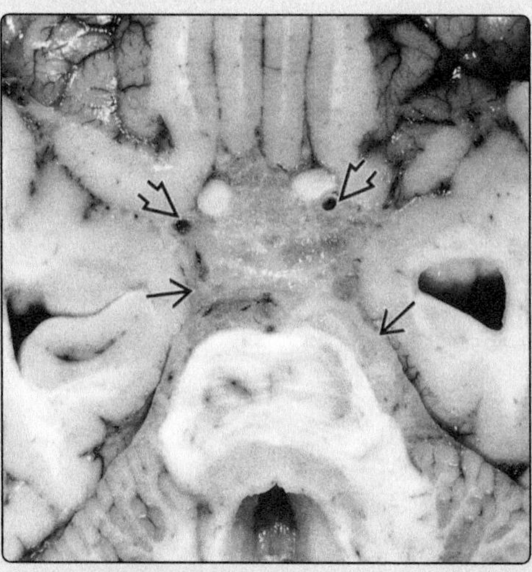

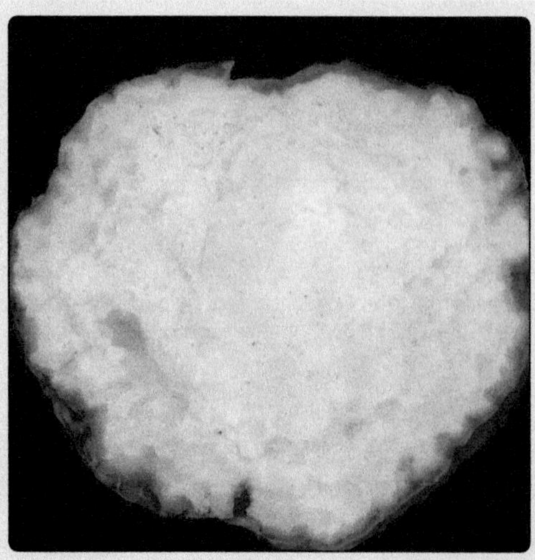

deteriorate within six weeks. Overall mortality is 25-30% and is even higher in drug-resistant TB.

Multidrug-resistant TB (MDR TB) is resistant to at least two of the first-line anti-TB drugs (isoniazid and rifampin). **Extensively drug-resistant TB (XDR TB)** is defined as TB that is resistant to first-line drugs, any fluoroquinolone, and at least one of three injectable second-line drugs (i.e., amikacin, kanamycin, or capreomycin).

Common complications of CNS TB include hydrocephalus (70%) and stroke (up to 40%).

CNS TB: ETIOLOGY, PATHOLOGY, AND CLINICAL ISSUES

Etiology

- Most caused by *Mycobacterium tuberculosis*
- Hematogeneous spread from extracranial site (e.g., lung)

Pathology

- TB meningitis (70-80%)
  - Basal cisterns > convexity sulci
- Tuberculoma (TB granuloma) (20-30%)
  - Caseating necrosis (hemispheres, basal ganglia)

Clinical Issues

- All ages, but 60-70% in children < 20 years
- 10-30% of brain parenchymal masses in endemic areas!
- Overall mortality: 25-30% (worse with MDR/XDR TB)

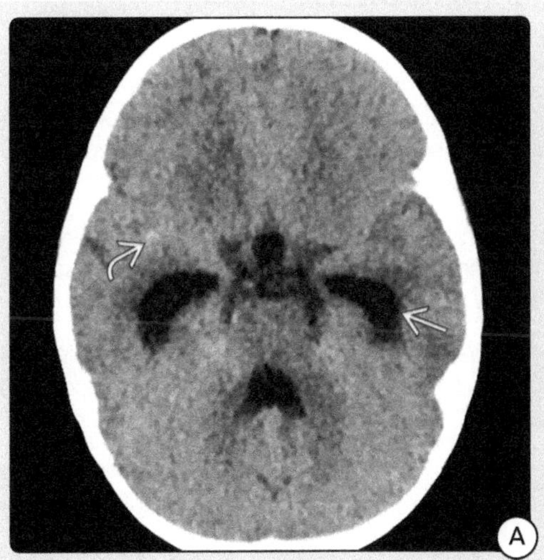

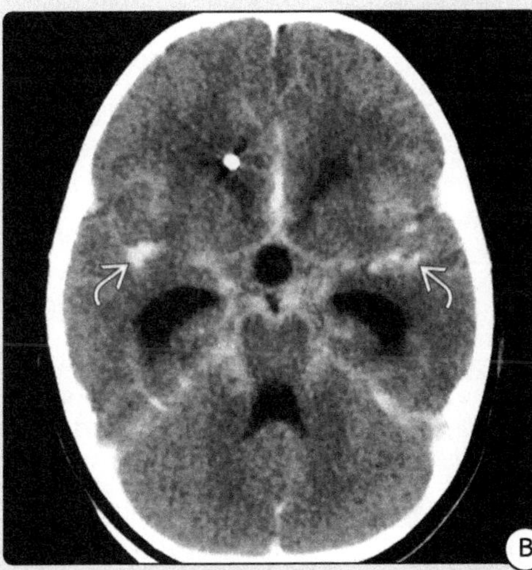

***(13-5A)** NECT in a 6-month-old child with TBM shows acute obstructive hydrocephalus with dilated temporal horns ➡ and effacement of the sylvian fissures with slightly hyperdense exudate ➡. **(13-5B)** CECT in the same case shows thick enhancing exudates throughout the basilar cisterns but most striking in the sylvian fissures ➡.*

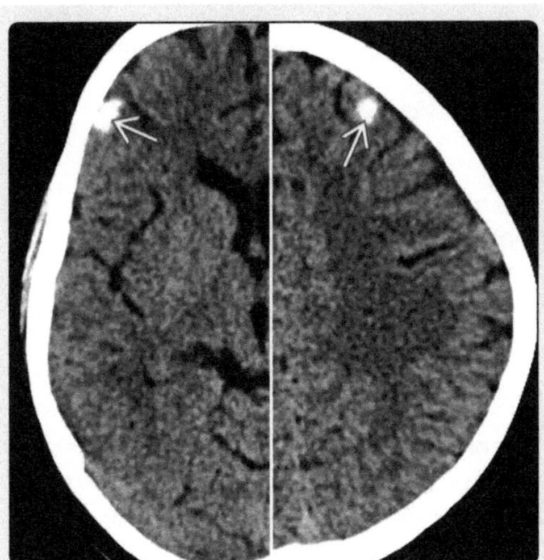

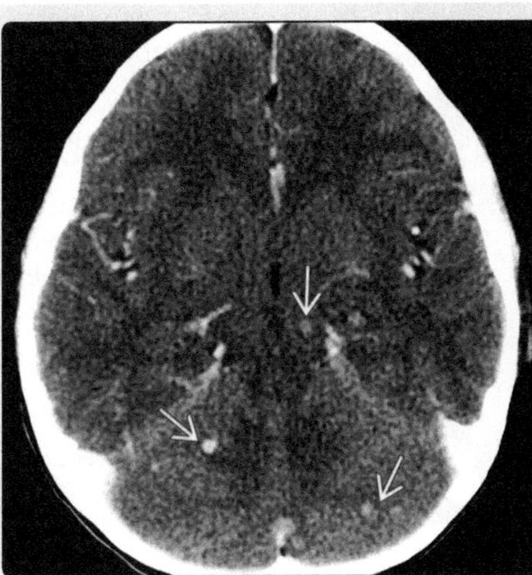

***(13-6)** Two different axial images from a NECT scan in a patient with CNS TB shows 2 calcified healed granulomas ➡. There was no evidence of active TBM. (Courtesy R. Ramakantan, MD.) **(13-7)** CECT scan in a 6-year-old immunocompetent boy shows multiple small punctate-enhancing tuberculomas ➡.*

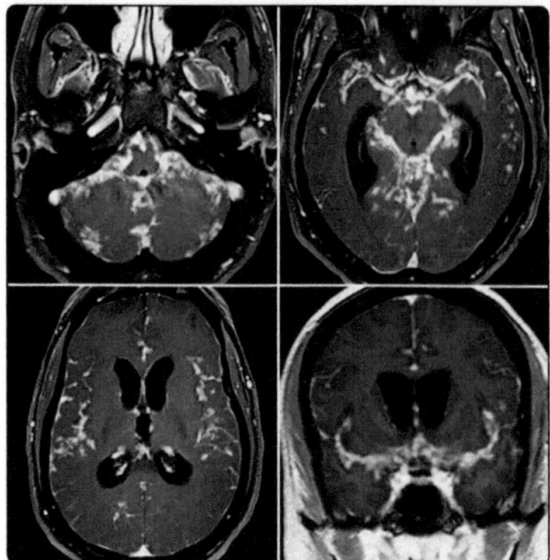

***(13-8)** T1 C+ FS MR scans show TBM with hydrocephalus, enhancing exudate throughout the basal cisterns and subarachnoid spaces.*

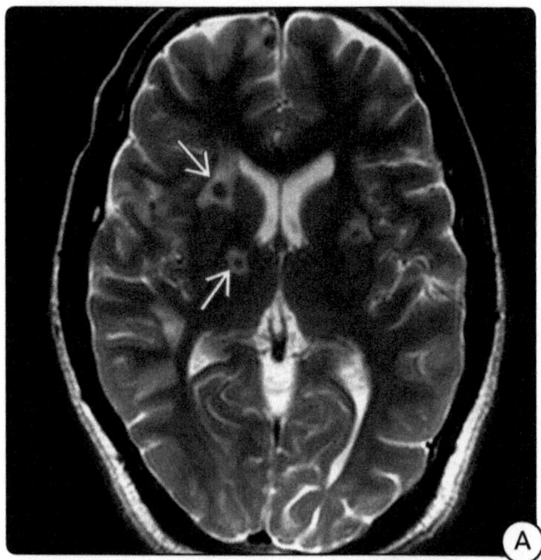

***(13-9A)** T2 MR demonstrates multifocal tuberculomas as hypointense foci surrounded by edema ➡.*

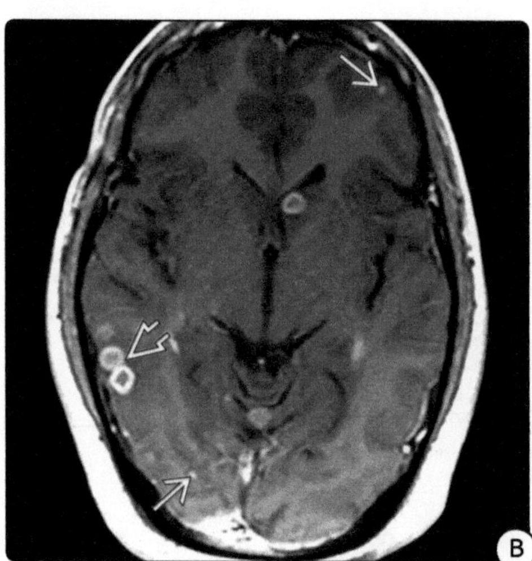

***(13-9B)** T1 C+ MR in the same case illustrates additional lesions with punctate ➡, ring enhancement ➡. (Courtesy R. Ramakantan, MD.)*

Imaging

CT Findings

TB Meningitis. Nonspecific hydrocephalus is the most frequent finding on NECT. "Blurred" ventricular margins indicate extracellular fluid accumulation in the subependymal white matter. As the disease progresses, iso- to mildly hyperdense basilar and sulcal exudates replace and efface the normal hypodense CSF **(13-5A)**. CECT usually shows intense enhancement of the basilar meninges and subarachnoid spaces **(13-5B)**.

Tuberculoma. NECT scans show one or more iso- to slightly hyperdense round, lobulated, or crenated masses with variable perilesional edema. Calcification can be seen in healed granulomas **(13-6)**. CECT scans demonstrate punctate, solid, or ring-like enhancement **(13-7)**.

MR Findings

TB Meningitis. Basilar exudates are isointense with brain on T1WI, giving the appearance of "dirty" CSF. FLAIR scans show increased signal intensity in the sulci and cisterns. Marked linear or nodular meningeal enhancement is seen on T1 C+ FS sequences **(13-8)**. Tuberculous exudates may extend into the brain parenchyma along the perivascular spaces, causing a meningoencephalitis.

Vascular complications occur in 20-50% of cases. The "flow voids" of major arteries may appear irregular or reduced. Penetrating artery infarcts with enhancement and restricted diffusion are common.

Cranial nerve (CN) involvement is seen in 17-40% of cases. The optic nerve and CNs III, IV, and VII are most commonly affected. The affected CNs appear thickened and enhance intensely on postcontrast images.

Tuberculoma. Most TB granulomas are solid caseating, necrotizing lesions that appear hypo- or isointense with brain on T1WI and hypointense on T2WI **(13-9A)**. Liquefied areas may be T2 hyperintense with a hypointense rim and resemble abscess.

Enhancement is variable, ranging from small punctate foci to multiple rim-enhancing lesions. Mild to moderate round or lobulated ring-like enhancement around a nonenhancing center is the most typical pattern **(13-9B)**.

MRS can be very helpful in characterizing tuberculomas and distinguishing them from neoplasm or pyogenic abscess. A large lipid peak with absence of other metabolites, such as amino acids and succinate, is seen in 85-90% of cases.

Differential Diagnosis

The major differential diagnosis of *TBM* is **pyogenic or carcinomatous meningitis**, as their imaging findings can be indistinguishable. **Carcinomatous meningitis** is usually seen in older patients with a known systemic or primary CNS neoplasm.

Neurosarcoidosis can also mimic TBM. Infiltration of the pituitary gland, infundibulum, and hypothalamus is common.

The major differential diagnosis of multiple parenchymal *tuberculomas* is **neurocysticercosis** (NCC). NCC usually shows multiple lesions in different stages of evolution. Tuberculomas can also resemble pyogenic **abscesses** or **neoplasms**. Abscesses restrict on DWI. Tuberculomas have a large lipid peak on MRS and lack the elevated Cho typical of neoplasm.

CNS TUBERCULOSIS: IMAGING AND DIFFERENTIAL DIAGNOSIS

General Features
- Best procedure = contrast-enhanced MR
- Findings vary with pathology
  - Tuberculosis meningitis (TBM)
  - Tuberculoma
  - Abscess
- Combination of findings (usually TBM, tuberculoma)

CT Findings
- TBM
  - Can be normal in early stages!
  - Nonspecific hydrocephalus common
  - "Blurred" ventricular margins
  - Effaced basilar cisterns, sulci
  - Iso-/mildly hyperdense exudates
  - Thick, intense pia-subarachnoid space enhancement
  - Can cause pachymeningopathy with diffuse dura-arachnoid enhancement
  - Look for secondary parenchymal infarcts
- Tuberculoma
  - Iso-/hyperdense parenchymal mass(es)
  - Round, lobulated > irregular margins
  - Variable edema
  - Punctate, solid, or ring enhancement
  - May cause focal enhancing dural mass
  - Chronic; healed may calcify
- Abscess
  - Hypodense mass
  - Perilesional edema usually marked
  - Ring enhancement

MR Findings
- TBM
  - Can be normal
  - "Dirty" CSF on T1WI
  - Hyperintense on FLAIR
  - Linear, nodular pia-subarachnoid space enhancement
  - May extend via perivascular spaces into brain
  - Vasculitis, secondary infarcts common
  - Penetrating arteries > large territorial infarcts
- Tuberculoma
  - Hypo-/isointense with brain on T1WI
  - Most are hypointense on T2WI
  - Rim enhancement
  - Rare = dural-based enhancing mass
  - Large lipid peak on MRS
- Abscess
  - T2/FLAIR hyperintense
  - Striking perilesional edema
  - Rim, multiloculated enhancement

Differential Diagnosis
- TBM
  - Pyogenic, carcinomatous meningitis
  - Neurosarcoid
- Tuberculoma
  - Neurocysticercosis
  - Primary or metastatic neoplasm
  - Pyogenic abscess
  - Dural-based mass can mimic meningioma

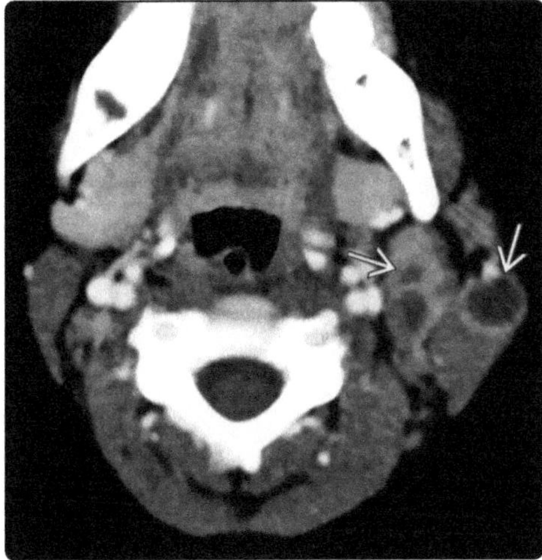

***(13-10)** CECT in a 2y girl shows multiple ring-enhancing lymph nodes ➡ with low-attenuation centers; this is non-TB mycobacterial adenitis.*

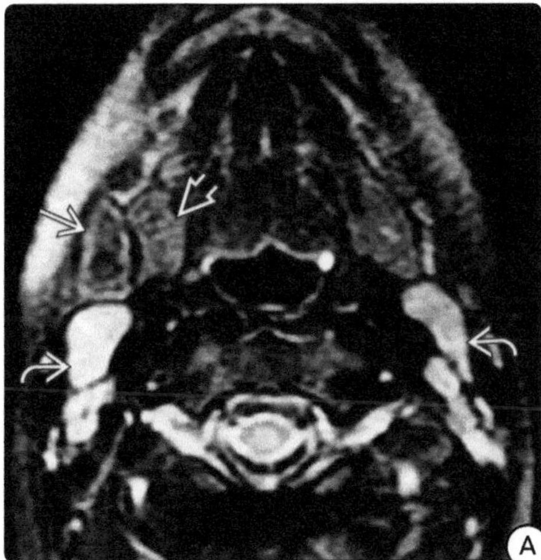

***(13-11A)** T2 FS in a 2y boy shows enlarged lymph nodes ➡, heterogeneous, less hyperintense node ➡ next to right submandibular gland ➡.*

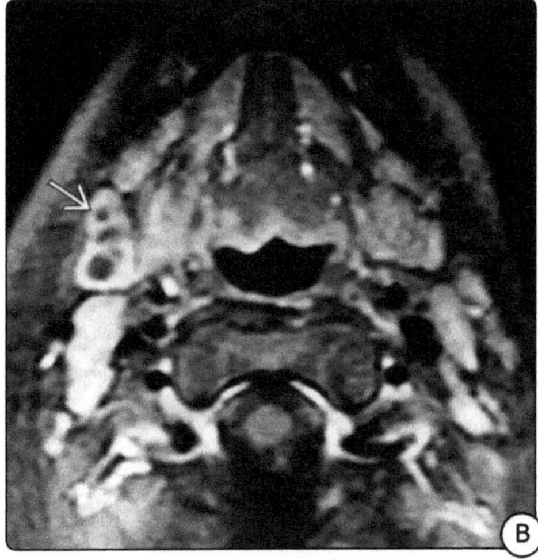

***(13-11B)** T1 C+ FS shows peripheral enhancement in nodal mass ➡. Enlarged level II nodes enhance homogeneously. Non-TB mycobacterial adenitis.*

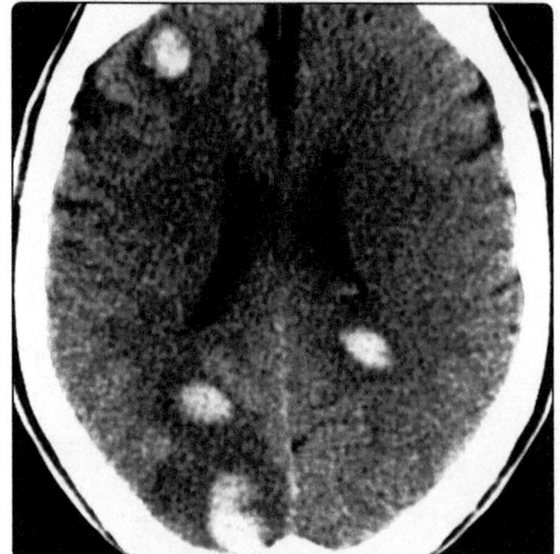

(13-12) NECT scan shows multifocal hemorrhages. Angioinvasive aspergillosis was documented at surgery.

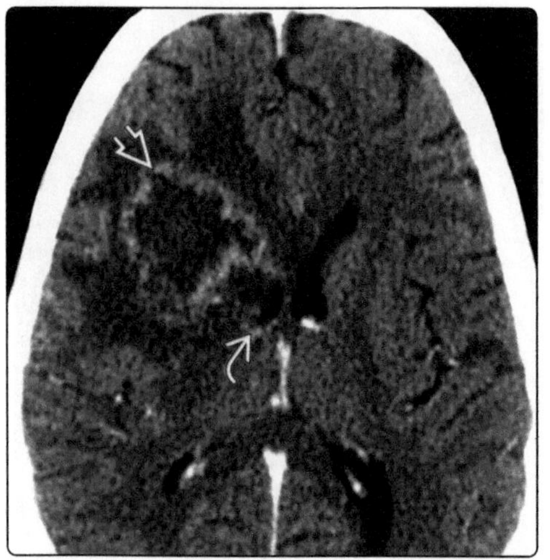

(13-13) CECT scan shows an irregular, crenulated enhancing lesion ➡ with edema, ventriculitis ➡. This is a solitary aspergilloma.

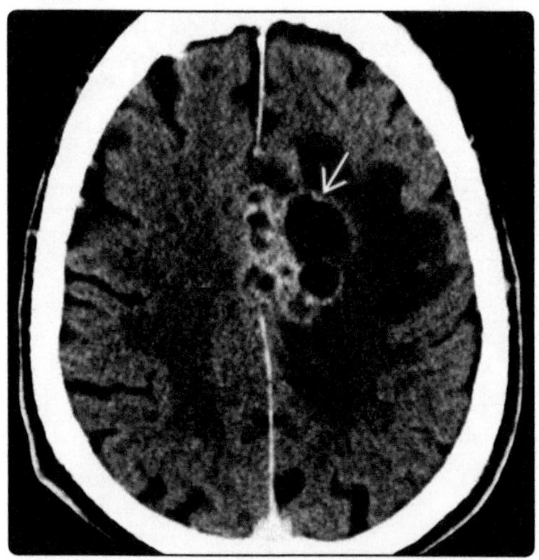

(13-14) CECT shows multiloculated ring-enhancing mass lesion ➡ with edema. Nocardia abscess was found at surgery.

Nontuberculous Mycobacterial Infections

Nontuberculous mycobacteria (NTM) are ubiquitous organisms that are widely distributed in water and soil. The most prevalent NTM capable of causing disease in humans is *Mycobacterium avium* complex. Human disease is usually caused by environmental exposure, not human-to-human spread.

Compared with *M. tuberculosis*, NTM infections are uncommon. The most common manifestation in the head and neck is cervical lymphadenitis, typically occurring in children younger than 5 years old **(13-10)** **(13-11)** and immunocompromised patients.

CNS involvement is rare. When it occurs, it is usually a manifestation of an immune reconstitution inflammatory syndrome (IRIS).

Fungal Infections

Fungi are ubiquitous organisms with worldwide distribution. Most CNS fungal infections are opportunistic, resulting from inhalation of fungal spores and pulmonary infection followed by hematogeneous dissemination. Once uncommon, their prevalence is rising as the number of immunocompromised patients increases worldwide.

Terminology

CNS fungal infections are also called cerebral mycosis. A focal "fungus ball" is also called a mycetoma or fungal granuloma.

Etiology

Fungal Pathogens. The specific agents vary with immune status. Candidiasis, mucormycosis, and cryptococcal infections are usually opportunistic infections. They occur in patients with predisposing factors, such as diabetes, hematologic malignancies, and immunosuppression. Coccidioidomycosis and aspergillosis affect both immunocompetent (often elderly) and immunocompromised patients.

Aside from *Candida albicans* (a normal constituent of human gut flora), most fungal infections are initially acquired by inhaling fungal spores in contaminated dust and soil.

Environmental Exposure. Coccidioidomycosis occurs in areas with low rainfall and high summer temperatures (e.g., Mexico, southwestern United States, some parts of South America), whereas histoplasmosis and blastomycosis occur in watershed areas with moist air and damp, rotting wood (e.g., Africa, around major lakes and river valleys in North America).

Systemic and CNS Infections. Hematogeneous spread from the lungs to the CNS is the most common route of infection, and cryptococcal meningitis is the most common fungal disease of the CNS.

Fungal sinonasal infections may invade the skull base and cavernous sinus directly. Sinonasal disease with intracranial extension (rhinocerebral disease) is the most common pattern of *Aspergillus* and *Mucor* CNS infection.

Disseminated fungal disease usually occurs only in immunocompromised patients.

Pathology

CNS mycoses have four basic pathologic manifestations: Diffuse meningeal disease, solitary or multiple focal parenchymal lesions, disseminated nonfocal parenchymal disease (rare), and focal dura-based masses (rarest).

The most common gross finding is basilar meningitis with congested meninges. Parenchymal fungal infections can be either focal or disseminated. Fungal abscesses are encapsulated lesions with a soft tan or thick mucoid-appearing center, an irregular reddish margin, and surrounding edema. Disseminated disease is less common and causes a fungal cerebritis with diffusely swollen brain.

Hemorrhagic infarcts, typically in the basal ganglia or at the gray matter-white matter junction, are common with angioinvasive fungi. On rare occasions, fungal infections can produce dura-based masses that closely resemble meningioma.

Clinical Issues

Epidemiology. Epidemiology varies with the specific fungus. Many infections are both common and asymptomatic (e.g., ~ 25% of the entire population in the USA and Canada are infected with *Histoplasma*).

Candidiasis is the most common nosocomial fungal infection worldwide. Aspergillosis accounts for 20-30% of fungal brain abscesses and is the most common cerebral complication following bone marrow transplantation. *Mucor* is ubiquitous but generally infects only immunocompromised patients.

Demographics and Presentation. Immunocompetent patients have a bimodal age distribution with fungal infections disproportionately represented in children and older individuals. There is a slight male predominance. Immunocompromised patients of all ages and both sexes are at risk.

Nonspecific symptoms, such as weight loss, fever, malaise, and fatigue, are common. Many patients initially have symptoms of pulmonary infection. CNS involvement is presaged by headache, meningismus, mental status changes, &/or seizure.

Imaging

General Features. Findings vary with the patient's immune status. Well-formed fungal abscesses are seen in immunocompetent patients. Imaging early in the course of a rapidly progressive infection in an immunocompromised patient may show diffuse cerebral edema more characteristic of encephalitis than fungal abscess.

CT Findings. Findings on NECT include hypodense parenchymal lesions caused by focal granulomas or ischemia. Hydrocephalus is common in patients with fungal meningitis. Patients with coccidioidal meningitis may demonstrate thickened, mildly hyperdense basal meninges.

Disseminated parenchymal infection causes diffuse cerebral edema. Multifocal parenchymal hemorrhages are common in patients with angioinvasive fungal species **(13-12)**.

Diffuse meningeal disease demonstrates pia-subarachnoid space enhancement on CECT. Multiple punctate or ring-enhancing parenchymal lesions are typical findings of parenchymal mycetomas **(13-13)** **(13-14)**.

Mycetoma in the paranasal sinuses is usually seen as a single opacified hyperdense sinus that contains fine round to linear calcifications. Fungal sinusitis occasionally becomes invasive, crossing the mucosa to involve blood vessels, bone, orbit, cavernous sinuses, and intracranial cavities. Focal or widespread bone erosion with adjacent soft tissue infiltration can mimic neoplasm. Bone CT with reconstructions in all three standard planes is helpful to assess skull base involvement, and T1 C+ FS MR is the best modality to delineate disease spread beyond the nose and sinuses **(13-17)**.

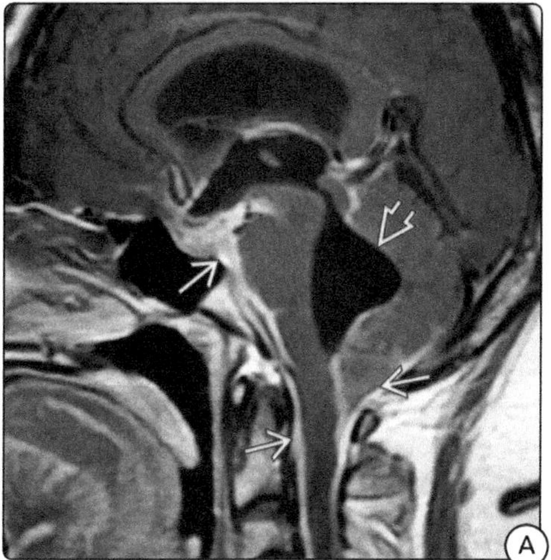

***(13-15A)** Sagittal T1 C+ MR of cocci meningitis shows thick enhancing basilar exudate ➡, obstructive hydrocephalus ➡.*

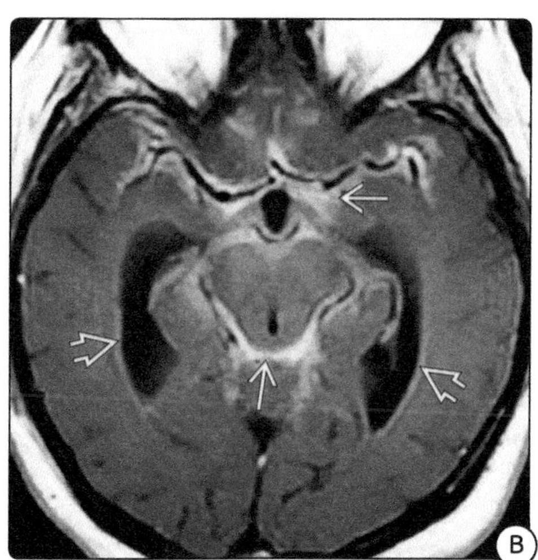

***(13-15B)** Axial T1 C+ MR in the same patient shows extensive enhancement in the basal and ambient cisterns ➡. Note ependymitis ➡.*

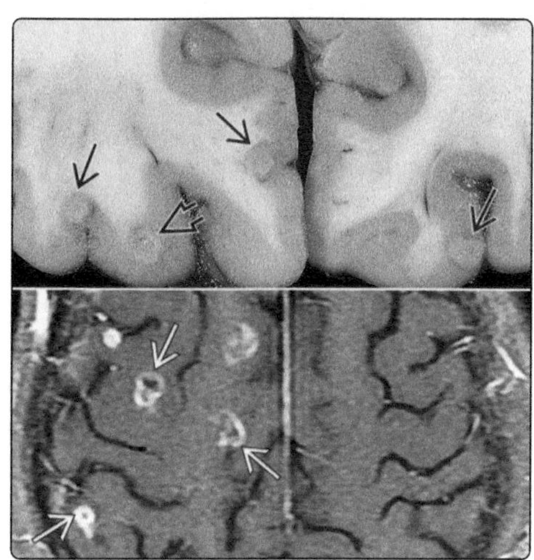

***(13-16)** (Top) Autopsy shows typical solid ➡, necrotic ➡ Nocardia abscesses. (Bottom) Note multiple ring-enhancing ➡ fungal abscesses.*

MR Findings. Fungal meningitis appears as "dirty" CSF on T1WI. Parenchymal lesions are typically hypointense on T1WI but demonstrate T1 shortening if subacute hemorrhage is present. Irregular walls with nonenhancing projections into the cavity are typical.

T2/FLAIR scans in patients with fungal cerebritis show bilateral but asymmetric cortical/subcortical white matter and basal ganglia hyperintensity. Focal lesions (mycetomas) show high-signal foci that typically have a peripheral hypointense rim, surrounded by vasogenic edema. T2* scans may show "blooming" foci caused by hemorrhages or calcification. Focal paranasal sinus and parenchymal mycetomas usually restrict on DWI **(13-17D)**.

T1 C+ FS scans usually show diffuse, thick, enhancing basilar leptomeninges **(13-15)**. Angioinvasive fungi may erode the skull base, cause plaque-like dural thickening, and occlude one or both carotid arteries **(13-18)** **(13-19)**. Parenchymal lesions show punctate, ring-like, or irregular enhancement **(13-16)**.

MRS shows mildly elevated Cho and decreased NAA. A lactate peak is seen in 90% of cases, whereas lipid and amino acids are identified in ~ 50%. Multiple peaks resonating between 3.6 and 3.8 ppm are common and probably represent trehalose.

Differential Diagnosis

The major differential is **pyogenic abscess(es)** and **tuberculoma**. **TB** can appear similar to fungal abscesses on standard imaging studies. Gross hemorrhage is more common with fungal than either pyogenic or tubercular abscesses. Fungal abscesses have more irregularly shaped walls and internal nonenhancing projections. Resonance between 3.6 and 3.8 ppm on MRS is typical.

Other mimics of fungal abscesses are primary **neoplasm** (e.g., glioblastoma with central necrosis) or metastases.

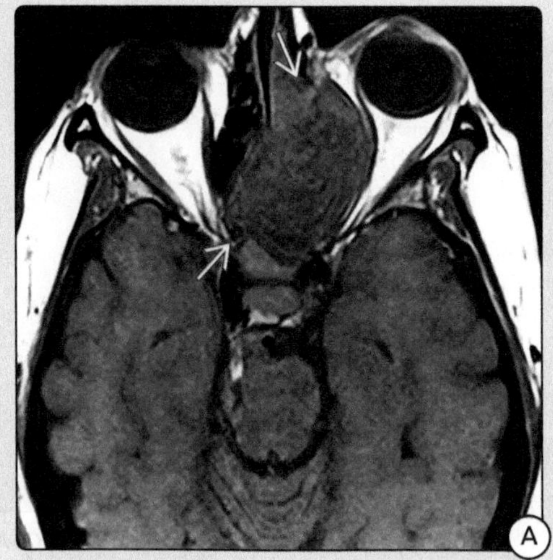

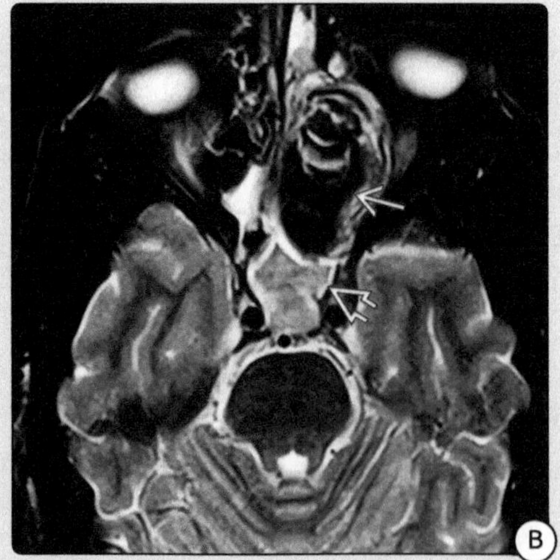

***(13-17A)** Series of images demonstrates a focal sinonasal mycetoma. Axial T1 MR shows an expansile, destructive isointense mass ➡ in the nose and ethmoid sinus. The lesion invades the left orbit and extends posteriorly, obstructing the sphenoid sinus. **(13-17B)** The lesion is of somewhat mixed signal intensity on T2 FS but mostly appears profoundly hypointense ➡. Note obstructive changes in the sphenoid sinus ➡.*

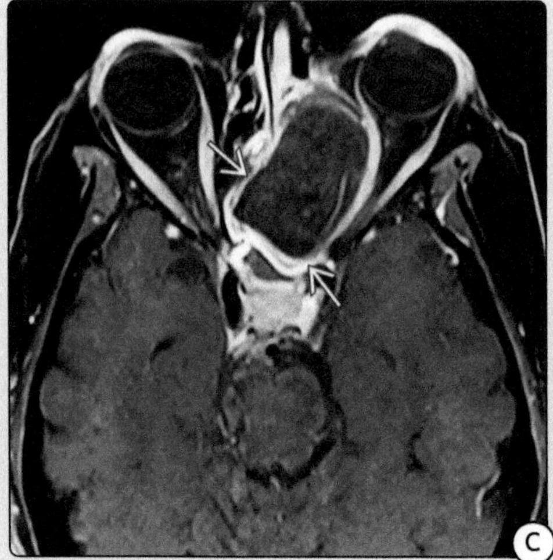

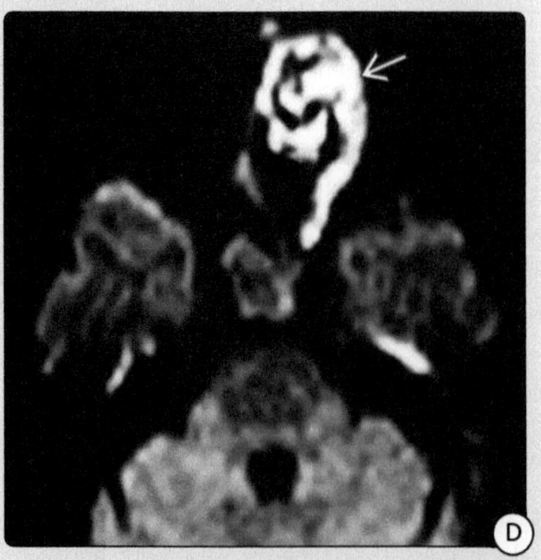

***(13-17C)** T1 C+ FS MR shows peripheral enhancement around the margins of the mass ➡. **(13-17D)** The mass shows diffusion restriction ➡.*

Parasitic Infections

Once considered endemic only in countries with poor sanitation and adverse economic conditions, parasitic diseases have become a global health concern, exacerbated by widespread travel and immigration. With the exception of neurocysticercosis, CNS parasitic diseases are rare.

Neurocysticercosis

Cysticercosis is the most common parasitic infection in the world, and CNS lesions eventually develop in 60-90% of patients with cysticercosis.

Terminology

When cysticercosis infects the CNS, it is termed neurocysticercosis (NCC). A "cysticercus" cyst in the brain is actually the secondary larval form of the parasite. The "scolex" is the head-like part of a tapeworm, bearing hooks and suckers. In the larval form, the scolex is invaginated into one end of the cyst, which is called the "bladder."

Etiology

Most NCC cases are caused by encysted larvae of the pork tapeworm *Taenia solium* and are acquired through fecal-oral contamination. Humans become infected by ingesting *T. solium* eggs. The eggs hatch and release their larvae that then disseminate via the bloodstream to virtually any organ in the body.

Pathology

Location. *T. solium* larvae are most common in the CNS, eyes, muscles, and subcutaneous tissue. The intracranial subarachnoid spaces are the most common CNS site followed by the brain parenchyma and ventricles (fourth > third > lateral ventricles) **(13-20)**. NCC cysts in the depths of sulci may

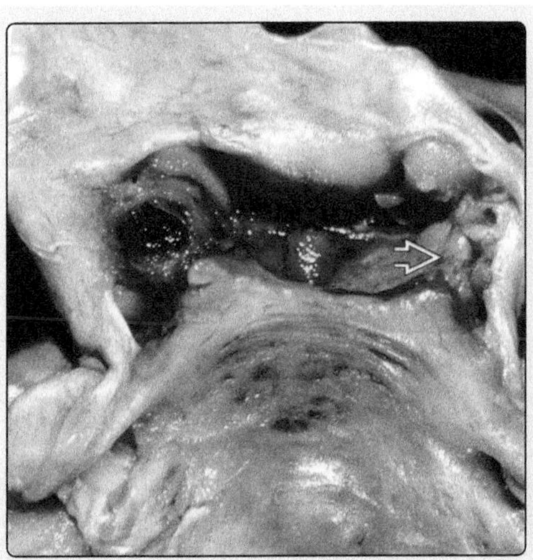

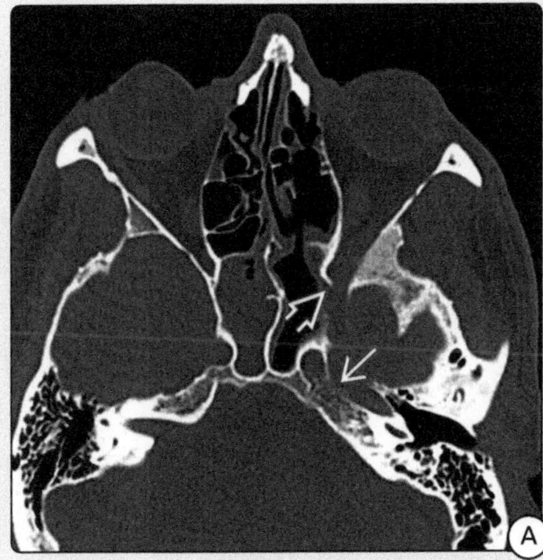

***(13-18)** Close-up view shows autopsied cavernous sinus with invasive fungal sinusitis occluding the left cavernous internal carotid artery ➡. (Courtesy R. Hewlett, MD.) **(13-19A)** Bone CT is of a patient with poorly controlled diabetes and invasive mucormycosis. Note bone invasion, destruction around orbital fissure and sphenoid sinus ➡, left petrous apex ➡.*

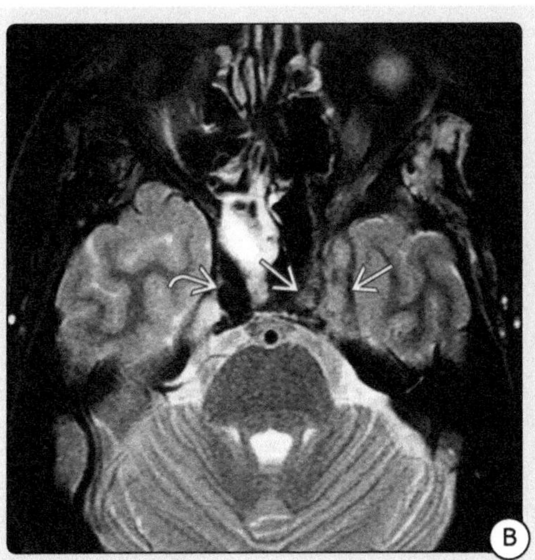

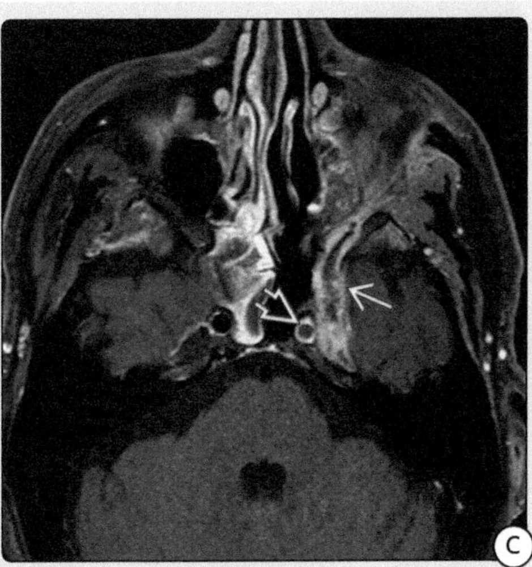

***(13-19B)** Axial T2 FS MR shows normal right cavernous internal carotid artery "flow void" ➡ with left cavernous sinus mass and occluded internal carotid artery ➡. **(13-19C)** T1 C+ FS MR in the same patient shows the left cavernous sinus invasion ➡ and occluded carotid artery ➡.*

incite an intense inflammatory response, effectively "sealing" the sulcus over the cysts and making them appear intraaxial.

Size and Number. Most parenchymal NCC cysts are small (a few millimeters to 1 cm). Occasionally, multiple large NCC cysts up to several centimeters can form in the subarachnoid space (the "racemose" form of NCC that resembles a bunch of grapes). Either solitary (20-50% of cases) or multiple small cysts may occur.

Gross Pathology. Four stages of NCC development and regression are recognized. Patients may have multiple lesions at different stages of evolution.

In the **vesicular stage**, viable larvae (the cysticerci) appear as translucent, thin-walled, fluid-filled cysts with an eccentrically located, whitish, invaginated scolex **(13-21)** **(13-22)**.

In the **colloidal vesicular stage**, the larvae begin to degenerate. The cyst fluid becomes thick and turbid. A striking inflammatory response is incited and characterized by a collection of multinucleated giant cells, macrophages, and neutrophils. A fibrous capsule develops, and perilesional edema becomes prominent.

The **granular nodular stage** represents progressive involution with collapse and retraction of the cyst into a granulomatous nodule that will eventually calcify. Edema persists, but pericystic gliosis is the most common pathologic finding at this stage.

In the **nodular calcified stage**, the entire lesion becomes a fibrocalcified nodule **(13-23)**. No host immune response is present.

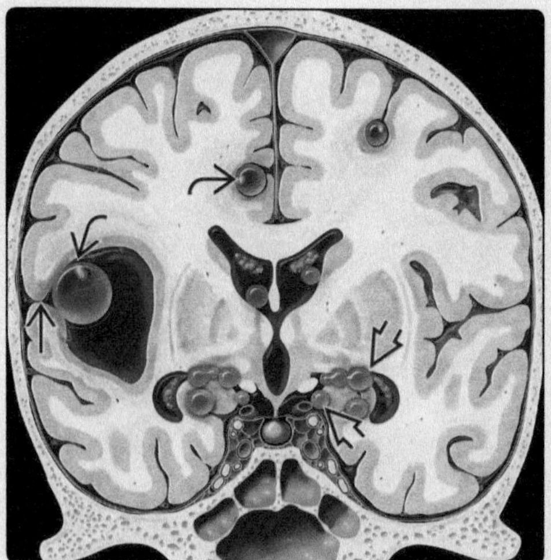

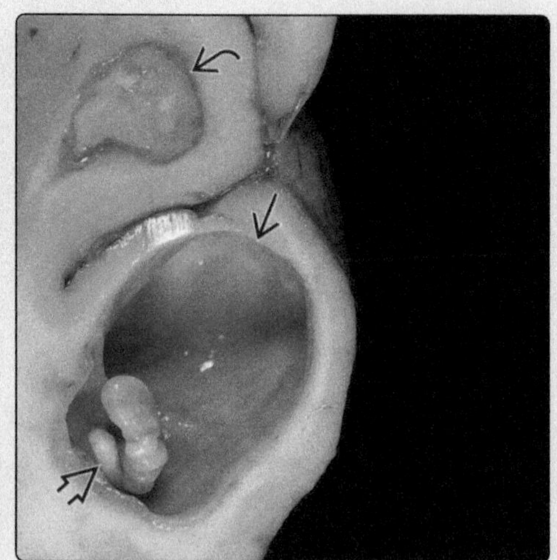

***(13-20)** This is NCC. Convexity cysts have scolex and surrounding inflammation, which, around the largest cyst, "seals" the sulcus, making it appear parenchymal. "Racemose" cysts without scolices are seen in basal cisterns. **(13-21)** NCC in the vesicular stage has a clear fluid-filled cyst and white eccentrically positioned scolex. Note the 2nd granular nodular lesion. (Courtesy R. Hewlett, MD.)*

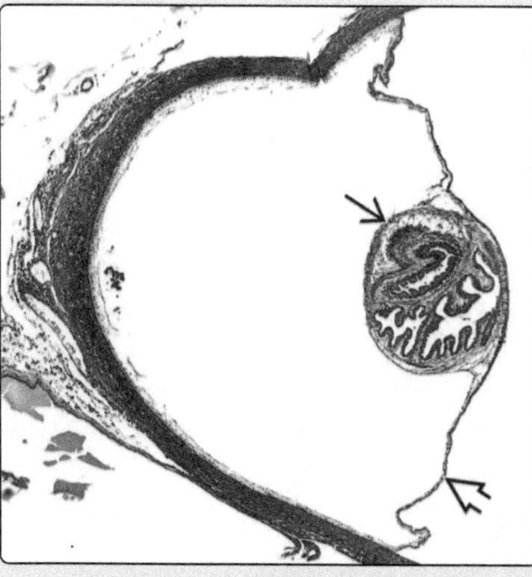

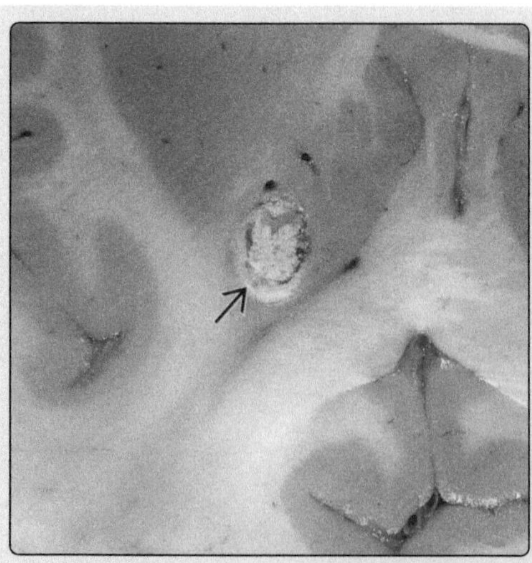

***(13-22)** Low-power photomicrograph of cysticercus shows the invaginated scolex lying within the thin-walled cyst a.k.a. the bladder. (Courtesy B. K. DeMasters, MD.) **(13-23)** Close-up view shows a nodular calcified NCC cyst. Note the lack of inflammation and lack of mass effect. (Courtesy R. Hewlett, MD.)*

NEUROCYSTICERCOSIS: GROSS PATHOLOGY

Location, Size, Number
- Subarachnoid > parenchyma > ventricles
- Usually < 1 cm
  - Subarachnoid ("racemose") cysts can be giant
- Multiple > solitary
  - Can have multiple innumerable tiny ("miliary") cysts

Development Stages
- Vesicular (quiescent, viable larva) = cyst + scolex
- Colloidal vesicular (dying larva)
  - Intense inflammation, edema
- Granular nodular (healing) = cyst involutes, edema ↓
- Nodular calcified (healed)
  - Quiescent, fibrocalcified nodule
  - No edema

Clinical Issues

Epidemiology. In countries where cysticercosis is endemic, calcified NCC granulomas are found in 10-20% of the entire population. Of these, ~ 5% (400,000 out of 75 million) will become symptomatic.

Demographics. NCC occurs at all ages, but peak symptomatic presentation is between 15 and 40 years. There is no sex or race predilection.

Presentation. NCC has a range of clinical manifestations. Signs and symptoms depend on the number and location of larvae, developmental stage, infection duration, and presence or absence of host immune response.

Seizures/epilepsy are the most common symptoms (80%) and are a result of inflammation around degeneration cysts. Headache (35-40%) and focal neurologic deficit (15%) are also

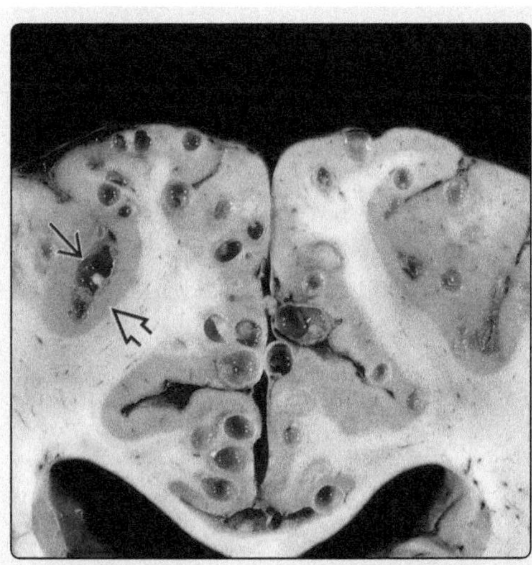

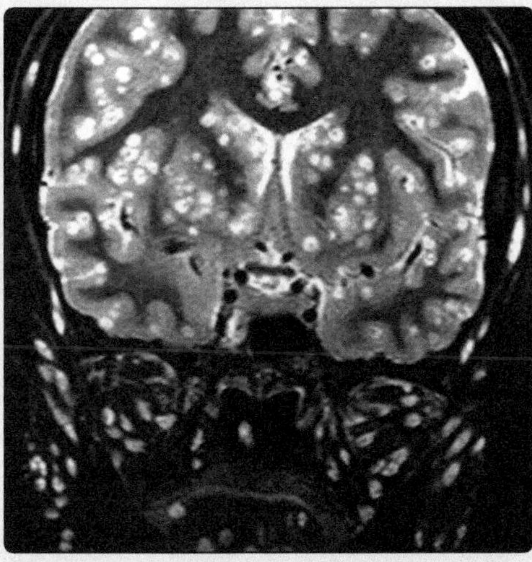

(13-24) Disseminated NCC with many cysts, mostly in the subarachnoid space, shows cyst with scolex in the depth of frontal sulcus ➡ surrounded by cortex ➡, making a subarachnoid cyst appear intraparenchymal. (13-25) T2 MR shows disseminated vesicular NCC with "salt and pepper." Innumerable tiny hyperintense cysticerci with scolices (seen as small black dots inside cysts) are present; perilesional edema is absent.

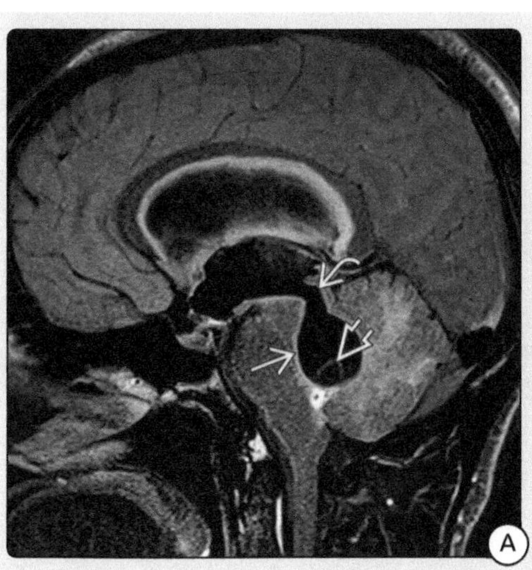

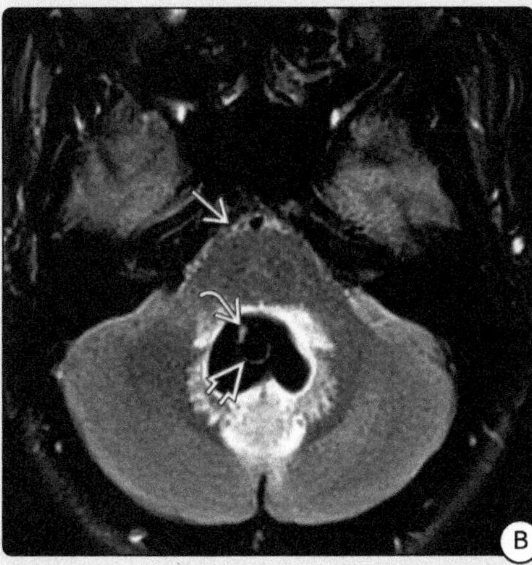

(13-26A) Sagittal FLAIR in a 26-year-old woman w/ headaches shows obstructive hydrocephalus w/ enlargement of lateral, 3rd, & 4th ventricles ➡ as well as aqueduct ➡. A solitary NCC cyst ➡ is visible in the bottom of the 4th ventricle. (13-26B) Axial FLAIR MR shows cyst wall ➡, scolex ➡, and interstitial fluid around the obstructed 4th ventricle. FLAIR hyperintensity ➡ in the basal cisterns indicates meningitis.

common. Between 10-12% of patients exhibit signs of elevated intracranial pressure.

NCC—particularly the subarachnoid forms—can also cause cerebral vascular diseases. These include cerebral infarction, transient ischemic attacks, and cerebral hemorrhage.

Natural History. During the early stages of the disease, patients are frequently asymptomatic. Many patients remain asymptomatic for years. The average time from initial infestation until symptoms develop is 2-5 years. The time to progress through all four stages varies from 1-9 years with a mean of 5 years.

Treatment Options. Oral albendazole with or without steroids, excision/drainage of parenchymal lesions, and endoscopic resection of intraventricular lesions are treatment options.

Imaging

General Features. Imaging findings depend on several factors: (1) Life cycle stage of *T. solium* at presentation, (2) host inflammatory response, (3) number and location of parasites, and (4) associated complications, such as hydrocephalus and vascular disease.

Vesicular (Quiescent) Stage. NECT shows a smooth thin-walled cyst that is isodense to CSF. There is no surrounding edema and no enhancement on CECT.

MR shows that the cyst is isointense with CSF on T1 and T2/FLAIR. The scolex is discrete, nodular, and hyperintense ("target" or "dot in a hole" appearance) and may restrict on DWI. Enhancement is typically absent. Disseminated or "miliary" NCC has a striking "salt and pepper brain" appearance **(13-24)** **(13-25)** with notable lack of perilesional edema.

(13-27A) NECT scan in a patient with NCC shows multiple nodular calcified lesions ➡. A few demonstrate adjacent edema ➡. (13-27B) FLAIR scan shows a few hypointense foci ➡ caused by quiescent NCC in the nodular calcified stage. Several foci of perilesional edema are apparent around lesions in the colloidal vesicular stage ➡, whereas minimal residual edema surrounds lesions in the granular nodular stage ➡.

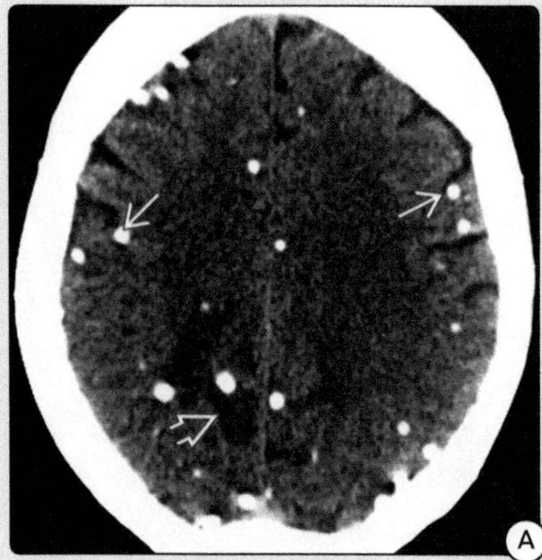

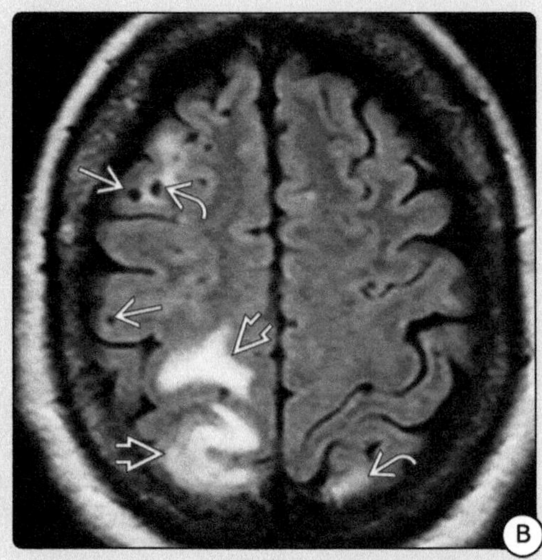

(13-27C) T2 GRE MR shows multiple "blooming black dots" characteristic of nodular calcified NCC. (13-27D) T1 C+ FS MR shows faint ring-like ➡ and nodular ➡ enhancement of healing granular nodular NCC cysts. "Shaggy" enhancement with adjacent edema ➡ is characteristic of degenerating larvae in the colloidal vesicular stage. Multiple lesions in different stages of evolution are characteristic of NCC.*

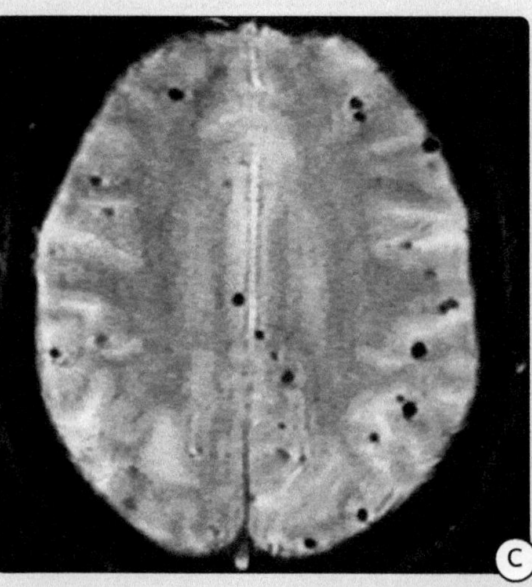

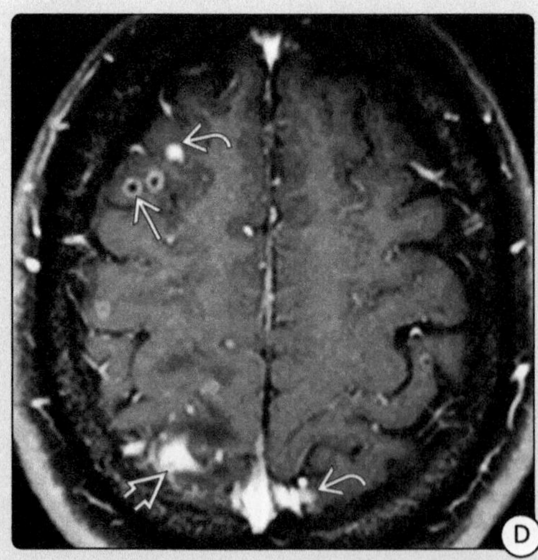

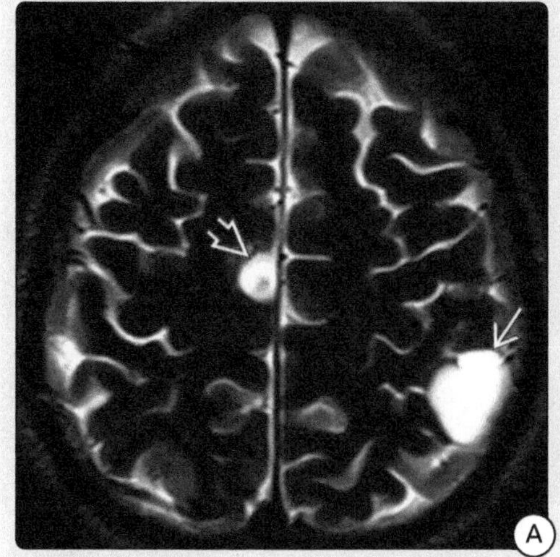

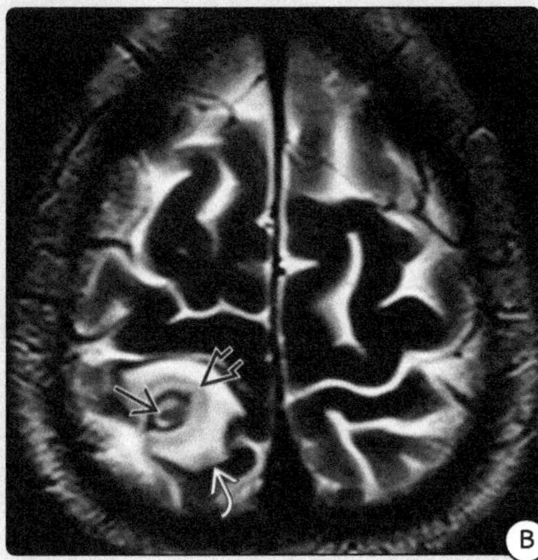

***(13-28A)** Series of images in a 41-year-old Hispanic man with seizures show NCC cysts in different stages. Axial T2 MR demonstrates a vesicular (cyst + scolex, no edema) ➡ and a cyst in the granular nodular stage ➡. **(13-28B)** More cephalad scan shows an intrasulcal NCC cyst in colloidal vesicular stage with a nodule (scolex) ➡ and thick, mixed hypo- and hyperintense intense cyst wall ➡. The surrounding edema ➡ is striking.*

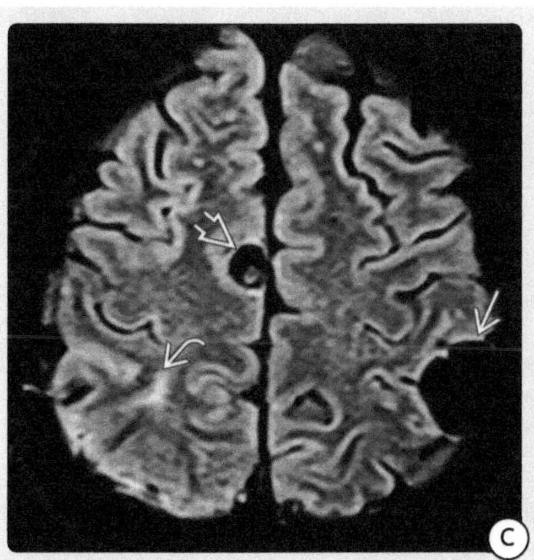

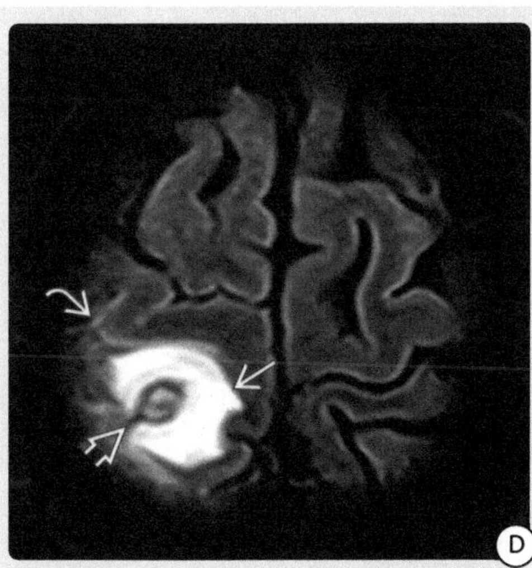

***(13-28C)** Axial FLAIR MR shows the vesicular NCC cyst with its scolex ➡. The granular nodular cyst ➡ has minimal residual edema. Group of FLAIR hyperintense sulci ➡ represents leptomeningeal inflammation from the colloidal vesicular cyst above. **(13-28D)** More cephalad FLAIR MR shows that the colloidal vesicular cyst + nodule ➡ has striking edema ➡ and adjacent hyperintense sulci ➡.*

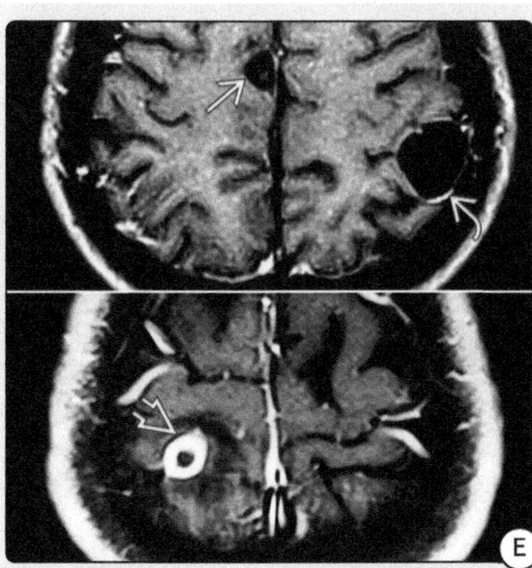

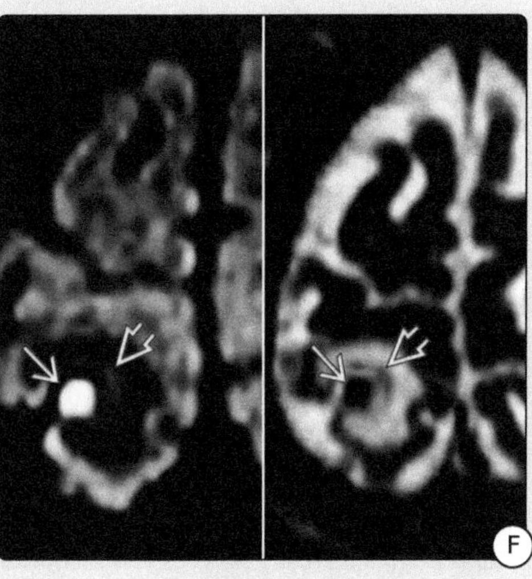

***(13-28E)** (Top) Axial T1 C+ FS MR shows no enhancement of vesicular NCC cyst ➡, faint rim enhancement of granular nodular cyst wall ➡. (Bottom) More cephalad scan shows the granular nodular cyst has thick, intense rim enhancement ➡. **(13-28F)** Axial DWI MR (L) and ADC map (R) through the colloidal vesicular cyst show that the central viscous cavity of the cyst restricts strongly ➡. Mild restriction in the enhancing capsule ➡ is present.*

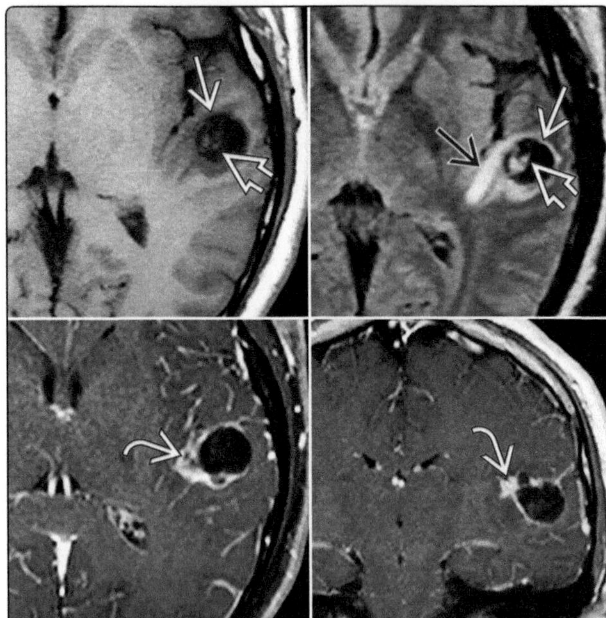

(13-29) Solitary degenerating colloidal vesicular NCC cyst with scolex demonstrates perilesional edema and "shaggy" enhancement.

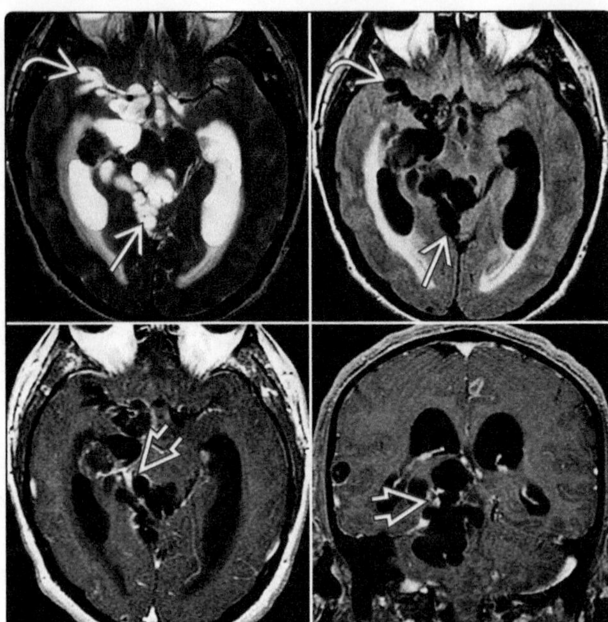

(13-30) "Racemose" NCC shows numerous variable-sized cysts filling the ambient cistern and sylvian fissure. Note the hydrocephalus, meningeal reaction with mild/moderate rim enhancement around the "bunch of grapes" cysts.

Colloidal Vesicular Stage (Dying Scolex). Cyst fluid is hyperdense relative to CSF on NECT and demonstrates a ring-enhancing capsule on CECT. Moderate to marked edema surrounds the degenerating dying larvae.

MR shows that the cyst fluid is mildly hyperintense to CSF on T1WI and that the scolex appears hyperintense on FLAIR **(13-26)**. Moderate to marked surrounding edema is present **(13-27B)** and may even progress to a diffuse encephalitis.

Enhancement of the cyst wall is typically intense, ring-like, and often slightly "shaggy" **(13-27D)** **(13-29)**. Restricted diffusion in the scolex and viscous degenerating cyst can be present **(13-28)**.

Granular Nodular (Healing) Stage. NECT shows mild residual edema. CECT demonstrates a progressively involuting, mildly to moderately enhancing nodule.

The cyst wall appears thickened and retracted, and the perilesional edema diminishes substantially, eventually disappearing. Nodular or faint ring-like enhancement is typical at this stage **(13-27D)**.

Nodular Calcified (Inactive) Stage. A small calcified nodule without surrounding edema or enhancement is seen on CT **(13-27A)**. Shrunken, calcified lesions are seen as hypointensities on T1WI and T2WI. Perilesional edema is absent.

"Blooming" on T2* GRE is seen and may show multifocal "blooming black dots" if multiple calcified nodules are present **(13-27C)**. Quiescent lesions do not enhance on T1 C+.

Special Features. "Racemose" NCC shows multilobulated, variably sized, grape-like lesions in the basal cisterns. Most cysts lack an identifiable scolex. Arachnoiditis with fibrosis and scarring demonstrates rim enhancement around the cysts and along the brain surfaces. Obstructive hydrocephalus is common **(13-30)**.

NCC-associated vasculitis with stroke is a rare but important complication of "racemose" NCC that can mimic tuberculosis. Most infarcts involve small perforating vessels, although large territorial infarcts have been reported.

Intraventricular NCC is associated with poor prognosis. Intraventricular cysts may be difficult to detect on CT. FLAIR and CISS are the most sensitive sequences for detecting the cysts on MR. The fourth ventricle is the most common site (50-55%) **(13-26)** followed by the third ventricle (25-30%), lateral ventricle (10-12%), and aqueduct (8-10%).

Differential Diagnosis

The differential diagnosis of NCC depends on lesion type and location. Subarachnoid/cisternal NCC can resemble **TB meningitis**. In contrast to NCC, the thick purulent basilar exudates typical of TB are solid and lack the cystic features of "racemose" NCC. **Carcinomatous meningitis** and **neurosarcoid** are also rarely cystic.

Abscess and **multifocal septic emboli** can resemble parenchymal NCC cysts but demonstrate a hypointense rim on T2WI and restrict strongly on DWI. A succinate peak on MRS helps distinguish a degenerating NCC cyst from abscess.

A giant parenchymal colloidal-vesicular NCC cyst with ring enhancement can mimic **neoplasm, tuberculoma**, or **toxoplasmosis**. Differential diagnosis of intraventricular cyst includes **colloid cyst** (solid), **ependymal cyst** (cystic but lacks a scolex), and **choroid plexus cyst.**

NEUROCYSTICERCOSIS: IMAGING AND DIFFERENTIAL DIAGNOSIS

Imaging

- Varies with stage (may have lesions in different stages)
  - Vesicular: Cyst with "dot" (scolex), no edema, no enhancement
  - Colloidal vesicular: Ring enhancement, edema striking
  - Granular nodular: Faint rim enhancement, edema decreased
  - Nodular calcified: CT Ca^{++}, MR "black dots"

Differential Diagnosis

- Parenchymal (colloidal vesicular) cyst = neoplasm, toxoplasmosis, TB
- "Racemose" (subarachnoid) NCC = pyogenic/TB meningitis
- Intraventricular cyst = ependymal, choroid plexus cysts

Other Parasitic Infections

Brain involvement by parasites other than NCC is relatively uncommon. Several parasites that affect humans can invade the CNS, particularly if humans serve as intermediate or nonpermissive hosts. Echinococcosis, schistosomiasis, paragonimiasis, sparganosis, trichinosis, and trypanosomiasis are examples of potentially neuroinvasive parasites.

Many parasites cause very bizarre-looking masses that can mimic neoplasm **(13-31)**. A history of travel to—or residence in—an endemic area is key to the diagnosis.

"Parasitomas" usually present as mass-like lesions with edema and multiple "conglomerate" ring-enhancing foci **(13-32)**. CNS parasitic infestations can be mistaken for neoplasms like **metastasis** and **glioblastoma**. **Inflammatory granulomas** (e.g., TB granulomas) can also mimic parasitic granulomas and are often endemic in the same geographic areas.

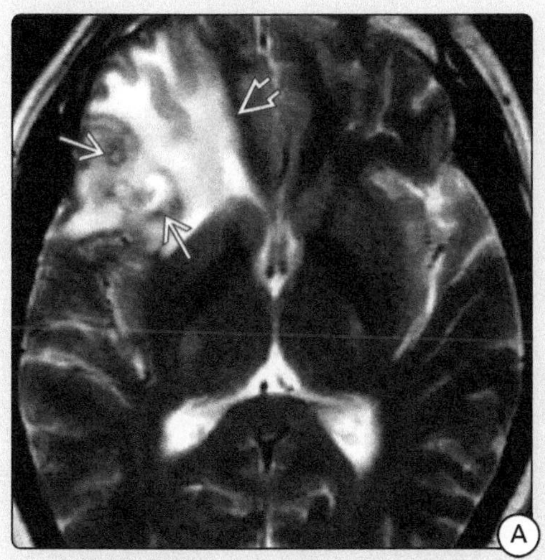

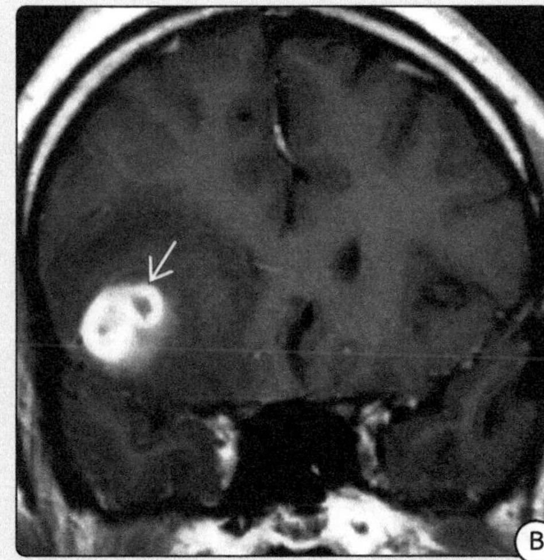

***(13-31A)** Axial T2 MR in a young man from Southeast Asia shows a heterogeneous right frontal lobe mass with intralesional hypointensities ➡, suggesting hemorrhage. Moderate perilesional edema ➡ is present. **(13-31B)** Coronal T1 C+ MR shows conglomerate ring-enhancing lesions ➡. Paragonimiasis granuloma was found at surgery.*

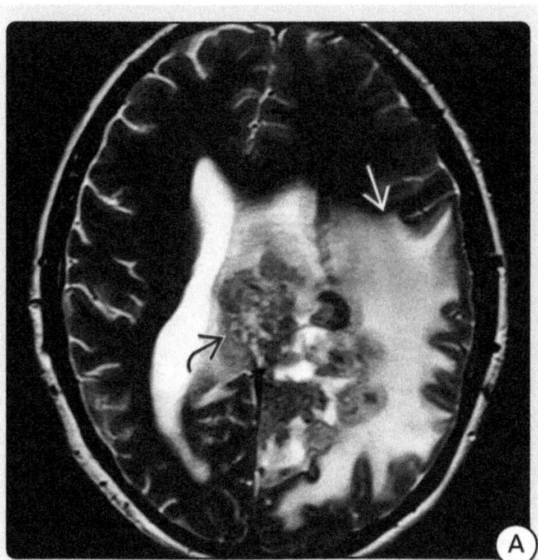

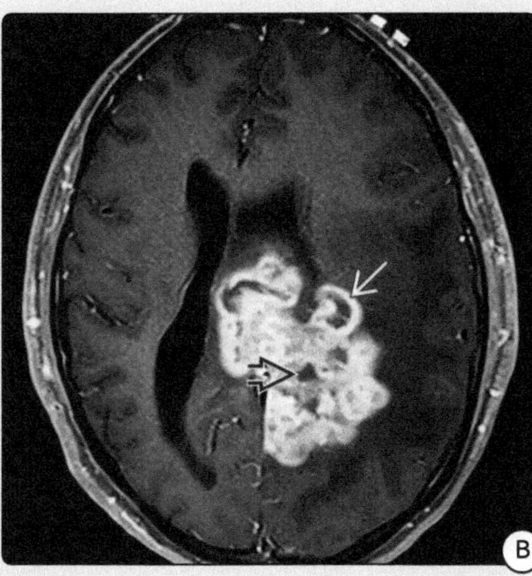

***(13-32A)** Axial T2 MR in a postpartum patient with seizures shows a very bizarre-appearing mixed signal intensity paraventricular mass ➡ with striking perilesional edema ➡. **(13-32B)** T1 C+ FS MR shows multiple conglomerate enhancing rings ➡ around presumed necrotic foci ➡. No definite causative agent was identified. Initially presumed TB, subsequent considerations include parasitic mass. Autopsy was declined.*

Miscellaneous and Emerging CNS Infections

Spirochete Infections of CNS

Two spirochete species can cause significant CNS disease: *Borrelia* (e.g., Lyme disease, relapsing fever borreliosis) and *Treponema* (neurosyphilis).

Lyme Disease

Lyme disease (LD) is also known as Lyme borreliosis. LD with neurologic disease is called Lyme neuroborreliosis (LNB) or neuro-Lyme disease. Lyme disease is a multisystem inflammatory disease caused by *Borrelia burgdorferi* in the United States and *Borrelia garinii* or *Borrelia afzelii* in Europe.

LD is a zoonosis maintained in animals, such as field mice and white-tailed deer.

LD is transmitted to humans by bite of *Ixodes* ticks and requires at least 36 hours of tick attachment as the spirochete moves from the tick midgut to the salivary glands to be transmitted. Most cases result from the bite of an infected nymph (about the size of a poppy seed) and may easily go unnoticed.

The clinical presentation and imaging features of CNS Lyme disease are protean and vary with location. Altered mental status and encephalopathy are the most common manifestations. Multiple small (2-8 mm) subcortical and periventricular white matter hyperintensities on T2/FLAIR are typical and identified in ~ 1/2 of all patients **(13-33)**. Enhancement varies from none to moderate. Multiple punctate and ring-enhancing lesions may be present **(13-35)**. Occasionally, "horseshoe" or incomplete ring enhancement occurs and can mimic demyelinating disease.

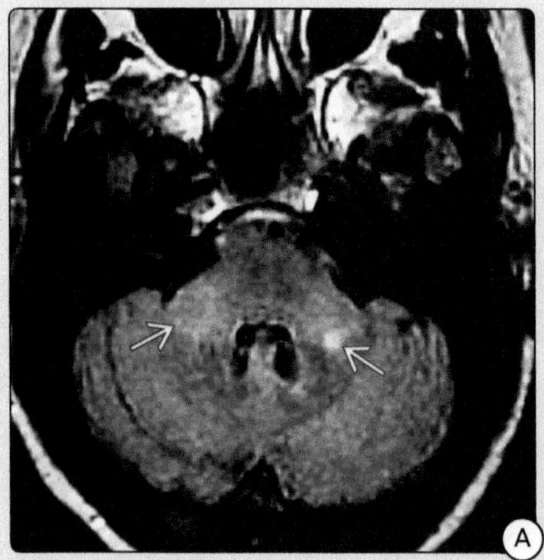

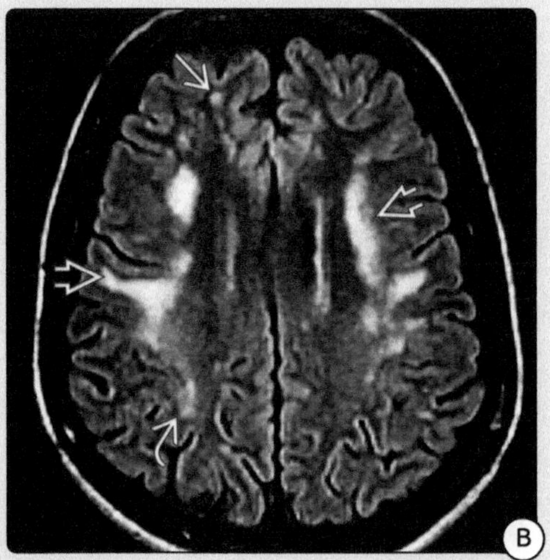

***(13-33A)** Series of axial FLAIR MR images demonstrates the multifocal T2/FLAIR white matter hyperintensities persisting 1 year after complete clinical response to treatment. Lesions are present in both middle cerebellar peduncles →. **(13-33B)** More cephalad scan in the same case shows multifocal punctate →, patchy →, and confluent → lesions in the subcortical and deep periventricular white matter.*

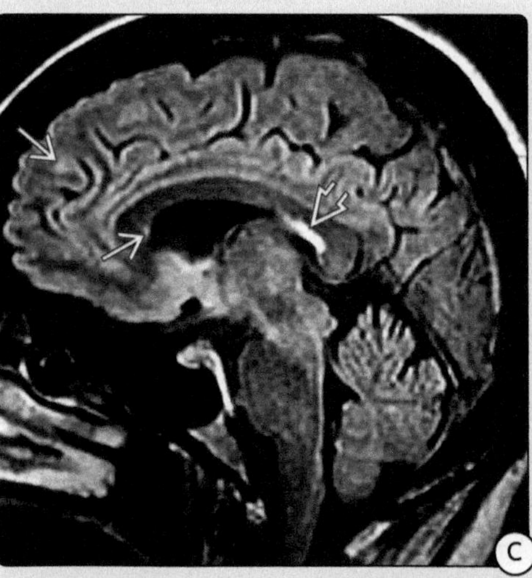

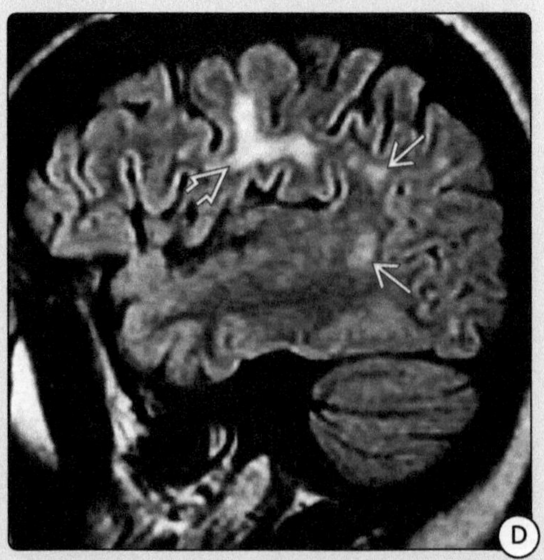

***(13-33C)** Midline sagittal FLAIR MR in the same case shows punctate lesions in the subcortical white matter and corpus callosum →. A larger confluent lesion in the corpus callosum → is present just anterior to the splenium. **(13-33D)** More lateral FLAIR MR in the same case shows multiple punctate → and confluent → lesions in the subcortical white matter. Note sparing of the subcortical U-fibers. This is documented Lyme disease.*

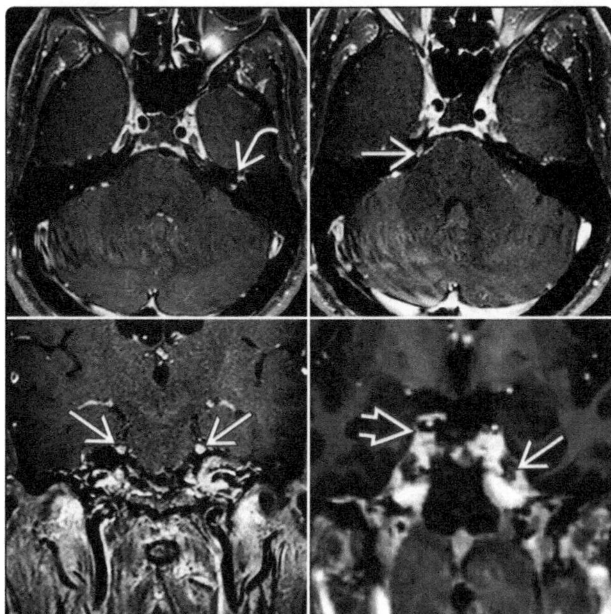

***(13-34)** Axial (top), coronal (bottom) T1 C+ FS MR scans in a patient with Lyme disease demonstrate left CNVII ➡, bilateral CNV ➡, and left CNIII ➡ enhancement. (Courtesy P. Hildenbrand, MD.)*

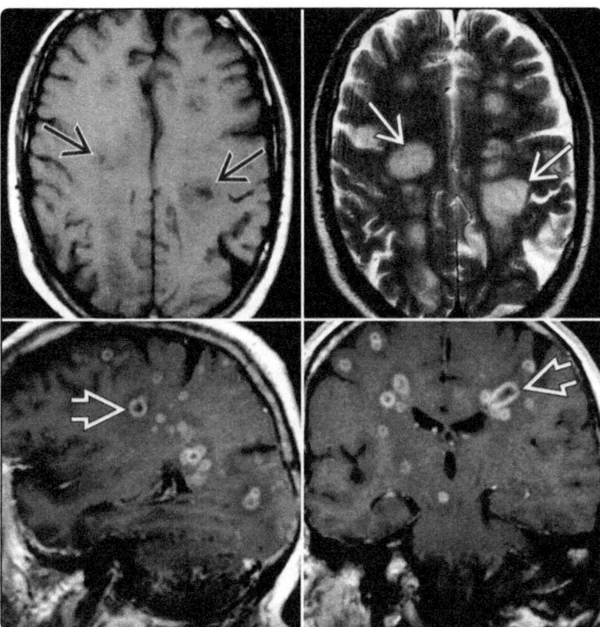

***(13-35)** (Upper L) T1 shows bilateral iso-/hypodense WM lesions ➡. (Upper R) T2 shows bilateral "fluffy" hyperintense lesions ➡ in the corona radiata. Sagittal (lower L) and coronal (lower R) show multifocal ring enhancement ➡; rickettsial encephalitis.*

Cranial nerve involvement is especially common in North American LNB **(13-34)**. CNVII is the most frequently involved followed by CNV and CNIII. Involvement of other cranial nerves is less common.

Myelitis and radiculitis are more common in European LD. Diffuse or multifocal hyperintense lesions on T2WI with patchy cord and linear nerve root enhancement are typical.

The major differential diagnosis of LNB is demyelinating disease. **Multiple sclerosis** (MS) frequently involves the periventricular white matter. Callososeptal involvement is more common in MS compared with LNB. Cranial nerve enhancement—especially CNVII—is less common than with LNB.

Neurosyphilis

Syphilis is a chronic systemic infectious disease caused by the spirochete *Treponema pallidum*. Syphilis is usually transmitted via sexual contact. Between 5-10% of patients with untreated syphilis develop neurosyphilis (NS).

Syphilitic gumma is the most common intracranial manifestation. Most are located along the brain subpial surfaces and consist of a dense inflammatory infiltrate surrounding a central caseous necrotic core. Imaging is that of a mixed-density/signal intensity mass with intense ring-like or diffuse enhancement. Because of their rarity, most syphilitic gummas are initially misdiagnosed as primary or metastatic neoplasms.

Emerging CNS Infections

Emerging infections are diseases that are literally emerging to infect humans. Some of these are zoonoses (i.e., diseases transmitted from animals to humans), whereas others are insect borne. Most rarely affect the CNS, but, when they do, the results can be disastrous. Examples of the latter include the hemorrhagic viral fevers, such as Korean hemorrhagic fever, Rift Valley fever, hantavirus, dengue, and Ebola.

Hemorrhagic Viral Fevers

The Centers for Disease Control and Prevention (CDC) has identified six biologic agents as "category A" (easily disseminated or transmitted from person to person, resulting in a high mortality rate and potential for major public health risk): Anthrax, smallpox, botulism, tularemia, viral hemorrhagic fever, and plague. Of these, the **viral hemorrhagic fevers** are the most likely to affect the CNS and cause multifocal brain bleeds **(13-36)**.

Filoviruses, such as **Ebola** and **Marburg**, are single-stranded RNA viruses that cause acute hemorrhagic fever with high mortality rates. Currently, there are no licensed vaccines or therapeutics to counter human filovirus infections.

During the 2015 Ebola epidemic in West Africa, it became apparent that many patients likely died from acute fulminant meningoencephalitis, which was not initially recognized because of multiorgan involvement. Most are never imaged.

The flaviviruses—primarily **dengue** and **Zika virus**—are some of the most important emerging viral infections with high global disease incidence and the potential for rapid spread beyond nonendemic regions.

Dengue is increasingly common. Transmitted by *Aedes* mosquitoes, ~ 40% of the world's population is at risk of infection.

The clinical spectrum of dengue ranges from asymptomatic infection to life-threatening dengue hemorrhagic fever and dengue shock syndrome. Approximately 10% of patients with serologically confirmed dengue infection develop neurologic complications. In endemic areas, dengue has become the most frequent cause of encephalitis, surpassing even herpes simplex virus.

Meningitis, encephalitis, ADEM, Guillain-Barré syndrome, and pituitary apoplexy have been reported in some cases.

Zika virus (ZIKV) is related to dengue, Chikungunya, West Nile, yellow fever, and Japanese encephalitis viruses. Brazil is the epicenter of the current ZIKV epidemic, which is rapidly spreading across the Americas. ZIKV is primarily a vector-borne disease carried by the *Aedes* mosquito. ZIKV can be transmitted congenitally, sexually, and through contaminated blood.

ZIKV causes severe microcephaly in infants born to infected mothers (congenital Zika syndrome). It has been reported to cause meningoencephalitis, myelitis, and Guillain-Barré syndrome in adults. To date, reported imaging findings are nonspecific.

Many patients with **hantavirus** or **Korean hemorrhagic fever** renal syndromes develop CNS symptoms, such as acute psychiatric disorders, epilepsy, and meningismus. Autopsy studies demonstrate pituitary hemorrhage in 37%, pituitary necrosis in 5%, and brainstem hemorrhage in nearly 70%. In the few reported cases, MR showed pituitary hemorrhage and reversible splenium lesion in the corpus callosum.

Selected References: The complete reference list is available on the Expert Consult™ eBook version included with purchase.

(13-36A) Axial FLAIR MR in a 38-year-old man with altered mental status, progressive decline, and a seizure shows bilateral hyperintense lesions ➡ in the white matter of both temporal lobes. (13-36B) SWI MIP obtained several days after the patient lapsed into a coma shows bilateral lobar hematomas ↷ and numerous scattered petechial microhemorrhages ➡.

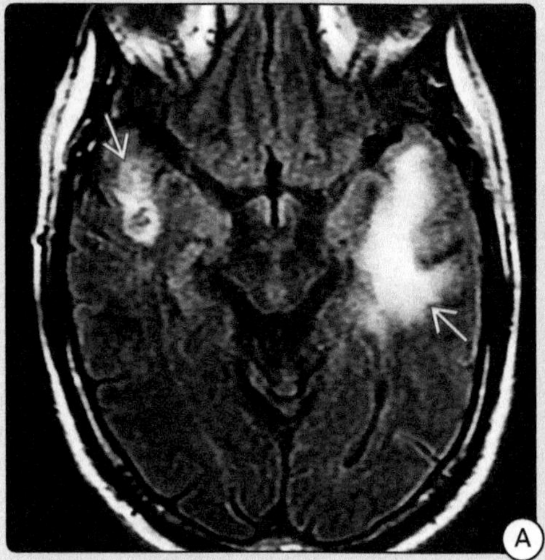

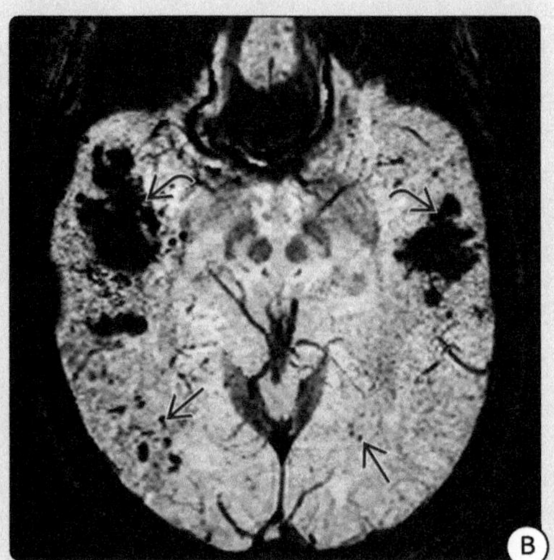

(13-36C) More cephalad T2 SWI MIP shows additional confluent hemorrhages ↷ and scattered microbleeds ➡. The basal ganglia are largely spared. (13-36D) More cephalad SWI shows numerous microhemorrhages. Fulminant hemorrhagic encephalitis is most likely viral. The inciting organism was not identified despite extensive laboratory investigation.*

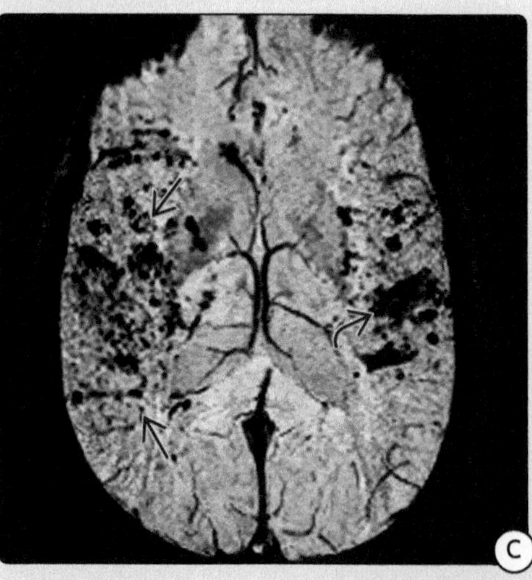

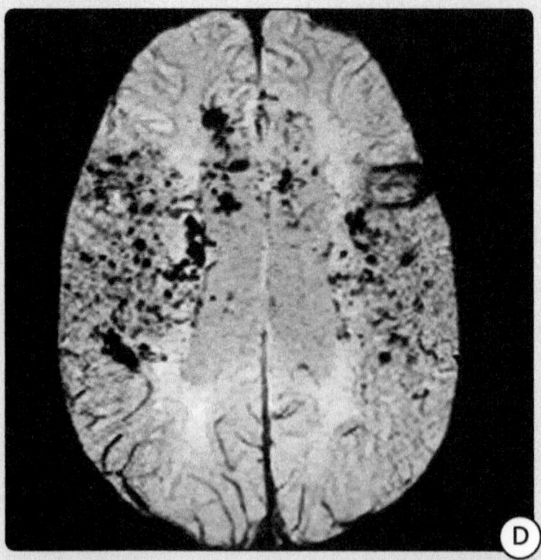

HIV/AIDS

In this chapter, we explore the "many faces" of HIV/AIDS as it affects the central nervous system (CNS). We begin by discussing the manifestations of HIV itself in the brain, i.e., HIV encephalitis. We follow with a consideration of unusual but important associated findings, such as HIV vasculopathy, HIV-associated bone marrow changes, and benign salivary gland lymphoepithelial lesions.

We then consider the broad spectrum of opportunistic infections that complicate HIV/AIDS and what happens when an HIV-positive patient is also coinfected with TB, another sexually transmitted disease, or malaria. Long-term survivors with treated AIDS and the phenomenon of immune reconstitution inflammatory syndrome (IRIS) are then presented. We conclude the chapter by discussing neoplasms that occur in the setting of HIV/AIDS (the so-called AIDS-defining malignancies).

HIV Infection

HIV is a neurovirulent infection that has both direct and indirect effects on the CNS. Neurologic complications can arise from the HIV infection itself, from opportunistic infections or neoplasms, and from treatment-related metabolic derangements.

In this section, we consider the effects of the HIV virus itself on the brain. Extracranial manifestations of HIV/AIDS may also be identified on brain imaging studies, so we discuss these as well.

HIV Encephalitis

Between 75-90% of HIV/AIDS patients have demonstrable HIV-induced brain injury at autopsy **(14-1)**. Although many patients remain asymptomatic for variable periods, brain infection is the initial presenting symptomatology in 5-10% of cases. Approximately 25% of treated HIV/AIDS patients develop moderate cognitive impairment despite good virologic response to therapy.

Terminology

HIV encephalitis (HIVE) and HIV leukoencephalopathy (HIVL) are the direct result of HIV infection of the brain. Opportunistic infections are absent early, although coinfections or multiple infections are common later in the disease course.

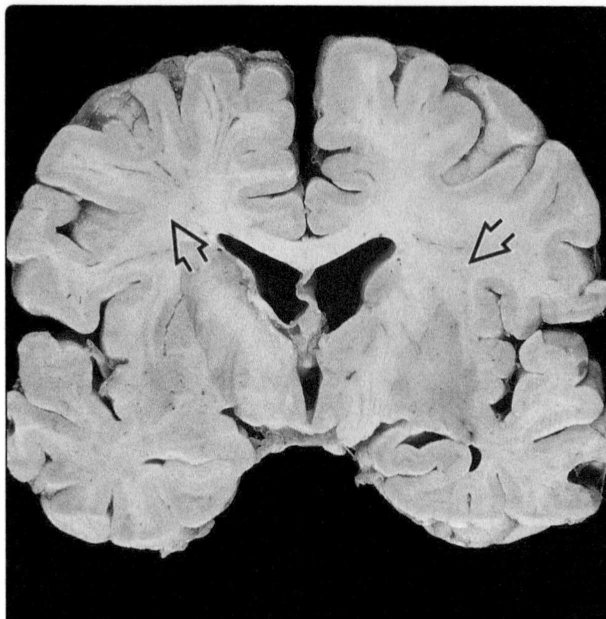

(14-1) Coronal autopsy of HIVE shows generalized volume loss with enlargement of the lateral ventricles, sylvian fissures. "Hazy," poorly defined abnormalities are present in WM ⇨ but spare the subcortical U-fibers. (Courtesy B. K. DeMasters, MD.)

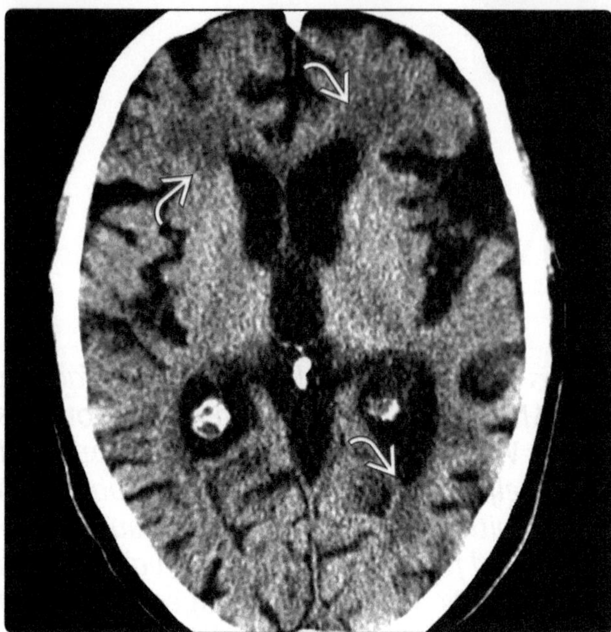

(14-2) Axial NECT in a 38-year-old man with longstanding HIV/AIDS shows gross cerebral atrophy and multifocal hypodensities ➡ in the subcortical WM.

Etiology

HIV is a pathogenic neurotropic human RNA retrovirus. **HIV-1** is responsible for most cases of HIV/AIDS. **HIV-2** infection is predominantly a disease of heterosexuals and is found primarily in West Africa. Unless otherwise noted in this discussion, "HIV" or "HIV infection" refers to HIV-1 infection.

The two major targets of viral infection are lymphoid tissue—especially T cells—and the CNS. HIV crosses the blood-brain barrier (BBB) both as cell-free virus and infected monocytes and T cells, which migrate across the intact BBB, penetrating the brain within 24-48 hours after initial exposure.

HIV infects astrocytes but does not directly infect neurons. However, once inside the brain, the HIV-infected monocytes and T cells produce proinflammatory cytokines, such as TNF and IL-1β, which, in turn, further activate resident microglia and astrocytes.

Pathology

In early stages, the brain appears grossly normal. Advanced HIVE results in generalized brain volume loss ("atrophy") with enlarged ventricles and subarachnoid spaces. Ill-defined, diffuse myelin pallor with poorly demarcated areas of myelin loss ensues. Lesions are most prominent in the deep periventricular white matter and corona radiata.

Microscopically, HIVE is characterized by gliosis, microglial activation, perivascular inflammation, and multinucleated giant cells containing viral antigens.

Clinical Issues

Epidemiology. Almost 60% of all AIDS patients eventually develop overt neurologic manifestations. Approximately 15-25% of treated patients develop moderate HIV-associated neurocognitive disorders (HANDs) cognitive impairment.

Presentation. Early brain infection with HIV is often asymptomatic, and cognitive and functional performances are both initially normal. HANDs develop as intermediate and long-term complications.

Imaging

CT Findings. NECT scans may be normal in the early stages. Mild to moderate atrophy with patchy or confluent white matter hypodensity develops as the disease progresses **(14-2)**. HIVE does not cause mass effect and does not enhance on CECT.

MR Findings. Generalized volume loss with enlarged ventricles and sulci is best appreciated on T1WI or thin-section inversion recovery sequences. White matter signal intensity is generally normal or near normal on T1WI.

T2/FLAIR initially shows bilateral, patchy, relatively symmetric white matter hyperintensities. With time, confluent "hazy," ill-defined hyperintensity in the subcortical and deep cerebral white matter develops, and volume loss ensues **(14-3)**. HIVE usually does not enhance on T1 C+ and usually shows no restriction on DWI. In fulminant cases, perivenular enhancement may indicate acute demyelination.

Differential Diagnosis

Progressive multifocal leukoencephalopathy (PML) has strikingly *asymmetric* hyperintensities on T2/FLAIR. Both the hemispheric and posterior fossa white matter (often both cerebral peduncles) are commonly affected. PML also often involves the subcortical U-fibers, which are usually spared in HIVE.

Coinfections with other infectious agents are common in HIVE and may complicate its classic imaging appearance. **Cytomegalovirus** (CMV) can also cause a similarly diffuse encephalitis but frequently exhibits ependymal enhancement. **Toxoplasmosis** causes multifocal punctate and "target" or ring-enhancing lesions that are most prominent in the basal ganglia.

Herpes encephalitis and **human herpesvirus-6 (HHV-6) encephalitis** both involve the temporal lobes, especially the cortex.

HIV ENCEPHALITIS: MR AND DDx

MR

- Volume loss with ↑ sulci, ventricles
- T2/FLAIR "hazy" white matter symmetric hyperintensity
  - Spares subcortical U-fibers
- No mass effect
- No enhancement (exception = acute fulminant HIVE)

Differential Diagnosis

- Progressive multifocal leukoencephalopathy (PML)
  - Coinfection with HIVE common
  - Usually asymmetric
  - Often involves U-fibers
- Opportunistic infections
  - CMV causes encephalitis, ependymitis
  - Toxoplasmosis: Multiple enhancing rings
  - Herpes, HHV-6 usually involve temporal lobes

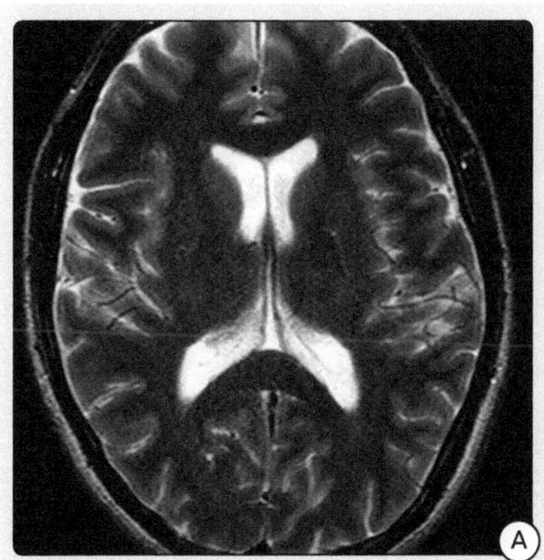

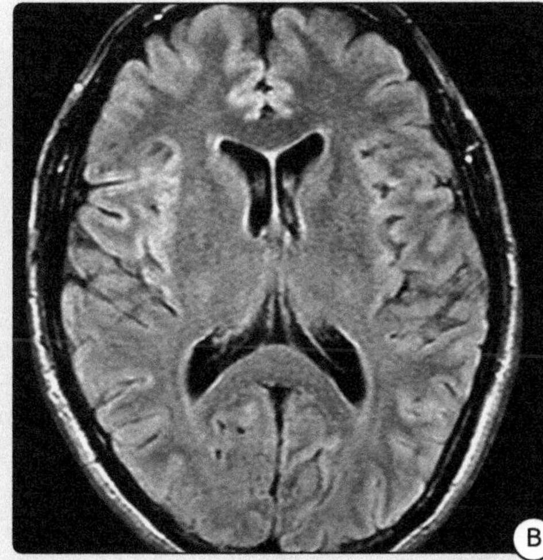

(14-3A) *Axial T2 MR in a 45-year-old man with early dementia shows minimal enlargement of the lateral ventricles and sulci.* ***(14-3B)*** *Axial FLAIR MR shows no evidence of WM hyperintensities.*

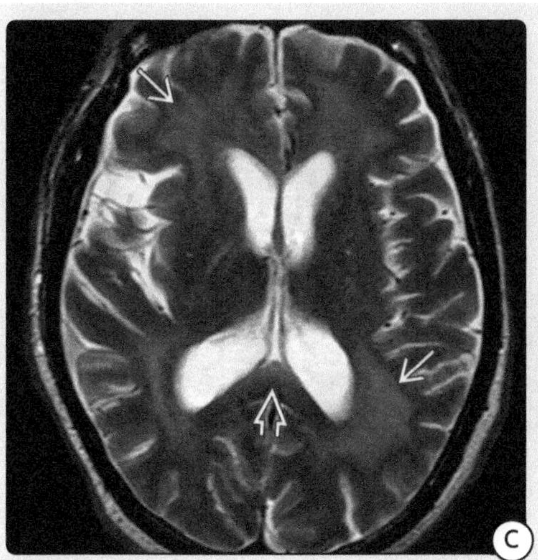

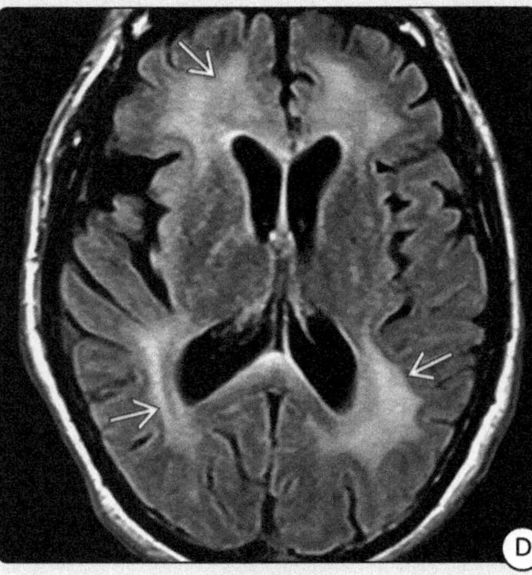

(14-3C) *Four years later, the same patient has developed severe HIV-associated dementia. Axial T2 MR shows significantly increased volume loss, reflected by the enlarged lateral ventricles and sulci. Symmetric confluent hyperintensities have developed in the cerebral WM ➡ and corpus callosum splenium ⇨.* ***(14-3D)*** *Axial FLAIR MR shows the dramatic interval WM changes of severe HIV encephalitis ➡. U-fibers are spared.*

Other Manifestations of HIV/AIDS

HIV/AIDS Bone Marrow Changes

Bone marrow alterations are common in HIV/AIDS patients. Fatty T1-hyperintense "yellow" marrow is replaced with T1-hypointense active hematopoietic tissue. The calvarium and clivus appear mottled or "gray." The affected vertebral bodies appear hypointense relative to the intervertebral discs (the "bright disc" sign).

Lymphoid Hyperplasia

Lymphoid hyperplasia of Waldeyer ring is the most common finding observed on brain MR. Unusually prominent tonsils and adenoids in a patient over 25-30 years of age should raise suspicion of HIV infection **(14-4)**.

Benign Lymphoepithelial Lesions

Benign lymphoepithelial lesions of HIV (BLL-HIV) are nonneoplastic cystic masses that enlarge salivary glands. Bilateral lesions are common. The parotid glands are most frequently affected.

NECT scans show multiple bilateral well-circumscribed cysts within enlarged parotid glands. A thin enhancing rim is present on CECT scans. The cysts are homogeneously hyperintense on T2WI and demonstrate rim enhancement on T1 C+ **(14-5)**.

Vasculopathy

Recurrent strokes are increasingly common in chronic HIV/AIDS. HIV-associated vasculopathy can cause striking fusiform dilatation of the circle of Willis and proximal middle cerebral arteries **(14-6)**.

__(14-4A)__ Sagittal T1 MR in a 43-year-old man with longstanding HIV/AIDS shows unusually prominent adenoids ➡. __(14-4B)__ Axial T1 MR in the same case shows that the upper nasopharynx is almost completely filled with enlarged adenoidal tissue ➡.

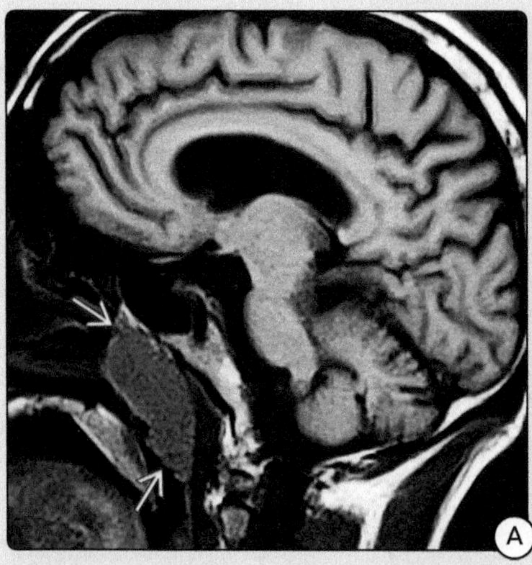

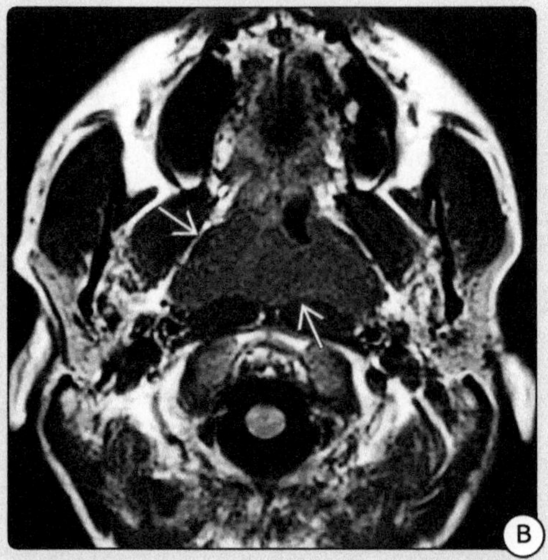

__(14-5)__ Axial T1 C+ FS MR in a 31-year-old HIV-positive man shows hyperplastic Waldeyer ring ➡ and classic lymphoepithelial lesions. Note rim-enhancing cysts in both parotid glands ➡ and enlarged deep cervical lymph nodes ➡. __(14-6)__ Axial T2 MR in a 13-year-old boy with congenital HIV/AIDS and multiple recurrent strokes shows markedly enlarged "flow voids" of both middle cerebral arteries ➡, characteristic of HIV fusiform arteriopathy.

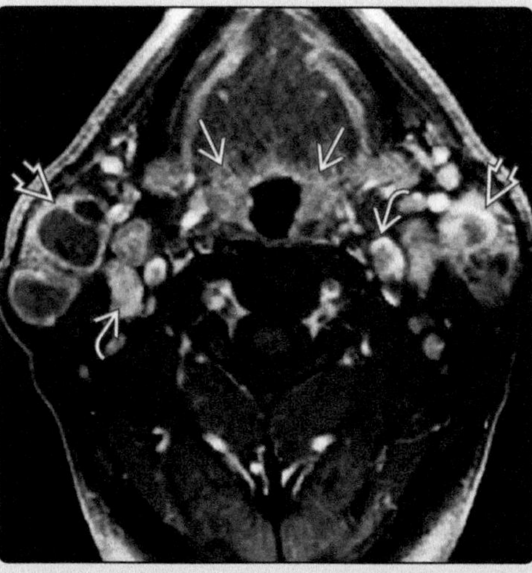

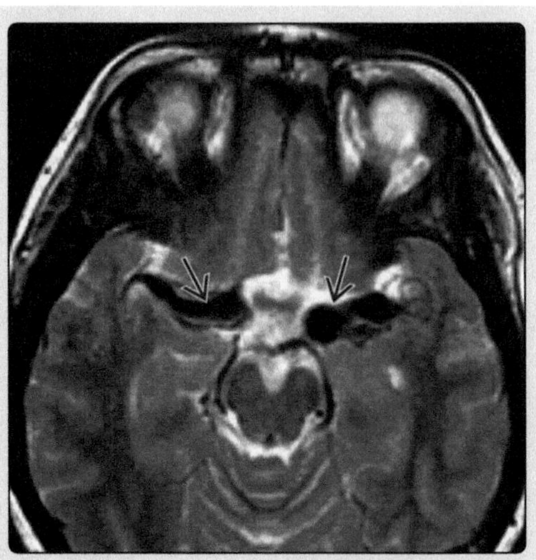

Opportunistic Infections

With the advent of highly active antiretroviral therapy (HAART), the prevalence of CNS opportunistic infections has decreased five- to tenfold. Nevertheless, these infections and HIV coinfections, such as tuberculosis, continue to create substantial morbidity.

Toxoplasmosis

Toxoplasmosis (toxo) is the most common opportunistic infection and overall cause of a mass lesion in patients with HIV/AIDS.

CNS toxo most commonly involves the basal ganglia, thalami, corticomedullary junctions, and cerebellum **(14-7)**. Multifocal lesions are more common than solitary ones. In contrast to lymphoma, only 15-20% of toxo lesions present as solitary masses. Although large lesions do occur, most lesions are small and average between 2-3 cm in diameter. The most common finding on NECT scan is multiple ill-defined hypodense lesions in the basal ganglia or thalamus with moderate to marked peripheral edema **(14-8A)**.

MR shows a T1-hypointense mass that occasionally demonstrates mild peripheral hyperintensity caused by coagulative necrosis or hemorrhage. One or more nodular and ring-enhancing masses are typical on T1 C+ **(14-8C)**. A ring-shaped zone of peripheral enhancement with a small eccentric mural nodule represents the "eccentric target" sign. The enhancing nodule is a collection of concentrically thickened vessels, whereas the rim enhancement is caused by an inflamed vascular zone that borders the necrotic abscess cavity.

The major differential diagnosis is **primary CNS lymphoma** (PCNSL). CNS toxo typically presents with multifocal lesions. AIDS-related CNS toxo also has positive findings on serology in 80% of cases, and CSF PCR is definitive.

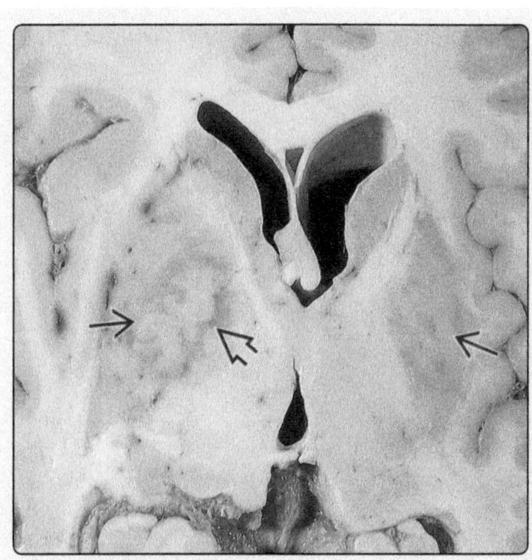

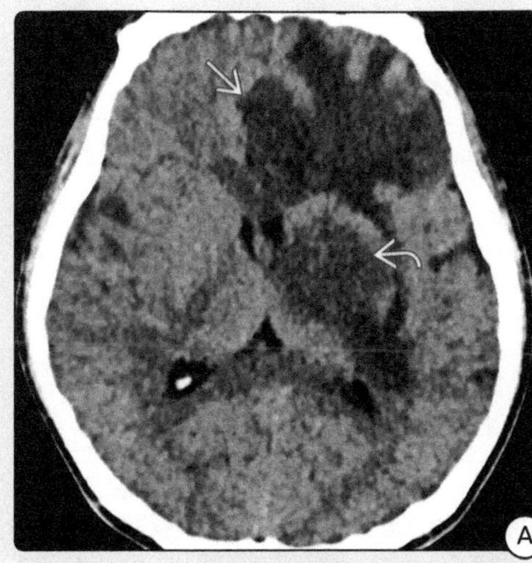

***(14-7)** Axial gross pathology from an HIV-positive patient shows ill-defined toxoplasmosis abscesses in both basal ganglia ➡. Note the hemorrhage ➡ surrounding the central necrosis in the right lesion. (Courtesy R. Hewlett, MD.) **(14-8A)** Axial NECT in a 33-year-old HIV-positive man in the ER with altered mental status shows hypodense masses in the left basal ganglia ➡ and frontal lobe ➡ with marked peripheral edema.*

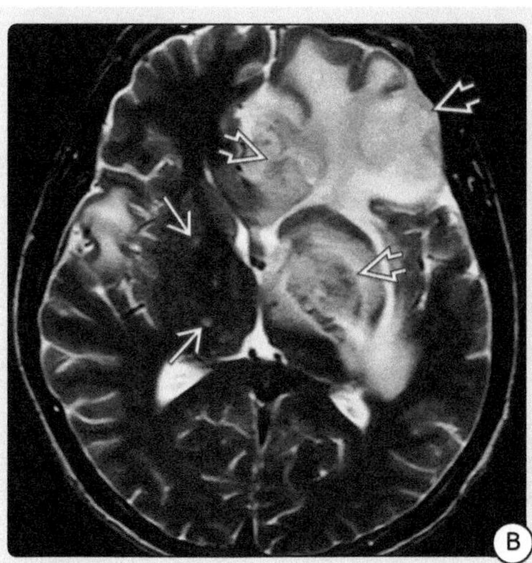

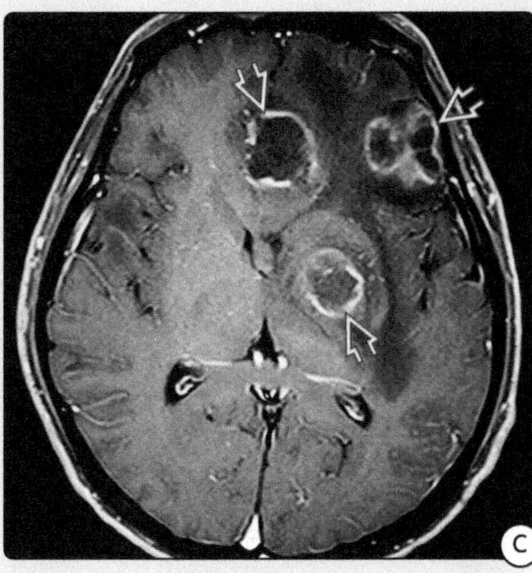

***(14-8B)** Axial T2 MR in the same case shows 3 separate masses ➡ that are surrounded by marked edema and appear very heterogeneous in signal intensity. Several small hyperintensities are also present in the right basal ganglia and thalamus ➡. **(14-8C)** Axial T1 C+ FS MR in the same case demonstrates irregular ring-enhancing lesions ➡.*

Solitary toxo lesions are uncommon. Approximately 70% of isolated CNS masses in HIV/AIDS patients are PCNSL.

Cryptococcosis

Fungal infections can be life threatening in immunocompromised patients, especially those with HIV/AIDS. Although many different fungi can cause CNS infection, the most common fungi to affect patients with HIV/AIDS are *Candida albicans, Aspergillus* species, and *Cryptococcus neoformans* (crypto). Crypto is the third most common CNS infectious agent in HIV/AIDS patients after HIV and *Toxoplasma gondii.* Prior to HAART, crypto CNS infections occurred in 10% of HIV patients, but it is now relatively rare in developed countries. Crypto usually occurs when CD4 counts drop below 50-100 cells/μL.

Gelatinous mucoid-like cryptococcal capsular polysaccharides and budding yeast may accumulate within dilated perivascular spaces (PVSs) **(14-9)**, especially in the basal ganglia **(14-10)**, midbrain, dentate nuclei, and subcortical white matter **(14-9)**. NECT scans show hypodensity in the basal ganglia. Cryptococcal gelatinous pseudocysts are hypointense to brain on T1WI and very hyperintense on T2WI **(14-12)**. The lesions generally follow CSF signal intensity and suppress on FLAIR. Perilesional edema is generally absent. Lack of enhancement on T1 C+ is typical, although mild pial enhancement is sometimes observed.

The differential diagnosis includes **prominent perivascular spaces**. Enlarged PVSs do not enhance. In HIV/AIDS patients with CD4 counts under 20, symmetrically enlarged PVSs should be considered cryptococcal infection and treated as such. **Toxoplasmosis** usually has multifocal ring- or "target"-like enhancing lesions with significant surrounding edema. **Tuberculosis** usually demonstrates strong enhancement in the basal meninges. Tuberculomas are generally hypointense on T2WI. **Primary CNS lymphoma** in HIV/AIDS patients often shows hemorrhage, necrosis, and ring

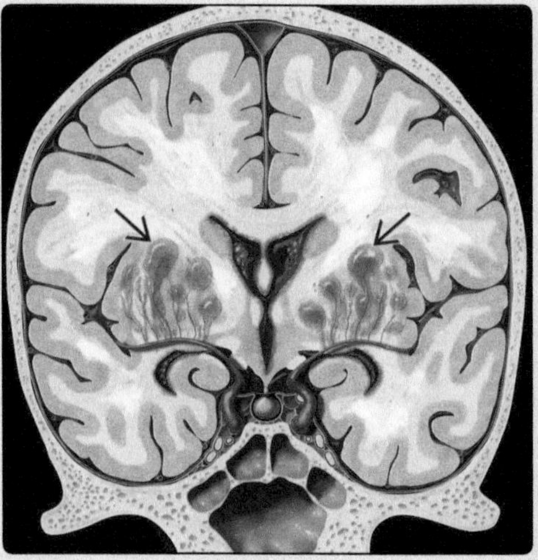

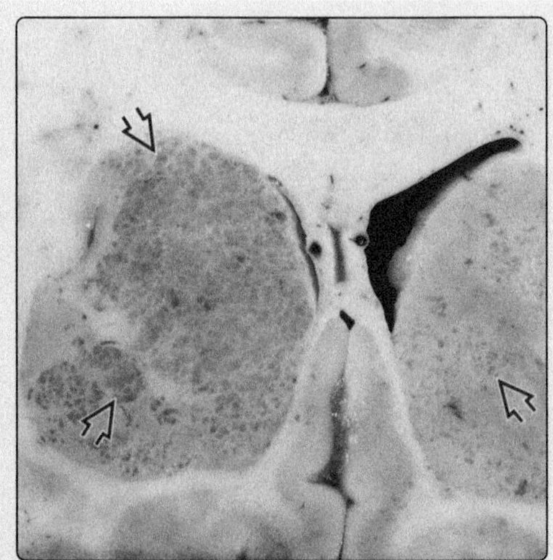

***(14-9)** Coronal graphic shows multiple dilated perivascular spaces ➔ filled with gelatinous mucoid-appearing material characteristic of cryptococcal infection in HIV/AIDS patients. **(14-10)** Coronal autopsied brain in HIV/AIDS shows innumerable tiny cryptococcal gelatinous pseudocysts in the basal ganglia ➔. (Courtesy A. T. Yachnis, Neuropathology, 2014.)*

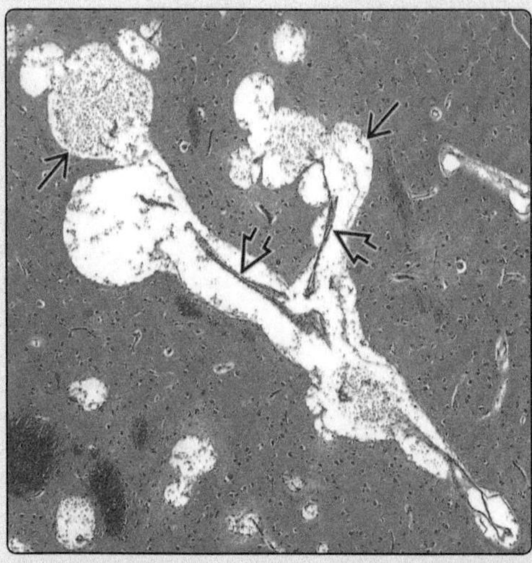

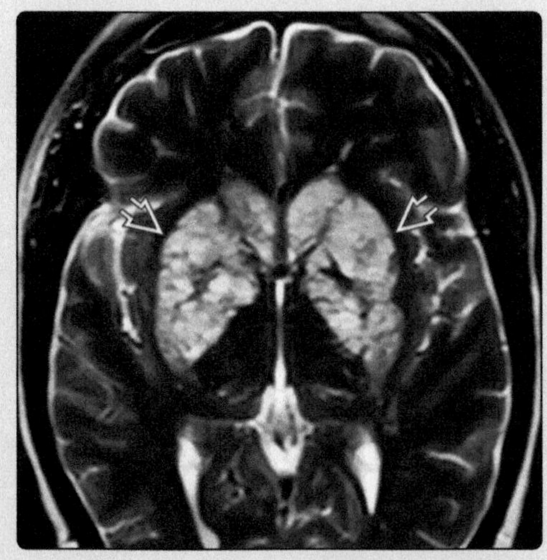

***(14-11)** Photomicrograph shows a branching vessel cut in a longitudinal section ➔ and surrounded by enlarged perivascular spaces stuffed full of cryptococcal gelatinous pseudocysts ➔. (Courtesy B. K. DeMasters, MD.) **(14-12)** T2 MR shows lentiform and nuclei and caudate nuclei are grossly expanded by innumerable hyperintense cysts ➔ characteristic of cryptococcal gelatinous pseudocysts. (Courtesy N. Omar, MD.)*

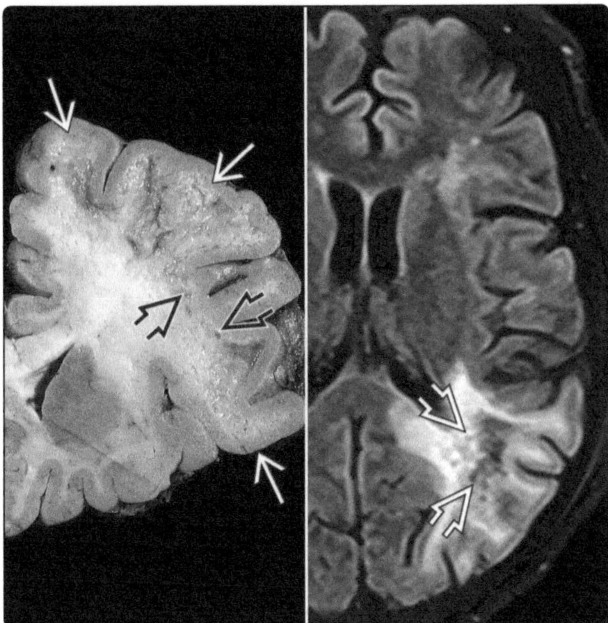

(14-13) (L) Autopsy of advanced PML shows coalescent subcortical demyelinated foci ➡ with multiple tiny cavities ⇨. (R) FLAIR of PML shows spongy-appearing hyperintense subcortical WM with multiple small hypointense cysts ➡.

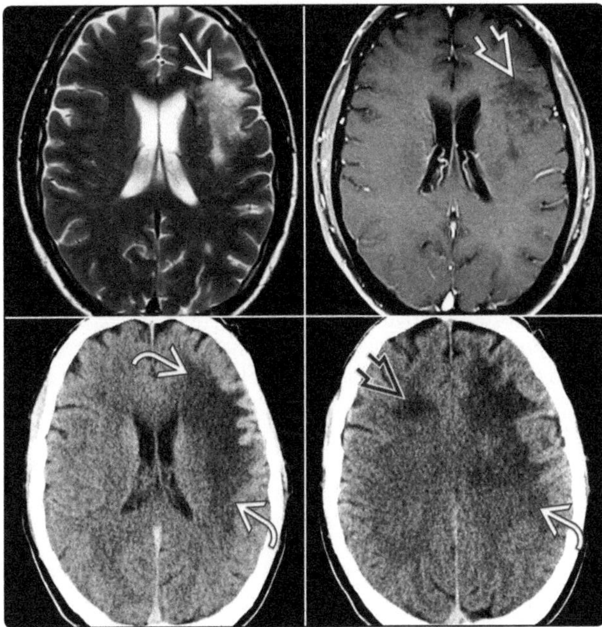

(14-14) cPML in a 32y HIV(+) man is shown. Confluent left frontal T2 hyperintensity ➡ spares cortex, does not enhance ➡. NECT 6 weeks later shows the left frontal lesion has increased in size ➡, and a new right frontal hypodensity is present ⇨.

enhancement. Solitary lesions are more common than multifocal involvement.

Progressive Multifocal Leukoencephalopathy

Progressive multifocal leukoencephalopathy (PML) is an opportunistic infection caused by the JC virus (JCV), a member of the Papovaviridae family. JCV is a ubiquitous virus that circulates widely. More than 85% of the adult population worldwide has antibodies against JCV. Asymptomatic infection is probably acquired in childhood or adolescence and remains latent until the virus is reactivated.

Pathologically, early lesions appear as small yellow-tan round to ovoid foci at the gray matter-white matter junction. The cortex remains normal. With lesion coalescence, large, spongy-appearing depressions in the cerebral and cerebellar white matter appear **(14-13)**.

Imaging plays a key role in the diagnosis and follow-up of JCV infections. cPML can appear as solitary or multifocal widespread lesions. Any area of the brain can be affected, although the supratentorial lobar white matter is the most commonly affected site. The posterior fossa white matter—especially the middle cerebellar peduncles—is the second most common location. In occasional cases, a solitary lesion in the subcortical U-fibers is present.

More than 90% of cPML cases show hypodense areas in the subcortical and deep periventricular white matter on NECT **(14-14)**; 70% are multifocal. Extent varies from small, scattered subcortical foci to large, bilateral but asymmetric confluent white matter lesions. In the early acute stage of infection, some mass effect with focal gyral expansion can be present. At later stages, encephaloclastic changes with atrophy and volume loss predominate. PML lesions generally do not enhance on CECT.

MR is the imaging procedure of choice in suspected PML. Multifocal, bilateral but asymmetric, irregularly shaped hypointensities on T1WI are typical. The lesions are heterogeneously hyperintense on T2WI **(14-13)** and typically extend into the subcortical U-fibers all the way to the undersurface of the cortex, which remains intact even in advanced disease. Smaller, almost microcyst-like, very hyperintense foci within and around the slightly less hyperintense confluent lesions represent the characteristic spongy lesions seen in more advanced PML.

Appearance on DWI varies according to disease stage. In newly active lesions, DWI restricts strongly. Slightly older lesions show a central core with low signal intensity and high mean diffusivity (MD) surrounded by a rim of higher signal intensity and lower MD. Chronic, "burned-out" lesions show increased diffusion due to disorganized cellular architecture **(14-15)**.

"Classic" PML generally does not enhance on T1 C+ scans, although faint, peripheral rim-like enhancement occurs in 5% of all cases. The exception is hyperacute PML in the setting of IRIS and in multiple sclerosis (MS) patients on natalizumab. In these cases, striking foci with irregular rim enhancement are frequently—but not invariably—present. Peripheral enhancement &/or mass effect decrease with corticosteroids.

The major differential diagnosis of cPML is **HIV encephalitis (HIVE)**. HIVE demonstrates more symmetric white matter disease while sparing the subcortical U-fibers. **IRIS** is usually more acute and demonstrates strong but irregular ring-like enhancement.

Cytomegalovirus

CNS CMV is a late-onset disease in immunocompromised patients. With increasing use of HAART, < 2% of HIV/AIDS patients develop overt symptoms of CMV infection.

Acquired CMV in the setting of HIV/AIDS most commonly manifests as meningoencephalitis **(14-16)** and ventriculitis/ependymitis. Typical imaging findings are those of underlying HIVE (atrophy, hazy white matter disease) with ependymal enhancement around the lateral ventricles **(14-17)**.

Tuberculosis

TB is one of the most devastating coinfections in immunocompromised patients and is the main cause of morbidity and mortality in HIV-infected patients worldwide.

HIV is the most powerful known risk factor for reactivation of latent TB to active disease. HIV patients who are coinfected with TB have 100x increased risk of developing active TB. In turn, TB coinfection exacerbates the severity and accelerates the progression of HIV.

Patients with prior TB who become HIV(+) may also reactivate their disease with old calcified tuberculomas developing new surrounding edema and mass effect **(14-18)**. In severely immunocompromised HIV patients with especially low CD4 counts, fulminant reactivated TB may develop multiple ring-enhancing pseudoabscesses **(14-19)**.

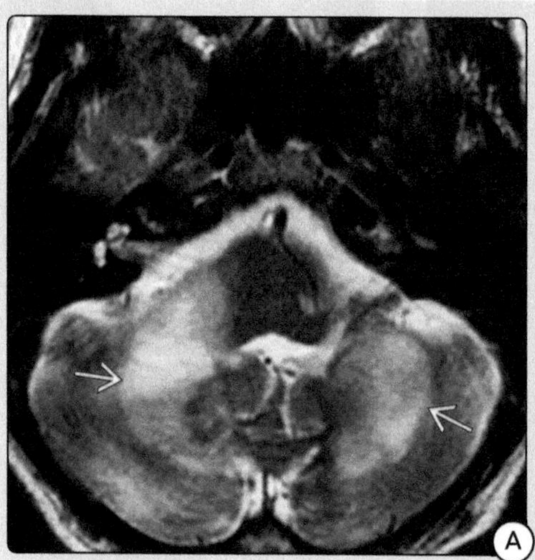

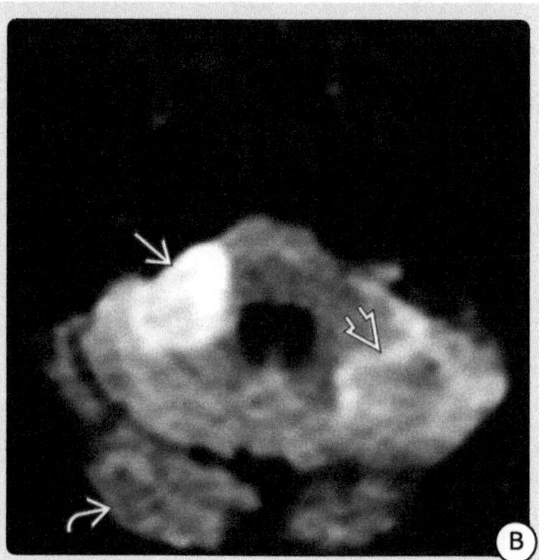

***(14-15A)** T2 MR in a 42-year-old HIV-positive woman with gait difficulties shows classic cerebellar PML with characteristic involvement of both middle cerebellar peduncles ➡. **(14-15B)** DWI shows cPML in different stages. The right posterior cerebellar lesion ➡ shows no restriction, the right middle cerebellar peduncle lesion ➡ restricts strongly and uniformly, and the left cerebellar lesion shows restriction around the lesion's rim ➡.*

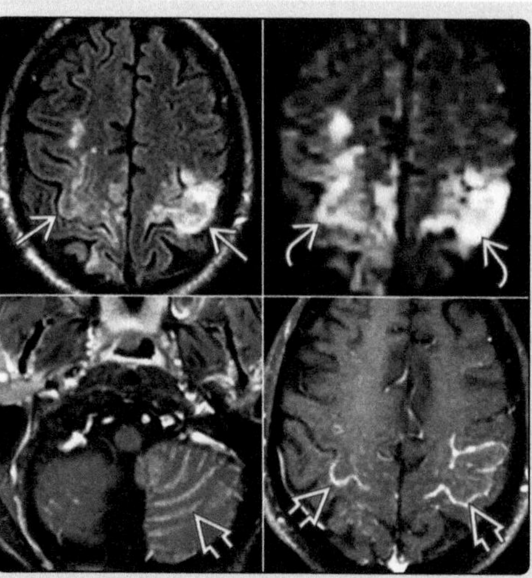

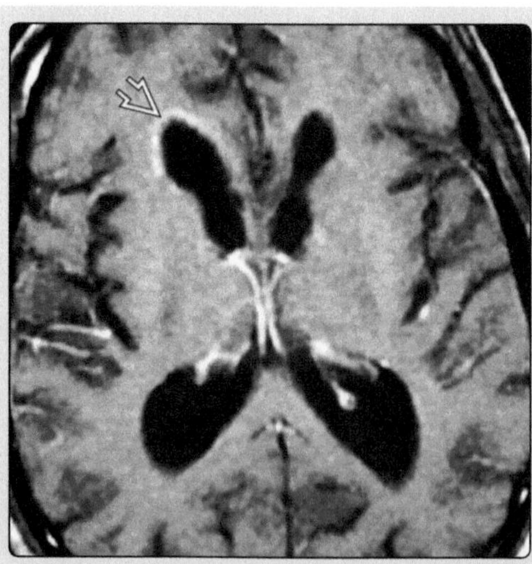

***(14-16)** MR was obtained in a 32-year-old HIV-positive man with acute CMV meningoencephalitis. FLAIR shows hyperintensity in both posterior frontal lobes ➡ that restricts on DWI ➡. T1 C+ MR shows pial enhancement ➡. **(14-17)** T1 C+ MR in a patient with HIV encephalitis shows generalized volume loss. Note striking ependymal enhancement ➡, atypical for HIV encephalitis. This is CMV ventriculitis.*

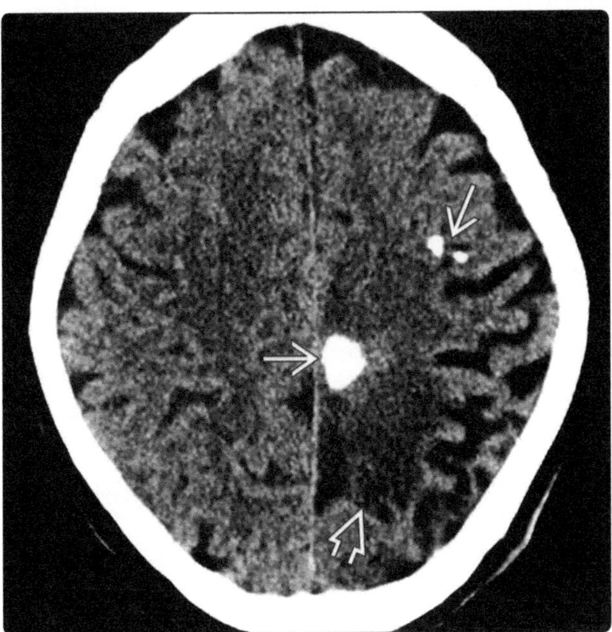

***(14-18)** A 30-year-old HIV-positive, TB-positive man treated with HAART developed increasing R-sided weakness. NECT shows multiple old calcified granulomas. Note edema surrounding the larger lesion. This is reactivation of latent tuberculosis.*

***(14-19)** HIV-positive man with a CD4 count < 50 had rapidly decreasing mental status. T1 C+ shows multiple rim-enhancing masses that were both granulomas and pseudoabscess. This is fulminant reactivated TB. (Courtesy S. Candy, MD.)*

Immune Reconstitution Inflammatory Syndrome

Terminology

CNS immune reconstitution inflammatory syndrome (IRIS) is a T-cell-mediated encephalitis that occurs in the setting of treated HIV or autoimmune disease (e.g., MS). CNS IRIS is also called neuro-IRIS.

Etiology

Most investigators consider neuro-IRIS a dysregulated immune response and pathogen-driven disease whose clinical expression depends on host susceptibility, the intensity and quality of the immune response, and the specific characteristics of the "provoking pathogen" itself.

IRIS occurs when forced immune reconstitution causes an exaggerated response to infectious (or sometimes noninfectious) antigens with massive destruction of virus-infected cells. IRIS develops in two distinct scenarios: "Unmasking" IRIS and "paradoxical" IRIS. Both differ in clinical expression, disease management, and prognosis, although their imaging manifestations are similar.

"Unmasking" IRIS occurs when antiretroviral therapy reveals a subclinical, previously undiagnosed opportunistic infection. Immune restoration leads to an immune response against a living pathogen. Here, brain parenchyma is damaged by both the replicating pathogen and the incited immune response.

"Paradoxical" IRIS occurs when a patient who has been successfully treated for a recent opportunistic infection unexpectedly deteriorates after initiation of antiretroviral therapy. Here, there is no newly acquired or reactivated infection. The recovering immune response targets persistent pathogen-derived antigens or self-antigens and causes tissue damage.

Several different underlying pathogens have been identified with IRIS. The most common are JC virus (PML-IRIS), tuberculosis (TB-IRIS), and fungal infections, especially *Cryptococcus* (crypto-IRIS). Some parasitic infections—such as toxoplasmosis—are relatively common in HIV/AIDS patients but rarely associated with IRIS.

Not all neurotropic viruses cause IRIS. HIV itself rarely causes neuro-IRIS. Herpesviruses (e.g., herpes simplex virus, varicella-zoster virus, cytomegalovirus) are all rarely reported causes of neuro-IRIS.

An unusual type of IRIS occurs in MS patients treated with natalizumab who subsequently develop PML. Natalizumab-related PML is managed by discontinuation of the drug and instituting plasmapheresis/immunoadsorption (PLEX/IA). Neurologic deficits and imaging studies in some patients worsen during subsequent immune reconstitution, causing **natalizumab-associated PML-IRIS**. Two types are recognized: Patients with early PML-IRIS (IRIS develops *before* institution of PLEX/IA) and patients with late PML-IRIS (IRIS develops *after* treatment with PLEX/IA). Neurologic outcome is generally worse in early PML-IRIS with a mortality rate approaching 25%.

Pathology

There are no specific histologic features or biomarkers for neuro-IRIS; rather, the diagnosis is established on the basis of clinical manifestations, exclusion of other disorders, and imaging or histopathologic evidence of inflammatory reaction.

Clinical Issues

Epidemiology. Between 15-35% of AIDS patients beginning HAART develop IRIS. Of these, ~ 1% develop neuro-IRIS. The two most important risk factors are a low CD4 count and a short time interval between treatment of the underlying infection and the commencement of antiretroviral therapy. The highest risk is in patients with a count < 50 cells/μL.

Epidemiology varies according to the specific "provoking pathogen." The most common cause of neuro-IRIS is JC virus. Latent virus is reactivated when patients become immunodeficient. The reactivated virus infects oligodendrocytes, causing the lytic demyelination characteristic of PML. Nearly 1/3 of patients with preexisting PML worsen after beginning HAART and are considered to have "unmasking" **PML-IRIS.**

TB-IRIS occurs in 15% of patients who are coinfected with TB if antiretroviral therapy is initiated before the TB is adequately treated. Inflammasome activation underlies the immunopathogenesis of TB-IRIS. Almost 20% of TB-IRIS patients develop neurologic involvement characterized by meningitis, tuberculomas, and radiculomyelopathies. TB-IRIS is associated with a mortality rate of up to 30%.

"Paradoxical" **crypto-IRIS** affects 20% of HIV-infected patients in whom antiretroviral therapy was initiated after treatment of neuromeningeal cryptococcosis. The major manifestation of crypto neuro-IRIS is aseptic recurrent meningitis. Parenchymal cryptococcomas are rare.

Despite the high prevalence of parasitic infestations in resource-poor countries, only a few cases of parasite-associated neuro-IRIS have been reported. All have been caused by *T. gondii.*

Natalizumab-associated IRIS is rare. To date, ~ 50 cases have been reported. Most are PML-IRIS.

(14-20A) Baseline T2 MR in a 40-year-old man with untreated HIV/AIDS for 8 years shows diffuse volume loss and bifrontal hyperintense subcortical WM lesions with both confluent ➡ and round ➡ "punctate" lesions. (14-20B) Axial T1 C+ MR shows that none of the lesions enhance. The patient was placed on combination antiretroviral treatment (cART).

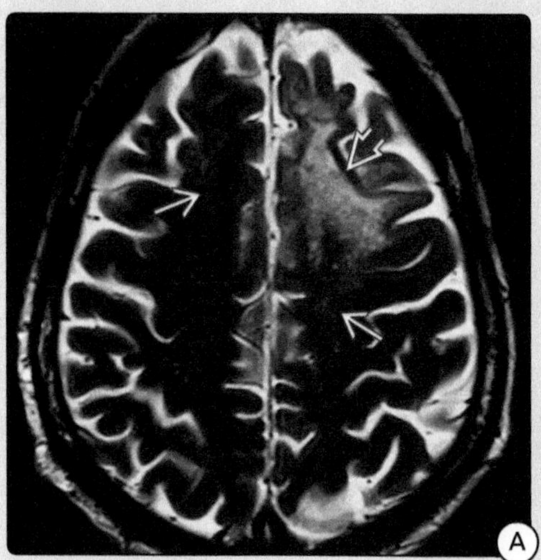

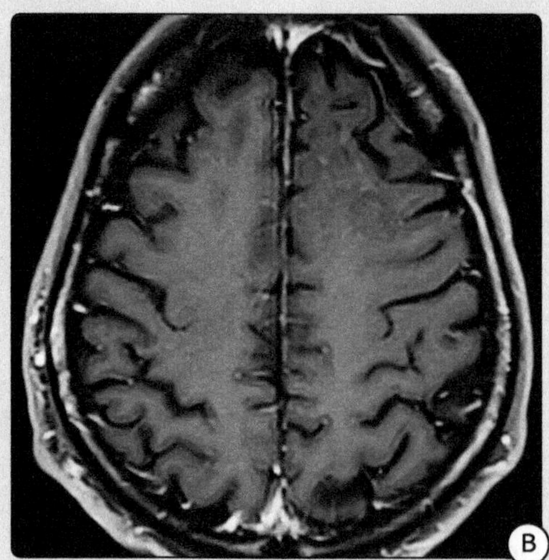

(14-20C) The patient deteriorated 5 weeks after beginning cART. Repeat T2 MR shows enlargement of the confluent left frontal lesion ➡ with interval appearance of innumerable punctate hyperintensities ➡ scattered throughout the subcortical and deep WM of both hemispheres. (14-20D) T1 C+ FS MR shows that the confluent ➡ and punctate lesions ➡ enhance. CSF was positive for JC virus. This is PML-IRIS.

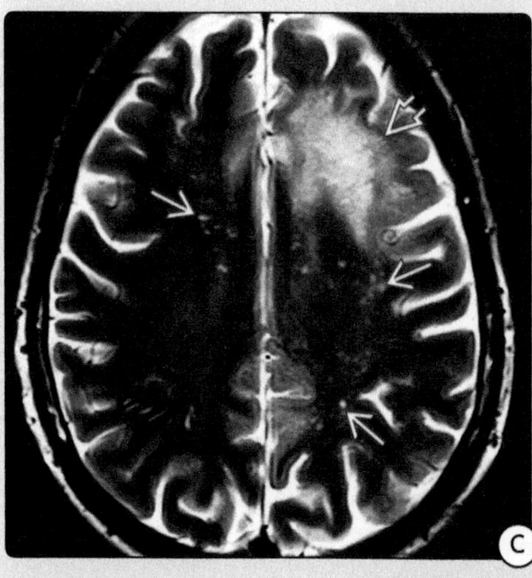

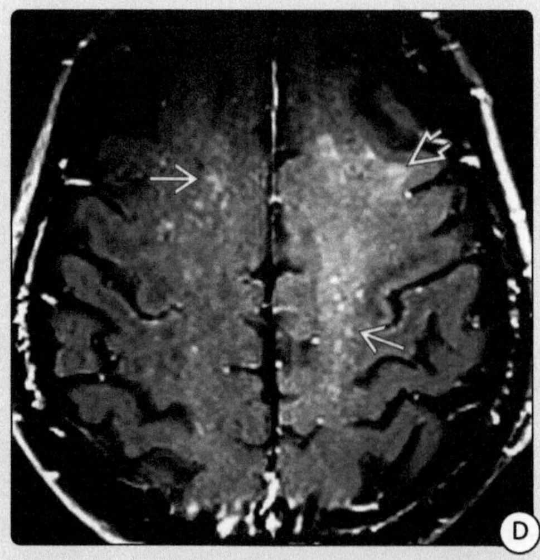

Presentation. Neuro-IRIS is a polymorphic condition with heterogeneous clinical manifestations. The most common presentation is clinical deterioration of a newly treated HIV-positive patient despite rising CD4 counts and diminishing viral loads.

Natural History and Treatment Options. Given that a low CD4 T-cell count is a major risk factor for developing IRIS, starting HAART at a count of > 350 cells/μL will prevent most cases.

Systemic IRIS is usually mild and self-limited. Prognosis in neuro-IRIS is variable. Corticosteroids and cytokine neutralization therapy have been used for treatment of neuro-IRIS with mixed results and are controversial.

Patients with neuro-IRIS may die within days to weeks. Mortality from PML-IRIS exceeds 40%, whereas that of crypto-IRIS is ~ 20%. TB-IRIS mortality is slightly lower (13%).

Imaging

A widespread pattern of confluent and linear or "punctate" perivascular hyperintensities on T2/FLAIR is virtually pathognomonic of PML-IRIS. A "punctate" pattern of enhancement is typical in the acute stage **(14-20)**.

Bizarre-looking parenchymal masses and progressively enlarging lesions can also occur in PML-IRIS. A rind of restricted diffusion and incomplete enhancement likely represent fulminant virus-induced demyelination **(14-21)**.

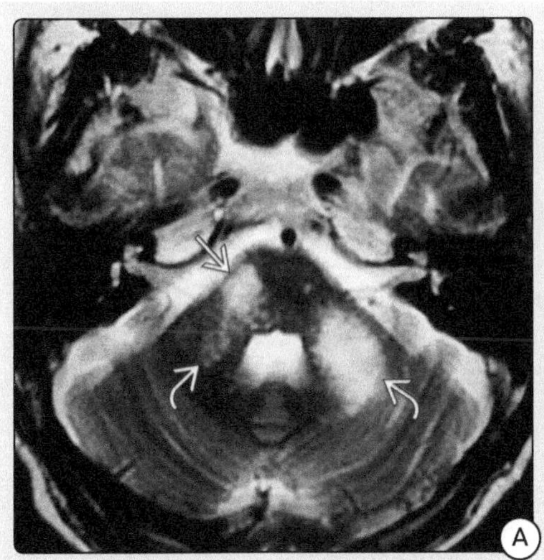

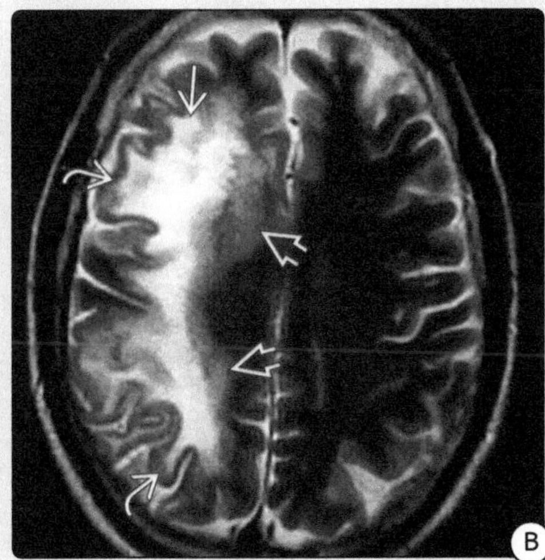

***(14-21A)** Axial T2 MR in a 56-year-old man with HIV/AIDS who deteriorated 8 weeks after HAART shows patchy hyperintense lesions in the pons ➡ and major cerebellar peduncles ➡. **(14-21B)** More cephalad T2 MR through the corona radiata shows a confluent hyperintense lesion ➡ surrounded by hazy, less hyperintensity ➡ in the right cerebral hemisphere. Note involvement of the subcortical U-fibers ➡.*

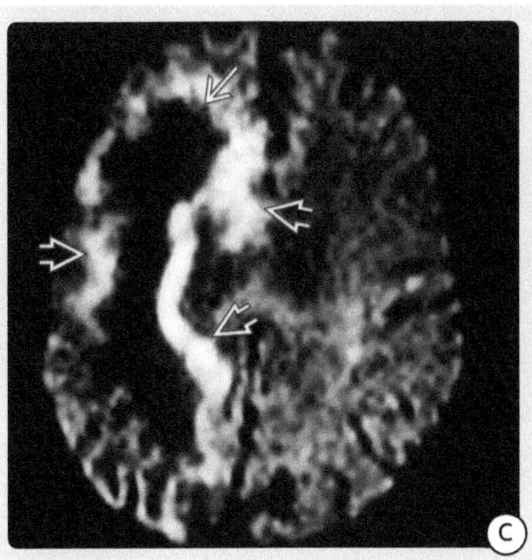

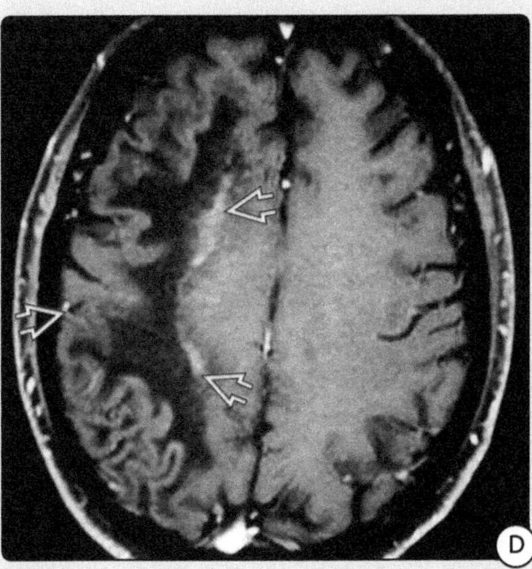

***(14-21C)** DWI MR in the same case shows a central area of T2 "black out" ➡ surrounded by an irregular area of restricted diffusion ➡ along the periphery of the lesion. **(14-21D)** More cephalad T1 C+ FS MR shows additional areas of strong contrast enhancement ➡. CSF PCR was positive for JC virus, so the imaging diagnosis of PML-IRIS was confirmed.*

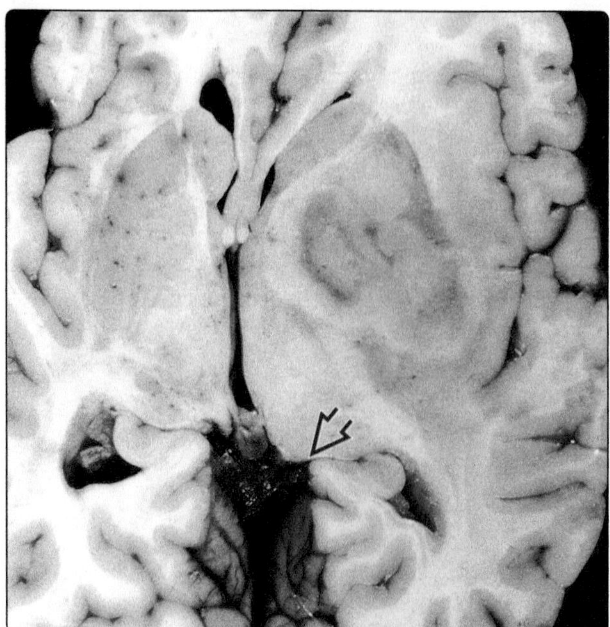

***(14-22)** Autopsy case of AIDS-related PCNSL shows a solitary mass in the basal ganglia with central necrosis and peripheral hemorrhage ➱. (Courtesy R. Hewlett, MD.)*

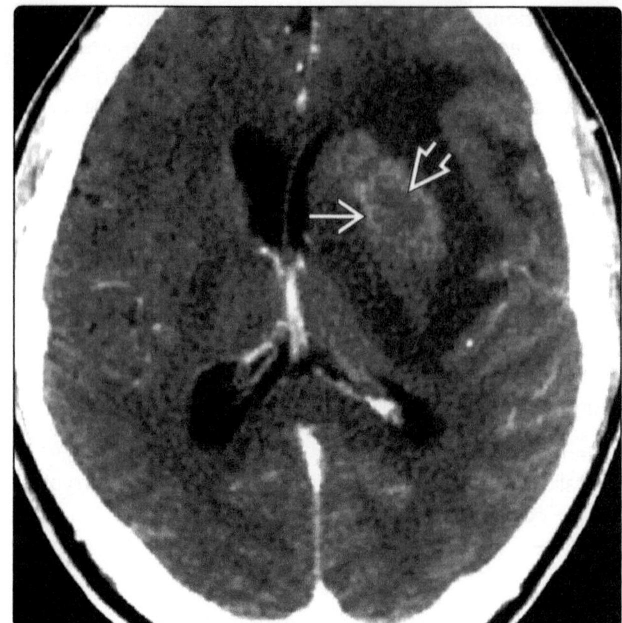

***(14-23)** Axial CECT in a different HIV-positive patient shows a solitary mass in the left basal ganglia with central necrosis ➱ and mild rim enhancement ➡. Perilesional edema is marked. Biopsy disclosed PCNSL.*

IMMUNE RECONSTITUTION INFLAMMATORY SYNDROME (IRIS)

Terminology and Etiology

- Neuro-IRIS
  - "Unmasking" IRIS (HAART "unmasks" existing subclinical opportunistic infection)
  - "Paradoxical" IRIS (treated infection worsens after HAART)
- Pathogens associated with neuro-IRIS
  - JC virus (PML-IRIS) most common
  - Tuberculosis (TB-IRIS) next most common
  - Fungi (crypto-IRIS)
  - Drugs (natalizumab-associated PML-IRIS)
  - Parasites (rare, except for toxo-IRIS)
  - Neurotropic viruses (e.g., HIV, herpesviruses) rarely cause IRIS

Epidemiology

- 15-35% of AIDS patients starting HAART develop IRIS
- Of these, 1% develop neuro-IRIS
- CD4 count < 50 cells/μL = sharply increased risk of IRIS

Imaging

- "Punctate" pattern of T2/FLAIR hyperintensities
  - "Punctate" pattern of enhancement on T1 C+
- Confluent disease extending into subcortical U-fibers
  - Variable mass-like enhancement, often bizarre and "wild"

Differential Diagnosis

- Non-IRIS-associated opportunistic infections
- AIDS-defining malignancies
  - Especially lymphoma

Differential Diagnosis

The major imaging differential diagnosis of neuro-IRIS is **non-IRIS-associated opportunistic infection**. Contrast enhancement in combination with mass effect is more typical of IRIS but may be absent early in the disease course.

Neoplasms in HIV/AIDS

In HIV-positive patients, both Epstein-Barr virus (EBV) and human herpesvirus-8 [HHV-8; a.k.a. Kaposi sarcoma-associated herpesvirus (KSHV)] have been implicated in the development of a wide range of tumors.

EBV is associated with several malignancies, including Hodgkin and non-Hodgkin lymphomas. EBV plays an especially prominent role in the development of lymphoma in patients with HIV or transplant-related immunosuppression.

KSHV-associated diseases include Kaposi sarcoma (KS), primary effusion lymphoma, and multicentric Castleman disease.

AIDS-defining malignancies (ADMs) include non-Hodgkin lymphomas, KS, and cervical cancer. The introduction of combination antiretroviral therapy (cART) has dramatically modified the natural history of HIV infection, causing a marked decline in the incidence of ADMs. In the United States and Europe, ADMs peaked in the mid-1990s and have since declined substantially. Recent statistics from South Africa show that, if cART is started before advanced immunodeficiency develops, the cancer burden in HIV-positive patients (especially children) can be substantially reduced.

In this text, we briefly discuss the two AIDS-defining malignancies that can affect the scalp, skull, and brain: Primary central nervous system lymphomas (PCNSLs) and KS.

HIV-Associated Lymphomas

Compared with other cancers, cART has had a substantial but relatively smaller impact on the prevalence of lymphoma, which remains the most common ADM in the cART era.

HIV-associated PCNSLs are typically the diffuse large B-cell non-Hodgkin type. Malignancy risk is linked to the patient's immune status and increases with CD4 counts < 50-100 cells/μL.

PCNSLs are the second most common cerebral mass lesion in AIDS (exceeded only by toxoplasmosis) and develop in 2-6% of patients. PCNSLs cause ~ 70% of all *solitary* brain parenchymal lesions in HIV/AIDS patients.

PCNSLs present as single or (less commonly) multiple masses. More than 90% are supratentorial with preferential location in the basal ganglia and deep white matter abutting the lateral ventricle. PCNSLs often cross the corpus callosum. Central necrosis and hemorrhage are common in AIDS-related lymphomas **(14-22)**, which is reflected in the imaging findings **(14-23)** **(14-24)**.

The major differential diagnosis is **toxoplasmosis**. Toxoplasmosis is more commonly multiple, and lesions often exhibit the "eccentric target" sign, i.e., an eccentrically located nodule within a ring-enhancing mass. DSC-pMR is helpful in distinguishing PCNSL from toxoplasmosis; lymphoma has typically increased relative cerebral blood volume (rCBV) whereas toxoplasmosis does not. PET and SPECT are also helpful imaging adjuncts, as lymphoma is "hot" but toxo is "not."

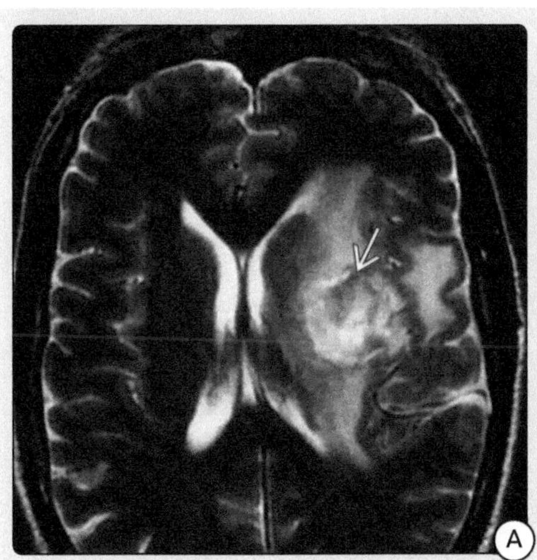

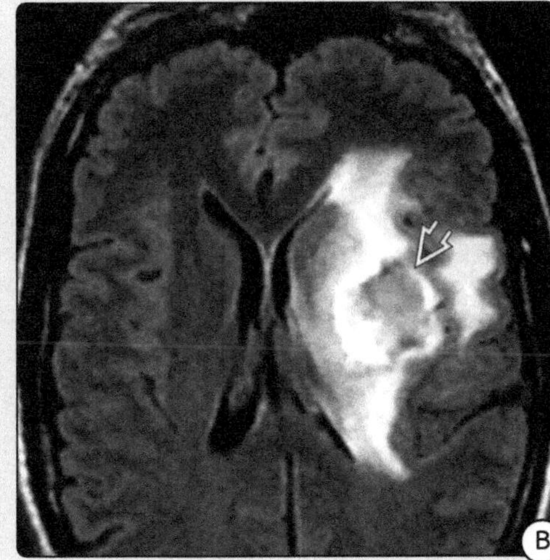

***(14-24A)** Axial T2 MR in an HIV/AIDS patient who developed right-sided weakness shows a solitary heterogeneous mass ➡ at the junction of the left basal ganglia and deep WM. **(14-24B)** The center of the lesion is isointense ➡ with brain on FLAIR MR.*

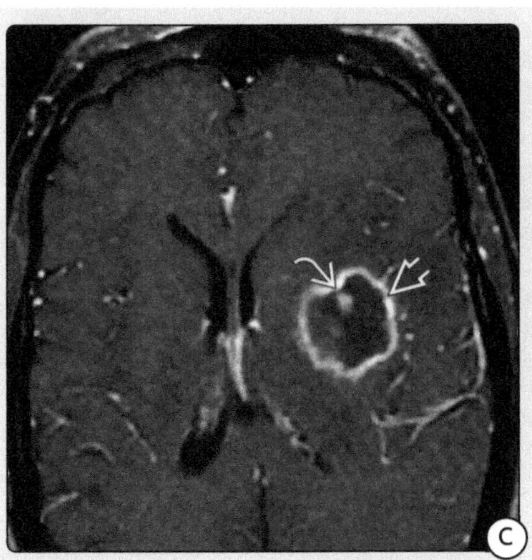

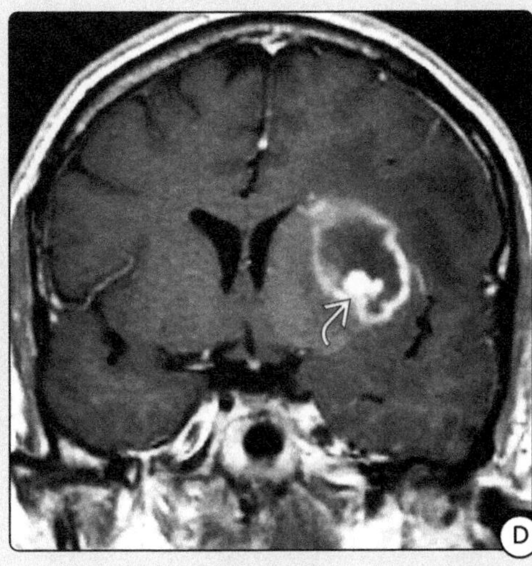

***(14-24C)** Axial T1 C+ FS MR shows an irregular rim of enhancement ➡ around the central necrotic area and an eccentric enhancing nodule ➡ within the necrotic mass. **(14-24D)** Because the coronal T1 C+ MR showed an "eccentric target" appearance ➡ of the lesion, imaging diagnosis was toxoplasmosis (even though a solitary lesion is statistically more likely to be PCNSL). Anti-toxo therapy was ineffective. Biopsy showed diffuse large B-cell lymphoma.*

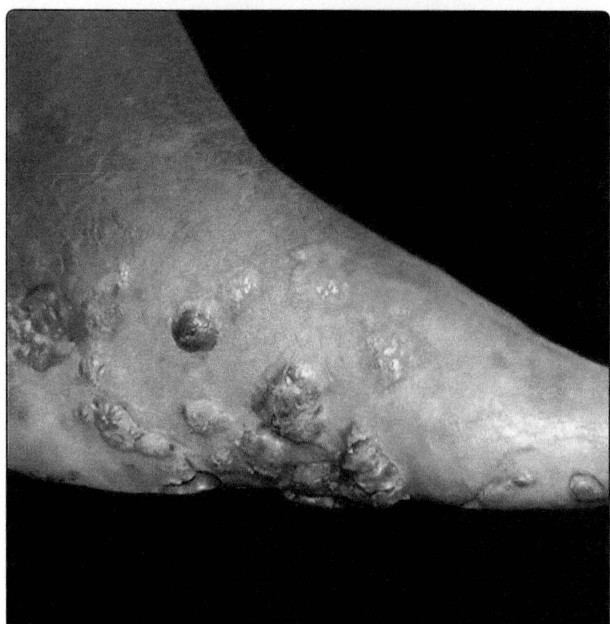

(14-25) *Clinical photograph shows classic Kaposi sarcoma (KS) presenting with multiple nodular skin lesions. (Courtesy T. Mentzel, MD.)*

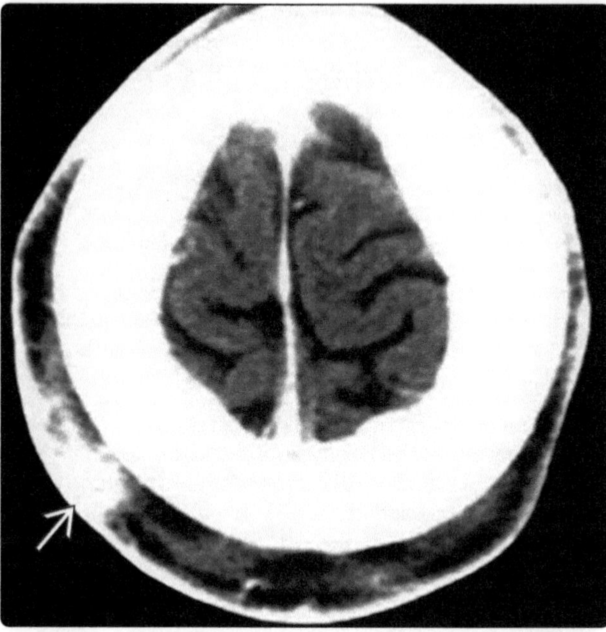

(14-26) *CECT demonstrates KS of the scalp in this AIDS patient. Note infiltration of the skin and subcutaneous tissues ➡.*

Kaposi Sarcoma

KS is the most common sarcoma in immunosuppressed patients. The next most frequent non-KS sarcoma is leiomyosarcoma followed by angiosarcoma and fibrohistiocytic tumors.

KS develops from a combination of factors: HHV-8 infection (a.k.a. KS-associated herpesvirus), altered immunity, and an inflammatory or angiogenic milieu. EBV infection is common in patients with HIV-associated leiomyosarcomas.

There has been a marked decline in the incidence of AIDS-related KS since the advent of antiretroviral therapy. Transplant-related KS often resolves after reduction of immunosuppression, highlighting the role of cellular immune response in the control of HHV-8 infection.

KS is the most common neoplasm in untreated AIDS patients. Overall, the most common site is the skin **(14-25)** followed by mucous membranes, lymph nodes, and viscera. Classic KS is an indolent tumor with purplish or dark brown plaques and nodules, usually on the extremities. AIDS-associated KS is much more aggressive. Lesions most commonly occur on the face, genitals, and mucous membranes.

Cranial KS is unusual and much less common than CNS lymphoma. When it occurs, cranial KS is typically seen as a localized scalp thickening **(14-26)** or an infiltrating soft tissue mass in the skin of the face and neck. Calvarial invasion is unusual. KS is isointense with muscle on T1WI, hyperintense on T2WI, and enhances strongly on CECT or T1 C+ MR.

AIDS-DEFINING MALIGNANCIES

HIV-Associated Lymphoma
- Etiology and pathology
  - Often associated with EBV
  - Most are diffuse large B-cell non-Hodgkin lymphoma type
- Clinical issues
  - 2nd most common mass lesion in AIDS
  - Occurs in 2-6% of HIV/AIDS patients
  - 70% of solitary CNS masses in HIV(+) patients
- Imaging
  - Hemorrhage, necrosis common
  - Supratentorial (90%)
  - Basal ganglia, deep white matter (often crosses corpus callosum)
  - Often ring enhancing
  - Increased rCBV

Kaposi Sarcoma
- Etiology and pathology
  - Associated with HHV-8
  - Most common sarcoma in immunosuppressed
- Clinical issues
  - Antiretrovirals seriously reduce prevalence
  - Skin, mucous membranes, lymph nodes, scalp
- Imaging
  - Localized scalp thickening
  - Infiltrating soft tissue mass in skin of face or neck

Selected References: The complete reference list is available on the Expert Consult™ eBook version included with purchase.

Demyelinating and Inflammatory Diseases

Once considered an "immune-privileged" site sequestered beyond the blood-brain barrier, we now know there is active and continuous immunologic surveillance in the CNS. A broad spectrum of noninfectious inflammatory, autoimmune/autoantibody-mediated disorders can affect the CNS.

In this chapter, we begin our discussion of autoimmune CNS disorders with **multiple sclerosis** (MS). We follow with a discussion of **neuromyelitis optica** and then turn our attention to postinfection and postvaccination inflammatory syndromes, specifically **acute disseminated encephalomyelitis (ADEM)**. Autoantibody-mediated diseases, such as **autoimmune encephalitis**, are then addressed.

This chapter concludes by discussing inflammatory-like disorders of unknown or uncertain etiology, such as neurosarcoidosis and idiopathic inflammatory pseudotumors.

Multiple Sclerosis and Variants

Multiple Sclerosis

Etiology

While the precise pathogenesis of MS remains unknown, the generally accepted hypothesis is that myelin antigens are presented by macrophages, microglia, and astrocytes to T cells. This leads to the release of proinflammatory cytokines and an immune attack on myelin-oligodendrocyte complexes that results in the destruction of myelin, axons, and neurons.

Epstein-Barr virus (EBV) exposure, chemicals, smoking, diet, and geographic variability all contribute to MS risk. MS occurs less often in nonwhites compared with whites. MS frequency also increases with increasing latitude and is most common in temperate climates.

Pathology

Location. Most MS plaques are supratentorial and are primarily (but not exclusively) located in the deep cerebral white matter, oriented perpendicular to the lateral ventricles **(15-1)**. The majority occur at or near the callososeptal interface. Centripetal perivenular extension is common, causing the appearance of so-called "Dawson fingers" radiating outward from the lateral ventricles **(15-2)**.

Other commonly affected areas include the subcortical U-fibers, brachium pontis, brainstem, and spinal cord. Gray matter (cortex and basal ganglia) lesions are seen in 10% of cases. Less than 10% occur in the posterior fossa.

Gross Pathology. Acute/subacute MS plaques are linear, round, or ovoid lesions with ill-defined margins. Chronic plaques have more defined borders with excavated, depressed centers.

Microscopic Features. Histopathologically, MS plaques typically demonstrate (1) relatively sharp borders **(15-3)**, (2) macrophage infiltrates (both interstitial and perivascular), and (3) perivascular chronic inflammation **(15-4)**. *Acute* lesions are often hypercellular with foamy macrophages and prominent perivascular T-cell lymphocytic cuffing **(15-9)**.

Chronic plaques range from chronic active to chronic silent lesions. Chronic active lesions have continuing inflammation around their outer borders. Chronic silent ("burned-out") lesions are characterized by hypocellular regions, myelin loss, absence of active inflammation, and glial scarring.

MULTIPLE SCLEROSIS

Location
- Supratentorial (90%), infratentorial (10%) (higher in children)
- Deep cerebral/periventricular white matter
- Predilection for callososeptal interface
- Perivenular extension (Dawson fingers)

Size and Number
- Multiple > solitary
- Mostly small (5-10 mm)
- Giant "tumefactive" plaques can be several centimeters
  - 30% of "tumefactive" MS lesions solitary

(15-1) Sagittal graphic illustrates MS plaques involving the corpus callosum, pons, and spinal cord. Note the characteristic perpendicular orientation of the lesions ➔ at the callososeptal interface along penetrating venules. (15-2) Axial autopsy section shows typical ovoid, grayish MS plaques oriented perpendicularly and adjacent to the lateral ventricles ➔, along medullary (deep WM) veins ➔. (Courtesy R. Hewlett, MD.)

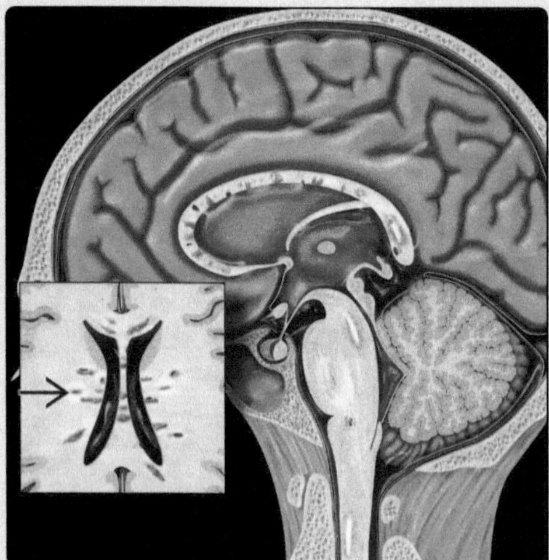

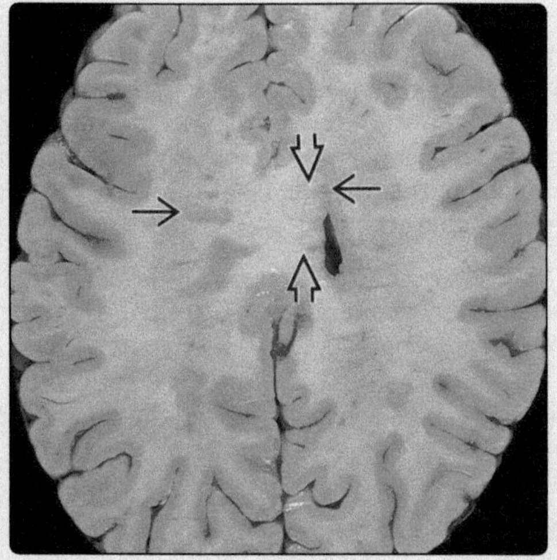

(15-3) Graphic of demyelinating plaque shows a sharp border with normal brain ➔ and interstitial and perivascular macrophages ➔. Perivascular chronic inflammation ➔ and scattered stellate reactive astrocytes ➔ are present. (15-4) H&E/Luxol fast blue stain of a demyelinating plaque emphasizes sharp interface ➔ between the lesion on the left (pale staining) and normal parenchyma on the right.

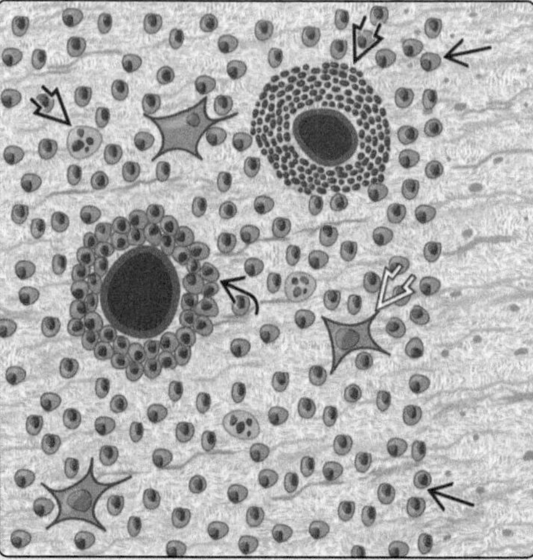

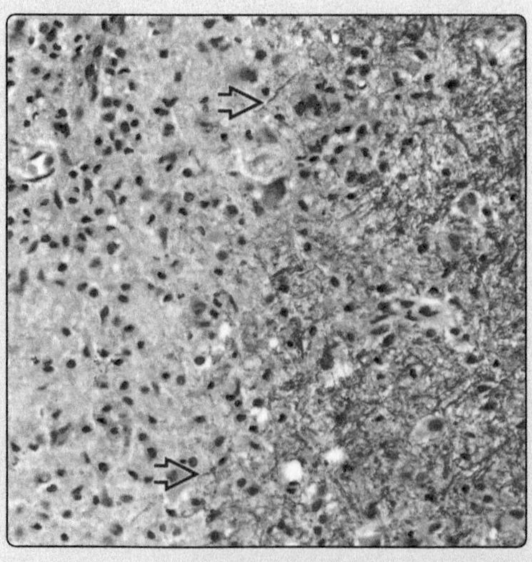

Clinical Issues

Demographics. MS is the most frequent primary demyelinating pathology in the CNS. Onset typically occurs in young to middle-aged adults from 20-40 years of age. Up to 10% of all patients with MS become symptomatic in childhood.

The overall F:M ratio is 1.77:1.00, but it is higher (3-5:1) in children. Caucasians of Northern European descent living in temperate zones are the most commonly affected ethnic group. MS is significantly less common in Asians and Africans.

Presentation. MS presentation varies with heterogeneous neurologic manifestations, evolution, and disability. Intermittent neurologic disturbances followed by progressive accumulation of disabilities is typical.

The first attack of MS (most commonly optic neuritis, transverse myelitis, or a brainstem syndrome) is known as a clinically isolated syndrome. Half of patients with optic neuritis eventually develop MS.

Clinical MS Subtypes. Several major MS subtypes are recognized. From least to most severe, they are as follows: Radiologically isolated syndrome (**RIS**), clinically isolated syndrome (**CIS**), relapsing-remitting MS (**RR-MS**), relapsing progressive MS (**RP-MS**), secondary-progressive MS (**SP-MS**), and primary-progressive MS (**PP-MS**).

Radiologically Isolated Syndrome. RIS is a new subtype described at the very mildest of the demyelinating disease spectrum. RIS refers to MR findings of T2/FLAIR lesions suggestive of MS in persons with no history of neurologic symptoms and with a normal neurologic examination.

By definition, patients with RIS have dissemination in space. When a clinical attack occurs in these patients, a diagnosis of MS can be made. Until that occurs, most experts agree that MS should *not* be diagnosed solely on the basis of MR findings.

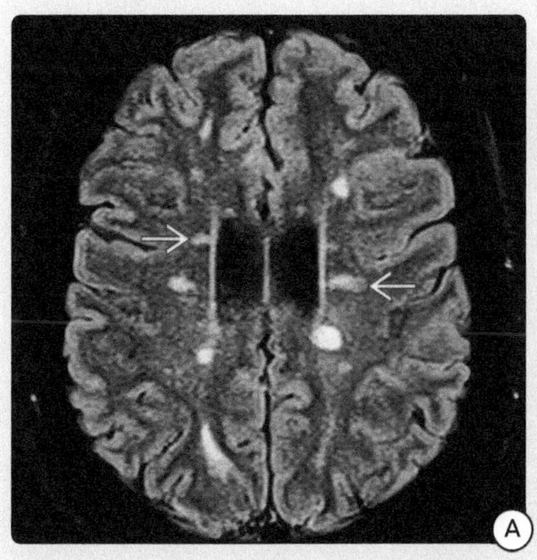

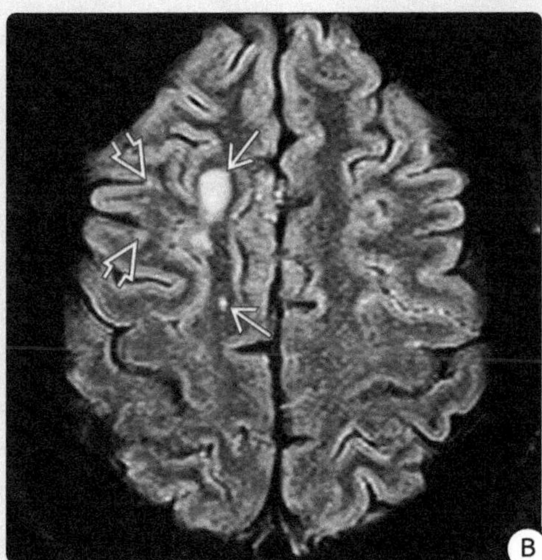

***(15-5A)** Axial FLAIR MR in a 30y woman with intermittent vague symptoms of numbness and tingling in her face and hands shows multiple ovoid subcortical and deep periventricular hyperintensities with several demonstrating a distinct perpendicular orientation to the lateral ventricles ➡ (Dawson fingers). **(15-5B)** More cephalad FLAIR in the same case shows additional lesions in the corona radiata ➡ and subtle lesions in the cortical gram ➡.*

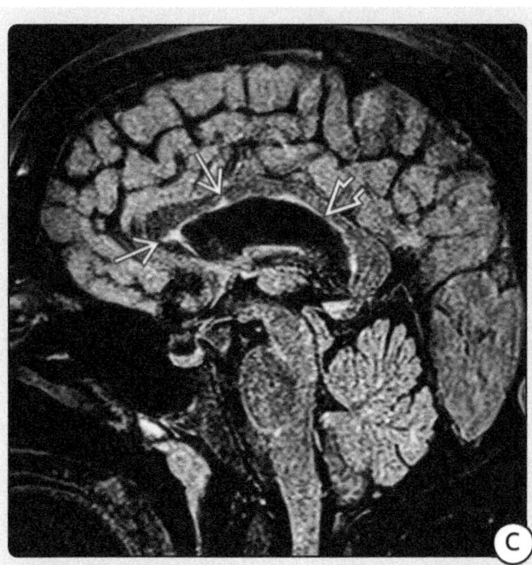

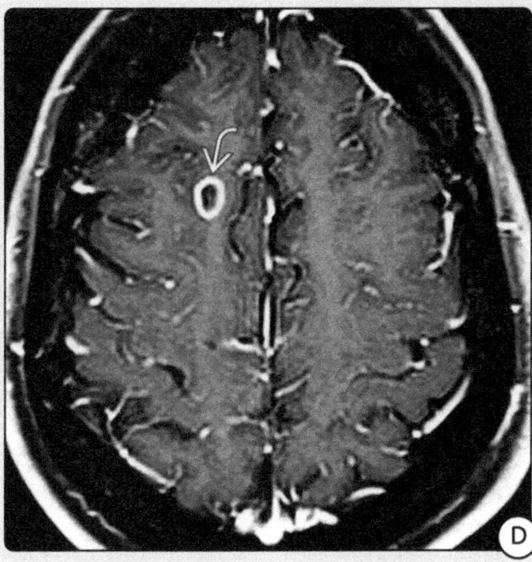

***(15-5C)** Sagittal FLAIR MR demonstrates several triangle-shaped hyperintensities ➡ at the callososeptal interface and a "dot-dash" appearance ➡ along the ventricle. **(15-5D)** T1 C+ FS MR in the same case shows a solitary ring-enhancing lesion ➡. The imaging appearance satisfies the additional data required by the revised 2017 McDonald criteria for the diagnosis of MS.*

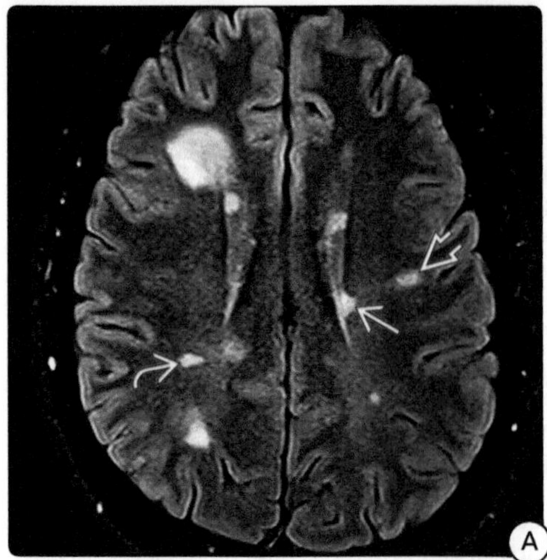

(15-6A) FLAIR shows typical MS hyperintensities ➡ with triangle shape ➡ and perpendicular orientation ➡ along deep medullary veins.

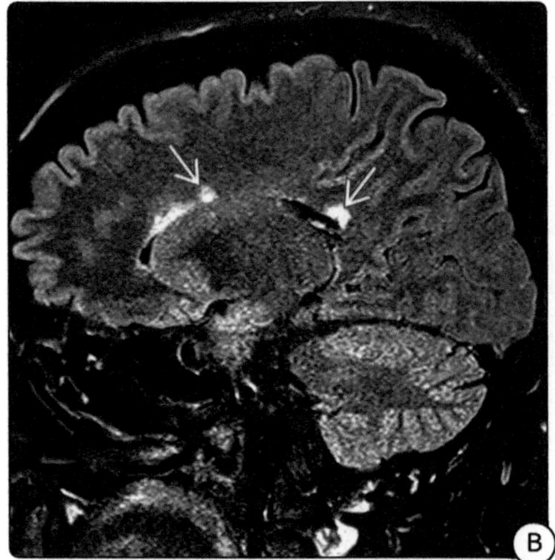

(15-6B) Sagittal FLAIR MR in the same case demonstrates the triangle shape of the periventricular lesions ➡.

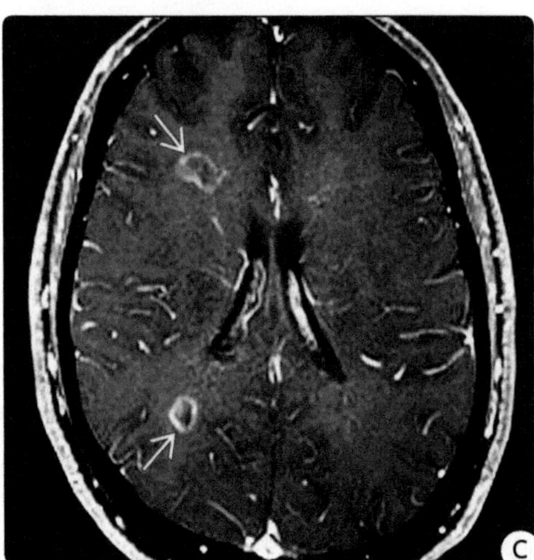

(15-6C) T1 C+ FS MR shows irregular rim enhancement ➡ of some—but not all—of the lesions. This is acute-onset MS.

Clinically Isolated Syndrome. The first attack of MS (most commonly optic neuritis, transverse myelitis, or a brainstem syndrome) is known as a clinically isolated syndrome. Half of patients with optic neuritis eventually develop MS.

Disease progression to MS varies. Patients with MR-negative CIS have a 20% chance of developing MS. If patients with CIS have MR evidence for typical brain lesions, the chance of developing clinically definite MS is 60-80%. If imaging demonstrates old lesions in a different location, dissemination in time is established, and the criteria for establishing MS are fulfilled (see below).

Relapsing-Remitting MS. The vast majority—about 85%—of all MS patients experience relapses alternating with remission phases and are classified as having RR-MS. Attacks ("relapses" or "exacerbations") are followed by periods of partial or complete recovery. New MR lesions often occur as part of a relapse but may also occur without symptoms.

Relapsing-Progressive MS. RP-MS is also known as secondary-progressive MS. In RP-MS, there is progressive worsening of neurologic function (accumulation of disability) over time.

Almost 1/2 of RR-MS patients enter an RP-MS stage within 10 years. By 25 years following initial diagnosis, 90% of RR-MS cases become the RP-MS subtype.

Primary-Progressive MS. PP-MS is characterized by worsening neurologic function from the outset and lacks periods of remission. Approximately 5-10% of patients have PP-MS. Patients with PP-MS tend to have fewer brain lesions but more lesions in the spinal cord.

Diagnosis. The diagnosis of MS requires (1) elimination of more likely diagnoses and (2) demonstration of dissemination of CNS lesions in space and time. The 2017 revised McDonald diagnostic criteria incorporate clinical presentation (such as clinical presentation in a person with typical attack/CIS at onset) and additional data (e.g., MR evidence for dissemination in space and dissemination in time, characteristic CSF findings) to establish the diagnosis.

2017 REVISED McDONALD CRITERIA FOR MS DIAGNOSIS

Clinical Presentation

- In a person with typical attack/CIS at onset
  - Varies with number of attacks, objective clinical evidence
  - May or may not require additional data
  - MR or CSF specific (oligoclonal bands)

MR: Dissemination in Space (DIS)

- ≥ 1 T2-hyperintense lesion(s)
  - Can be symptomatic or asymptomatic
- In ≥ 2 areas
  - Periventricular
  - Juxtacortical/cortical
  - Infratentorial
  - Spinal cord

MR: Dissemination in Time (DIT)

- *Simultaneous* presence of both enhancing, nonenhancing MS-typical lesions
  - Can be symptomatic or asymptomatic
- *New* T2 or enhancing lesion on follow-up MR
  - Compared to baseline scan (without regard to timing of baseline scan)

Imaging

General Features. Most MS plaques are small—between 5 mm and 10 mm—although large lesions can reach several centimeters. Plaques are usually multiple, although 30% of giant "tumefactive" plaques initially occur as solitary lesions and are relatively more common in children and young adults.

CT Findings. NECT is often normal early in the disease course, especially with mild cases. Solitary or multiple ill-defined white matter hypodensities may be present. Acute or subacute lesions may show mild to moderate punctate, patchy, or ring enhancement on CECT.

MR Findings. Over 95% of patients with clinically definite MS have positive findings on MR scans. Therefore, MR is the procedure of choice for both initial evaluation and treatment follow-up. The 2017 revised McDonald criteria for MS diagnosis allow MR to demonstrate dissemination in both space (DIS) and time (DIT).

T1WI. Most MS plaques are hypo- or isointense on T1WI. A faint, poorly delineated peripheral rim of mild hyperintensity secondary to lipid peroxidation and macrophage infiltration often surrounds sharply delineated hypointense "black holes." This gives many subacute and chronic lesions a characteristic "beveled" or "lesion-within-a-lesion" appearance **(15-7)**.

Chronic and severe cases typically show moderate volume loss and generalized atrophy. The corpus callosum becomes progressively thinner and is best delineated on sagittal T1WI.

T2/FLAIR. T2WI shows multiple hyperintense linear, round, or ovoid lesions surrounding the medullary veins that radiate centripetally away from the lateral ventricles **(15-5)**. Larger lesions often demonstrate a very hyperintense center surrounded by a slightly less hyperintense peripheral area and variable amounts of perilesional edema.

MS plaques often assume a distinct triangular shape with the base adjacent to the ventricle on sagittal FLAIR or T2WI images **(15-7C)**.

T1 C+. Punctate, nodular, linear **(15-10)**, and rim patterns are seen during active demyelination **(15-6)**. A prominent incomplete rim ("horseshoe") of enhancement with the "open" nonenhancing segment facing the cortex can be present, especially in large "tumefactive" lesions **(15-8)** **(15-11)**.

Enhancement disappears within 6 months in > 90% of lesions. *Steroid administration significantly reduces lesion enhancement and conspicuity and may render some lesions virtually invisible!*

DWI and MRS. Although occasionally acute MS plaques can demonstrate restricted diffusion, such an appearance is atypical and should not be considered a reliable biomarker of plaque activity. MRS shows elevated MI in acute lesions. "Tumefactive" MS shows nonspecific findings (elevated choline, decreased NAA, and high lactate).

Differential Diagnosis

Multifocal nonenhancing T2/FLAIR "white spots" are nonspecific imaging findings and have a broad differential diagnosis. It is helpful to suggest whether such lesions do or do not meet the revised 2017 McDonald criteria for multiple sclerosis.

Multifocal enhancing white matter lesions can be caused by **acute disseminated encephalomyelitis** (ADEM), **vasculitis**, and **Lyme disease**. **Susac syndrome** (see later discussion) is often mistaken for MS on imaging studies, as both have multifocal T2/FLAIR white matter hyperintensities and

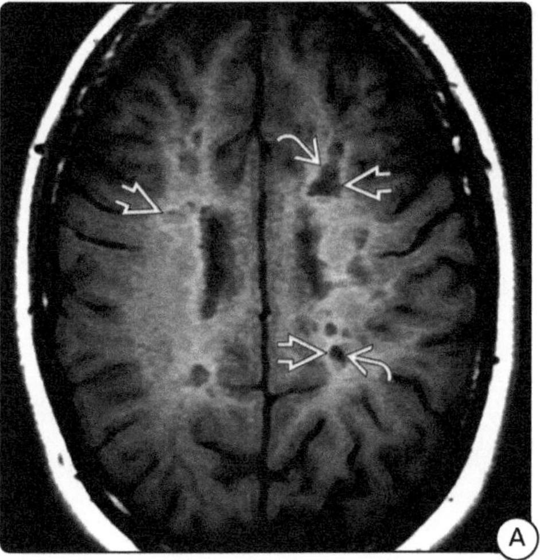

***(15-7A)** T1 MR in chronic MS shows hyperintense rims surrounding deep WM plaques, giving the distinct "lesion-within-a-lesion" appearance.*

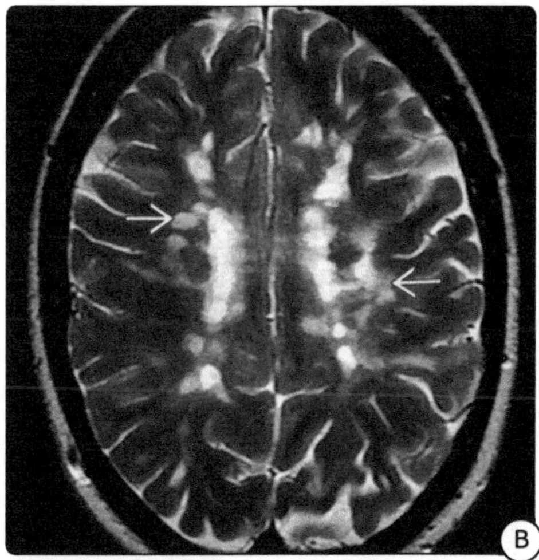

***(15-7B)** T2 MR shows the ovoid perivenular plaques that are oriented perpendicular to the lateral ventricles, as seen in the axial plane.*

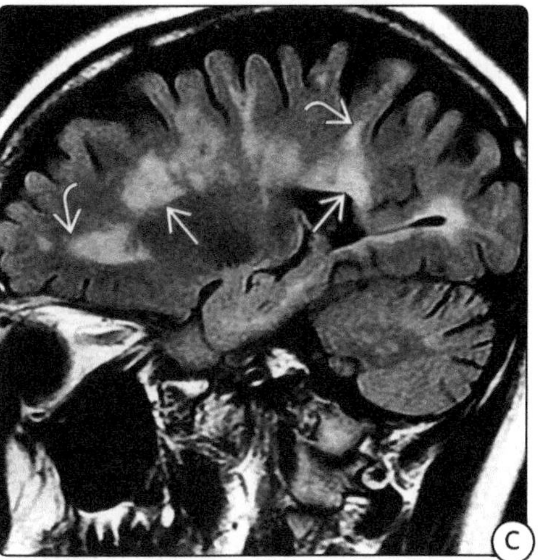

***(15-7C)** FLAIR MR shows broad-based lesions oriented toward ventricular surface with their apices pointing toward the cortex.*

both commonly affect young adult women. Lesions in Susac syndrome preferentially involve the *middle* of the corpus callosum, not the callososeptal interface **(15-24)**.

"Tumefactive" MS can mimic **abscess** or **neoplasm** (**glioblastoma** or **metastasis**). *"Tumefactive" demyelination often has an incomplete or "horseshoe" pattern of enhancement.*

MULTIPLE SCLEROSIS: IMAGING

CT

- Patchy/confluent hypodensities
- Mild/moderate, patchy, ring enhancement

MR

- Hypointense on T1WI ± faint hyperintense rim
- Very hyperintense center on T2WI, slightly less hyperintense rim
  - Callososeptal interface
  - Triangular on sagittal
  - Ovoid, perivenular on axial
  - Subpial, intracortical lesions common
- Active plaques enhance ("tumefactive" partial rim)
- Steroids suppress enhancement!

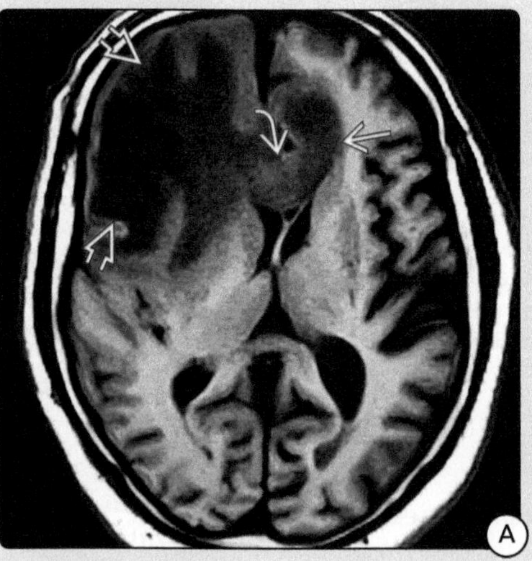

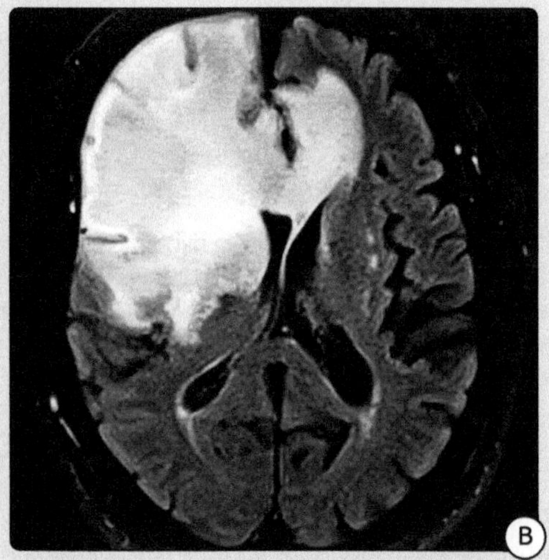

***(15-8A)** Axial T1 MR in a 77-year-old man with 2 days of progressive confusion shows a large hypointense right frontal lobe mass ➡ that thickens and crosses the corpus callosum ➡ and extends into the white matter of the left frontal lobe ➡. **(15-8B)** FLAIR MR in the same case shows that the huge mass is heterogeneously hyperintense. Note that, compared with the size of the lesion, the mass effect is relatively minor.*

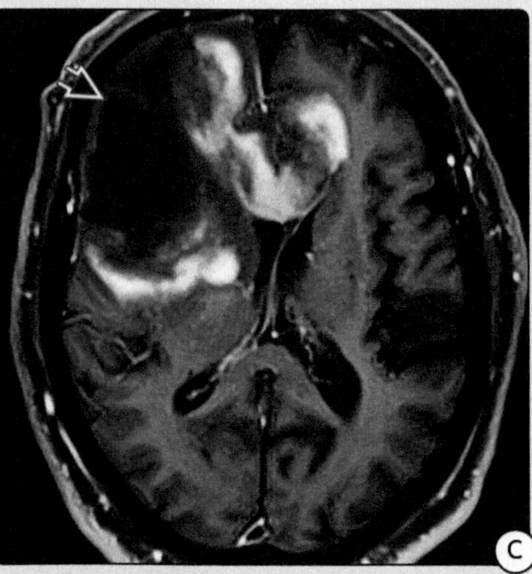

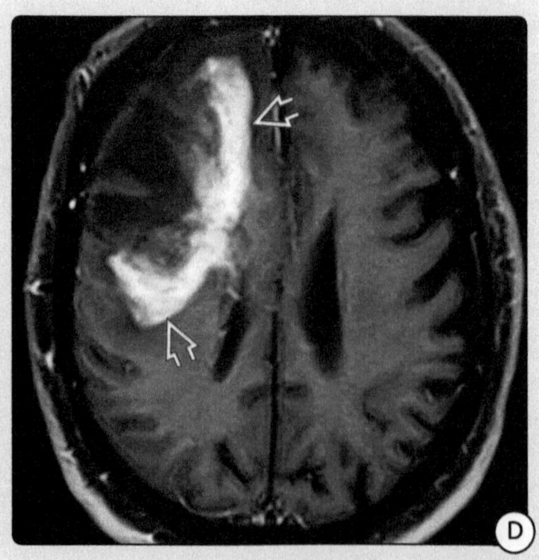

***(15-8C)** T1 C+ FS MR shows that the mass enhances strongly but very heterogeneously with significant nonenhancing areas ➡ near the cortex of the right frontal lobe. **(15-8D)** More cephalad T1 C+ MR shows a thick, incomplete rim of enhancement ➡. Imaging diagnosis was tumefactive demyelination. Because of the patient's age and location of the mass, biopsy was performed. Pathologic diagnosis was tumefactive demyelination.*

Multiple Sclerosis "Variants"

The relationship of atypical demyelinating disorders, such as Marburg disease (**MD**), Schilder disease (**SD**), Balo concentric sclerosis (**BCS**), and progressive solitary sclerosis (**SS**) as well as atypical idiopathic inflammatory demyelinating disorders (**IIDDs**), to the acute-onset MS spectrum remains uncertain.

Marburg Disease

MD is generally considered as an acute fulminant MS variant characterized by rapid, relentless progression and an exceptionally severe clinical course that usually leads to death within 1 year. Patients are typically young adults.

Marked lymphocytic infiltrates **(15-9)** with inflammatory changes in the perivenular spaces can lead to hyperacute, fulminant demyelination with a "centrifugal" pattern of contrast leakage from medullary veins on T1 C+ imaging **(15-10)**. The presence of developmental venous anomalies (DVAs) seems to predispose to "tumefactive" demyelination centered around the "Medusa head" **(15-11)**.

Imaging shows multifocal diffusely disseminated disease with focal and confluent white matter hyperintensities on T2/FLAIR. Strong patchy enhancement on T1 C+ is typical, and large, cavitating, incomplete, ring-enhancing, "tumefactive" lesions are common **(15-12)**.

Schilder Disease

SD—a.k.a. myelinoclastic diffuse sclerosis—is a rare subacute or chronic demyelinating disorder characterized by one or more inflammatory demyelinating white matter plaques. SD is typically a disease of childhood and young adults. Median age at presentation is 18 years with a slight female predominance.

Although SD is considered to be a variant of MS, clinical features are atypical for MS, and the disease is usually monophasic with a low rate of recurrence. Signs of increased

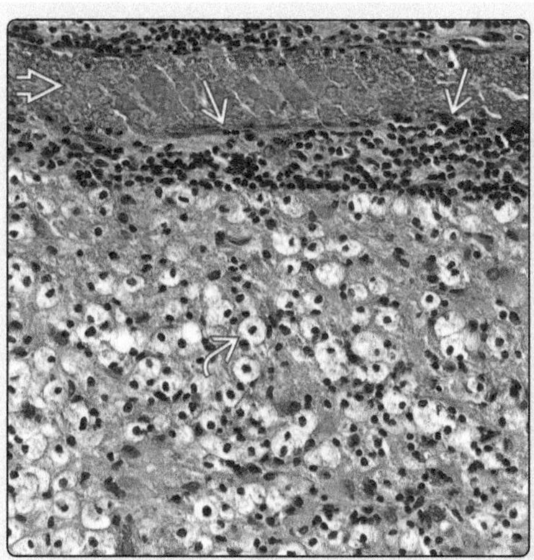

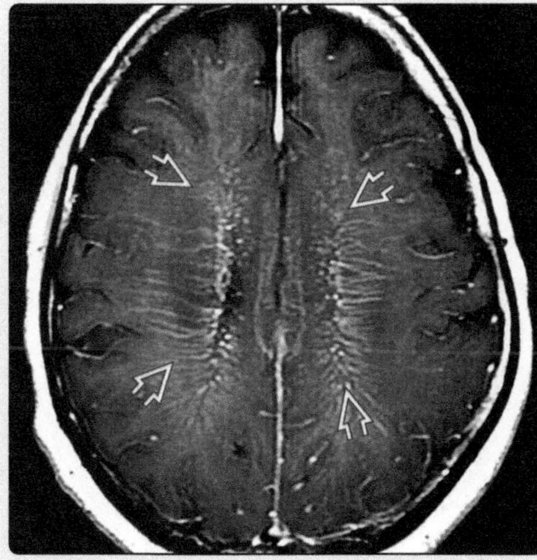

***(15-9)** H&E shows venule ➡ with marked perivascular lymphocytic cuffing ➡, striking macrophage infiltrates ➡ in acute, fulminant "tumefactive" demyelination. **(15-10)** T1 C+ FS MR in hyperacute demyelination (from fulminant MS or ADEM, PML-IRIS, etc.) can show striking enhancement, enlargement of deep medullary veins ➡. Findings can mimic vasculitis and intravascular lymphoma.*

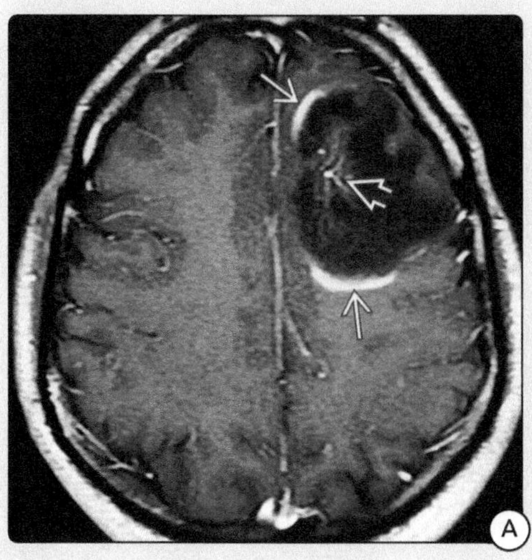

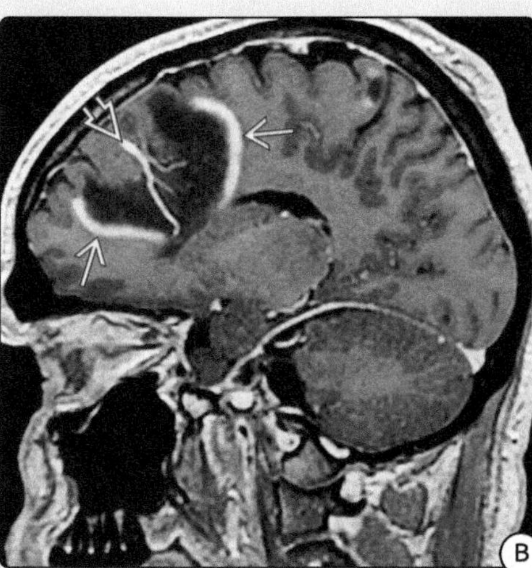

***(15-11A)** T1 C+ MR in a 38-year-old man with optic neuritis shows tumefactive demyelination with partial rim enhancement ➡. Note that the lesion surrounds a classic DVA ➡. **(15-11B)** Sagittal T1 C+ MR shows the DVA ➡ surrounded by the incompletely enhancing rim of tumefactive MS ➡.*

intracranial pressure, aphasia, and behavioral symptoms are typical. CSF is usually normal, and there is no history to suggest acute disseminated encephalomyelitis (ADEM) (i.e., no fever, infection, or preceding vaccination). Approximately 15% of cases progress to MS.

MR shows a hypointense lesion on T1WI that is hyperintense on T2/FLAIR. Rim enhancement—often the incomplete or "open ring" pattern—is seen during the acute inflammatory stage. The lesion rim usually restricts on DWI during the acute phase.

The differential diagnosis of SD can be difficult. **"Tumefactive" MS** can appear identical to SD on imaging studies. SD often mimics intracranial neoplasm or abscess both in clinical presentation and on imaging studies. **Pyogenic abscess** generally shows strong diffusion restriction in the lesion core. Perfusion MR may be helpful in distinguishing SD from **metastasis** and **glioblastoma**.

Balo Concentric Sclerosis

BCS is generally considered an atypical or variant form of MS and occurs as a discrete, concentrically layered white matter lesion. It is often described as having an "onion ring" or "whorled" appearance caused by its peculiar pattern of alternating rims of demyelination and myelin preservation.

BCS is usually characterized by acute onset and rapid clinical deterioration. Peak presentation is between 20 and 50 years. The F:M ratio is ~ 2:1 and is most common in patients of east Asian origin.

Imaging studies reflect the distinctive gross pathology of BCS and vary with disease stage. Acute lesions have significant surrounding edema **(15-13A)**. The actively demyelinating layers enhance on T1 C+ sequences. Other more typical MS-like plaques can also be present. Lesions in subacute/chronic BCS exhibit alternating bands of differing signal intensities on T2WI and resemble a "whirlpool" of concentric rings **(15-13B)**.

(15-12A) T1 C+ FS MR through the ventricles shows the necrotic, cavitating, acutely enhancing right parietal "tumefactive" mass ➡. Other enhancing foci are present ➡. (15-12B) Coronal T1 C+ MR shows extension around the left ventricle ➡ in addition to other enhancing foci ➡. This is the Marburg variant of MS.

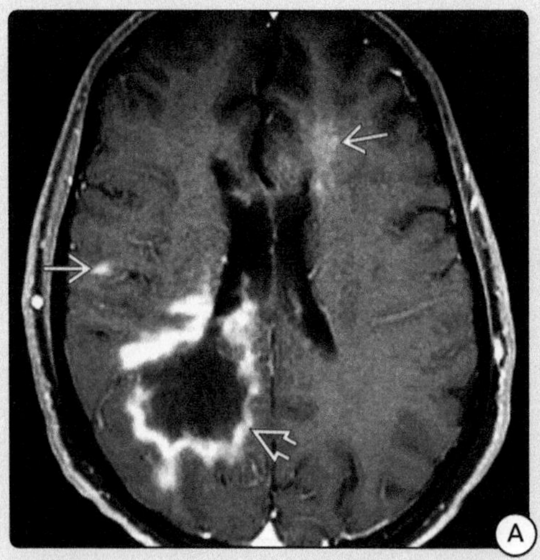

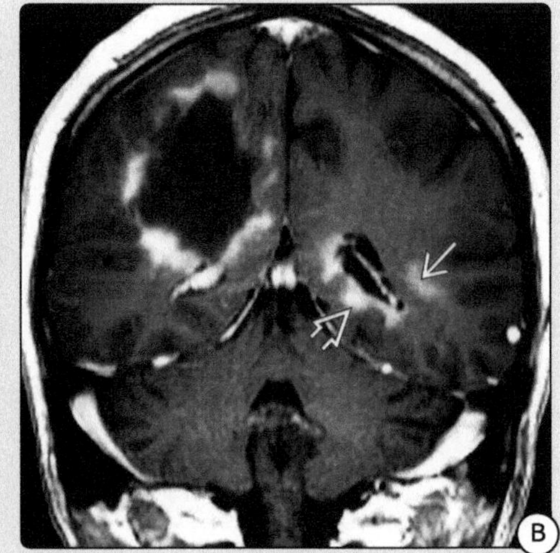

(15-13A) Acute Balo concentric sclerosis lesions are hyperintense on FLAIR ➡, restrict on DWI ➡, and show concentric "onion bulb" enhancement ➡. (15-13B) Follow-up scans show alternating rings of iso- and hyperintensity on T1 ➡ and T2WI ➡, no enhancement ➡. (Courtesy P. Rodriguez, MD.)

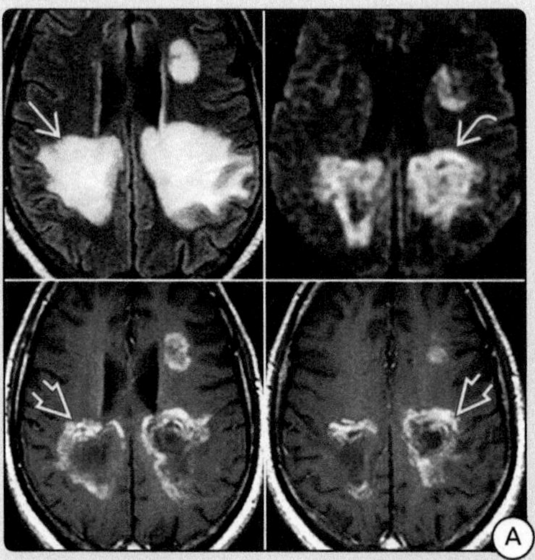

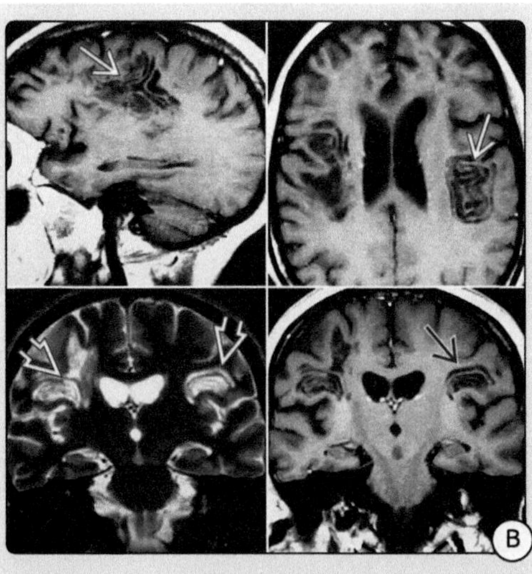

Postinfection and Postimmunization Demyelination

Postinfectious demyelinating disorders, **acute disseminated encephalomyelitis (ADEM)** and **acute hemorrhagic leukoencephalopathy (AHLE)**, are considered part of the inflammatory demyelinating disease spectrum. A serious, potentially life-threatening type of acute encephalopathy in children, **acute necrotizing encephalopathy (ANE)**, is also included in this discussion.

Acute Disseminated Encephalomyelitis

Terminology

ADEM is a postinfection, postimmunization disorder that is also called parainfectious encephalomyelitis. Once considered a purely monophasic illness, recurrent and **multiphasic forms (MDEM)** of ADEM are now recognized.

Etiology

The immunohistopathologic features of ADEM mimic those of experimental allergic encephalitis, an induced autoimmune disease precipitated by myelin antibodies. Therefore, most investigators consider ADEM an immune-mediated CNS demyelinating disorder.

Pathology

Location. As the name implies, ADEM can involve both the brain and spinal cord. White matter lesions usually predominate, but basal ganglia involvement is seen in nearly 1/2 of all cases. Spinal cord lesions are found in 10-30% of cases.

A rare ADEM variant, acute infantile bilateral striatal necrosis, occurs 1-2 weeks following a respiratory illness. Viral and streptococcal infections have been implicated and cause enlarged hyperintense basal ganglia, caudate nuclei, and internal/external capsules.

Size and Number. Lesion size varies from a few millimeters to several centimeters ("tumefactive" ADEM), and lesions have a punctate to flocculent configuration. Multiple lesions are more common than solitary lesions.

Gross Pathology. Small lesions are often inapparent on gross examination. Large "tumefactive" lesions cause a gray-pink white matter discoloration and often extend all the way to the cortex-white matter junction **(15-14)**. Mass effect is minimal compared with lesion size. Gross intralesional hemorrhage is rare and more characteristic of AHLE than ADEM.

Microscopic Features. "Sleeves" of pronounced perivenular demyelination with macrophage-predominant inflammatory infiltrates are typical. The outer margins of ADEM lesions are indistinct compared with the relatively well-delineated edges of MS plaques. Viral inclusion bodies are generally absent, unlike viral encephalitis.

Clinical Issues

Epidemiology and Demographics. ADEM is second only to MS as the most common acquired idiopathic inflammatory demyelinating disease. Unlike MS, there is no female predominance. ADEM occurs most commonly in spring and autumn.

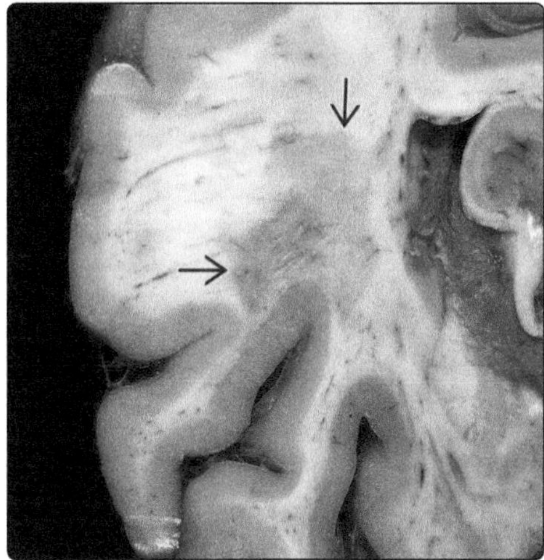

***(15-14)** Autopsy shows necrotizing demyelination ⇨ typical of post-infection, post-vaccination disorders. (Courtesy R. Hewlett, MD.)*

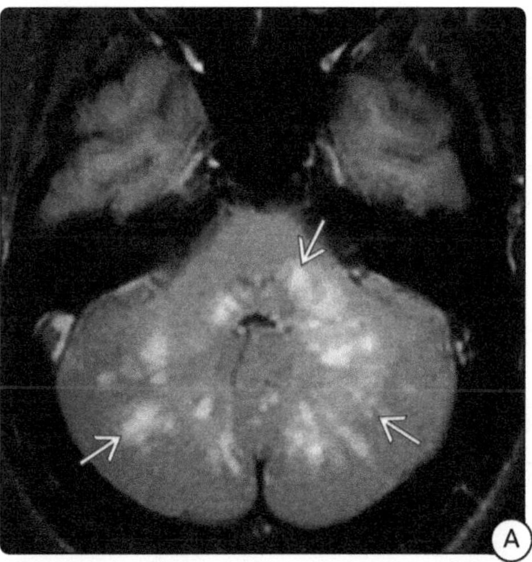

***(15-15A)** T1 C+ FS of 37y woman with headache, unsteady gait 2 weeks after URI shows multifocal patchy enhancing foci in pons, cerebellum ➡.*

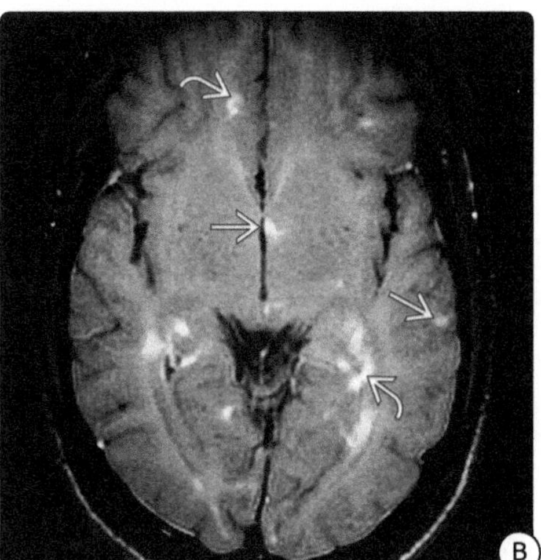

***(15-15B)** Axial T1 C+ FS MR shows several punctate ➡ and incomplete ring-enhancing lesions ➡ in both hemispheres. This is ADEM.*

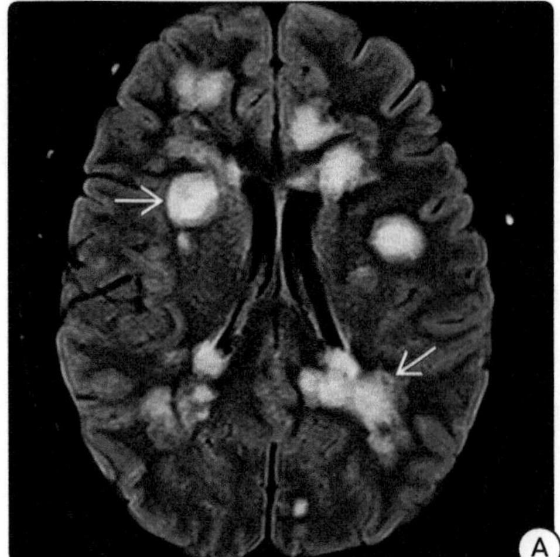

***(15-16A)** FLAIR MR following viral infection shows bilateral white matter lesions with a "fluffy" appearance and "fuzzy" margins ➡.*

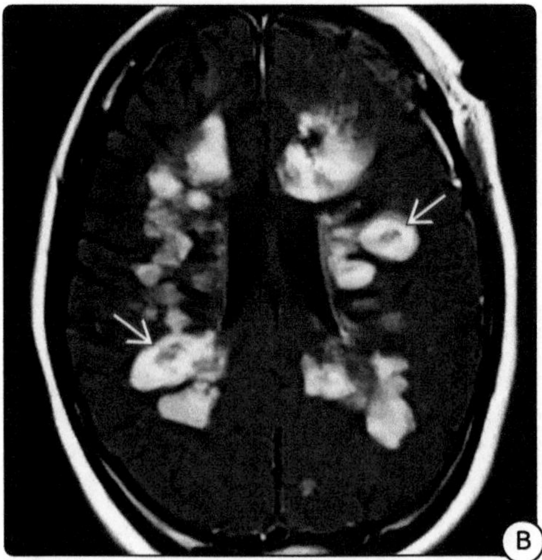

***(15-16B)** T1 C+ MR shows that the lesions enhance intensely but heterogeneously. Some have a ring-like appearance ➡.*

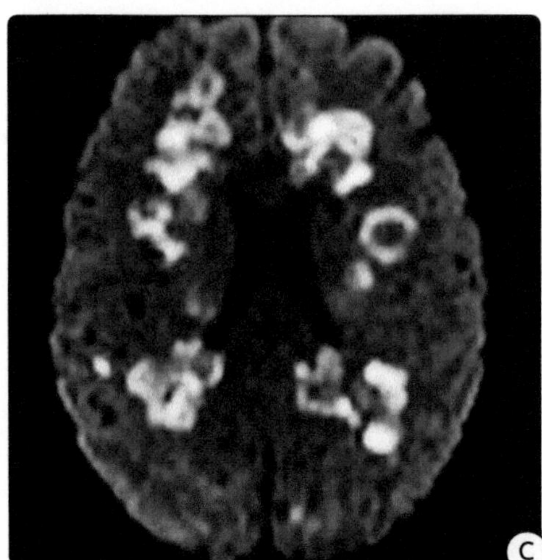

***(15-16C)** DWI MR shows acute diffusion restriction in the lesions. Biopsy disclosed demyelinating disease, most likely ADEM.*

ADEM can occur at any age but—perhaps because of the frequency of immunizations and antigen exposure—is more common in childhood with peak occurrence between 5 and 8 years of age. The overall estimated incidence is 0.8 per 100,000 persons annually. The incidence of childhood ADEM is estimated at 2-10 cases per million children per year. Between 10-25% of children with ADEM are eventually diagnosed with MS.

Presentation. Symptoms typically occur a few days to a few weeks following antigenic challenge (e.g., infection or vaccination). The majority of children with ADEM have a nonspecific febrile illness preceding onset. Viral exanthema is usually absent. Unlike MS, optic neuritis is rare.

Natural History. Disease course and outcome vary. **Monophasic ADEM** is the most common type. However, the disease sometimes follows an atypical course, waxing and waning over a period of several months.

Approximately 25% of patients initially diagnosed with ADEM experience a relapse**. Recurrent ADEM** is characterized by a second episode occurring within two years after the initial illness and involving the *same* anatomic area(s) as the original illness.

Multiphasic ADEM (MDEM) is characterized by one or more subsequent events that involve a *different* anatomic area as demonstrated by a new lesion on MR or a new focal neurologic deficit. MDEM is more common in children and is frequently associated with myelin oligodendrocyte glycoprotein (MOG) seropositivity.

More than 1/2 of all patients recover completely within one or two months after onset, whereas ~ 20% experience some residual functional impairment. Overall mortality in recent series is low.

ACUTE DISSEMINATED ENCEPHALOMYELITIS (ADEM)

Etiology and Pathology
- Postinfection, postimmunization
- Immune-mediated perivenular demyelination

Clinical Issues
- 2nd only to MS as acquired demyelinating disease
- No female predominance
- Occurs at all ages, but children 5-8 years old most affected
- Course, outcome vary
  - Monophasic ADEM: Most common (> 70%)
  - Recurrent ADEM: 2nd episode, same site (10%)
  - Multiphasic ADEM: Multiple episodes, different sites (10%)
- Recover completely (> 50%)
- Mortality (1-2%)

Imaging

CT Findings. NECT is usually normal. CECT may show multifocal punctate or partial ring-enhancing lesions.

MR Findings. Multifocal hyperintensities on T2/FLAIR are the most common findings and vary from small round/ovoid foci **(15-15)** to flocculent "cotton ball" lesions with very hyperintense centers surrounded by slightly less hyperintense areas with "fuzzy" margins **(15-16A)**. Bilateral but asymmetric involvement is typical. Basal ganglia and posterior fossa lesions are common.

Enhancement varies from minimal to striking. Punctate, linear, ring, and incomplete "horseshoe" patterns all occur **(15-16B)** **(15-17C)**. Large "tumefactive" lesions with horseshoe-shaped enhancement resemble "tumefactive" MS. Cranial nerve enhancement is relatively common. Acute lesions may show restriction on DWI **(15-16C)**.

Differential Diagnosis

The major differential diagnosis of ADEM is **MS**. "Tumefactive" lesions—including those with incomplete ring enhancement—occur in both disorders. ADEM is more common in children and often has a history of viral infection or immunization. MS more commonly involves the callososeptal interface and typically has a relapsing-remitting course, whereas most (but not all!) cases of ADEM are monophasic.

Neuromyelitis optica spectrum disorder (NMOSD) may be difficult to distinguish from recurrent ADEM. **MOG antibody-associated demyelination** may overlap with some forms of NMOSD.

Although very rare, **treatment-associated demyelinating diseases** with TNF-α inhibitors, such as etanercept, can mimic ADEM and NMOSD on imaging studies **(15-17)**. Demyelination associated with anti-TNF agents typically develops from one week to 12 months after treatment initiation.

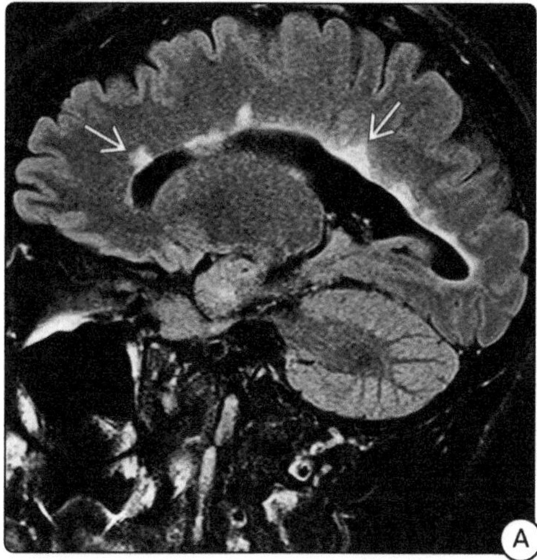

***(15-17A)** FLAIR in 44yF on etanercept shows classic triangle-shaped demyelinating lesions ➡ along the callososeptal interface, ependyma.*

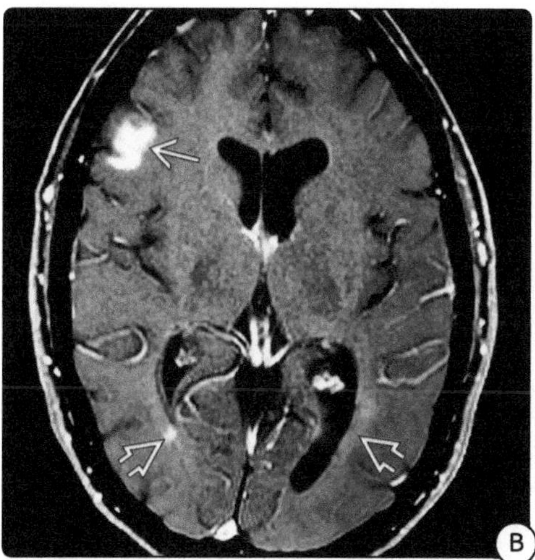

***(15-17B)** T1 C+ FS MR shows a large enhancing lesion in the left frontal subcortical white matter ➡, additional ependymal enhancing foci ⮕.*

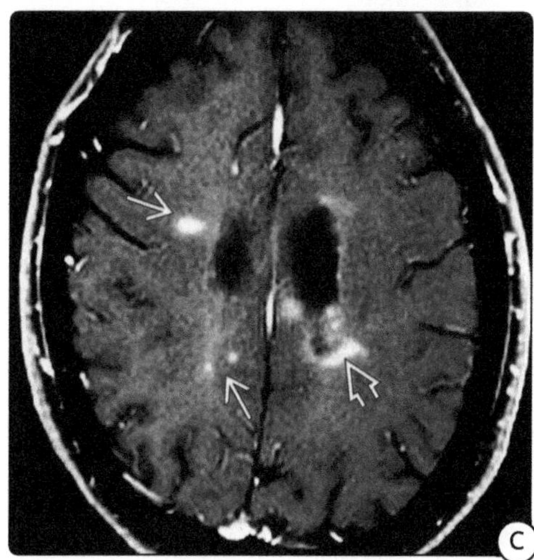

***(15-17C)** T1 C+ FS MR shows additional lesions ➡, partial ring-enhancing mass ⮕. This is anti-TNF treatment-associated demyelination.*

ADEM: IMAGING

Brain
- Multifocal T2/FLAIR hyperintensities
  - Bilateral but asymmetric white matter lesions
  - Most lesions small, round/ovoid
  - Hazy flocculent "cotton balls" (> 2 cm, usually in children)
  - ± basal ganglia, posterior fossa, cranial nerves
- Enhancement varies from none to striking
  - Multifocal punctate, linear, partial ring
  - Can be perivenular
  - Large lesions ("tumefactive") less common

Spinal Cord
- Patchy/longitudinally extensive T2 hyperintensity
- Strong but patchy enhancement

Acute Hemorrhagic Leukoencephalitis

Terminology

AHLE is also known as acute hemorrhagic leukoencephalopathy, acute hemorrhagic encephalomyelitis (AHEM), and Weston Hurst disease. Some investigators include AHLE as part of the ADEM spectrum—as a hyperacute, exceptionally severe variant of ADEM.

Pathology

Location. AHLE predominantly affects the white matter. Both the cerebral hemispheres and cerebellum are typically affected. Despite its name, AHLE may affect the gray matter; basal ganglia involvement is common, but the cortical gray matter is generally spared.

Size and Number. AHLE has two distinct manifestations: Innumerable petechial microbleeds and macroscopic parenchymal hemorrhages. Some cases have features of both.

Gross Pathology. The typical gross appearance is that of marked brain swelling with diffuse confluent **(15-20)** &/or petechial hemorrhages **(15-18)**. Hemorrhages are typically present in the cerebral hemispheres (predominately the white matter) and cerebellum. Fibrinoid necrosis of vessel walls with perivascular hemorrhages and mononuclear inflammatory cell cuffing are the microscopic hallmarks of fulminant AHLE.

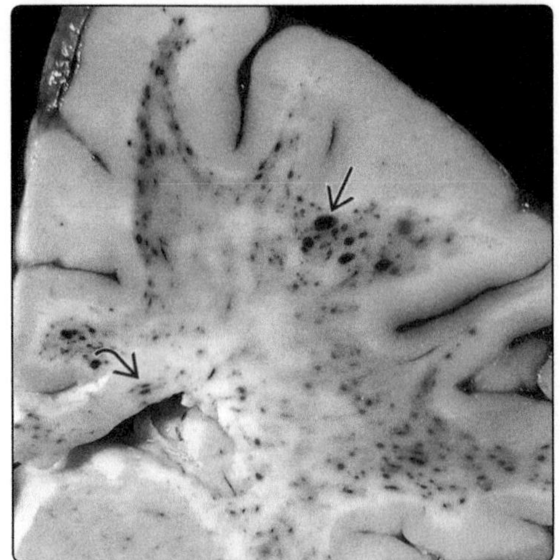

(15-18) *Autopsied AHLE shows innumerable tiny subcortical WM hemorrhages ➡ extending into the corpus callosum ➡. Cortex is spared.*

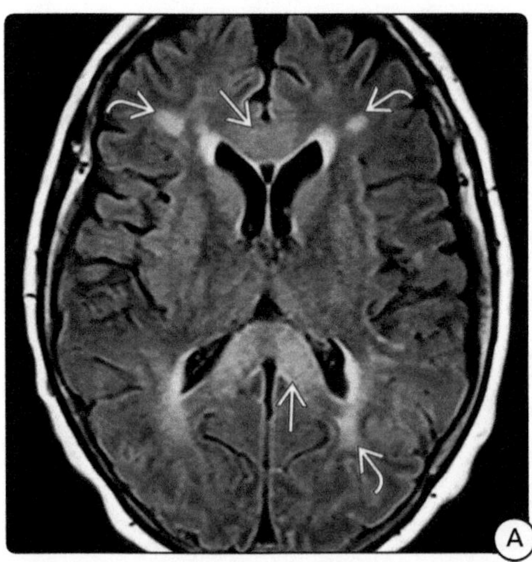

(15-19A) *FLAIR in a 69yF with postviral altered mental status shows confluent hyperintensity in corpus callosum ➡ and hemispheric WM ➡.*

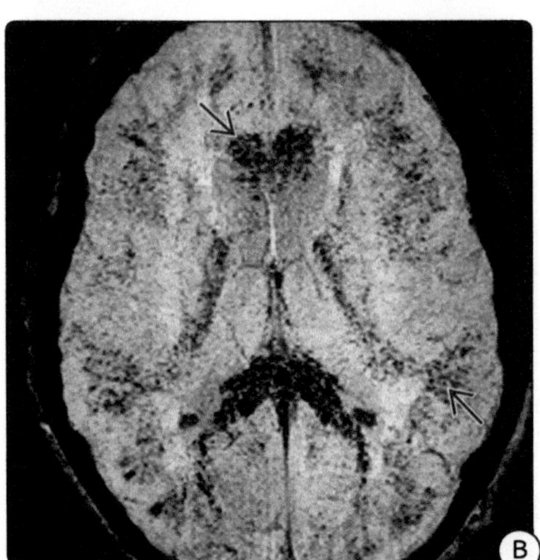

(15-19B) *SWI 2 weeks later shows "blooming" hypointensities throughout WM ➡. AHLE was diagnosed on imaging and confirmed with biopsy.*

Clinical Issues

Epidemiology and Demographics. AHLE is considerably less common than ADEM. Approximately 2% of all ADEM cases are of the hyperacute hemorrhagic type that could be considered consistent with AHLE. Although AHLE occurs at all ages, most patients are children and young adults.

Presentation and Natural History. History of a viral prodrome or flu-like illness followed by rapid neurologic deterioration is typical. Fever and lethargy with increasing somnolence, decreased mental status, impaired consciousness, and long-tract signs are the most common clinical symptoms.

Untreated AHLE has a very poor prognosis. Clinical deterioration and death usually occur within days to a week after symptom onset. Mortality is 60-80%.

AHLE is almost always fatal if untreated. Aggressive treatment with decompressive craniectomy, intravenous high-dose corticosteroids, and plasmapheresis has been associated with survival and even favorable outcome in a few cases.

Imaging

CT Findings. NECT may be normal unless confluent lobar hemorrhages are present **(15-21A)**. Petechial microhemorrhages are generally invisible on CT but white matter edema with diffuse, relatively asymmetric hypodensity in one or both hemispheres may be present.

MR Findings. T1 scans are often normal unless lobar hemorrhage is present. T2/FLAIR findings vary from subtle to striking. Multifocal scattered or confluent hyperintensities as well as bilateral confluent hyperintensity of the cerebral white matter are typical but nonspecific findings **(15-19A)**.

T2* scans are the key to diagnosis; SWI sequences are more sensitive than GRE **(15-21B)**. Multifocal punctate and linear "blooming" hypointensities in the corpus callosum that extend through the full thickness of the hemispheric white matter to the subcortical U-fibers are typical findings on T2* **(15-19B)**. Striking sparing of the overlying cortex is common. Additional lesions are frequently present in the basal ganglia, midbrain, pons, and cerebellum.

Enhancement on T1 C+ occurs in 50% of cases and ranges from linear perivascular space enhancement to larger patchy or confluent foci.

Differential Diagnosis

The major differential diagnosis of AHLE is **ADEM**. Both share a number of similar features. However, ADEM usually follows a much less fulminant course and does not demonstrate the characteristic lobar or perivascular hemorrhages of AHLE.

Petechial microhemorrhages similar to those seen in AHLE can be found in a number of other disorders, including disseminated intravascular coagulopathy, fat emboli, thrombotic thrombocytopenic purpura, sepsis, vasculitis, hemorrhagic viral fevers, malaria, and rickettsial diseases. A recently described entity, **critical illness-associated microbleeds**, may be seen in the setting of acute respiratory failure and appear indistinguishable from AHLE.

ACUTE HEMORRHAGIC LEUKOENCEPHALITIS (AHLE)

Terminology
- Also called acute hemorrhagic encephalomyelitis (AHEM), Weston Hurst disease

Etiology and Pathology
- Similar to ADEM (viral/postviral autoimmune-mediated condition)
- May represent fulminant form of ADEM

Clinical Issues
- Rare; 2% of ADEM cases
- All ages affected, especially children/young adults
- Fever, lethargy, impaired consciousness
- Rapidly progressive, often lethal course

Imaging
- General features
  - White matter edema
  - Focal macroscopic hemorrhages or multifocal microbleeds
- MR procedure of choice
  - Multifocal scattered or confluent lesions on T2/FLAIR
  - Corpus callosum, cerebral white matter, pons, cerebellum ± basal ganglia
  - Cortical gray matter generally spared
  - T2* (GRE, SWI) depicts microbleeds
  - 50% show variable enhancement

Differential Diagnosis
- Severe ADEM
- Critical illness-associated microbleeds

Other Autoimmune Disorders

In this section, we consider other autoimmune CNS disorders, such as autoimmune encephalitis and neuromyelitis optica spectrum disorder. Susac syndrome—often mistaken for multiple sclerosis—is also considered here.

Autoimmune Encephalitis

Autoimmune encephalitis (AE) is a family of closely related disease processes in which an antibody-mediated attack causes a localized CNS inflammatory response. The prevalence and incidence of AE has been underestimated in the past but may be nearly equal to infectious encephalitis.

Autoimmune encephalitides share overlapping clinical features and imaging findings and are differentiated by specific antibody subtypes. Most—but not all—are characterized by limbic dysfunction and varying involvement of the temporal lobes and neocortex.

In addition to paraneoplastic and non-tumor-associated disorders, the autoimmune encephalitides are further subdivided according to the cellular location of their neuronal antigens.

Group I antibodies target intracellular antigens, whereas group II antibodies target cell surface antigens. Group I antibodies are more closely associated with underlying malignancy, although **anti-glutamic acid decarboxylase (GAD)** disease targets intracellular antigens but is most commonly associated with nonneoplastic conditions, such as type 1 diabetes mellitus.

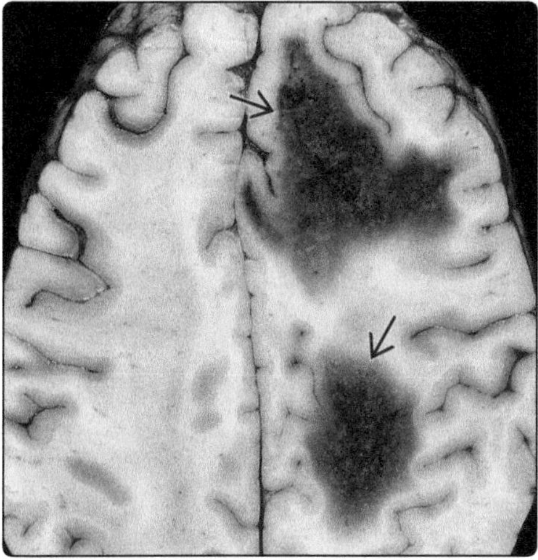

***(15-20)** Autopsied fulminant AHLE shows 2 confluent areas of WM hemorrhagic necrosis ➡ with cortical sparing. (Courtesy R. Hewlett, MD.)*

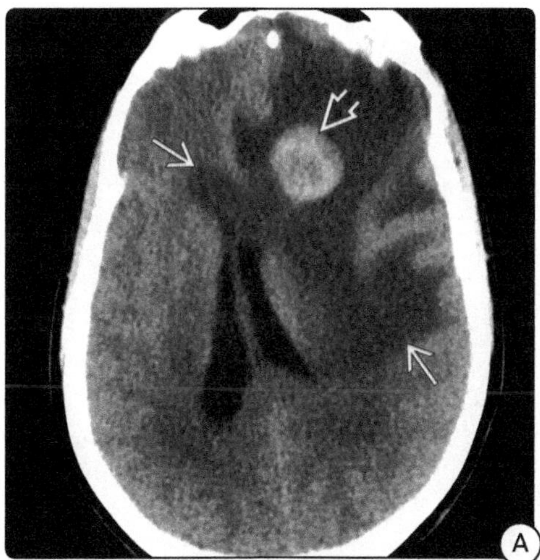

***(15-21A)** NECT in a 26y woman with biopsy-proven AHLE shows left frontal hematoma ➡ with mass effect, striking perilesional edema ➡.*

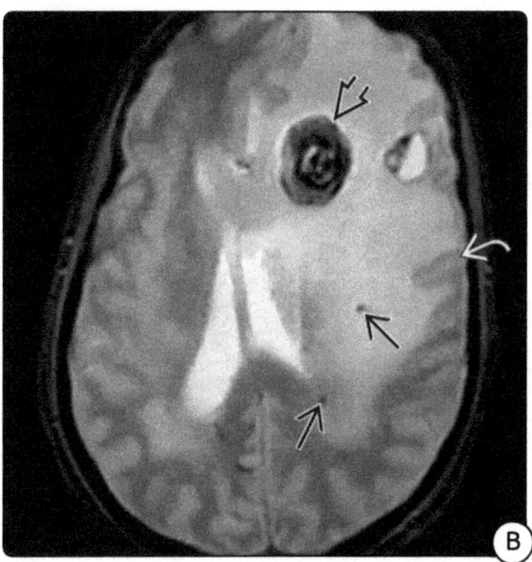

***(15-21B)** T2* GRE shows focal hematoma ➡, several "blooming black dots" ➡. Note cortical sparing ➡. (Courtesy M. Preece, MD.)*

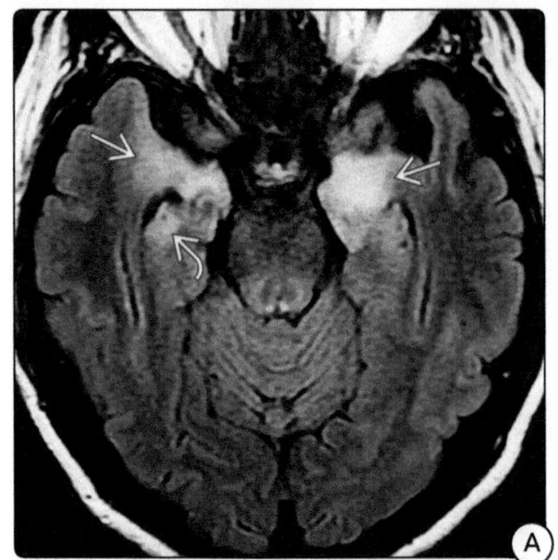

(15-22A) 71yF with subacute encephalopathy shows FLAIR hyperintensity in anteromedial temporal lobes ➡, right hippocampus ➡.

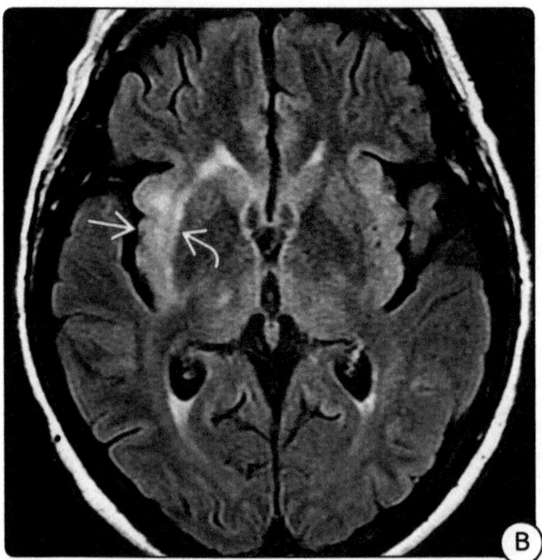

(15-22B) More cephalad FLAIR in the same case shows hyperintensity in the right insular cortex ➡ and external capsule ➡.

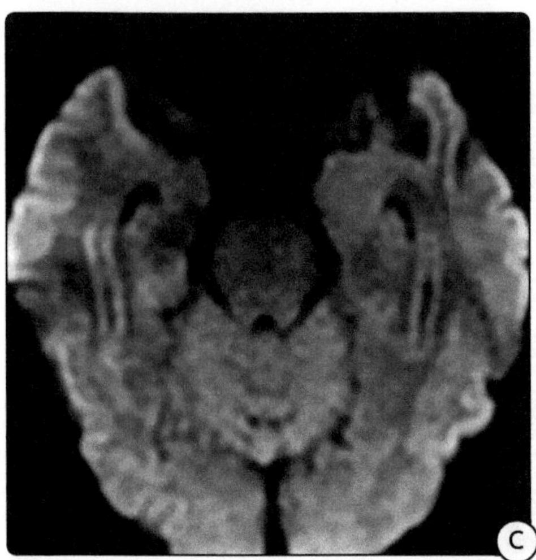

(15-22C) DWI shows no evidence for restricted diffusion. Anti-LGI1 (VKGC) autoantibodies were later detected in her CSF.

Terminology

The autoimmune encephalitides are differentiated by—and named according to—specific antibody subtypes that cause immune-mediated attacks on the CNS.

AE can be paraneoplastic or nonparaneoplastic. Paraneoplastic-associated disorders, such as anti-Hu and anti-Ma encephalitis, are discussed in Chapter 27. Nonneoplastic AE is discussed here. Because of its unique imaging findings, aquaporin-4 (AQP4) and neuromyelitis optica spectrum disorder (NMOSD) are discussed separately in this section.

Etiology

The major antigens responsible for inciting AE are an ever-expanding group of antibodies that is shown in the box below.

Antibodies against cell-surface antigens, such as **AQP4** and **leucine-rich glioma inactivated 1 (LGI1)**, are among the most common autoantibodies in patients with nonneoplastic autoimmune-mediated CNS disease.

Another common group of autoimmune disorders are those with ion channel antigens. These include the most common AE, **N-methyl, D-aspartate receptor (NMDAR or NMDAr)** and **γ-aminobutyric acid receptor (GABAr)** encephalitis (which has a higher association with malignancies, such as small cell lung cancer) than other group II autoantibodies.

Less common subtypes include **anti-glutamate receptor 3 (GluR3)** autoantibodies (associated with Rasmussen encephalitis) and **voltage-gated calcium channel (VGCC)** encephalitis.

NONNEOPLASTIC AUTOIMMUNE ENCEPHALITIS

Group I
- Intracellular antigens
- Often associated with underlying malignancy
- Examples
  - Anti-Hu (75% small cell lung cancer), anti-Ma
  - Anti-Ri (breast, small cell lung), anti-Yo (ovarian, breast)
  - Anti-GAD (usually *not* associated with malignancy)

Group II
- Cell-surface antigens
- Malignancy less common
- Examples
  - NMDAr, GABAr
  - LGI1 (VGKC), VGCC
  - GluR3 (Rasmussen)

Pathology

Regardless of the etiology and antibody profile, the autoimmune encephalitides have a distinct predilection for the limbic system.

Clinical Issues

Antigenic specificities appear to determine the associated clinical syndromes. Onset is typically *subacute*. The most common presentation is cognitive dysfunction and altered mental status. Seizures and medically intractable epilepsy are also common.

The definitive diagnosis of AE is established by the identification of specific autoantibodies in the CSF &/or sera. **Up to 50% of AE cases are negative as typical screening panels do not detect all potential autoantibodies!**

Imaging

Imaging findings are variable; a subset of patients will have no neuroimaging findings despite severe neuropsychiatric dysfunction or subacute cognitive decline.

The most common identifiable pattern is that of limbic encephalitis. T2/FLAIR hyperintensity in one or both medial temporal lobes is typical **(15-22)**. Extralimbic involvement with structures, such as the cortex, striatum, and diencephalon, varies.

Diffusion restriction is variable but usually absent **(15-22C)**. Enhancement on T1 C+ occurs in ~ 25% of cases and is frequently associated with subsequent development of mesial temporal sclerosis.

Differential Diagnosis

The differential diagnosis of AE includes **herpes simplex encephalitis, HHV-6 encephalitis**, and systemic autoimmune disorders, such as SLE, antiphospholipid antibody syndrome, and thyroid encephalopathy.

Neuromyelitis Optica Spectrum Disorder

Neuromyelitis optica (NMO) is an autoimmune inflammatory demyelinating disease of the CNS. The diagnostic criteria for NMO have recently been broadened and the disease renamed **NMO spectrum disorder (NMOSD)**.

Etiology

The most common form of NMOSD is an autoimmune-mediated water channelopathy characterized by the presence of autoantibodies to **aquaporin-4 (AQP4)**. AQP4 is located in the foot processes of astrocytes and is the most abundant water channel in the CNS. It is especially highly expressed in the circumventricular organs surrounding the third and fourth ventricles.

A specific biomarker of the disease, AQP4-IgG, is 90% specific and 70-75% sensitive for NMOSD. NMOSD can be AQP4-IgG seropositive *or* seronegative (less common).

Pathology

Location. In classic NMOSD, one or both optic nerves are involved together with the spinal cord **(15-23)**. The cervical cord is most commonly affected. Lesions usually surround the central canal and classically extend over three or more consecutive segments.

Brain lesions occur in the optic chiasm/hypothalamus. They also cluster around the periependymal surfaces of the ventricles, corpus callosum, cerebral aqueduct, and dorsal midbrain.

Microscopic Features. It is the *immunohistochemistry* of AQP4-IgG that is diagnostic. AQP4-IgG binds to the abluminal face of microvessels at sites of immune complex deposition. The active demyelination in NMOSD is characterized by astrocytic injury, vessel hyalinization, and eosinophilic infiltration, findings not typically present in either MS or ADEM.

Clinical Issues

Epidemiology and Demographics. NMOSD is a worldwide disease and does not exhibit the characteristic geographic gradient of MS. Patients with NMOSD are, on average, 10 years older than patients with MS. Mean age at initial diagnosis is around 40 years. Pediatric-onset NMOSD does occur and represents 3-5% of cases. The F:M ratio for AQP4-positive NMOSD is 8-9:1.

Between 10-25% of NMOSD patients are seronegative for AQP4. Seronegative NMO is equally distributed among the sexes.

Presentation and Natural History. In adults, NMOSD is classically characterized by severe uni- or bilateral optic neuritis and longitudinally extensive transverse myelitis (LETM). Involvement of other CNS regions (either by clinical presentation or MR findings) is now recognized as part of the NMOSD spectrum (see box below).

AQP4-seropositive NMOSD patients usually have more severe clinical disease and worse outcome than individuals who are seronegative. The vast majority of cases (85-90%) are relapsing, although monophasic illness may occur.

Almost 30% of NMOSD patients are initially misdiagnosed with MS. Some patients also develop clinical features of anti-NMDAr encephalitis.

Treatment Options. Accurate diagnosis is essential because some drugs used for MS can worsen NMOSD. Recent studies suggest that the therapeutic options in NMO should be immunosuppressive rather than immunomodulatory drugs. Plasma exchange can be used in severe cases.

2015 REVISED NMOSD DIAGNOSTIC CRITERIA: AQP4-IgG POSITIVITY

AQP4-IgG positivity plus 1 core clinical characteristic

- Optic neuritis
- Acute myelitis
- Area postrema syndrome
    - Unexplained hiccups or nausea and vomiting
- Acute brainstem syndrome
- Symptomatic narcolepsy or diencephalic clinical syndrome
    - With NMOSD-typical diencephalic MR lesions
- Symptomatic cerebral syndrome
    - With NMOSD-typical brain lesions

2015 NMOSD CRITERIA: AQP4-IgG NEGATIVITY

If AQP4-IgG negative
- At least 2 core clinical characteristics; 1 must be
  - Optic neuritis, longitudinally extensive transverse myelitis, or area postrema syndrome
- *If acute optic neuritis*, MR with
  - Normal brain or nonspecific WM lesions or
  - T2-hyperintense or T1 C+ enhancing optic nerve lesion involving optic chiasm or > 50% of optic nerve
- *If acute myelitis*, MR with
  - Intramedullary lesion over 3 contiguous segments
  - Or focal atrophy of at least 3 contiguous segments
- *If area postrema* syndrome, MR with
  - Dorsal medulla/area postrema lesion(s)
- *If acute brainstem* syndrome, MR with
  - Periependymal brainstem lesions

Imaging

MR imaging has become an essential tool for NMOSD diagnosis, particularly for recognition of AQP4-IgG seronegative patients. Radiologists may be the first to recognize the disease.

The most common MR findings are (1) bilateral, longitudinally extensive optic nerve hyperintensity &/or enhancement consistent with acute optic neuritis **(15-23)** and (2) hyperintense, enhancing LETM (three or more contiguous vertebral segments). So-called "short transverse myelitis" occurs in ~ 15% of patients.

The presence of brain lesions varies. **Between 30-60% of NMOSD patients have nonspecific T2/FLAIR hyperintensities in the cerebral white matter, so this finding per se does not exclude the diagnosis.** However, if lesions are found in areas where AQP4 is highly expressed (e.g., undersurface of the corpus callosum, dorsal brainstem,

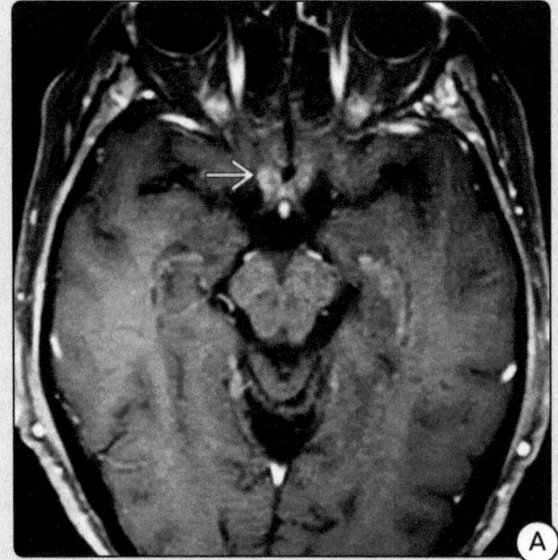

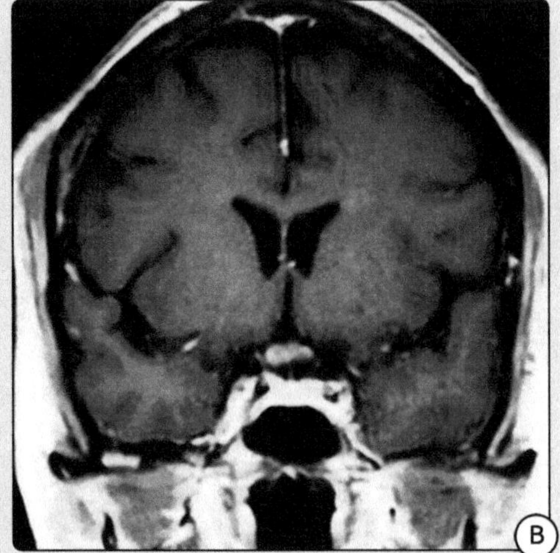

***(15-23A)** Axial T1 C+ FS MR in a patient with serologically proven neuromyelitis optica (NMO) shows optic chiasm enhancement ➡. **(15-23B)** Coronal T1 C+ MR in the same patient confirms the optic chiasm enhancement. T2/FLAIR scans (not shown) showed no evidence of other lesions.*

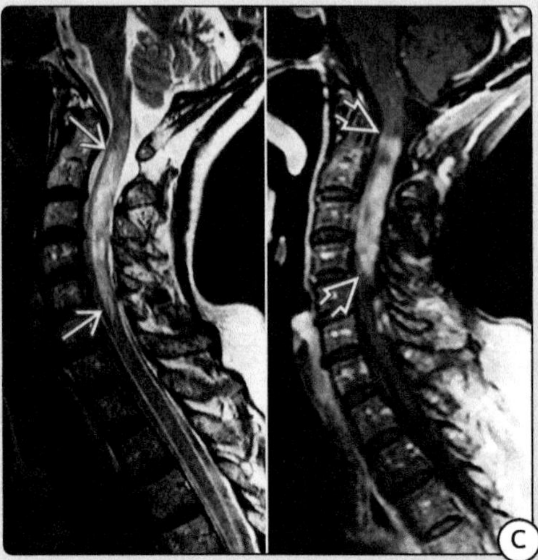

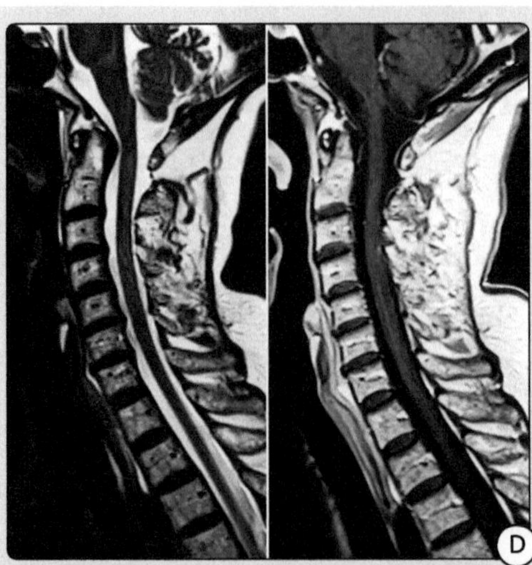

***(15-23C)** (L) Sagittal T2 MR in the same case shows a swollen cord with confluent hyperintense lesion extending from C1-C5 ➡. (R) T1 C+ MR shows patchy enhancement ➡. **(15-23D)** Repeat study after 3 months of immunosuppressive therapy shows that the lesions have completely resolved.*

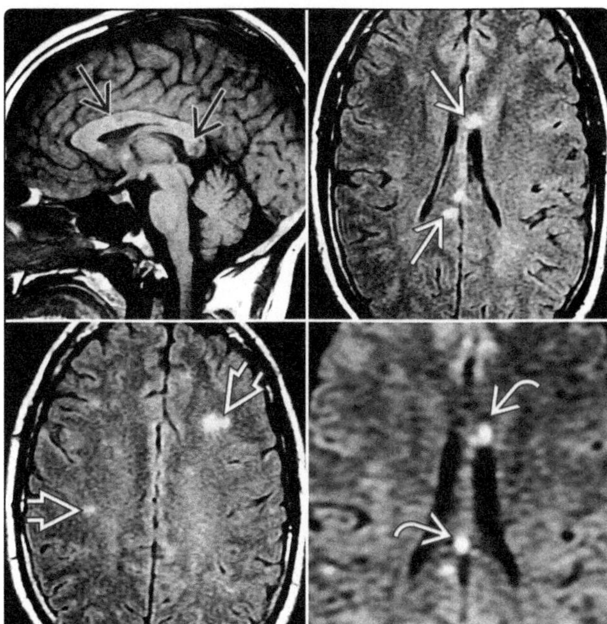

(15-24) Classic findings of Susac syndrome (SuS) are middle callosal "holes" on sagittal T1WI ⇨, multifocal ovoid callosal ➡ and WM hyperintensities ⇨ on FLAIR, and diffusion restriction on DWI ➡. (Courtesy P. Rodriguez, MD.)

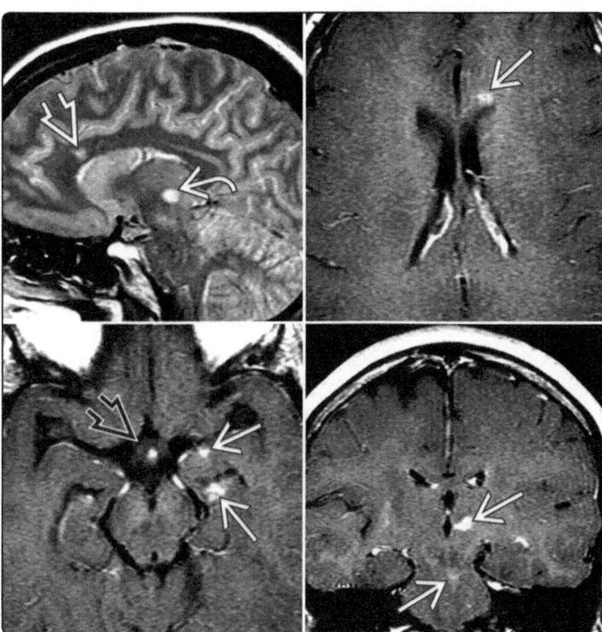

(15-25) MR in a 27y woman with SuS shows T2-hyperintense lesions in the midbrain ➡, middle layers of corpus callosum ➡. T1 C+ images show several discrete enhancing foci ➡. Optic chiasm ⇨, undersurface of corpus callosum are spared.

and periependymal surfaces around the third ventricle) or so-called "pencil-thin" ependymal enhancement is present, NMOSD should be considered.

Differential Diagnosis

While there are numerous differential diagnoses, the major differential diagnosis of NMOSD is **MS**. Bilateral, long-segment optic nerve involvement and LETM are more characteristic of NMOSD. The brain is more involved in MS. The presence of a cortical or juxtacortical U-fiber lesion is much more characteristic of MS than NMOSD. AQP4-IgG is almost always negative in MS.

Some AQP4-IgG seronegative patients have antibodies to myelin oligodendrocyte glycoprotein (MOG). **MOG antibody-associated disease** targets oligodendrocytes, not astrocytes, and is also found in other demyelinating disorders, such as MS.

ADEM can have LETM that is identical to NMOSD. "Tumefactive" lesions and gray matter involvement are also more suggestive of ADEM. Primary CNS **vasculitis** is often multifocal, frequently "blooms" on T2* SWI, and causes cortical/subcortical and basal ganglia infarcts.

Susac syndrome is characterized classically by bilateral sensorineural hearing loss, branch retinal artery occlusions, and subacute encephalopathy. It involves the middle layers of the corpus callosum, not the periependymal surfaces.

Susac Syndrome (SuS)

SuS is an autoimmune endotheliopathy that causes microvascular occlusions in the brain. Most patients are young adult females who present with the classic clinical triad of subacute encephalopathy, branch retinal artery occlusions, and sensorineural hearing loss. In 50% of cases, migraine-like headache is a heralding symptom.

Imaging

SuS is often initially mistaken for MS on imaging studies. Sagittal T1WI in patients with chronic SuS may show typical "punched-out" lesions in the middle layers of the corpus callosum **(15-24)**. T2/FLAIR shows multiple deep white matter hyperintensities in over 90% of cases. Basal ganglia lesions occur in 70% of cases and brainstem lesions in nearly 1/3 of cases. Acute SuS lesions show punctate enhancement on T1 C+ **(15-25)**.

Differential Diagnosis

MS preferentially involves the undersurface of the corpus callosum, which is usually spared in SuS. **ADEM** and **Lyme disease** also rarely involve the middle layers of the corpus callosum. ADEM is generally monophasic, preceded by a viral prodrome or history of vaccination. **Primary arteritis of the CNS (PACNS)** rarely affects the corpus callosum, whereas cortical lesions and hemorrhages are common.

CLIPPERS

CLIPPERS is the acronym for **c**hronic **l**ymphocytic **i**nflammation with **p**ontine **p**erivascular **e**nhancement **r**esponsive to **s**teroids.

Pathology

CLIPPERS is characterized histopathologically by widespread foci of CD4(+) T-cell perivascular inflammation in the brainstem and cerebellum.

Clinical Issues

Patients typically present with subacute pontocerebellar dysfunction (e.g., gait ataxia) with or without other CNS symptoms (e.g., cognitive dysfunction or myelopathy). Mean age at onset is 40-50 years. Dramatic response to glucocorticosteroids (GCSs) as well as worsening following corticosteroid withdrawal is a hallmark feature of CLIPPERS but does not exclude non-CLIPPERS pathology.

Imaging

Multifocal T2/FLAIR homogeneously hyperintense lesions with ≤ 3-mm punctate or curvilinear "peppering" enhancement on T1 C+ ("peppering") are typical **(15-26)**. Ring enhancement and mass effect are absent, and the area of T2 signal abnormality typically does not significantly exceed that of the T1 C+ enhancement.

Lesions *outside* the pons and cerebellum are present in 60% of cases and occur in the midbrain, medulla, subcortical white matter, cerebral hemispheres, and spinal cord. There is a clear geographic gradient of lesser inflammation with increasing distance from the brainstem and cerebellum.

Foci of restricted diffusion may occur in the acute phase. Punctate microbleeds in the affected areas are sometimes identified on T2* SWI sequences. Posttreatment atrophy is common.

Differential Diagnosis

Lesion-associated mass effect and lesions with T2/FLAIR signal abnormality much larger than the enhancing foci should

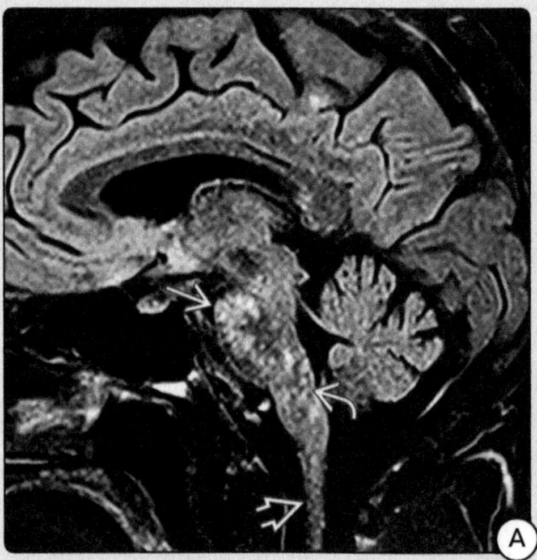

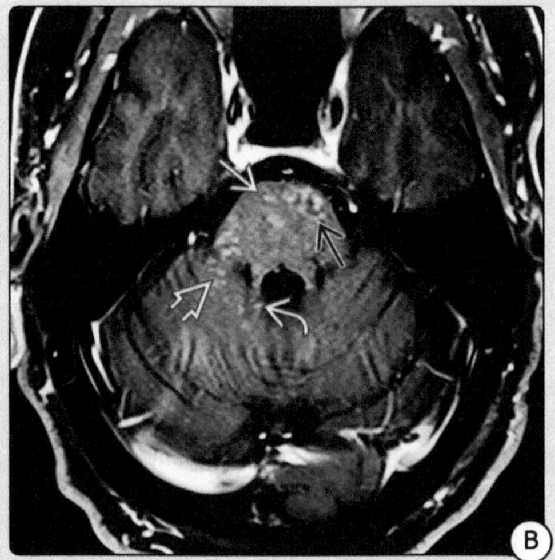

***(15-26A)** Sagittal FLAIR MR in a 52-year-old man with diplopia, dysarthria, and facial numbness shows multiple punctate hyperintensities "peppering" the pons ➡, medulla ➡, and extending into the upper cervical spinal cord ➡. **(15-26B)** T1 C+ FS MR shows punctate ➡ and curvilinear ➡ foci of contrast enhancement. Note extension into the cerebellum ➡ and superior cerebellar peduncle ➡.*

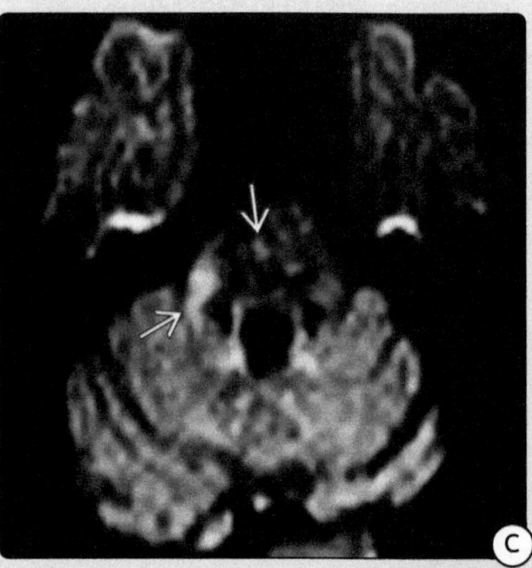

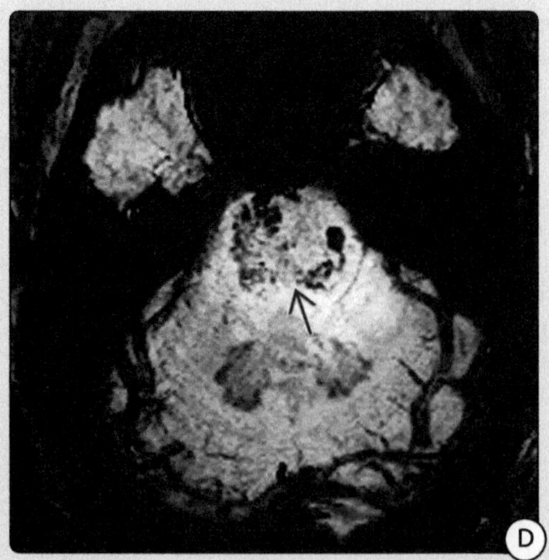

***(15-26C)** DWI MR shows scattered foci of restricted diffusion ➡. **(15-26D)** Axial T2* SWI MIP shows multiple hemorrhagic foci ➡ in the pons. The patient responded dramatically to steroids, but cessation of GCS treatment resulted in disease recurrence. CLIPPERS was diagnosed on the basis of imaging findings and GCS responsiveness.*

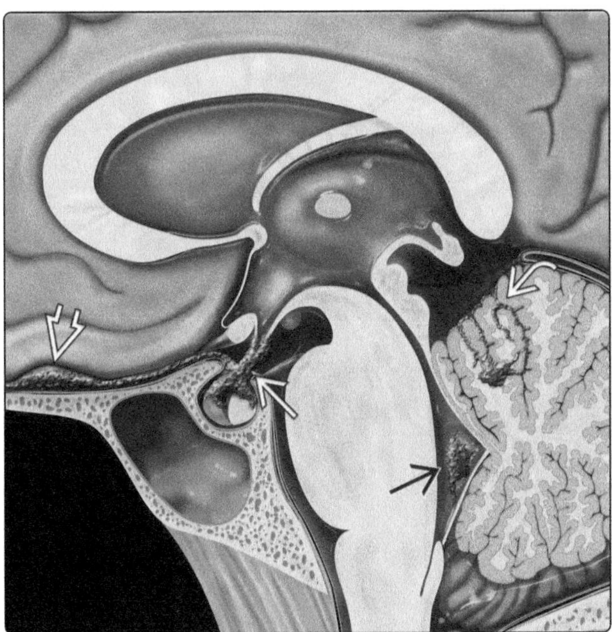

***(15-27)** Graphic illustrates common neurosarcoid locations: (1) Infundibulum, extending into the pituitary ➡, (2) plaque-like dura-arachnoid thickening ➡, and (3) synchronous lesions of the superior vermis ➡ and 4th ventricle choroid plexus ➡.*

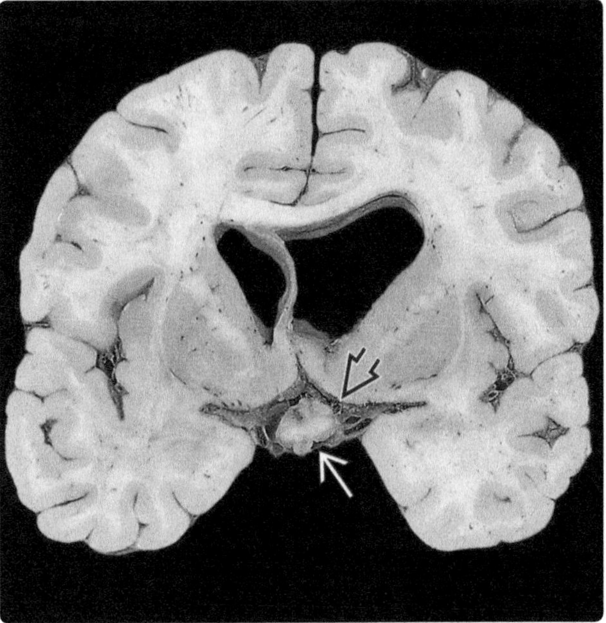

***(15-28)** Autopsy of neurosarcoidosis demonstrates gelatinous infiltration of the leptomeninges ➡ around the thickened hypothalamus and optic chiasm ➡. (Courtesy Ellison, Neuropathology, 3e.)*

suggest non-CLIPPERS etiology, such as **intravascular lymphoma**, **vasculitis**, **neurosarcoidosis**, and **MS** or **NMOSD**. GCS therapy failure with lack of complete resolution of enhancing abnormalities should also strongly suggest an alternative diagnosis.

Inflammatory-Like Disorders

Neurosarcoidosis

Terminology

Sarcoidosis ("sarcoid") is a multisystem inflammatory disorder characterized by discrete noncaseating epithelioid granulomas. When sarcoidosis affects the CNS, it is termed "neurosarcoidosis" (NS).

Etiology

The etiology of sarcoidosis remains unknown, but the prevailing view is that genetically susceptible individuals develop sarcoidosis following exposure to presently unidentified antigens. A reactive inflammatory cascade ensues that appears to be driven primarily through CD4(+) T cells.

Pathology

Location. The CNS is involved in ~ 5% of cases, usually in combination with disease elsewhere. Only 5-10% of NS cases are confined to the CNS and occur without evidence of systemic sarcoidosis.

Sarcoid can involve any part of the nervous system or its coverings. Lesions vary in size, from tiny granulomas that infiltrate along the pia and perivascular spaces.

The most common location is the meninges, especially around the base of the brain. Diffuse leptomeningeal thickening with or without more focal nodular lesions is seen in ~ 40% of cases **(15-27)**. Large dura-based masses may occur, resembling meningiomas.

The hypothalamus and infundibulum are also favored intracranial sites **(15-28)**. NS can involve cranial nerves, eye and periorbita, bone, the ventricles and choroid plexus, and the brain parenchyma itself. Sarcoid can also involve the spinal leptomeninges, cord, and nerve roots.

Clinical Issues

Epidemiology and Demographics. NS is a worldwide disorder that has a bimodal age distribution. The largest peak occurs during the third and fourth decades with a second smaller peak in patients—especially women—over the age of 50 years.

Presentation. Symptoms vary with location. The most common presentation of NS is isolated or multiple cranial nerve deficits seen in 50-75% of patients. The facial and optic nerves are the most frequently affected. Symptoms of pituitary/hypothalamic dysfunction, such as diabetes insipidus or panhypopituitarism, are seen in 10-15% of cases.

Diagnosing NS may be difficult because the clinical features can be nonspecific, and elevated serum angiotensin-converting enzyme (ACE) levels are seen in < 1/2 of all cases.

Treatment Options. Most patients with NS respond to corticosteroids. Second-line treatment with immunosuppressive agents and third-line treatment with monoclonal antibodies against TNF-α have been tried with variable success.

Imaging

CT Findings. Depending on the amount of fibrosis present, NS can appear slightly hyperdense relative to normal brain parenchyma on NECT scan. Well-circumscribed "punched-out" lesions with nonsclerotic margins can be seen on bone CT.

Leptomeningeal disease may enhance on CECT, resembling tuberculosis or pyogenic meningitis. Dura-based masses are typically modestly hyperdense and enhance strongly and uniformly on CECT.

MR Findings. NS is isointense with brain on T1WI and hyperintense relative to CSF. Sulci filled with leptomeningeal infiltrates appear effaced, and the border between the sarcoid and brain is indistinct. Dura-based masses resemble meningiomas.

Parenchymal infiltration along the perivascular spaces causes a vasculitis-like reaction with edema, mass effect, and hyperintensity on T2/FLAIR.

The most common finding on T1 C+ scans is nodular or diffuse pial thickening, found in ~ 1/3 to 1/2 of all cases **(15-29)**.

1/2 of NS patients eventually develop parenchymal disease. Hypothalamic and infundibular thickening with intense enhancement is seen in 5-10% of cases. Multifocal nodular enhancing masses or more diffuse perivascular infiltrates may develop. Solitary parenchymal or dura-based masses are less common. In rare cases, coalescing granulomas form a focal expansile mass ("tumefactive" NS).

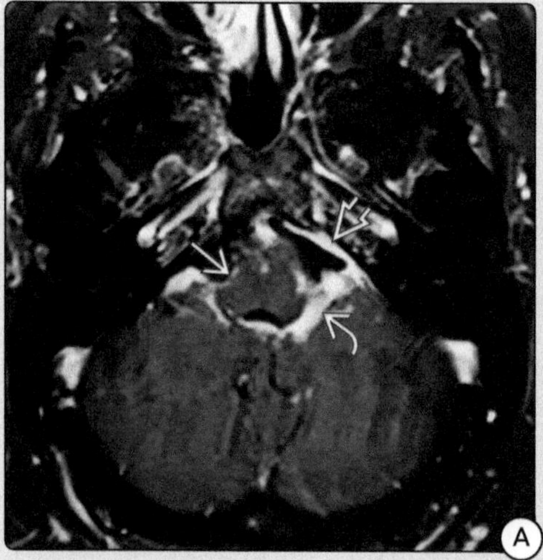

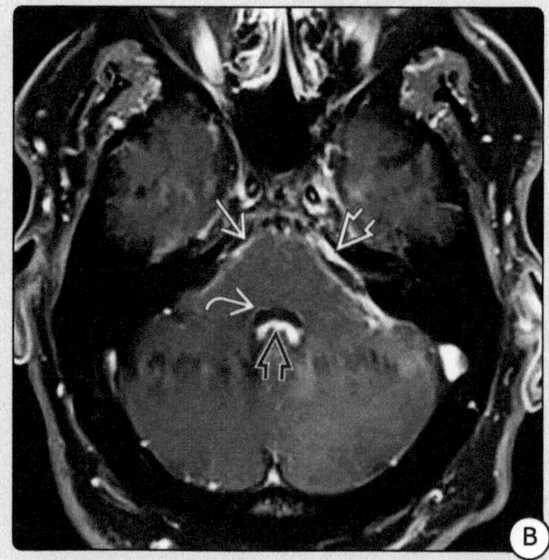

(15-29A) Axial T1 C+ FS MR in a 56-year-old woman with proven neurosarcoid shows thickening and enhancement along the choroid plexus ➡, dura ➡, and pial surface of the medulla ➡. (15-29B) More cephalad T1 C+ FS MR shows a thickened, enhancing dural plaque ➡. Lesions are also present along the pial surface of the pons ➡, the choroid plexus of the 4th ventricle ➡, and the ventricular ependyma ➡.

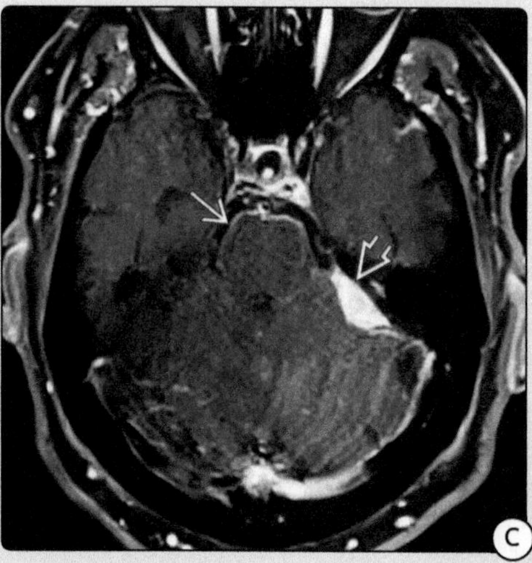

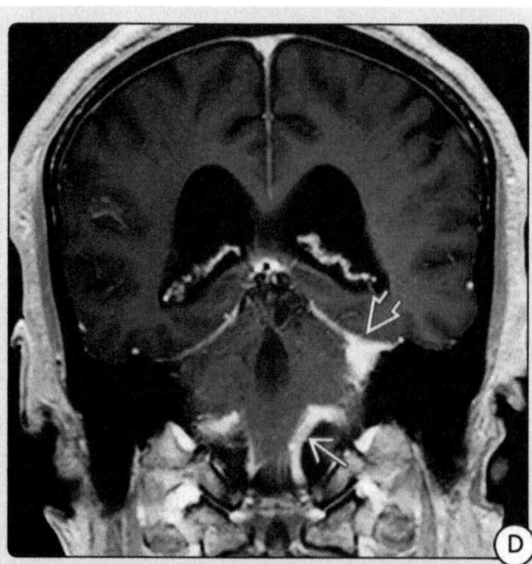

(15-29C) More cephalad axial T1 C+ FS MR shows the pial involvement ➡. A mass-like enhancing dural plaque at the left cerebellopontine angle (CPA) cistern ➡ resembles a meningioma. (15-29D) Coronal T1 C+ MR in the same case shows the extensive leptomeningeal enhancement ➡ and the CPA dural plaque ➡.

NS may cause solitary or multifocal thickened enhancing cranial nerves as well as enhancing masses in the ventricles and choroid plexus.

Differential Diagnosis

The differential diagnosis of NS depends on lesion location. **Meningitis** can look very similar to NS of the basilar leptomeninges. Dura-based NS may resemble **meningioma** or **lymphoma**; hypothalamic/infundibular/pituitary NS may look like **histiocytosis** or lymphocytic **hypophysitis**.

Multifocal parenchymal enhancing lesions can resemble **MS**, **metastases**, and **intravascular lymphoma**. The differential diagnosis of solitary or multiple cranial NS includes infection, demyelinating disease, and neoplasm.

IgG4-Related Disease

IgG4-related disease (IgG4-RD) is a multisystem, multifocal fibrosclerotic inflammatory disorder that is primarily tumefactive or "mass-like." IgG4-RD most frequently involves the lung and retroperitoneal spaces. The most common head and neck sites are the orbit and salivary glands **(15-30C)** where IgG4-RD can closely resemble orbital lymphoproliferative disorders.

Intracranial IgG4-RD has been described in the pituitary gland and stalk, cranial nerves, cavernous sinus, and dura **(15-30)**. Isolated intracranial disease occurs but is uncommon.

Selected References: The complete reference list is available on the Expert Consult™ eBook version included with purchase.

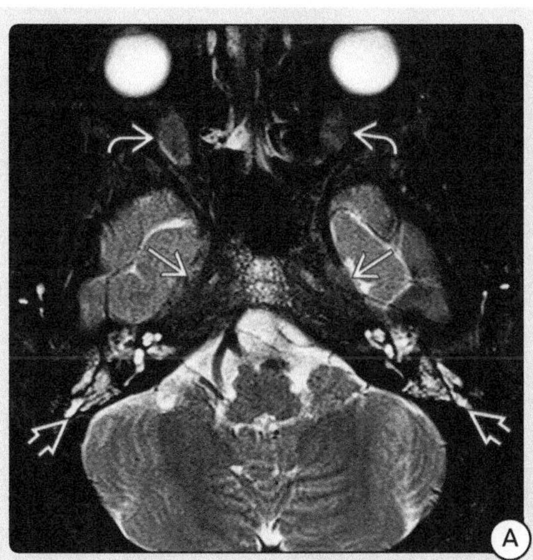

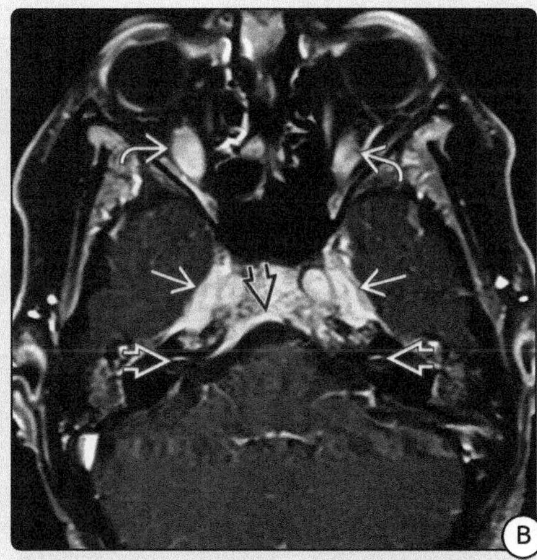

***(15-30A)** Axial T2 FS MR in a 26y woman with headache, proptosis, and right CNVI palsy shows hypointense diffusely infiltrating mass in both cavernous sinuses ➡ and orbital apices ➡. Bilateral serous otitis media is present ➡. **(15-30B)** T1 C+ FS MR in the same case shows that the cavernous sinus ➡ and orbital apex ➡ masses enhance strongly. Also note clival dura-arachnoid ➡ thickening with linear enhancement in both internal auditory canals ➡.*

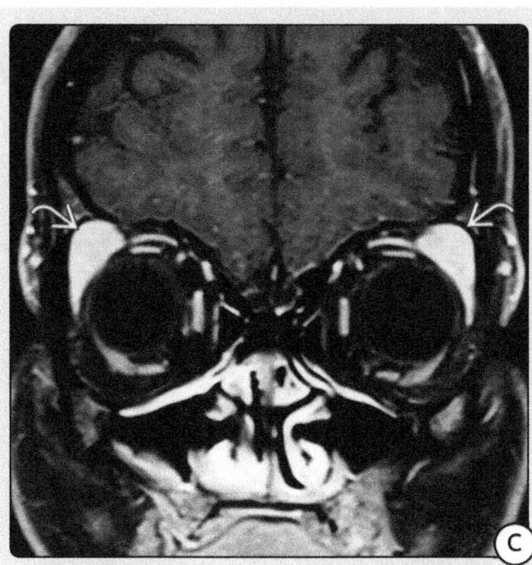

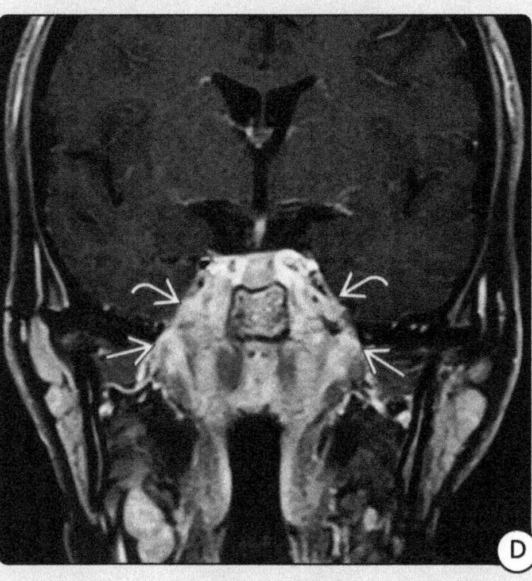

***(15-30C)** Coronal T1 C+ FS MR shows markedly enlarged, intensely enhancing lacrimal glands ➡. **(15-30D)** More posterior T1 C+ FS MR shows that the cavernous sinus infiltrating mass involves both Meckel caves ➡ and extends through the foramen ovale ➡ into the nasopharynx, obstructing the eustachian tubes. This is biopsy-proven IgG4-related disease (IgG4-RD).*

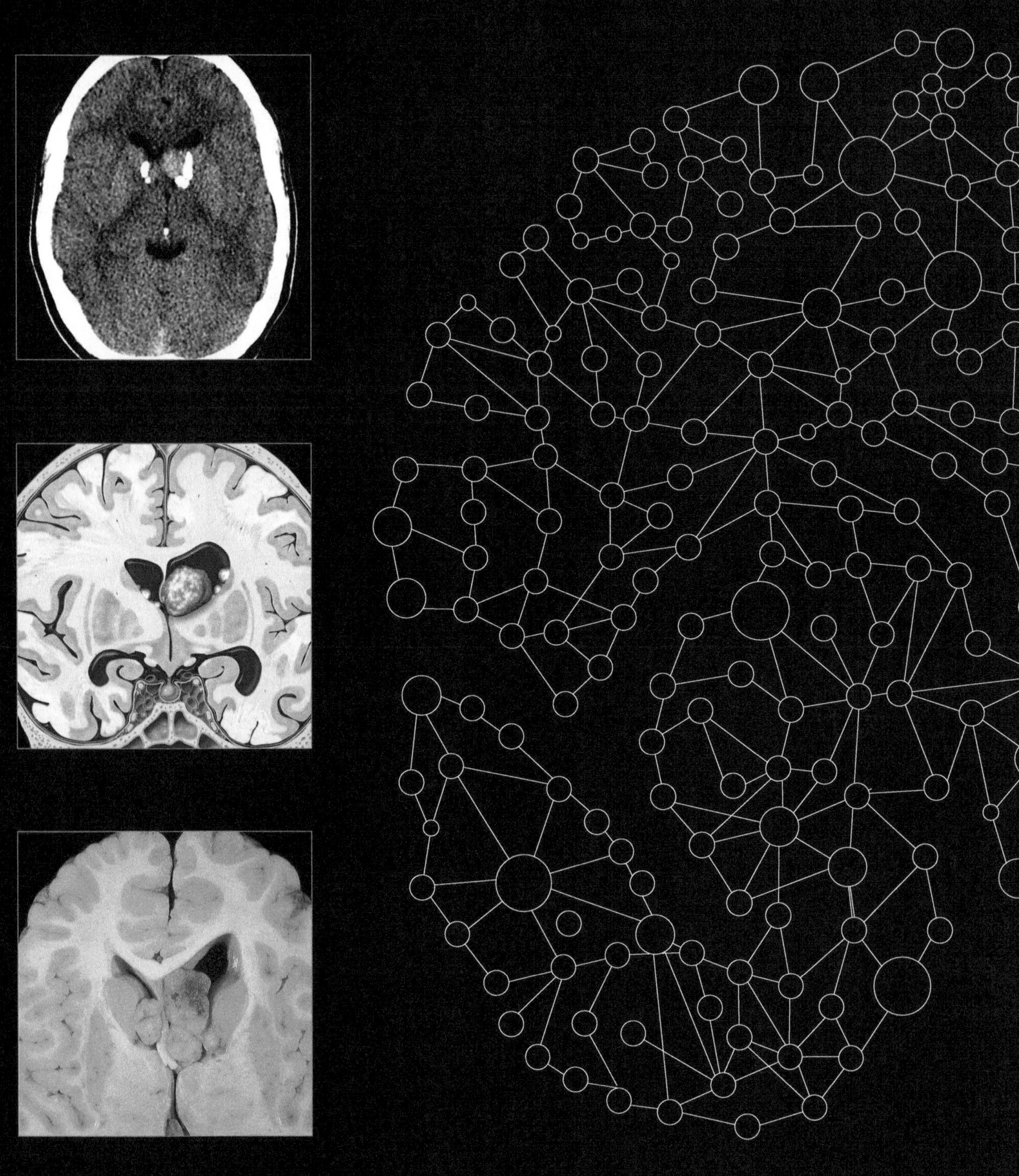

Section 4

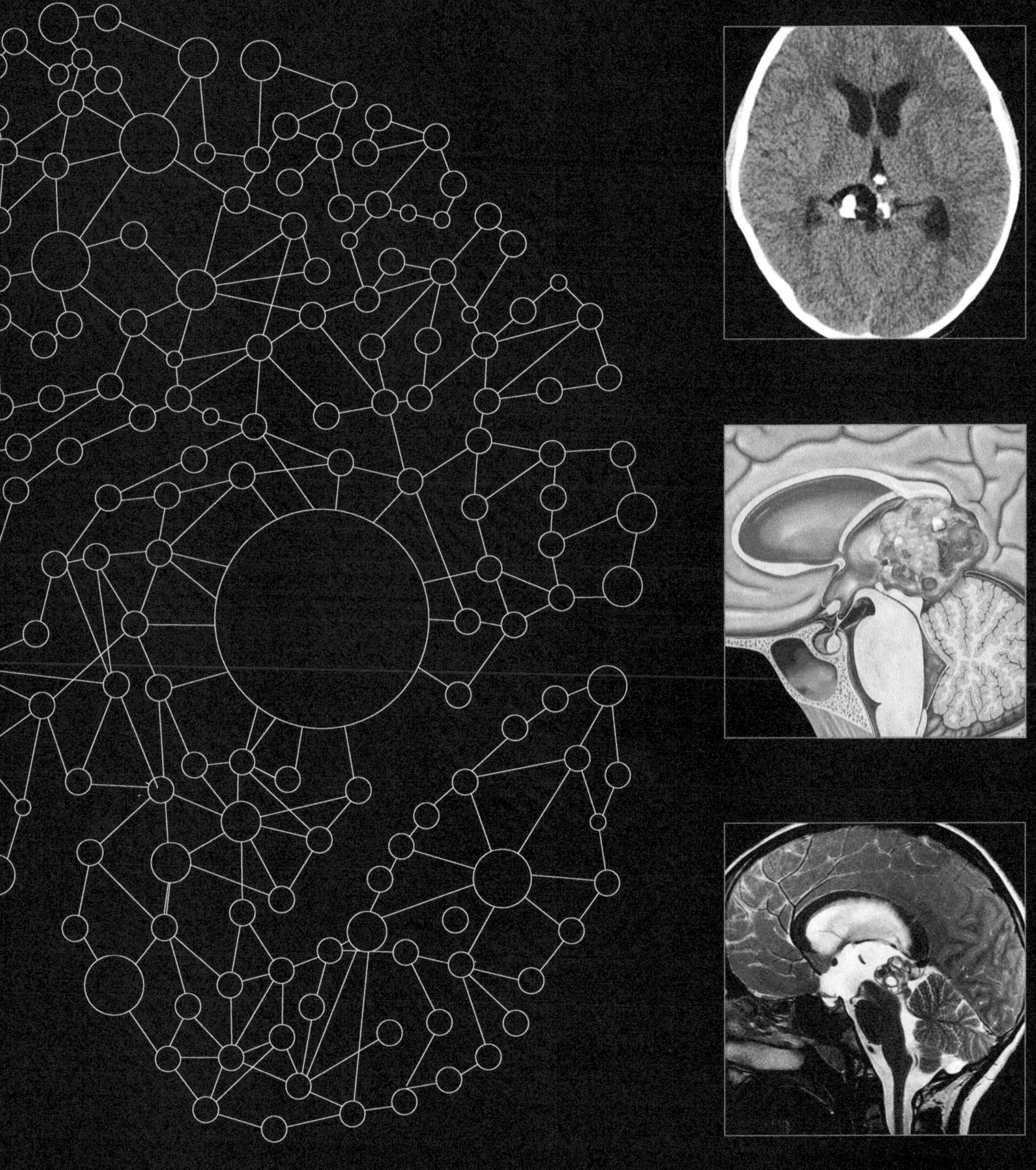

Section 4

Neoplasms, Cysts, and Tumor-Like Lesions

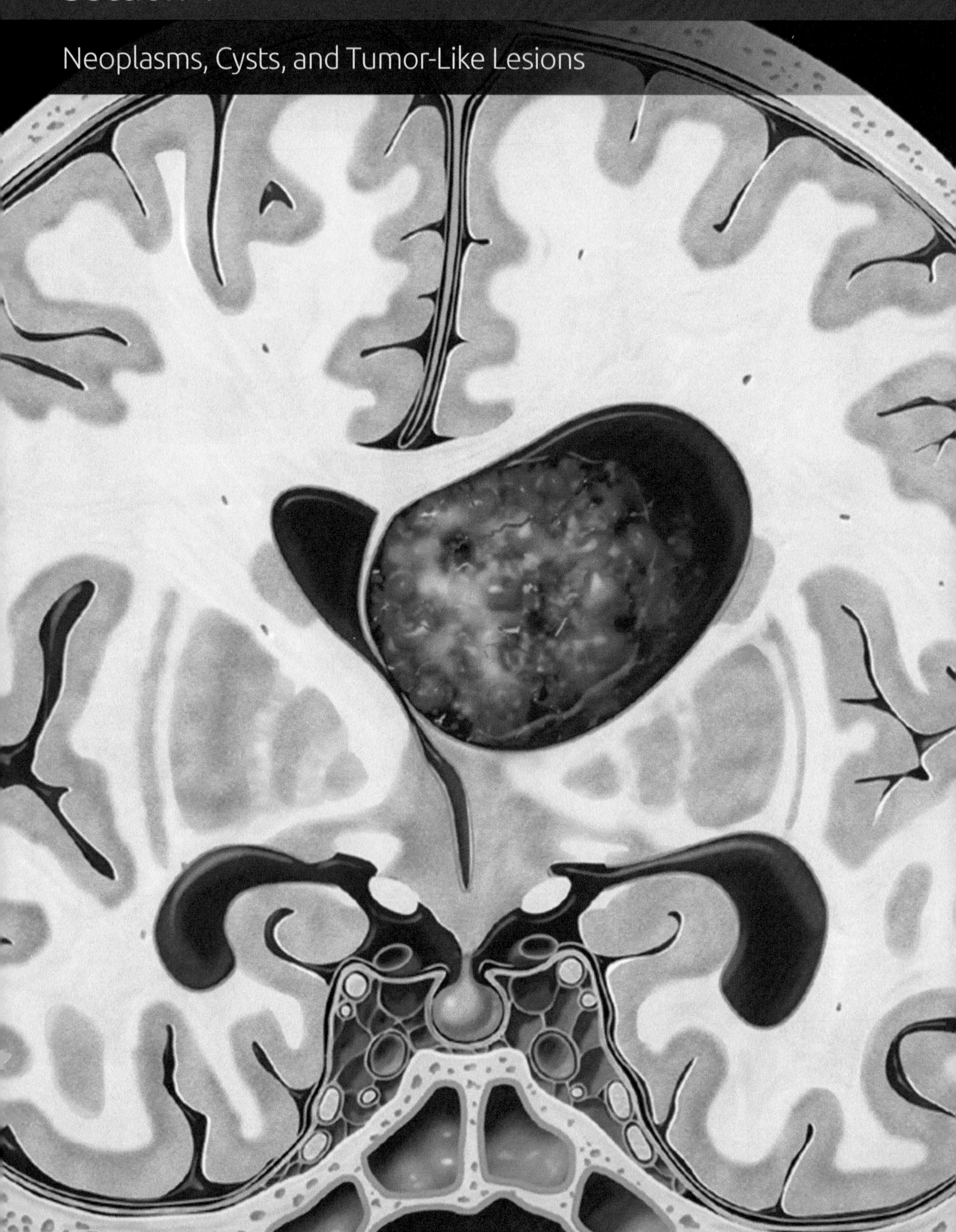

Introduction to Neoplasms, Cysts, and Tumor-Like Lesions

CNS neoplasms are both (1) classified and (2) graded. The universally accepted classification of brain neoplasms is sponsored by the World Health Organization (WHO). The 2016 WHO Classification of Tumours of the Central Nervous System—the version followed in this text and the second edition of Osborn's Brain—represented a dramatic paradigm shift in the way brain tumors are classified. The 2016 WHO integrates both genotypic and phenotypic (i.e., histologic) parameters, incorporating both into the newly updated classification schema.

Rapid, continued progress in elucidating tumor genetics fundamentally altered the classification of CNS neoplasms. The increasing availability of immunohistochemical surrogates for identifying molecular genetic alterations in CNS neoplasms made applying the new 2016 WHO criteria an integral part of modern neuropathology and neuroradiology.

For a variety of reasons, formal WHO classification updates, such as the 2016 CNS WHO, occur only every decade or so. Interim updates on the 2016 WHO are published by a consensus panel of internationally recognized neuropathologists dubbed **cIMPACT-NOW** (the Consortium to Inform Molecular and Practical Approaches to CNS Tumor Taxonomy), and these continuing updates have been incorporated into this text.

Classification and Grading of CNS Neoplasms

Brain tumors are both classified and graded. **Classification** traditionally assigned CNS neoplasms to discrete categories based on the histologic similarity of tumor cells to normal or embryonic constituents of the nervous system.

The identification of distinct genetic, epigenomic profiles and cellular heterogeneity has led to newly updated classifications of adult and pediatric brain tumor subtypes, affording insights into molecular and lineage-specific groupings for treatment.

Grading has been used as a means of predicting the biologic behavior of primary CNS neoplasms and stratifying patients for treatment. The 2016 WHO tumor grade determinations were made largely on the basis of traditional histologic criteria. This introduced some inconsistencies, e.g., an IDH-wild-type diffuse astrocytoma was designated a grade II neoplasm but its biologic behavior is more like that of an anaplastic astrocytoma (grade III)

Selected CNS Glial Neoplasms and WHO Grades

Neoplasm	Grade
DIFFUSE ASTROCYTIC AND OLIGODENDROGLIAL TUMORS	
Diffuse astrocytoma, IDH-mutant	II
Diffuse astrocytoma, IDH-wild-type	II*
Anaplastic astrocytoma, IDH-mutant	III
Anaplastic astrocytoma, IDH-wild-type	III*
Glioblastoma, IDH-wild-type	IV
Glioblastoma, IDH-mutant	IV
Diffuse midline glioma, *H3 K27M*-mutant	IV
Oligodendroglioma, IDH-mutant and Ip/19q-codeleted	II
Anaplastic oligodendroglioma, IDH-mutant and Ip/19q-codeleted	III
OTHER ASTROCYTIC TUMORS	
Pilocytic astrocytoma	I
Pilomyxoid astrocytoma	N/A
Subependymal giant cell astrocytoma	I
Pleomorphic xanthoastrocytoma	II
Anaplastic pleomorphic xanthoastrocytoma	III
EPENDYMAL TUMORS	
Subependymoma	I
Myxopapillary ependymoma	I
Ependymoma	II
Ependymoma, *RELA* fusion-positive	II/III
Anaplastic ependymoma	III

Neoplasm	Grade
OTHER GLIOMAS	
Choroid glioma of the 3rd ventricle	II
Angiocentric glioma	I
Astroblastoma	N/A
CHOROID PLEXUS TUMORS	
Choroid plexus papilloma	I
Atypical choroid plexus papilloma	II
Choroid plexus carcinoma	III
NEURONAL AND MIXED NEURONAL-GLIAL TUMORS	
Dysembryoplastic neuroepithelial tumor	I
Gangliocytoma	I
Multinodular and vacuolated tumor (pattern)	I
Ganglioglioma	I
Anaplastic ganglioma	III
Dysplastic cerebellar gangliocytoma (Lhermitte-Duclos disease)	I
Desmoplastic infantile astrocytoma and ganglioma	I
Rosette-forming glioneuronal tumor	I
Diffuse leptomeningeal glioneuronal tumor	N/A
Central neurocytoma	II

(Table 16-1) *N/A = tumor not assigned a grade by the World Health Organization. Modified from Louis DN: WHO classification and grading of tumors of the central nervous system. In Louis DN et al: WHO Classification of Tumors of the Central Nervous System. Lyon: IARC. 12-13, 2016. *Behaves more like IDH-wild-type GBM. cIMPACT-NOW update 3, 2018 allows for diagnosis of "diffuse astrocytic glioma, IDH-wild-type, with molecular features of glioblastoma, WHO grade IV." Acta Neuropathol 136: 805-10, 2018.*

or even glioblastoma (IV) **(Table 16-1)**. The recent cIMPACT-NOW update on IDH-wild-type astrocytoma designates some of these tumors as "molecular glioblastoma" with WHO grade IV (see Chapter 17).

Demographics of CNS Neoplasms

The incidence of CNS tumors is bimodal. It peaks among young children (those younger than 5 years old) **(16-1)** and then again in the fifth to seventh decades of life. Primary CNS tumors are the most common of all solid neoplasms in children and adolescents (0-19 years) and the second leading cause of cancer mortality in individuals younger than 20 years old.

Prevalence of tumor type varies with location. The most common anatomic location of all intracranial tumors is the meninges followed by the cerebral hemispheres, sellar region, cranial nerves, brainstem, and cerebellum **(16-3)**.

Meningiomas are the most common histologic subtype of primary CNS neoplasm followed by gliomas and pituitary adenomas **(16-4)**.

Tumor prevalence also varies significantly with age. Approximately 1/2 of all adult brain tumors are primary neoplasms, while 1/2 represent metastatic spread from extra-CNS tumors **(16-5)**. Overall, the most common primary brain tumor in adults is meningioma followed by astrocytomas and pituitary neoplasms **(16-4)**. However, the most common *malignant* CNS neoplasm is glioblastoma **(16-6)**, which represents ~ 1/2 of all malignant brain tumors and > 55% of all CNS gliomas **(16-7)**.

The most common overall childhood cancers (ages 0-19 years) are pilocytic astrocytoma and embryonal tumors (2/3 of which are medulloblastoma) **(16-8)**. In children ≤ 5 years old, the most frequently reported tumor type is embryonal neoplasm.

The incidences of primary CNS neoplasms by location, histologic group, and age are illustrated in the pie charts and shaded boxes. Statistics are from the Central Brain Tumor Registry in the USA (CBTRUS) statistical report and, because of rounding, may not add up to 100%.

BRAIN TUMOR INCIDENCE BY AGE GROUP

Children (0-14 Years Old)

- Pilocytic astrocytoma: 18%
- Embryonal neoplasms: 15%
  - 2/3 = medulloblastoma
- Malignant glioma, NOS: 15%
- Diffuse astrocytoma: 11%
- Neuronal/mixed glioneuronal: 6%
- Ependymal: 6%
- Nerve sheath: 5%
- Pituitary: 4%
- Craniopharyngioma: 4%
- Germ cell: 4%
- Glioblastoma: 3%
- Meningioma: 2%
- Oligodendroglioma: 1%
- All others: 5%

Adolescents (15-19 Years Old)

- Pituitary: 27%
- Pilocytic astrocytoma: 10%
- Other astrocytomas: 8%
- Neuronal, mixed glioneuronal: 8%
- Nerve sheath: 6%
- Meningioma: 5%
- Germ cell: 4%
- Ependymal: 4%
- Embryonal tumors: 4%
- Glioblastoma: 3%
- Craniopharyngioma: 2%
- Oligodendroglioma: 2%
- Lymphoma: 1%

Adults (20+ Years Old)

- Metastatic: 50%
- Primary: 50%
  - Meningioma: 18%
  - Glioblastoma: 7%
  - Pituitary: 7%
  - Nerve sheath tumor: 4%
  - Other astrocytomas: 3%
  - Lymphoma: 2%
  - Oligodendroglioma: 2%
  - All others: 7%

Gliomas

Glial neoplasms (often referred to as "gliomas") constitute one of the most heterogeneous groups of brain tumors and are the most common overall group of malignant brain tumors. Gliomas are classified histologically by the WHO according to the glial tissue lineage they most resemble (primarily astrocytomas and oligodendrogliomas) and molecularly by their mutational profiles.

The origin of gliomas is controversial. Multipotent neural stem cells (NSCs) exist in the adult subventricular zone and can self-renew throughout life. Their high proliferation rate makes them prone to genetic errors.

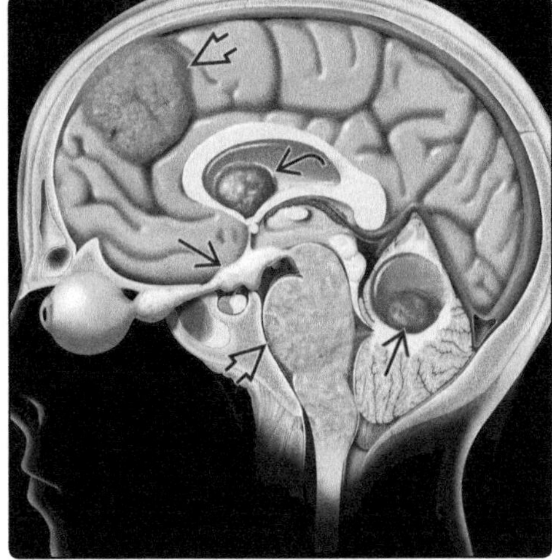

***(16-1)** Childhood astrocytomas are mostly pilocytic ➙. Diffuse astrocytomas ➙ are less common. SEGA in TS is shown ➙.*

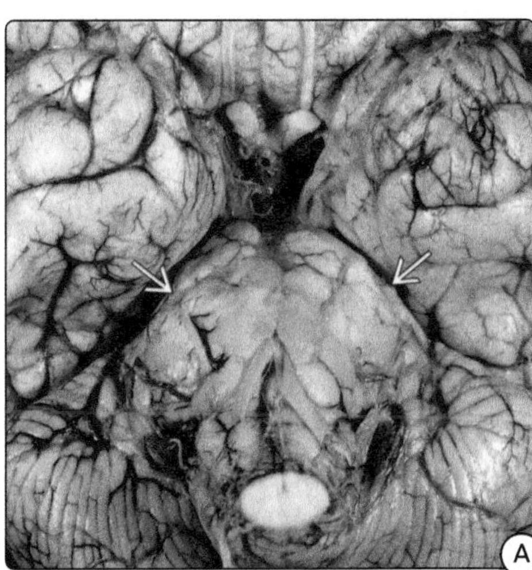

***(16-2A)** Autopsy shows pediatric diffuse intrinsic pontine glioma with "fat" pons ➙. Most are IDH-wild-type histone-mutant tumors.*

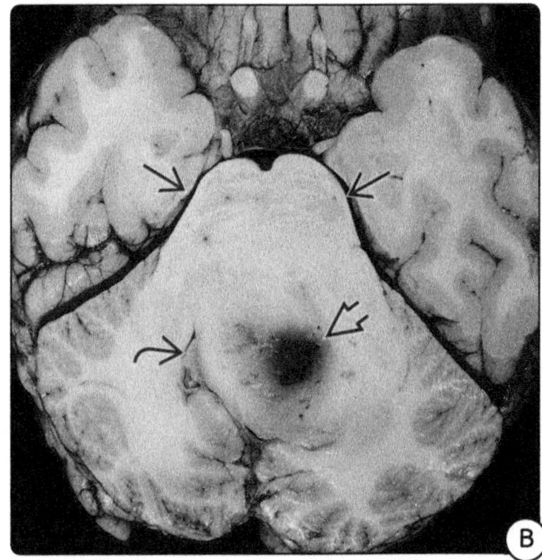

***(16-2B)** DIPG shows enlarged pons ➙ & tumor compressing the 4th ventricle ➙. Hemorrhagic focus ➙ was GBM. (Courtesy R. Hewlett, MD.)*

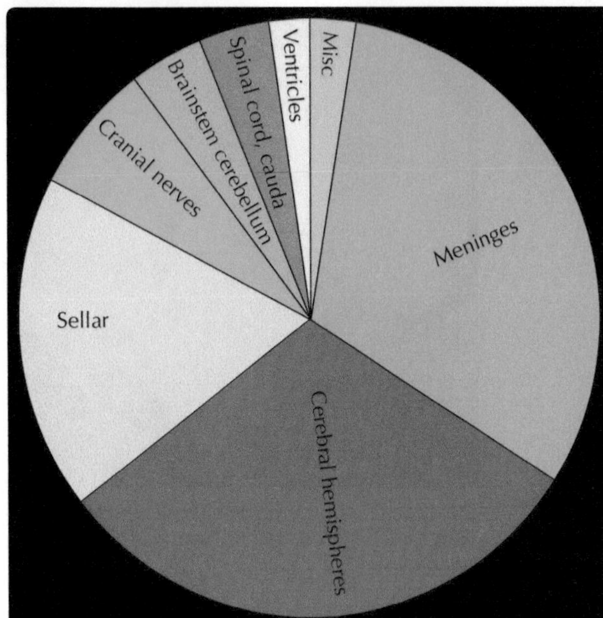

(16-3) Graph indicates percentage of primary brain tumors by location. The most common overall site is the cranial meninges followed by the cerebral hemispheres and sellar region. All other locations account for < 25% of primary CNS neoplasms.

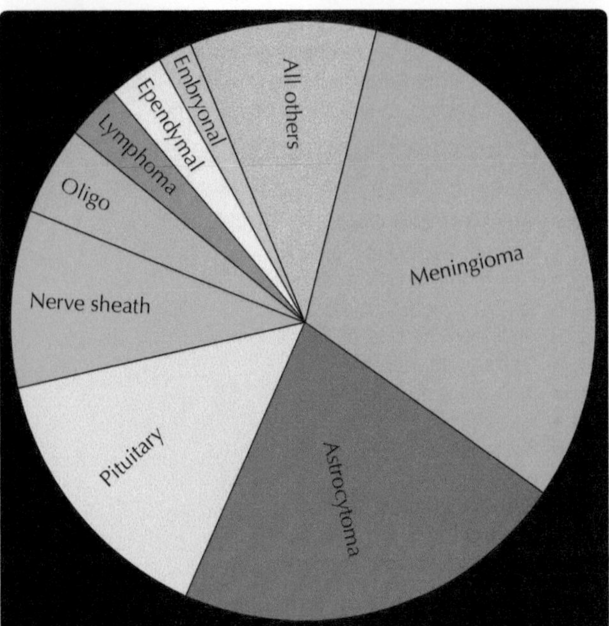

(16-4) Graph represents primary CNS neoplasms by histologic subtypes. Meningiomas are the most common group followed by astrocytomas and pituitary tumors. All other histologic groups comprise ~ 1/3 of the total.

NSCs can differentiate into different fate-restricted progenitors, such as neuron precursor cells (NPCs), oligodendrocyte precursor cells (OPCs), and astrocyte progenitor cells (APCs). All have the ability to accumulate mutations that can induce tumorigenesis.

The existence of any specific dedicated cancer stem cell in brain tumors has yet to be defined, although low-level glioblastoma (GBM) driver mutations have been identified in normal subventricular zone tissue. However, to date, there is no evidence that NSCs are necessary or exclusive players in gliomagenesis. Fate-committed cells like OPCs can also dedifferentiate and behave like facultative stem cells. As malignant gliomas are very heterogeneous neoplasms, their cells of origin may be NSCs, OPCs, other stem-like progenitors, or even astrocytes.

Data from The Cancer Genome Atlas identified a mutation in **isocitrate dehydrogenase (IDH)** as an early "driver mutation" in gliomagenesis. Mutated IDH converts a normal metabolite, α-ketoglutarate, to D-2-hydroxyglutarate (2-HG). 2-HG is an "oncometabolite" that alters cellular epigenetic profiles and induces "broad metabolic reprogramming." In the 2016 WHO, IDH status—which can be reliably determined using IHC—is the major (but not the only) characteristic identifying diffusely infiltrating astrocytic and oligodendroglial tumors.

In the 2016 WHO, astrocytomas that have a more circumscribed growth pattern (e.g., pilocytic astrocytoma, pleomorphic xanthoastrocytoma, and subependymal giant cell astrocytomas) are now separated from the diffusely infiltrating gliomas (e.g., astrocytomas and oligodendrogliomas). The latter are nosologically more similar than are diffuse astrocytoma and pilocytic astrocytoma. The "family trees" in the "new WHO" have been redrawn to reflect this new understanding.

Entity-defining glioma mutations may also differ in children vs. adults. In prior WHO classifications, pediatric diffuse gliomas were grouped together with their adult counterparts despite long-recognized differences in biologic behavior. Although they look the same under the microscope, they have distinct and very different underlying genetic abnormalities.

The 2016 WHO has therefore designated a narrowly defined group of diffusely infiltrating tumors that are characterized by a specific mutation in histone H3 genes as a new, separate entity (H3 K27M-mutant diffuse midline glioma). In time, other pediatric gliomas that appear similar to adult neoplasms may be given separate diagnostic categories (e.g., pediatric oligodendrogliomas, which often lack the entity-defining 1p19q codeletion of adult oligodendrogliomas).

Astrocytomas

There are many histologic types and subtypes of astrocytomas. Astrocytomas can be relatively localized (and generally behave more benignly) or diffusely infiltrating with an inherent tendency to malignant degeneration **(16-2)**.

The most common astrocytomas are diffusely infiltrating neoplasms in which no distinct border between tumor and normal brain is present (even though the tumor may look discrete on imaging studies). Diffuse astrocytomas are now divided into IDH-mutant and IDH-wild-type tumors. Diffuse astrocytomas are generally designated as WHO grade II neoplasms. However, IDH-wild-type grade II and grade III astrocytomas behave more like a grade IV astrocytoma (i.e., glioblastoma). In the presence of certain other mutations,

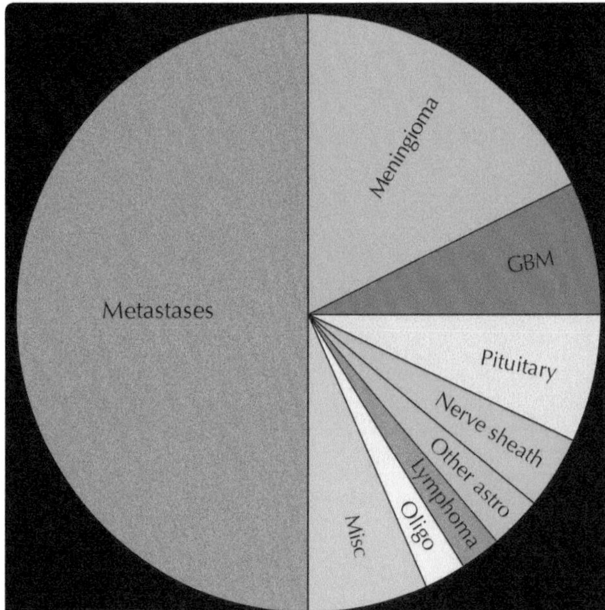

***(16-5)** Graph depicts the relative prevalence of all intracranial tumors in adults. Roughly 1/2 are metastases from systemic cancers; the other 1/2 are primary neoplasms.*

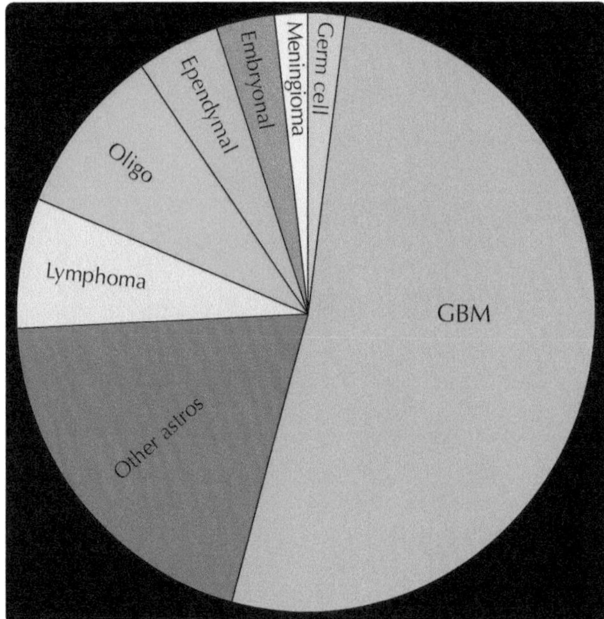

***(16-6)** When all malignant primary CNS neoplasms are grouped together regardless of age, glioblastoma and other malignant astrocytomas (diffuse fibrillary, anaplastic astrocytomas) far outweigh all other types combined.*

these tumors can now be designated as "molecular glioblastoma, WHO grade IV" for treatment purposes.

Anaplastic astrocytomas are also subdivided into IDH-mutant or wild-type and designated as WHO grade III, whereas all glioblastomas are grade IV neoplasms [the rare IDH(+) GBM behaves better than its wild-type counterpart but is still designated as grade IV].

All diffusely infiltrating astrocytomas have an inherent tendency to malignant progression, but, grade for grade, IDH-mutant neoplasms behave better than IDH-wild-type tumors. *Note that there is no such thing as a grade I diffusely infiltrating astrocytoma.*

The more localized astrocytic tumors are less common than the diffusely infiltrating astrocytomas. Two of the localized tumors, pilocytic astrocytoma (PA) and subependymal giant cell astrocytoma (SEGA), are designated WHO grade I neoplasms. Neither displays a tendency to malignant progression, although a variant of PA, pilomyxoid astrocytoma, may behave more aggressively.

Patient age has a significant effect on neoplasm type and location. This is especially true for astrocytomas. Astrocytomas in adults tend to be malignant (e.g., anaplastic astrocytomas, glioblastomas) and to affect the cerebral hemispheres. In contrast, PAs are tumors of children and young adults. They are common in the cerebellum and around the third ventricle but rarely occur in the hemispheres **(16-1)**.

Nonastrocytic Glial Neoplasms

Oligodendrogliomas, ependymomas, and choroid plexus tumors are all considered nonastrocytic glial neoplasms.

Oligodendroglial Tumors. Adult oligodendroglial tumors are nearly always IDH-mutant and have a category-defining mutation, 1p19q codeletion. Two grades are recognized: A well-differentiated WHO grade II neoplasm (oligodendroglioma) and a WHO grade III neoplasm (anaplastic oligodendrogliomas).

Ependymal Tumors. Ependymal tumors vary from WHO grade I to III. Subependymoma, a benign-behaving neoplasm of middle-aged and older adults that occurs in the frontal horns and fourth ventricle, is a WHO grade I tumor; as is myxopapillary ependymoma, a tumor of young and middle-aged adults that is almost exclusively found at the conus, cauda equina, and filum terminale of the spinal cord.

Ependymoma, generally a slow-growing tumor of children and young adults, is a WHO grade II neoplasm that may arise anywhere along the ventricular system and in the central canal of the spinal cord. Anaplastic ependymomas are biologically more aggressive, have poorer prognosis, and are designated WHO grade III neoplasms.

Infratentorial ependymomas, typically arising within the fourth ventricle, occur predominantly in children. Supratentorial ependymomas are more common in the cerebral hemispheres than the lateral ventricle and are usually tumors of young children.

Each ependymoma subtype is developmentally and molecularly distinct, has a predilection for a specific anatomic location, and has specific identifiable genetic mutations. Ependymomas and a newly described tumor, *RELA* fusion-positive ependymoma, are discussed in detail in Chapter 18.

Choroid Plexus Tumors. Choroid plexus tumors are papillary intraventricular neoplasms derived from choroid plexus

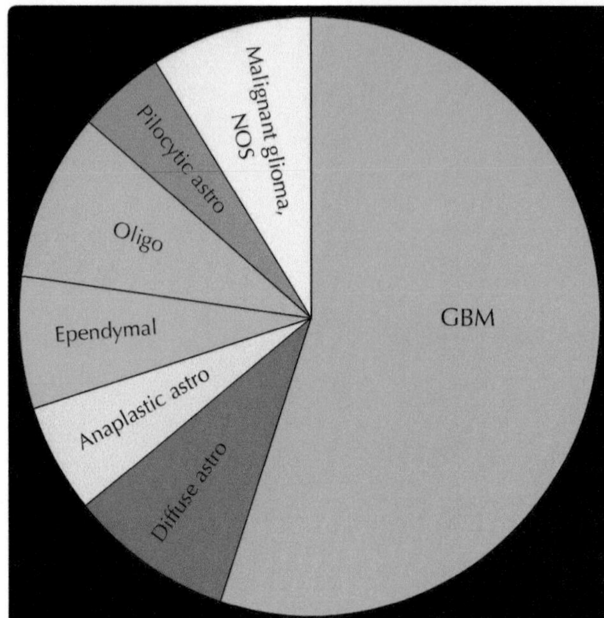

(16-7) ***More than 1/2 of all CNS glial neoplasms are glioblastomas. Of the nonastrocytic gliomas, oligodendrogliomas are the most common subtype.***

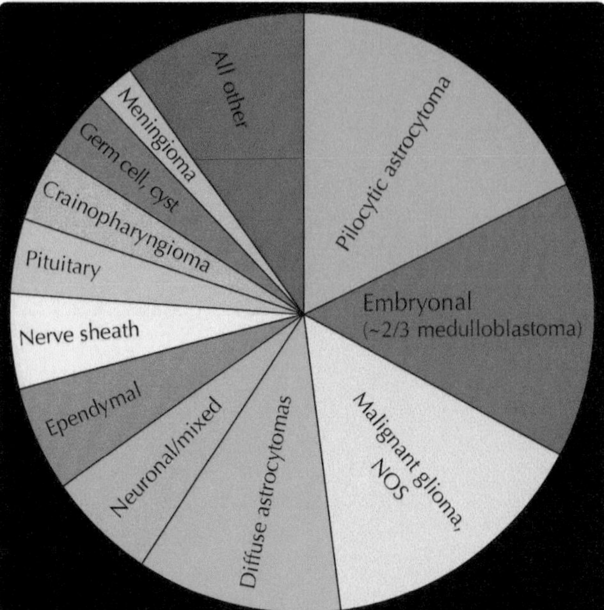

(16-8) ***This graph depicts brain tumors in children from newborn to age 14. Pilocytic astrocytoma and embryonal neoplasms are the most common types. Compared with adults, malignant gliomas are rare, and metastases are insignificant.***

epithelial cells. Almost 80% of choroid plexus tumors are found in children and are one of the most common brain tumors in children under the age of 3 years.

Choroid plexus tumors are divided into choroid plexus papillomas (CPPs), which are WHO grade I tumors, atypical choroid plexus papilloma (WHO grade II), and choroid plexus carcinomas (CPCas), designated WHO grade III. CPPs are five to ten times more common than CPCas. Both CPPs and CPCas can spread diffusely through the CSF, so the entire neuraxis should be imaged before surgical intervention.

Other Gliomas. Other gliomas include chordoid glioma of the third ventricle, angiocentric glioma, and astroblastoma.

CNS GLIOMAS

- Glioblastoma: 55%
- Diffuse astrocytoma: 9%
- Anaplastic astrocytoma: 6%
- Oligodendroglial tumors: 9%
- Ependymal tumors: 7%
- Pilocytic astrocytoma: 5%
- Malignant glioma, NOS: 9%

Neuronal and Mixed Neuronal-Glial Tumors

Neuroepithelial tumors with ganglion-like cells, differentiated neurocytes, or poorly differentiated neuroblastic cells are characteristic of this heterogeneous group.

This group includes dysembryoplastic neuroepithelial tumor (DNET), and ganglion cell neoplasms include gangliocytoma, ganglioglioma, and dysplastic cerebellar gangliocytoma (Lhermitte-Duclos disease). Other tumors in this category are desmoplastic infantile astrocytoma and ganglioglioma, neurocytoma, papillary glioneuronal tumor, rosette-forming glioneuronal tumor, and cerebellar liponeurocytoma.

One new tumor entity—diffuse leptomeningeal glioneuronal tumor—and one pattern, multinodular and vacuolating neuronal tumor of the cerebrum (considered a distinct pattern of gangliocytoma), have been added to the 2016 WHO classification.

Tumors of the Pineal Region

Pineal region neoplasms account for < 1% of all intracranial neoplasms and can be germ cell tumors or pineal parenchymal tumors. Pineal parenchymal tumors are less common than germ cell tumors. Germ cell neoplasms do occur in other intracranial sites but are discussed together with pineal parenchymal neoplasms.

Pineocytoma is a very slowly growing, well-delineated pineal parenchymal tumor that is usually found in adults. Pineocytomas are WHO grade I. Pineal parenchymal tumor of intermediate differentiation (PPTID) is intermediate in malignancy. PPTIDs can be either WHO grade II or III neoplasms **(Table 16-2)**.

Pineoblastoma is a highly malignant primitive embryonal tumor mostly found in children. Highly aggressive and associated with early CSF dissemination, pineoblastomas are WHO grade IV neoplasms.

Papillary tumor of the pineal region (PTPR) is a rare neuroepithelial tumor of adults. PTPRs are designated as WHO grade II or III neoplasms.

Pineal, Embryonal, and Selected Mesenchymal CNS Neoplasms

Neoplasm	Grade
PINEAL PARENCHYMAL TUMORS	
Pineocytoma	I
Pineal parenchymal tumor of intermediate differentiation	II/III
Pineoblastoma	IV
EMBRYONAL NEOPLASMS	
Medulloblastomas, genetically defined *Medulloblastoma, WNT-activated* *Medulloblastoma, SHH-activated* *Medulloblastoma, group 3* *Medulloblastoma, group 4*	IV IV IV IV
Embryonal tumors with multilayered rosettes, *C19MC*-altered	IV
Medulloepithelioma	IV
CNS embryonal tumor, NOS	IV
Atypical teratoid/rhabdoid tumor	IV
TUMORS OF CRANIAL/PARASPINAL NERVES	
Schwannoma	I
Neurofibroma	I
Perineurioma	I
Malignant peripheral nerve sheath tumor (MPNST)	II/III/IV

Neoplasm	Grade
MENINGIOMAS	
Meningioma	I
Atypical meningioma	II
Anaplastic (malignant) meningioma	III
MESENCHYMAL, NONMENINGOTHELIAL TUMORS	
Solitary fibrous tumor/hemangiopericytomas *Grade 1* *Grade 2* *Grade 3*	I II III
Hemangioblastoma	I
Hemangioma	I
Inflammatory myofibroblastic tumor	N/A
Benign/malignant fibrous histiocytoma	N/A
Lipoma	I
Sarcomas (many types)	III/IV
Chondroma	N/A
Chondrosarcoma	N/A

(Table 16-2) *N/A = tumor not assigned a grade by the World Health Organization.*
Modified from Louis DN: WHO classification and grading of tumors of the central nervous system. In Louis DN et al: WHO Classification of Tumors of the Central Nervous System. Lyon: IARC. 12-13, 2016.

Embryonal Tumors

The embryonal tumor group includes medulloblastoma, embryonal tumors, and atypical teratoid/rhabdoid tumors (AT/RTs). All are highly malignant invasive tumors. All are WHO grade IV and mostly tumors of young children.

Embryonal tumors have undergone major restructuring in the 2016 WHO. Two alternative ways of looking at medulloblastoma—as genetically defined or histologically defined—are included. Some of the genetically defined and recognized histologic variants are associated with dramatically different prognoses and therapeutic implications.

The term "primitive neuroectodermal tumor" has been eliminated, and a new tumor, embryonal tumor with multilayered rosetted, C19MC-altered, has been recognized.

Meningeal Tumors

Meningeal tumors are the second largest category of primary CNS neoplasms. They are divided into meningiomas and mesenchymal, nonmeningothelial tumors (i.e., tumors that are *not* meningiomas).

Meningiomas

Meningiomas arise from meningothelial (arachnoidal) cells. Most are attached to the dura but can occur in other locations (e.g., choroid plexus of the lateral ventricles).

Although meningiomas have many histologic subtypes (e.g., meningothelial, fibrous, psammomatous), each with a different ICD-O code, the current WHO schema classifies them rather simply. Most meningioma subtypes are benign, have a low risk of recurrence &/or aggressive growth, and are grouped together as WHO grade I neoplasms.

Atypical meningiomas, as well as the chordoid and clear cell variants, are WHO grade II tumors. Anaplastic (malignant) meningiomas, including the papillary and rhabdoid subtypes, correspond to WHO grade III.

Both WHO grade II and III meningiomas have a greater likelihood of recurrence &/or aggressive behavior. The WHO classification also notes that meningiomas of any subtype or grade with a high proliferation index &/or brain invasion have a greater likelihood of aggressive behavior.

Miscellaneous Selected CNS Primary Neoplasms and WHO Grades

Neoplasm	Grade
LYMPHOMAS	
Diffuse large B-cell lymphoma of CNS	N/A
Immunodeficiency-associated CNS lymphomas	
AIDS-related (large B cell)	
EBV-positive (large B cell)	
Lymphomatoid granulomatosis	
Intravascular large B-cell lymphoma	N/A
MALT lymphoma of the dura	N/A
HISTIOCYTIC TUMORS	
Langerhans cell histiocytosis	
Erdheim-Chester disease	
Rosai-Dorfman disease	N/A
Juvenile xanthogranuloma	N/A

Neoplasm	Grade
GERM CELL TUMORS	
Germinoma	
Embryonal carcinoma	
Teratoma	N/A
Mature	
Immature	
Malignant	
Mixed germ cell tumor	
SELLAR REGION TUMORS	
Craniopharyngioma	I
Adamantinomatous craniopharyngioma	
Papillary craniopharyngioma	
Granular cell tumor	I
Pituicytoma	I
Spindle cell oncocytoma	I

(Table 16-3) *N/A = tumor not assigned a grade by the World Health Organization. Modified from Louis DN: WHO classification and grading of tumors of the central nervous system. In Louis DN et al: WHO Classification of Tumors of the Central Nervous System. Lyon: IARC. 12-13, 2016.*

Mesenchymal Nonmeningothelial Tumors

Both benign and malignant nonmeningothelial mesenchymal tumors can originate in the CNS. Most correspond to tumors of soft tissue or bone. Generally, both a benign and malignant (sarcomatous) type occur. Lipomas and liposarcomas, chondromas and chondrosarcomas, osteomas and osteosarcomas are examples.

A major change in 2016 is consolidating solitary fibrous tumor (SFT) and hemangiopericytoma (HPC) into a single entity (SFT/HPC) with three grades. Grade I corresponds to the low cellularity, spindle cell lesion traditionally diagnosed as SFT. Grade II corresponds to the tumor previously diagnosed in the CNS as hemangiopericytoma, and grade III is used to designate SFT/HPCs with malignant features.

Primary melanocytic neoplasms of the CNS are rare. They arise from leptomeningeal melanocytes and can be diffuse or circumscribed, benign or malignant.

Tumors of Cranial (and Spinal) Nerves

Schwannoma

Schwannomas are benign encapsulated nerve sheath tumors that consist of well-differentiated Schwann cells. They can be solitary or multiple. Multiple schwannomas are associated with neurofibromatosis type 2 (NF2) and schwannomatosis, a syndrome characterized by multiple schwannomas but lacking other features of NF2.

Intracranial schwannomas are almost always associated with cranial nerves (CNVIII is by far the most common) but occasionally occur as parenchymal lesions. Schwannomas do not undergo malignant degeneration and are thus designated WHO grade I neoplasms **(Table 16-3)**.

Neurofibroma

Neurofibromas (NFs) are diffusely infiltrating extraneural tumors that consist of Schwann cells and fibroblasts. Solitary scalp neurofibromas occur, and multiple NFs or plexiform NFs occur as part of neurofibromatosis type 1. NFs correspond histologically to WHO grade I. Plexiform NFs may degenerate into malignant peripheral nerve sheath tumors (MPNSTs). MPNSTs are graded from WHO II to IV, the same three-tiered system used for soft tissue sarcomas.

WHO Changes

Changes to the 2007 WHO include recognizing melanotic schwannoma as a distinct entity rather than a schwannoma variant, recognition of hybrid nerve sheath tumors, and designation of two histologic subtypes of MPNST.

Lymphomas and Histiocytic Tumors

With the onset of the HIV/AIDS era and increasing drug-induced immunocompromised states, some neuropathologists predicted that lymphoma would soon become the most common malignant intracranial neoplasm, surpassing glioblastoma. Although their incidence has increased slightly over the past two decades, lymphomas are still significantly less common than glioblastoma and other malignant astrocytomas.

The 2016 CNS WHO has expanded the classification of systemic lymphomas and histiocytic neoplasms to parallel those in the corresponding hematopoietic/lymphoid WHO classification **(Table 16-3)**.

MALIGNANT PRIMARY CNS NEOPLASMS

- Glioblastoma: 46%
- All other astrocytomas: 17%
- Lymphoma: 6%
- Oligodendroglioma: 7%
- Ependymal neoplasms: 4%
- Embryonal neoplasm: 3%
- Meningioma: 1%
- Germ cell neoplasm: 1%

Germ Cell Tumors

Intracranial germ cell tumors (GCTs) are morphologic and immunophenotypic homologs of germinal neoplasms that arise in the gonads and extragonadal sites. From 80-90% occur in adolescents. Most occur in the midline (pineal region, around the third ventricle).

Germinomas are the most common intracranial GCT. Teratomas differentiate along ectodermal, endodermal, and mesodermal lines. They can be mature, immature, or occur as teratomas with malignant transformation. Other miscellaneous GCTs include the highly aggressive yolk sac tumor, embryonal carcinoma, and choriocarcinoma.

Germ cell tumors are discussed in detail with tumors of the pineal region.

Sellar Region Tumors

The sellar region is one of the most anatomically complex areas in the brain. However, the official WHO classification of sellar region tumors includes only craniopharyngioma and rare tumors, such as granular cell tumor of the neurohypophysis, pituicytoma, and spindle cell oncocytoma of the adenohypophysis.

The sellar region contains many structures besides the craniopharyngeal duct and infundibular stalk that give rise to masses seen on imaging studies. The most common of these masses—pituitary adenoma—is not part of the WHO classification but is included here, as are variants (such as pituitary hyperplasia) and nonneoplastic tumor-like masses (e.g., hypophysitis and hypothalamic hamartoma) that can mimic neoplasms.

Pituitary Adenoma

Pituitary adenomas account for the majority of sellar/suprasellar masses in adults and the third most common overall intracranial neoplasm in this age group. Pituitary adenomas are classified by size as microadenomas (≤ 10 mm) and macroadenomas (≥ 11 mm).

Craniopharyngioma

Craniopharyngioma is a benign (WHO grade I), often partially cystic neoplasm that is the most common nonneuroepithelial intracranial neoplasm in children. It shows a distinct bimodal age distribution with the cystic adamantinomatous type seen mostly in children and a smaller peak in middle-aged adults. The less common papillary type is usually solid and found almost exclusively in adults.

Miscellaneous Sellar Region Tumors

Granular cell tumor of the neurohypophysis, also called choristoma, is a rare tumor of adults that usually arises from the infundibulum. Pituicytomas are glial neoplasms of adults that also usually arise within the infundibulum. Spindle cell oncocytoma of the adenohypophysis is an oncocytic nonendocrine neoplasm. All of these rare tumors are WHO grade I. The diagnosis is usually histologic, as differentiating these tumors from each other and from other adult tumors, such as macroadenoma, can be problematic.

Metastatic Tumors

Metastatic neoplasms represent nearly 1/2 of all CNS tumors. In Chapter 27, we consider the "many faces" of CNS metastatic disease as well as the intriguing topic of paraneoplastic syndromes.

Paraneoplastic neurologic syndromes (PNSs) are rare nervous system dysfunctions in cancer patients that are not due to metastases or local effects of a tumor. Classic PNSs with "onconeural" antibodies and several recently described nonparaneoplastic encephalitides are likewise included in Chapter 27.

Intracranial Cysts

Cysts are common findings on neuroimaging studies and, for purposes of discussion, included in this part of the text. Although our focus is primarily neoplasms, nonneoplastic CNS cysts can sometimes be confused with "real" brain tumors and are often considered in the differential diagnosis of mass lesions in specific anatomic locations.

We therefore take an anatomic- and imaging-based approach to intracranial cysts. Here, the key consideration is not cyst wall histopathology (as in brain neoplasms) but anatomic location **(16-9)**.

There are four key anatomy-based questions to pose when considering the imaging diagnosis of an intracranial cyst. (1) Is the cyst extra- or intraaxial? (2) Is it supra- or infratentorial? (3) Is it midline or off-midline? (4) If the cyst is intraaxial, is it in the brain parenchyma or inside the ventricles?

Although many cysts can be found in multiple locations, each type has its own "preferred" (i.e., most common) site. The three major anatomic sublocations are the extraaxial spaces (including the scalp and skull), the brain parenchyma, and the cerebral ventricles.

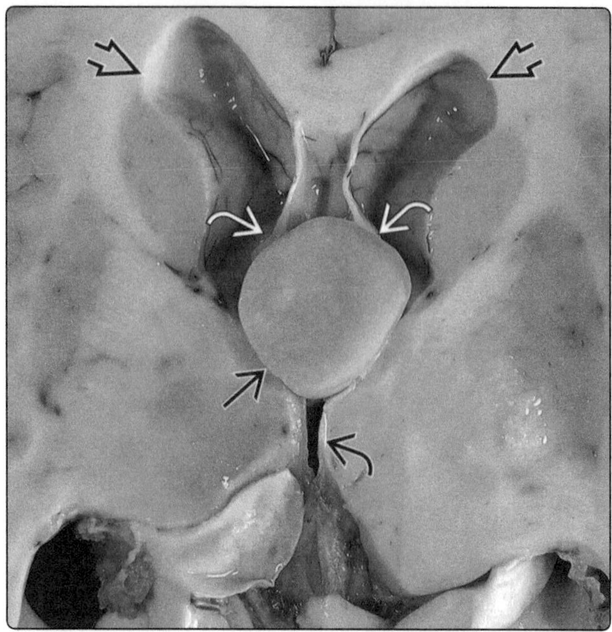

(16-9) A gelatinous cyst ➡ at the foramen of Monro splays the fornices ➡ and enlarges the lateral ventricles ➡, whereas the 3rd ventricle ➡ is normal. Location is virtually pathognomonic for colloid cyst. (Courtesy R. Hewlett, MD.)

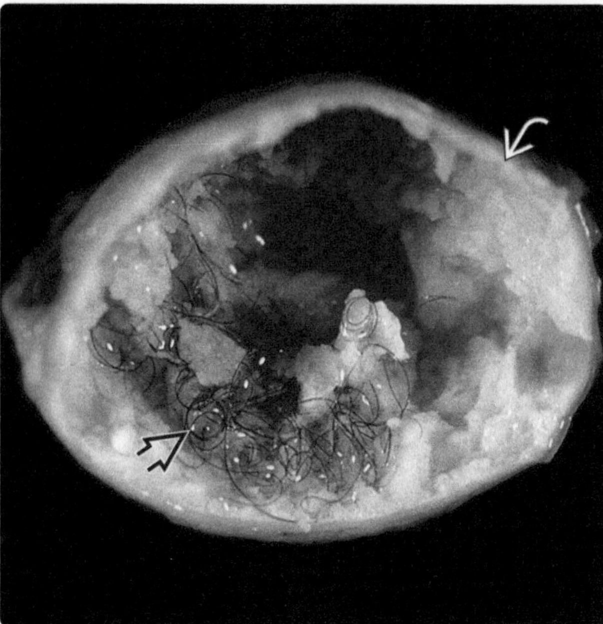

(16-10) Gross pathology of a resected dermoid cyst shows thick, greasy sebaceous and keratin debris ➡. Note tangles of hair ➡ within the well-delineated cyst.

Extraaxial Cysts

This is the second largest group of nonneoplastic cysts. The chapter on nonneoplastic cysts considers these first, beginning from the scalp and skull and proceeding inward to the arachnoid. The uncommon but important "neoplasm-associated cysts" that are sometimes seen around extraaxial tumors, such as macroadenoma, meningioma, and vestibular schwannoma, are probably a form of arachnoid cyst. Epidermoid and dermoid cysts **(16-10)** are also included in this discussion.

Intraaxial (Parenchymal) Cysts

The most common parenchymal cysts are enlarged perivascular spaces and hippocampal sulcus remnants followed by porencephalic (encephaloclastic) cysts. Neuroglial cysts—parenchymal cysts lined by nonneoplastic gliotic brain—are relatively uncommon.

Intraventricular Cysts

Intraventricular cysts are less common than cysts in the brain parenchyma. The most common intraventricular cysts are choroid plexus cysts, which are almost always incidental findings on imaging studies. Colloid cysts are the second most common cyst but the most important to diagnose because they can suddenly and unexpectedly obstruct the foramen of Monro **(16-9)**. Acute obstructive hydrocephalus and even death can result.

INTRACRANIAL CYSTS

Extraaxial Cysts
- Arachnoid cyst
  - Choroid fissure cyst
- Epidermoid cyst
- Dermoid cyst
- Neurenteric cyst
- Pineal cyst
- Nonneoplastic tumor-associated cyst

Intraaxial (Parenchymal) Cysts
- Enlarged perivascular spaces
- Hippocampal sulcus remnants
- Neuroglial cyst
- Porencephalic cyst

Intraventricular Cysts
- Choroid plexus cyst
- Colloid cyst
- Ependymal cyst

Selected References: The complete reference list is available on the Expert Consult™ eBook version included with purchase.

Astrocytomas

Gliomas account for slightly less than 1/3 of all intracranial neoplasms and over 80% of the primary malignant ones. Almost 3/4 of gliomas are astrocytomas. Astrocytomas are the single largest group of neoplasms that arise within the brain itself.

Astrocytomas form a surprisingly diverse group of neoplasms with many different histologic types and subtypes. These fascinating tumors differ widely in preferential location, peak age, clinical manifestations, morphologic features, biologic behavior, and prognosis.

General Features of Astrocytomas

Introduction

We introduce astrocytomas with a brief discussion of their putative origin, classification (by both histologic phenotype and genotype), grading, and importance of age and location in determining astrocytoma tumor subtypes.

For purposes of our discussion, astrocytomas are organized into two general categories: A relatively "localized," comparatively more benign-behaving group and a "diffusely infiltrating," more biologically aggressive group. This distinction is somewhat arbitrary and imperfect, as some "circumscribed" astrocytomas occasionally become more aggressive and infiltrate adjacent structures despite their low-grade histology.

Origin of Astrocytomas

Astrocytomas were originally named for their putative origin from the stellate-shaped cells—"astrocytes"—that are the dominant component of the neuropil (vastly outnumbering neurons). It was once assumed that astrocytes could undergo both hyperplasia (nonneoplastic "reactive astrocytosis") and neoplastic transformation.

There is now considerable evidence that diffuse astrocytomas do *not* arise from neoplastic transformation of normal mature astrocytes. Instead, they probably develop from precursor "glioma-initiating" cells that possess stem cell properties.

Classification and Grading of Astrocytomas

Although tumor staging is commonly used for neoplasms elsewhere in the body, CNS neoplasms are first classified (into specific tumor types) and then graded (a measure of malignancy).

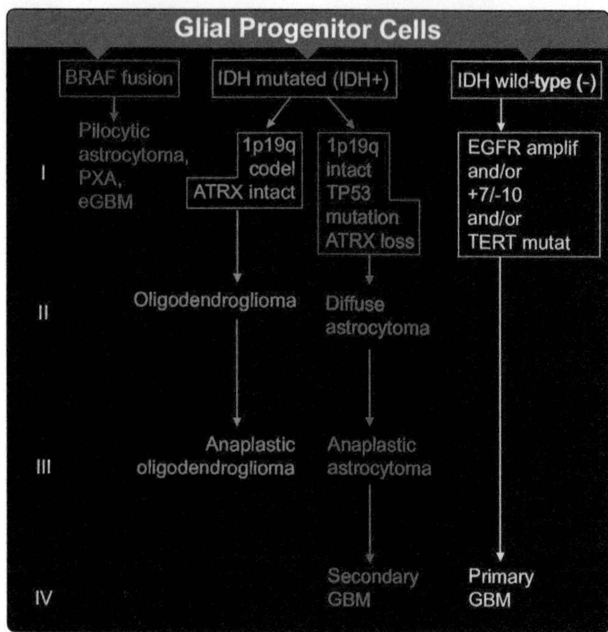

(17-1) Glioma "families" with "driver" mutations, WHO grades. IDH1 mutation leads to astrocytoma (blue) or oligodendroglioma (green) depending on subsequent mutations. IDH(-) gliomas with different mutations (yellow) are "molecular" GBMs.

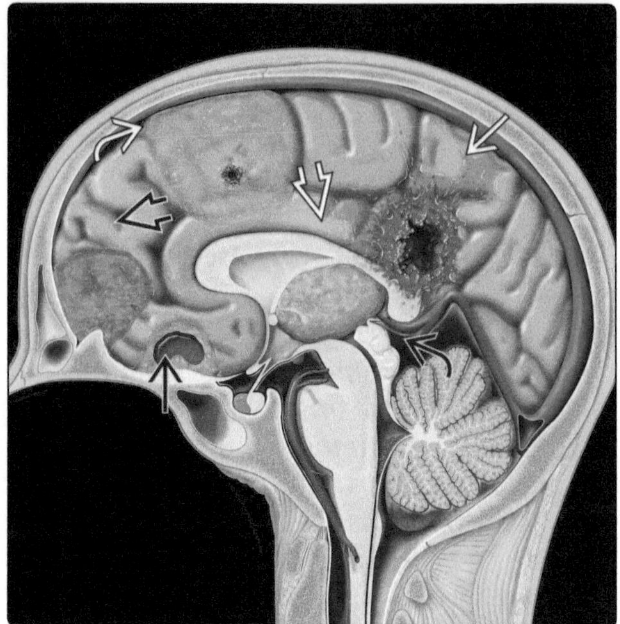

(17-2) Adult GBM and AA are common in cerebral hemispheres, corpus callosum; DA is in frontal lobe, brainstem/tectum. PXA with cyst, meningeal reaction, thalamic H3 K27M-mutant midline glioma are shown.

Classification

The two major types of diffuse glioma are astrocytomas and oligodendrogliomas. The initial entity-defining genetic marker in adult diffuse gliomas is **isocitrate dehydrogenase (IDH)** mutation status. IDH1 and IDH2 are a key part of the citric acid cycle. IDH metabolizes isocitrate to α-ketoglutarate (α-KG). *Mutated* IDH converts α-KG to D-2-hydroxyglutarate (2-HG), which is an oncometabolite.

In the 2016 WHO "family tree" **(17-1)**, IDH-mutant gliomas are then separated by other, mutually exclusive genetic mutations into **astrocytomas (IDH-mutated, 1p19q intact, ATRX loss of nuclear expression &/or p53 immunopositivity)** and **oligodendrogliomas (IDH-mutated, 1p19q codeleted, ATRX intact).** We discuss astrocytomas in this chapter; oligodendrogliomas are grouped with other nonastrocytic glial neoplasms and discussed in Chapter 18.

Localized Astrocytomas. Astrocytomas with a more circumscribed or localized growth pattern (e.g., pilocytic astrocytoma, pleomorphic xanthoastrocytoma, and subependymal giant cell astrocytoma) lack IDH mutations and often exhibit *BRAF* fusion. This group represents between 10% and 15% of astrocytomas.

IDH-Mutant Astrocytomas. The vast majority of astrocytomas grow more rapidly than localized astrocytomas, diffusely infiltrate adjacent tissues, and display an inherent propensity to undergo malignant degeneration. Approximately 85% of diffusely infiltrating astrocytomas are IDH-mutant.

IDH-Wild-Type Astrocytomas. The less common adult IDH-wild-type astrocytomas lack IDH mutation and are characterized by a different group of genetic abnormalities (e.g., *EGFR* amplification, *TERT* promoter mutation, etc.). Childhood diffuse gliomas have different sets of mutations, including *BRAF* V600E mutation, *FGFR1* alteration, or *MYB* or *MYBL1* rearrangements.

Histone H3-Mutant Gliomas. A fourth "family" of gliomas lacks IDH mutation and is characterized by mutations in histone H3 genes, a diffuse growth pattern, and midline location. These tumors are more common in children but occasionally occur in adults.

Grading

Astrocytomas are graded from I to IV. Only two relatively circumscribed astrocytoma subtypes—pilocytic and subependymal giant cell astrocytomas—are designated as **WHO grade I**.

Diffuse ("low grade") astrocytomas are **WHO grade II**. Anaplasia and mitotic activity are characteristic of **WHO grade III** (i.e., anaplastic astrocytoma). **WHO grade IV** neoplasms (i.e., glioblastoma) exhibit neovascularity and necrosis.

A subset of IDH(-) gliomas do not exhibit microvascular proliferation &/or necrosis, so traditionally they would be designated WHO grade II or III. However, some of these tumors follow a clinical course that approximates that of glioblastoma. The cIMPACT-NOW interim updates specify that with certain molecular criteria (*EGFR* amplification, &/or whole chromosome 7 gain and whole chromosome 10 loss, i.e., +7/-10, &/or *TERT* promoter mutation), these tumors should be designated as "diffuse astrocytic glioma, IDH-wild-type, with molecular features of glioblastoma, WHO grade IV."

Age and Location in Astrocytomas

Astrocytomas in children are typically localized tumors that occur most commonly in the posterior fossa or optic pathway (see Fig. 16-1 in Chapter 16). The highly lethal H3 K27M-mutant diffuse midline glioma occurs in the pons or thalamus. Hemispheric diffuse astrocytomas are relatively less uncommon. The vast majority of adult astrocytomas are diffusely infiltrating (grades II-IV), almost exclusively supratentorial, and located in the cerebral hemispheres **(17-2)**.

Localized Astrocytomas

Only two localized astrocytomas, **pilocytic astrocytoma** (PA) and **subependymal giant cell astrocytoma**, are designated as WHO grade I neoplasms. WHO grade I tumors have low proliferative potential, can often be cured with surgical resection alone, and do not display an inherent tendency to malignant progression.

Pilocytic Astrocytoma

Terminology

PA, sometimes termed "juvenile pilocytic astrocytoma" or "cystic cerebellar astrocytoma," is a well-circumscribed, typically slow-growing glioma of young patients.

Etiology

Genetics of PA. PAs can be sporadic or syndromic. Nearly all sporadic PAs have a *BRAF* gene fusion. Approximately 15% of neurofibromatosis type 1 (NF1) patients develop syndromic PAs, most commonly in the optic nerves/tracts ("optic pathway gliomas"). PAs in patients with NF1 have a biallelic

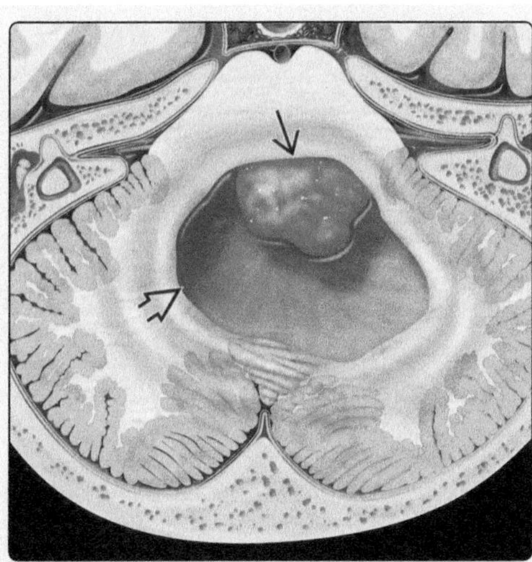

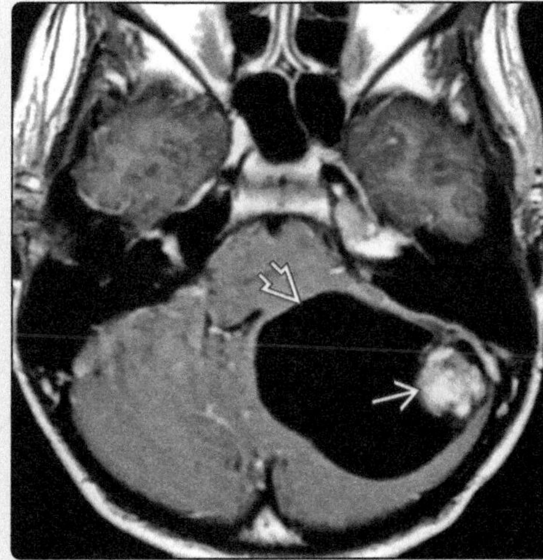

***(17-3)** Graphic shows typical cerebellar pilocytic astrocytoma with a vascular-appearing tumor nodule ➡ and large nonneoplastic cyst ⇨. Cyst wall consists of compressed but otherwise histologically normal brain parenchyma. **(17-4)** T1 C+ MR shows a classic PA in the cerebellum with an enhancing mural nodule ➡, nonenhancing cyst wall ⇨, little peritumoral edema.*

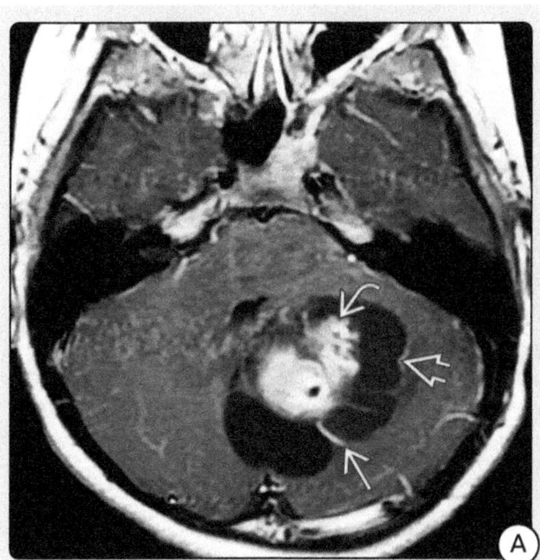

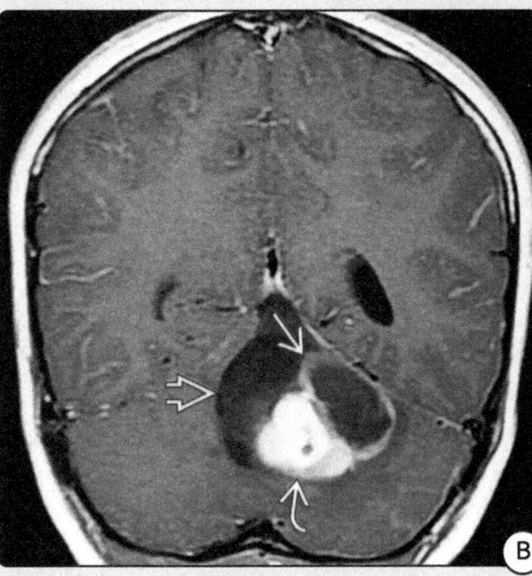

***(17-5A)** Axial T1 C+ MR in a child with headaches shows a cerebellar mass with a cyst nodule ↗ that enhances strongly but heterogeneously. Some enhancement of the cyst wall ⇨ and internal septations ➡ is present. **(17-5B)** Coronal T1 C+ MR shows that the cyst wall is mostly nonenhancing ⇨, while the cyst nodule ↗ and some internal septations ➡ enhance strongly. Pathology disclosed pilocytic astrocytoma, BRAF V600E mutation.*

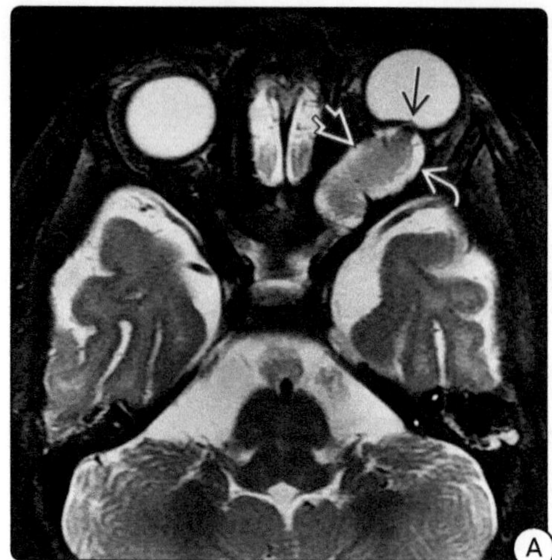

***(17-6A)** T2 MR in a 6m infant shows thickened, tortuous left optic nerve ➡, dilated sheath ➡ with protrusion of the optic nerve head ➡.*

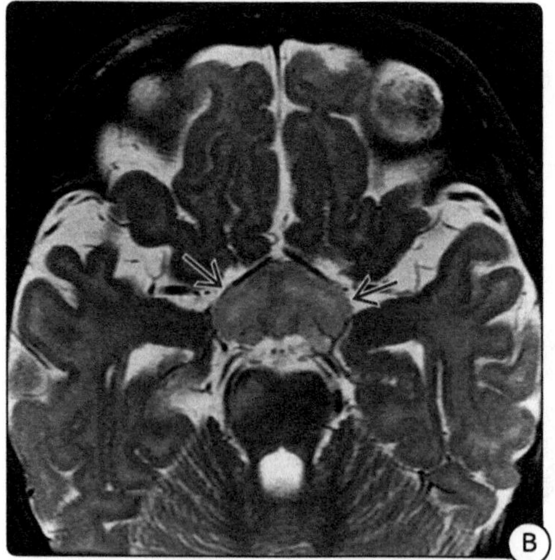

***(17-6B)** More cephalad T2 MR shows that the optic chiasm is enlarged, infiltrated by tumor ➡.*

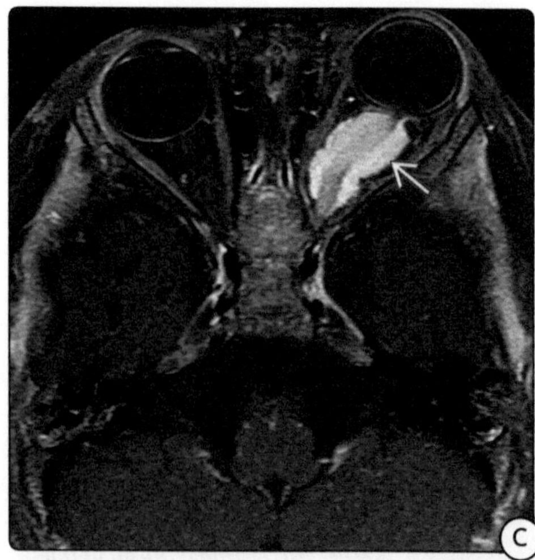

***(17-6C)** T1 C+ FS shows that the left optic nerve is enlarged, infiltrated with enhancing tumor ➡. This is NF1-associated pilocytic astrocytoma.*

mutational inactivation on chromosome 17 that encodes neurofibromin, resulting in overactivity of the RAS and MAPK pathways.

Pathology

Location. The cerebellum is the most common location, accounting for nearly 60% of all PAs **(17-3)**. The second most common site is in and around the optic nerve/chiasm and hypothalamus/third ventricle. The third most common location is the pons and medulla. PAs also occur in the tectum, where they may cause aqueductal stenosis.

The cerebral hemispheres are a reported but uncommon location of PA. When they occur outside the posterior fossa, optic pathway, or suprasellar region, PAs tend to be cortically based cysts with a tumor nodule.

Gross Pathology. Sometimes PAs form a mural nodule in association with a cyst. The walls of most PA-associated cysts usually consist of compressed but otherwise normal brain parenchyma with the neoplastic element confined to the mural tumor nodule. Cyst contents are typically a protein-rich xanthochromic fluid.

PA is a WHO grade I tumor. Tumor dissemination occasionally occurs but is rare.

Clinical Issues

Demographics. More than 80% of PAs occur in patients under 20. Peak incidence is between 5 and 15 years. There is no sex predilection.

Presentation. Cerebellar PAs often present with headache, morning nausea, and vomiting, as intraventricular obstructive hydrocephalus is common. Ataxia, visual loss, and cranial nerve palsies also occur. Optic pathway PAs typically present with visual loss.

Natural History. PAs generally grow slowly. Ten-year survival exceeds 90%, even with partially resected tumors. Almost 1/2 of residual tumors show spontaneous regression or arrested long-term growth. Dissemination occurs but is rare.

Imaging

Imaging findings vary with PA location. The most common appearance of a posterior fossa PA is a well-delineated cerebellar cyst with a mural nodule. PAs in and around the optic nerve, chiasm, third ventricle, and tectum tend to be solid, infiltrating, and less well marginated. PAs in the tectum expand the collicular plate and may cause aqueductal obstruction. The rare hemispheric PA typically presents as a cortically based lesion, usually a cyst with a mural nodule.

CT Findings. NECT scans show a mixed cystic/solid or solid mass with focal mass effect and little, if any, adjacent edema. Calcification occurs in 10-20% of cases.

MR Findings. Cystic PAs are usually well delineated and appear slightly hyperintense to CSF on both T1- and T2WI. They do not suppress completely on FLAIR. The mural nodule is iso-/hypointense on T1WI and iso-/hyperintense on T2WI. Solid PAs appear iso- or hypointense to parenchyma on T1WI and hyperintense on T2/FLAIR. Posterior extension along the optic radiations is not uncommon with a suprasellar PA and does not denote malignancy.

Intense but heterogeneous enhancement of the nodule in a cystic PA is typical on T1 C+ **(17-4)**. Enhancement of the cyst wall itself varies from none

(17-4) to moderate **(17-5)**. A variant pattern is a solid mass with central necrosis and a thick peripherally enhancing "rind" of tumor **(17-7)**.

PAs in the optic nerve, optic chiasm, and hypothalamus/third ventricle show variable enhancement (from none to striking) **(17-6)**, whereas hemispheric PAs generally present with a cyst plus an enhancing mural nodule **(17-8)**.

MRS in PAs often shows elevated Cho, low NAA, and a lactate peak—paradoxical findings that are more characteristic of malignant neoplasms than this clinically benign-behaving tumor. pMR shows low to moderate rCBV.

Differential Diagnosis

Posterior fossa PAs can resemble **medulloblastoma**, especially when they are mostly solid midline tumors. Medulloblastomas typically restrict on DWI, whereas PAs do not.

Ependymoma is a plastic-appearing tumor that extrudes out of the foramen of Magendie and lateral recesses. The imaging appearance of **hemangioblastoma** (HGBL) can resemble PA, but HGBLs are tumors of middle-aged adults rather than children. HGBLs have significant peritumoral edema and markedly elevated rCBV.

The differential diagnosis of a hemispheric PA with a "nodule plus cyst" appearance is **ganglioglioma**. Gangliogliomas are generally cortically based and often calcify.

Pilomyxoid astrocytoma (PMA) is a rare but more aggressive PA variant. PMAs occur at a younger age and are heterogenous, bulky "H-shaped" tumors that are most common in the hypothalamus/optic chiasm **(17-9)**. Lateral extension into the temporal lobes is common.

Subependymal Giant Cell Astrocytoma

Terminology

Subependymal giant cell astrocytoma (SEGA) is a localized, circumscribed, WHO grade I astrocytic tumor predominately associated with tuberous sclerosis complex (TSC).

Etiology

The vast majority of SEGAs occur in patients with TSC. Biallelic inactivation of the *TSC1* or *TSC2* genes that encode the tumor suppressor proteins hamartin and tuberin is present.

Between 10% and 20% of patients with SEGA do not have other features of TSC. SEGAs with low levels of *TSC1* somatic mosaicisms may occur. Isolated nonsyndromic SEGAs have also been reported in patients *without* demonstrable germline or tumor mutations in *TSC1* or *TSC2* on sequencing.

Pathology

Location. Nearly all SEGAs are located in the lateral ventricles, adjacent to the foramen of Monro **(17-10)**. SEGAs vary in size from tiny to lesions measuring several centimeters in diameter. The average tumor size is 10-15 mm. Most SEGAs are solitary lesions. So-called double SEGAs occur in up to 20% of cases.

Gross Pathology. SEGAs are well-circumscribed, multilobulated solid intraventricular masses that rarely hemorrhage or undergo necrosis **(17-11)**. Calcification is common.

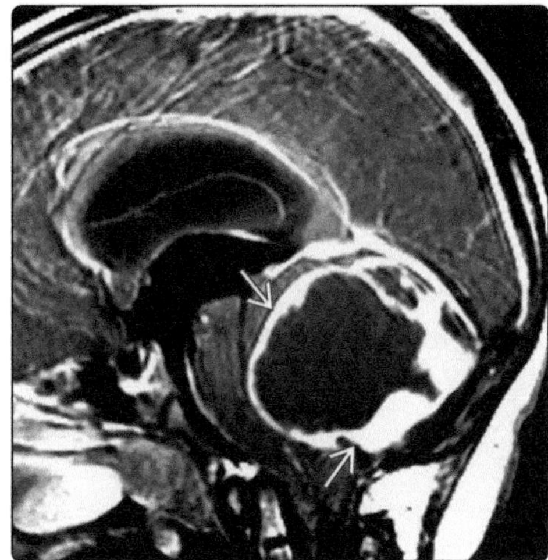

***(17-7)** Sagittal T1 C+ MR shows variant appearance of cerebellar PA with thick, nodular enhancing rim ➡.*

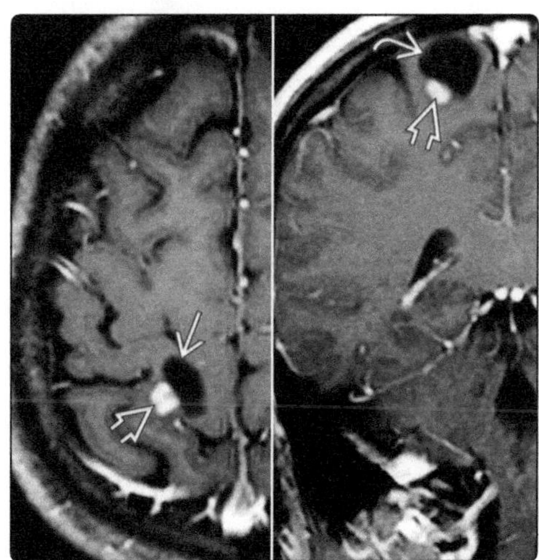

***(17-8)** T1 C+ MR shows hemispheric cyst ➡ with enhancing nodule ➡. The cyst wall ➡ does not enhance. Pilocytic astrocytoma, WHO grade I.*

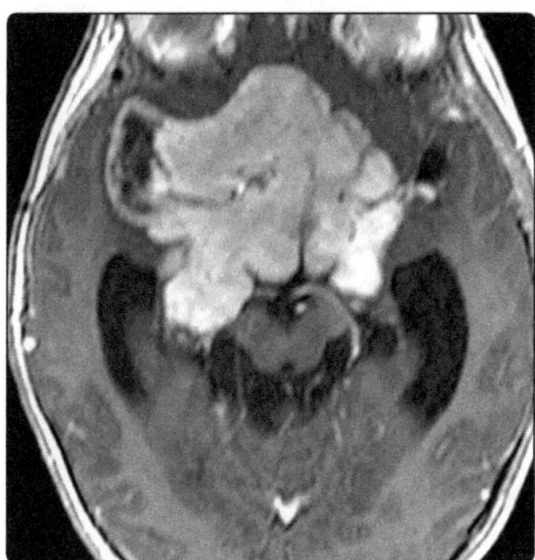

***(17-9)** T1 C+ MR shows typical intensely enhancing H-shaped configuration of a hypothalamic PMA. (Courtesy M. Thurnher, MD.)*

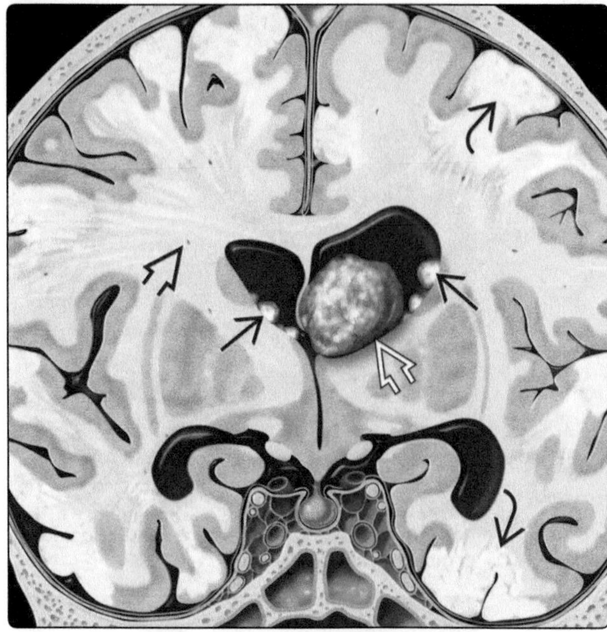

(17-10) Coronal graphic shows a SEGA in a patient with tuberous sclerosis. Note subependymal nodules and cortical tubers with "blurring" of the gray-white interface. Prominent radial glial bands are also present in the medullary WM.

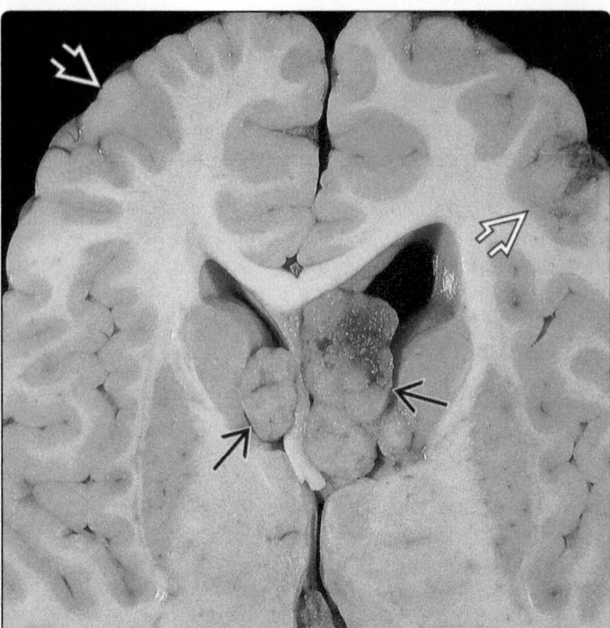

(17-11) Axial autopsy in a patient with tuberous sclerosis shows cortical tubers and bilateral SEGAs. Note that the left frontal horn is enlarged, but the tumor remains circumscribed and noninvasive. (Courtesy R. Hewlett, MD.)

Microscopic Features. SEGA tumor cells display a wide spectrum of astroglial phenotypes that may be indistinguishable from subependymal nodules (SENs).

Although there are histologic similarities between SEGAs and subependymal nodules, mitotic figures are found only in SEGAs. Mitoses are generally few in number so MIB-1 is low.

Staging, Grading, and Classification. SEGAs are WHO grade I neoplasms.

Clinical Issues

Demographics. SEGAs generally occur in the setting of TSC and typically develop during the first two decades of life. Mean age at diagnosis is 11 years.

Presentation. Epilepsy in tuberous sclerosis patients is related to cortical tubers, not SEGA. SEGAs are generally asymptomatic until they cause obstructive hydrocephalus, which may develop suddenly and result in rapidly rising intracranial pressure.

Natural History. Prognosis is generally good, as SEGAs are benign lesions that grow slowly and rarely infiltrate the adjacent brain. Many patients with SEGAs have small lesions that may remain relatively stable. Median growth rate generally ranges from 2.5-5.6 mm per year.

Treatment Options. When imaging findings are indeterminate and a lesion near the foramen of Monro cannot be clearly identified as an SEN or SEGA, close interval follow-up imaging (initially every 6 months, then annually if there is no evidence of growth) is recommended. A lesion in this location should be treated as soon as it shows evidence of enlargement.

Surgical resection has been the treatment of choice, as regrowth rates after complete tumor removal are very low. However, not all SEGAs can be resected completely. Biologically targeted pharmacotherapy with mTOR inhibitors, such as sirolimus and everolimus, has provided a safe and efficacious treatment option.

Imaging

The most important ancillary imaging findings to identify are those of TSC (see Chapter 39). In the absence of a known family history, mental retardation, epilepsy, or cutaneous stigmata, imaging may provide the first clues to the diagnosis of TSC.

CT Findings. SEGAs are hypo- to isodense, variably calcified lesions near the foramen of Monro **(17-12A)**. Calcified SENs may be seen along the lateral ventricle margins, especially the caudothalamic grooves. Hydrocephalus is present in 15% of cases. "Blurred" lateral ventricle margins indicate severe obstructive hydrocephalus with transependymal CSF migration.

SEGAs demonstrate strong but heterogeneous enhancement. An enhancing lesion at the foramen of Monro on CECT scan should be considered SEGA until proven otherwise.

MR Findings. SEGAs are hypo- to isointense compared with cortex on T1WI and heterogeneously iso- to hyperintense on T2WI. Larger SEGAs may have prominent "flow voids." Strong but heterogeneous enhancement is typical.

FLAIR is especially useful for detecting subtle CNS features of TSC, such as SENs, cortical tubers, and white matter radial migration lines. Streaky linear hyperintensities extending through the white matter to the subjacent ventricle or wedge-shaped hyperintensities underlying expanded ("clubbed") gyri are typical **(17-12B)**.

SEN enhancement is much more visible on MR than on CT. Between 30-80% of SENs enhance following contrast administration **(17-12C)**, so enhancement alone is insufficient to distinguish an SEN from a SEGA. Although a mass at the foramen of Monro larger than 10-12 mm in diameter is usually a SEGA, only progressive enlargement is sufficient to differentiate a SEGA from an SEN.

SUBEPENDYMAL GIANT CELL ASTROCYTOMA

Etiology, Genetics
- 5-15% of patients with TSC develop SEGA
- 80-90% of SEGAs are associated with TSC

Pathology
- Circumscribed, multinodular mass at foramen of Monro
- Does not infiltrate brain
- WHO grade I

Clinical Issues
- Mean age = 11 years
- Seizures, ↑ intracranial pressure

Imaging Findings
- Ca^{++} on NECT, enhance on CECT
- T1 iso-/hypointense, T2/FLAIR hyperintense
- May have prominent vascular "flow voids"
- Strong, heterogeneous enhancement
- Look for signs of TSC

Differential Diagnosis

The major differential diagnosis of SEGA in a patient with TSC is a benign nonneoplastic **SEN**. SENs remain stable and do not need to be treated, whereas SEGAs gradually enlarge and eventually require surgical treatment. SEGAs arise only near the foramen of Monro, whereas SENs can be located anywhere around the ventricular wall, especially along the caudothalamic groove. Although SENs are much more common than SEGAs, a partially calcified enhancing lesion at the foramen of Monro > 5 mm is more likely to be a SEGA than an SEN.

Other lateral ventricle masses that should be included in the differential diagnosis are **subependymoma** (a tumor of middle-aged and elderly patients) and **central neurocytoma** (a "bubbly" tumor that arises in the lateral ventricle body). Low-grade **diffusely infiltrating astrocytoma** can arise in the septi pellucidi or fornices, but these tumors typically neither calcify nor enhance.

Pleomorphic Xanthoastrocytoma

Terminology

Pleomorphic xanthoastrocytoma (PXA) is a rare astrocytic glioma occurring mostly in children and young adults.

Etiology

PXAs lack IDH and H3 histone mutations. Between 1/3 and 1/2 have *BRAF* V600E point mutations, a feature they share with pilocytic astrocytoma and ganglioglioma. Other reported mutations are *FANCA/D1/I/M*, *PRKDC*, *NF1*, and *NOTCH2* somatic gene mutations. Copy number variations of

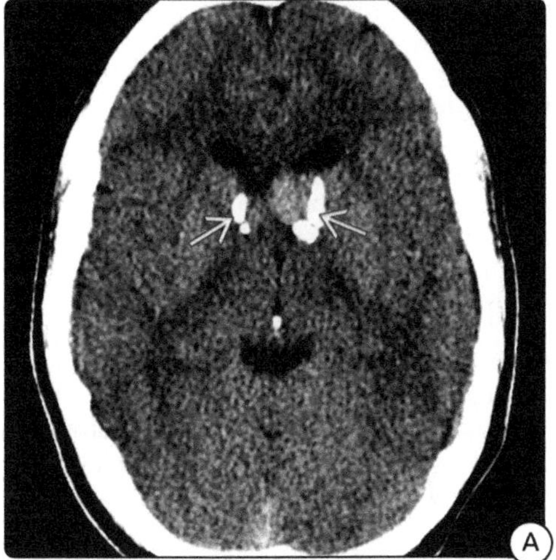

***(17-12A)** NECT in child with TSC shows hyperdense calcified masses in the frontal horns of both lateral ventricles ➡.*

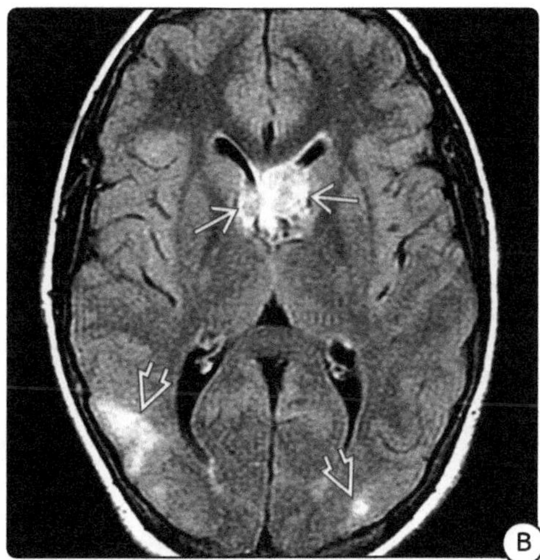

***(17-12B)** FLAIR MR in the same patient shows that the masses ➡ are heterogeneously hyperintense. Note the cortical tubers ➡.*

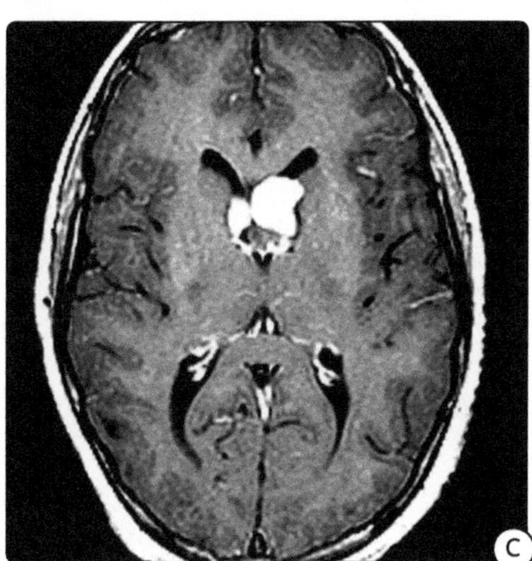

***(17-12C)** T1 C+ MR shows intense enhancement of the masses. These are subependymal giant cell astrocytomas in TSC.*

CDKN2A/B are more frequent than in glioblastoma. *PTEN* and *EGFR* mutations are absent.

Pathology

Location. Over 95% of PXAs are supratentorial hemispheric masses. Most are superficial, cortically based, seizure-associated neoplasms. The temporal lobe is the most common site (40-50%), and involvement of the adjacent leptomeninges is common. Most are small, solitary lesions ≤ 3 cm.

Gross Pathology. PXAs are relatively discrete, partially cystic masses with a mural nodule that abuts or is attached to the leptomeninges **(17-13)**. Deep tumor margins may be indistinct with focal parenchymal infiltration into the adjacent subcortical white matter.

PXAs are WHO grade II tumors. PXAs that display anaplastic features, including higher cellularity and increased mitoses, are designated WHO grade III tumors **(17-15)**.

Clinical Issues

Epidemiology. PXA is a rare tumor, accounting for slightly < 1% of all astrocytomas. Mean age at diagnosis is 22 years.

Presentation and Natural History. Because of its characteristic superficial cortically based location, the most common presentation is longstanding epilepsy. Recurrence following gross total resection is uncommon. Overall 5-year survival is ~ 80%, and the 10-year survival rate is 70%.

Imaging

CT Findings. NECT scans show a well-delineated, peripheral, cortically based "cyst + nodule" that contacts the leptomeninges. Calcifications are present in 40% of cases, but gross intratumoral hemorrhage is rare. The overlying skull may be thinned and remodeled on bone CT. The mural nodule of a PXA shows moderate to intense enhancement on CECT.

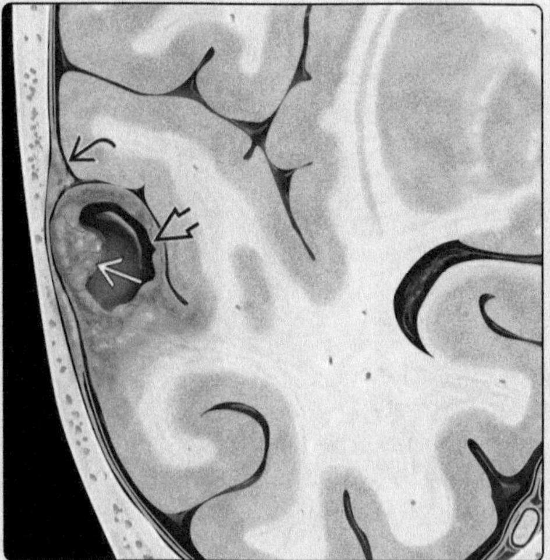

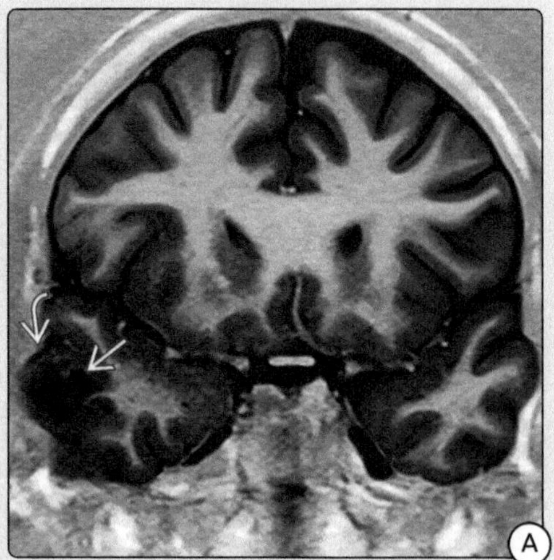

***(17-13)** Coronal graphic depicts pleomorphic xanthoastrocytoma with a cyst ➩, a nodule abutting the pial surface ➡, and reactive thickening of the adjacent dura-arachnoid ➩. **(17-14A)** Coronal inversion recovery scan in a 19-year-old man with longstanding temporal lobe epilepsy shows a partially cystic right temporal lobe mass ➡ that remodels the adjacent calvarium ➩.*

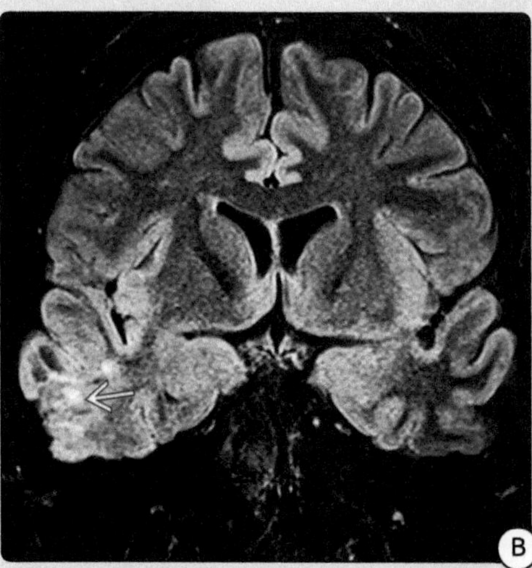

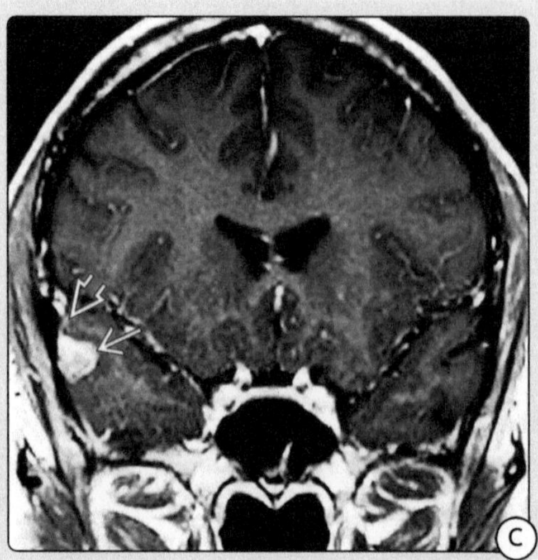

***(17-14B)** Coronal FLAIR MR shows that the lesion is heterogeneously hyperintense ➡. **(17-14C)** Coronal T1 C+ MR demonstrates an enhancing nodule ➡ that abuts the dura, causing minimal thickening and enhancement ➩. WHO grade II pleomorphic xanthoastrocytoma was removed at surgery.*

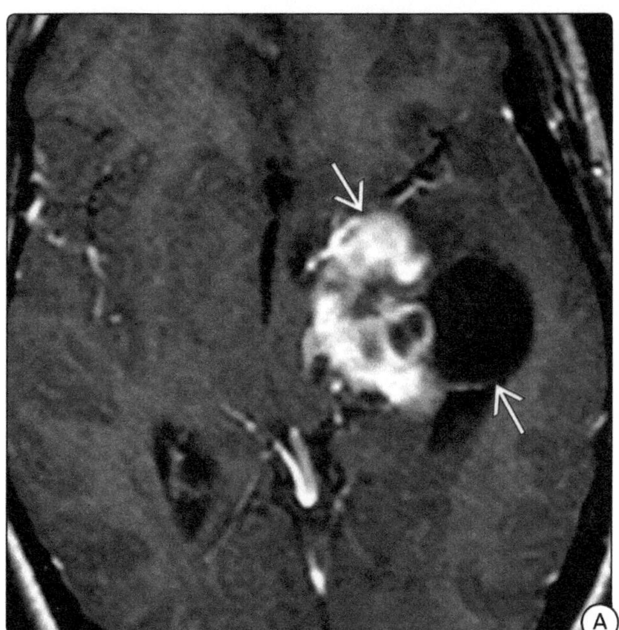

***(17-15A)** T1 C+ FS MR in a 27-year-old woman with seizures shows a mixed solid, cystic mass in the left medial temporal lobe ➡. Histopathology disclosed PXA with anaplastic features.*

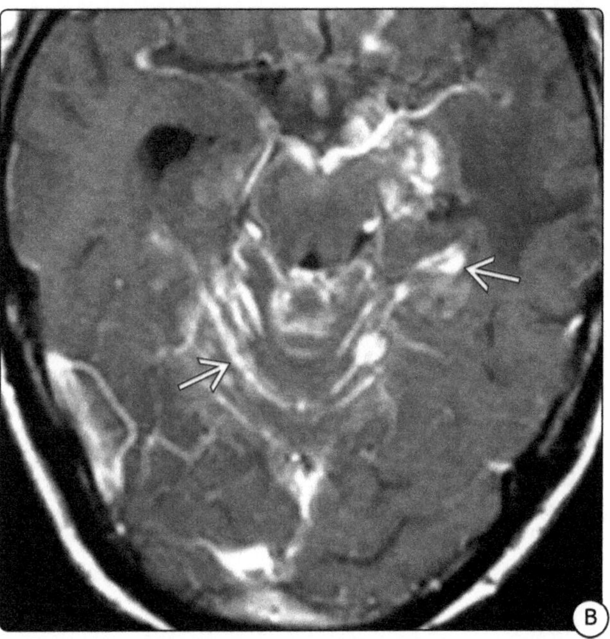

***(17-15B)** The patient was lost to follow-up but returned 18 months later with severe headaches, multiple cranial nerve palsies. T1 C+ MR shows diffuse CSF metastases ➡. She expired 2 years after initial diagnosis. This was PXA, WHO grade III.*

MR Findings. The solid component of a PXA is heterogeneously hypo- or isointense relative to cortex on T1WI **(17-14A)**. Over 90% of the tumor nodules demonstrate heterogeneous hyperintensity on T2WI and FLAIR. The cystic portions of PXA are usually hyperintense relative to CSF **(17-14B)**.

Moderate enhancement of the tumor nodule is typical following contrast administration **(17-14C)**. Over 90% of PXAs abut the pia and may incite reactive thickening of the adjacent dura. A "dural tail" sign was seen in 15-50% of cases in reported series.

Differential Diagnosis

The major differential diagnosis of PXA is **ganglioglioma**, another cortically based tumor that often causes epilepsy. Other less common tumors with a "cyst + nodule" appearance can mimic PXA, including hemispheric **pilocytic astrocytoma. Dysembryoplastic neuroepithelial tumor (DNET)** has a similar presentation and age range but typically has a multicystic "bubbly" appearance.

Diffuse (low-grade) fibrillary astrocytoma usually involves the white matter and does not involve the meninges. **Oligodendroglioma** can present as a slow-growing cortical-white matter junction lesion that remodels the adjacent calvarium, but the "cyst + nodule" pattern is usually absent.

CORTICALLY BASED TUMORS WITH "CYST + NODULE"

Common
- Ganglioglioma
- Metastasis

Less Common
- Pilocytic astrocytoma
- Pleomorphic xanthoastrocytoma
- Glioblastoma multiforme

Rare
- Hemangioblastoma
- Desmoplastic infantile astrocytoma/ganglioglioma
- Papillary glioneuronal tumor
- Schwannoma

Anaplastic Pleomorphic Xanthoastrocytoma

A PXA that has anaplastic features (> 5 mitoses per 10 HPFs) is classified as anaplastic pleomorphic xanthoastrocytoma (aPXA), WHO grade III.

Few aPXAs with imaging findings have been reported. Large, more heterogeneous-appearing masses are typical. As leptomeningeal spread is common with these more aggressive tumors, complete craniospinal imaging should be obtained either at the time of diagnosis or on short interval follow-up **(17-15)**.

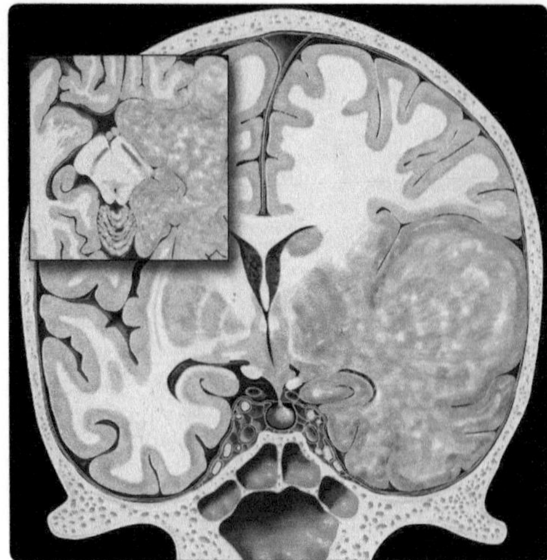

(17-16) Diffusely infiltrating astrocytoma (WHO grade II) is shown expanding the temporal lobe, infiltrating cortex/subcortical WM.

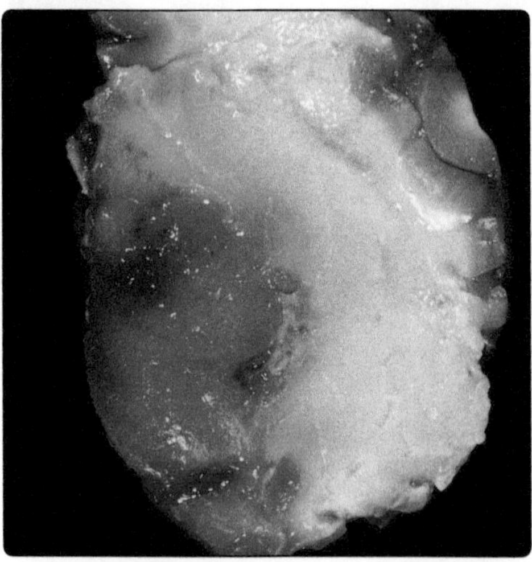

(17-17) Grade II diffuse astrocytoma infiltrates cortex, subcortical WM; no clear border between normal, abnormal brain. (R. Hewlett, MD.)

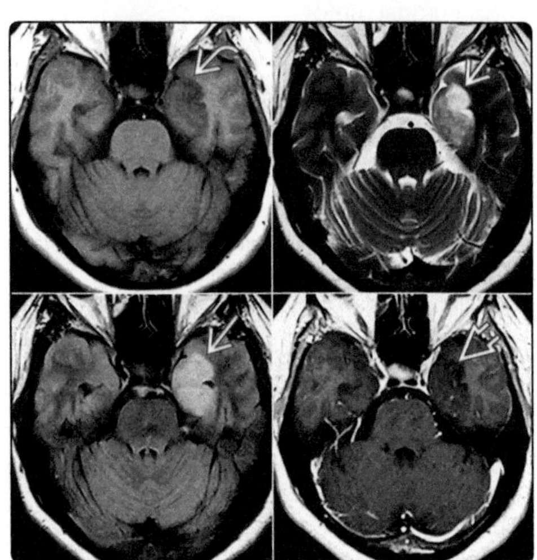

(17-18) 27yF with seizures shows T1-hypo ➡ T2/FLAIR-hyperintense ➡ nonenhancing ➡ mass. IDH(+) diffuse astrocytoma, WHO grade II.

Diffuse Astrocytomas

WHO grade II diffuse astrocytomas, WHO grade III anaplastic astrocytomas, and WHO grade IV glioblastomas are each divided into two subtypes depending on the presence or absence of IDH1/2 mutation.

We begin the section with a discussion of IDH-mutant [IDH(+)] astrocytomas. **IDH-mutant** [IDH(+)] tumors account for ~ 90% of grade II and III astrocytomas but only 5-10% of grade IV lesions. We then follow with **IDH-wild-type** [IDH(-)] astrocytomas.

We conclude this chapter with a discussion of pediatric brainstem tumors and the newly recognized, highly malignant **diffuse midline glioma, H3 K27M-mutant.**

Diffuse Astrocytoma, IDH-Mutant [IDH(+)]

Terminology

Diffuse astrocytoma, IDH-mutant [IDH(+) DA] is a diffusely infiltrating astrocytoma with a mutation in either the *IDH1* or *IDH2* gene that corresponds histologically to WHO grade II.

Etiology

In addition to *IDH1* mutation, IDH(+) DAs also typically harbor other "class-defining" mutations. These include loss of *ATRX* nuclear expression &/or *TP53* mutation. If tested, 1p/19q codeletion is absent.

Pathology

Location. Although IDH-mutant DAs can arise anywhere, the cerebral hemispheres are the most common overall site **(17-16)** with a preferential location in the frontal lobes. Almost 20% involve the deep gray nuclei.

Gross Pathology. Diffuse astrocytomas are infiltrating lesions with ill-defined borders. Enlargement and distortion of invaded structures are typical. Gray-white matter interfaces are blurred **(17-17)**. Occasional cysts and calcification may be present. Hemorrhage is rare. IDH-mutant DAs are WHO grade II neoplasms.

Clinical Issues

Epidemiology. DAs (the vast majority of which are IDH-mutant) account for between 10% and 15% of astrocytomas in adults.

Presentation. Mean age at presentation is mid-30s (range: 20-50 years). Symptoms are location dependent. Seizure is the most common presentation of hemispheric lesions.

Natural History. IDH(+) DAs grow slowly but have an intrinsic tendency for malignant progression to IDH-mutant anaplastic astrocytoma [IDH(+) AA] and (eventually) IDH-mutant glioblastoma [IDH(+) GBM]. Recurrence following surgical resection is common. Mean survival is nearly 11 years, almost identical with IDH-mutant AAs.

Imaging

CT Findings. NECT shows a hypodense, relatively homogeneous mass **(17-19A)**. Calcification is seen in 20% of cases. Gross cystic change and hemorrhage are rare. CECT shows no enhancement.

MR Findings. Most IDH-mutant DAs are frontal or temporal lobe predominant and tend to infiltrate the white matter with relative sparing of the overlying cortex. Moderate mass effect with adjacent gyral expansion is common.

DAs are typically hypointense on T1WI and hyperintense on T2/FLAIR **(17-18)**. Although diffusely infiltrating astrocytomas often appear relatively well-circumscribed on MR **(17-19B)**, neoplastic cells infiltrate adjacent normal-appearing brain.

T2* scans may show "blooming" foci if calcification is present. IDH-mutant DAs rarely enhance following contrast administration **(17-19C)** and do not restrict on DWI.

MRS shows elevated choline, low NAA, and a high mI:Cr ratio. 3T MRS may exhibit an elevated 2-hydroxyglutarate (2-HG) peak resonating at 2.25 ppm. Dynamic contrast-enhanced (DCE) MR perfusion shows relatively low rCBV. Foci of increased rCBV may represent areas of early malignant degeneration.

Differential Diagnosis

The definitive diagnosis of IDH-mutant DA requires histologic confirmation and molecular profiling. The major *imaging* differential diagnoses are other astrocytomas and oligodendroglioma.

IDH-mutant anaplastic astrocytoma, a WHO grade III neoplasm, is indistinguishable from grade II DA on the basis of imaging findings. **Oligodendroglioma** is generally cortically based, more often calcifies, and frequently has enhancing foci.

Nonneoplastic masses that can mimic IDH-mutant DA include acute stroke and encephalitis. **Acute cerebral ischemia-infarction** typically involves both cortex and subcortical white matter and occurs in specific vascular distribution. **Encephalitis** with T2/FLAIR hyperintensity shows enhancement on T1 C+. *Both acute strokes and encephalitis typically exhibit restricted diffusion on DWI sequences.*

IDH-MUTANT [IDH(+)] DIFFUSE ASTROCYTOMAS

Terminology
- Formerly known as low-grade astrocytoma

Etiology
- Molecular genetics
  - *IDH1/2* mutated
  - *ATRX* nuclear loss
  - *TP53* mutated
  - 1p/19q intact (not codeleted)

Pathology
- Supratentorial (frontal lobe most common)
- Infiltrating, ill-defined borders
- WHO grade II
- Inherent tendency to undergo malignant degeneration

Clinical Issues
- 10-15% of astrocytomas
- Age = 20-45 years (mean = 38 years)
- Overall survival = 11 years
  - Not significantly different from IDH(+) anaplastic astrocytoma

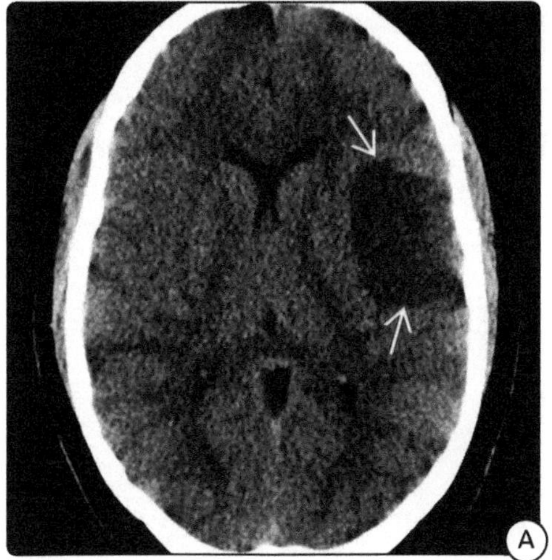

***(17-19A)** Emergent NECT for "stroke" shows a hypodense L temporal lobe mass ➡. CTA (not shown) was normal.*

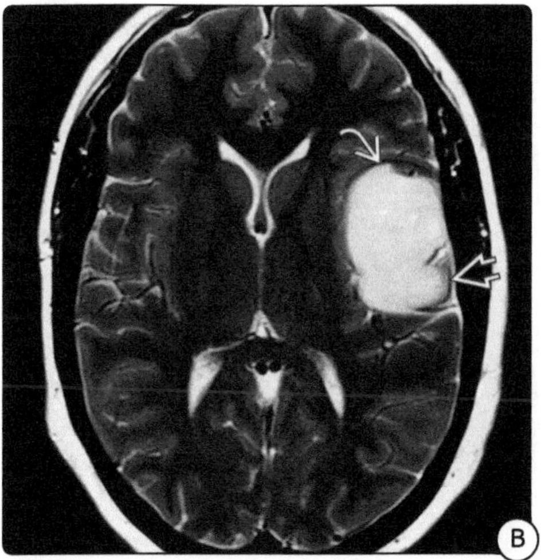

***(17-19B)** T2 MR shows the hyperintense, well-demarcated mass ➡. A thin, compressed layer of cortex ➡ overlies the mass.*

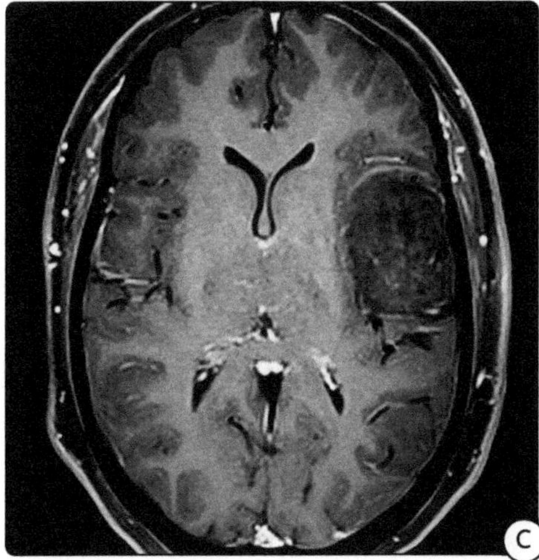

***(17-19C)** T1 C+ FS MR shows no enhancement. This is WHO grade II astrocytoma, IDH-mutated, both p53 and PTEN positive.*

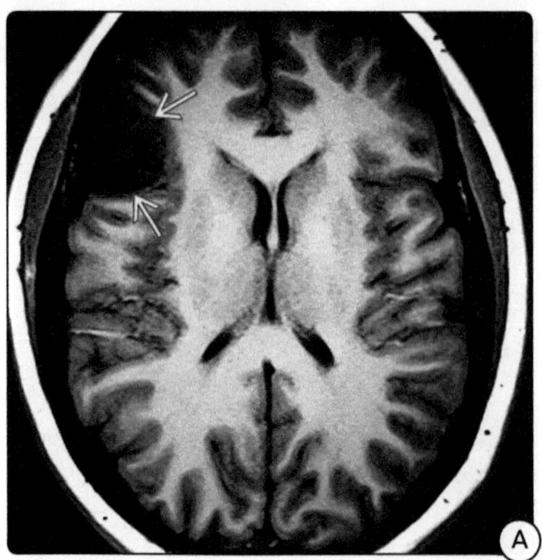

(17-20A) T1 MR in a 45-year-old woman with seizure shows well-delineated hypointense mass in right frontal lobe cortex, subcortical WM ➡.

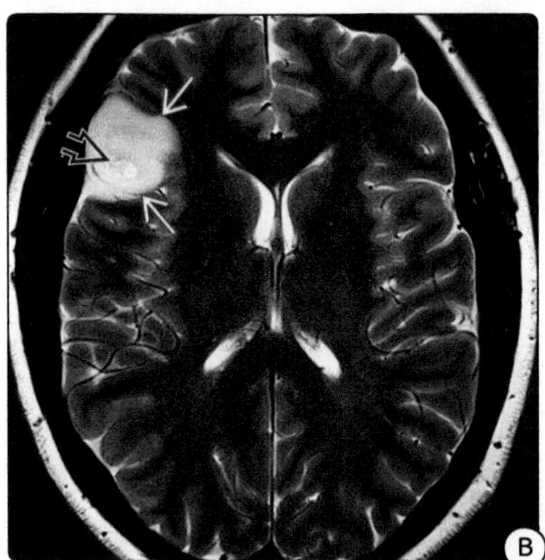

(17-20B) The mass appears hyperintense ➡, relatively well circumscribed. Note small central focus of heterogeneous signal intensity ⇨.

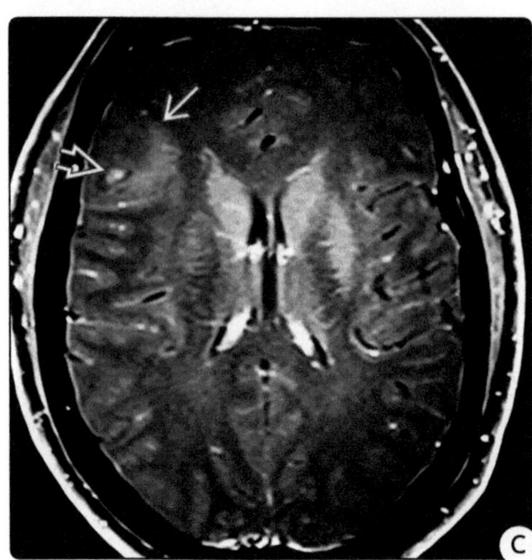

(17-20C) T1 C+ FS MR shows enhancement ⇨ in center of mass ➡. WHO grade III IDH-mutated AA was resected. Patient is alive 3 years later.

IMAGING OF IDH-MUTANT DIFFUSE ASTROCYTOMAS

Imaging Features

- Hypodense on NECT
- No enhancement on CECT
- Hypointense on T1, hyperintense on T2/FLAIR
- No enhancement, hemorrhage
- MRS shows 2-HG peak at 2.25 ppm
- Low rCBV
    - Foci of ↑ rCBV suspicious for malignant degeneration

Differential Diagnosis

- IDH-mutant anaplastic astrocytoma
- Pilocytic astrocytoma
- Oligodendroglioma
- Nonneoplastic
    - Acute cerebral ischemia-infarction
    - Encephalitis

Anaplastic Astrocytoma, IDH-Mutant

Terminology

Anaplastic astrocytoma, IDH-mutant [**IDH(+) AA**] is a diffusely infiltrating astrocytoma with anaplasia, significant proliferative activity, and a mutation in either the *IDH1* or *IDH2* gene.

Etiology

IDH(+) AAs rarely arise de novo and typically originate as IDH(+) diffuse astrocytomas (WHO grade II). IDH(+) DA/AAs exhibit an inherent tendency for malignant progression to IDH(+) glioblastoma (WHO grade IV).

The basic molecular features of IDH(+) AAs are similar to those of IDH(+) DAs. IDH(+) tumors do not change their IDH status with malignant degeneration. *TP53* mutation and *ATRX* loss are present in the majority of IDH(+) AAs. 1p/19q are not codeleted.

Pathology

Gross expansion of the affected brain without frank tissue destruction is typical. The adjacent gyri are enlarged, and tumor often extends into the basal ganglia. Cysts and intratumoral hemorrhage are rare.

The principal histopathologic features of IDH-mutant AA are those of a diffusely infiltrating astrocytoma that has increased mitotic activity. Proliferation indices are usually in the 5-10% range. IDH(+) AA corresponds histologically to WHO grade III.

Clinical Issues

The symptoms, mean age at diagnosis, and length of progression-free survival are similar to those of IDH(+) diffuse astrocytomas, WHO grade II.

Imaging

Imaging features and differential diagnosis of WHO grade III IDH(+) AAs are similar to—and generally indistinguishable from—those of WHO grade II IDH(+) diffuse astrocytomas.

CT Findings. IDH(+) AAs are ill-defined low-density lesions on NECT. The majority do not enhance on CECT. When present, enhancement is usually focal, patchy, poorly delineated, and heterogeneous.

MR Findings. Most IDH(+) AAs are hypointense on T1WI **(17-20A)** and hyperintense on T2/FLAIR **(17-20B)**. The margins may appear grossly discrete, but tumor cells invariably infiltrate adjacent brain. Hemorrhage and calcification are uncommon, so T2* "blooming" is typically absent.

Contrast enhancement varies from none to moderate. Between 50-70% show some degree of enhancement. Focal **(17-20C)**, nodular, homogeneous, patchy, or even ring-enhancing patterns may be seen.

IDH(+) AAs generally do not restrict on DWI. MRS shows elevated choline, decreased NAA, and a 2-HG peak at 2.25 ppm. DTI can be helpful in delineating early WM tract invasion. Perfusion MR shows increased rCBV in the most malignant parts of the tumor. Color choline maps are helpful in guiding stereotactic biopsy, improving diagnostic accuracy with decreased sampling error.

Differential Diagnosis

The major differential diagnosis of IDH(+) AA (WHO grade III) is **IDH(+) diffuse astrocytoma** (WHO grade II). The two may be indistinguishable on imaging studies, although recent studies show that contrast enhancement in IDH(+) lower grade gliomas is associated with decreased overall survival.

IDH-MUTANT ANAPLASTIC ASTROCYTOMA

Etiology
- Begins as IDH(+) diffuse astrocytoma, WHO grade II
- Undergoes malignant degeneration to anaplastic astrocytoma
  - Maintains IDH(+) status (IDH status does not change)

Pathology
- WHO grade III
  - IDH(+), *ATRX* loss
- Hypercellular
- Anaplasia
- Increased mitoses
- Lacks necrosis, microvascular proliferation

Clinical Issues
- Overall survival not statistically different from IDH(+) diffuse astrocytoma (DA)

Imaging
- Similar to IDH(+) DA
- Contrast-enhancing foci variable, associated with ↓ overall survival
- Areas of ↑ rCBV may represent malignant degeneration

Glioblastoma, IDH-Mutant

Terminology

IDH-mutant GBMs [**IDH(+) GBMs**] are also called **"secondary GBMs."**

Etiology

IDH(+) GBMs almost always develop from malignant degeneration of lower grade IDH(+) astrocytic tumors. IDH mutation persists throughout the progression from diffuse and anaplastic astrocytoma to GBM. *TP53* mutations and *ATRX* loss are common, but *EGFR* amplification is absent. Methylation profiles resemble those of IDH(+) DA/AA.

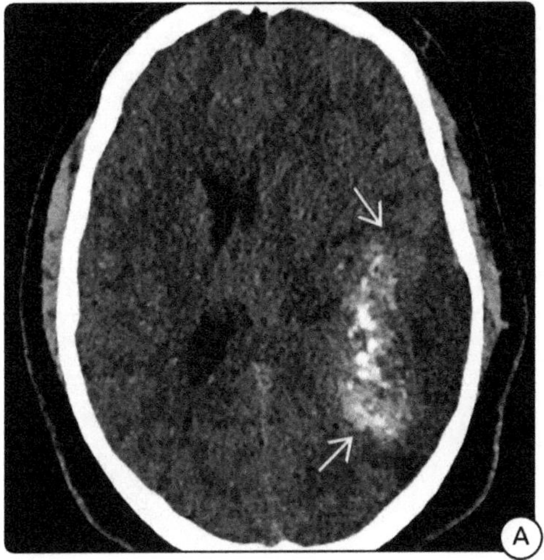

***(17-21A)** NECT scan in a 26-year-old man shows a partially calcified mixed-density mass ➡ in the left temporoparietal region.*

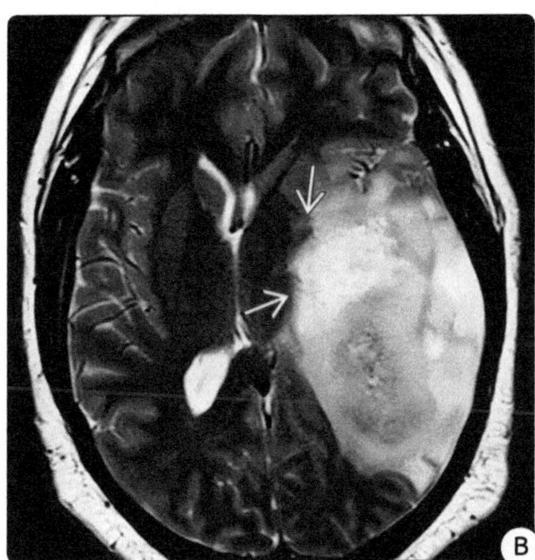

***(17-21B)** T2 MR shows the mass involves virtually all of the temporal and parietal lobes, extending medially into the basal ganglia and thalamus ➡.*

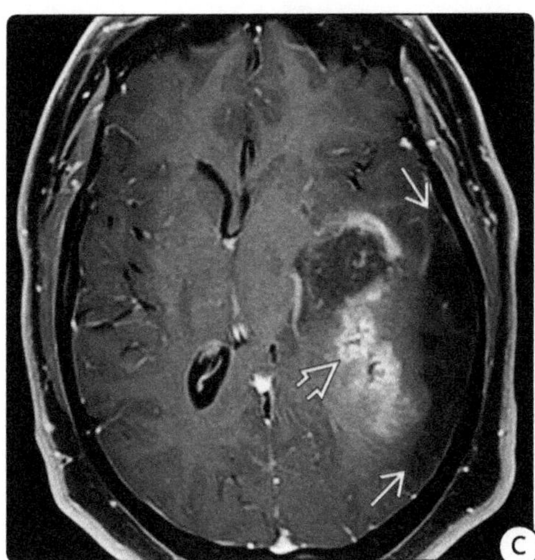

***(17-21C)** T1 C+ FS shows patchy enhancement ➡ but majority of mass is nonenhancing ➡. IDH(+) GBM arising from lower grade astrocytoma.*

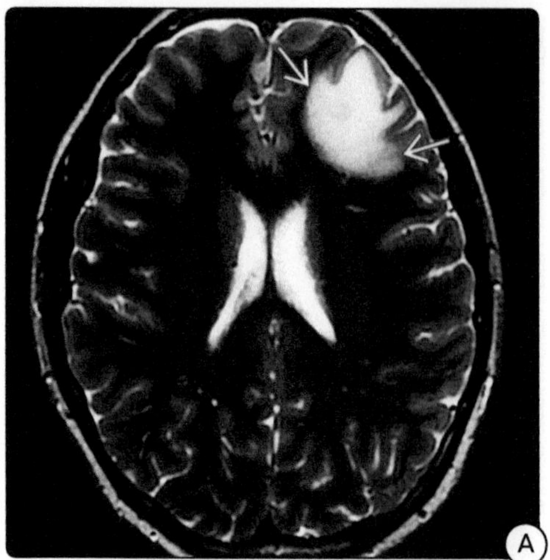
(17-22A) T2 MR in a 15-year-old girl shows a hyperintense mass ➡ predominately involving the subcortical and deep WM.

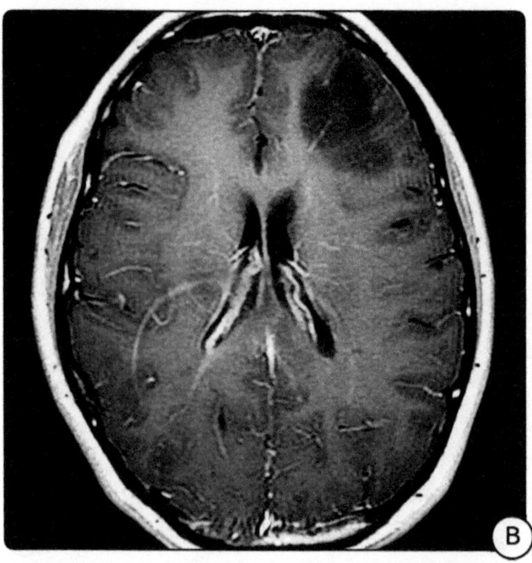
(17-22B) T1 C+ FS MR shows no enhancement. Surgery disclosed IDH(-) AA, WHO grades II/III.

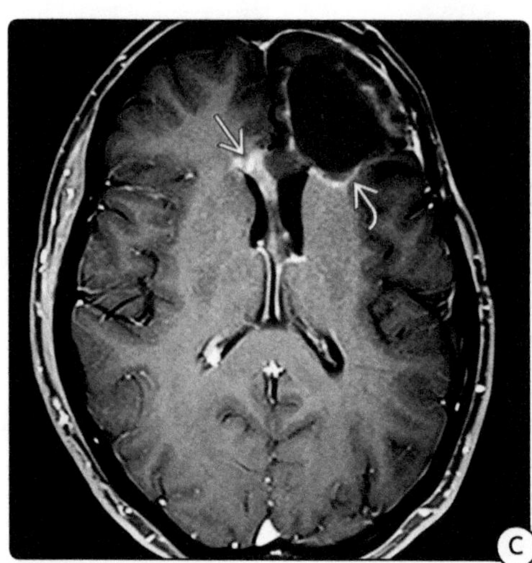
(17-22C) MR 3 years later shows nodular enhancement around resection site ➡, corpus callosum ➡. Reoperation disclosed IDH(-) GBM.

Pathology

IDH(+) GBMs have a strong predilection for the frontal lobe, similar to the preferential localization of WHO grade II diffuse astrocytomas. IDH-mutant GBMs diffusely infiltrate the brain but hemorrhage, and the large regions of central necrosis that are so characteristic of IDH-wild-type GBMs are usually absent.

With some exceptions, histologic features of IDH-mutant GBMs resemble those of IDH-wild-type tumors. IDH(+) GBMs correspond histologically to WHO grade IV.

Clinical Issues

IDH(+) GBM is much less common than IDH(-) GBM, accounting for only 5-10% of all cases. IDH(+) GBMs arise at a significantly younger age (mean = 45 years) and have a better prognosis compared with their IDH-wild-type counterparts. Mean overall survival is 2-3 years.

Imaging

IDH(+) GBMs show a distinct (but not exclusive) predilection for the frontal lobes **(17-21)**. Significant nonenhancing areas are often present and the classic thick tumor rind surrounding a large central necrotic core that characterizes IDH-wild-type GBMs (see below) is generally absent. Exceptions are common, so molecular profiling is still necessary to establish the definitive diagnosis.

GLIOBLASTOMA, IDH-MUTANT [IDH(+) GBM]

Terminology, Etiology
- Also called "secondary" GBM
- Malignant degeneration of lower grade IDH(+) neoplasm
- IDH1 mutated [IDH(+)], *TP53* mutated, *ATRX* loss

Pathology
- WHO grade IV

Clinical
- 5-10% of GBMs
- Younger age than IDH(-) GBMs (mean = 45 years)
- Better survival (2-3 years vs. < 1 year)

Imaging
- Frontal lobe predominance
- Often significant nonenhancing areas
- MRS may show 2-HB peak at 2.25 ppm

Diffuse and Anaplastic Astrocytomas, IDH-Wild-Type

Terminology

IDH-wild-type diffuse astrocytomas [IDH(-) DAs] and anaplastic astrocytomas [IDH(-) AAs] are diffusely infiltrating astrocytomas without *IDH* gene mutations.

Etiology

IDH(-) DAs and AAs arise from a line of glioma progenitor cells that is genetically distinct from the IDH(+) line. More than 75% carry mutations similar to those of IDH(-) GBMs.

If standard immunohistochemistry of a diffuse astrocytoma is *IDH1* negative, next-generation sequencing is recommended to detect a "noncanonical" *IDH1* mutation (~ 5% of cases) or any *IDH2* mutation.

Pathology

Microscopically, IDH(-) DAs and AAs appear to be WHO grade II or III neoplasms. Most have an identical gross/microscopic and imaging appearance to their IDH(+) counterparts, i.e., they lack the histologically defining features of glioblastoma, such as microvascular proliferation &/or necrosis.

The cIMPACT-NOW interim updates provide that if certain molecular criteria are present (see box below), these tumors correspond to WHO grade IV biological behavior **(17-22)** and can be referred to as **"diffuse astrocytic glioma, IDH-wild-type, with molecular features of glioblastoma, WHO grade IV."**

DIFFUSE/ANAPLASTIC ASTROCYTIC GLIOMAS, IDH-WILD-TYPE

If any/all of the following 3 molecular criteria are present
- *EGFR* amplification &/or
- Whole chromosome gain and whole chromosome 10 loss (+7/-10) &/or
- *TERT* promoter mutation

These correspond to WHO grade IV behavior; can be designated as "molecular glioblastoma" for treatment stratification, clinical trials.

Clinical Issues

Grade for grade, IDH-wild-type astrocytomas generally carry a worse prognosis than their IDH-mutated counterparts. With many IDH(-) DA/AAs, histologic WHO grade does not correlate well with biologic behavior. If features of "molecular GBM" are present, malignant degeneration to frank GBM may occur relatively rapidly.

Imaging

Standard imaging findings and differential diagnosis are similar to those of IDH-mutant DA. An infiltrating expansile mass that predominantly involves the hemispheric white matter is typical **(17-22)** **(17-23)**. MRS shows absence of a 2-HG peak.

In the past, some diffusely infiltrating gliomas with a unique pattern of widespread brain invasion were designated as **gliomatosis cerebri** (GC). By definition, ≥ 3 lobes with frequent bihemispheric, basal ganglionic, &/or infratentorial extension were involved.

Although IDH-mutant tumors occasionally exhibit this widespread infiltrative pattern, the majority of adult tumors that would once have been designated as GCs are IDH-wild-type AAs or GBM **(17-33A)**. GC does not represent a distinct molecular entity and is no longer considered a separate diagnosis.

Glioblastoma, IDH-Wild-Type

IDH-wild-type glioblastoma (GBM) is the most common and most malignant of all astrocytomas, accounting for > 95% of GBMs.

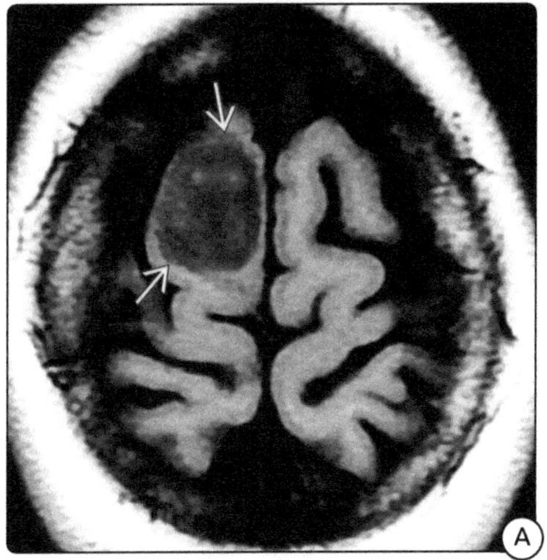

***(17-23A)** Axial T1 MR in a 24-year-old woman with seizures shows a hypodense mass in the right frontal lobe ➡.*

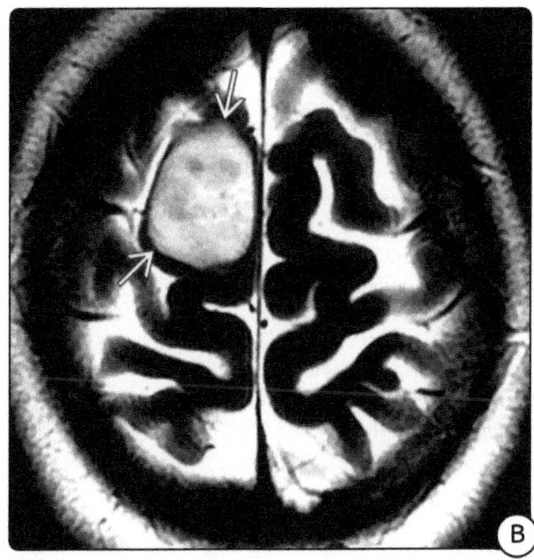

***(17-23B)** T2 MR in the same case shows that the mass is heterogeneously hyperintense with sharply delineated borders ➡.*

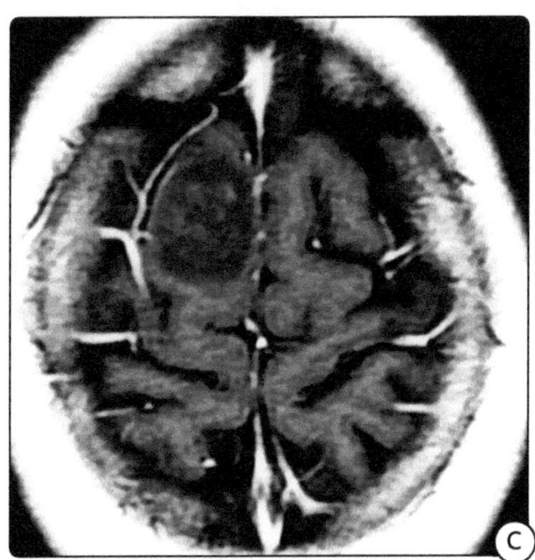

***(17-23C)** T1 C+ shows no enhancement. Resected mass is IDH(-) WHO grade II diffuse astrocytoma. Tumor recurred 4 years later as GBM.*

Terminology

IDH-wild-type GBM is sometimes called **"IDH-wild-type primary glioblastoma"** to distinguish it from IDH-mutant GBMs, which arise from lower grade IDH-mutant astrocytomas.

Etiology

IDH-wild-type GBMs are putative de novo lesions with no recognizable lower grade precursor tumor. Recent studies show that characteristic driver mutations are acquired by losses or gains of parts of chromosomes. Chromosome 7 gain, 9p loss, or 10 loss are tumor-initiating events that occur several years before diagnosis. *TERT* promoter mutations often follow later as a prerequisite for rapid growth.

Three inherited cancer syndromes—namely **neurofibromatosis type 1** (NF1), **Li-Fraumeni**, and **Turcot syndrome**—demonstrate an enhanced propensity to develop IDH-wild-type GBMs.

Pathology

Location. In contrast to IDH-mutant GBMs, IDH-wild-type GBMs are distributed throughout the cerebral hemispheres. They preferentially involve the subcortical and deep periventricular white matter, easily spreading across compact tracts, such as the corpus callosum and corticospinal tracts. Symmetric involvement of the corpus callosum is common, the so-called "butterfly glioma" pattern **(17-26)**.

Size and Number. IDH-wild-type GBMs vary widely in size. Because they spread quickly and extensively along compact white matter tracts, up to 20% appear as multifocal lesions at the time of initial diagnosis. Between 2-5% of multifocal GBMs are true synchronous, independently developing tumors.

__(17-24)__ Autopsy specimen shows classic primary glioblastoma multiforme with hemorrhage and viable "rind" of tumor ➡ surrounding a necrotic core. (Courtesy R. Hewlett, MD.) __(17-25)__ Axial T1 C+ FS MR shows thick, irregular enhancing "rind" of tumor surrounding the necrotic center. This is classic IDH-negative GBM.

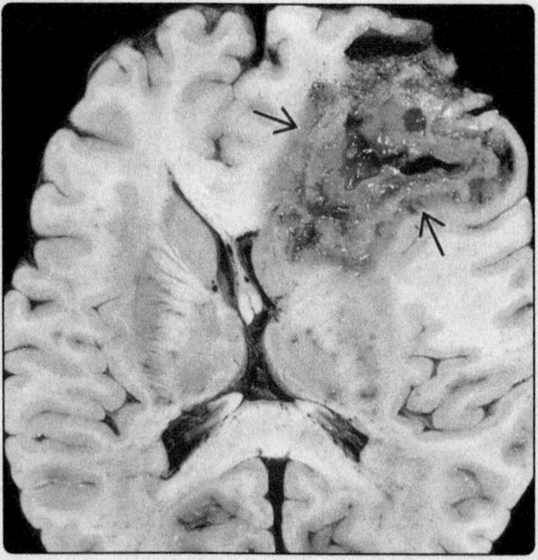

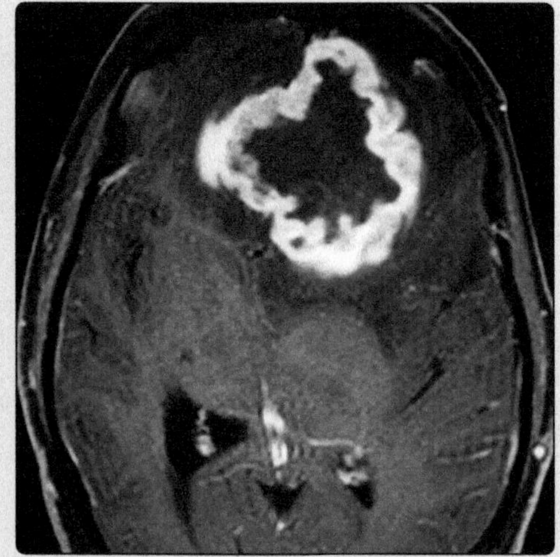

__(17-26)__ Autopsy specimen shows "butterfly" glioblastoma multiforme ➡ crossing the corpus callosum genu, extending into and enlarging the fornix ⇨. (Courtesy R. Hewlett, MD.) __(17-27)__ T1 C+ FS MR shows classic "butterfly" IDH(-) GBM spreading across the corpus callosum. Note the solid rim enhancement around the necrotic center.

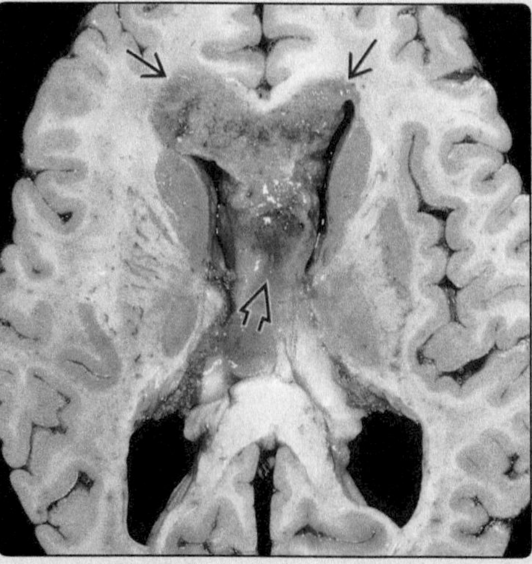

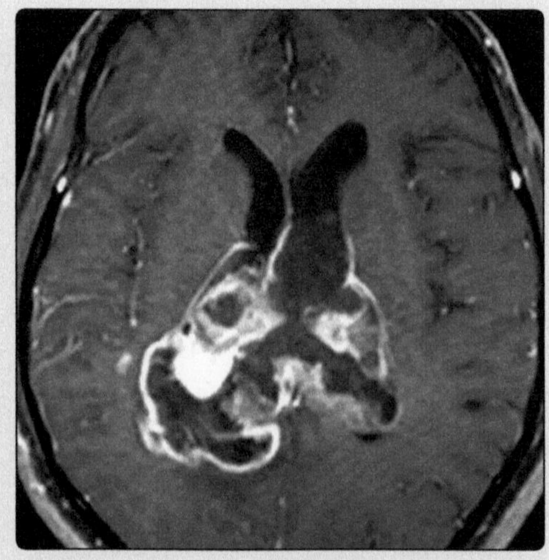

Gross Pathology. The most frequent appearance is a reddish-gray tumor "rind" surrounding a central necrotic core **(17-24)**. Mass effect and peritumoral edema are marked and intratumoral hemorrhage is common.

Microscopic Features. Necrosis and microvascular proliferation are the histologic hallmarks of GBMs that distinguish them from anaplastic astrocytomas. GBMs generally have a high proliferation index (MIB-1), almost always > 10%.

GBMs are WHO grade IV neoplasms.

Clinical Issues

Demographics. GBM is the most common malignant brain tumor in adults, representing between 12% and 15% of all intracranial neoplasms and 60-75% of astrocytomas.

GBMs can occur at any age (including in neonates and infants), but peak age is 55-85 years. IDH(-) GBMs tend to occur in older adults (peaking between 60 and 75 years) whereas IDH(+) GBMs occur a decade or two earlier.

Presentation. Seizure, focal neurologic deficits, and mental status changes are the most common symptoms. Headache from elevated intracranial pressure is also common. Approximately 2% of GBMs present with sudden stroke-like onset caused by acute intratumoral hemorrhage.

Natural History. Mean survival in patients with IDH(-) GBM is under 1 year from symptom onset. **MGMT promoter methylation** ("methylated" tumor) is a strong predictor for a positive response to alkylating agents and correlates with longer term survival.

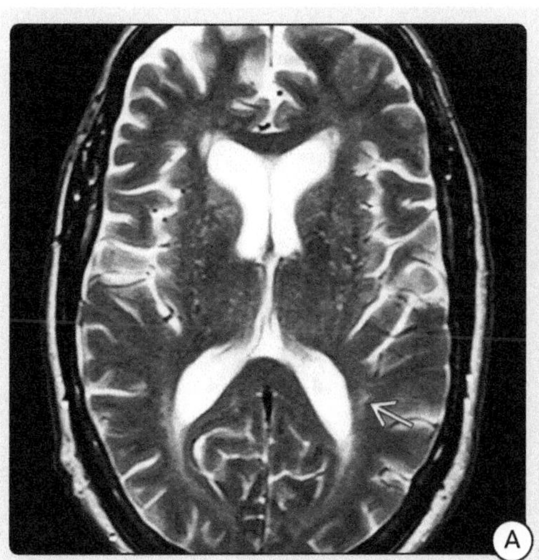

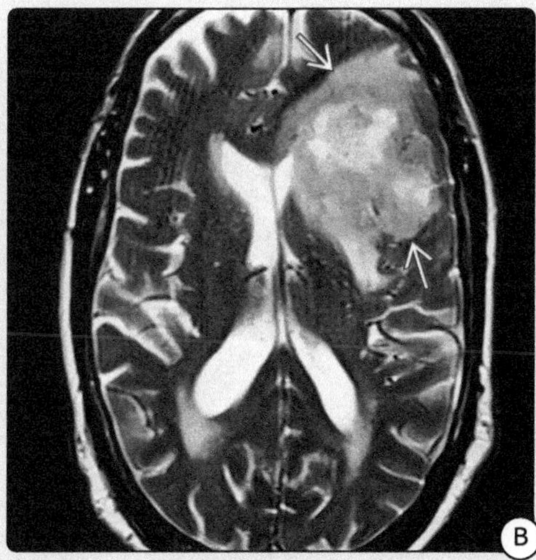

***(17-28A)** Axial T2 MR in a 69-year-old man with headaches, normal neurologic examination shows some prominent perivascular spaces and a few scattered white matter hyperintensities ➡, but the MR is otherwise normal. **(17-28B)** 2 years later, the patient developed left-sided weakness. T2 MR shows interval appearance of an inhomogeneously hyperintense left frontal mass ➡.*

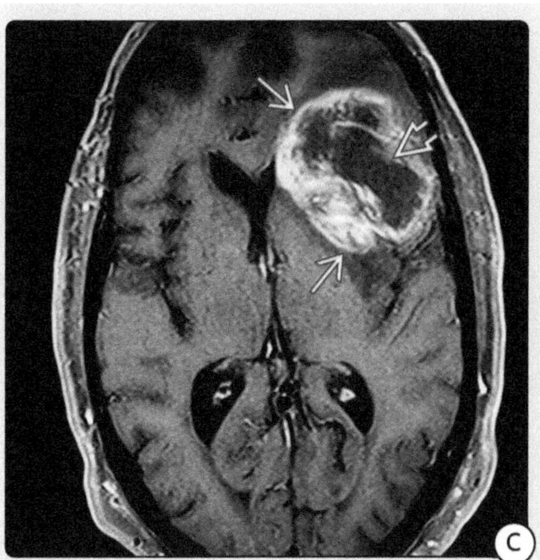

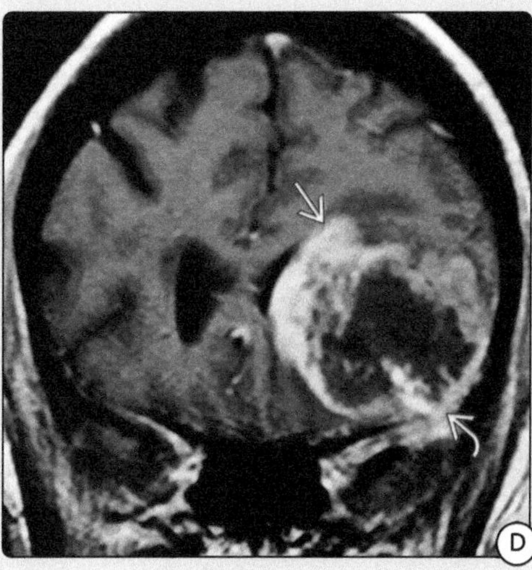

***(17-28C)** T1 C+ FS MR shows a thick, irregular rind of contrast enhancement ➡ surrounding a nonenhancing necrotic center ➡. **(17-28D)** Coronal T1 C+ MR shows the rim-enhancing mass ➡. Note erosion into/through the skull, dura ➡. This is IDH(-) GBM, WHO grade IV, and the patient expired 8 months later.*

Imaging

CT Findings. Most IDH(-) GBMs demonstrate a hypodense central mass surrounded by an iso- to moderately hyperdense rim on NECT. Hemorrhage is common, but calcification is rare. Marked mass effect and significant hypodense peritumoral edema are typical ancillary findings.

CECT shows strong but heterogeneous irregular rim enhancement. Prominent vessels in highly vascular GBMs are seen as linear enhancing foci adjacent to the mass.

MR Findings. T1WI shows a poorly marginated mass with mixed signal intensity. Subacute hemorrhage is common. T2/FLAIR shows heterogeneous hyperintensity with indistinct tumor margins and extensive vasogenic edema **(17-28)**. Necrosis, cysts, hemorrhage at various stages of evolution, fluid/debris levels, and "flow voids" from extensive neovascularity may be seen. T2* imaging often shows foci of susceptibility artifact.

T1 C+ shows strong but irregular ring enhancement surrounding a central nonenhancing core of necrotic tumor **(17-25)**. Nodular, punctate, or patchy enhancing foci outside the main mass represent macroscopic tumor extension into adjacent structures. Microscopic foci of viable tumor cells are invariably present far beyond any demonstrable areas of enhancement or edema on standard imaging sequences.

Most GBMs do not restrict on DWI. DTI may show reduced fractional anisotropy and disrupted white matter tracts from tumor invasion. MRS usually shows elevated choline, decreased NAA and mI, and a lipid/lactate peak resonating at 1.33 ppm. pMR shows elevated rCBV in the tumor "rind" and increased vascular permeability.

Patterns of GBM Spread. GBMs are notorious for their ability to spread via multiple routes, including "brain-to-brain" metastases **(17-30)**.

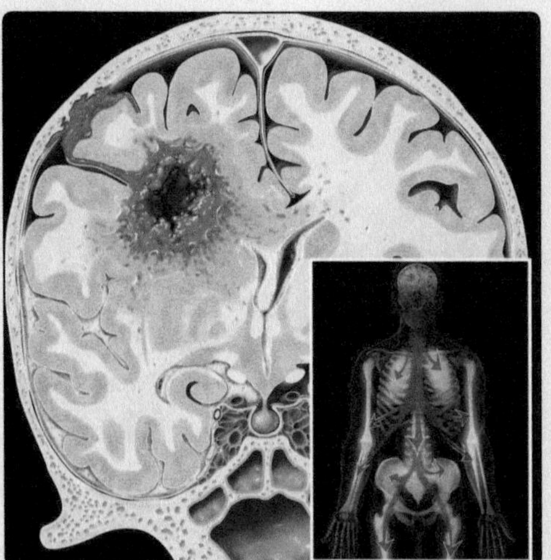

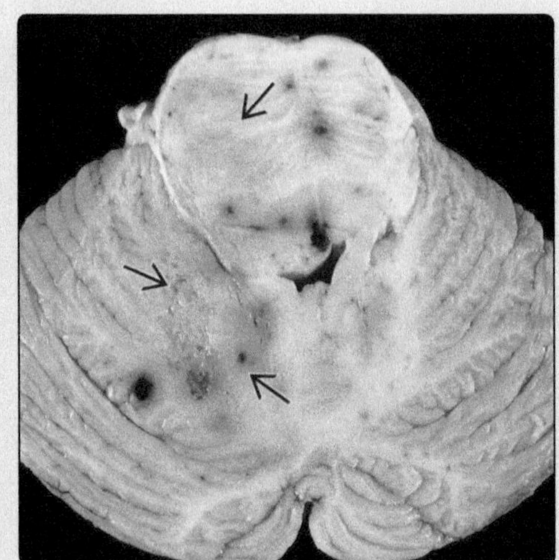

***(17-29)** Graphic shows potential GBM routes of spread. Preferential tumor spread is along compact WM tracts but can be ependymal, subpial, diffuse CSF ("carcinomatous meningitis"). Dural, skull invasion, extracranial metastases rarely occur. **(17-30)** Autopsy shows patterns of GBM dissemination. Axial section through pons and cerebellum shows multiple discrete foci of parenchymal tumor ➙. (Courtesy E. T. Hedley-Whyte, MD.)*

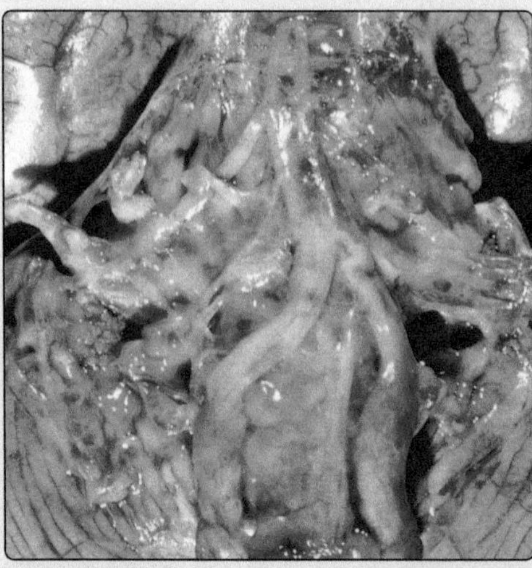

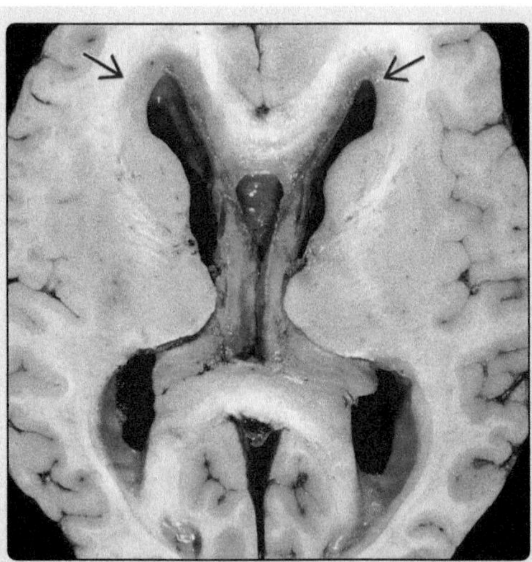

***(17-31)** "Carcinomatous meningitis" from GBM coats the surface of the brainstem and cerebellum, basilar artery, and cranial nerves. Gross appearance is virtually indistinguishable from that of pyogenic meningitis. (Courtesy R. Hewlett, MD.) **(17-32)** Glioblastoma has spread around both lateral ventricles in a thick band of subependymal tumor ➙. (Courtesy R. Hewlett, MD.)*

White Matter Spread. The most common route of GBM spread is through the white matter **(17-29) (17-33)**. Dissemination along compact white matter tracts, such as the corpus callosum **(17-27)**, fornices, anterior commissure, and corticospinal tract, can result in tumor implantation in geographically remote areas, such as the pons, cerebellum, medulla, and spinal cord **(17-30)**. Viable tumor cells are dispersed into (and beyond) the visible peritumoral edema.

CSF Dissemination. GBM often seeds the CSF, filling the sulci and cisterns **(17-34)**. Diffuse coating of cranial nerves and the pial surface of the brain is also common. This appearance of "carcinomatous meningitis" may be indistinguishable on imaging studies from pyogenic meningitis **(17-31) (17-34B)**. Direct invasion of the dura-arachnoid is rare **(17-28D)**.

Ependymal and Subependymal Spread. GBM spread along the ventricular ependyma occurs but is less common than diffuse CSF dissemination **(17-34A)**. Subependymal tumor spread produces a thick neoplastic "rind" as tumor "creeps" and crawls around the ventricular margins **(17-32)**.

Extra-CNS Metastases. Hematogeneous spread of GBM to systemic sites occurs but is rare. Bone marrow (especially the vertebral bodies), liver, lung, and even lymph node metastases can occur.

Differential Diagnosis

Anaplastic astrocytomas generally do not enhance, although some do and may be difficult to distinguish from GBM on imaging alone. The major neoplasm that should be distinguished from GBM is **metastasis**. Metastases are typically round or ovoid, not infiltrating like GBM.

Gliosarcoma (GS) is a rare IDH(-) GBM variant characterized by a biphasic tissue pattern with areas of glial (gliomatous) and mesenchymal (sarcomatous) differentiation. The most common appearance is a peripherally located,

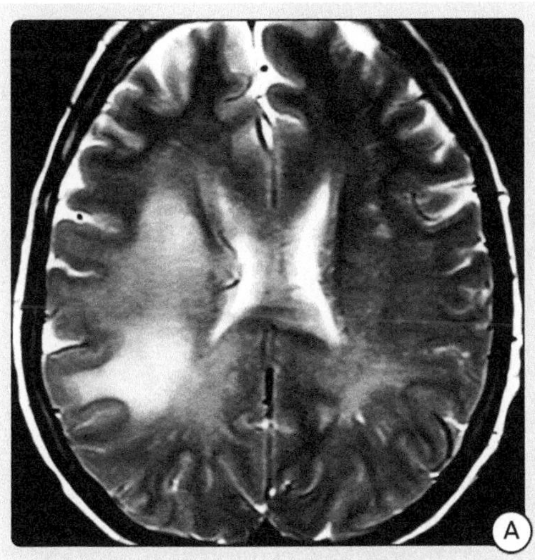

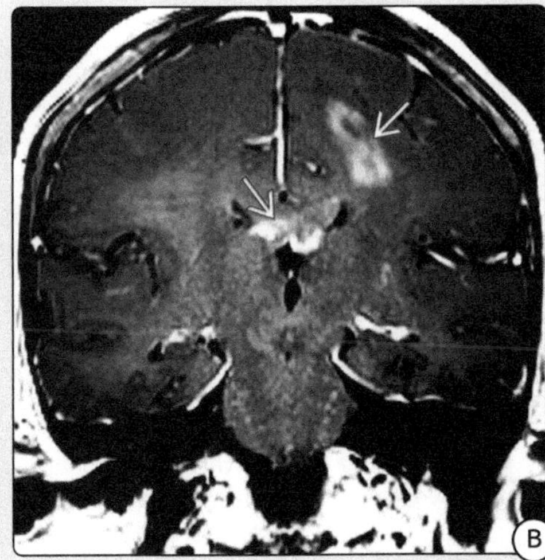

(17-33A) T2 MR shows diffuse confluent and patchy WM hyperintensity in this elderly patient with increasing confusion and left-sided weakness. (17-33B) Coronal T1 C+ MR in the same patient shows enhancement in the left hemispheric WM and corpus callosum ➡. Biopsy disclosed diffusely infiltrating GBM.

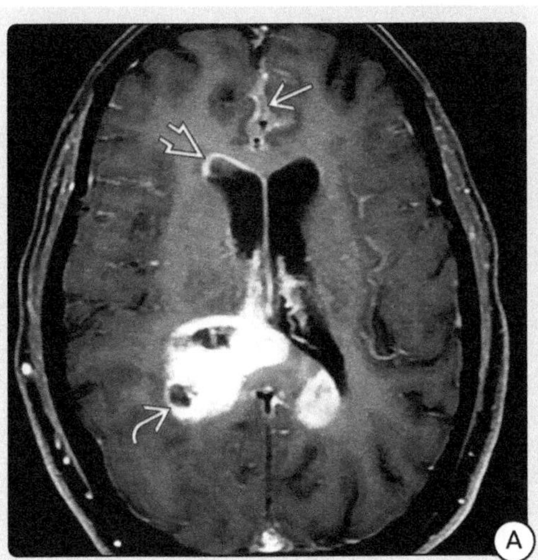

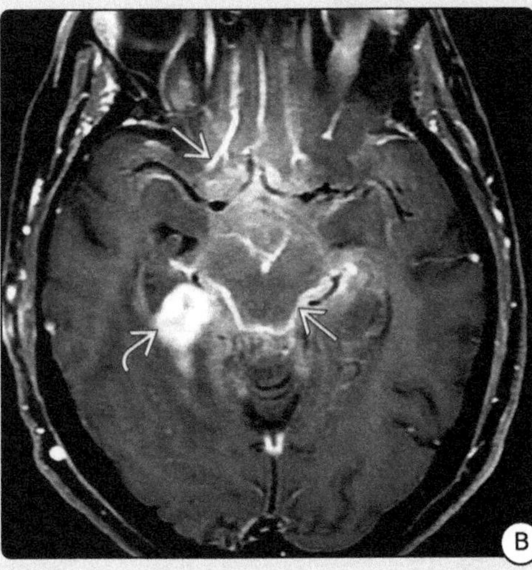

(17-34A) Series of T1 C+ FS MR scans demonstrates GBM ➡ with widespread CSF dissemination. Note ependymal ➡, sulcal-cisternal ➡ enhancement. (17-34B) Lower T1 C+ FS MR shows the primary tumor ➡ together with a diffuse coating of midbrain, enhancement throughout the suprasellar cistern extending into both sylvian fissures and olfactory sulci ➡.

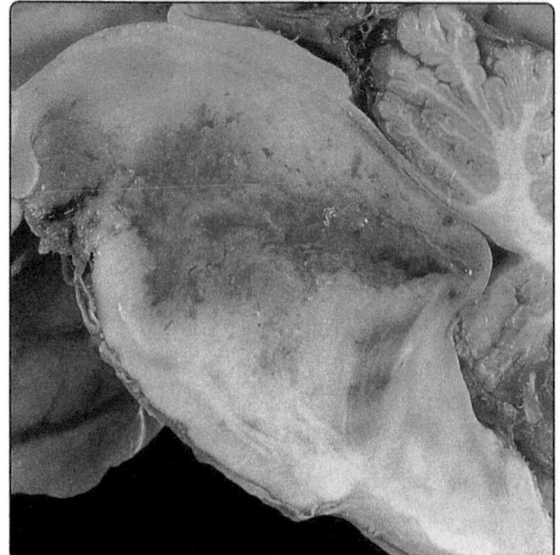

(17-35) Autopsied case of pediatric DIPG shows diffusely expanded pons, CSF metastases. (From Ellison, Neuropathology, 2013.)

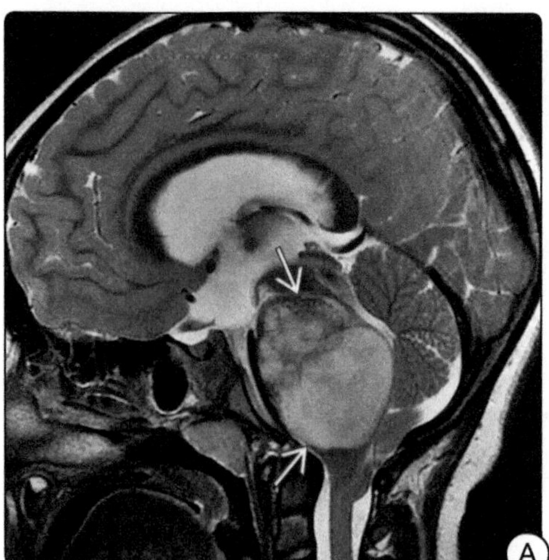

(17-36A) Sagittal T2 MR in a 5y girl with multiple cranial nerve palsies shows heterogeneous hyperintense tumor ➡ expanding entire pons.

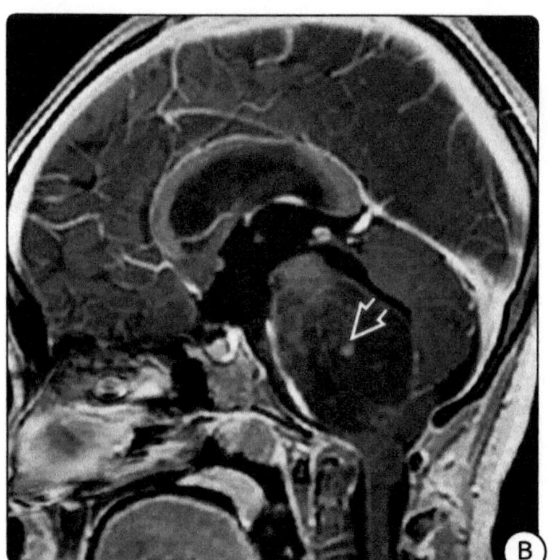

(17-36B) Sagittal T1 C+ FS MR shows single focus of mild enhancement in the tumor ➡. This is proven diffuse midline glioma, H3 K27M-mutant.

heterogeneously enhancing solid mass with moderate to marked surrounding edema. GSs often abut the meninges but may not demonstrate dural attachment or obvious invasion.

The major nonneoplastic differential diagnosis of GBM is **abscess**. Abscesses typically have thinner, more regular rims and restrict on DWI. MRS often shows succinate and cytosolic amino acids, which are rare in GBM.

"Tumefactive" demyelination in the subcortical white matter may demonstrate peripheral rim enhancement and mimic GBM. A "horseshoe" pattern with an incomplete enhancing rim and the open segment pointing toward the cortex is typical for "tumefactive" demyelination.

GLIOBLASTOMA: IDH-WILD-TYPE

Terminology, Etiology

- Also called "primary" GBM
  - Arises de novo [different progenitor than IDH(+) gliomas]

Pathology

- > 95% of all GBMs
- Necrosis, microvascular proliferation
- *IDH1* negative, *PTEN* mutated, *EGFR* amplified
- WHO grade IV

Clinical

- Peak age = 55-85 years
  - Survival < 1 year

Imaging

- Anywhere in hemispheres
- Hemorrhage, necrosis common
- Thick, irregular enhancing tumor "rind" around central necrotic core

Pediatric Diffuse Gliomas

In the past, diffusely infiltrating gliomas in children were lumped together with their adult counterparts. Although microscopically similar, their molecular profiles and biologic behaviors are often very different. For example, pediatric oligodendrogliomas frequently lack the 1p19q codeletions that characterize adult tumors. Most pediatric high-grade gliomas also lack *IDH1* mutation.

Unlike adult high-grade astrocytomas, pediatric high-grade astrocytomas frequently arise in the midline (pons, thalamus, and spinal cord). A newly defined entity that is characterized by midline location and mutations in the histone H3 gene includes tumors that were previously referred to as diffuse intrinsic pontine glioma (DIPG) and is now officially recognized as **diffuse midline glioma, H3 K27M-mutant**.

Pediatric brainstem gliomas (BSGs) account for 10% of pediatric brain tumors and can involve the midbrain, pons, or medulla. *Not all pediatric BSGs are the same—geography, molecular profile, tumor grade, and patient outcome are remarkably variable!*

Pathology

Pediatric BSGs are divided into two groups by location. The most common location is the pons (2/3 of cases). These pontine gliomas are called **DIPGs (17-35)**. Approximately 80% are high-grade tumors. Intrapontine histologic variation is common. Different areas of WHO grade II, III, and IV astrocytoma can all occur within the densely tumor-packed pons. Most of these DIPGs exhibit histone mutations **(17-36)** and are IDH-wild-type.

Midline nonbrainstem diffuse high-grade gliomas are less common. They involve the midbrain (15%) or the medulla/pontomedullary junction (20%). These tumors share many clinical and biologic features with DIPGs and have a similarly dismal prognosis.

The second group of midline gliomas consists of focal, much less aggressive tumors that are confined predominately to the tectal plate/periaqueductal region and often remain stable over long periods of time.

Tectal gliomas are frequently found in older children and young adults, typically presenting with symptoms of obstructive hydrocephalus rather than cranial neuropathy. Most tectal gliomas are pilocytic astrocytomas (WHO grade I neoplasms) or IDH-mutant diffuse WHO grade II astrocytomas (10-20%).

BRAINSTEM GLIOMAS

Pathology
- Children (10% of childhood brain tumors)
  - 2/3 in pons [diffusely infiltrating pontine glioma (DIPG)]
  - Most are H3 (histone) mutant, IDH-wild-type
- Adults (uncommon)
  - 60% medulla, 30% pons, 10% midbrain/tectum
  - Low grade > high grade

Prognosis
- Children
  - Among most lethal of childhood cancers
  - H3 mutant DIPG = poor prognosis; < 10% survive 2 years
  - WHO grade varies (poor correlation with survival)
- Adults: Generally better prognosis

Imaging
- "Fat" pons, tectum, or medulla
  - T2/FLAIR hyperintensity
  - Enhancement often absent/minimal in pediatric brainstem gliomas (BSGs)
  - Enhancement common in adult BSGs

Differential Diagnosis
- Brainstem encephalitis
- Demyelinating disease
- Metabolic disease (e.g., osmotic demyelination)
- Intracranial hypotension
  - Brainstem "sagging" → "fat" pons

Clinical Issues

DIPGs are among the most lethal of all childhood cancers. Overall, median survival is < 1 year despite multimodal therapies. Adult DIPGs are rare. Most are IDH-wild-type anaplastic astrocytomas or GBMs. Survival is similar to supratentorial IDH-wild-type tumors of similar grade and histology.

Imaging

DIPGs expand and diffusely infiltrate the pons. They have indistinct margins and are hypointense on T1WI and hyperintense on T2/FLAIR. DIPGs often expand anteriorly, enfolding and sometimes almost completely engulfing the basilar artery. Foci of necrosis and even intratumoral hemorrhage may be present. Most DIPGs show either no or relatively little patchy enhancement **(17-36)**.

Tectal gliomas are discrete, well-marginated lesions that focally enlarge the colliculi or midbrain tegmentum and often obstruct the cerebral aqueduct.

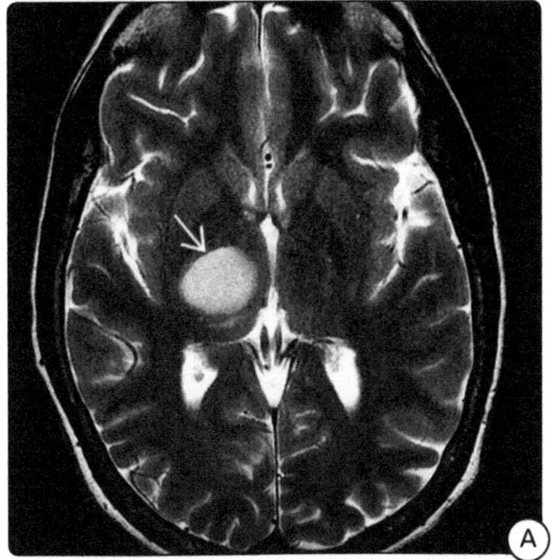

***(17-37A)** T2 MR shows a hyperintense right thalamic mass ➡. The mass did not enhance on T1 C+ FS MR and no biopsy was performed.*

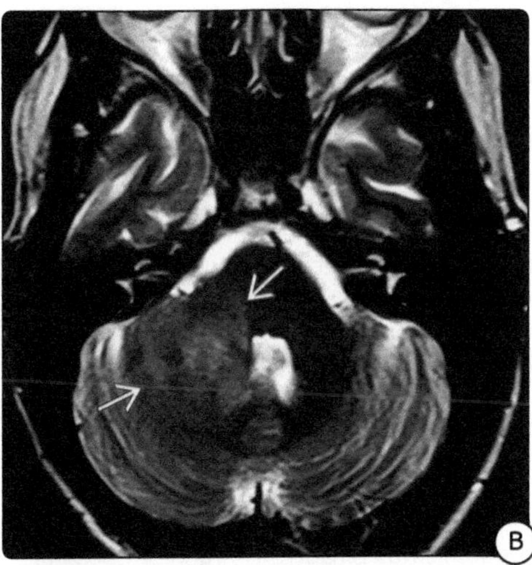

***(17-37B)** 18 months later, T2 MR shows a mildly hyperintense mass in the right brachium pontis and cerebellar hemisphere ➡.*

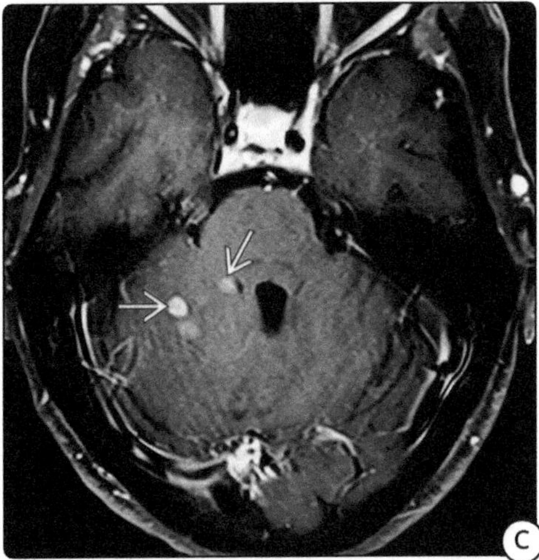

***(17-37C)** T1 C+ FS MR shows multiple metastases ➡ identified as H3 K27M mutation, seen in 2/3 of unilateral high-grade thalamic astrocytomas.*

They are iso- to hypointense on T1WI and hyperintense on T2/FLAIR. Contrast enhancement is minimal or absent. Tectal gliomas are indolent lesions that typically remain stable in size over many years.

Differential Diagnosis

The general differential diagnosis of pediatric BSG is **brainstem encephalitis, demyelinating disease** (MS, ADEM), **neurofibromatosis type 1** (NF1), and **osmotic demyelination**. A "fat" pons can be mimicked by **intracranial hypotension**. Brain "sagging" can make the midbrain and pons look abnormally large on axial images but T2/FLAIR signal intensity is normal.

Diffuse Midline Glioma, H3 K27M-Mutant

Terminology

An H3 K27M-mutant diffuse midline glioma is an infiltrative, high-grade glioma with predominantly astrocytic differentiation and a K27M mutation.

Etiology

This molecularly defined set of neoplasms is characterized by K27M mutations in the histone H3 gene *H3F3A*. The K27M mutation appears to be mutually exclusive with *IDH1* mutation and *EGFR* amplification. *BRAF* mutation is rare.

Pathology

Gross Pathology. Symmetric or asymmetric fusiform enlargement of the pons is typical for DIPGs **(17-35)**. The thalami are the second most common intracranial site. Other reported locations include the spinal cord, third ventricle, hypothalamus, pineal region, and cerebellum.

Pontine tumors may extend superiorly into the thalami or inferiorly into the upper cervical cord. Occasionally, H3-mutant tumors exhibit diffuse spread with a gliomatosis cerebri pattern. Leptomeningeal dissemination occurs in ~ 40% of cases.

Microscopic Features. The vast majority of H3 midline gliomas exhibit astrocytic morphology, but a wide spectrum of morphologic variations has been reported. Focal areas of necrosis, hemorrhage, and microvascular proliferation may be present. Mitotic figures are high.

H3 K27M-mutant diffuse midline gliomas are WHO grade IV neoplasms.

Clinical Issues

H3 K27M-mutant diffuse midline glioma is mostly a tumor of children but can also occur in adults. Median age at diagnosis with pontine tumors is 7 years, whereas nonbrainstem (primarily thalamic and spinal) histone-mutant gliomas average two decades older. Diffuse high-grade gliomas with H3 K27M mutations carry a dismal prognosis independent of tumor location.

Imaging

Imaging features of H3 K27M-mutant brainstem gliomas are those described previously for DIPGs.

Thalamic diffuse H3-mutant gliomas show an enlarged thalamus with T2/FLAIR hyperintensity. Enhancement is variable but typically minimal or patchy and usually involves < 25% of the tumor. Leptomeningeal dissemination and "brain-to-brain" metastases are common in all H3 K27M-mutant midline glioma **(17-37)**, so the entire neuraxis should be visualized on initial evaluation.

Differential Diagnosis

The differential diagnosis for pontine diffuse midline gliomas, H3 K27M-mutant, is the same as delineated previously for DIPGs.

The differential diagnosis for unilateral thalamic H3 K27M-mutant glioma is the same for other IDH-wild-type WHO grade II and III astrocytomas. Bithalamic tumors can resemble nonneoplastic disorders, such as internal cerebral vein thrombosis, artery of Percheron infarct, and Wernicke encephalopathy.

Selected References: The complete reference list is available on the Expert Consult™ eBook version included with purchase.

Nonastrocytic Glial Neoplasms

Nonastrocytic gliomas represent a broad spectrum of neoplasms derived from progenitor cells that maintain glial characteristics. This group of neoplasms is significantly smaller than the astrocytomas but nevertheless comprises an important class of tumors that range from relatively well-circumscribed and biologically indolent neoplasms (e.g., choroid plexus papilloma) to highly malignant tumors, such as anaplastic oligodendroglioma and ependymoma.

Oligodendrogliomas

Tumors that morphologically resemble oligodendrocytes—oligodendrogliomas (OGs)—are the third most common type of glial neoplasm (after anaplastic astrocytoma and glioblastoma). OGs are currently classified into two types: A well-differentiated tumor (OG) and a malignant variant (anaplastic OG).

Oligodendroglioma

Terminology

OGs are diffusely infiltrating, slow-growing gliomas with specific entity-defining molecular markers, i.e., *IDH1* or *IDH2* mutation plus deletion of chromosomal arms 1p and 19q (termed 1p/19q codeletion). Hence the full pathologic name of OG is **oligodendroglioma, IDH-mutant and 1p/19q codeleted.**

Etiology

Genetics. OGs and diffuse astrocytomas share the same early "driver" IDH mutation. OGs then diverge, undergoing subsequent genetic alterations (1p and 19q losses) that distinguish them from astrocytomas as well as from other gliomas **(18-1)**. Childhood tumors that histologically resemble OG are rare. They are often IDH(-) and do not exhibit 1p/19q codeletion.

Pathology

Location. Most OGs arise at the gray matter-white matter junction **(18-2)**. The vast majority (85-90%) are supratentorial. The most common site is the frontal lobe (50-65%) followed by the parietal, temporal, and occipital lobes.

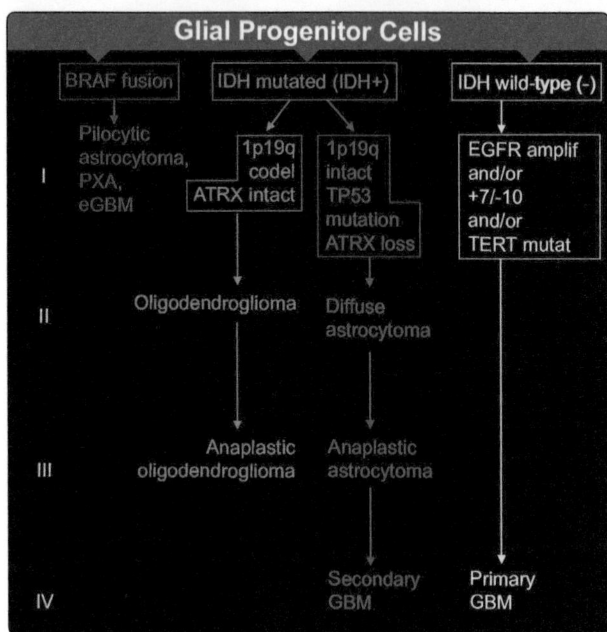

(18-1) After the "driver" IDH mutation in gliomagenesis, sequential mutations (1p19q) give rise to oligodendrogliomas. Oligodendrogliomas (OGs) are WHO grade II neoplasms; anaplastic oligodendrogliomas are WHO grade III.

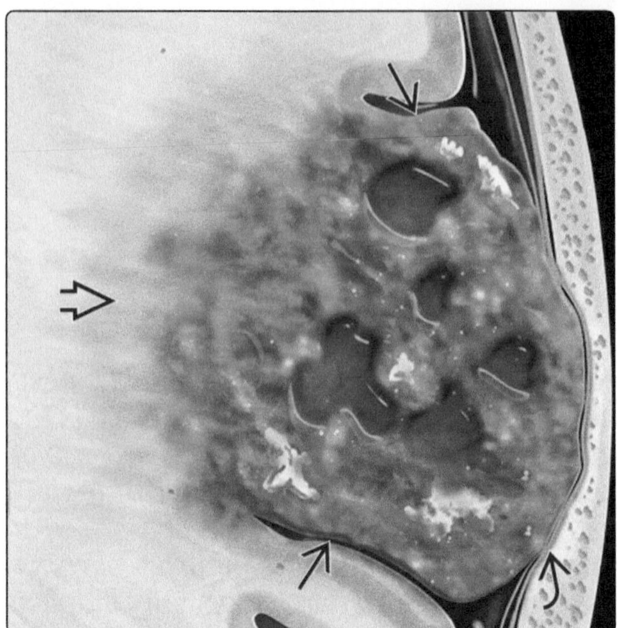

(18-2) OGs are poorly demarcated, cortically based "fleshy" masses ⇨ that infiltrate cortex and subcortical white matter →. Remodeling of adjacent bone ↗ is common.

Primary leptomeningeal OGs have been reported but are now considered a newly recognized and codified entity, diffuse leptomeningeal glioneuronal tumor (discussed in the next chapter).

Gross Pathology. OGs are typically solid, soft, "fleshy," cortically based tan-to-pink masses. They are poorly circumscribed and blend gradually into adjacent structures, blurring the gray matter-white matter boundary and expanding one or more gyri. Calcification is frequent and intratumoral hemorrhage may be present.

Oligodendrogliomas are defined by IDH mutation and deletion of both the short arm of chromosome 1 (1p) and the long arm of chromosome 19 (19q). OGs are designated as WHO grade II neoplasms.

Clinical Issues

Epidemiology. OGs account for 2-5% of all primary CNS neoplasms and 5-20% of gliomas. Approximately 1/2 of oligodendroglial tumors are WHO grade II neoplasms, and 1/2 are grade III (anaplastic OG, discussed later).

OGs are primarily tumors of adults with only 1-5% occurring in children. Most OGs arise between the ages of 35 and 55 years with a peak incidence between 40 and 45 years.

Natural History. OGs are slow-growing but locally aggressive neoplasms that often present clinically with seizures. The 5-year survival rate is nearly 80%, and median survival time is 10-12 years. OGs are relatively indolent tumors, but local recurrence following resection is common.

Imaging

CT Findings. OGs are most often peripheral and cortically based. Focal gyral expansion with thinning and remodeling of the overlying calvarium is common. Almost 2/3 are hypodense on NECT scan **(18-3A)**, while 1/3 exhibit mixed-density patterns.

Coarse nodular or clumped calcification is seen in 70-90% of cases. Gyriform Ca^{++} is very suggestive. Cystic degeneration occurs in 20%. Gross hemorrhage and peritumoral edema are less common and do not indicate malignant degeneration.

Enhancement varies from none to moderate; ~ 50% of OGs demonstrate some degree of enhancement. A patchy multifocal pattern is typical.

MR Findings. OGs often appear relatively well delineated and are usually hypointense relative to gray matter on T1WI. They are typically heterogeneously hyperintense on T2/FLAIR **(18-3B)** **(18-3C)**. Vasogenic edema is uncommon. Calcification is seen as "blooming" foci on T2* sequences.

Many OGs do not enhance on T1 C+ **(18-3D)**. Moderate heterogeneous enhancement is seen in ~ 1/2 of all cases. OGs do not restrict on DWI. Because of their relative vascularity, OGs may display high rCBV foci on pMR. Therefore, *an elevated rCBV in an OG does not necessarily indicate high-grade histopathology!*

Differential Diagnosis

The major differential diagnosis of OG is **diffuse astrocytoma**. Diffusely infiltrating astrocytomas more commonly involve the white matter—less often the cortex—and do not enhance.

Differentiation of a WHO grade II OG from **anaplastic oligodendroglioma** (AO) may be difficult on the basis of imaging alone. Hemorrhage and necrosis are more common in AO than OG but are not definitive.

Other cortically based, slow-growing tumors that typically present with seizures include **ganglioglioma** and **dysembryoplastic neuroepithelial tumor (DNET)**. Both are more common in children and young adults. Gangliogliomas are more common in the temporal lobe with a "cyst + nodule" appearance. DNETs are typically "bubbly" and may have associated cortical dysplasia.

Central neurocytoma is indistinguishable from OG on light microscopy and requires immunohistochemical stains (e.g., synaptophysin) for diagnosis. Most central neurocytomas are intraventricular, whereas OGs are lobar, typically cortically based masses.

OLIGODENDROGLIOMA

Pathology
- Defined by IDH(+), 1p/19q codeletion
- 85-90% in hemispheres (most common = frontal lobes)
- Cortical based, extension into deep WM
- Poorly circumscribed, infiltrating

Clinical Issues
- Third most common primary brain tumor (2-5%)
  - Mostly middle-aged adults (rare in children)
- Grows slowly; survival: 10-12 years

Imaging
- Ca^{++} 70%; hemorrhage, edema uncommon
- Very heterogeneous on MR; 50% enhance

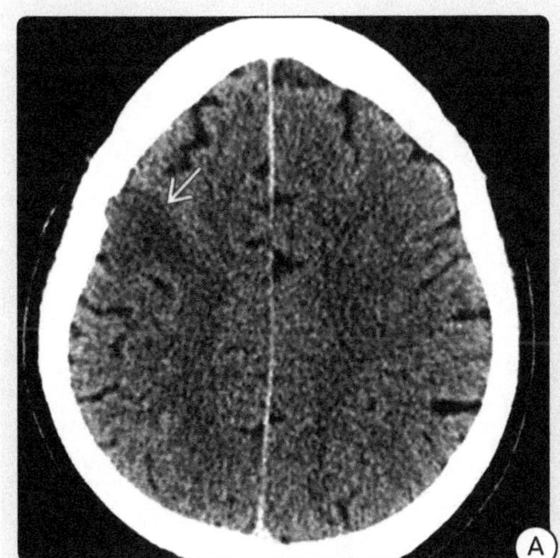

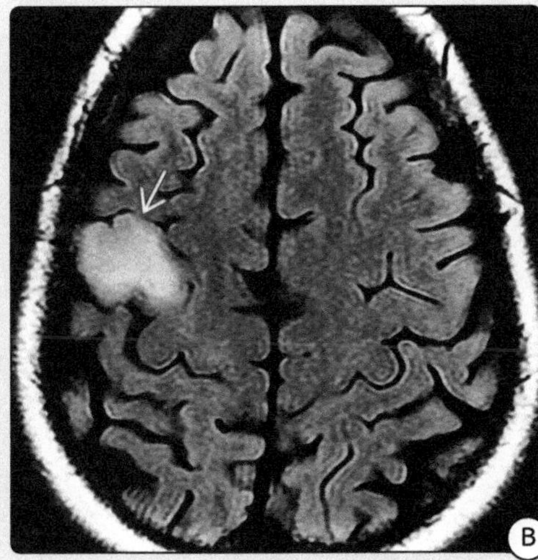

***(18-3A)** NECT in a 31-year-old woman with a 1st-time seizure shows a wedge-shaped hypodensity ➡ in the right posterior frontal lobe. **(18-3B)** Axial FLAIR MR in the same case shows that the mass is hyperintense ➡ and involves the cortex, infiltrating the underlying white matter and expanding the overlying gyrus.*

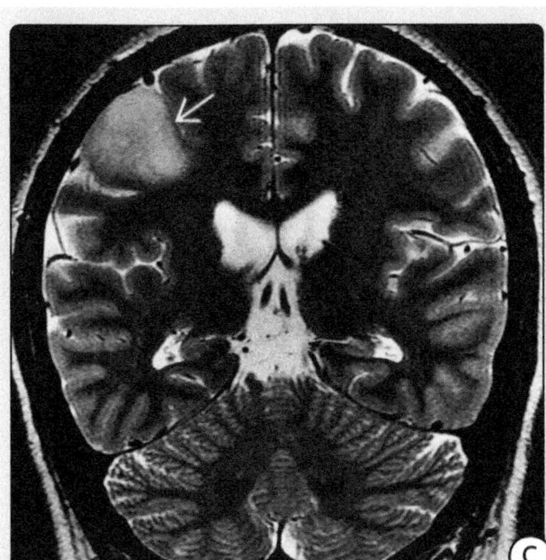

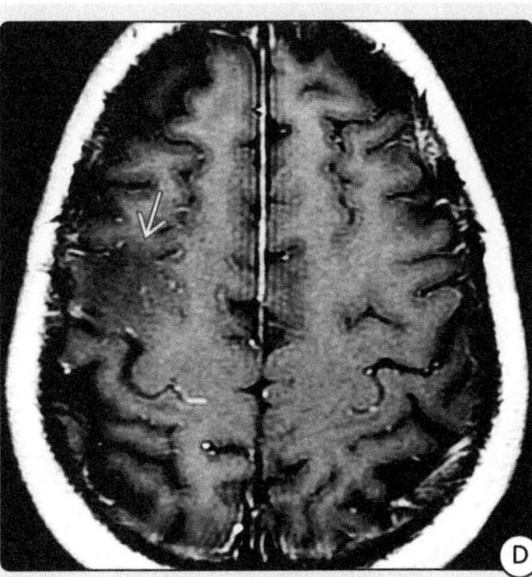

***(18-3C)** Coronal T2 MR shows that the heterogeneously hyperintense mass ➡ extends to the cortical surface and deep into the subcortical white matter. **(18-3D)** T1 C+ MR shows that the mass ➡ is hypointense and does not enhance. WHO grade II OG, IDH-mutant 1p/19q codeleted was found at histopathology.*

Anaplastic Oligodendroglioma, IDH-Mutant and 1p/19q Codeleted

Terminology

An IDH-mutant and 1p/19q codeleted OG with focal or diffuse histologic features of anaplasia is designated as anaplastic oligodendroglioma (AO), WHO grade III.

Etiology

AOs can develop either de novo or arise from progression of a preexisting WHO grade II OG. Mean time to progression from a WHO grade II OG to WHO grade III AO is ~ 6-7 years.

AOs have the same basic immunoprofile as WHO grade II OGs. In addition to the IDH mutations, 1p/19q codeletion, and *TERT* promoter mutations, AOs usually have additional subsequent genetic alterations. 9p LOH and polysomies are common, whereas *EGFR* amplification is absent.

A small subset of classic OGs and AOs lack IDH mutation and 1p/19q codeletions. Most of these "oligodendroglial-like" tumors in children and adolescents are biologically as well as genetically distinct from their adult counterparts. *BRAF* fusions are common.

Pathology

Between 25-35% of all oligodendroglial tumors are anaplastic. AOs demonstrate the same preference for the frontal lobe as do OGs. Other than the presence of necrotic foci, the macroscopic features of AO are similar to those of grade II OGs.

Focal or diffuse features of malignancy are present. AOs have higher cell density with more nuclear pleomorphism and

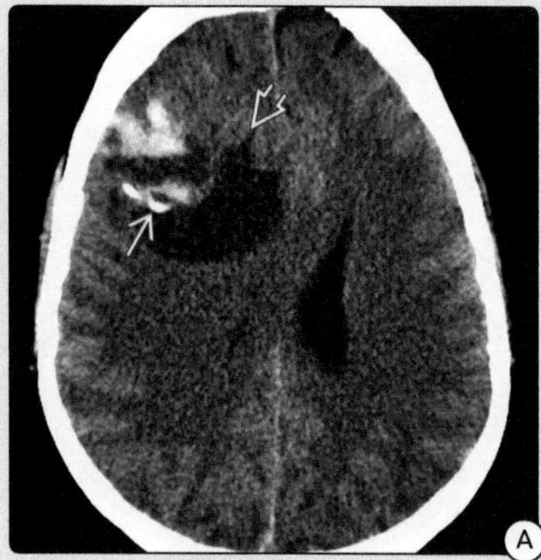

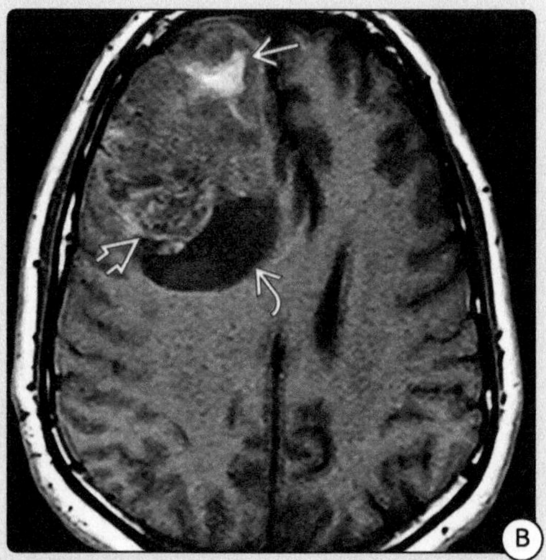

***(18-4A)** NECT in a 39-year-old man with headache shows a mixed-density right frontal mass ➡ with prominent calcifications ➡. **(18-4B)** T1 MR shows a very heterogeneous tumor that extends from the cortex into the deep white matter. Note hemorrhage ➡ and solid ➡ and cystic-appearing portions ➡ of the mass.*

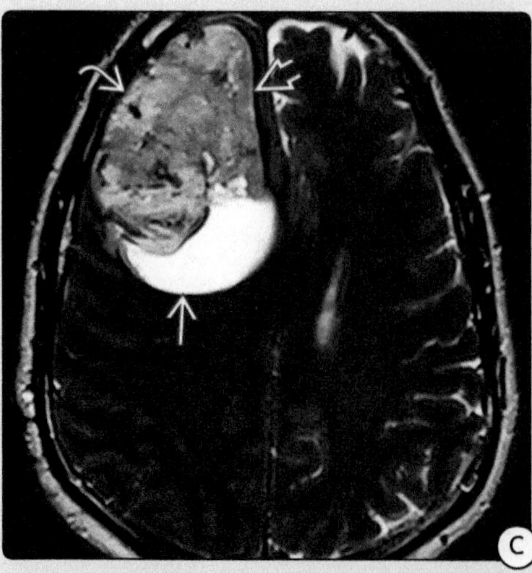

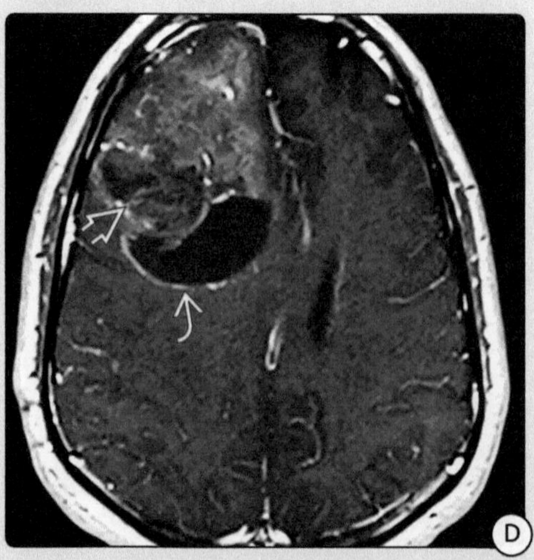

***(18-4C)** T2 MR shows bright fluid in the cystic portion ➡ and heterogeneous signal intensity in the solid part of the mass ➡. The mass extends to the cortical surface of the frontal lobe ➡. **(18-4D)** T1 C+ MR shows patchy, heterogeneous enhancement in the solid tumor ➡ with rim enhancement around the cyst ➡. This is an anaplastic OG, WHO grade III, IDH-mutant 1p/19q codeleted.*

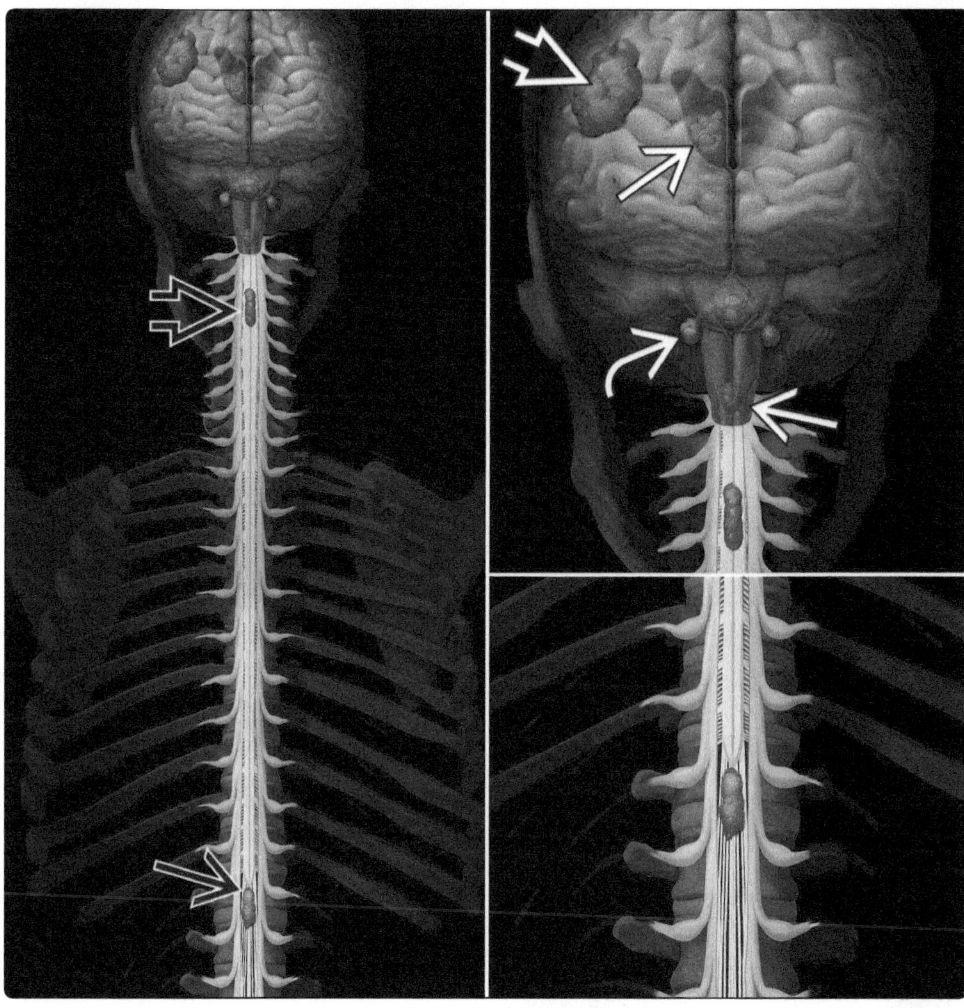

(18-5) Graphic shows ependymoma subtype and correlation with geographic localization. Subependymomas are found in the frontal horn of the lateral ventricle (ST-SE) and obex (PF-SE) ➡. Supratentorial EPNs ➡ are most often RELA- or YAP-fusion tumors. Posterior fossa ependymomas ➡ are PF-EPN-A or B. Spinal ependymomas can be myxopapillary ➡ (SP-MPE), which occur almost exclusively in the conus/filum terminale, or cellular/anaplastic ependymomas ➡ (SP-EPN), which occur in the central canal of the spinal cord and are intramedullary neoplasms.

hyperchromatism than OGs. Proliferative activity is higher, usually > 5%. AOs are WHO grade III tumors.

Clinical Issues

Patients are ~ 6 years older than patients with OGs. Mean age at presentation is 50 years. Survival time varies from a few months to as much as a decade.

Imaging

The general imaging features of AO are very similar to those of OG and do not reliably predict tumor grade. Peritumoral edema, hemorrhage, and foci of cystic degeneration are more common **(18-4)**. Enhancement is variable, ranging from none to striking. Cho:Cr ratio > 2.33 on MRS is suggestive of AO.

Differential Diagnosis

The major differential diagnosis of AO is **oligodendroglioma**. Tumor contrast enhancement is not helpful in distinguishing AO from low-grade OG. **Anaplastic astrocytoma** or even **glioblastoma** may also be difficult to differentiate from AO on the basis of imaging findings alone.

Ependymal Tumors

Ependymal tumors are a heterogeneous group of neoplasms that can arise anywhere in the neuraxis. The 2016 WHO classifies tumors that exhibit ependymal differentiation into several distinct tumor types: Subependymoma (SE), myxopapillary ependymoma, ependymoma, *RELA* fusion-positive ependymoma, and anaplastic ependymoma **(18-5)**.

The molecular biology of ependymoma is heterogeneous and varies with anatomic location. *Supratentorial and posterior fossa ependymomas are distinct diseases* with distinct genetic, transcriptional, and epigenetic alterations.

We begin our discussion with **ependymoma** (including anaplastic ependymoma and supratentorial ependymomas), primarily—but not exclusively—a childhood neoplasm. The most common histopathologic subtype that occurs in middle-aged and older adults is **subependymoma**. **Myxopapillary ependymoma** is almost exclusively a tumor of the conus medullaris, cauda equina, and filum terminale of the spinal cord.

Ependymoma

Posterior fossa (PF) ependymomas can be either subependymomas or "classic" ependymomas. Two PF ependymoma groups can be distinguished and are designated **PF-EPN-A** and **PF-EPN-B**. Although they appear similar at gross pathology and on imaging studies, they differ in both age and biologic behavior.

Pathology

Location. Approximately 60% of ependymomas are *infratentorial*. Of these, 95% are found in the fourth ventricle. The remainder occur as cerebellopontine angle (CPA) lesions.

Between 30-40% of ependymomas are *supratentorial*. Most supratentorial ependymomas are large, bulky neoplasms that exceed 4 cm in diameter. The majority arise from the lateral or third ventricles. In 40% of cases, they arise in the cerebral hemispheres without a visible connection to the ventricular system.

Gross Pathology. PF-EPNs have a well-delineated, lobulated "plastic" appearance, extruding through the foramina of Luschka and Magendie into the cerebellopontine cisterns **(18-6) (18-7)**. Calcification, cyst formation, and hemorrhage are common.

Clinical Issues

Demographics and Natural History. Ependymoma is the third most common PF tumor of childhood (after medulloblastoma and astrocytoma). PF-EPN-A ependymomas occur almost exclusively in children < 3 years. PF-EPN-Bs are primarily seen in adolescents and young adults (median age = 30 years). Progression-free survival for the PF-EPN-A subgroup at 4 years is ~ 70%, whereas it is 85-90% for the PF-EPN-B group.

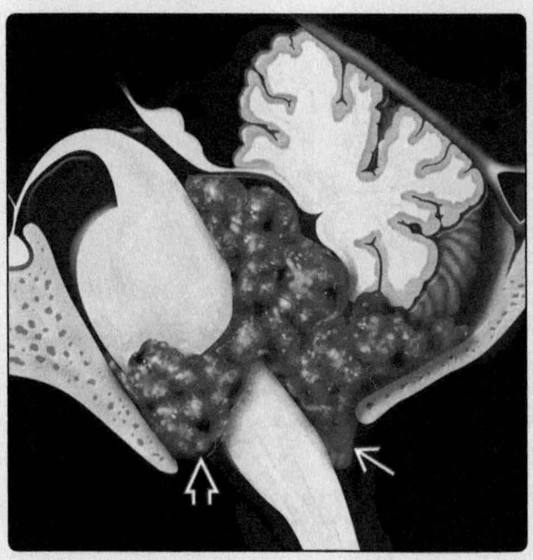

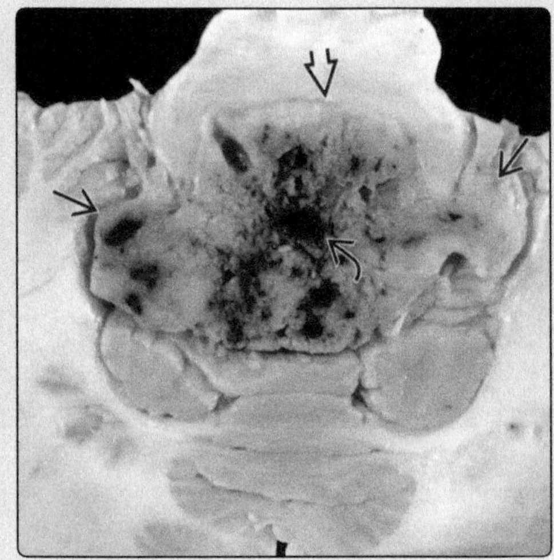

***(18-6)** Graphic depicts "classic" cellular ependymoma of the 4th ventricle extending through the foramen of Magendie into the cisterna magna ➔, around the pons under the brachium pontis, and through the lateral recesses into the cerebellopontine angle cisterns ➔. **(18-7)** Classic ependymoma fills the 4th ventricle ➔, extends through lateral recesses to foramina of Luschka ➔. Note multiple hemorrhagic foci ➔. (Courtesy E. Ross, MD.)*

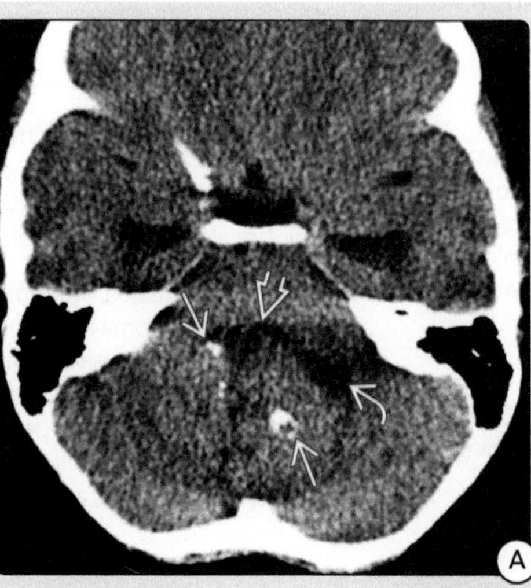

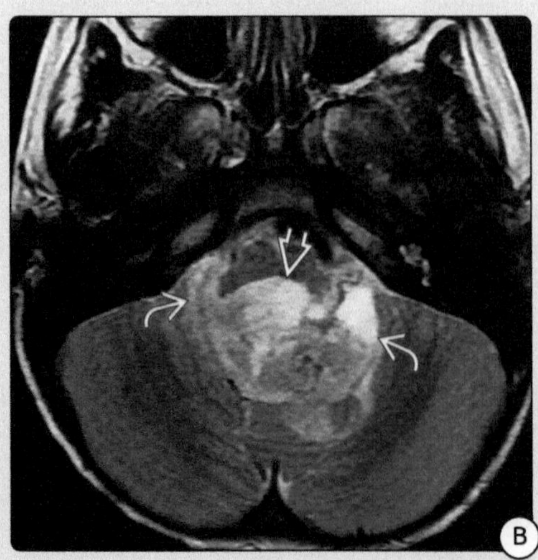

***(18-8A)** Axial NECT in a 3-year-old boy with seizures and vomiting shows a heterogeneous mass ➔ filling and expanding the 4th ventricle ➔. Note intratumoral calcifications ➔. **(18-8B)** T2 MR shows that the mass fills the 4th ventricle ➔ and extends laterally through both foramina of Luschka ➔. This is the classic "plastic" appearance of ependymoma.*

EPENDYMOMA

Location
- 60-70% posterior fossa
- 30-40% supratentorial

Pathology
- From 4th ventricle → cisterna magna, CPA
- WHO grade II or III

Clinical Issues
- 10% of childhood brain tumors
- PF-EPN-A
  - Median age: 3 years, M:F = 2:1
  - Ataxia, hydrocephalus
  - 4-year, progression-free survival: 70%
- PF-EPN-B
  - Older children, adults (median age: 30 years)
  - 5-year survival: 85-90%

Imaging

General Features. *Infratentorial* ependymomas are relatively well-delineated "plastic" tumors that typically arise from the floor of the fourth ventricle and extrude through the outlet foramina. They extend laterally through the foramina of Luschka toward the CPA cistern **(18-8)** and posteroinferiorly through the foramen of Magendie into the cisterna magna.

Sagittal images disclose a mass that fills most of the fourth ventricle and extrudes inferiorly into the cisterna magna **(18-9B)**. Axial and coronal images show lateral extension toward or into the CPA cisterns **(18-8B)**.

Obstructive hydrocephalus is a frequent accompanying feature of infratentorial ependymoma. Extracellular fluid often accumulates around the ventricles, giving the appearance of "blurred" margins.

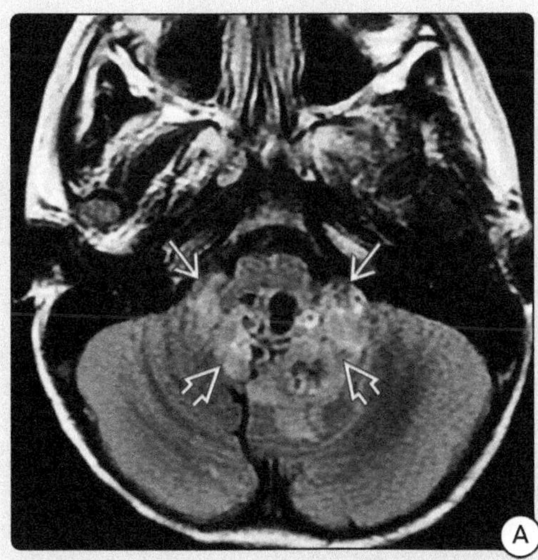

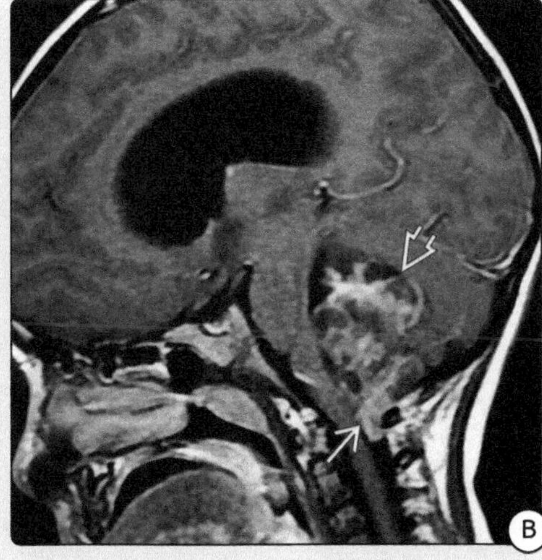

***(18-9A)** FLAIR MR in a 3-year-old boy shows a mixed signal intensity mass ➡ in the inferior 4th ventricle that extends anterolaterally through both foramina of Luschka into the cerebellopontine angle cisterns ➡. **(18-9B)** Sagittal T1 C+ MR in the same patient shows the heterogeneously enhancing 4th ventricle mass ➡ extruding posteroinferiorly through the foramen of Magendie into the cisterna magna ➡.*

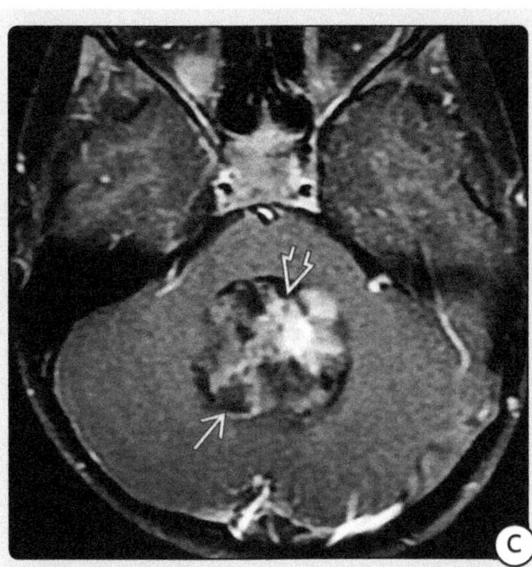

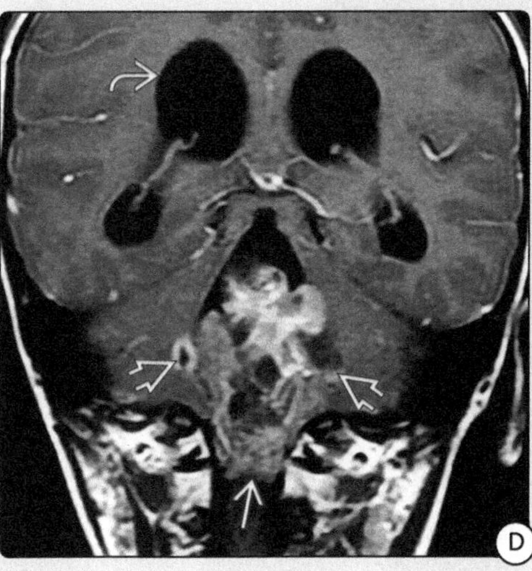

***(18-9C)** Axial T1 C+ FS MR in the same patient shows mixed cystic, solid enhancing tumor ➡ that expands and fills the 4th ventricle ➡. **(18-9D)** Coronal T1 C+ MR shows tumor extending inferiorly from the 4th ventricle into the cisterna magna ➡, laterally through the foramina of Luschka ➡. Note obstructive hydrocephalus ➡. Histopathology showed anaplastic ependymoma (WHO grade III), PF-EPN-A. The child survived for 2 years.*

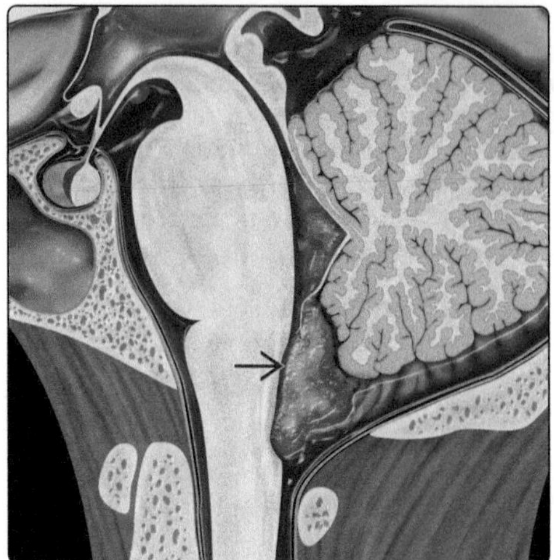

(18-10) Graphic depicts subependymoma of the inferior 4th ventricle ⇒ at the level of the obex.

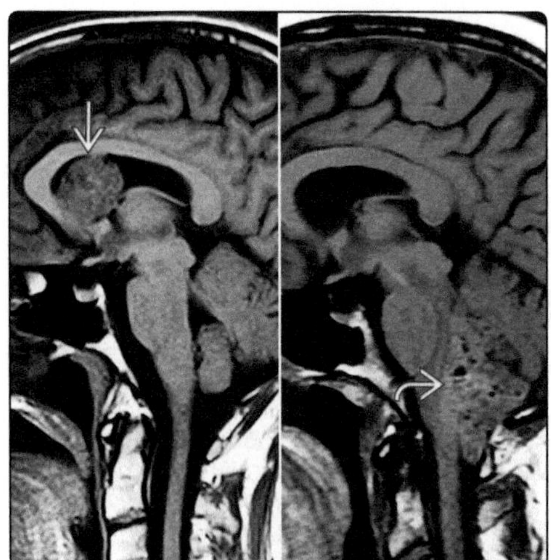

(18-11) Sagittal T1 MRs show locations of subependymoma in the frontal horn of the lateral ventricle ➡ (L), obex of 4th ventricle ➡ (R).

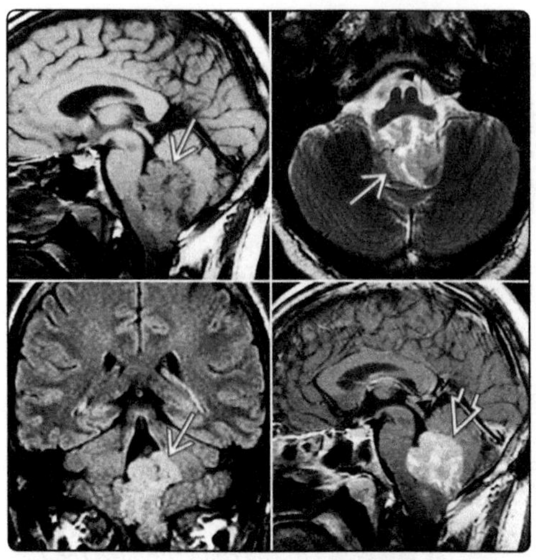

(18-12) Large subependymoma has 4th ventricle mass ➡ with T1 iso-/hypointensity, T2/FLAIR hyperintensity, strong enhancement ➡.

CSF dissemination is a key factor in staging, prognosis, and treatment so *preoperative imaging of the entire cranial-spinal axis should be performed in any child with a posterior fossa neoplasm*, especially if medulloblastoma or ependymoma is suspected.

Supratentorial ependymomas are relatively rare and generally present as large, bulky, aggressive-looking hemispheric tumors. Gross cyst formation, calcification, and hemorrhage are more common compared with their infratentorial counterparts.

CT Findings. Ependymomas are generally of mixed density on NECT scans with hypodense intratumoral cysts intermixed with iso- and hyperdense soft tissue portions. Coarse calcification occurs in ~ 1/2 of all ependymomas. Hemorrhage occurs in 10% of cases. Most ependymomas show mild to moderate heterogeneous enhancement on CECT.

MR Findings. Ependymomas are typically heterogeneously hypointense relative to brain parenchyma on T1WI and hyperintense on T2/FLAIR **(18-9)**. Most enhance with areas of strong, relatively homogeneous enhancement intermixed with foci of minimal or no enhancement. T2* imaging (GRE, SWI) commonly demonstrates "blooming" foci that can be caused by calcification &/or old hemorrhage.

Supratentorial ependymomas (often *RELA*- or *YAP*-fusion) are large, mixed solid/cystic-appearing masses that occur almost exclusively in the cerebral hemispheres. Imaging shows a heterogeneous mass with variable enhancement and little or no surrounding edema.

EPENDYMOMA: IMAGING

Infratentorial Ependymoma
- Fills 4th ventricle
- Extends into CPA, cisterna magna
- Obstructive hydrocephalus
- Cysts, Ca^{++} (50%), hemorrhage (10%) on NECT
- Mixed signal intensity, strong enhancement on MR
- "Blooming" foci on T2* common
- Usually does not restrict on DWI

Supratentorial Ependymoma
- Most are *RELA* fusion-positive ependymoma
- Usually large, bulky, aggressive-looking
  - Gross cysts, Ca^{++}, hemorrhage common
- Poor prognosis

Differential Diagnosis

The differential diagnosis of ependymoma is location dependent. The major differential diagnosis of *infratentorial* ependymoma is **medulloblastoma**. Cysts, hemorrhage, and calcification are more common in ependymoma, while restricted diffusion is more characteristic of medulloblastoma. **Pilocytic astrocytoma** is a common PF tumor in children and young adults but is more often found in the cerebellar hemispheres.

The major differential diagnosis of *supratentorial* ependymoma is **anaplastic astrocytoma** or **glioblastoma**. In very young children, **primitive neuroectodermal tumor** and **atypical teratoid/rhabdoid tumor** can cause hemispheric masses that closely resemble parenchymal ependymoma.

Subependymoma

Terminology

Subependymomas (SEs) are rare, benign, slow-growing, noninvasive tumors that are often found incidentally at imaging or autopsy.

Pathology

Location. SEs are usually located within or adjacent to an ependyma-lined space. Nearly 1/2 of all cases occur in the frontal horn of the lateral ventricle, near the foramen of Monro, where they are often attached to the septi pellucidi **(18-13)**. The fourth ventricle is the second most common site **(18-10)**.

Gross Pathology. SEs are solid, round to somewhat lobulated, well-delineated masses. Calcification, cysts, and hemorrhage are common in larger lesions. SEs are WHO grade I neoplasms.

Clinical Issues

Presentation. SEs are tumors of middle-aged and older adults. The majority of SEs are discovered incidentally on imaging studies. Approximately 40% cause symptoms, mostly related to CSF obstruction or mass effect.

Natural History. SEs exhibit an indolent growth pattern, expanding slowly into a ventricular space. Larger tumors may cause obstructive hydrocephalus, but they rarely invade adjacent brain.

Treatment Options. "Watchful waiting" with serial imaging is appropriate in asymptomatic patients. Complete surgical resection of symptomatic SEs is the procedure of choice. Recurrence is rare.

Imaging

General Features. SEs are well-demarcated nodular masses that may expand the ventricle but usually cause little mass effect. Large lesions may cause obstructive hydrocephalus.

CT Findings. SEs are iso- to slightly hypodense compared with brain on NECT scans. Calcification and intratumoral cysts may be present, especially in larger lesions. Hemorrhage is rare. Little or no enhancement is seen on CECT.

MR Findings. SEs are hypo- to isointense compared with brain on T1WI **(18-11)**. Intratumoral cysts are common in larger lesions. SEs are heterogeneously hyperintense on T2/FLAIR **(18-12)**. Peritumoral edema is usually absent. T2* (GRE, SWI) may show "blooming" foci, probably secondary to calcification. Hemorrhage is seen in 10-12%. Enhancement varies from none or mild to moderate **(18-14)**.

SEs do not restrict on DWI. MRS shows normal choline with mildly decreased NAA.

Differential Diagnosis

The differential diagnosis of SE varies with age and SE location. In older patients, the major differential is intraventricular **metastasis**. In young to middle-aged adults, **central neurocytoma** should be considered, although it more commonly involves the body—not the frontal horn—of the lateral ventricle. **Choroid plexus papilloma** usually occupies the body, not the inferior fourth ventricle.

In children, **ependymoma** and (in patients with tuberous sclerosis) **subependymal giant cell astrocytoma** are

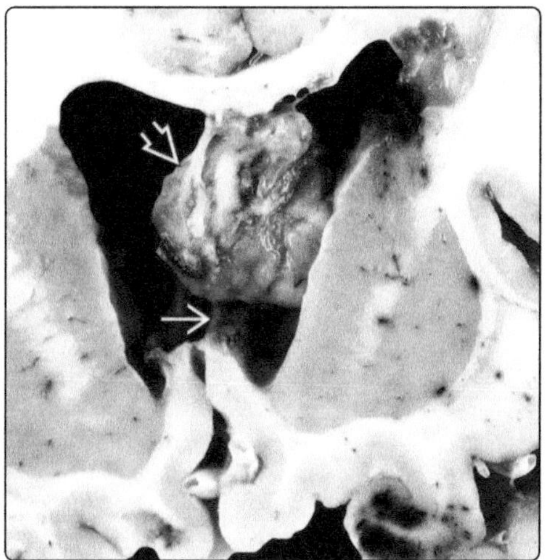

***(18-13)** Pathology shows well-delineated frontal horn mass ➡ attached to the septum pellucidum ➡. This is subependymoma (ST-SE).*

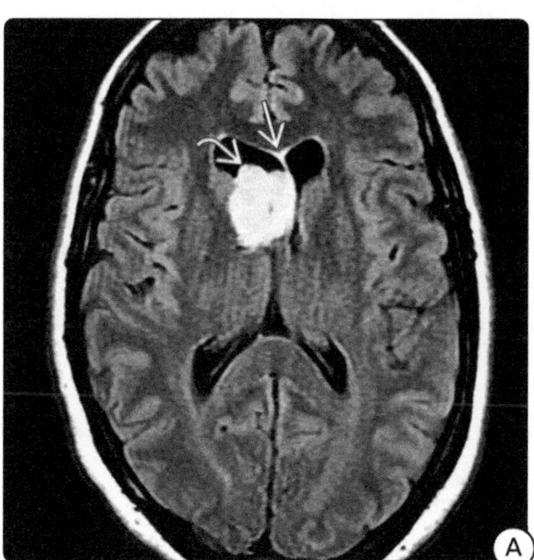

***(18-14A)** FLAIR shows hyperintense frontal horn mass ➡ attached to septum pellucidum ➡. No evidence for periventricular fluid accumulation.*

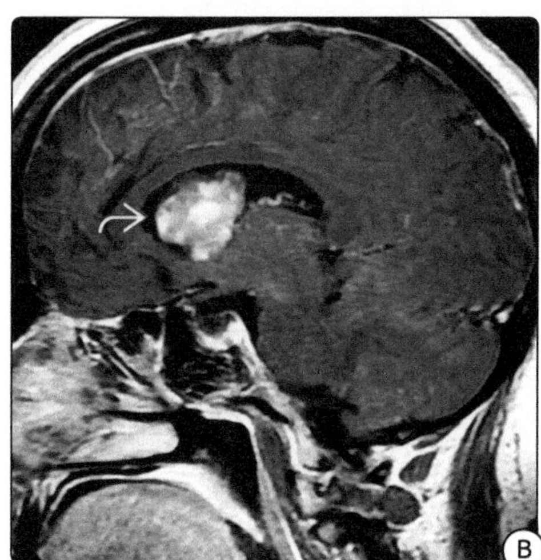

***(18-14B)** Sagittal T1 C+ MR shows lobulated heterogeneous mass ➡ confined to frontal horn. Subependymoma (ST-SE), WHO grade I.*

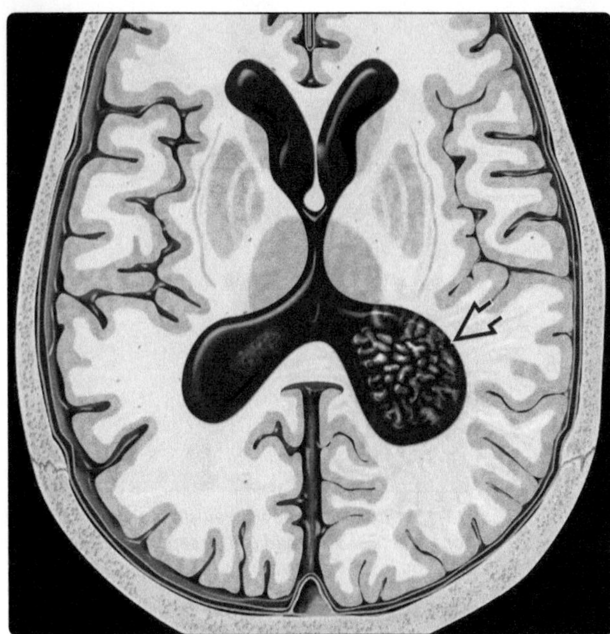

***(18-15)** Axial graphic depicts a frond-like mass ➡ in the atrium of the left lateral ventricle. The ventricles are moderately enlarged from overproduction of CSF. This is a choroid plexus papilloma.*

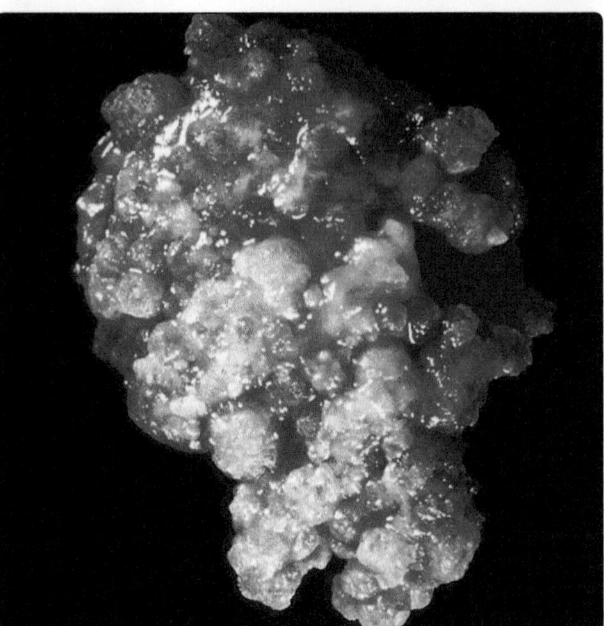

***(18-16)** Resected choroid plexus papilloma exhibits classic "cauliflower-like" gross appearance. Multiple vascular papillary excrescences are typical. (From Perry et al: Practical Neuropathy: A Diagnostic Approach, 2nd ed, 2018.)*

considerations. **Choroid plexus papillomas** in children are usually in the atrium of the lateral ventricle. Choroid plexus papilloma also has a frond-like appearance and typically shows intense uniform enhancement.

SUBEPENDYMOMA

Pathology

- Can be found in all 3 anatomic compartments
  - Posterior fossa (4th ventricle) > supratentorial (frontal horn) > spine
  - WHO grade I

Clinical Issues

- Middle-aged, older adults
- Often asymptomatic, discovered incidentally

Imaging Features

- Often Ca^{++}; hemorrhage rare
- Iso-/hypointense on T1WI, hyperintense on T2WI
- Variable enhancement

Myxopapillary Ependymoma

Myxopapillary ependymoma (MPE) is a very slow-growing type of ependymoma that occurs mostly in young adults. It is almost exclusively a tumor of the conus medullaris, cauda equina, and filum terminale of the spinal cord.

Primary intracranial myxopapillary ependymomas are exceptionally rare but have been reported in the ventricles and brain parenchyma. Imaging findings are nonspecific but generally those of a cyst with enhancing nodule.

Choroid Plexus Tumors

Choroid plexus epithelium shares a common embryologic origin with ependymal cells. Hence choroid plexus tumors are considered tumors of neuroepithelial tissue and comprise an important subgroup of the nonastrocytic gliomas.

Three histologic subtypes of choroid plexus neoplasms are recognized: Choroid plexus papilloma (CPP), atypical choroid plexus papilloma (aCPP), and choroid plexus carcinoma (CPCa).

In addition to histopathology in the diagnosis of choroid plexus tumors, recent methylation profiling studies have revealed three clinically distinct molecular subgroups of choroid plexus tumors: Pediatric low-risk choroid plexus tumors (cluster 1), adult low-risk choroid plexus tumors (cluster 2), and pediatric high-risk choroid plexus tumors (cluster 3). Cluster 1 (young age, mainly supratentorial location) and cluster 2 (adult age, mainly infratentorial location) are characterized by low risk of tumor progression. Cluster 3 (young age, supratentorial location) is characterized by choroid plexus tumors with a higher risk of progression and includes many aCPPs and basically all CPCas.

In this section, we discuss each of these types with the major focus on choroid plexus papilloma—the most common primary choroid plexus tumor.

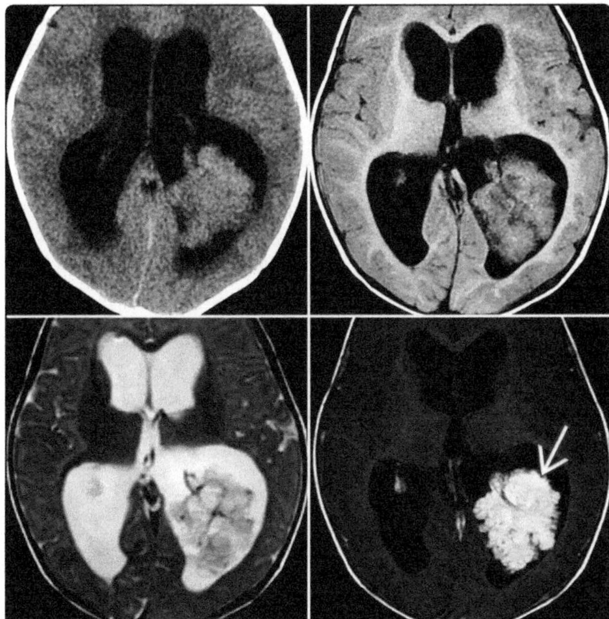

***(18-17)** NECT and a series of MRs demonstrate the typical appearance of choroid plexus papilloma. The lobulated intraventricular mass enhances strongly ➡. Note hydrocephalus caused by overproduction of CSF.*

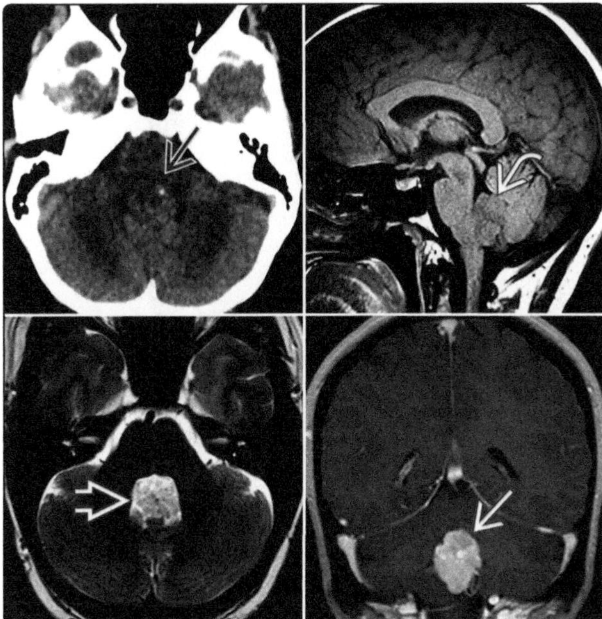

***(18-18)** A 39-year-old woman had a calcified 4th ventricular mass ➡ discovered incidentally on a head CT for trauma. The mass is well demarcated on T1 ➡, hyperintense on T2 ➡, and enhances intensely ➡; choroid plexus papilloma (WHO grade I).*

Choroid Plexus Papilloma

Terminology

Choroid plexus papilloma (CPP) is the most benign of the choroid plexus neoplasms.

Etiology

Genetics. Recurrent focal chromosomal gains are common to all sporadic CPPs, most commonly genes involved in the development and biology of plexus epithelium (i.e., *OTX2* and *TRPM3*).

Syndromic choroid plexus tumors—especially carcinomas—occur in patients with **Li-Fraumeni syndrome**, a cancer predisposition syndrome caused by *TP53* germline mutation. *SMARCB1* mutations with INI1 protein alterations and CPPs have been described in the **rhabdoid predisposition syndrome**. Both mutations are very rarely identified in sporadic CPPs.

CPPs also occur as part of **Aicardi syndrome**, an X-linked dominant syndrome that occurs almost exclusively in female patients. The prevalence of CPPs in Aicardi syndrome is estimated at 3-5%. Bilateral and triventricular CPPs occur in 1% of cases.

Pathology

Location. CPPs arise wherever choroid plexus is normally found, occurring in proportion to the amount of choroid plexus normally present in each location. Therefore, the vast majority arise in the lateral (50%) and fourth (40%) ventricles. The trigone is the most common overall site **(18-15)**.

Only 5-10% of all CPPs occur in locations other than the lateral and fourth ventricles. Just 5% are found in the third ventricle. CPPs are occasionally found as primary cerebellopontine angle (CPA) tumors in which tufts of choroid plexus extrude through the foramina of Luschka into the adjacent CPA cisterns.

There is a strong effect of age on CPP location. More than 80% of all CPPs in infants arise in the atrium of the lateral ventricle. The fourth ventricle and CPA cisterns are more typical locations in adults. The lateral ventricles are an exceptionally rare site of CPP in older patients.

Gross Pathology. CPPs vary in size from small to huge masses. CPPs are well-circumscribed papillary or cauliflower-like masses **(18-16)** that may adhere to—but usually do not invade through—the ventricular wall. Cysts and hemorrhage are common.

Mitotic activity is very low, usually < 1%. CPPs are generally confined to the ventricle of origin and rarely exhibit an infiltrative growth pattern. CPPs are WHO grade I neoplasms.

Clinical Issues

Demographics. CPPs are rare lesions, accounting for < 1% of all primary intracranial neoplasms. However, CPPs represent 10-20% of brain tumors occurring in the first year of life. Median age at presentation is 1.5 years for lateral and third ventricular CPPs, 22.5 years for fourth ventricular CPPs, and 35.5 years for CPA CPPs.

Presentation and Natural History. CPPs tend to obstruct normal CSF pathways. Infants present with increased head size and raised intracranial pressure. Children and adults may experience headache, nausea, and vomiting.

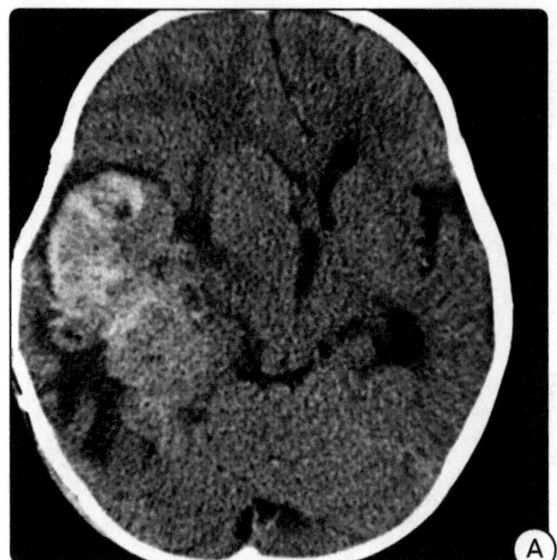

***(18-19A)** NECT in 2y girl with papilledema shows a predominantly hyperdense lobulated mass in right lateral ventricle invading adjacent brain.*

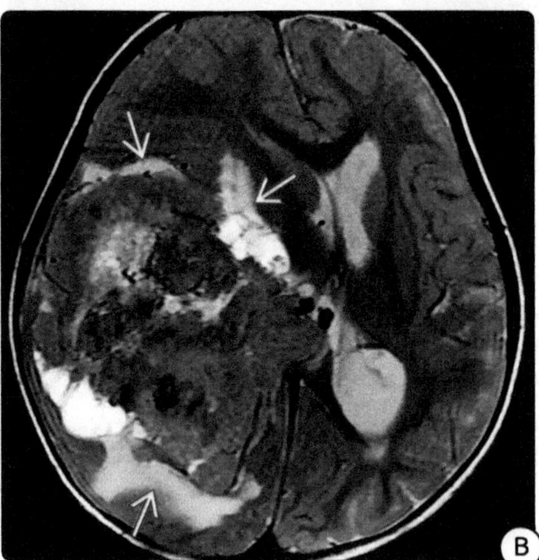

***(18-19B)** T2 MR shows extremely heterogeneous mass. Tumor invasion of the brain parenchyma with surrounding edema ➡ is present.*

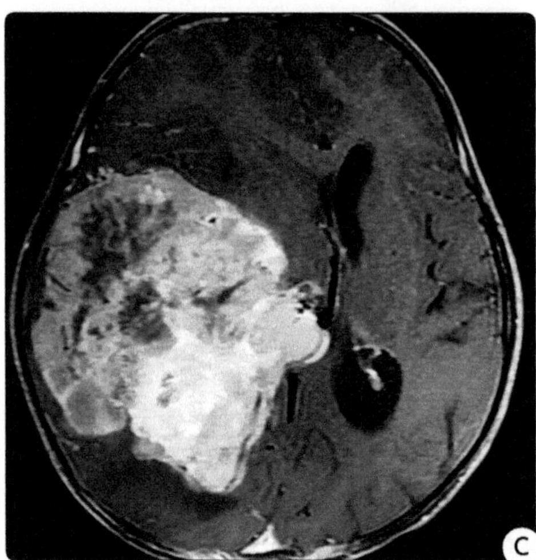

***(18-19C)** T1 C+ FS MR shows that the mass enhances intensely but heterogeneously. This is choroid plexus carcinoma.*

Surgical resection is usually curative. The recurrence rate following gross total resection is low, only ~ 5-6%. Malignant progression of CPP to choroid plexus carcinoma has been reported but is rare.

Imaging

General Features. A well-delineated, lobulated intraventricular mass with frond-like papillary excrescences is typical. *Diffuse leptomeningeal dissemination is uncommon but does occur with histologically benign CPPs, so preoperative imaging of the entire neuraxis is recommended!*

CHOROID PLEXUS PAPILLOMA

Pathology

- Lateral ventricle (50%, usually children)
- 4th ventricle, CPA cistern (40%, usually adults)
- 3rd ventricle (10%, children)
- Lobulated, frond-like configuration
- WHO grade I

Clinical Issues

- 13% of brain tumors in 1st year of life
- Mean age = 1.5 years for CPPs in lateral, 3rd ventricle
- Symptoms of obstructive hydrocephalus common
- Occurs with Aicardi, Li-Fraumeni, rhabdoid predisposition syndromes

Imaging Findings

- CT
  - Iso-/hyperdense lobulated mass
  - Hydrocephalus common
  - Ca^{++} (25%)
  - CECT shows intense enhancement
- MR
  - Iso-/hypointense on T1
  - Iso-/hyperintense on T2/FLAIR
  - "Flow voids" common
  - May show "blooming" foci on T2*
  - Intense enhancement, no restriction
  - Occasionally demonstrates CSF dissemination (image entire neuraxis preoperatively!)

CT Findings. Most CPPs are iso- to hyperdense compared with brain on NECT scans **(18-17)**. Calcification is seen in 25% of cases **(18-18)**. Hydrocephalus—either obstructive or caused by CSF overproduction—is common. CECT scans show intense homogeneous enhancement.

MR Findings. A sharply marginated lobular mass that is iso- to slightly hypointense relative to brain is seen on T1WI. CPPs are iso- to hyperintense on T2WI and FLAIR. Linear and branching internal "flow voids" reflect the increased vascularity common in CPPs. T2* (GRE, SWI) may show hypointense foci secondary to calcification or intratumoral hemorrhage. Intense homogeneous enhancement is seen following contrast administration **(18-17)**.

Differential Diagnosis

The major differential diagnosis of CPP is **atypical choroid plexus papilloma**. Both share similar imaging features. **Choroid plexus xanthogranulomas** are benign incidental lesions that occur commonly in the lateral ventricular choroid plexus, mostly in middle-aged and older patients. **Choroid plexus metastasis** occurs in middle-aged and older adults and is not in the differential diagnosis of a pediatric CPP.

Atypical Choroid Plexus Papilloma

Atypical choroid plexus papilloma (aCPP) is intermediate in malignancy between CPP (WHO grade I neoplasm) and choroid plexus carcinoma (WHO grade III neoplasm). aCPPs represent ~ 15% of all choroid plexus tumors.

Imaging characteristics overlap with those of CPP so the definitive diagnosis depends on histopathology. Large mass, irregular or "fuzzy" internal morphology, necrosis, and edema have been reported as suggestive of higher grade tumors.

Choroid Plexus Carcinoma

Etiology

Choroid plexus carcinoma (CPCa) is a rare malignant tumor that occurs almost exclusively in young children. Nearly 1/2 of all CPCas harbor *TP53* mutations.

Pathology

Gross Pathology. CPCa almost always arises in the lateral ventricle. This heterogeneous, bulky intraventricular tumor often displays gross hemorrhage and necrotic foci. Invasion into adjacent brain parenchyma is common. Frank features of malignancy include frequent mitoses, increased cellularity, nuclear pleomorphism, and necrosis.

CPCa is a WHO grade III neoplasm.

Clinical Issues

Demographics. CPCa represents 20-40% of all primary choroid plexus neoplasms. Between 70-80% of CPCas arise in children younger than 3 years. Median age at diagnosis is 18 months.

Presentation and Natural History. The most common symptoms—nausea, vomiting, headache, and obtundation—are caused by obstructive hydrocephalus. Prognosis in patients with these aggressive tumors is generally dismal, especially those with incomplete resection of a *TP53*-mutated genotype.

Imaging

CPCa often invades through the ventricular ependyma into adjacent brain. Edema, necrosis, intratumoral cysts, and hemorrhage are common **(18-19)**. Enhancement is typically strong but heterogeneous. CSF dissemination is common.

Differential Diagnosis

The major differential diagnoses are **choroid plexus papilloma (CPP)** and **atypical choroid plexus papilloma (aCPP)**. Imaging features of all three primary choroid plexus tumors overlap. CSF spread occurs with both benign and malignant varieties.

Other Neuroepithelial Tumors

"Other neuroepithelial tumors" is an eclectic group of uncommon neoplasms in the 2016 WHO that included astroblastoma, chordoid glioma of the third ventricle, and angiocentric glioma.

Astroblastoma

Astroblastoma (AB) is a rare glial neoplasm that mainly affects children, adolescents, and young adults. Mutations in genes that are commonly altered in infiltrating astrocytoma (e.g., *IDH1*, *ATRX*, or *TP53*) are absent.

"Astroblastoma" seems to be a histomorphologic pattern that can be seen across a spectrum of molecularly distinct tumor entities. Some exhibit features consistent with a recently identified **CNS high-grade neuroepithelial tumor with MN1 alteration**.

Imaging findings are nonspecific. Astroblastoma is almost exclusively a supratentorial, often superficially located hemispheric tumor that is typically well demarcated. Surrounding edema is minimal or absent. Most exhibit both solid and cystic components, frequently giving them a "bubbly" appearance **(18-20)**.

Chordoid Glioma of the Third Ventricle

Chordoid glioma (CG) is a rare slow-growing noninvasive adult tumor that is distinguished by its location (third ventricular region), stereotypical histology (both glial and chordoid elements), and characteristic imaging features.

CGs are solid, round, or slightly lobulated masses that arise in the anterior aspect of the third ventricle **(18-21)**. Microscopically, CGs resemble chordomas or chordoid meningiomas and are strongly positive for the glial marker GFAP but negative for IDH-1 immunostaining. CGs are WHO grade II neoplasms.

Radiologic features of reported CGs are remarkably consistent. Most are well-demarcated ovoid masses that are confined to the anterior third ventricle and are clearly separate from the pituitary gland and infundibulum **(18-22)**. Gross brain invasion is rare. CGs are typically isointense with brain on T1WI and iso- to slightly hyperintense on T2WI. Strong uniform enhancement is typical.

Primary third ventricular tumors in adults are all uncommon so the differential diagnosis is limited. As CGs are clearly separate from the pituitary gland, macroadenoma is usually not in the differential diagnosis, although a few purely third ventricular **pituitary macroadenomas** and **craniopharyngiomas** have been reported. **Chordoid meningioma** can look just like a CG, but the third ventricle is a rarely reported site for a rare meningioma variant. **Metastases** rarely occur in the third ventricle.

Tuber cinereum (TC) hamartomas are most common in preadolescent male patients with precocious puberty. Although TC hamartomas are isointense with brain on T1- and T2WI, they do not enhance. As CGs are tumors of adults, childhood hypothalamic tumors, such as adamantinomatous **craniopharyngioma** and **pilocytic astrocytoma**, are not diagnostic considerations.

Angiocentric Glioma

Angiocentric glioma (AG), a.k.a. "angiocentric neuroepithelial tumor," is an epilepsy-associated low-grade glioma. Because of its uncertain histogenesis, the WHO groups AG together with astroblastoma and chordoid glioma in the "other gliomas" category.

AG—a.k.a. "angiocentric neuroepithelial tumor"—is an epilepsy-associated WHO grade I glioma. The most common location is the cortex of the frontal and temporal lobes.

AGs are typically tumors of children and young adults. More than 95% of patients present with intractable focal epilepsy. Surgical excision is generally curative.

MR demonstrates a diffusely infiltrating expansile cortical mass without sharply demarcated borders. Most AGs are hyperintense on T2/FLAIR. A subtle rim of T1 shortening and stalk-like extension toward the ventricle have been described in some cases. Enhancement is generally absent. Focal cortical dysplasia can often be identified adjacent to the tumor.

Selected References: The complete reference list is available on the Expert Consult™ eBook version included with purchase.

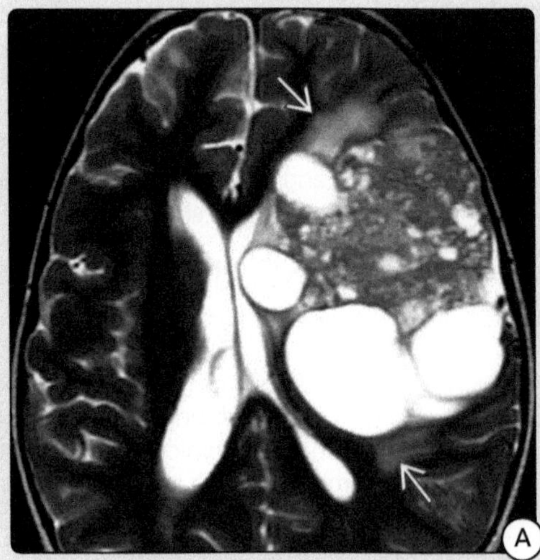

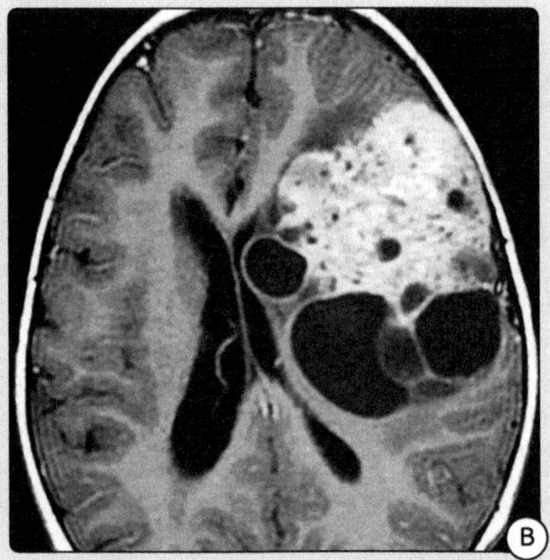

***(18-20A)** T2 MR shows typical findings of astroblastoma with innumerable tiny and multiple large cysts. Relative to the size of the mass, there is little peritumoral edema ➡.* ***(18-20B)** T1 C+ MR shows that the solid portions of the mass enhance, whereas the cysts do not.*

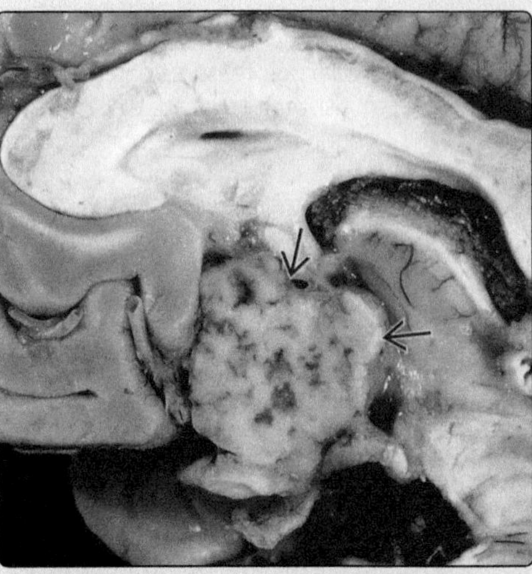

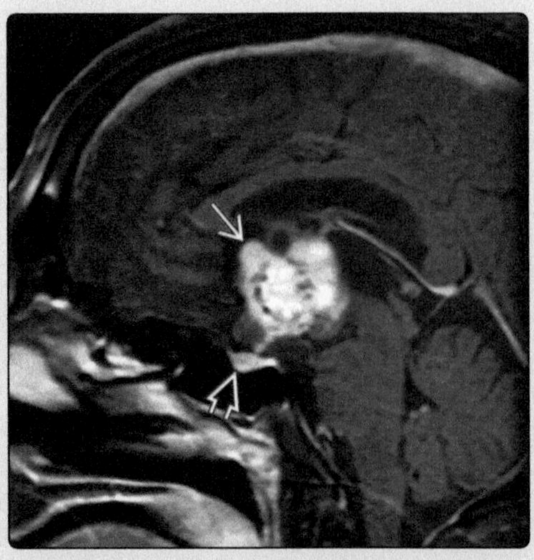

***(18-21)** Midline sagittal autopsy specimen shows chordoid glioma as a lobulated mass ➡ that fills the 3rd ventricle. (Courtesy P. Burger, MD.)* ***(18-22)** Sagittal T1 C+ MR shows a well-marginated, intensely but somewhat heterogeneously enhancing mass in the 3rd ventricle ➡. The infundibular stalk and pituitary gland ➡ appear entirely normal. Chordoid glioma of the 3rd ventricle was the histopathologic diagnosis.*

Neuronal and Glioneuronal Tumors

Neuronal and mixed glioneuronal tumors are much less common than astrocytomas and oligodendrogliomas, accounting for only 1-2% of all primary brain tumors. However, glioneuronal neoplasms are important as are relatively benign, slow-growing tumors that are frequently associated with epilepsy.

Glioneuronal Tumors

We begin this section by discussing the most common histologically mixed glioneuronal neoplasm, **ganglioglioma**. We then consider **dysembryoplastic neuroepithelial tumor (DNET)**, now recognized as one of the more common causes of temporal lobe epilepsy.

Overview of Ganglion Cell Tumors

Ganglion cell tumors are benign, well-differentiated neoplasms characterized by the presence of dysplastic ganglion cells. Two types of ganglion cell tumors are recognized: Gangliogliomas and gangliocytomas. Gangliocytomas—ganglion cell tumors that demonstrate *exclusive* ganglion cell composition—are relatively rare and discussed in the following section together with neuronal neoplasms and tumor-like lesions.

The vast majority of ganglion cell tumors are histologically mixed lesions that contain *both* neoplastic ganglion cell and glial elements. These neoplasms are called **gangliogliomas** and designated as WHO grade I. More aggressive tumors (i.e., those with substantial mitotic activity, microvascular proliferation, and occasional necrosis), called **anaplastic gangliomas**, are assigned WHO grade III.

Ganglioglioma

Terminology

Ganglioglioma (GG) is a well-differentiated, slow-growing tumor composed of dysplastic ganglion cells and neoplastic glial cells.

Etiology

The neuronal and glial components in GGs both likely derive from a common precursor cell. The most frequent genetic alterations are *BRAF* V600E mutation (40-60%). *H3F3A* mutations occur in midline pediatric grade 1 GGs but have a better outcome than the diffuse pontine gliomas.

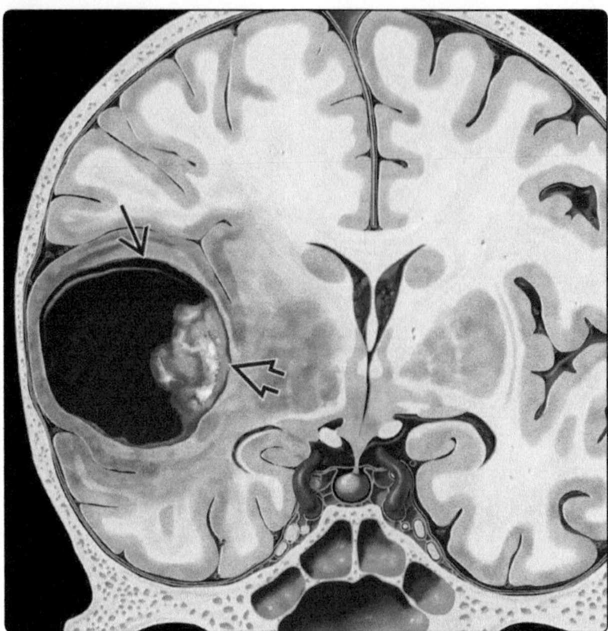

(19-1) Coronal graphic depicts a typical ganglioglioma (GG) of the temporal lobe with a cyst ➔ and a partially calcified mural nodule ➔.

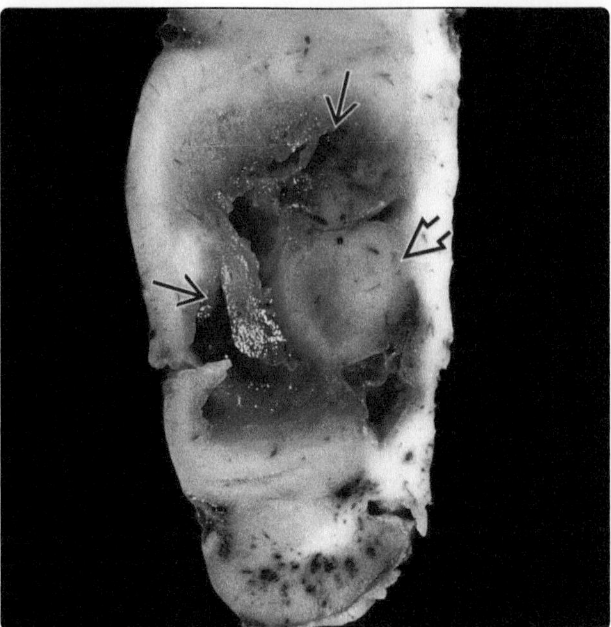

(19-2) Partial temporal lobectomy specimen with GG shows tumor nodule ➔, partially collapsed cysts ➔. Hemorrhage is primarily surgical. (Courtesy R. Hewlett, MD.)

Pathology

GGs occur throughout the CNS. Most are solitary and > 75% arise in the temporal lobe. The next most common site is the frontal lobe, the location for 10% of GGs. Approximately 15% of GGs are found in the posterior fossa, usually either in the brainstem or cerebellum. GGs vary in size from 1-6 cm and virtually never metastasize.

GGs are superficially located, well-delineated neoplasms that often expand the cortex. The most common appearance is that of a cyst with mural nodule **(19-1)** or a solid tumor. Calcification is common, but gross hemorrhage and frank necrosis are rare.

The histologic hallmark of GG is its combination of neuronal and glial elements, which can be intermixed or geographically separated. Varying numbers of dysplastic neurons are interspersed with the glial component, which constitutes the proliferative and neoplastic element of the tumor. Astrocytic cells with pilocytic or fibrillary-like features are the most common glial element.

GGs are benign and designated as WHO grade I neoplasms. GGs with anaplastic features correspond histologically to WHO grade III. Malignant features in GGs are uncommon but—when present—almost invariably involve the glial component. Malignant degeneration is uncommon, occurring in 1-5% of cases.

Clinical Issues

GG is predominantly a tumor of children and young adults; 80% of patients are younger than 30 years old. Peak presentation is 15-20 years old. Chronic, pharmacologically resistant temporal lobe epilepsy is present in the majority of cases. Seizures are generally the complex partial type.

GGs are typically very slow-growing neoplasms. Complete surgical resection is generally curative with 80% of patients becoming seizure free after tumor removal.

Imaging

General Features. GGs are cortically based superficial parenchymal lesions that have two general imaging patterns: (1) A well-defined solid or partially cystic mass with mural nodule **(19-2)** and (2) a diffusely infiltrating, less well-delineated mass with ill-defined borders and patchy enhancement uncommonly occurring.

CT Findings. GGs display varying attenuation on NECT. A cystic component is seen in nearly 60% of cases. Approximately 30% have a well-circumscribed hypodense cyst with isodense mural nodule **(19-3A)**, whereas 40% are primarily hypodense. Between 30-50% of GGs calcify. Hemorrhage is rare. Only 50% of GGs enhance following contrast administration. Patterns vary from solid, rim, or nodular to cystic with an enhancing nodule.

MR Findings. GGs are hypo- to isointense relative to cortex on T1WI and hyperintense on T2/FLAIR **(19-3B)**. Surrounding edema is generally absent. Focal cortical dysplasia (FCD) adjacent to the tumor occurs in some cases.

Enhancement varies from none or minimal to moderate but heterogeneous. The classic pattern is a cystic mass with an enhancing mural nodule **(19-3C)**. Homogeneous solid enhancement also occurs. Ill-defined, patchy enhancement is atypical and associated with a worse clinical outcome **(19-4)**.

Differential Diagnosis

Diffuse astrocytoma is typically infiltrating, not well circumscribed, and does not enhance. A supratentorial hemispheric **pilocytic astrocytoma** can present as a cyst with an enhancing nodule. Calcification is rare compared with GG. **Pleomorphic xanthoastrocytoma** (PXA) often has a "cyst + mural nodule" and can resemble GG but often has a dural "tail."

Dysembryoplastic neuroepithelial tumor (DNET) is a superficial cortical neoplasm that typically has a multicystic "bubbly" appearance. A hyperintense rim surrounding the mass on FLAIR scan is common. In contrast to GG, enhancement is rare. **Oligodendroglioma** commonly involves the cortex but is typically more diffuse and less well delineated than GG. Oligodendrogliomas with a "cyst + mural nodule" configuration are uncommon.

CAUSES OF TEMPORAL LOBE EPILEPSY

Most Common = Mesial Temporal Sclerosis

Tumor-Associated Temporal Lobe Epilepsy

- Ganglioglioma (40%)
- DNET (20%)
- Diffuse low-grade astrocytoma (20%)
- Other (20%)
  - Pilocytic astrocytoma
  - Pleomorphic xanthoastrocytoma
  - Oligodendroglioma

Anaplastic Ganglioglioma

Anaplastic ganglioglioma (AGG) is rare, representing only 5-6% of all GGs. Most occur as malignant transformation of previously diagnosed GGs **(19-4)** and almost invariably involve the glial component. AGGs are WHO grade III neoplasms.

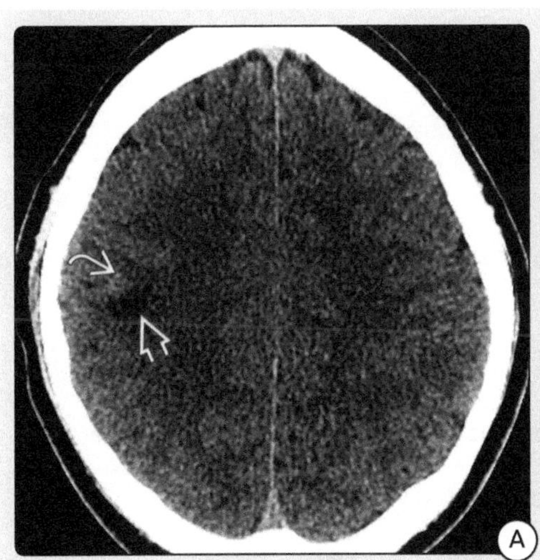

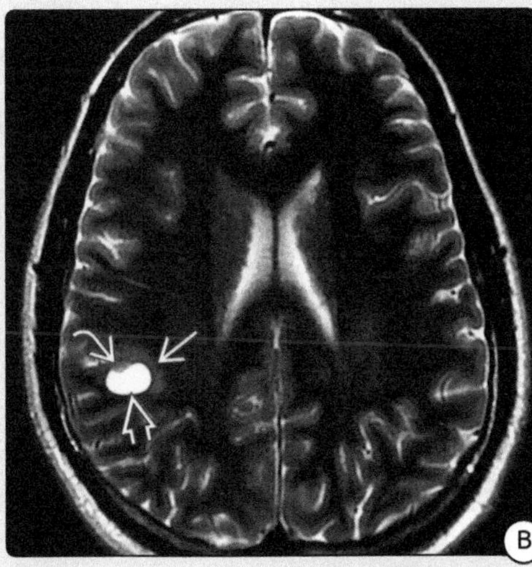

***(19-3A)** NECT in a 24-year-old man with intractable seizures shows a right posterior frontal cyst ➡ with a slightly hyperdense nodule ➡. Lesion is located at the cortex in the bottom of a sulcus. **(19-3B)** T2 MR shows that the cyst ➡ is extremely hyperintense. The small mural nodule ➡ is isointense with cortex ➡, which surrounds the mass completely.*

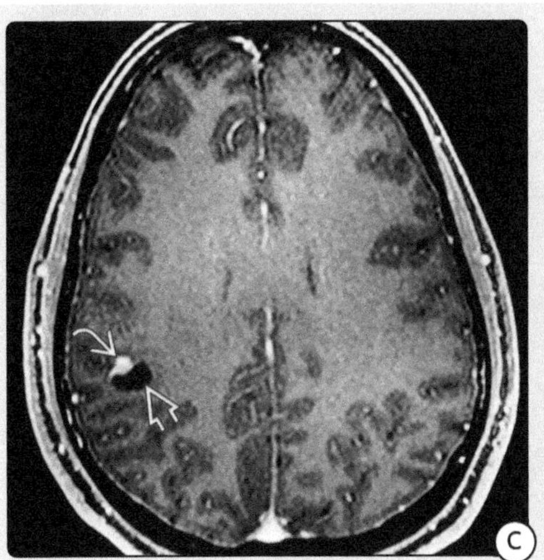

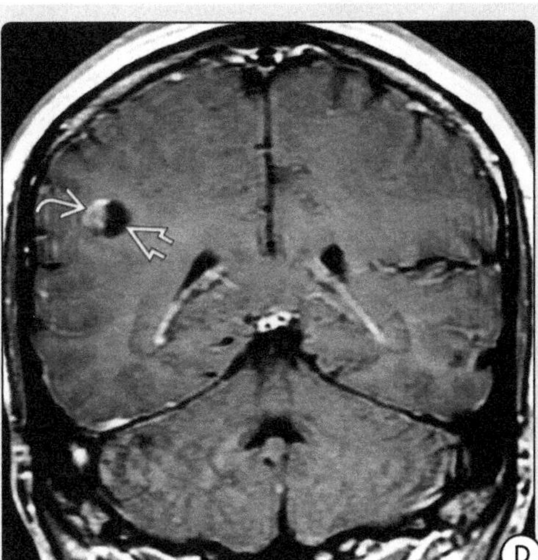

***(19-3C)** T1 C+ SPGR shows that the nodule ➡ enhances intensely while the cyst wall ➡ does not. **(19-3D)** Coronal T1 C+ MR nicely depicts the classic configuration of a GG with cyst ➡, enhancing mural nodule ➡. GG was completely resected and the patient's longstanding epilepsy resolved.*

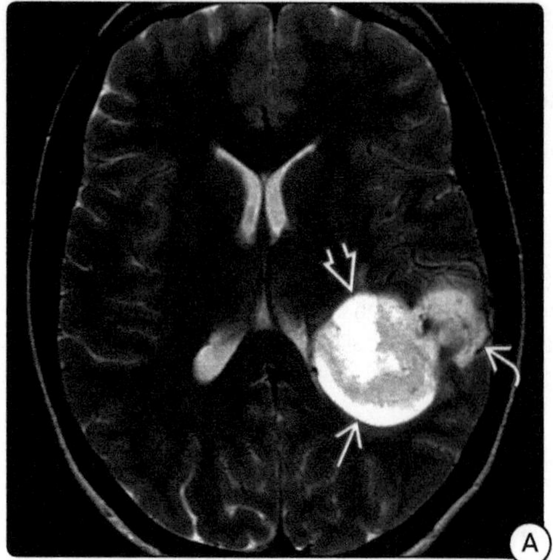

***(19-4A)** T2 MR shows a heterogeneously hyperintense left parietal mass and cyst extending superficially toward the cortex.*

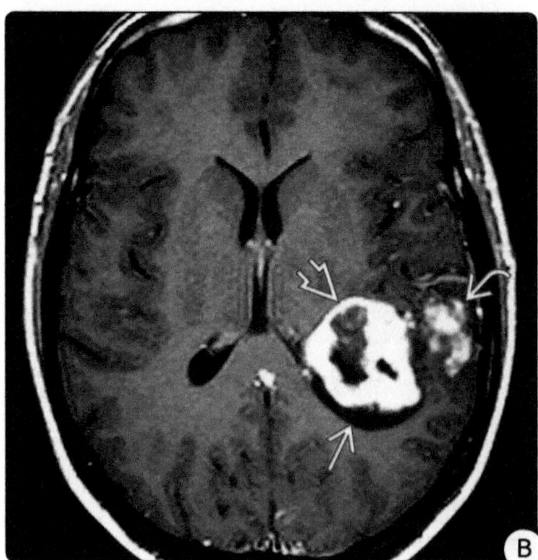

***(19-4B)** T1 C+ shows cystic, solid enhancing mass, patchy enhancement in the cortex; GG WHO grade I but with "atypical" features.*

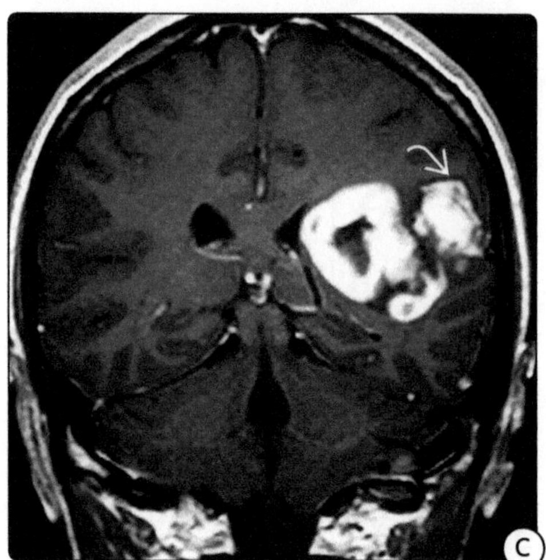

***(19-4C)** T1 C+ MR shows deep tumor, ill-defined enhancement. Subtotal resection; recurred later with anaplastic features, WHO grade III.*

GANGLIOGLIOMAS

Ganglioglioma

- Terminology
  - Well-differentiated, slow-growing tumor
  - Variable combination of neuronal, glial elements
- Etiology and genetics
  - *BRAF* V600E mutation
  - IDH1(-), 1p/19q not codeleted
- Pathology
  - Dysplastic ganglion cells + neoplastic glial cells
  - Superficial, corticocentric
  - Solid or mixed cystic/solid, usually noninfiltrative
  - Temporal, frontal lobes > parietal > brainstem, ventricles
  - WHO grade I
- Clinical issues
  - Most common mixed glial-neuronal neoplasm
  - Children, young adults
  - Common presentation = seizures
- Imaging findings
  - Well-delineated (often temporal lobe) mass
  - Cyst + enhancing nodule most common

Anaplastic Ganglioglioma

- Pathology
  - Usually malignant transformation of benign GG
  - Dysplastic ganglion cells + anaplastic glial component
  - WHO grade III
- Imaging findings
  - Atypical location common (i.e., deep rather than cortical)
  - Often larger, more infiltrative/poorly demarcated

DNET

Ganglioglioma and dysembryoplastic neuroepithelial tumor (DNET) are the two most common long-term epilepsy-associated tumors (so-called "LEATs"). The 2016 WHO classification includes DNET in the category of "neuronal and mixed neuronal-glial tumors."

Terminology

DNET is a benign, usually cortically based lesion characterized by a multinodular architecture **(19-5)**. Because DNET is often associated with cortical dysplasia, some neuropathologists believe it may be a congenital malformation rather than a true neoplastic lesion.

Etiology

Although the exact histogenesis remains unknown, *FGFR1* alterations and MAP kinase pathway activation are key events in the pathogenesis of DNET. *BRAF* V600E mutations occur in 30-60% of cases. *TP53* and IDH mutations as well as 1p/19q codeletions are absent.

Pathology

DNETs are cortically based neoplasms. Between 45-50% are located in the temporal lobes, whereas 1/3 occur in the frontal lobes. Other locations, such as the lateral ventricle, are rare. An unusual "diffuse" form of DNET has also been described.

Grossly, DNETs thicken and expand the gyri. Most are solitary, varying in size from millimeters to several centimeters **(19-7)**. The adjacent cortex is dysplastic in nearly 80% of DNETs. DNETs are WHO grade I neoplasms.

Clinical Issues

DNET is a tumor of children and young adults. The vast majority present before the age of 20 years, typically with pharmacologically resistant partial complex seizures. Although DNETs account for only 1% of all neuroepithelial tumors, they are second only to ganglioglioma as a cause of temporal lobe epilepsy.

DNETs exhibit little or no growth, but because cortical dysplasia is frequently associated with DNET, a more aggressive resection is often performed. Long-term clinical follow-up usually demonstrates no tumor recurrence, even in patients with subtotal resection.

DNET: ETIOLOGY AND PATHOLOGY

Etiology

- *FGFR1*, *BRAF* mutations

Pathology

- Benign (WHO grade I)
- Rare (< 1% of all neuroepithelial tumors)
- Location
  - Supratentorial, superficial
  - Intracortical
  - Temporal lobe most common site
- Frequently associated with cortical dysplasia
  - Classified as ILAE FCD type IIIb

Imaging

DNET has a distinct appearance on neuroimaging studies. A well-demarcated, triangular, "pseudocystic" or "bubbly" cortical/subcortical mass in a young patient with longstanding complex partial epilepsy is highly suggestive of the diagnosis **(19-6)**.

NECT scans disclose a hypodense cortical/subcortical mass. Calcification is seen in 20% of cases. Gross intratumoral hemorrhage is rare. Focal bony scalloping or calvarial remodeling is common with tumors adjacent to the inner table of the skull.

A multicystic or septated appearance is typical on MR **(19-8A)**. DNETs are strikingly hyperintense on T2WI **(19-8B)**. A FLAIR hyperintense rim along the tumor periphery is present in 75% of cases **(19-8C)**. Peritumoral edema is absent. "Blooming" on T2* (GRE, SWI) occurs in a few cases, more likely related to calcification than to hemorrhage.

DNETs generally show little or no enhancement on T1WI C+. When present, enhancement is generally limited to a mild nodular or punctate pattern.

Differential Diagnosis

The main differential diagnoses are **focal cortical dysplasia** (often associated), **ganglioglioma**, and **multinodular and vacuolating neuronal tumor of the cerebrum** (MVNT). The "bubbly" appearance of DNET and FLAIR hyperintense rim are helpful distinguishing features. MVNTs are typically multifocal and occur in the deep layers of the cortex and white matter, not superficially located like DNET. **Angiocentric glioma** closely resembles DNET on imaging but a hyperintense rim is seen on T1WI, not FLAIR.

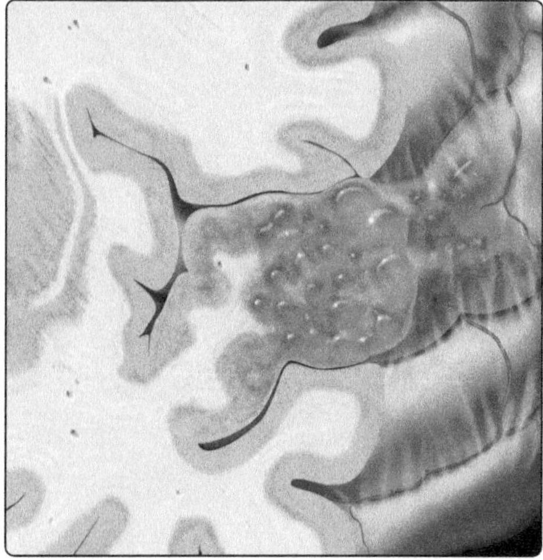

***(19-5)** Graphic depicts DNET with multicystic and multinodular components.*

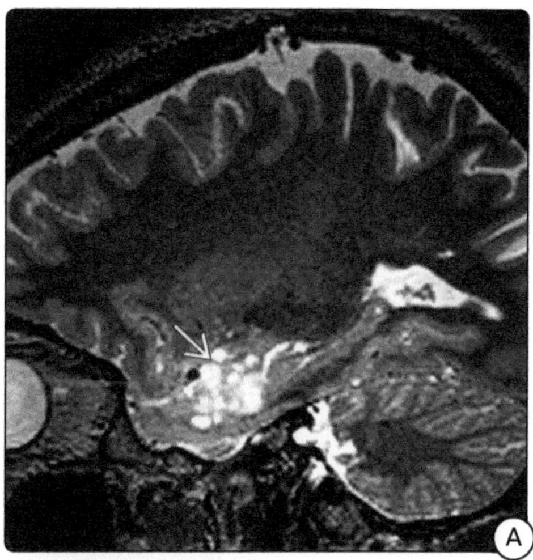

***(19-6A)** Sagittal T2 MR shows a "bubbly" temporal lobe mass ➡.*

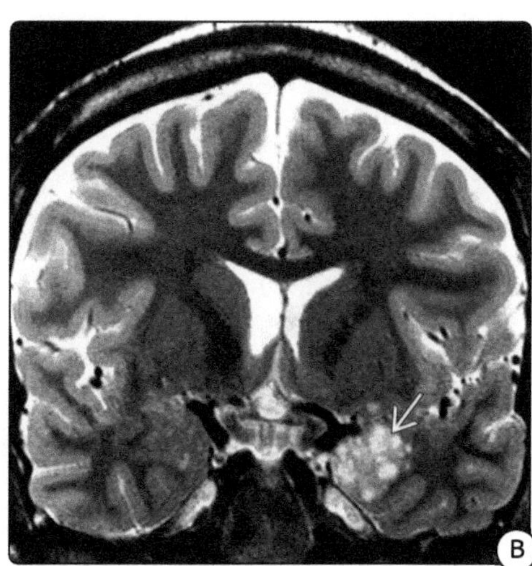

***(19-6B)** Coronal T2 MR in the same patient shows a cortically based, "bubbly" mass with the typical appearance of a DNET ➡.*

DNET: CLINICAL ISSUES AND IMAGING

Clinical Issues

- Most patients < 20 years old
- Intractable epilepsy common
- Grows slowly; surgery usually curative

Imaging

- Wedge-shaped cortical/subcortical mass
- Tip "points" toward ventricle
- Multicystic/septated "bubbly" appearance
  - Hyperintense on T2WI
  - FLAIR hyperintense rim
  - Edema absent
  - Usually no enhancement

Neuronal Tumors

Tumors that exhibit exclusive ganglion cell or neurocytic differentiation are rare. Two general categories of neuronal tumors are recognized: Gangliocytoma and neurocytoma.

We begin our discussion of ganglion cell tumors with the pure ganglion cell neoplasm, **gangliocytoma**, and its most common presentation, cerebellar gangliocytoma [better known as **Lhermitte-Duclos disease** (LDD)]. We close this section with a unique, newly described pattern of ganglion cell tumor called **multinodular and vacuolating neuronal tumor of the cerebrum**.

(19-7) Resected surgical specimen shows the typical nodular, somewhat "mucinous-appearing" cysts ➡ of a DNET. (Courtesy R. Hewlett, MD.) (19-8A) Sagittal T1 C+ MR in a 14-year-old boy with longstanding right body complex partial seizures shows a wedge-shaped, superficially located "bubbly" mass ➡. The mass is hypointense and shows no enhancement. Note the adjacent calvarial remodeling ➡.

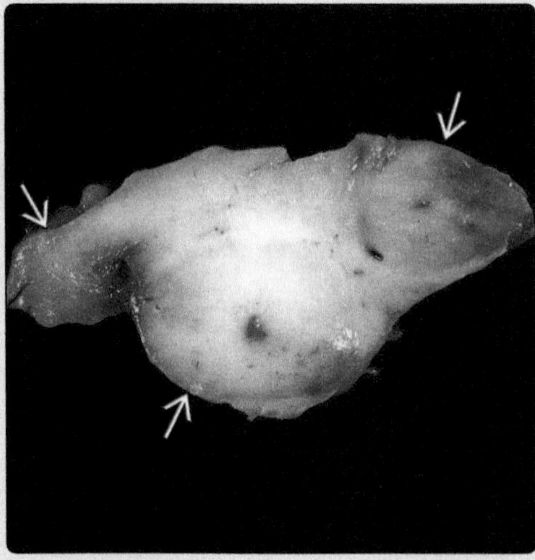

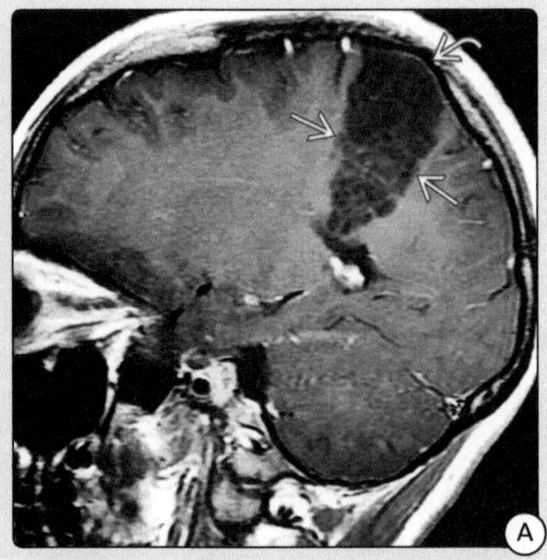

(19-8B) T2 MR in the same case shows that the "bubbly appearing" mass ➡ is very hyperintense and sharply demarcated. There is no surrounding edema. (19-8C) FLAIR MR in the same case shows that the mass is heterogeneously hypointense with a hyperintense rim ➡. Classic DNET was found at surgery.

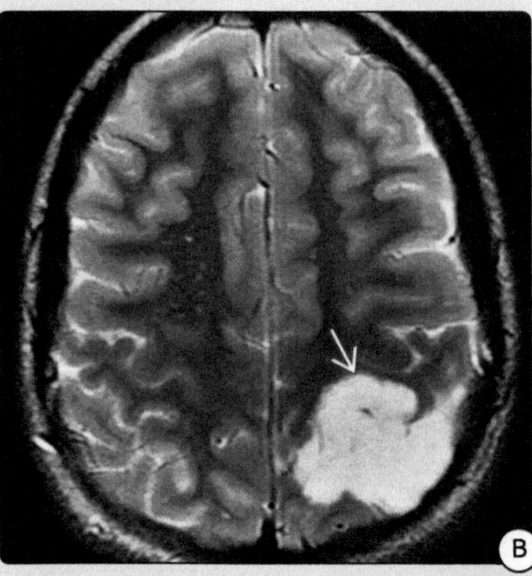

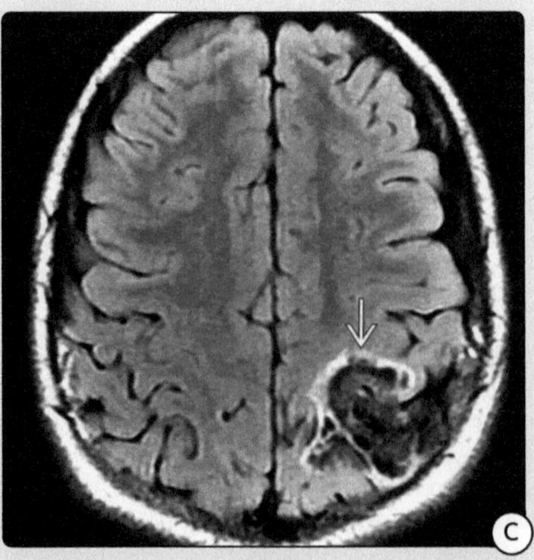

Cerebral Gangliocytoma

Terminology

Gangliocytoma (GCyt) is a benign, well-circumscribed neoplasm that contains only differentiated ganglion cells. No glial component is present. Cerebral hemisphere GCyts are very rare.

Pathology

GCyts can be solid or mixed solid and cystic lesions that consist of bizarre-appearing but mature ganglion cells. Mitoses are few or absent. GCyts are WHO grade I neoplasms.

Clinical Issues

GCyt occurs most frequently in children and young adults under the age of 30 years. Most patients present with pharmacoresistant epilepsy. GCyts grow slowly, if at all. Surgical resection is generally curative.

Imaging

GCyts are of mixed density on NECT, often containing both cystic and solid components **(19-9A)**. Calcification is common, occurring in ~ 1/3 of cases. Hemorrhage and necrosis are absent.

GCyts are hypo- to isointense relative to cortex on T1WI and hyperintense on T2/FLAIR. Enhancement varies from none to striking homogeneous enhancement in the solid portions of the tumor **(19-9)**.

Differential Diagnosis

The major differential diagnosis of GCyt is **ganglioglioma**. Gangliogliomas are far more common and may be indistinguishable from GCyt on imaging studies.

Cortical dysplasia, another common cause of refractory epilepsy in young patients, follows gray matter on all sequences and does not enhance.

Dysplastic Cerebellar Gangliocytoma

Terminology

Dysplastic cerebellar gangliocytoma is a rare benign cerebellar mass composed of dysplastic ganglion cells that is better known as **Lhermitte-Duclos disease** (LDD).

LDD may occur as part of the multiple hamartoma syndrome called **Cowden syndrome** (CS). When LDD and CS occur together, they are sometimes called Cowden-Lhermitte-Duclos or **COLD syndrome**. CS is also known as **multiple hamartoma-neoplasia syndrome** or **PTEN hamartoma tumor syndrome**.

CS is an autosomal dominant phacomatosis. The vast majority of patients have hamartomatous neoplasms of the skin combined with neoplasms and hamartomas of multiple other organs. Breast, thyroid, endometrium, and gastrointestinal cancers are the most prevalent other neoplasms in CS.

Etiology

Whether LDD constitutes a neoplastic, malformative, or hamartomatous lesion is debated. The majority of cases are sporadic but the association of LDD with CS favors a hamartomatous origin.

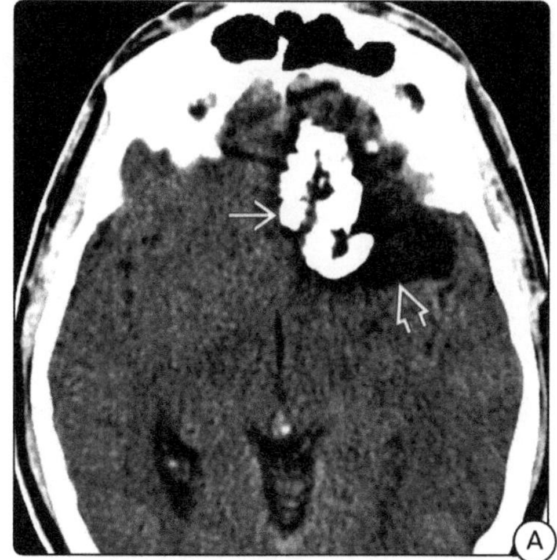

***(19-9A)** NECT scan in a 29-year-old man with seizures shows a partially calcified ➡, partially cystic ➡ left frontal lobe mass.*

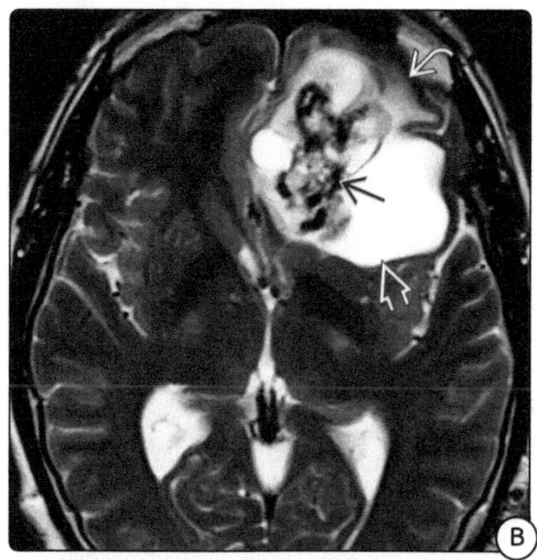

***(19-9B)** T2 MR shows that the solid portion of the mass ➡ is very heterogeneous, the adjacent cyst ➡ is hyperintense, and edema ➡ is minimal.*

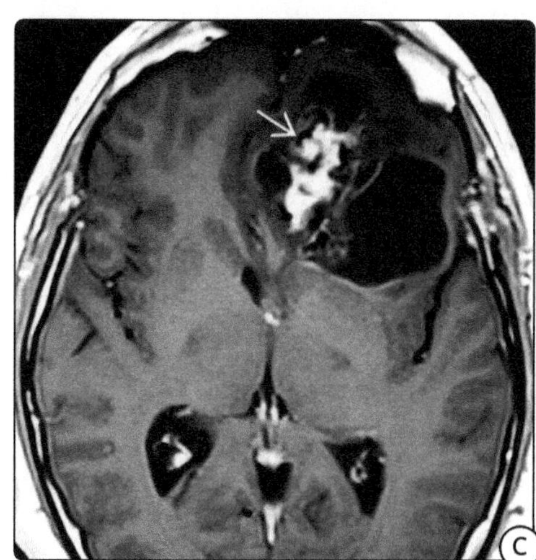

***(19-9C)** Tumor nodule shows mild patchy enhancement ➡. This was pathologically proven gangliocytoma. (Courtesy N. Agarwal, MD.)*

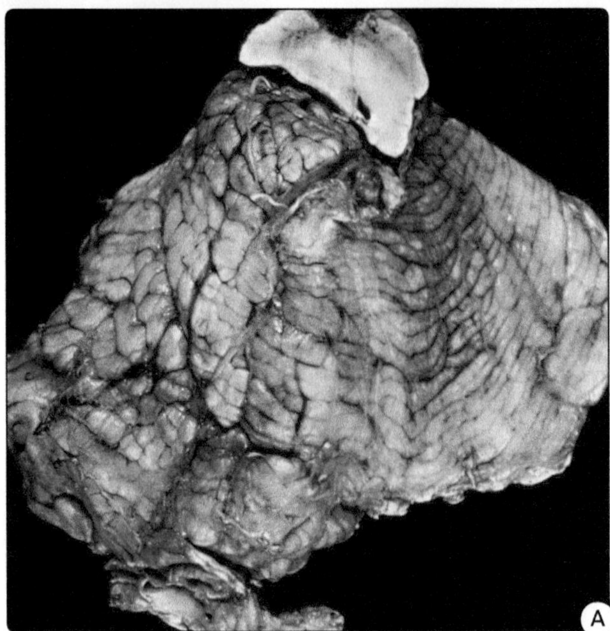

(19-10A) Autopsy specimen shows dysplastic cerebellar gangliocytoma expanding the cerebellar hemisphere. (Courtesy AFIP Archives.)

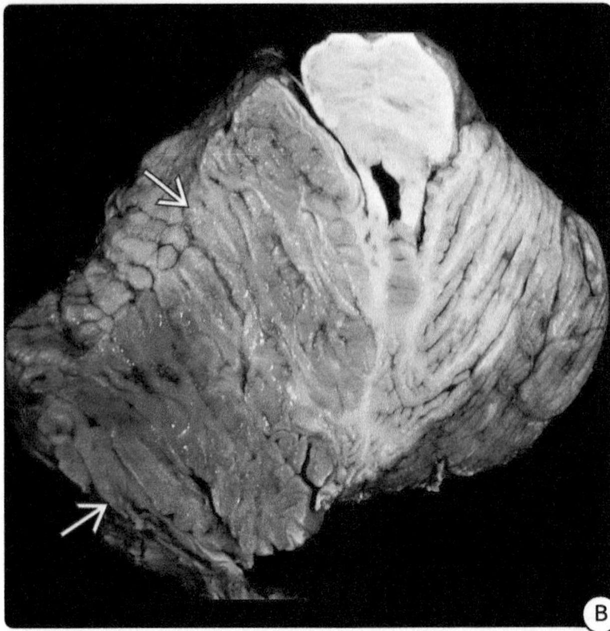

(19-10B) Cut section through the mass shows grossly thickened cerebellar folia ➡. (Courtesy AFIP Archives.)

Approximately 40% of dysplastic cerebellar gangliocytomas occur as part of CS. CS is caused by a *PTEN* germline mutation that results in multiple hamartomas and malignant neoplasms.

Pathology

LDD is always infratentorial, usually involving the cerebellar hemisphere or the vermis. Dysplastic cerebellar gangliocytomas often become very large, displacing the fourth ventricle and causing obstructive hydrocephalus.

The gross appearance of LDD is a tumor-like mass that expands and replaces the normal cerebellar architecture **(19-10A)**. On cut section, the cerebellar folia are markedly widened and have a grossly "gyriform" appearance **(19-10B)**.

Microscopically, LDD is characterized by marked disruption of the normal cerebellar cortical layers. Diffuse hypertrophy of the granular cell layer with absence of the Purkinje layer of the cerebellum is typical. Mitoses and necrosis are absent.

It is unclear whether dysplastic cerebellar gangliocytoma (LDD) is neoplastic or hamartomatous. If neoplastic, LDD corresponds to WHO grade I.

Clinical Issues

LDD occurs in all age groups, but most cases occur in adults between 20-40 years. The average age at diagnosis is 34 years. Patients may be asymptomatic or present with symptoms of increased intracranial pressure, such as headache, nausea, and vomiting. Cranial nerve palsies, gait disturbance, and visual abnormalities are also common.

LDD enlarges very slowly over many years. No cases of metastatic spread or CSF dissemination have been reported. Shunting or surgical debulking are options for symptomatic patients with hydrocephalus.

Imaging

General Features. A nonenhancing unilateral cerebellar mass in a middle-aged patient that demonstrates a prominent "tiger stripe" pattern **(19-11)** on MR is typical of LDD.

CT Findings. Most cases of LDD are hypodense on NECT. Mass effect with compression of the fourth ventricle, effacement of the cerebellopontine angle cisterns, and obstructive hydrocephalus is common. Calcification is rare. CECT generally shows no appreciable enhancement.

MR Findings. An expansile cerebellar mass with linear hypointense bands on T1WI is typical. T2WI shows the nearly pathognomonic "tiger stripe" pattern of alternating inner hyperintense and outer hypointense layers in enlarged cerebellar folia **(19-12)**.

T2* (GRE, SWI) demonstrates prominent venous channels surrounding the grossly thickened folia. T1 C+ shows striking linear enhancement of these abnormal veins in between the folia.

DWI may show restricted diffusion, probably reflecting the hypercellularity and increased axonal density characteristic of LDD. PWI shows increased relative cerebral blood volume, reflecting the prominent enlarged interfolial veins, not malignancy. MRS shows normal or slightly reduced NAA and normal Cho:Cr ratios. A lactate doublet may be present.

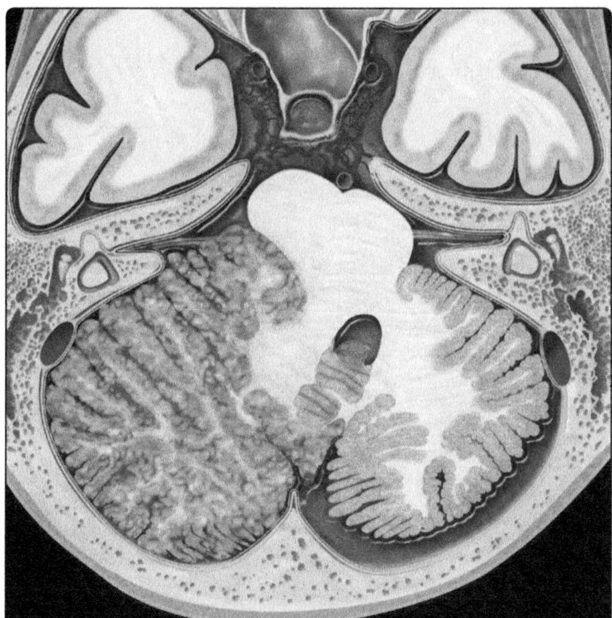

(19-11) *Graphic depicts dysplastic cerebellar gangliocytoma (Lhermitte-Duclos disease).*

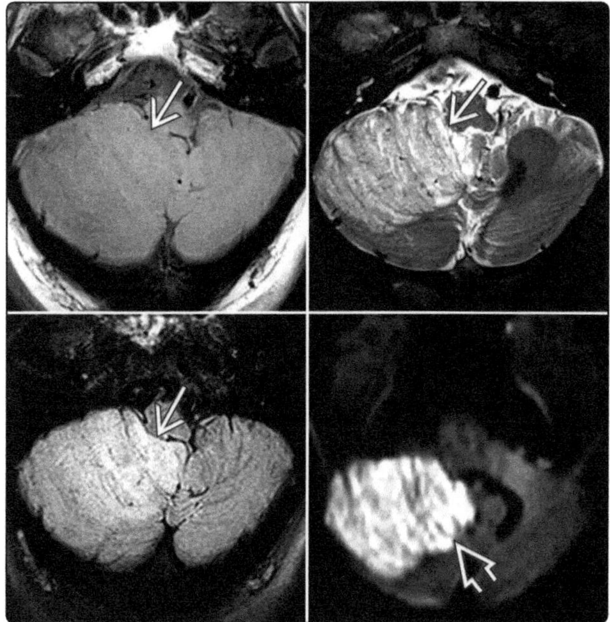

(19-12) *Series of MRs in a patient with LDD shows typical findings of thickened cerebellar folia and mass effect ➡. LDD is cellular and may show restricted diffusion ➡.*

Differential Diagnosis

Imaging findings of LDD are so characteristic that the diagnosis can usually be established without biopsy confirmation.

Medulloblastoma, especially the Shh desmoplastic variant, may present as a lateral cerebellar mass but usually occurs in younger patients and rarely displays the "tiger stripes" so characteristic of LDD. **Cerebellar infarction** is confined to a specific vascular territory, and symptom onset is acute or subacute rather than chronic. Occasionally, **ganglioglioma** occurs in the posterior fossa and may mimic LDD. Gangliogliomas typically enhance and, although sometimes bizarre-appearing, rarely demonstrate prominent "tiger stripes."

A few rare **cerebellar cortical dysplasias** can mimic LDD. However, these malformations do not demonstrate progressive enlargement and rarely cause mass effect with hydrocephalus.

A few cases of posterior fossa **tuberous sclerosis complex** (TSC) that mimic LDD have been reported. However, these patients are generally younger and have other stigmata of TSC.

CEREBRAL GANGLIOCYTOMAS

Gangliocytoma
- Pathology
  - Rare tumor composed of differentiated ganglion cells
  - Temporal lobe (75%)
  - WHO grade I
- Clinical issues
  - Most patients < 30 years
  - Epilepsy
- Imaging findings
  - "Cyst + nodule" or solid
  - No hemorrhage, necrosis
  - Ca^{++} frequent, enhancement variable

Dysplastic Cerebellar Gangliocytoma
- Terminology
  - Lhermitte-Duclos disease (LDD)
  - LDD + multiple hamartomas = Cowden-Lhermitte-Duclos (COLD)
- Pathology
  - Enlarged, thick "gyriform" cerebellar folia
  - Hypertrophied granular layer, absent Purkinje
  - WHO grade I
- Imaging findings
  - Mass with laminated, "tiger stripe" appearance
  - Linear enhancement of veins around thickened folia

Multinodular and Vacuolating Tumor of the Cerebrum
- Unique pattern of gangliocytoma (see next box)
- T2-/FLAIR-hyperintense "bubbles" along inner surface of cortex

Multinodular and Vacuolating Tumor of the Cerebrum

Terminology

Multinodular and vacuolating neuronal tumor (MVNT) of the cerebrum is a recently described clinicopathologic lesion with uncertain class assignment. The 2016 WHO includes MVNT as a "pattern" of gangliocytoma.

Etiology

It was initially unclear whether MVNT represents a true neoplasm or is a hamartomatous/malformative process ("quasi-tumor"). Recent analyses have demonstrated that MVNT is a clonal neoplasm defined by genetic alterations that activate the MAP kinase signaling pathway.

Pathology

MVNTs consist of multiple discrete and coalescent nodules exhibiting varying degrees of matrix vacuolization. They are located primarily within the deep cortical ribbon and superficial subcortical white matter, although separate nodules sometimes occur in the deep and periventricular white matter **(19-13)**.

Histopathologically, MVNTs are characterized by ambiguous to recognizably neuronal cells &/or dysplastic ganglion cells with cytoplasmic vacuoles. *IDH1/2*, *BRAF*, and 1p19q mutations are absent.

Clinical Issues

Most cases of MVNT are discovered incidentally on imaging studies. Seizures and headache are the principal clinical manifestations.

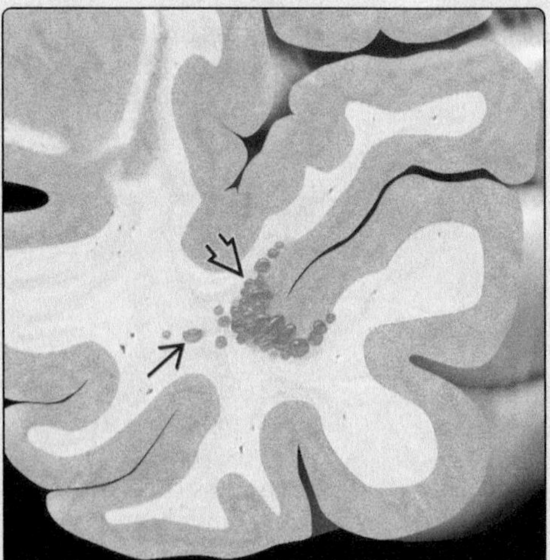

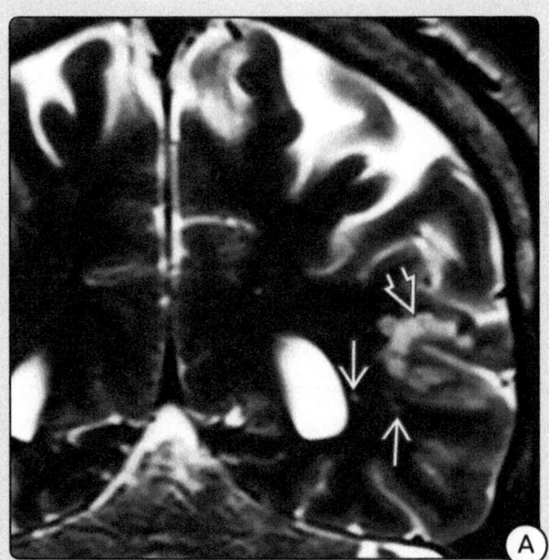

***(19-13)** Graphic depicts MVNT pattern of gangliocytoma seen as clustered ⇨ and scattered ⇨, variably sized, cystic-appearing nodules on the inner cortex, superficial white matter. **(19-14A)** Coronal T2 MR shows a cluster of variably sized cysts in the superficial white matter that hugs the inner cortex in a distinct U-shaped configuration ➡. Note similar-appearing scattered nodules in the deep white matter ➡, a typical pattern of MVNT.*

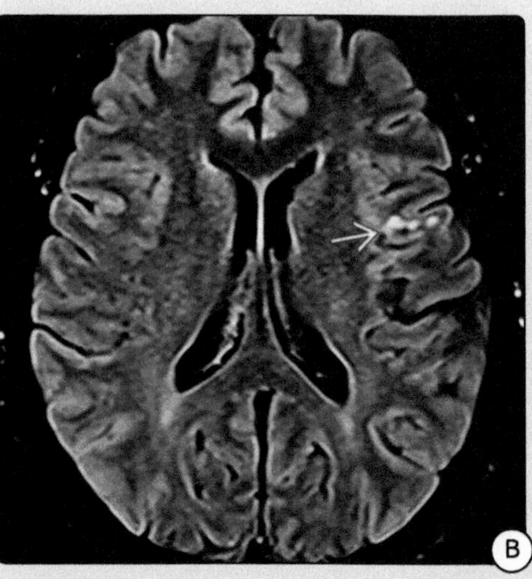

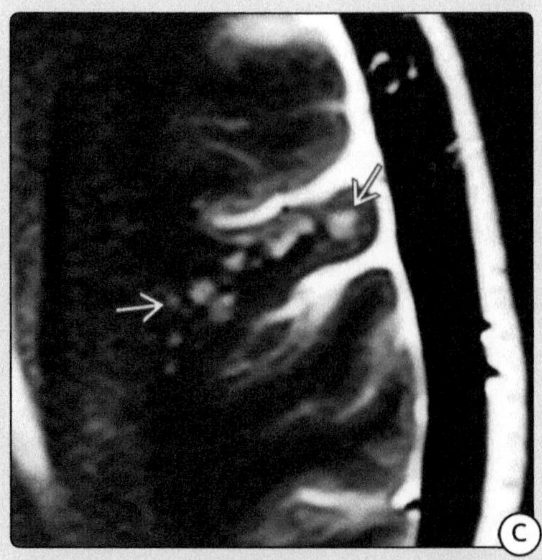

***(19-14B)** Axial FLAIR MR in a patient with headache and a nonfocal neurologic examination shows several discrete subcortical nodules ➡ that do not suppress and do not cause mass effect. **(19-14C)** Close-up view of the T2WI in the same case shows that the scattered hyperintense nodules ➡ are variably sized, located along the deep margin of the cortical ribbon and subcortical white matter. This was presumed MVNT.*

Imaging

MVNTs are benign, nonaggressive-appearing lesions that remain stable over serial imaging. CT scans are typically normal. Large coalescent collections may appear as ill-defined subcortical hypodensities **(19-15)** without evidence for calcification, hemorrhage, or mass effect **(19-15A)**.

MR scans show a unique, virtually pathognomonic pattern of multiple, variably sized (usually small) discrete and coalescent nodules along the inner cortical ribbon and subcortical white matter **(19-14A)** **(19-14C)**. The nodules are isointense with gray matter on T1WI and hyperintense on T2WI.

MVNTs do not suppress on FLAIR **(19-14B)** and may be embedded in FLAIR-hyperintense white matter. A characteristic appearance is that of a ribbon-like or nodular pattern that "cups" the undersurface of the cortex in a U-shaped configuration **(19-14A)**. Occasionally, more diffuse confluent gyriform or "tiger stripe" T2/FLAIR hyperintensity infiltrates the cortex. Mass effect and edema are absent. Enhancement is rare.

Differential Diagnosis

MVNTs are often misdiagnosed on imaging studies as "atypical perivascular spaces." PVSs suppress on FLAIR while MVNTs remain hyperintense.

The major differential diagnoses of MVNT include dysembryoplastic neuroepithelial tumor (DNET) and focal cortical dysplasia. **DNET** typically involves the whole cortical ribbon and extends to the surface. The nodules of MVNT are typically smaller with multiple scattered discrete nodules rather than the solid coalescent mass of DNET. Most foci of **cortical dysplasia** are isointense with gray matter on all sequences.

MULTINODULAR AND VACUOLATING TUMOR OF THE CEREBRUM (MVNT)

Terminology
- 2016 WHO considers MVNT a "pattern" of gangliocytoma
- Malformation vs. neoplasm?
  - True clonal neoplasm with MAP kinase alterations

Pathology
- Discrete, coalescent vacuolated nodules
- Deep cortical ribbon/subcortical white matter
- Benign, nonaggressive (WHO grade I)

Clinical Issues
- Usually found incidentally on imaging
- Most common = headache, seizure

Imaging Features
- Multiple discrete small T2-/FLAIR-hyperintense nodules
  - Tiny "bubbles"
- Along undersurface of cortex
  - Form "cup" around cortex
  - Ribbon of U-shaped hyperintensity
- Can be imbedded in FLAIR-hyperintense white matter
- Normal MRS, DWI

Differential Diagnosis
- DNET (larger, surface of cortex)
- Cortical dysplasia/hamartoma

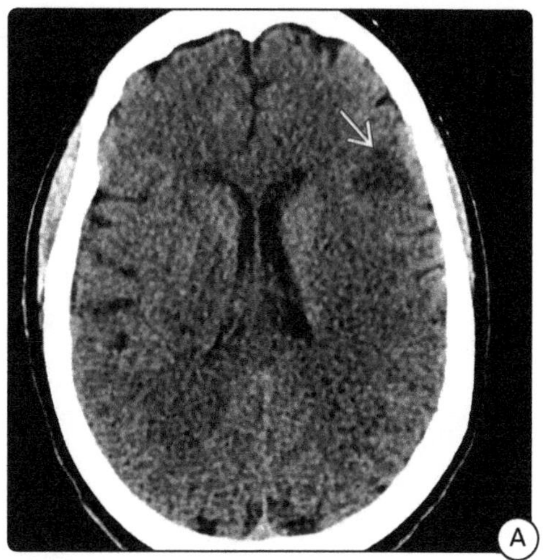

***(19-15A)** NECT in a 63-year-old woman with headaches shows wedge-shaped subcortical hypodensity ➡ in the left frontal lobe.*

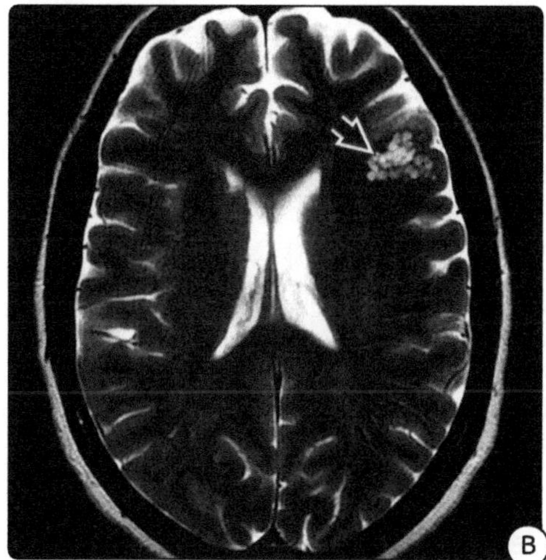

***(19-15B)** T2 MR shows collection of hyperintense nodules ➡ under the cortex extending into the white matter. Nodules did not suppress on FLAIR.*

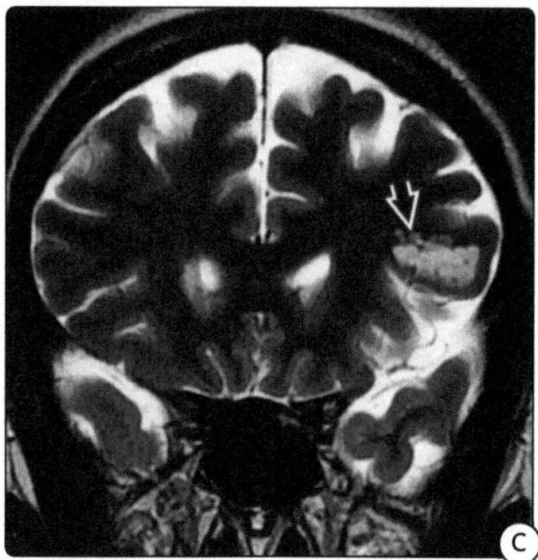

***(19-15C)** Coronal T2 MR shows superficial cortex is spared and clustered nodules ➡ are located along deep margin. This is presumed MVNT.*

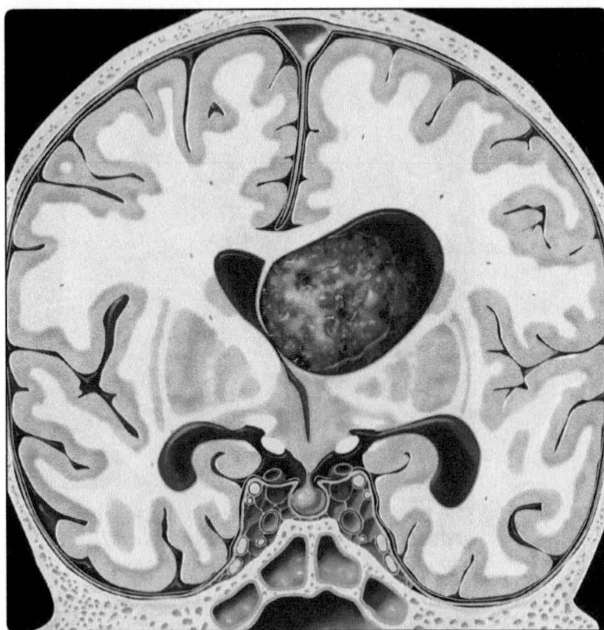

(19-16) Coronal graphic depicts central neurocytoma as a multicystic, relatively vascular, occasionally hemorrhagic mass in the body of the lateral ventricle.

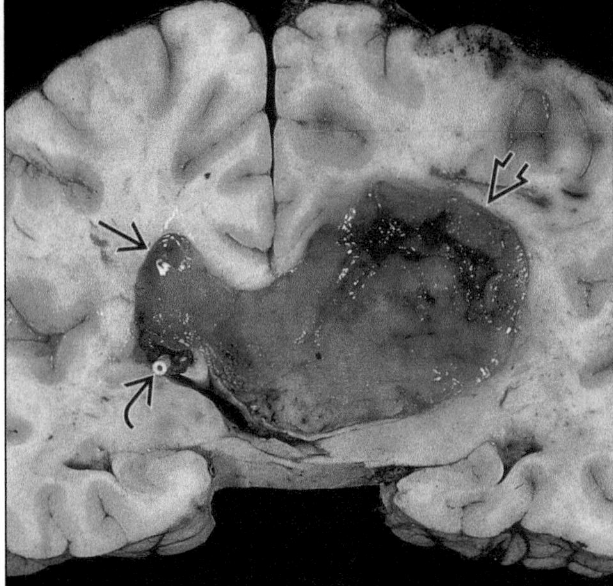

(19-17) Coronal autopsy shows a vascular, flesh-appearing central neurocytoma expanding the left lateral ventricle ⇨, crossing through the foramen of Monro to fill the right lateral ventricle →. Note ventricular shunt ↗. (Neuropathology, 2013.)

Central Neurocytoma

An unusual benign-acting intraventricular neoplasm of young adults, originally thought to be an oligodendroglioma subtype, is now recognized as a tumor of neuronal lineage and has been given the name **central neurocytoma (CNC)**. Similar-appearing neoplasms in the brain parenchyma are less common and termed **extraventricular neurocytoma**.

Terminology

CNC is a well-differentiated neuroepithelial tumor with mature neurocytic elements.

Pathology

CNCs are tumors of the lateral ventricle body, usually attached to the septi pellucidi and arising near the foramen of Monro **(19-16)**. They vary in size from small to huge lesions that extend through the foramen of Monro to involve the contralateral ventricle **(19-17)**.

The gross appearance of CNC is similar to that of oligodendroglioma. A well-defined, lobulated, moderately vascular intraventricular mass is characteristic. CNCs rarely invade the adjacent brain parenchyma. Immunohistochemistry is positive for synaptophysin and negative for OLIG2.

MIB-1 is generally < 2%. CNCs are WHO grade II neoplasms.

Clinical Issues

Epidemiology. CNC is the most common primary intraventricular neoplasm of young and middle-aged adults, accounting for nearly 1/2 of all cases. They are rarely diagnosed in children or the elderly. Overall, they are rare neoplasms that represent between 0.25-0.50% of intracranial neoplasms and 10% of all intraventricular tumors.

Presentation. Symptoms are usually those of increased intracranial pressure. Headache, mental status changes, and visual disturbances are common while focal neurologic deficits are rare. Sudden ventricular obstruction or acute intratumoral hemorrhage may cause abrupt clinical deterioration and even death.

Natural History. CNCs are slow-growing neoplasms that rarely recur following complete surgical resection. Five-year survival rate is 90%.

Imaging

General Features. A "bubbly" mass in the body or frontal horn of the lateral ventricle is classic for CNC.

CT Findings. NECT shows a mixed-density solid and cystic intraventricular neoplasm attached to the septi pellucidi **(19-18A)**. Obstructive hydrocephalus is common. Calcification is present in 50-70% of cases. Gross intratumoral hemorrhage occurs but is rare. CNCs show moderately strong but heterogeneous enhancement on CECT.

MR Findings. CNCs are heterogeneous masses that are mostly isodense with gray matter on T1WI. Intratumoral cysts and prominent vascular "flow voids" are common. A "bubbly" appearance on T2WI is typical. CNCs are heterogeneously hyperintense on FLAIR **(19-18B)** and demonstrate moderate to strong but "bubbly" heterogeneous enhancement following contrast administration **(19-18D)**.

Decreased NAA and modestly elevated Cho are present on MRS. The presence of some NAA and glycine along with an inverted alanine peak at 1.5 ppm with a TE of 135 ms is highly suggestive of neurocytoma.

Differential Diagnosis

The major differential diagnosis of CNC is **subependymoma**. Supratentorial subependymomas are typically located adjacent to the foramen of Monro and may appear very similar. CNCs are tumors of younger adults, whereas subependymoma is more common in older adults.

Subependymal giant cell astrocytoma also occurs in a similar location, adjacent to the foramen of Monro. Clinical and other imaging stigmata of tuberous sclerosis (i.e., subependymal nodules and cortical tubers) are usually present.

An intraventricular **metastasis** usually occurs in older patients. Choroid plexus is a more common site than the lateral ventricle body. **Meningioma** is also more common in the ventricular trigone (choroid plexus glomus) than the frontal horn or body.

True intraventricular **oligodendroglioma** is rare. As the imaging appearance is indistinguishable from CNC, the diagnosis of intraventricular oligodendroglioma is established on the basis of immunohistochemistry and genetic studies. Oligodendrogliomas are synaptophysin negative and often show mutations of *OLIG2* and 1p,19q.

Extraventricular neurocytoma is histologically identical to CNCs. These unusual tumors vary widely in imaging appearance; some resemble CNCs or DNETs with a T2-hyperintense "bubbly" appearance.

Selected References: The complete reference list is available on the Expert Consult™ eBook version included with purchase.

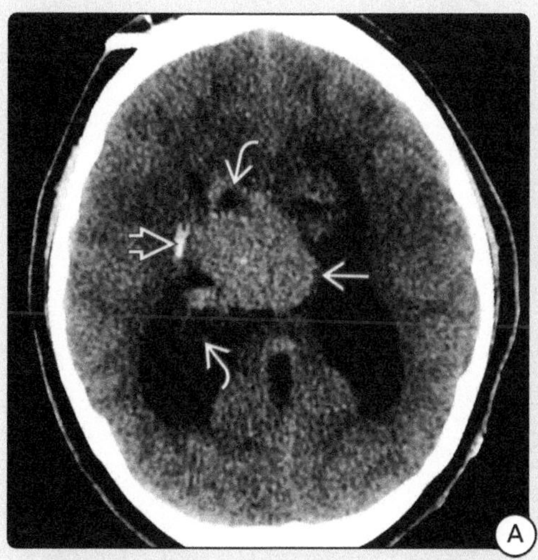

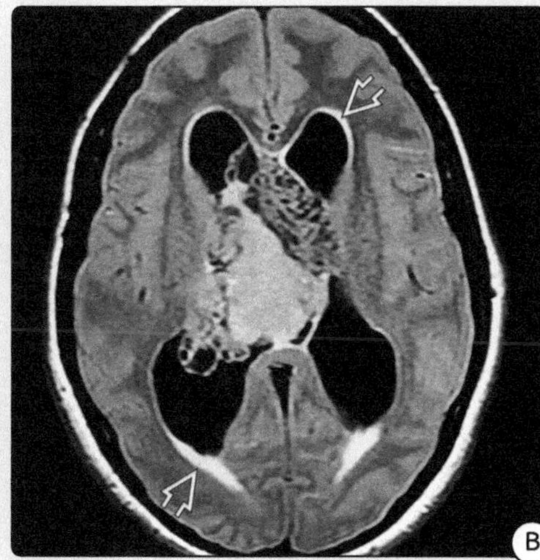

***(19-18A)** NECT in an 18-year-old woman in the emergency room with 1 month of increasingly severe headaches shows a biventricular mass with hyperdense ➡ and hypodense ➡ components with focal calcifications ➡. **(19-18B)** FLAIR MR shows periventricular fluid accumulation ➡ and multiple cysts with fluid that suppresses incompletely.*

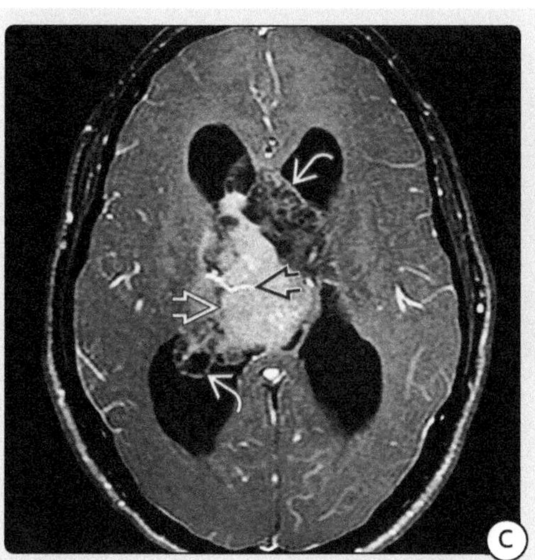

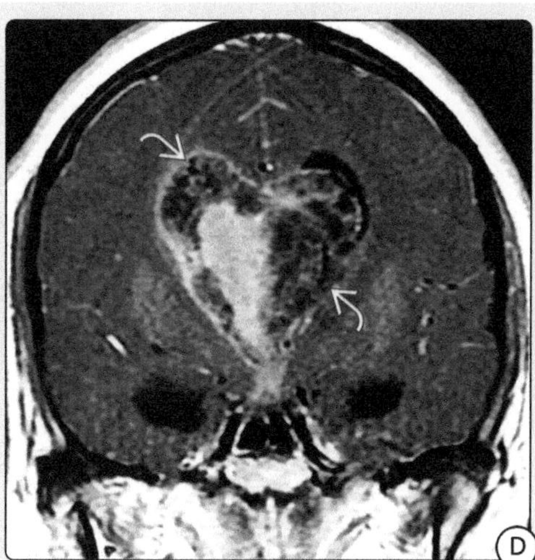

***(19-18C)** T1 C+ FS MR shows that the solid portion of the mass enhances intensely ➡, as do the walls of the variably sized cysts ➡. Note the prominent vessel ➡ supplying the solid portion of the mass. **(19-18D)** Coronal T1 C+ MR shows the typical "soap bubble" appearance ➡ of central neurocytoma.*

Pineal and Germ Cell Tumors

The region in and around the pineal gland is one of the most anatomically complex intracranial sites. A broad spectrum of both neoplasms and nonneoplastic entities can arise from the pineal gland itself or structures that are in its vicinity.

Overall, pineal region tumors are rare, accounting for 1-3% of all intracranial neoplasms. Neoplasms in this region can be grouped into three simple overarching categories. The two most important groups arise from cells within the pineal gland itself: (1) Germ cell tumors (GCTs) and (2) tumors of pineal parenchymal cells. We begin our discussion with these two major types of pineal neoplasms, then close with a brief discussion of (3) so-called "other cell" tumors in the pineal gland.

Germ Cell Tumors

Overview of Germ Cell Tumors

The most common pineal gland neoplasms are GCTs, accounting for 40%. GCTs are divided into two basic groups, **germinomas** and **nongerminomatous GCTs**.

Germinomas represent ~ 2/3 of all GCTs. 1/3 are *non*germinomatous GCTs (NGGCTs). NGGCTs include both teratomas and a heterogeneous group of miscellaneous nongerminomatous malignant germ cell neoplasms.

Germinoma

Etiology

The normal mature pineal gland does not contain germ cells. Once thought to arise from "aberrant migration" of primordial germ cell layers, recent studies show that activation of the MAPK &/or PI3K-AKT signalling pathway is the genetic driver of pure GCTs as well as NGGCTs.

Pathology

Location. Intracranial germinomas have a distinct predilection for midline structures **(20-1)**. Between 80-90% "hug" the midline, extending along the midline axis from the pineal gland to the suprasellar region. 1/2 to 2/3 are found in the pineal region with the suprasellar region the second most frequent location, accounting for 1/4 to 1/3 of germinomas.

Off-midline germinomas occur in only 5-10% of cases. The basal ganglia and thalami are the most common off-midline sites.

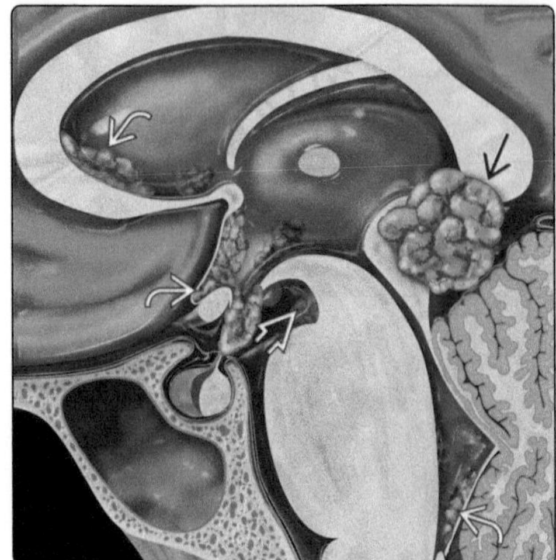

(20-1) Pineal germinoma ⇒ is shown with CSF dissemination ➡ to the 3rd, lateral, and 4th ventricles ➡.

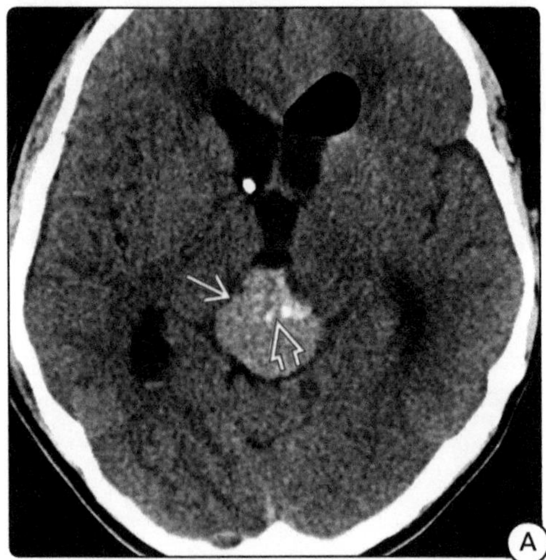

(20-2A) Postventriculostomy NECT in a 19-year-old man shows hyperdense pineal mass ➡ "engulfing" pineal gland calcifications ➡.

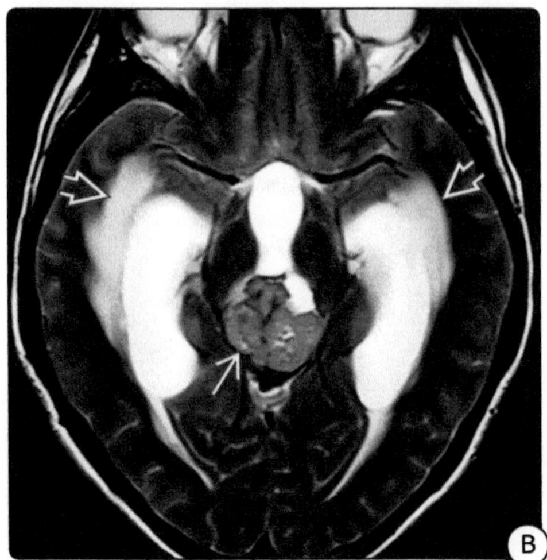

(20-2B) T2 MR shows mixed signal intensity ➡, severe hydrocephalus with "halo" of fluid around both temporal horns ➡. This is germinoma.

Size and Number. Pineal germinomas that do not invade the tectum or cause hydrocephalus can be as large as several centimeters at the time of initial diagnosis. Infundibular stalk germinomas may become symptomatic (usually causing central diabetes insipidus) before they can be detected on high-resolution contrast-enhanced MRs.

Approximately 20% of intracranial germinomas are multiple. The most frequent combination is a pineal plus a suprasellar ("bifocal" or "double midline") germinoma **(20-1)**.

Gross Pathology. Germinomas are generally solid masses that often infiltrate adjacent structures. Intratumoral cysts, small hemorrhagic foci, and CSF dissemination are common.

Microscopic Features. A biphasic pattern of neoplastic germinoma cells mixed with benign lymphocytes is typical. Some tumors exhibit such a florid immune cell infiltrate that it can obscure the neoplastic elements. Mitotic activity is common and may even be conspicuous, but frank necrosis is rare.

Clinical Issues

Demographics. Germinoma is the most common intracranial GCT and accounts for 1-2% of all primary brain tumors. More than 90% of patients are younger than 20 years of age at initial diagnosis. Peak presentation is 10-14 years. The M:F ratio for pineal germinoma is 10:1. Suprasellar germinomas have no sex predilection.

Presentation. Pineal germinomas typically present with headache and Parinaud syndrome. The most common presentation for suprasellar germinoma is central diabetes insipidus.

CSF cytology is rarely positive for tumor cells. Elevated serum or CSF markers (α-fetoprotein, β-HCG) are rare in pure germinomas but common with mixed GCTs.

Natural History. CSF dissemination and invasion are common, but pure germinomas have a very favorable response to radiation therapy. The five-year survival for treated patients with pure germinoma is > 90%.

Treatment Options. Histologic documentation followed by radiation therapy is the standard first-line treatment. Adjuvant chemotherapy is reserved for disseminated or recurrent tumors.

Imaging

General Features. CSF dissemination is common, so MR imaging of the entire neuraxis should be performed in patients with suspected germinoma. Caution: Some suprasellar germinomas may present with diabetes insipidus long before lesions are visible on MR. In such cases, serial imaging should be performed.

CT Findings. Germinomas are typically hyperdense on NECT. Pineal calcifications can appear "engulfed" and surrounded by tumor **(20-2A)**. Obstructive hydrocephalus is common. Strong uniform enhancement on CECT is typical.

MR Findings. Germinomas are iso- to slightly hyperintense to cortex on T1- and T2WI **(20-2B)**. Variably sized intratumoral cysts are common, especially in larger and "ectopic" lesions. Hemorrhage is generally uncommon except in basal ganglionic germinomas. T2* (GRE, SWI) may show "blooming" due to intratumoral calcification. Because of their high cellularity, germinomas may show restricted diffusion **(20-2E)**.

Enhancement is strong and usually homogeneous **(20-2D)**. Nearly 20% of germinomas are multiple, so look carefully for a second lesion in the suprasellar region (anterior third ventricle recesses, infundibular stalk) **(20-2C)**!

"Inflammatory" germinomas may show extensive, nonenhancing peritumoral T2/FLAIR hyperintensity that extends into adjacent structures, such as the midbrain and thalami. In such cases, biopsies—especially small stereotaxic samples—may disclose only granulomatous reaction and be mistaken for tuberculosis or neurosarcoid.

Differential Diagnosis

The major differential diagnosis of pineal germinoma is **mixed GCT** as well as **NGGCTs**. NGGCTs tend to be larger and more heterogeneous than germinomas. Bifocal lesions are almost always germinomas.

Some **pineoblastomas** may appear similar to germinoma but "explode" rather than "engulf" pineal calcifications. **Pineal parenchymal tumor of intermediate differentiation** usually occurs in middle-aged and older adults.

The major differential diagnosis of suprasellar germinoma is **Langerhans cell histiocytosis** (LCH). Both are common in children, often cause diabetes insipidus, and may be indistinguishable on imaging studies alone. However, LCH does not produce oncoproteins. **Neurosarcoidosis** in an adult can cause a suprasellar mass that resembles germinoma.

GERMINOMA: IMAGING AND DDx

CT

- NECT: Hyperdense, "engulfs" pineal Ca^{++}
- CECT: Enhances strongly, uniformly

MR

- T1 iso-/hypointense, T2 iso-/hyperintense
- Inflammatory germinomas may have extensive peritumoral T2/FLAIR hyperintensity
- GRE shows Ca^{++}, hemorrhage
- Often restricts on DWI
- Enhances intensely, heterogeneously
- CSF spread common (look for other lesions)
  - Anteroinferior 3rd ventricle, infundibular stalk
- Image entire neuraxis before surgery!

Differential Diagnosis

- Nongerminomatous GCT
- Pineal parenchymal tumors (pineoblastoma, pineal parenchymal tumor of intermediate differentiation)
- Histiocytosis (stalk lesion in child)
- Neurosarcoidosis (stalk lesion in adult)

Teratoma

Teratomas are tridermic masses that originate from "misenfolded" or displaced embryonic stem cells. Teratomas recapitulate somatic development and differentiate along ectodermal, mesodermal, and endodermal cell types **(20-3)**.

There are three recognized types of teratoma. These range from a benign well-differentiated "mature" teratoma to an immature teratoma to a teratoma with malignant differentiation. All three share some imaging features, such as complex masses with striking heterogeneity in density &/or signal intensity. Cysts and hemorrhage are common.

Although they may originate anywhere in the body, teratomas are most commonly found in sacrococcygeal, gonadal, mediastinal, retroperitoneal,

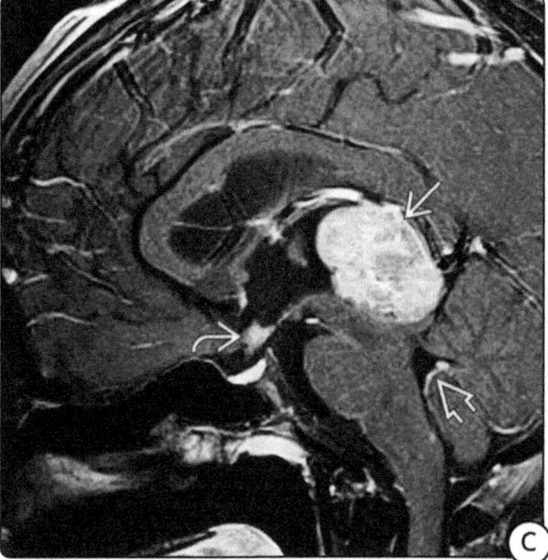

(20-2C) Same patient as Fig. 20-2 shows mass ➡ enhancing intensely. Note tumor in 3rd ventricle ➡ and along floor of 4th ventricle ➡.

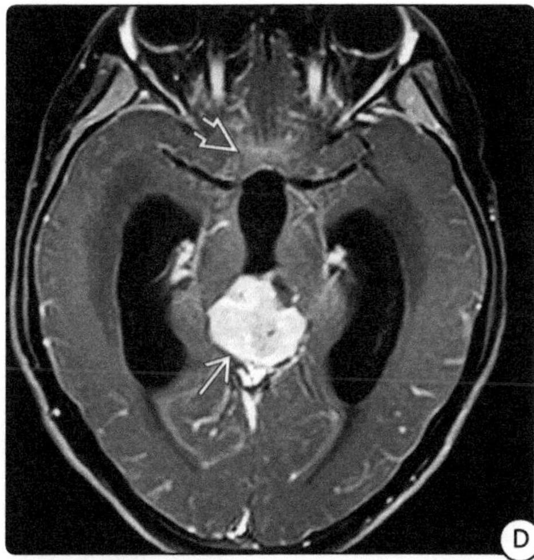

(20-2D) Axial T1 C+ FS MR shows the enhancing mass ➡ and sulcal-cisternal enhancement ➡ suggesting CSF dissemination.

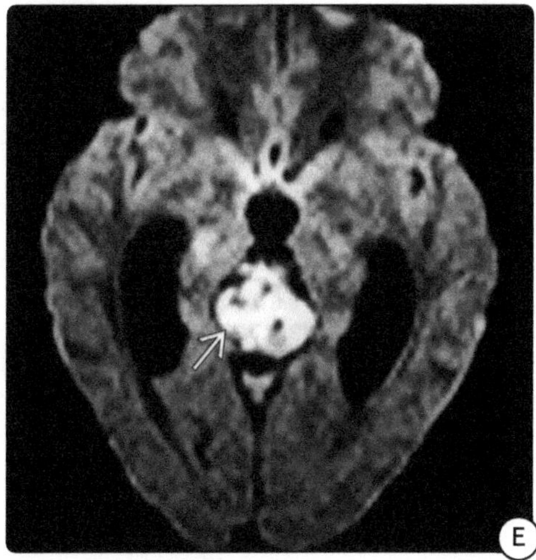

(20-2E) DWI MR shows diffusion restriction ➡. This is typical germinoma.

cervicofacial, and intracranial locations. Teratomas preferentially involve the midline; intracranial lesions most often arise in the pineal or suprasellar region.

Teratomas account for 2-4% of primary brain tumors in children and almost 1/2 of all congenital (perinatal) brain tumors. Teratomas are more common in Asians and male patients.

Imaging of mature teratomas shows a complex-appearing multiloculated lesion with fat, calcification, numerous cysts, and other tissues **(20-4)**. Hemorrhage is common. Enhancement is variable.

Immature teratomas contain a complex admixture of at least some fetal-type tissues from all three germ cell layers in combination with more mature tissue elements. It is common to have cartilage, bone, intestinal mucous, and smooth muscle intermixed with primitive neural ectodermal tissue. Hemorrhage and necrosis are common. CT or MR demonstrate almost complete replacement of brain tissue by a complex mixed-density or signal intensity mass.

Teratomas with malignant transformation generally arise from immature teratomas and contain somatic-type cancers, such as rhabdomyosarcoma or undifferentiated sarcoma.

Other Germ Cell Neoplasms

Germinomas are by far the most common of the germ cell neoplasms. Nongerminomatous malignant germ cell tumors (NGMGCTs) are rare neoplasms that contain undifferentiated epithelial cells and are often mixed with other germ cell elements (most often germinoma). These include **yolk sac (endodermal sinus) tumor, embryonal carcinoma, choriocarcinoma**, and **mixed germ cell tumor**.

NGMGCTs generally occur in adolescents with a peak incidence at 10-15 years of age. Prognosis is usually poor with overall survival of < 2 years.

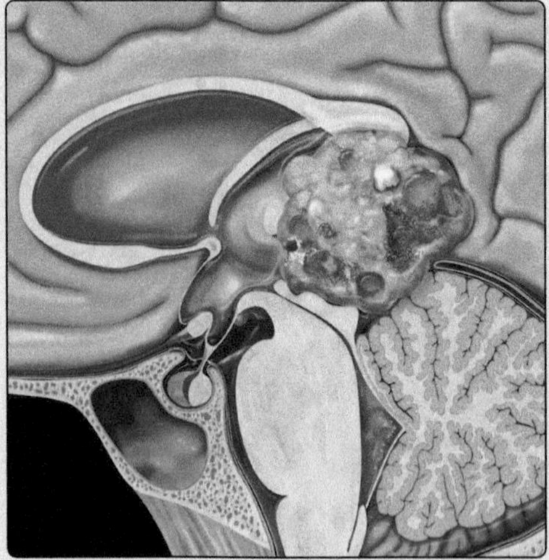

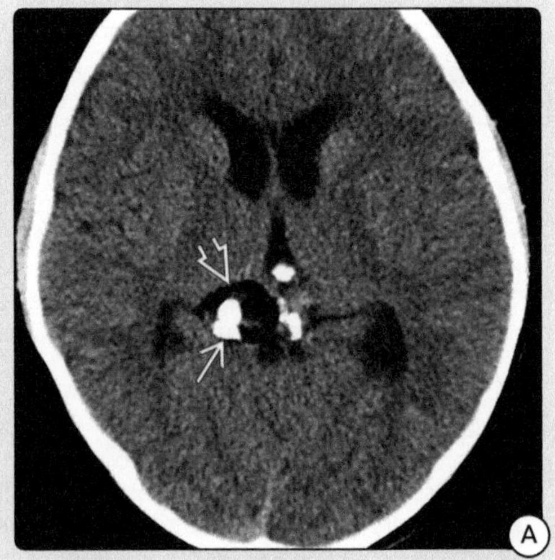

***(20-3)** Graphic showcases a pineal teratoma with the typical heterogeneous tissue components (cysts, solid tumor, calcifications, fat, etc.). **(20-4A)** Axial NECT in an 8-year-old boy with headaches, nausea, and vomiting shows a very heterogeneous mass in the pineal region. Hypodense fat-attenuation tissue ➡ surrounds a densely calcified component ➡ that grossly resembles a tooth.*

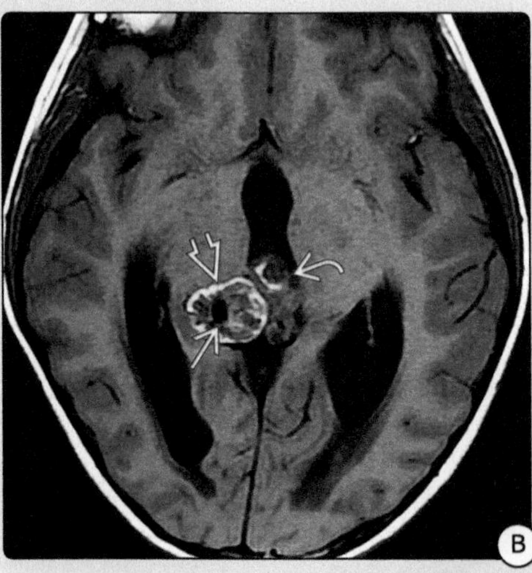

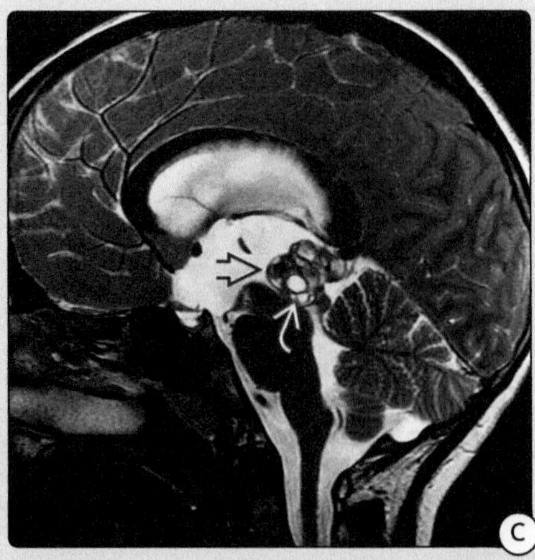

***(20-4B)** Axial T1 MR shows T1 shortening around the periphery of the mass ➡ consistent with fat. The internal signal void ➡ is caused by the densely calcified component. A lobulated mixed signal intensity component is present in the posterior 3rd ventricle ➡. **(20-4C)** Sagittal T2 MR shows that the heterogeneous-appearing mass ➡ also contains numerous cysts ➡.*

Differentiating intracranial germ cell neoplasms on the basis of imaging studies alone is problematic. All intracranial GCTs—whether benign or malignant—tend to "hug" the midline.

Serum and CSF biomarkers can be helpful in the preoperative evaluation of a pineal mass. Embryonal carcinomas, immature teratomas, and endodermal sinus tumors can cause elevated α-fetoprotein. Choriocarcinomas and germinomas are associated with elevated β-hCG. Germinomas are also associated with elevated lactate dehydrogenase and placental alkaline phosphatase.

Many pineal neoplasms express different oncoproteins, so immunohistochemical profiling of biopsied tissue is an essential part of the diagnosis.

Pineal Parenchymal Tumors

Pineal parenchymal tumors (PPTs) are intrinsic primary tumors that arise from pinealocytes or their precursors. PPTs account for < 0.2% of all brain tumors but cause ~ 15-30% of pineal gland tumors.

Three grades are recognized: (1) **Pineocytoma**, (2) **pineal parenchymal tumor of intermediate differentiation (PPTID)**, and (3) **pineoblastoma**, the most malignant parenchymal cell tumors.

In the most recent epidemiologic studies, pineocytomas account for 13-15% of pineal parenchymal neoplasms (probably an underrepresentation, as many presumed cases are not resected or biopsied). PPTIDs represent nearly 2/3 of cases, and pineoblastomas account for ~ 20%.

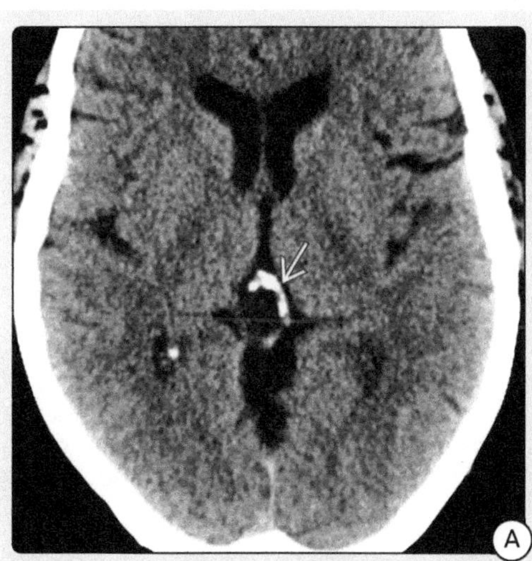

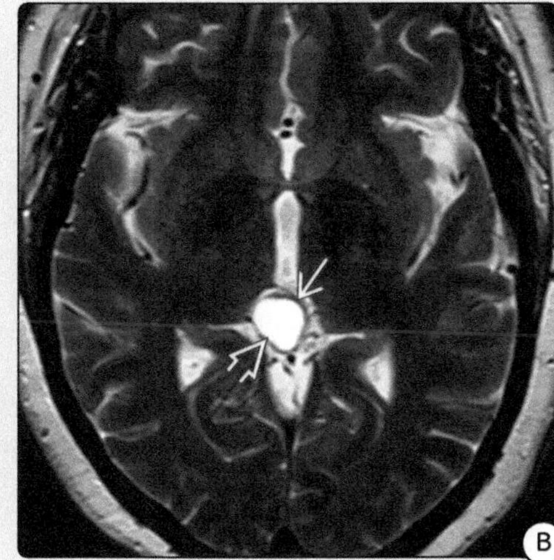

***(20-5A)** NECT shows the typical findings of pineocytoma. The cystic-appearing pineal mass "explodes" calcifications toward the periphery of the lesion ➡. **(20-5B)** T2 MR in the same patient shows a cyst ➡ surrounded by a thin rim of solid tissue ➡.*

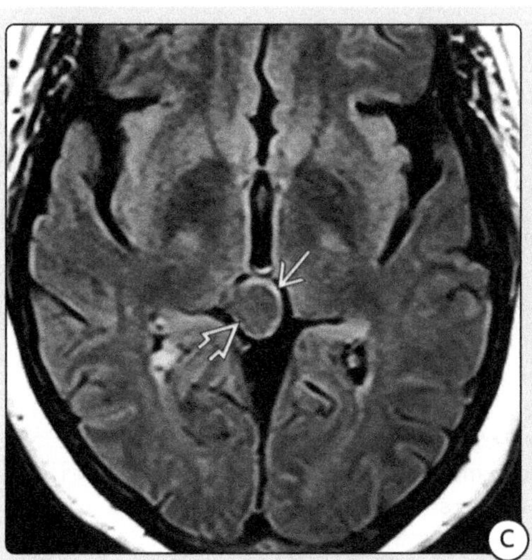

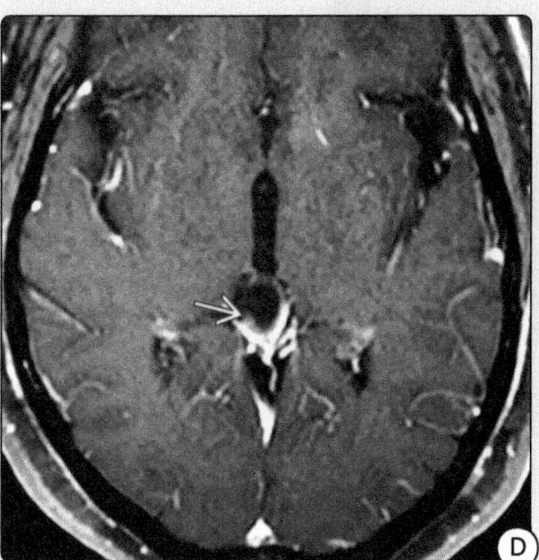

***(20-5C)** FLAIR MR shows that the cyst wall ➡ is mildly hyperintense and that the cyst fluid ➡ does not suppress. **(20-5D)** T1 C+ FS MR demonstrates that the cyst wall enhances ➡. This is pathologically proven pineocytoma, WHO grade I.*

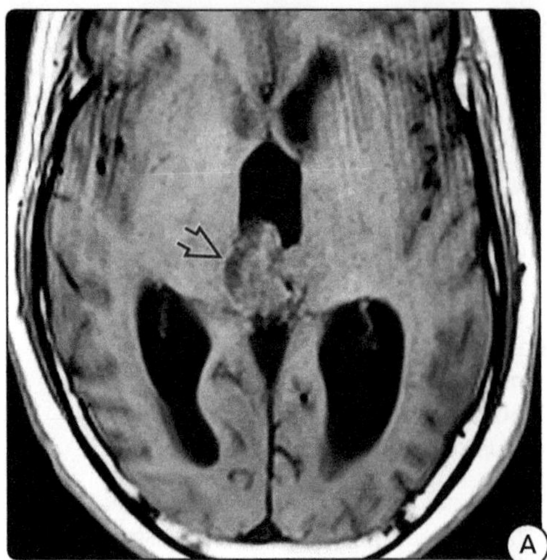

***(20-6A)** Axial T1WI in a 57y man with headaches shows a lobulated mixed iso-/hypointense pineal mass ⇒ causing obstructive hydrocephalus.*

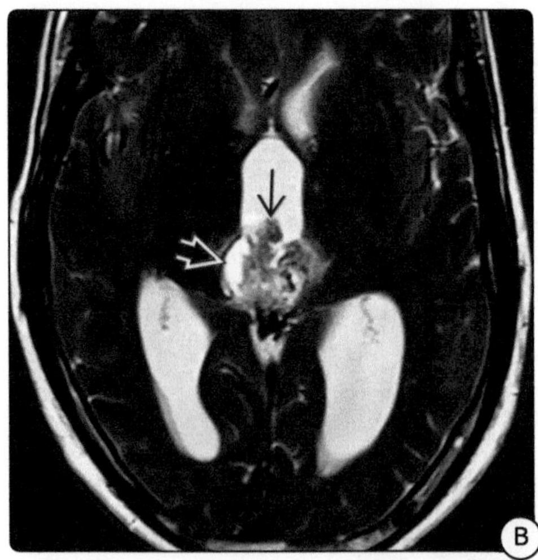

***(20-6B)** Axial T2 MR in the same case shows both solid ⇒ and cystic ➡ portions of the mass.*

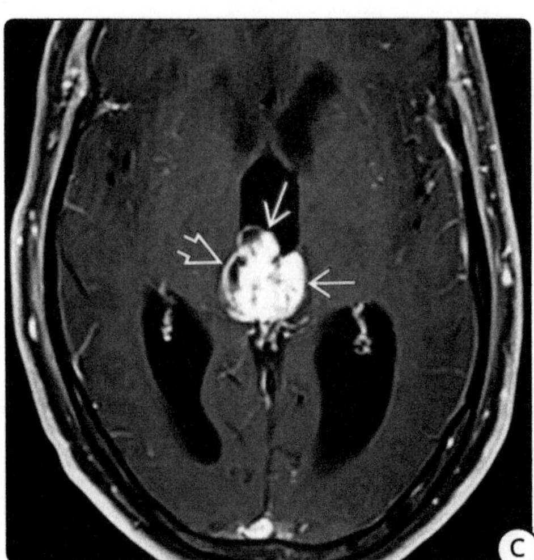

***(20-6C)** Axial T1 C+ FS MR shows the solid portions of the mass ➡ and cyst ➡ enhancing strongly. This is PPTID, WHO grade II.*

At present, the genetic alterations that drive PPTs are largely unknown except for the subset of pineoblastomas that arise in patients with germline mutations in either *RB1* or as part of their eponymous tumor predisposition syndromes.

Pineocytoma

In the most recent epidemiologic studies, pineocytomas account for 13-15% of pineal parenchymal neoplasms (probably an underrepresentation, as many presumed cases are not resected or biopsied).

Pathology

Grossly, pineocytomas are well-circumscribed, round or lobular, gray-tan masses that are located behind the third ventricle and rarely invade adjacent structures. Although "giant" tumors have been reported, most are < 3 cm in diameter.

Pineocytomas are composed of small uniform cells that resemble pinealocytes and are positive for both synaptophysin and neurofilament. Large "pineocytomatous rosettes" are the most characteristic feature. Mitoses are absent. Pineocytomas are designated as WHO grade I neoplasms.

Clinical Issues

Pineocytomas occur at all ages but are mostly tumors of adults. Mean age at diagnosis is 43 years. There is a slight female predominance (M:F = 0.6:1).

Many small pineocytomas are discovered incidentally on imaging studies. Larger lesions may compress adjacent structures or cause hydrocephalus. Headache and Parinaud syndrome (paralysis of upward gaze) are common in symptomatic patients.

Pineocytomas grow very slowly and often remain stable in size over many years. "Watchful waiting" is common with small lesions. Imaging is usually obtained only if the patient's symptoms change. Complete surgical resection is generally curative without recurrence or metastatic tumor spread.

Imaging

Pineocytomas are globular, well-delineated masses that are mixed iso- to hypodense on NECT scans. Calcifications typically appear "exploded" toward the periphery of the pineal gland **(20-5A)**.

Pineocytomas are well-demarcated round or lobular masses that are iso- to hypointense on T1WI and hyperintense on T2WI and FLAIR **(20-5C)**. T2* GRE may show "blooming" foci secondary to calcification or hemorrhage. Pineocytomas typically enhance avidly with solid, rim, or even nodular patterns **(20-5D)**.

Differential Diagnosis

The major differential diagnosis of pineocytoma is a benign, nonneoplastic **pineal cyst**. Pineal cysts may be indistinguishable from pineocytomas on imaging studies.

Germinoma typically "engulfs" rather than "explodes" the pineal calcifications, is most common in male adolescents, and enhances intensely and uniformly. **Pineal parenchymal tumor of intermediate differentiation** (PPTID) is a tumor of middle-aged and older patients. The imaging appearance of PPTIDs is more "aggressive" than that of pineocytoma.

PINEOCYTOMA

Pathology
- Most are 1-3 cm
- Well demarcated, round/lobulated
- WHO grade I

Clinical Issues
- Adults (mean = 40 years)
- Grows very slowly, often stable for years

Imaging
- CT
  - Mixed iso-/hypodense
  - Pineal Ca^{++} "exploded"
- MR
  - Iso-/hypointense on T1, hyperintense on T2
  - Cysts common, may hemorrhage
  - Variable enhancement (solid, rim, nodular)

Differential Diagnosis
- Benign pineal cyst (may be indistinguishable)
- Germinoma ("engulfs" Ca^{++}, male adolescents)
- PPTID (more "aggressive-looking")

Pineal Parenchymal Tumor of Intermediate Differentiation

Pineal parenchymal tumor of intermediate differentiation (PPTID) is intermediate in malignancy between pineocytoma and pineoblastoma. PPTID supersedes the terms "atypical" or "aggressive" pineocytoma.

Pathology

Grossly, PPTID is a large, heterogeneous mass with peripheral calcification and variable cystic changes. Microscopically, PPTIDs are moderate to highly cellular tumors that exhibit dense lobular architecture. Two morphologic subtypes, small cell and large cell, have been recently described.

PPTIDs can be either WHO grade II or III, although definite histologic grading criteria remain to be defined.

Clinical Issues

PPTIDs are the most common pineal parenchymal tumor, representing between 1/2 and 2/3 of all cases. PPTIDs can occur at any age but are typically tumors of middle-aged adults.

Diplopia, Parinaud syndrome, and headache are the most common presenting symptoms. Biologic behavior is variable and clinical progression can be seen in both grades II and III PPTIDs. Tumors tend to enlarge slowly and recur locally, although CSF dissemination may occur. Malignant degeneration into pineoblastoma has been reported in a few cases.

No serum or CSF biomarkers are currently available that inform the diagnosis or treatment of PPTIDs.

Imaging

PPTIDs have a more "aggressive" imaging appearance than pineocytoma **(20-6)**. Extension into adjacent structures (e.g., the ventricles and thalami) is common. Size varies from < 1 cm to large masses that are 4-6 cm in

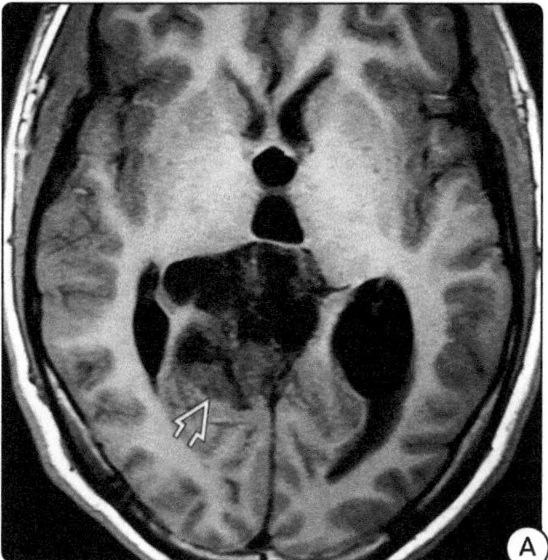

***(20-7A)** Axial T1 MR in a 21y man with Parinaud syndrome shows a large heterogeneous mass ➡ causing moderate obstructive hydrocephalus.*

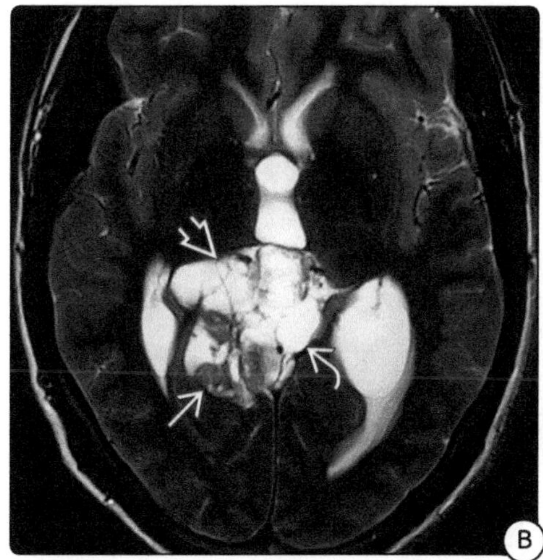

***(20-7B)** T2 MR shows numerous hyperintense cysts ➡ and solid isointense nodules ➡ comprising the mass ➡.*

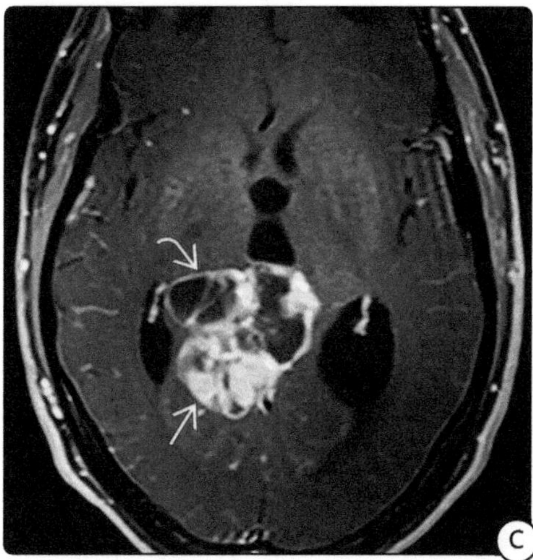

***(20-7C)** T1 C+ FS MR shows strong enhancement of the solid portions of the mass ➡ and cyst walls ➡. Pathology was PPTID, WHO grade III.*

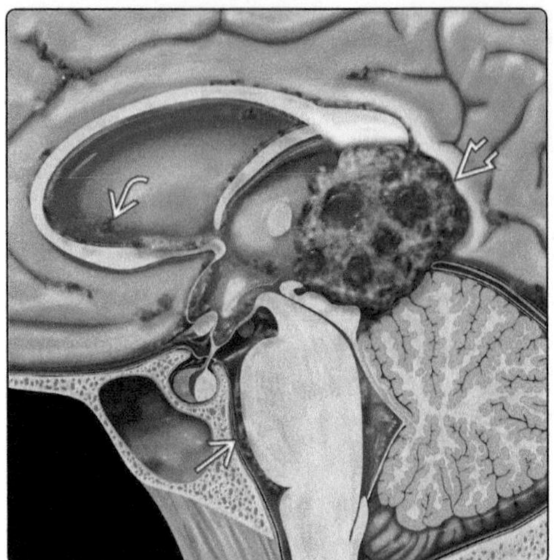

***(20-8)** Sagittal graphic depicts pineoblastoma ➡ with CSF dissemination into ventricles ➡, subarachnoid spaces ➡.*

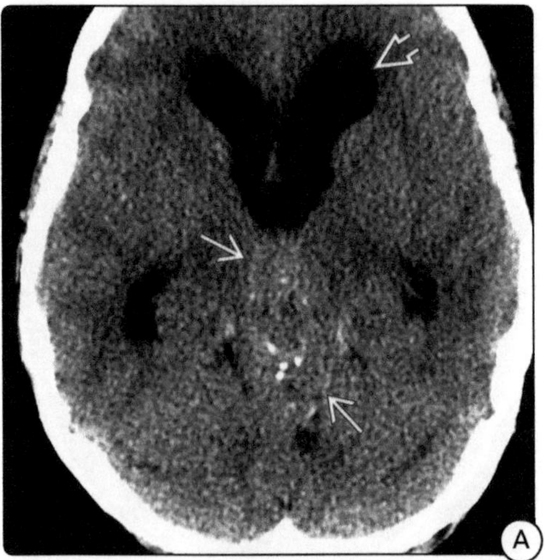

***(20-9A)** NECT of pineoblastoma shows a large ill-defined, slightly hyperdense pineal region mass ➡ causing obstructive hydrocephalus ➡.*

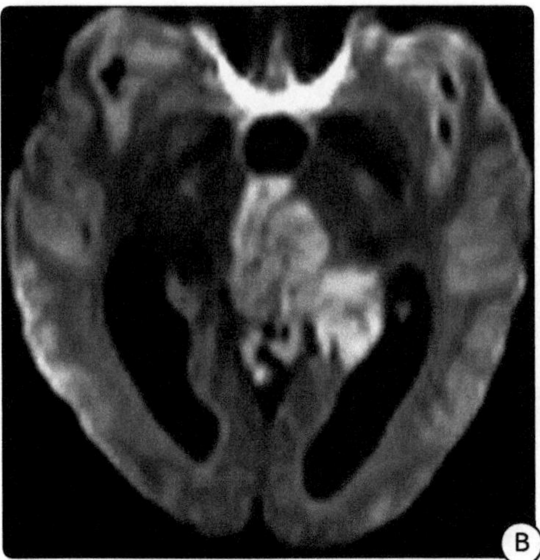

***(20-9B)** DWI in same patient shows moderate diffusion restriction, consistent with high cellularity. This is pineoblastoma, WHO grade IV.*

diameter. CSF dissemination is uncommon but does occur, so imaging evaluation of the entire neuraxis should be performed prior to surgical intervention.

NECT scans show a hyperdense mass that "engulfs" pineal gland calcifications. PPTIDs generally enhance strongly and uniformly.

PPTIDs are mixed iso- and hypointense on T1-weighted MR, isointense with gray matter on T2WI, and hyperintense on FLAIR. T2* (GRE, SWI) scans may show hypointense "blooming" foci. Enhancement is generally strong but heterogeneous on T1 C+ **(20-7)**.

Differential Diagnosis

The major differential diagnosis of PPTID is **pineocytoma**. A more aggressive-appearing pineal mass in a middle-aged or older adult is most consistent with PPTID. **Pineoblastoma** is typically a tumor of younger patients. **Germinoma** is more common in male adolescents. **Papillary tumor of the pineal region** can appear identical on imaging studies but is very rare.

PINEAL PARENCHYMAL TUMOR OF INTERMEDIATE DIFFERENTIATION

Pathology
- 50-68% of pineal parenchymal tumors
- WHO grade II or III

Clinical Issues
- Middle-aged adults

Imaging
- Appears more "aggressive" than pineocytoma
- Usually larger, more heterogeneous
- May disseminate via CSF

Differential Diagnosis
- Pineocytoma > > pineoblastoma
- Germinoma

Pineoblastoma

Pineoblastomas (PBs) are the most primitive and biologically aggressive of all pineal parenchymal tumors.

PBs are known to occur in patients with *RB1* gene abnormalities. PBs also occur in patients with familial (bilateral) retinoblastoma (the so-called "trilateral retinoblastoma syndrome"), and cases have been reported in familial adenomatous polyposis. Patients with **DICER1 syndrome** are at increased risk for developing PBs.

Pathology

Grossly, a soft, friable, diffusely infiltrating tumor that invades adjacent brain and obstructs the cerebral aqueduct is typical. Necrosis and intratumoral hemorrhage are common, as is CSF dissemination with sheet-like coating of the brain and spinal cord **(20-8)**.

Microscopically, PBs are poorly differentiated, highly malignant tumors consisting of undifferentiated small round blue cells with hyperchromatic nuclei that exhibit a high nuclear:cytoplasmic ratio. PBs are designated as WHO grade IV neoplasms.

Clinical Issues

Epidemiology. PBs comprise 0.5-1.0% of primary brain tumors, 15% of pineal region neoplasms, and 20-35% of pineal parenchymal tumors. They can occur at any age, including adults, but PBs are decidedly more prevalent in children.

Presentation and Natural History. Symptoms of elevated intracranial pressure, such as headache, nausea, and vomiting, are typical. Parinaud syndrome is common.

Surgical debulking with adjuvant chemotherapy and craniospinal radiation comprise the typical regimen. Prognosis is poor with a median survival of 16-25 months. CSF dissemination is frequent and the most common cause of death.

Imaging

PBs are large, bulky, aggressive-looking pineal region masses that invade adjacent brain and usually cause obstructive hydrocephalus. CSF dissemination is common, so the entire neuraxis should be imaged prior to surgical intervention.

NECTs show a large, hyperdense, inhomogeneously enhancing mass with obstructive hydrocephalus **(20-9A)**. If pineal calcifications are present, they appear "exploded" toward the periphery of the tumor.

PBs are heterogeneous tumors that frequently demonstrate necrosis and intratumoral hemorrhage on MR. They are usually mixed iso- to hypointense compared with brain on T1WI and mixed iso- to hyperintense on T2WI. They enhance strongly but heterogeneously **(20-10)**. Because they are densely cellular tumors, restriction on DWI is common **(20-9B)**.

PINEOBLASTOMA

Pathology
- Most primitive, malignant of all PPTs
- Diffusely infiltrates adjacent structures
- Early, widespread CSF dissemination common
- WHO grade IV
- Some exhibit *RB1*, *DICER1* mutation

Clinical Issues
- 15% of pineal region tumors
- 20-35% of PPTs
- All ages but primarily children (< 20 years old)
- Prognosis generally poor

Imaging
- CT
  - Inhomogeneously hyperdense
  - Ca^{++} "exploded"
- MR
  - Large, bulky, aggressive-looking
  - Necrosis, intratumoral hemorrhage common
  - Enhances strongly, heterogeneously
  - Restricts on DWI (densely cellular)
  - Look for CSF spread (image entire neuraxis)

Differential Diagnosis

The major differential diagnosis of PB is **PPTID**. PBs tend to occur in children, and CSF dissemination at diagnosis is more common. **Germinoma** also frequently demonstrates CSF spread but is more common in adolescent and

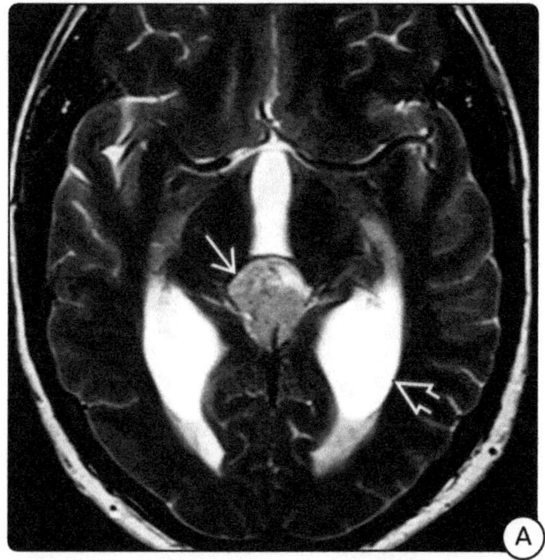

(20-10A) T2 MR in 43y man w/ headache, nausea, vomiting for 11 days shows hyperintense pineal mass ➡, acute obstructive hydrocephalus ➡.

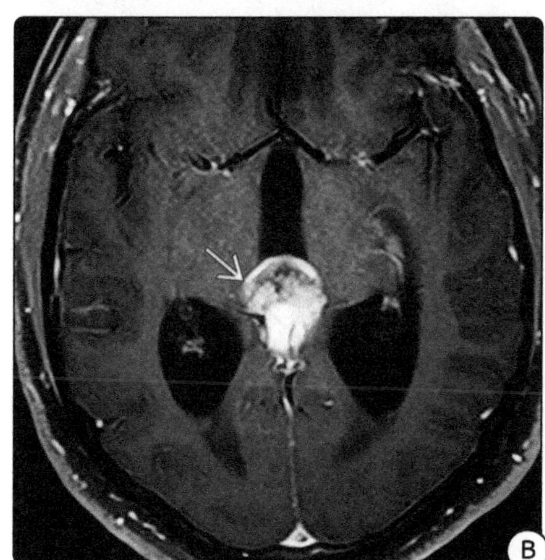

(20-10B) T1 C+ FS MR shows mass ➡ enhancing intensely, heterogeneously with no evidence for CSF spread. Imaging diagnosis was PPTID.

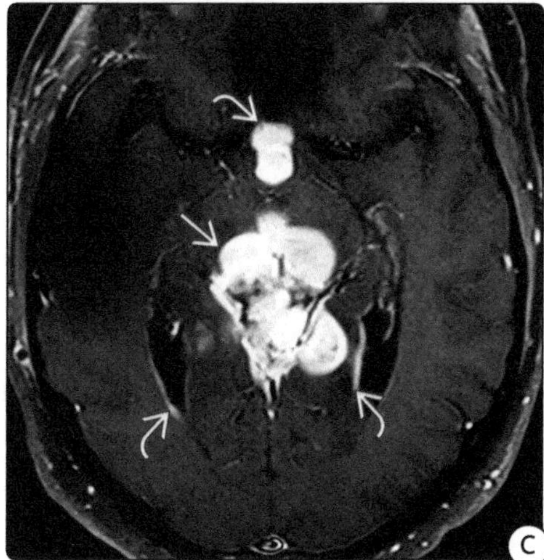

(20-10C) T1 C+ FS MR 5 weeks later shows mass ➡ has increased significantly, and there is CSF dissemination ➡. Pineoblastoma, WHO grade IV.

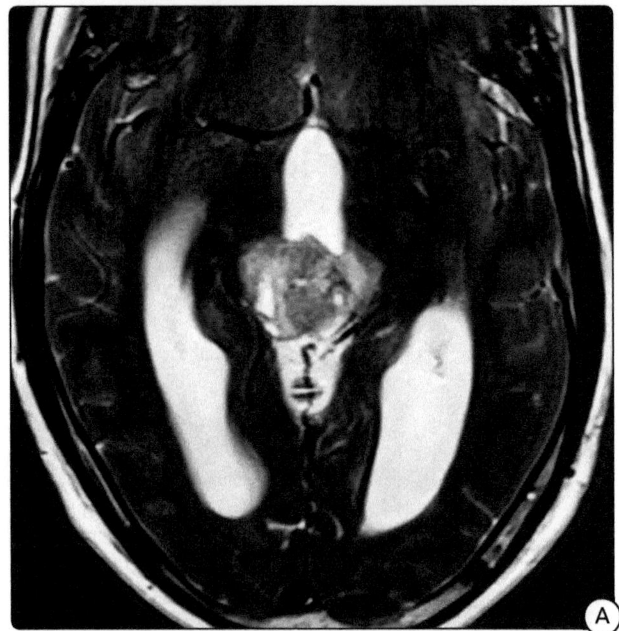

***(20-11A)** Axial T2 MR in a 56-year-old man with a 4-week history of headache and diplopia shows a mixed iso- and hyperintense mass in the posterior 3rd ventricle/pineal region.*

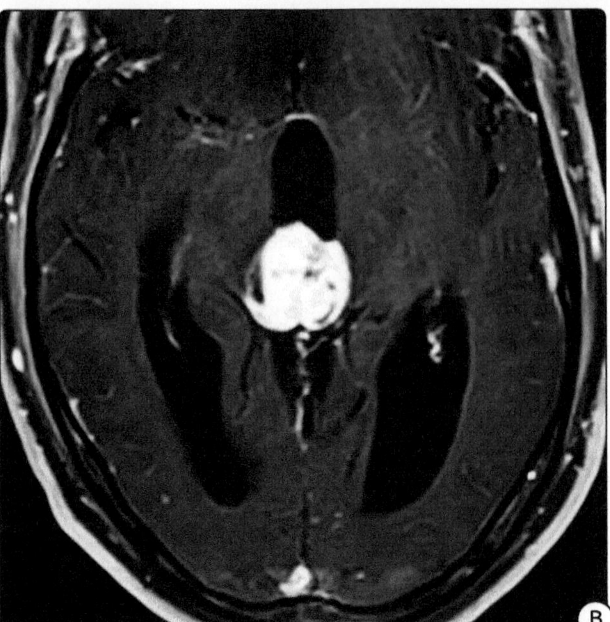

***(20-11B)** T1 C+ FS MR in the same case shows that the mass enhances strongly. Preoperative diagnosis was PPTID. Anaplastic astrocytoma, IDH-wild-type was found at histopathology.*

young adult males. **Nongerminomatous malignant germ cell tumors** are a heterogeneous group of tumors that may be indistinguishable on imaging studies from PBs.

"Other Cell" Pineal and Pineal Region Neoplasms

Miscellaneous Pineal Neoplasms

Rarely, tumors arising within the pineal gland are composed of neoplastic elements other than parenchymal or germ cells. Primary glial neoplasms, such as astrocytoma (including glioblastoma) **(20-11)** and oligodendroglioma, can occur within the pineal gland itself as can melanoma arising from pineal melanocytes. Metastases from extracranial sources also occasionally present as pineal masses.

In general, imaging findings with intrinsic pineal gland masses are nonspecific and often do not permit differentiation between the broad spectrum of histologic types. A general approach to the differential diagnosis is outlined in the accompanying box.

Selected References: The complete reference list is available on the Expert Consult™ eBook version included with purchase.

APPROACH TO PINEAL MASSES

Key Questions to Consider
- Is the mass in the pineal gland or adjacent to it?
- What is the patient's age, sex?
- Is there serum or CSF evidence for oncoproteins?
- Are additional lesions present?

Pineal Gland Mass
- Most common = benign, nonneoplastic cyst!
- Less common
  - Pineocytoma
  - Germinoma
  - PPTID
- Rare but important
  - Pineoblastoma
  - Teratoma
  - Rare pineal tumors (e.g., papillary tumor of pineal region)
  - Other (e.g., glioma, metastasis)

Pineal Region Mass
- Adjacent to—but not in—the pineal gland
  - Arachnoid cyst
  - Dermoid or epidermoid cyst
  - Meningioma
  - Lipoma (quadrigeminal plate)
  - Astrocytoma (e.g., tectal glioma)
  - Metastasis
  - Aneurysm (basilar tip, PCA)

Embryonal Neoplasms

The rapidly evolving molecular classification of brain tumors has fundamentally changed the understanding of embryonal neoplasms. In the 2016 World Health Organization schema, the classification of the largest group of embryonal neoplasms—medulloblastoma—was revised to reflect clinically relevant molecular subgroups.

The 2016 WHO classification recognizes three general categories of embryonal tumors: (1) Medulloblastoma, (2) other (nonmedulloblastoma) embryonal tumors, and (3) atypical teratoid/rhabdoid tumor. The term "primitive neuroectodermal tumor (PNET)" has been removed from the diagnostic lexicon, and the tumors formerly included in this category have been redefined using molecular data.

Medulloblastoma

Medulloblastoma: Histology and Genetics

Medulloblastoma (MB) is the most common malignant CNS neoplasm of childhood and the second most common overall pediatric brain tumor (after astrocytoma). As a group, MBs accounts for ~ 20% of childhood CNS neoplasms.

MB is not a single tumor entity but a heterogeneous cluster of multiple distinct, clinically relevant molecular subgroups. International consensus now recognizes four molecular subgroups, each differing in its demographics, recommended treatments, and clinical outcomes.

Histologically Defined Classification of Medulloblastoma

MBs consist of densely packed small round undifferentiated ("blue") cells. Moderate nuclear pleomorphism and a high mitotic index (MIB-1 or Ki-67) are characteristic.

The 2016 WHO classification recognizes **classic medulloblastoma** and three histopathologic variants: (1) **Desmoplastic/nodular medulloblastoma**, (2) **medulloblastoma with extensive nodularity**, and (3) **large cell/anaplastic medulloblastoma**. All MBs are currently designated as WHO grade IV neoplasms.

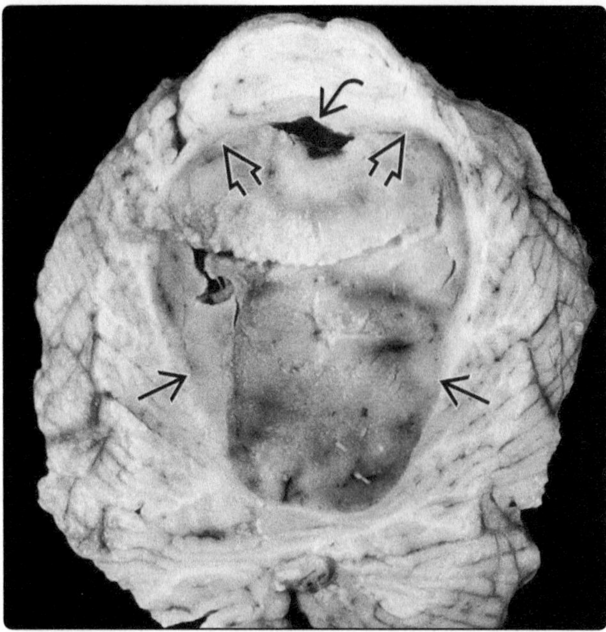

(21-1) Autopsy specimen demonstrates a large medulloblastoma (MB) ⇒ nearly filling the 4th ventricle with some sparing of the uppermost aspect of the ventricle ⇒. Pons is compressed anteriorly ⇒. (Courtesy R. Hewlett, MD.)

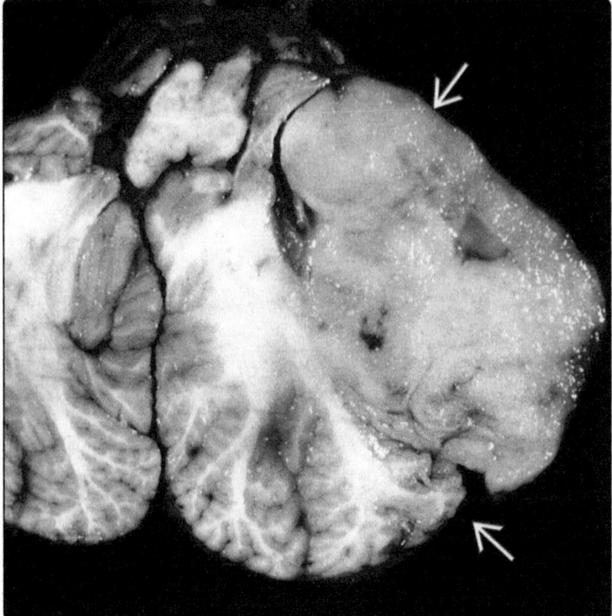

(21-2) Cut section shows the classic desmoplastic MB located in the lateral cerebellar hemisphere ⇒. Most tumors in this location are SHH activated. (Courtesy R. Hewlett, MD.)

Genetically Defined Classification of Medulloblastomas

MB is a genetically heterogeneous disease with four main molecular subgroups. All four MB subtypes have different origins, preferred anatomic locations, and demographics, as well as dramatically different prognosis and therapeutic implications. Each of these four subtypes has been further subdivided into distinctive molecular subgroups, adding more precision to patient-based risk stratification.

The two named pathways are the WNT-activated and SHH-activated pathways. Two non-WNT, non-SHH groups are designated as simply "group 3" and "group 4."

Wingless or WNT-Activated Medulloblastomas. WNT-activated medulloblastoma (WNT MB) is the smallest molecular subgroup (10%) and appears strikingly different from the other MBs in origin, appearance, and prognosis. WNT MBs are lateralized tumors that arise from the lower rhombic lip in the dorsolateral primitive brainstem around the foramen of Luschka **(21-3)**.

WNT MBs are very rare in infants and usually affect older children and young adults. They almost always exhibit classic histology. Childhood patients with WNT MBs have a favorable prognosis (5-year survival > 90%) and reduced intensity risk-adapted therapies are often utilized.

Germline mutations in the WNT pathway inhibitor, *APC*, predispose individuals to develop MB in the setting of **Turcot syndrome**.

SHH-Activated MBs. The SHH subgroup accounts for 25-30% of MBs. **SHH-activated MB** (SHH MB) arises from granule neuron precursor cells, which are found in the external granular layer of the cerebellum. SHH MBs are often located laterally within the cerebellar hemispheres **(21-2)**. Compared with all other subgroups, SHH MBs more often have desmoplastic or nodular pathology.

Mutational status and prognosis vary with age. *PTCHD1* mutations occur across all age groups while *SUFU* mutation is more common in infants and *SMO* in adults. Individuals with germline mutations in the SHH receptor *PTCHD1* have **basal cell nevus (Gorlin) syndrome** and are predisposed to develop SHH-activated MBs.

Four clinically significant subtypes of SHH MB have been identified with two infant subgroups associated with poor (SHHβ) and good (SHHγ) prognoses. SHHα MBs in children have *TP53* mutations and are associated with poor prognosis even when treated with high-dose craniospinal radiation and adjuvant chemotherapy. SHHΔ MBs occur in adults with *TERT* mutations.

Non-WNT/Non-SHH Medulloblastoma. Non-WNT/non-SHH MBs cluster into two groups ("group 3" and "group 4").

Group 3 is the third largest MB subgroup (20-25%) and has the worst outcome. Group 3 tumors are common in infants but exceedingly rare in adults. *MYC* amplification is common, and ~ 50% of patients present with metastases **(21-5)**. NOTCH1 has been identified as a pivotal driver of group 3 MB metastasis and self-renewal.

Group 4 is the largest (~ 35%) of the four molecular MB subgroups. Most group 4 MBs exhibit classic histology. Group 4 MBs affect all ages but are most common in children. The M:F ratio is 2:1. A minority of group 4 MBs present with

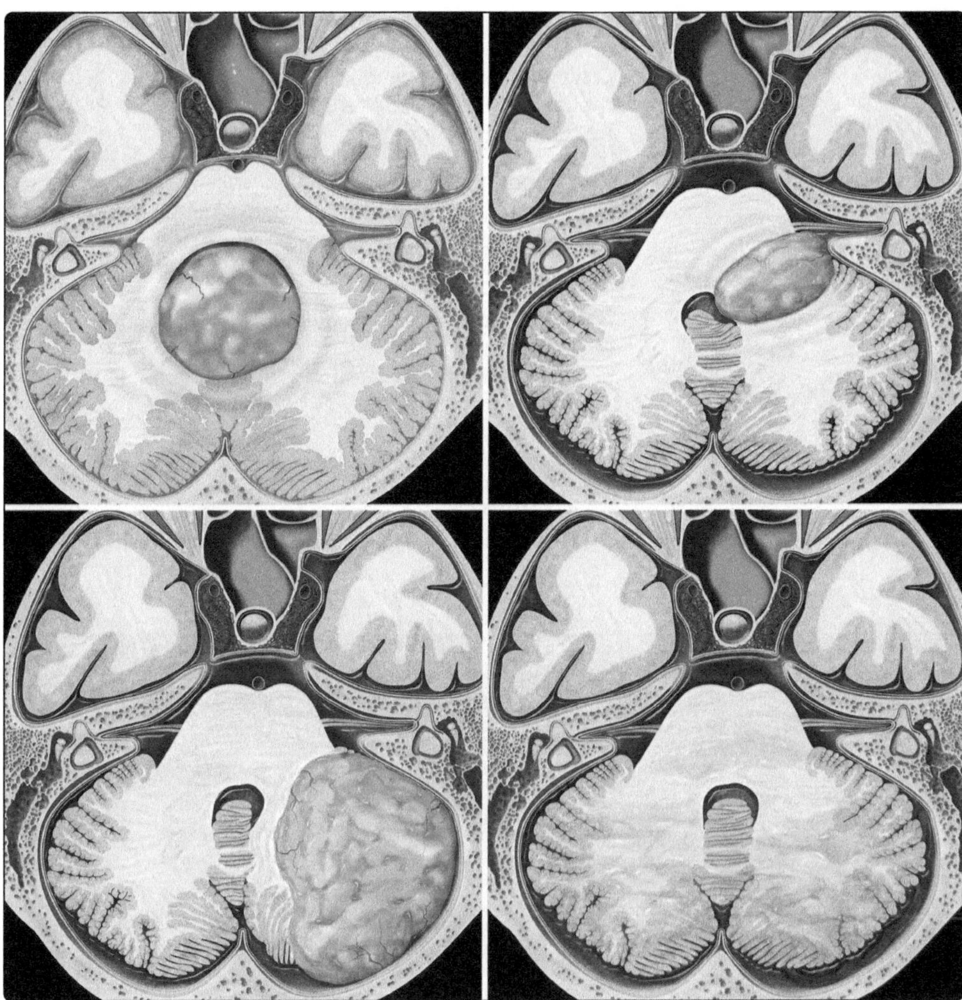

(21-3) (Upper left) Graphic depicts classic MB in the midline 4th ventricle with CSF spread. All molecular subgroups and all histologies can be located here, but the most common subtypes are groups 3 and 4 (compare to Fig. 21-9). (Upper right) Graphic depicts an MB in the cerebellar peduncle/CPA cistern. This location is classic for WNT MB (compare to Figs. 21-10 and 21-12). (Lower left) Graphic depicts an MB in the lateral cerebellar hemisphere. This is the classic location for desmoplastic MB, SHH molecular subtype (compare to Fig. 21-11). (Lower right) Graphic depicts a nonfocal, diffusely infiltrating MB (compare to Fig. 21-13). Groups 3 and 4 can be diffusely infiltrating with no dominant mass. Group 4 MBs are sometimes characterized by exhibiting minimal or no enhancement on T1 C+ FS (compare to Fig. 21-9).

metastasis. Overall prognosis is intermediate but poor in adults.

MEDULLOBLASTOMA CLASSIFICATION

Histologically Defined Medulloblastomas
- Classic medulloblastoma
- Medulloblastoma variants
  - Desmoplastic/nodular medulloblastoma
  - Medulloblastoma with extensive nodularity
  - Large cell/anaplastic medulloblastoma

Genetically Defined Medulloblastomas
- WNT-activated medulloblastoma
- SHH-activated medulloblastomas
  - *TP53* mutant
  - *TP53* wild-type
- Non-WNT/non-SHH medulloblastomas
  - Group 3 medulloblastoma
  - Group 4 medulloblastoma

Medulloblastoma: Pathology, Clinical, and Imaging Features

Pathology

Location. While any histologic type can be found in any location, > 85% of classic, group 3 and group 4 MBs arise in the midline. They typically fill the fourth ventricle, displacing and compressing the pons anteriorly **(21-1)**. Posteroinferior extension into the cisterna magna is common. Unlike ependymoma, lateral extension into the cerebellopontine angle is rare.

WNT MBs are also found at the cerebellopontine angle and along the lateral recess of the fourth ventricle. SHH MBs are most often located in the lateral cerebellum. Occasionally, MB occurs as a diffusely infiltrating lesion without a focal dominant mass.

Microscopic Features. MBs are highly cellular tumors ("small round blue cell tumor"). Neuroblastic (Homer Wright) rosettes—radial arrangements of tumor cells around fibrillary processes—are found in 40% of cases.

MEDULLOBLASTOMA: PATHOLOGY AND CLINICAL

Etiology
- All 4 molecular subtypes represented
  - Almost all WNT-activated MBs are CMBs

Pathology
- Midline (> 85%, 4th ventricle)
- "Small round blue cell tumor"
- Neuroblastic (Homer Wright) rosettes
- WHO grade IV

Clinical Features
- MB = 20% of all pediatric brain tumors
- Most common malignant posterior fossa childhood neoplasm
- Most CMBs in patients < 10 years
  - 2nd peak in patients 20-40 years

Clinical Issues

Epidemiology and Demographics. Most MBs occur before the age of 10 years old. There is a second, smaller peak in adults aged 20-40 years.

Presentation. The most common clinical manifestations of MB are vomiting (90%) and headache (80%). Because of their location, MBs tend to compress the fourth ventricle and cause obstructive hydrocephalus.

Natural History. Risk varies with the molecular subgroup. For example, almost all WNT-activated MBs exhibit classic histology and are considered low-risk neoplasms.

Imaging

The three main standard imaging phenotypes that can help predict MB molecular subgroups are (1) anatomic location **(21-3)**, (2) enhancement pattern, and (3) metastasis.

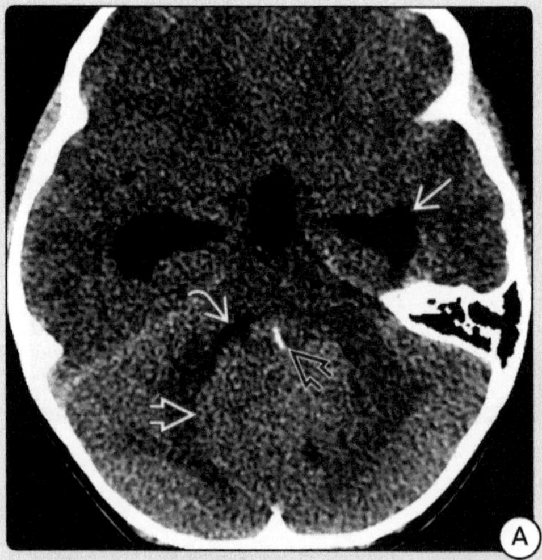

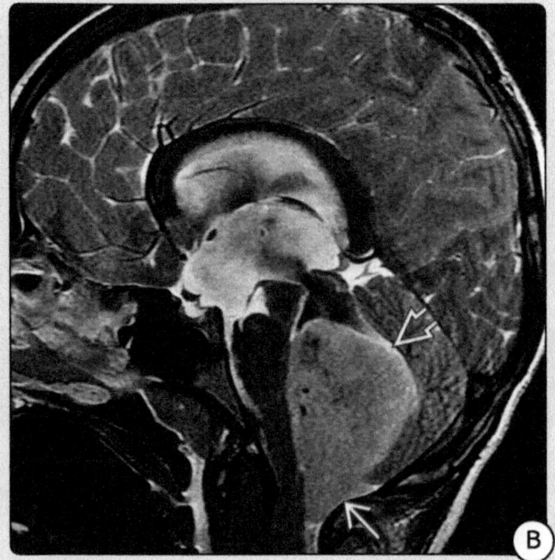

***(21-4A)** NECT in an 8y boy with confusion, headache, and 3 weeks of vomiting shows a mildly hyperdense mass ➡ in the midline posterior fossa that fills the 4th ventricle ➡. Obstructive hydrocephalus ➡ and a small focus of calcification ➡ in the mass are present. **(21-4B)** Sagittal T2 MR shows that the mass ➡ fills the 4th ventricle and extends posteroinferiorly through the foramen of Magendie into the cisterna magna ➡.*

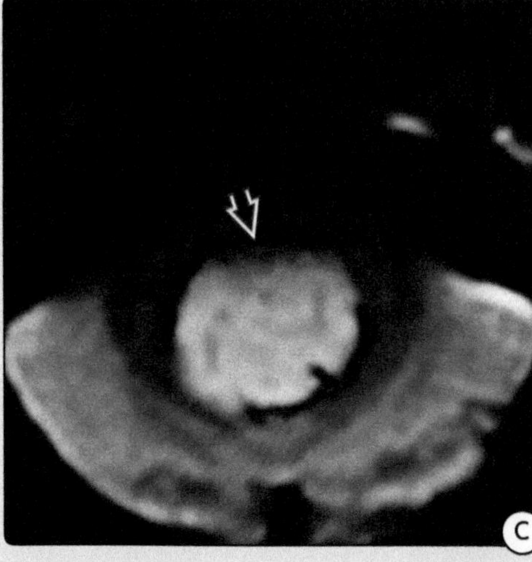

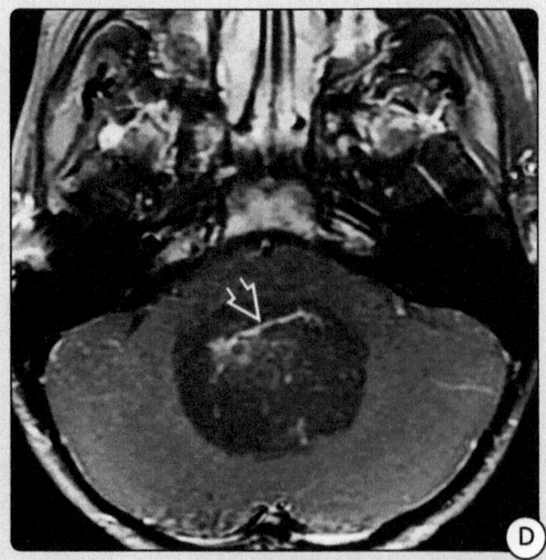

***(21-4C)** Axial DWI MR in the same case shows that the mass ➡ exhibits uniformly restricted diffusion. **(21-4D)** Axial T1 C+ FS MR shows mild irregular enhancement ➡ in the center of the mass. This is group 4, classic histology, WHO grade IV, standard risk.*

Radiomics and machine learning approaches have recently been reported as significantly improving the prediction of the MB subgroup in individual cases.

As 40-50% of MBs have CSF dissemination at the time of initial diagnosis, preoperative contrast-enhanced MR of the entire neuraxis is recommended.

CT Findings. NECT scans show a moderately hyperdense, relatively well-defined mass in the midline posterior fossa (classic MB) **(21-4A)**, around the foramen of Luschka (WNT-subgroup MB) **(21-7)** or lateral cerebellum (SHH) **(21-6)**. Cyst formation (40%) and calcification (20-25%) are common **(21-4A)**. Gross hemorrhage is rare. Strong but heterogeneous enhancement is seen on CECT.

If dense tentorial or falcine calcifications are present, the patient should be evaluated for basal cell nevus (Gorlin) syndrome.

MR Findings. Almost all MBs are hypointense relative to gray matter on T1WI and hyperintense on T2WI **(21-4B)**. Peritumoral edema is present in 1/3 of cases. Obstructive hydrocephalus with periventricular accumulation of CSF is common and best delineated on FLAIR.

Because of their dense cellularity, MBs often show moderate restriction on DWI **(21-4C)**. pMR shows low rCBV and increased permeability.

Enhancement patterns show striking variation. 2/3 of MBs show marked enhancement, whereas 1/3 show only subtle, marginal, or linear enhancement **(21-4D)**. Multifocal grape-like tumor masses that enhance strongly and uniformly can be seen in MBs with extensive nodularity.

Group 4 MBs typically exhibit minimal or no enhancement. Enhancing CSF metastases at initial diagnosis are common ("sugar icing") and typically occur with groups 3 and 4 **(21-5)**.

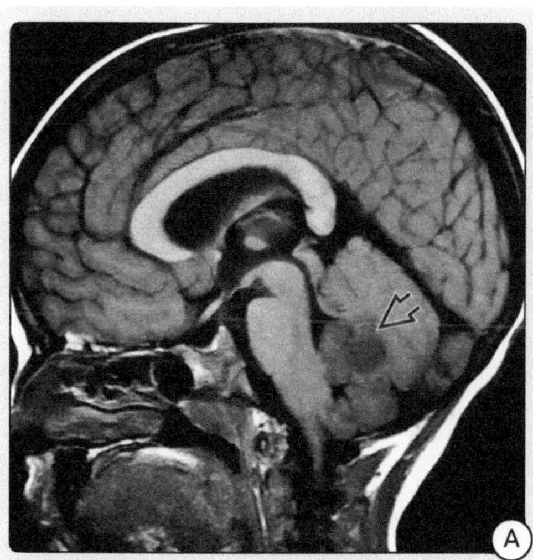

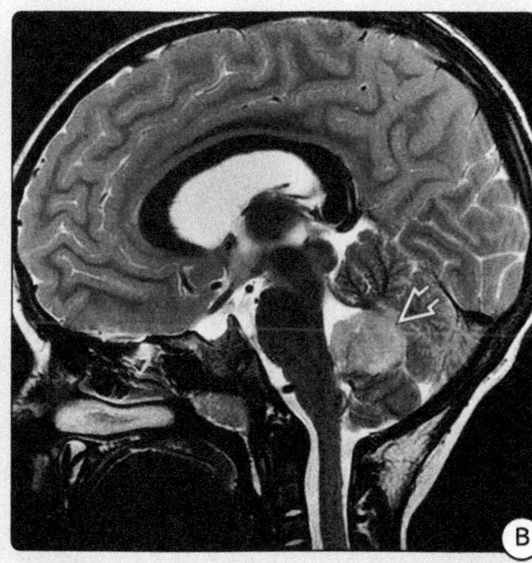

***(21-5A)** Sagittal T1 MR in a 4-year-old boy with vomiting and bulging fontanelle shows a mixed iso- and hypointense mass ➡ in the midline posterior fossa. **(21-5B)** Sagittal T2 MR in the same case shows that the mass ➡ bulges into the 4th ventricle and is iso- to mildly hyperintense compared with gray matter.*

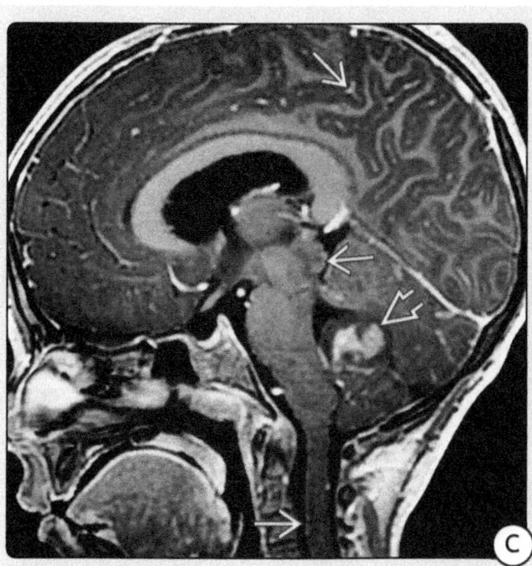

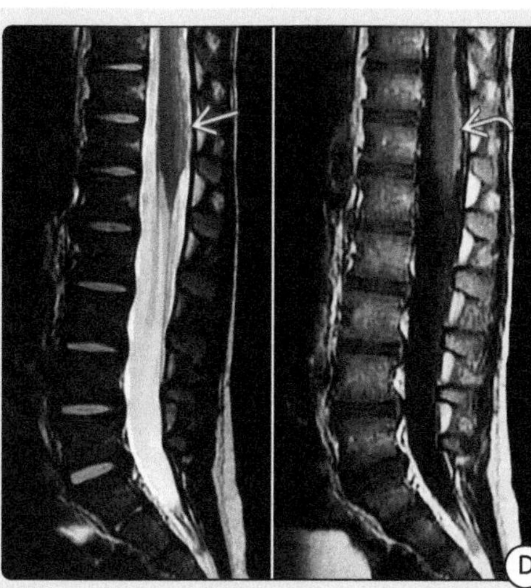

***(21-5C)** Sagittal T1 C+ MR shows strong but patchy enhancement ➡ in the mass. Note subtle pial enhancement along the tectum, in the hemispheric sulci, and coating the spinal cord ➡. **(21-5D)** (L) Sagittal T2 MR shows thickened nodular "lumpy-bumpy" hyperintensity ➡ along the distal spinal cord. (R) Sagittal T1 C+ MR shows that these are enhancing pial metastases ➡. This is group 3 MB with CSF dissemination at initial presentation.*

MEDULLOBLASTOMA IMAGING

CT

- Hyperdense on NECT
- Cysts (40%)
- Ca^{++} (20-25%)
- Hemorrhage rare

MR

- Hypointense on T1, hyperintense on T2
- Often restricts on DWI
- Enhancement: None to strong
  - Strong but heterogeneous common
  - Little/no enhancement characteristic of group 4

Differential Diagnosis

- Atypical teratoid/rhabdoid tumor
- Lhermitte-Duclos disease (adults)
- Metastasis (adult)

Differential Diagnosis

The major differential diagnosis of MB in children is **atypical teratoid/rhabdoid tumor (AT/RT)**. AT/RT may be indistinguishable from CMB on imaging studies alone.

Lhermitte-Duclos disease (LDD) can be seen in children but is more common in young adults. LDD and SHH-activated desmoplastic MB may resemble one another, although the striated pattern of LDD is quite characteristic.

The differential diagnosis of MB in adults differs. The most common parenchymal posterior fossa mass in adults is **metastasis**.

(21-6A) Axial T1 MR in a 24-year-old woman with headaches and dizziness shows a mildly hypointense mass ➡ in the right cerebellar hemisphere. (21-6B) T2 MR in the same case shows that the mass ➡ is hyperintense compared with cortex.

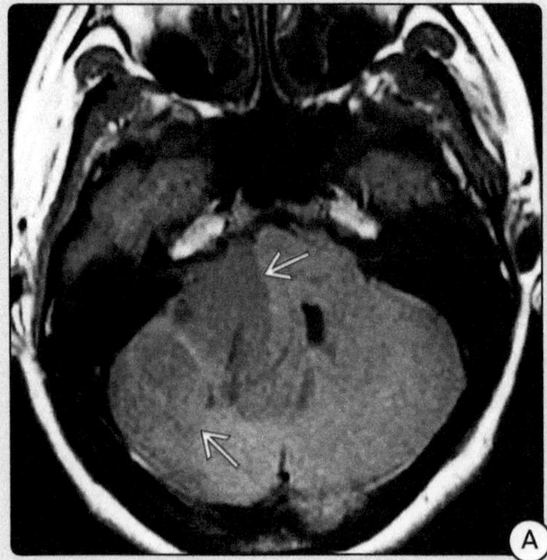

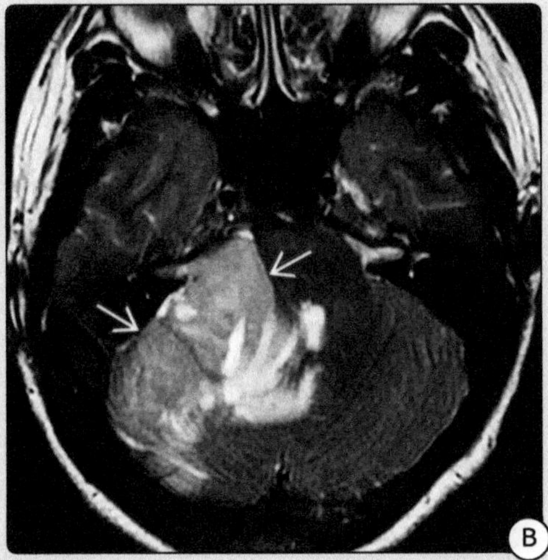

(21-6C) T1 C+ FS MR in the same case shows strong, uniform enhancement in the solid, lobulated-appearing mass ➡. (21-6D) DWI MR shows that the mass restricts strongly and uniformly ➡. Desmoplastic MB was found at surgery. Most desmoplastic MBs in the lateral cerebellum are SHH-activated, low-risk tumors of children and adults.

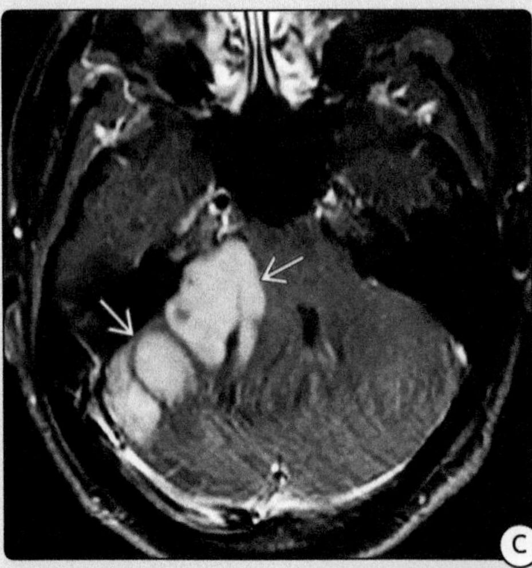

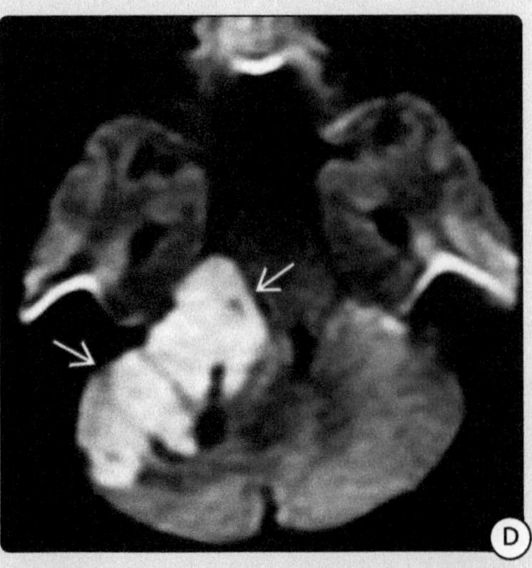

Other CNS Embryonal Tumors

CNS embryonal neoplasms other than medulloblastoma (MB) are a heterogeneous group of poorly differentiated tumors. Classification of these non-MB embryonal tumors has changed with the deletion of the term "primitive neuroectodermal tumor (PNET)" and the addition of a new entity, **embryonal tumor with multilayered rosettes (ETMR)**.

In addition to many pediatric CNS embryonal tumors that were formerly designated as PNETs, the new group of ETMRs also includes entities variously called ETANTR (**e**mbryonald **t**umor with **a**bundant **n**europil and **t**rue **r**osettes), ependymoblastoma, and medulloepithelioma. An embryonal tumor that does not correspond to known genetically defined entities is now designated as **CNS embryonal tumor, not otherwise specified (NOS)**.

Embryonal Tumor With Multilayered Rosettes

Terminology

ETMRs are aggressive CNS embryonal tumors that are characterized histologically by multilayered rosettes. ETMR also includes entities previously called ETANTR (**e**mbryonal **t**umor with **a**bundant **n**europil and **t**rue **r**osettes), ependymoblastoma, and medulloepithelioma. All share a common molecular signature, C19MC locus amplification, and therefore comprise a single clinicopathologic entity.

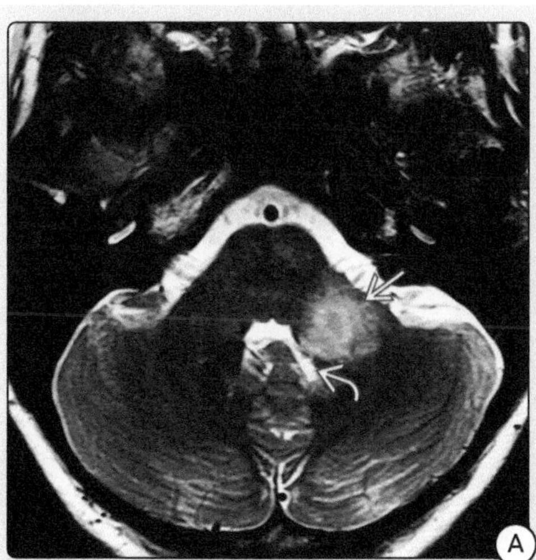

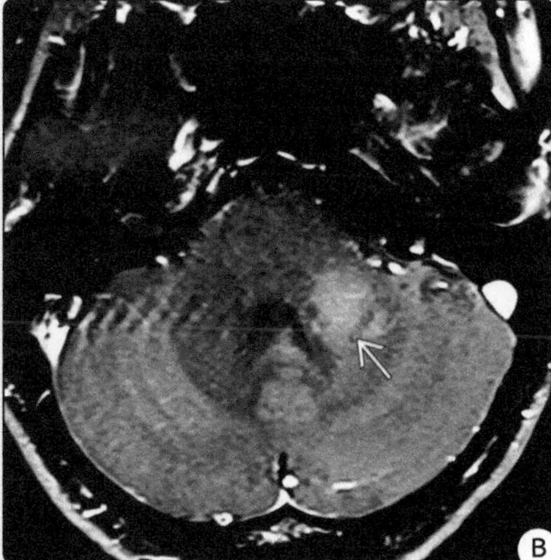

***(21-7A)** T2 MR in a 22-year-old woman with headaches shows a heterogeneously hyperintense mass in the left cerebellar peduncle ➡ that compresses and displaces the lateral recess of the 4th ventricle ➡. **(21-7B)** Axial T1 C+ FS MR shows mild enhancement in the brachium pontis mass ➡.*

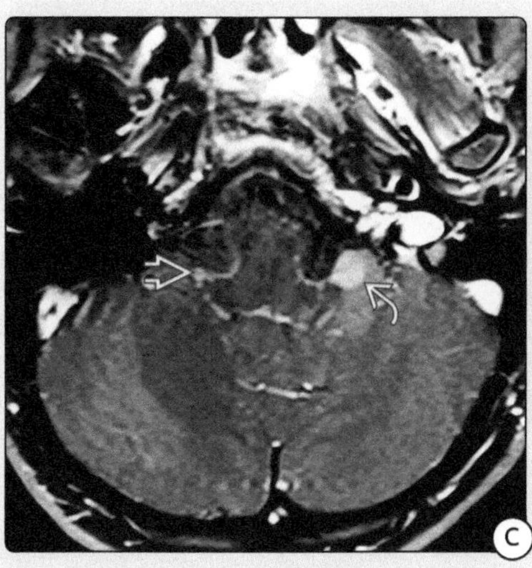

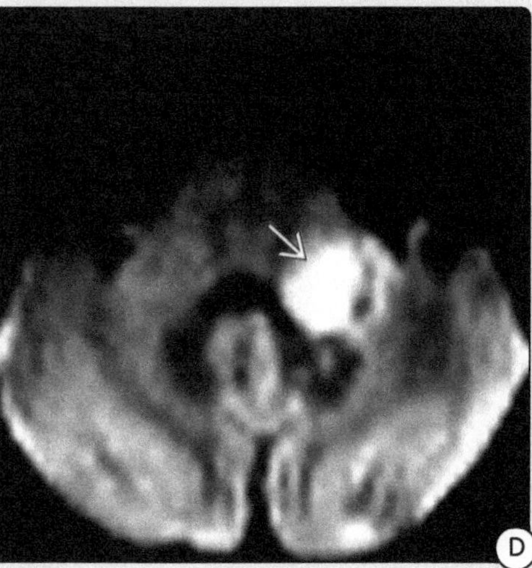

***(21-7C)** More inferior axial T1 C+ FS MR shows an enhancing mass ➡ near the left foramen of Luschka. Note pial enhancement ➡, suggesting CSF metastases. **(21-7D)** Axial DWI MR in the same case shows that the mass ➡ restricts strongly. Surgery disclosed classic histology, WNT activated. This is considered a low-risk tumor. Despite CSF spread, the patient is alive and well 5 years later.*

Pathology

Approximately 70% of ETMRs are supratentorial masses that appear relatively well demarcated with little surrounding edema. Tumors are often > 5 cm in diameter, and some are massive lesions that occupy much of the cerebral hemispheres **(21-8)**. The cerebellum and brainstem are the primary site in 30% of cases.

Microscopically, ETMRs contain abundant neuropil and true rosettes with a pseudostratified neuroepithelium surrounding a central round or slit-like lumen. Mitoses are frequent, and CSF dissemination is common. C19MC-altered ETMR corresponds histologically to WHO grade IV.

Clinical Issues

Almost all ETMRs occur under the age of 4 years with the majority occurring in the first 2 years of life. Increasing head circumference and signs of elevated intracranial pressure are common. ETMRs are extremely aggressive neoplasms, and the clinical prognosis is dismal.

Imaging

General Features. ETMRs grow rapidly and are often very large, heterogeneous-appearing masses that cause gross distortion and effacement of the underlying brain architecture **(21-9)**.

CT Findings. A complex, heterogeneously iso- to hyperdense mass with mixed cystic and solid components is typical on NECT. Necrosis and intratumoral hemorrhages are common, as are dystrophic calcifications. CECT scans show moderate but heterogeneous enhancement.

MR Findings. All sequences exhibit heterogeneous signal intensity with T1 shortening **(21-9A)** and T2* blooming secondary to intratumoral hemorrhage. T2/FLAIR hyperintensity in cystic or necrotic segments and isointensity

(21-8) Autopsy (L) and antemortem FLAIR scan (R) in an 8m infant with a supratentorial embryonal neoplasm show a large, aggressive-looking hemispheric mass with confluent areas of necrosis and hemorrhage. There is relatively little peritumoral edema. (Courtesy R. Hewlett, MD.) (21-9A) Axial T1 MR in an infant with macrocephaly shows a very large right frontal mass ➡ with areas of necrosis ⇨ and hemorrhage ↪.

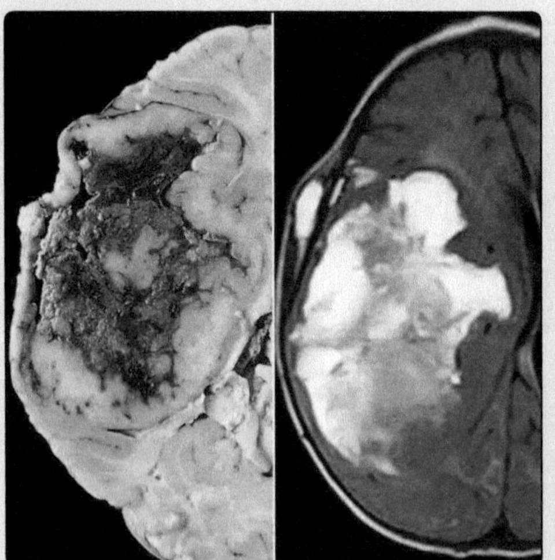

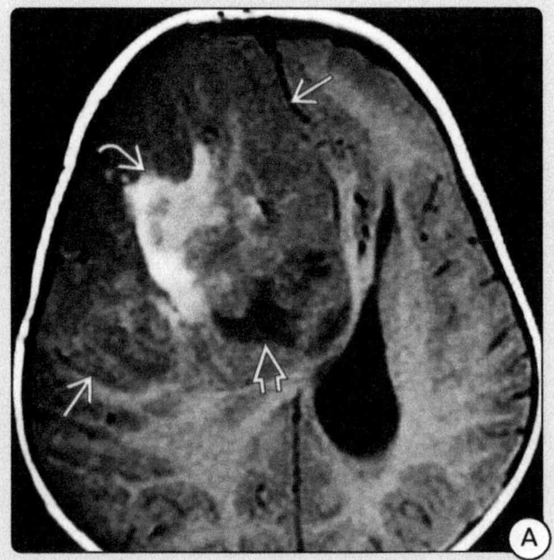

(21-9B) T2 MR in the same patient shows that the mass is relatively well demarcated ➡ and mostly hyperintense with heterogeneously hypointense foci of hemorrhage ↪. (21-9C) The lesion restricts on DWI ➡. This is a supratentorial embryonal neoplasm (formerly designated as primitive neuroectodermal tumor). (Courtesy G. Hedlund, DO.)

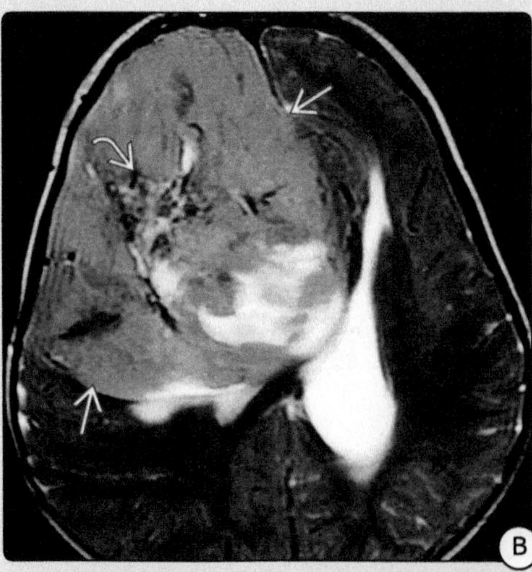

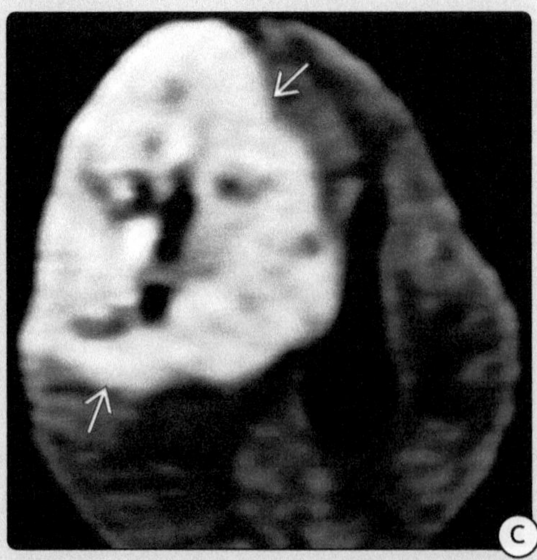

in the solid portions of the mass are typical. Peritumoral edema is typically minimal or absent **(21-9B)**.

Because of their relatively dense cellularity, C19MC-altered ETMRs may show foci of moderately restricted diffusion **(21-9C)**. pMR shows areas of elevated rCBV and vascular permeability.

Heterogeneous enhancement with solid and rim enhancement is typical **(21-10)**.

Differential Diagnosis

The differential diagnosis of C19MC-altered ETMR in infants and children includes other bulky hemispheric masses, including **AT/RT, RELA fusion-positive ependymoma, astroblastoma, glioblastoma**, and the rare **CNS neuroblastoma** or **ganglioneuroblastoma**.

Malignant Rhabdoid Tumors

Malignant rhabdoid tumors (MRTs) are aggressive tumors that were first described in the kidneys and soft tissues of infants and young children. Cranial rhabdoid tumors were subsequently recognized as a distinct pathologic entity and termed atypical teratoid/rhabdoid tumor (AT/RT). AT/RTs are separated from other CNS embryonal neoplasms and non-CNS MRTs by distinct immunohistochemical, histopathologic, and molecular features.

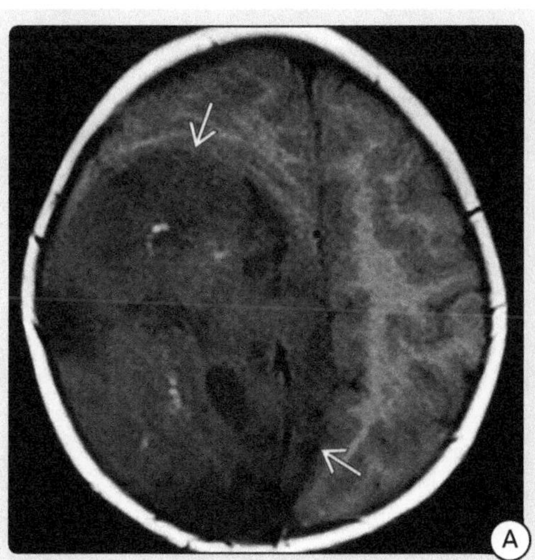

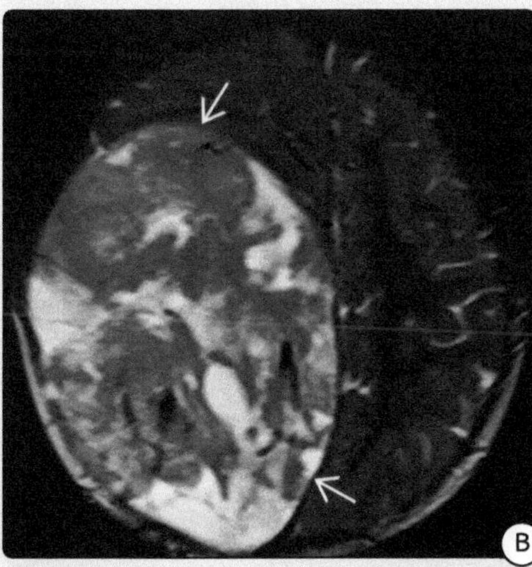

(21-10A) Axial T1 MR in a 2-year-old girl shows a large mass of mixed signal intensity ➡ that occupies most of the right cerebral hemisphere. (21-10B) Axial T2 FS MR in the same case shows that the mass is very heterogeneously hyperintense ➡ and relatively well demarcated. There is no discernible surrounding edema.

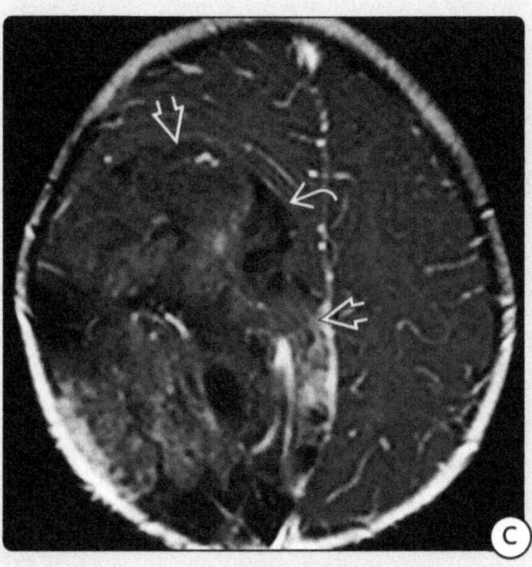

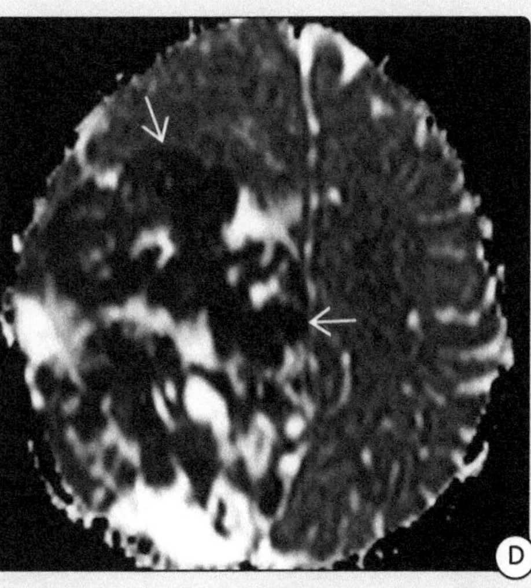

(21-10C) Axial T1 C+ MR shows mild to moderate patchy enhancement ➡ in some portions of the mass, whereas others show little or no enhancement ➡. (21-10D) ADC map shows that solid portions of the tumor ➡ exhibit restricted diffusion. Embryonal tumor with multilayered rosettes, C19MC altered, was documented. (Courtesy M. Warmuth-Metz, MD.)

Atypical Teratoid/Rhabdoid Tumor

Terminology

AT/RT is a rare, highly malignant CNS embryonal tumor composed of poorly differentiated elements and malignant rhabdoid cells.

Etiology

AT/RT is now a genetically defined tumor characterized by deletions and biallelic inactivating mutations of the *SMARCB1/*SNF5 gene. Loss of the SMARCB1 protein in AT/RT results in unopposed expression of *LIN28B* (a key gene in embryonic development and for maintaining pluripotency in stem cells).

Molecular profiling has identified three epigenetically and clinically distinct AT/RT subgroups, currently designated as ATRT-TYR, ATRT-SHH, and ATRT-MYC.

Pathology

Location. AT/RTs occur in both the supra- and infratentorial compartments. Location is strongly correlated with molecular subgroup.

Slightly more than 1/2 of AT/RTs are supratentorial, usually occurring in the cerebral hemispheres **(21-11)**, although cases in other sites (including the suprasellar cistern, ventricles, and pineal gland) have been reported. Most supratentorial AT/RTs are ATRT-MYC or ATRT-SHH subtypes.

Posterior fossa AT/RTs preferentially occur in the cerebellar hemispheres **(21-12)**, although they can occur in the fourth ventricle where they mimic medulloblastoma. Although ATRT-MYC and ATRT-SHH subtypes occasionally occur here, the posterior fossa is the site of ~ 75% of ATRT-TYR neoplasms.

*(**21-11A**) NECT in an 18-month-old girl with vomiting for 1-2 weeks shows a mixed, mostly hyperdense right frontal mass ➡ with marked vasogenic edema ➡. (**21-11B**) T2 MR shows that the mass has mixed, mostly hypo- and isointense signal intensity.*

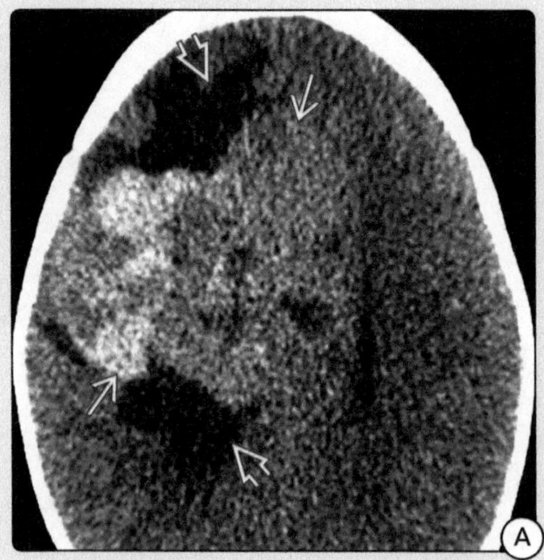

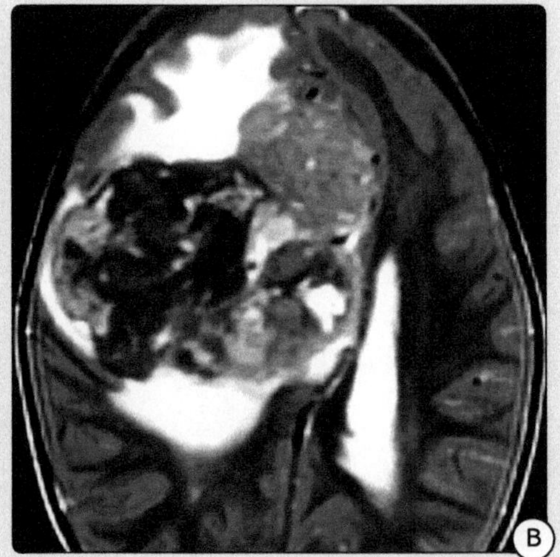

*(**21-11C**) T1 C+ MR shows diffuse but very heterogeneous enhancement. (**21-11D**) ADC map shows marked diffuse restriction ➡ due to the high cellularity of the tumor. MRS (not shown) demonstrated elevated Cho and lactate. Histologic diagnosis was atypical teratoid/rhabdoid tumor (AT/RT). (Courtesy B. Jones, MD.)*

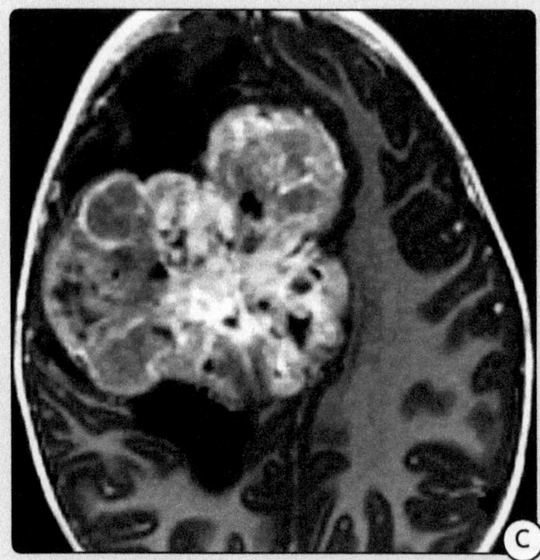

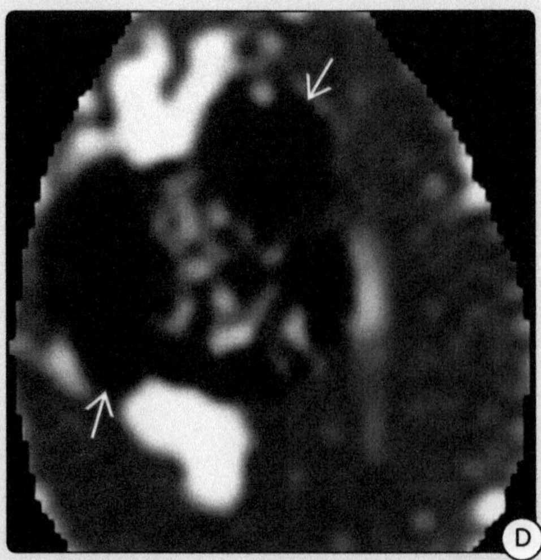

AT/RT: ETIOLOGY AND PATHOLOGY

Etiology
- Loss of expression of *SMARCB1* protein (INI1) required for diagnosis
- 3 epigenetically distinct AT/RT subgroups
  - ATRT-TYR, ATRT-SHH, ATRT-MYC

Pathology
- Supratentorial: ~ 50%
  - Most are ATRT-MYC or ATRT-SHH
- Infratentorial: ~ 50%
  - All 3 subgroups (75% of ATRT-TYR)
- Poorly differentiated neuroepithelial elements + rhabdoid cells
- WHO grade IV

Gross Pathology. The gross appearance—a large, soft, fleshy, hemorrhagic, necrotic mass—is similar to that of other CNS embryonal neoplasms.

Microscopic Features. AT/RTs are composed of poorly differentiated neural, epithelial, and mesenchymal elements together with prominent rhabdoid cells. Loss of nuclear staining for INI1 is diagnostic of AT/RT.

Clinical Issues

Epidemiology. AT/RT accounts for 1-2% of all pediatric brain tumors and up to 20% of patients < 3 years of age. AT/RT does occur in adults but is rare. There is a moderate male predominance.

AT/RT can occur sporadically or in **rhabdoid tumor predisposition syndrome** (RTPS). RTPS is a familial cancer syndrome characterized by a markedly increased risk of developing MRTs—including AT/RT—caused by loss or

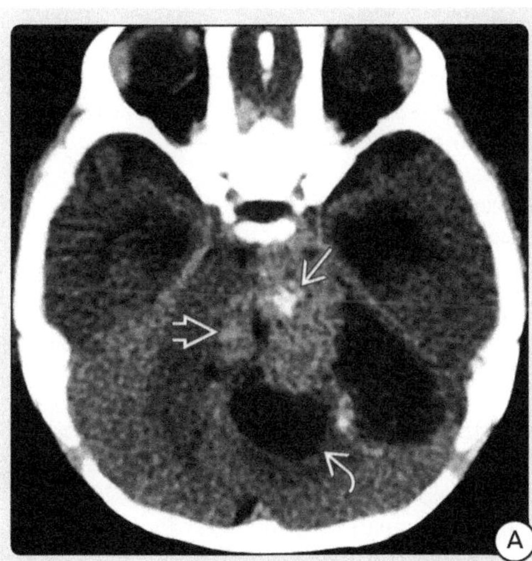

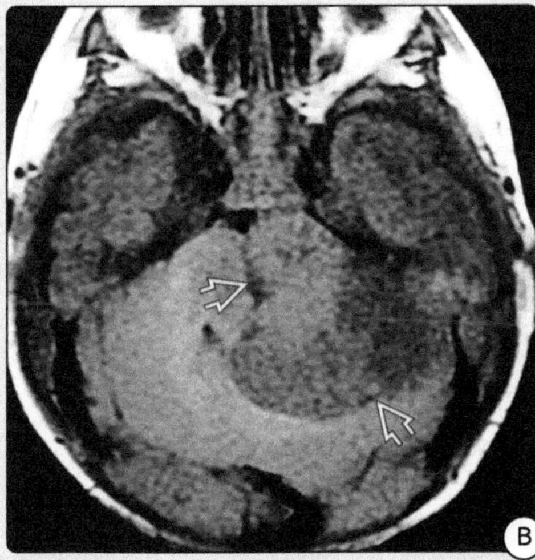

(21-12A) NECT in a 4-month-old boy with vomiting, head tilt, and bulging fontanelle shows a partially solid ➡, partially cystic-appearing ➡ posterior fossa mass that exhibits focal calcifications ➡. (21-12B) Axial T1 MR in the same case shows that the mass ➡ is mixed iso-/hypointense compared with gray matter.

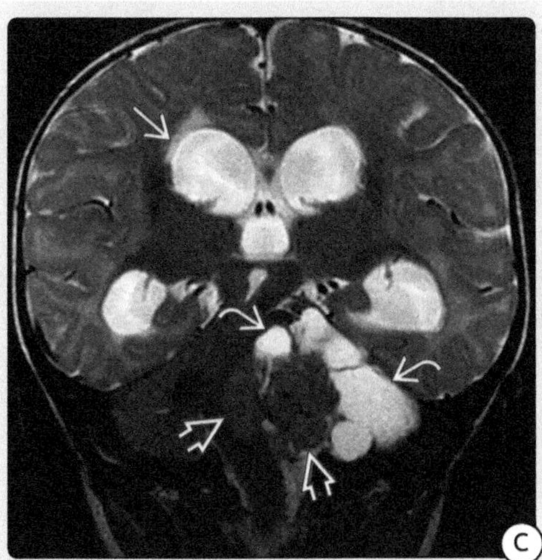

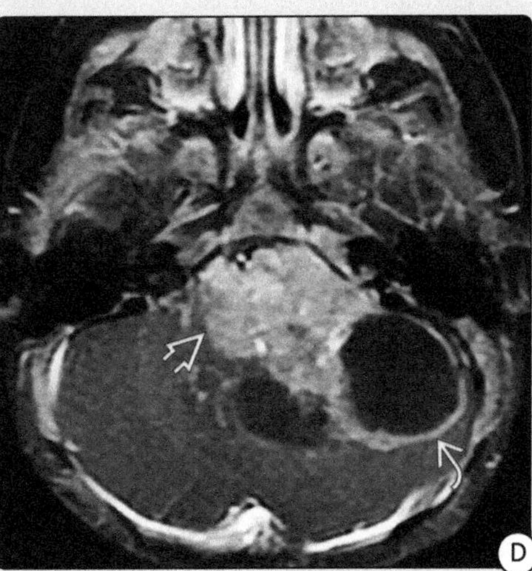

(21-12C) Coronal T2 MR in the same case shows that the mixed solid ➡, cystic ➡ mass is causing severe obstructive hydrocephalus ➡. (21-12D) Axial T1 C+ FS MR shows the solid components ➡ of the mass enhancing strongly but heterogeneously. The cysts exhibit rim enhancement ➡. This is AT/RT, WHO grade IV.

inactivation of the *SMARCB1* gene (less commonly, the mutation involves the *SMARCA4* gene).

Children with RTPS and AT/RT are even younger, have more extensive disease, and experience more rapid progression compared to sporadic tumors. Other CNS tumors associated with RTPS include choroid plexus carcinoma and rhabdoid meningioma.

Natural History. AT/RT is a highly malignant tumor with generally poor prognosis. Median survival is around 17 months. Most children die within 6-8 months despite aggressive therapy. Survival in adults is somewhat better, averaging two years.

AT/RT: CLINICAL ISSUES

Epidemiology
- 1-2% of pediatric brain tumors
    - Children < 5 years, most < 2 years
    - 10% of CNS neoplasms in infants
    - Occasionally occur in adults (rare)

Rhabdoid Tumor Predisposition Syndrome
- Malignant rhabdoid tumors
- Choroid plexus carcinoma

Imaging

General Features. AT/RT shares many imaging features with other embryonal tumors, i.e., they are densely cellular neoplasms that frequently contain hemorrhage, necrosis, cysts, and calcifications. A moderately large, bulky tumor with mixed solid and cystic components and heterogeneous density/signal intensity is typical.

CSF dissemination is common, so the entire neuraxis should be imaged prior to surgical intervention.

CT Findings. NECT scan shows a mildly to moderately hyperdense mass with cysts and hemorrhagic foci **(21-11A)**. Peripheral cysts can be found in all molecular subgroups independent of location but occur most frequently in ATRT-TYR. Calcification and obstructive hydrocephalus—especially with posterior fossa AT/RT—are common. Enhancement is typically strong but heterogeneous.

MR Findings. AT/RTs are heterogeneously hypo- to isointense to brain on T1WI and iso- to hyperintense on T2WI **(21-11)**. "Blooming" foci on T2* (GRE, SWI) are common. Mild to moderate diffusion restriction is seen in the majority of cases **(21-11D)**. MRS shows elevated Cho and decreased or absent NAA.

Enhancement on T1 C+ is strong but heterogeneous, especially in ATRT-TYR and ATRT-MYC tumors. Although not present in the majority of AT/RTs, a distinct and unusual pattern of a "wavy" band-like enhancement surrounding a central hypointensity has been described in 38% of AT/RTs and is found throughout all molecular subgroups. Leptomeningeal spread at initial imaging is present in 15% of cases and occurs equally across all subgroups.

Differential Diagnosis

The major differential diagnosis for supratentorial AT/RT includes **C19MC-altered embryonal neoplasm, RELA-fusion ependymoma, teratoma**, and **malignant astrocytoma**. As all of these may be bulky—even massive—tumors with very heterogeneous imaging appearance, definitive diagnosis requires biopsy and *SMARCB1* (INI1) staining.

The major differential diagnosis for posterior fossa AT/RT is **medulloblastoma**. These tumors can look virtually identical on imaging studies.

AT/RT: IMAGING AND DIFFERENTIAL DIAGNOSIS

Imaging
- Heterogeneous, hyperdense on NECT
- Heterogeneous on both T1, T2
- Enhances strongly but heterogeneously
- CSF spread in 15-20% at diagnosis
- Restricts on DWI

Differential Diagnosis
- DDx of *supratentorial* AT/RT
    - CNS embryonal tumor, C19MC-altered
    - *RELA*-fusion ependymoma, teratoma, malignant astrocytoma
- DDx of *posterior fossa* AT/RT
    - Medulloblastoma (midline AT/RT may be indistinguishable)

Other CNS Neoplasms With Rhabdoid Features

CNS embryonal tumor with rhabdoid features is a highly malignant neoplasm composed of poorly differentiated elements and rhabdoid cells with *SMARCB1* or *SMARCA4* expression. These extremely rare tumors correspond histologically to WHO grade IV.

Rhabdoid meningioma is an uncommon WHO grade III meningioma subtype that contains sheets of rhabdoid cells. Most have high proliferative indices and exhibit other cytologic features of malignancy. Rhabdoid meningiomas are very rare in infants and retain INI1 staining, which differentiates them histopathologically from AT/RT.

Selected References: The complete reference list is available on the Expert Consult™ eBook version included with purchase.

Tumors of the Meninges

The cranial meninges give rise to a broad spectrum of neoplasms that usually occur as extraaxial masses (i.e., outside the brain parenchyma but inside the skull). The 2016 WHO classification divides tumors of the cranial meninges into two separate groups: (1) Meningiomas and meningioma variants and (2) mesenchymal nonmeningothelial tumors.

In this chapter, we focus on meningioma—the most common of all intracranial tumors and by far the largest group of meningothelial neoplasms. We then briefly consider nonmeningothelial mesenchymal tumors, CNS neoplasms that correspond to soft tissue or bone tumors found elsewhere in the body.

Meningomas

Meningiomas are the most common of all brain tumors, accounting for over 1/3 of all primary intracranial neoplasms. Meningioma is a benign lesion with nonaggressive growth and a low recurrence risk that corresponds histologically to WHO grade I.

Some histologic subtypes or meningiomas with various combinations of morphologic features and genomic instability are associated with more aggressive clinical behavior and less favorable outcomes. **Atypical meningioma** corresponds to WHO grade II. The most aggressive form of meningioma is **anaplastic ("malignant") meningioma**. Anaplastic meningiomas are WHO grade III neoplasms.

Meningioma

Terminology

Meningiomas comprise a group of relatively benign, slow-growing neoplasms that most likely arise from arachnoid meningothelial cells. They are sometimes called common or typical meningiomas (TM).

Etiology

Although meningiomas are physically attached to the dura **(22-1)** **(22-4)**, they actually arise from progenitors of arachnoid meningothelial ("cap") cells.

The mutational landscape of meningiomas is complex. Four distinct mutational subgroups have been proposed, defined by mutations in *NF2*, *TRAF7*, the hedgehog pathway, or *POLR21*. For purposes of this discussion, we divide meningiomas into NF2-mutant and non-NF2 meningiomas.

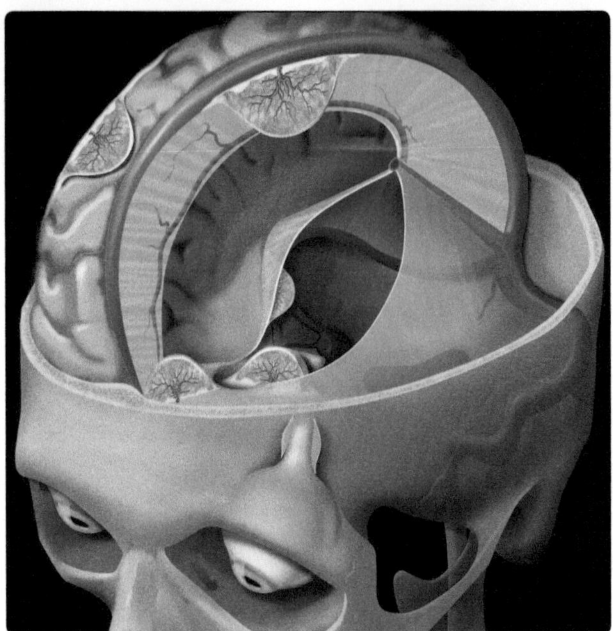

(22-1) The most common meningioma sites are convexity, parafalcine, followed by sphenoid ridge, olfactory groove, sella/parasellar region. 8-10% are infratentorial. Extracranial sites include optic nerve sheath, nose, and paranasal sinuses.

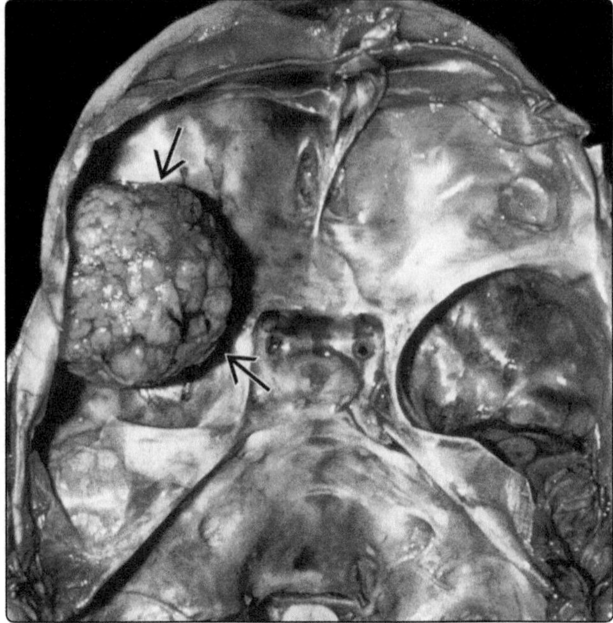

(22-2) Autopsy specimen demonstrates classic globose meningioma ⇒ as a round, "bosselated" mass with a flat surface toward the dura. (Courtesy R. Hewlett, MD.)

NF2-Mutant Meningiomas. The most common cytogenetic alteration in meningioma is biallelic mutation or loss of the tumor suppressor gene, neurofibromatosis 2 (*NF2*) on chromosome 22. This results in loss of its protein product Merlin (i.e., schwannomin), which modulates a wide variety of key signaling pathways (e.g., Ras/Raf/MEK) and serves as a tumor suppressor.

NF2 mutations are detected in most meningiomas associated with **type 2 neurofibromatosis (NF2)** and are found in 50% of sporadic meningiomas. *NF2* mutations occur in approximately equal frequency among all three WHO grades.

NF2-mutant meningiomas usually exhibit fibrous or transitional histology and originate along the posterior or superior cerebral hemispheres, the posterior and lateral skull base, and the spinal cord.

Non-NF2 Meningiomas. A number of other driver mutations, including *TRAF7*, *NOTCH2*, *SMARCB1*, and *SMO* (which modulates hedgehog pathway signaling), have been identified in 50% of meningiomas with wild-type *NF2*.

These non-NF2 meningiomas are usually benign and originate from the medial skull base and along the anterior cerebral hemispheres. Meningothelial, secretory, and microcystic subtypes are common.

Pathology

Location. Meningiomas can occur at virtually any site within the CNS **(22-1)**. Over 90% are supratentorial; 50% are parasagittal/convexity **(22-3)**. Between 15-20% are located along the sphenoid ridge **(22-2)**. Other common skull base locations are the olfactory groove and sellar/parasellar region (including the cavernous sinus). Less common supratentorial sites include the choroid plexus and tentorial apex.

The cerebellopontine angle is by far the most common infratentorial site followed by the jugular foramen and foramen magnum, usually from the clivus or craniocervical junction.

Between 1-2% of meningiomas are extracranial, e.g., orbit (optic nerve sheath) and paranasal sinuses. Calvarial vault ("intradiploic" or "intraosseous") meningiomas are seen in 1% of cases.

MENINGIOMA: LOCATION

General
- Supratentorial (90%), infratentorial (8-10%)
- Multiple (10%; NF2, meningiomatosis)

Sites
- Most common (60-70%)
  - Parasagittal (25%)
  - Convexity (25%)
  - Sphenoid ridge (15-20%)
- Less common (20-25%)
  - Posterior fossa (8-10%)
  - Olfactory groove (5-10%)
  - Parasellar (5-10%)
- Rare (2%)
  - Choroid plexus
  - Pineal region/tentorial apex
  - Extracranial (optic nerve sheath, sinuses)
  - Intraosseous (diploic space)

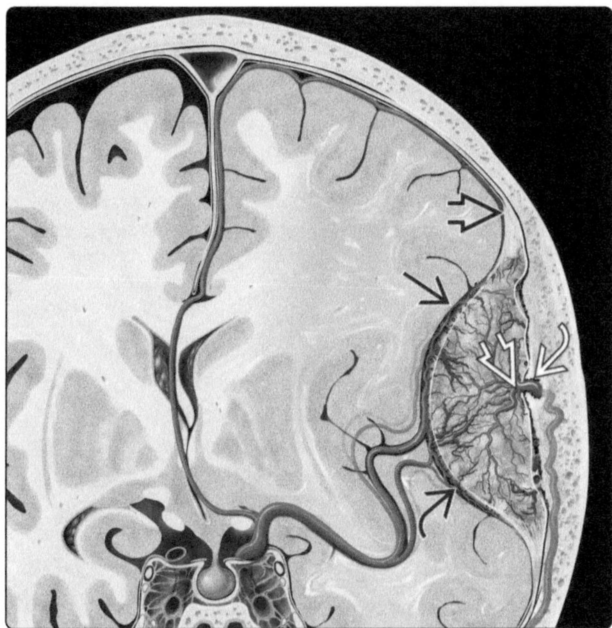

***(22-3)** Classic meningioma has a broad base toward dura, reactive dural thickening (dural "tail") ➡, enostotic "spur" ➡, CSF-vascular "cleft" ➡. MMA supplies tumor core in "sunburst" pattern ➡; pial vessels supply periphery ➡.*

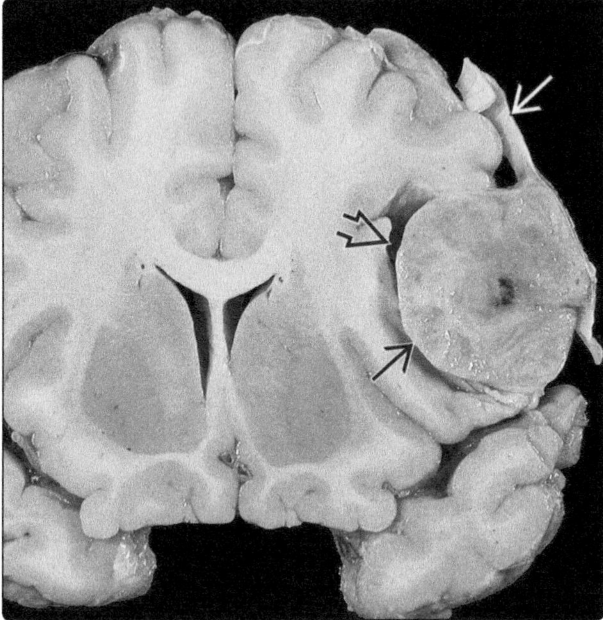

***(22-4)** Autopsy specimen shows classic globose meningioma ➡. Note prominent CSF-vascular cleft ➡ and reactive dural thickening ➡ ("dural tail" sign).*

Size and Number. Meningiomas vary widely in size. Most are small (< 1 cm) and found incidentally at imaging or autopsy. Some—especially those arising in the anterior fossa from the olfactory groove—attain large size before causing symptoms.

Meningiomas can be solitary (90%) or multiple. Multiple meningiomas occur in **NF2** as well as in **multiple meningiomatosis syndrome**.

Gross Pathology. Meningiomas have two general configurations: A round ("globose") **(22-2)** **(22-4)** and a flat, sheet-like or carpet-like ("en plaque") appearance. Most are well-demarcated masses that have a broad base of dural attachment. As they grow, meningiomas typically invaginate toward the adjacent brain. A CSF-vascular "cleft" is usually present between the tumor and underlying cortex **(22-3)** **(22-4)**. Histologically benign meningiomas rarely invade the brain.

Meningiomas often cause reactive nonneoplastic thickening of the adjacent dura ("dural tail" sign on imaging) **(22-6)** **(22-7)**. They commonly invade adjacent dural venous sinuses and may extend through the dura to involve the skull, inducing calvarial hyperostosis.

Although small "microcysts" are not uncommon in TMs, gross cystic change is rare. Frank hemorrhage is uncommon, occurring in only 1-2% of cases.

Rarely, metastasis from an extracranial primary to an intracranial meningioma occurs. Such **"collision tumors"** are typically lung or breast metastases to a histologically benign meningioma.

Microscopic Features. The 2016 WHO classification lists many meningioma subtypes. The most common are the **meningothelial, fibrous**, and mixed or **transitional** variants.

The vast majority of meningiomas are benign WHO grade I tumors and, by definition, carry a low risk of recurrence and aggressive growth. Their mitotic index is low with MIB-1 usually < 1%.

Histologically benign-appearing meningiomas that show gross or microscopic brain invasion are designated as grade II neoplasms.

Clinical Issues

Epidemiology. Meningioma is the most common primary brain tumor, accounting for over 1/3 of all reported CNS tumors. Between 90-95% are WHO grade I lesions.

Many meningiomas are small and discovered incidentally, often at imaging. The lifetime risk of developing meningioma is ~ 1% and meningiomas are found in 1-3% of autopsies.

Multiple meningiomas are common in patients with NF2 and non-NF2 hereditary multiple meningioma syndromes. Sporadic multiple (i.e., not syndromic) meningiomas occur in ~ 10% of cases.

Demographics. Meningiomas are classically tumors of middle-aged and older adults. Peak occurrence is in the sixth and seventh decades (mean = 65 years). Although meningioma accounts for slightly less than 3% of primary brain tumors in children, meningioma still represents the most common dura-based neoplasm in this age group. Many (but by no means all)

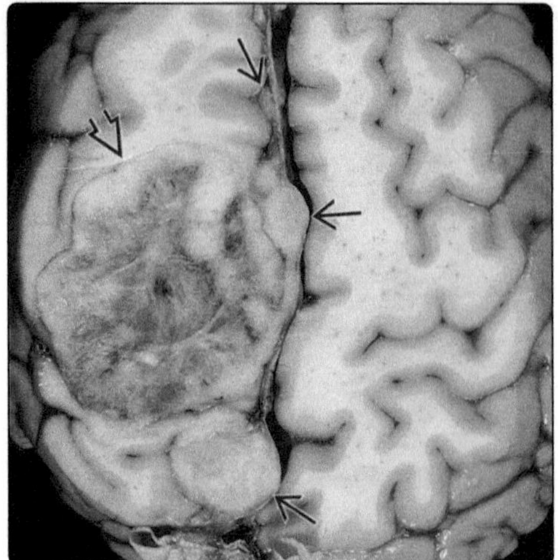

(22-5) Autopsied meningiomatosis shows meningioma invaginating into brain ⇒, multiple falcine meningiomas ⇒. (R. Hewlett, MD.)

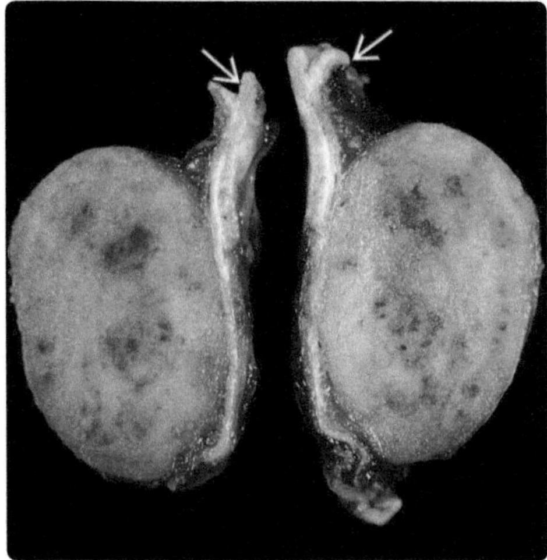

(22-6) Meningioma in cut section shows attachment to dura, reactive dural thickening ⇒ ("dural tail" sign). (Courtesy R. Hewlett, MD.)

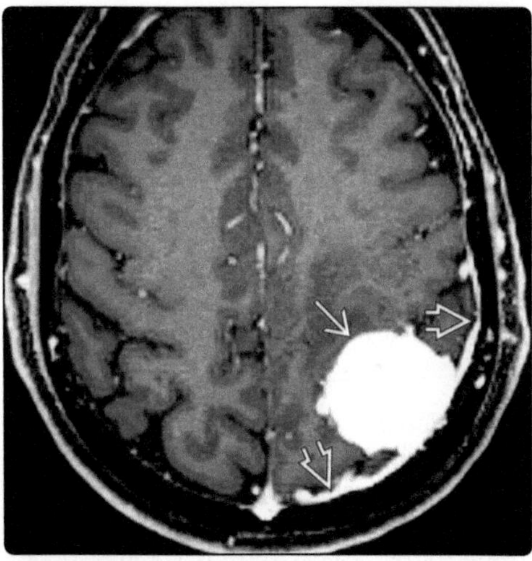

(22-7) Axial T1 C+ MR shows strongly enhancing typical meningioma ⇒. Adjacent dural thickening ⇒ ("dural tail" sign) is common.

are related to NF2. NF2-related meningiomas occur at a significantly younger age compared with nonsyndromic meningiomas.

Meningioma is one of the few brain tumors that exhibits a female predominance. The F:M ratio varies with age, peaking at 3.5-4.0:1.0 in premenopausal women in the 35- to 44-year age group.

Most WHO grade I meningiomas have progesterone receptors, and progesterone receptor expression is inversely associated with meningioma grade.

Presentation. Symptoms relate to tumor size and location. Less than 10% of meningiomas become symptomatic.

Natural History. Longitudinal studies have demonstrated that most small meningiomas (< 2.5 cm) grow very slowly—if at all—over five years. The majority of small, asymptomatic, incidentally discovered meningiomas show minimal growth and are usually followed with serial imaging.

Methylation class is important in prognosis; patients with WHO grade I meningiomas of intermediate methylation class have a less favorable outcome that is comparable to WHO grade II meningiomas. Malignant degeneration of a WHO grade I meningioma into an atypical or anaplastic meningioma is rare.

Treatment Options. Stratified treatment risk:benefit ratios vary, not just with tumor type, grade, and methylation status, but also with size and location, vascular supply, and presence or absence of a brain/tumor cleavage plane.

Image-guided surgery with resection of symptomatic lesions is generally curative. The major factor associated with meningioma recurrence is subtotal resection.

MENINGIOMA: CLINICAL ISSUES

Epidemiology
- Most common intracranial primary neoplasm
  - 36% of all primary CNS neoplasms
- Most are asymptomatic
  - Found incidentally at imaging/autopsy (1-3%)
- Solitary (> 90%)
  - Multiple in NF2, meningiomatosis

Demographics
- F:M = 2:1
  - Sex difference greatest prior to menopause
- Median age at diagnosis: 65 years
- Rare in children unless NF2

Natural History
- Grows slowly
- Rarely metastasizes
- Malignant degeneration is rare

Imaging

General Features. The general appearance of meningioma is a round or lobulated, sharply demarcated, extraaxial dura-based mass that buckles the cortex inward. A discernible CSF-vascular "cleft" is usually present, especially on MR. Parenchymal invasion is uncommon. When present, it indicates atypical meningioma, WHO grade II.

Meningioma-associated cysts are found in 4-7% of cases. These can be intra- or extra-/peritumoral. Occasionally, pools of CSF are trapped between the tumor and adjacent brain.

CT Findings

NECT. Almost 3/4 of meningiomas are mildly to moderately hyperdense compared with cortex **(22-10)**. About 1/4 are isodense **(22-11A)**. Hypodense meningiomas occur but are uncommon **(22-15A)**. Frank necrosis or hemorrhage is rare.

Peritumoral vasogenic edema, seen as confluent hypodensity in the adjacent brain, is present in ~ 60% of all cases.

Approximately 25% of meningiomas demonstrate calcification **(22-8)** **(22-9)**. Focal globular or more diffuse sand-like ("psammomatous") calcifications occur.

Bone CT may show hyperostosis that varies from minimal to striking **(22-12)**. Hyperostosis is often but not invariably associated with tumor invasion. Striking enlargement of an adjacent paranasal sinus may occur with skull base meningiomas **(22-13)**. Bone lysis or frank destruction can also occur. Bone involvement by meningioma occurs with both benign and malignant meningiomas and is not predictive of tumor grade.

CECT. The vast majority of meningiomas enhance strongly and uniformly **(22-10)**.

MR Findings

General Features. The majority of meningiomas are isointense with cortex on all sequences. Between 10-25% of cases demonstrate changes suggestive of cyst formation or necrosis, although frank hemorrhage is uncommon.

T1WI. Meningiomas are typically iso- to slightly hypointense compared with cortex. Predominant hypointensity on T1WI and hyperintensity on T2WI suggest the microcystic variant **(22-15)**.

T2WI. Most meningiomas are iso- to moderately hyperintense compared with cortex on T2WIs. T2-/FLAIR-hypointense tumors tend to be "hard" and somewhat gritty. Densely fibrotic and calcified meningiomas (appearing as "brain rocks" on NECT) can be very hypointense.

The CSF-vascular "cleft" **(22-3)** is especially well delineated on T2WI and is seen as a hyperintense rim interposed between the tumor and brain. A number of "flow voids" representing displaced vessels are often seen within the "cleft."

Sometimes a "sunburst" pattern that represents the dural vascular supply to the tumor can be identified radiating toward the periphery of the mass **(22-14B)**.

FLAIR. Meningioma signal intensity varies from iso- to hyperintense relative to brain. FLAIR is especially useful for depicting peritumoral edema, which is found with ~ 1/2 of all meningiomas. Peritumoral edema is related to the presence of pial blood supply and VEGF expression, *not* tumor size or grade.

Pools of CSF trapped in the cleft between tumor and brain (nonneoplastic "peritumoral cysts") are usually proteinaceous and may not suppress completely on FLAIR.

T1 C+. Virtually all meningiomas, including densely calcified "brain rocks" and intraosseous tumors, demonstrate at least some enhancement following

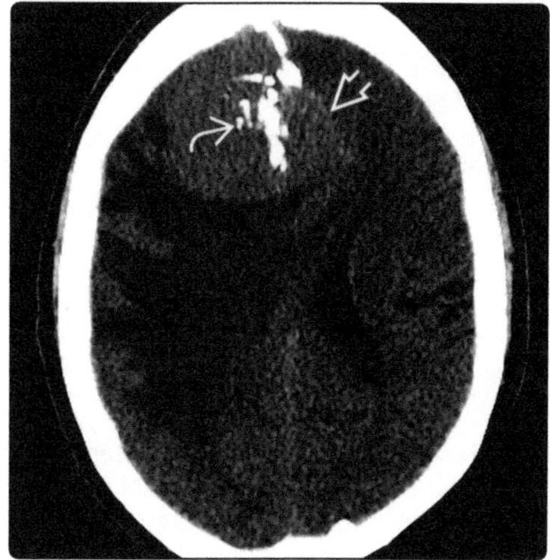

***(22-8)** Axial NECT in a 67-year-old woman with headaches shows a slightly hyperdense, heavily calcified right frontal mass.*

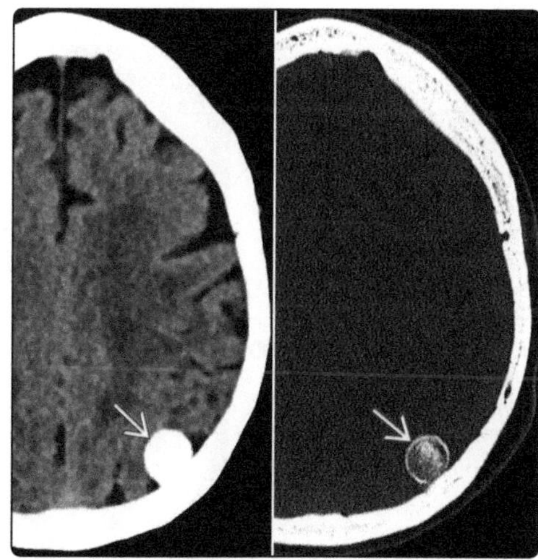

***(22-9)** NECT in an 88y woman with soft tissue (L), bone algorithm (R) shows densely calcified meningioma. This is an incidental finding.*

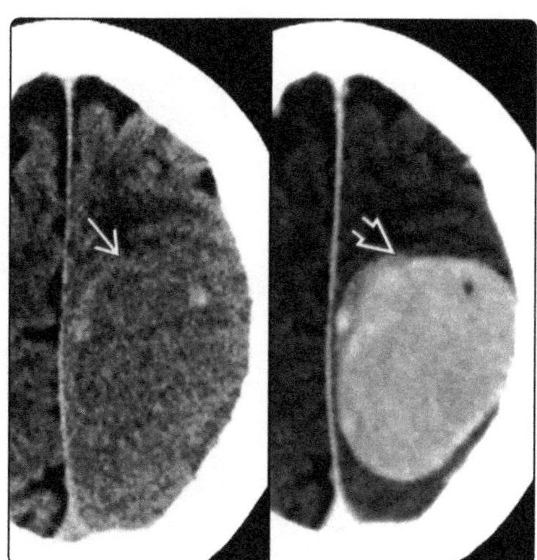

***(22-10)** NECT (L) and CECT (R) show isodense left convexity mass that enhances uniformly. This is classic meningioma, WHO grade I.*

contrast administration. Over 95% enhance strongly and homogeneously **(22-11B)**.

A dural "tail" is seen in the majority of meningiomas and varies from a relatively focal area adjacent to the tumor **(22-7)** to dural thickening and enhancement that extends far beyond the site of tumor attachment. The dural "tail" often enhances more intensely and more uniformly than the tumor itself. A "dural tail" sign is not pathognomonic of meningioma.

Most of the enhancing dural "tail" represents benign, reactive dural thickening. Tumor extending 1 cm beyond the base of the tumor is rare.

Nonenhancing *intratumoral* cysts are seen in 5% of cases. Nonneoplastic *peritumoral* cysts do not enhance. Enhancement around the rim of a cyst suggests the presence of marginal tumor in the cyst wall, so complete cyst resection is recommended if technically feasible.

Other Sequences. T2* sequences are helpful to depict intratumoral calcification. "Blooming" secondary to intratumoral hemorrhage is rare. Most meningiomas do not restrict on DWI.

Perfusion MR may be helpful in distinguishing TM from atypical/malignant meningiomas. High rCBV in the lesion or in the surrounding edema suggests a more aggressive tumor grade.

Alanine (Ala, peak at 1.48 ppm) is often elevated in meningioma, although glutamate-glutamine (Glx, peak at 2.1-2.6 ppm) and glutathione (GSH, peak at 2.95 ppm) may be more specific potential markers.

Angiography. CTA is very helpful in detecting dural venous sinus invasion or occlusion. Although it may be helpful in depicting the general status of the vascular supply to a meningioma, DSA is best for detailed delineation of tumor

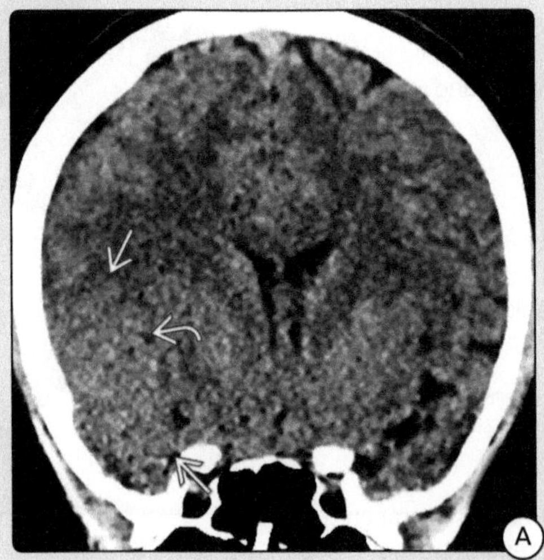

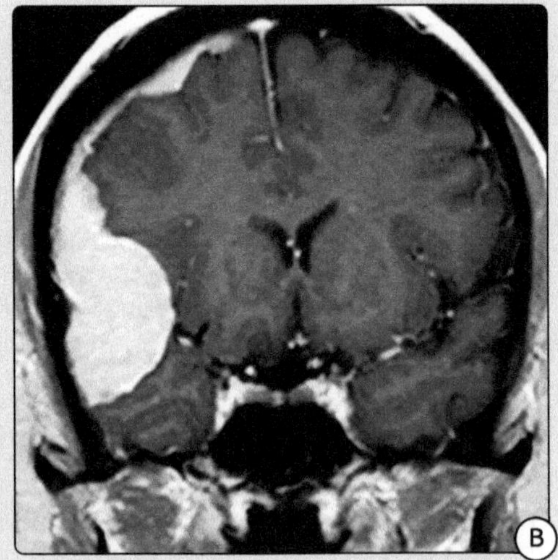

***(22-11A)** Coronal NECT in a 43-year-old woman with headaches shows subtle effacement of the right sylvian fissure ➔ by a mass ➔ that is isodense with cortex. **(22-11B)** Coronal T1 C+ MR in the same case shows extensive "en plaque" meningioma. Because they are often isodense with cortex, noncalcified meningiomas can be difficult to detect on NECT.*

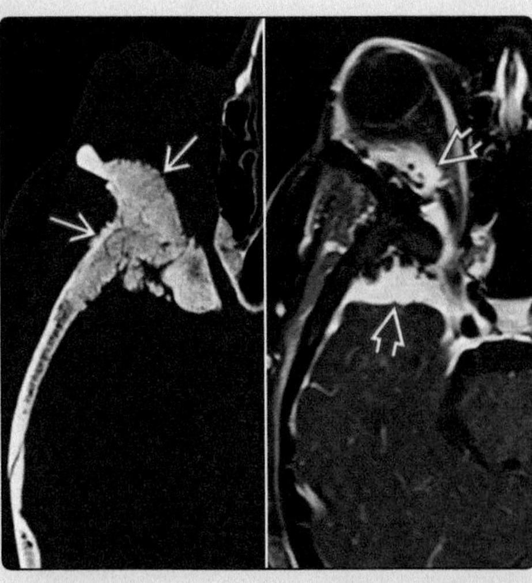

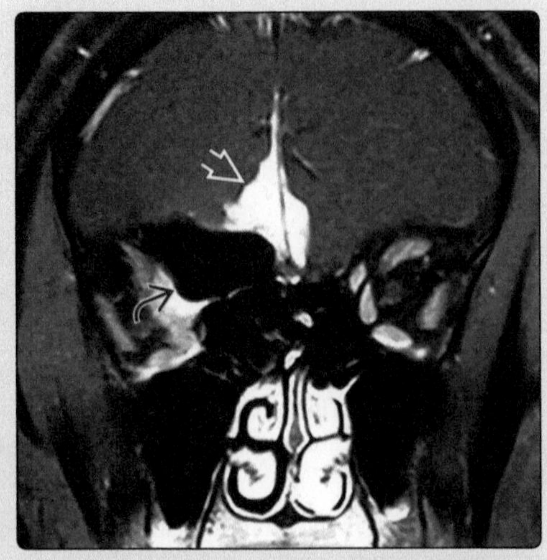

***(22-12)** (L) Bone CT shows striking hyperostosis of the sphenoid wing ➔ in a middle-aged woman with proptosis. (R) T1 C+ FS MR shows enhancing "en plaque" meningioma ➔. **(22-13)** Occasionally, skull base meningiomas adjacent to a paranasal sinus cause massive enlargement of the sinus, a condition known as pneumosinus dilatans. This relatively small meningioma ➔ caused massive enlargement of the frontal sinus ➔.*

vascularity prior to embolization or surgery. Tumor invasion of major dural venous sinuses is especially well depicted on MRV.

The classic appearance of meningioma on DSA is a radial "sunburst" of arteries extending from the base of the tumor toward its periphery. Dural vessels supply the core or center of the lesion, radiating outward from the vascular pedicle of the tumor **(22-16A)**. Pial vessels from internal carotid artery branches may become "parasitized" and supply the periphery of the mass **(22-16C)**.

A prolonged vascular "blush" that persists late into the venous phase is typical **(22-16B)**. In some cases, arteriovenous shunting with the appearance of "early draining" veins occurs **(22-16B)**. Careful examination of the venous phase should be conducted to detect dural sinus invasion or occlusion.

MENINGIOMA: IMAGING

CT
- Hyperdense (70-75%), calcified (20-25%)
- Cysts (peri- or intratumoral) (10-15%)
- Hemorrhage rare
- > 90% enhance

MR
- Usually isointense with gray matter
- CSF-vascular "cleft" ± vascular "flow voids"
- Strong, often heterogeneous enhancement (> 98%)
- Nonneoplastic dural "tail" (60%)

Angiography
- "Sunburst" vascularity
- Dural arteries to outside, pial to inside
- Prolonged, dense vascular "blush"
- Look for dural sinus invasion, occlusion

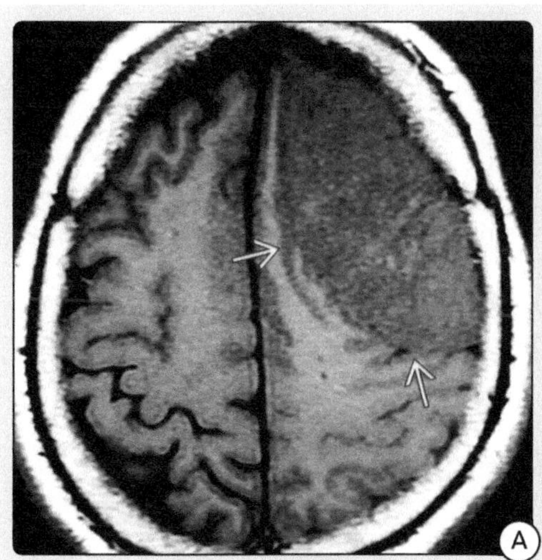

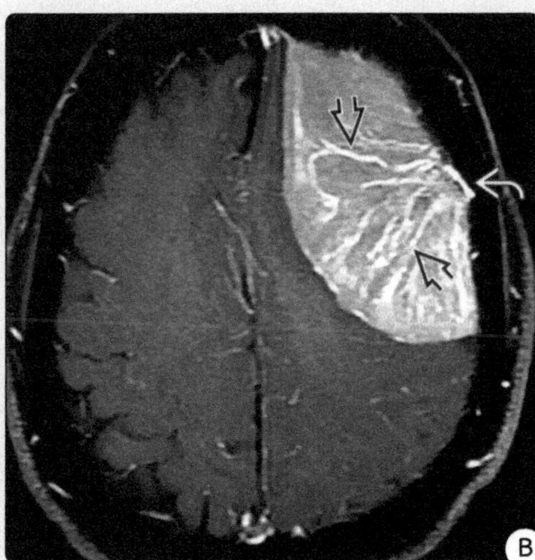

***(22-14A)** Large-convexity meningioma is shown with typical MR findings. The tumor has a flat base toward the dural surface and "buckles" the cortex and GM-WM interface inward ➡. Meningiomas are most commonly isointense with cortex on T1WI. **(22-14B)** T1 C+ FS MR shows that the tumor enhances intensely. Especially well seen is the even more hyperintense "sunburst" of vessels ➡ that supplies the tumor, radiating outward from the enostotic "spur" ➡.*

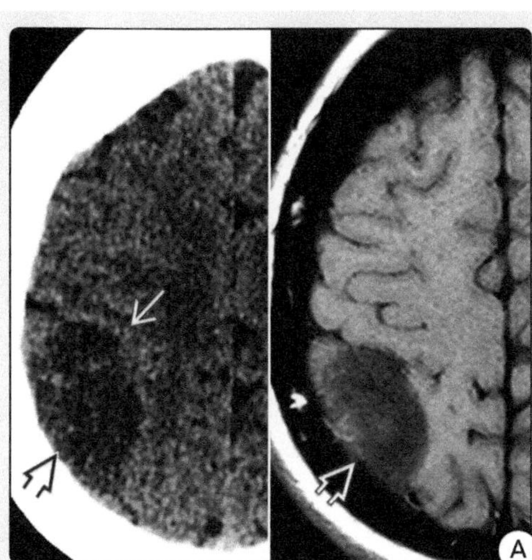

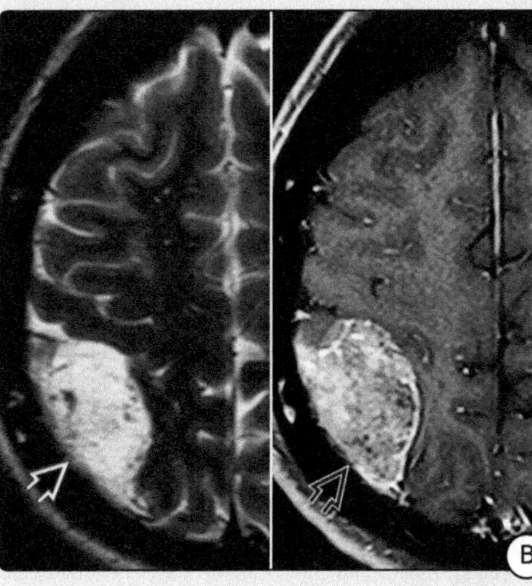

***(22-15A)** (L) NECT in a 48-year-old woman shows hypodense right parietal mass ➡ with inward displacement of the adjacent cortex ➡, suggesting that the mass is extraaxial. (R) Mass ➡ is hypointense on T1WI. **(22-15B)** (L) T2 MR in the same case shows that the mass ➡ is very hyperintense relative to the adjacent brain. (R) Mass ➡ enhances intensely and heterogeneously. This is WHO grade I microcystic meningioma.*

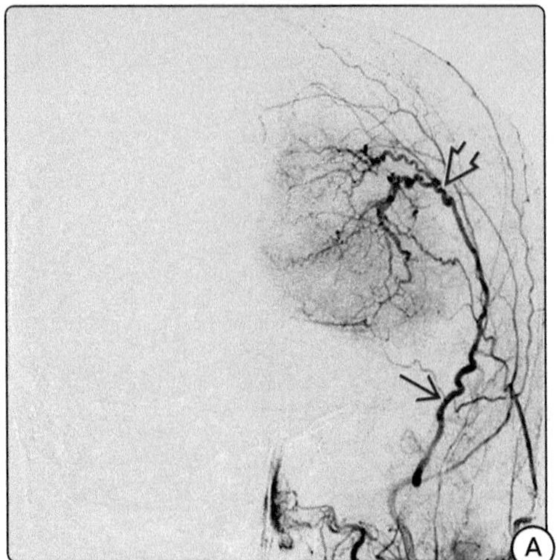

(22-16A) *AP DSA of ECA shows enlarged middle meningeal artery with "sunburst" of vessels supplying meningioma.*

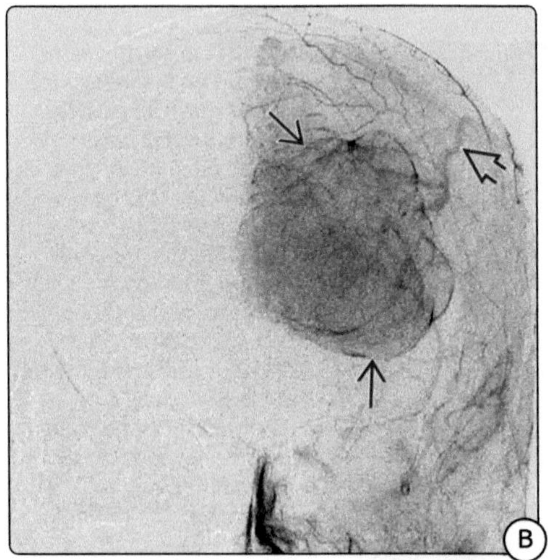

(22-16B) *Later phase of ECA DSA shows prolonged vascular "blush" characteristic of meningioma. "Early draining" vein is seen.*

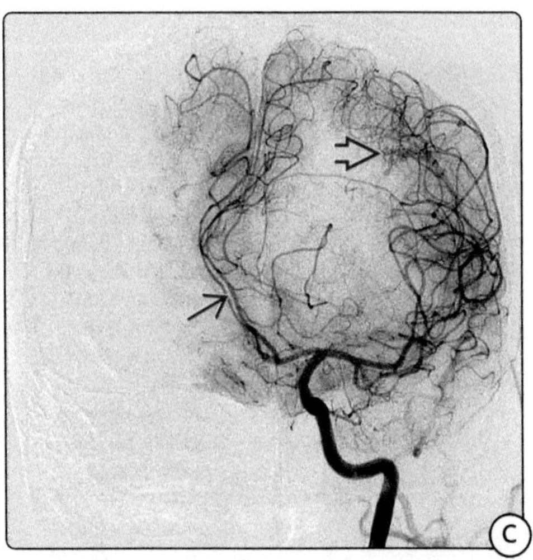

(22-16C) *ICA DSA shows mass effect with the ACA shifted. Only minimal supply to periphery of tumor is coming from pial MCA branches.*

Differential Diagnosis

The major differential diagnosis of typical meningioma is **atypical** or **malignant meningioma**. There are no pathognomonic imaging features that reliably distinguish benign meningioma from these more aggressive variants, but WHO grade I lesions are statistically far more common. Malignant meningiomas typically invade the brain and may exhibit a "mushrooming" configuration.

Dural metastasis, usually from a breast or lung primary, may be virtually indistinguishable from meningioma on imaging studies. Other meningioma mimics include **granuloma** (TB, sarcoid) and **inflammatory pseudotumors**. Neither has the intense vascularity of meningioma.

Rare entities that can closely resemble meningioma include hemangioma and solitary fibrous tumor/hemangiopericytoma. A **hemangioma of the dura** or **venous sinuses** is a true vasoformative neoplasm that can resemble meningioma. Most hemangiomas are very hyperintense on T2WI, whereas most meningiomas are iso- to mildly hyperintense. Delayed slow centripetal "filling in" of the mass on dynamic contrast-enhanced MR is suggestive of hemangioma.

Intracranial **solitary fibrous tumor/hemangiopericytoma** is relatively rare. Most are found adjacent to the dura and venous sinuses. Solitary fibrous tumor may be indistinguishable on imaging studies from typical meningioma.

Extramedullary hematopoiesis (EMH) can present as confluent or multifocal dura-based disease resembling "en plaque" solitary or multiple meningiomatosis. EMH occurs in the setting of chronic anemia or marrow depletion disorders.

MENINGIOMA MIMICS

Common
- Metastasis
  - Most common = breast, lung, colon, prostate
- Lymphoma

Less Common
- Granuloma
  - TB, sarcoid most common
  - Inflammatory pseudotumors

Rare but Important
- IgG4-related disease
- Dural/venous sinus hemangioma
- Solitary fibrous tumor/hemangiopericytoma
- Rosai-Dorfman disease
- Gliosarcoma, other sarcoma (e.g., Ewing)
- Extramedullary hematopoiesis

Atypical Meningioma

Terminology

Atypical meningioma (AM) is intermediate in grade between benign and malignant forms and is defined histopathologically.

Etiology

There is a significant correlation between the number of inactivating *NF2* mutations and tumor grade. Almost 60% of AMs show gain of chromosome arm 1q.

Pathology

Location. Most atypical and malignant meningiomas arise from the calvarium. The skull base is a relatively uncommon location for these more aggressive lesions.

Gross Pathology. Approximately 1/2 of all atypical meningiomas invade the adjacent brain. In such cases, there is no intervening layer of leptomeninges between the invading tumor and underlying parenchyma.

Microscopic Features. The 2016 WHO now recognizes brain invasion together with a mitotic count of four or more mitoses per high-power field as sufficient criteria for diagnosing atypical meningioma. Clusters or irregular finger-like protrusions of tumor cells infiltrating the underlying parenchyma are present. Brain invasion is also strongly correlated with the presence of other histopathologic criteria of atypia.

Atypical meningioma can also be diagnosed on the presence of three or more of the following histologic features: Foci of spontaneous necrosis, sheeting (loss of whorling or fascicular architecture with a patternless or sheet-like growth), prominent nucleoli, high cellularity, and small cells (tumor clusters with high nuclear:cytoplasmic ratio).

Some meningioma subtypes are classified as WHO grade II tumors simply because of their greater likelihood of recurrence &/or more aggressive behavior. These include the **chordoid** and **clear cell meningioma** subtypes.

All atypical meningiomas are WHO grade II neoplasms.

Clinical Issues

Epidemiology. AMs represent 10-15% of all meningiomas.

Demographics. AMs tend to occur in slightly younger patients compared with TMs. Pediatric meningiomas tend to be more aggressive. In contrast with TMs, AMs display a slight male predominance.

A new autosomal dominant tumor predisposition syndrome with heterozygous loss-of-function germline mutations in the *SMARCE1* tumor suppressor gene causes spinal and intracranial clear cell meningiomas. Symptomatic male patients develop tumors in childhood, whereas carrier female patients develop tumors in adolescence or early adulthood.

Natural History. AMs are generally associated with a higher recurrence rate (25-30%) and shorter recurrence-free survival compared with TMs. The Simpson and modified Shinsu grading systems are the best predictors of recurrence after resection. Grade I represents macroscopically complete tumor removal, including excision of its dural attachment and any abnormal bone. Grades II-IV represent progressively less complete resection, and grade V is simple decompression with or without biopsy.

Imaging

General Features. A good general rule is that it is difficult—if not impossible—to predict meningioma grade on the basis of imaging findings. However, because brain invasion is a frequent (but not always visible) feature of AMs, the CSF-vascular "cleft" typically seen in TMs is often compromised or absent.

CT Findings. AMs are usually hyperdense with irregular margins. Minimal or no calcification is seen, and frank bone invasion with osteolysis is common. Tumor may invade through the skull into the scalp.

MR Findings. Tumor margins are usually indistinct with no border between the tumor and the underlying cortex. A CSF-vascular "cleft" is often absent or

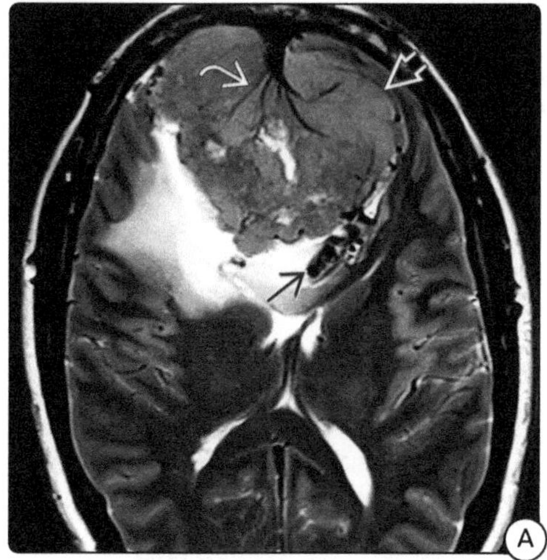

***(22-17A)** T2 MR shows bifrontal mass ➡ isointense mass. Note prominent "sunburst" vessels within mass ➡, CSF-vascular "cleft" ➡.*

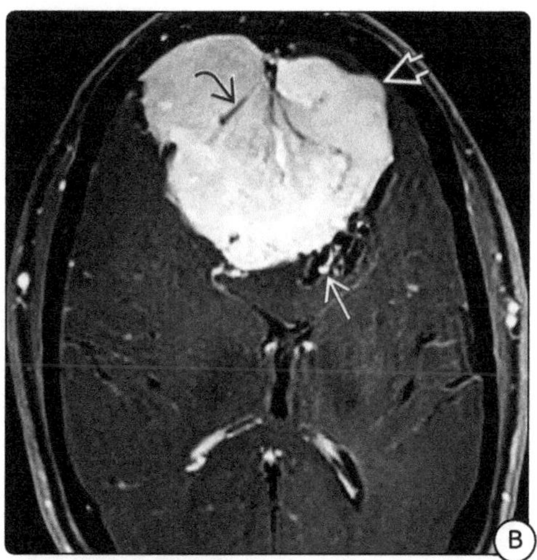

***(22-17B)** Mass ➡ enhances intensely, uniformly. Note prominent "flow voids" within the tumor ➡ as well as in the CSF-vascular cleft ➡.*

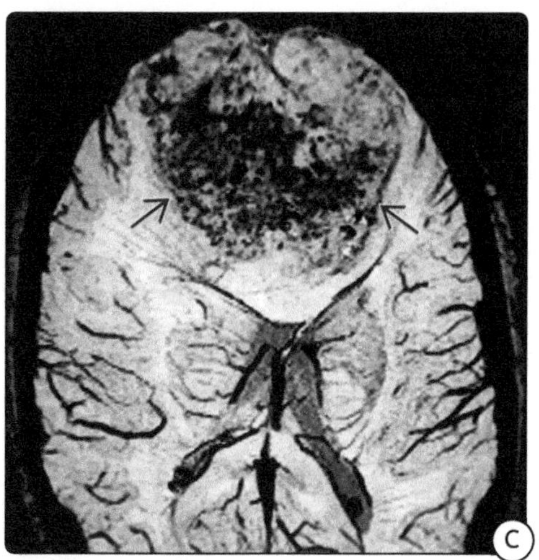

***(22-17C)** T2* SWI shows vascular tumor filled by enlarged vessels with slow flow causing susceptibility artifact ➡. Grade II meningioma.*

partially effaced. Peritumoral edema and cyst formation are common but nonspecific findings **(22-17)**. Contrast enhancement is strong but often quite heterogeneous **(22-17B)**.

With the exception of the chordoid meningioma histologic subtype (where it is elevated), ADC is significantly lower in atypical and malignant meningiomas compared with typical meningiomas. Perfusion MR may show elevated rCBV **(22-18)**. MRS often shows elevated alanine.

Differential Diagnosis

Because it is difficult to determine meningioma tumor grade on the basis of imaging findings alone, the major differential diagnosis of AM is **meningioma, WHO grade I. Dural metastasis** and **malignant meningioma** can also be indistinguishable from AM. **Sarcomas** may also be difficult to distinguish from biologically aggressive meningiomas.

Anaplastic Meningioma

Terminology

Anaplastic meningioma—also called malignant meningioma—exhibits overtly malignant cytology &/or markedly elevated mitotic activity.

Etiology

Chromosomal mutations are increased compared with AMs. Several genes have been associated with malignant progression in meningioma. Homozygous deletions or mutations of the tumor suppressor genes, *CDKN2A* (ARF) and *CDKN2B*, are found in most anaplastic meningiomas. A new meningioma-associated tumor suppressor gene, *NDRG2*, is downregulated in anaplastic meningioma and atypical meningiomas with aggressive clinical behavior.

(22-18A) T1 C+ FS MR shows lobulated, intensely enhancing mass ➡. Coronal T1 C+ (not shown) demonstrated that the mass was attached to the dura and exhibited a "dural tail" sign. (22-18B) MRS shows markedly elevated Cho, decreased NAA. Choline map shows the elevated Cho ➡ with the highest levels in the center of the lesion ➡. This is atypical meningioma, clear cell type, WHO grade II. (Courtesy M. Thurnher, MD.)

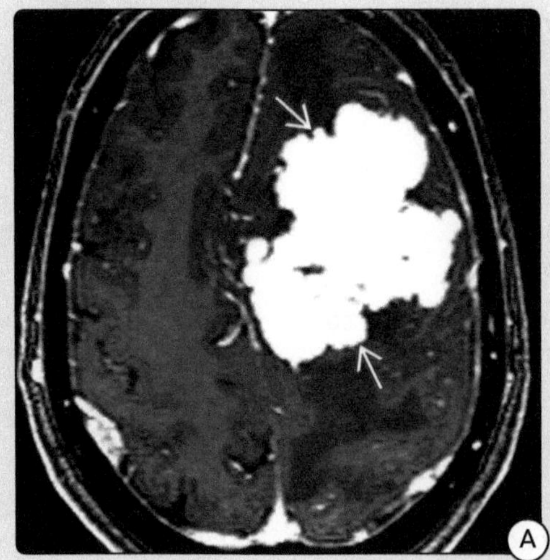

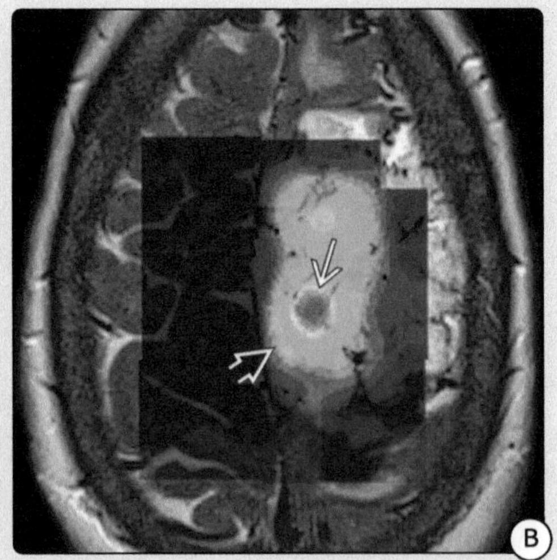

(22-19A) T2 MR in a 40-year-old man with headaches shows well-marginated, very hyperintense extraaxial mass ➡. Note displaced cortex around the mass ➡. (22-19B) The well-delineated mass ➡ enhances intensely. Mean ADC (not shown) was elevated. No brain invasion was seen at surgery, but this is a chordoid meningioma, which makes this a WHO grade II (atypical) meningioma.

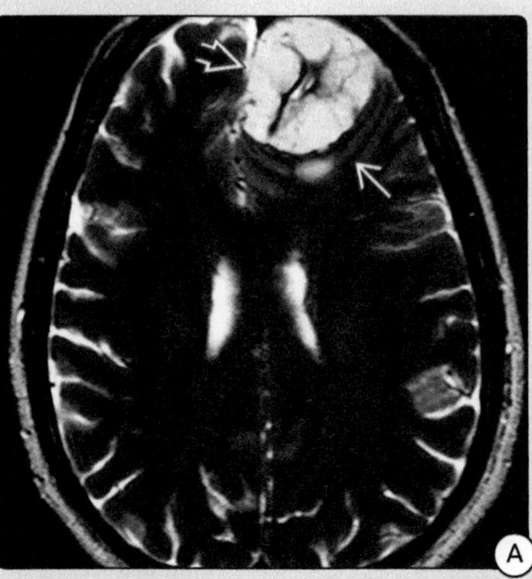

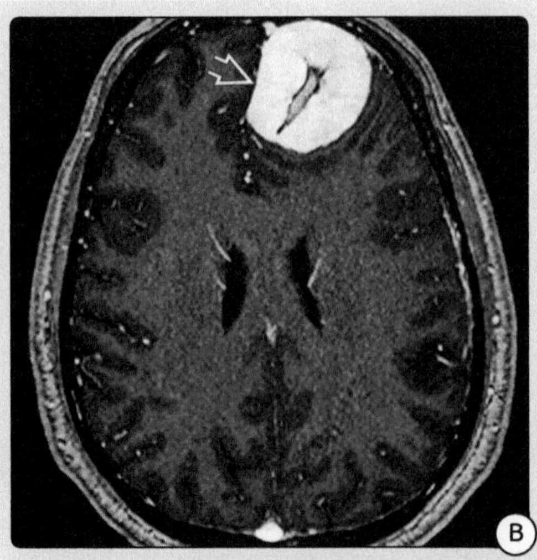

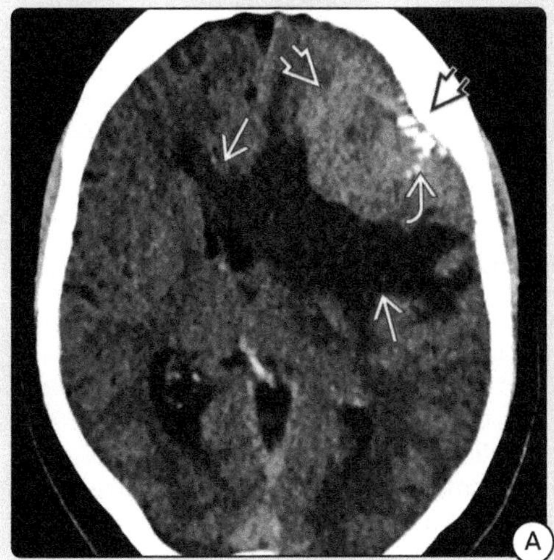

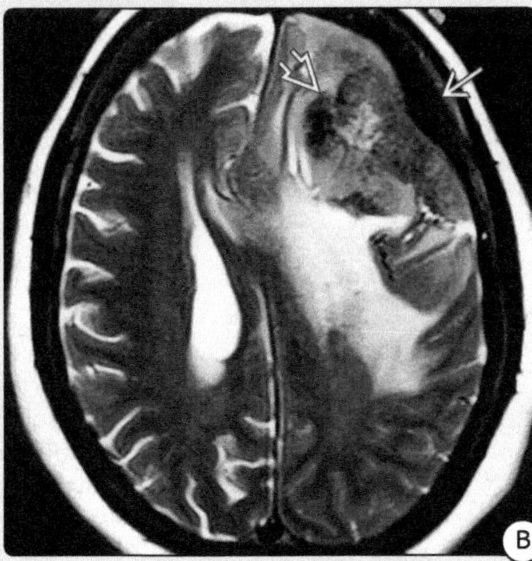

***(22-20A)** NECT shows a hyperdense left frontal mass ➡ with marked WM edema ➡. Note calcifications ➡ and adjacent calvarial hyperostosis ➡. **(22-20B)** T2 MR shows that the mass ➡ is very heterogeneous. Calvarial hyperostosis with thickening of the inner table ➡ is well seen. There is no clear cleft between the tumor and brain.*

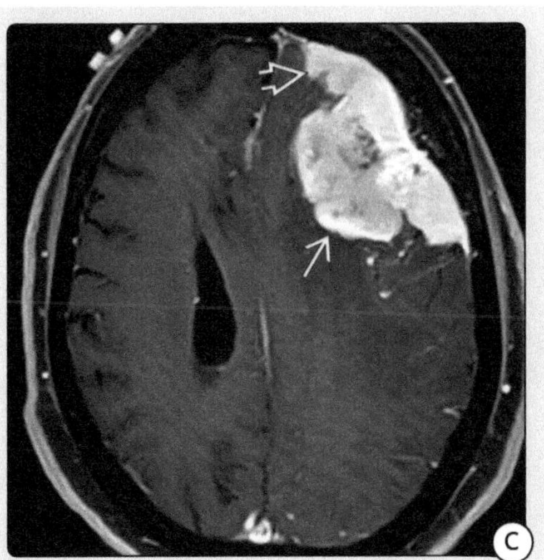

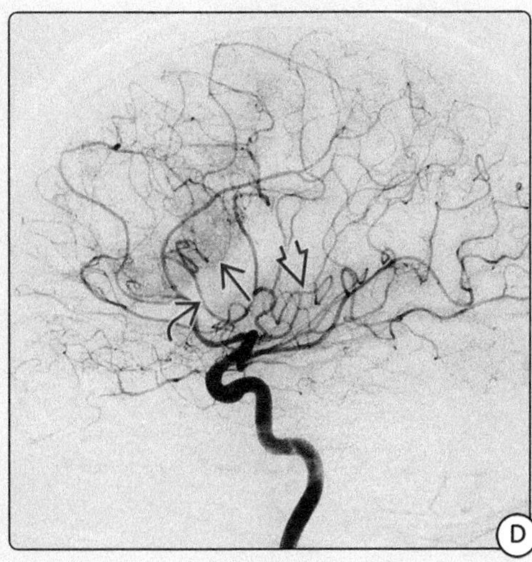

***(22-20C)** T1 C+ FS MR shows that a dural-based, intensely enhancing mass ➡ "mushrooms" into the brain ➡. **(22-20D)** Lateral view, arterial phase of a left ICA DSA shows mass effect displacing ➡, stretching MCA branches ➡. Note faint vascular "blush" ➡ around the periphery of the mass.*

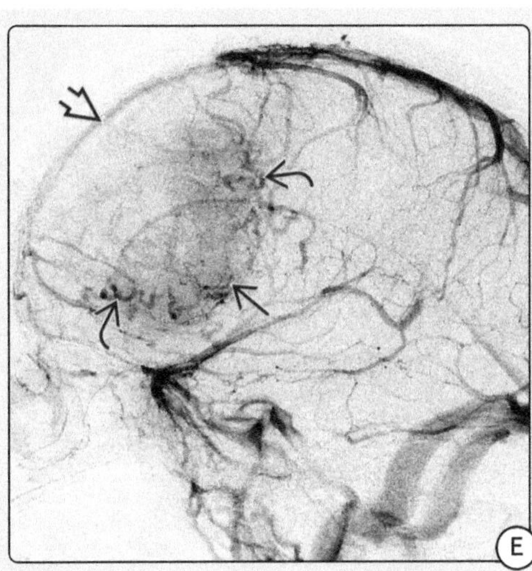

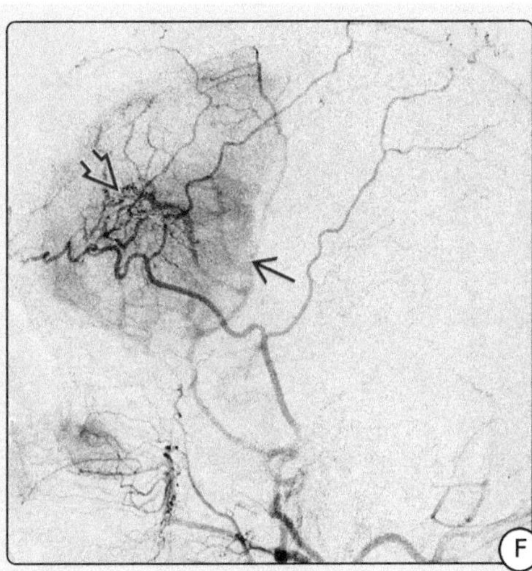

***(22-20E)** Venous phase of the left ICA DSA shows intense vascular "blush" ➡, tortuous draining veins ➡ around the periphery of the mass. The center of the mass ➡ is not vascularized by the ICA. **(22-20F)** Lateral view of an ipsilateral ECA shows enlarged middle meningeal, dural branches supplying the center ➡ of the vascular mass ➡. This is WHO grade II meningioma.*

Pathology

Most anaplastic meningiomas invade the brain and exhibit histologic features of frank malignancy **(22-21)**. These include increased cellular atypia with bizarre nuclei and markedly elevated mitotic index (> 20 mitoses per 10 high-power fields). Malignant meningioma subtypes include **papillary** and **rhabdoid** meningiomas as well as meningiomas of any histologic subtype with a high proliferation index.

Anaplastic meningioma corresponds histologically to WHO grade III.

Clinical Issues

Frankly malignant meningiomas are rare, representing only 1-3% of all meningiomas. Prognosis is poor. Recurrence rates following tumor resection range from 50-95%. Survival times range from 2-5 years and vary depending on resection extent.

Imaging

General Features. The imaging triad of extracranial mass, osteolysis, and "mushrooming" intracranial tumor is present in most—but not all—cases of anaplastic meningioma **(22-21) (22-22)**. Calcification is rare, and contrast enhancement is typically heterogeneous.

Differential Diagnosis

Atypical meningioma can be indistinguishable from malignant meningioma on imaging studies alone, as brain invasion occurs in both. The other major differential diagnosis of anaplastic meningioma is dura-arachnoid **metastasis.** Rare tumors, such as **solitary fibrous tumor (hemangiopericytoma)**, and **sarcomas**, such as meningeal fibrosarcoma, can all mimic anaplastic meningioma.

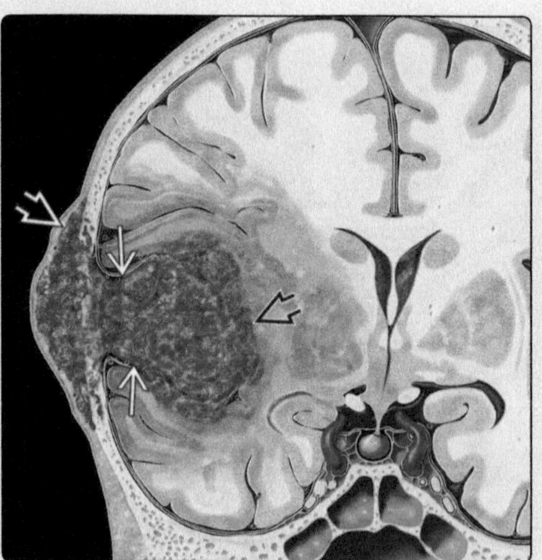

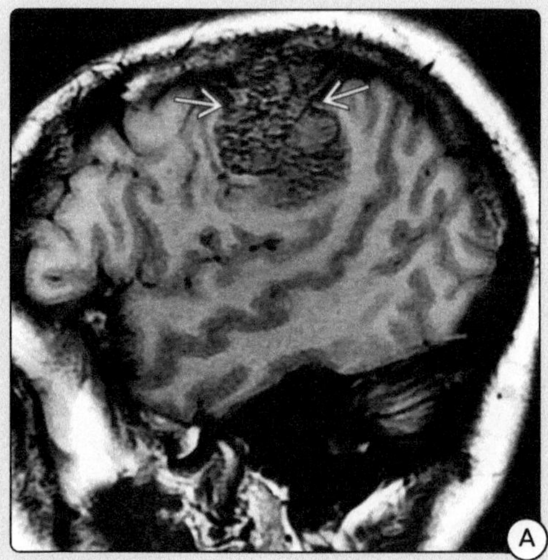

***(22-21)** Graphic shows malignant meningioma invading the brain ⇨ without CSF-vascular "cleft." The tumor also penetrates dura, invades calvarium, has a significant extracranial component ➡. Note "mushroom" configuration ➡, which may suggest more aggressive meningioma. **(22-22A)** Sagittal T1 MR in a 50-year-old man with left-sided weakness shows mixed iso-/hypointense extraaxial mass "mushrooming" ➡ into brain.*

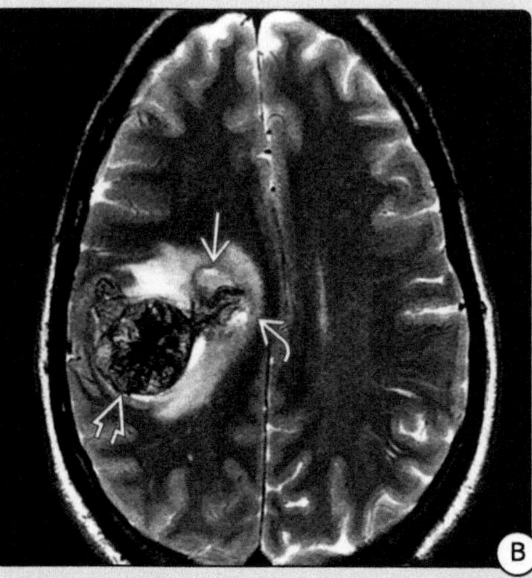

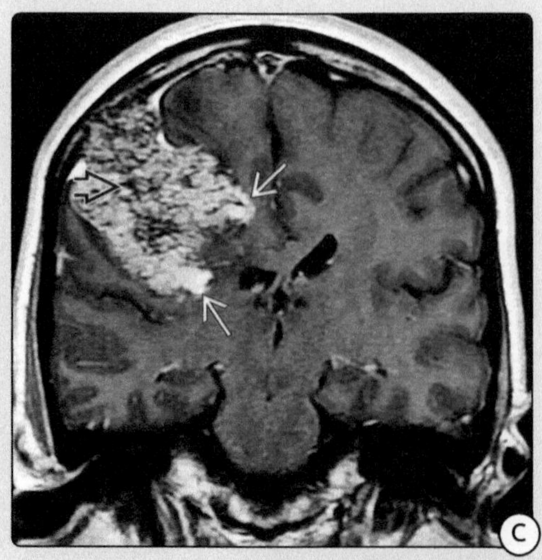

***(22-22B)** Axial T2 MR shows the very heterogeneous signal of the lesion ➡, "mushroom" of focal brain invasion ➡ with adjacent edema ➡. **(22-22C)** Coronal T1 C+ MR shows that an intensely enhancing lesion contains numerous "flow voids" ⇨ and invades adjacent brain ➡. This is papillary meningioma, WHO grade III.*

Solitary fibrous tumor/hemangiopericytoma, gliosarcoma, and **sarcomas**, such as meningeal fibrosarcoma, can all mimic anaplastic meningioma.

Nonmeningothelial Mesenchymal Tumors

Nonmeningothelial mesenchymal tumors rarely involve the CNS. When they do, they are usually extraaxial lesions that correspond to soft tissue or bone tumors found elsewhere in the body. Both benign and malignant varieties of each type occur, ranging from benign (WHO grade I) to highly malignant (WHO grade IV) sarcomatous neoplasms.

Benign Mesenchymal Tumors (BMTs)

With the exception of hemangiomas and lipomas, cranial mesenchymal nonmeningothelial tumors are all rare. Together, these BMTs account for < 1% of all intracranial neoplasms. Overall, **chondroma/enchondroma** is the most common benign osteocartilaginous tumor of the skull base **(22-23)**. **Osteoma** is the most common benign osseous tumor of the calvarium.

Solitary fibrous tumors (SFTs) can arise anywhere but are generally dura based. SFTs and hemangiopericytoma are now considered to constitute a continuous pathologic spectrum and are discussed separately.

Osteomas are benign tumors that arise from membranous bone. In the head, the paranasal sinuses and calvarium are the most common sites.

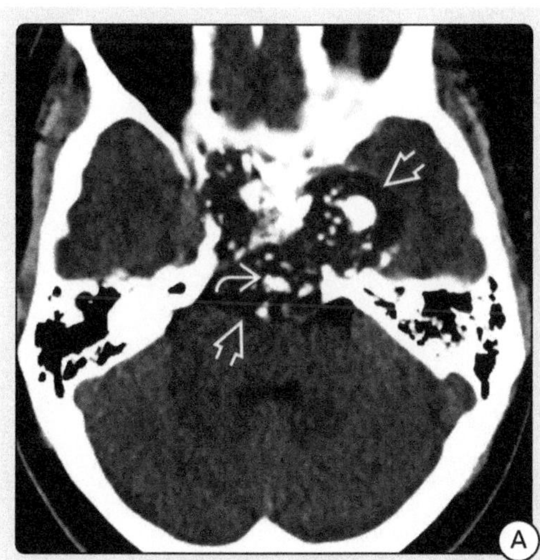

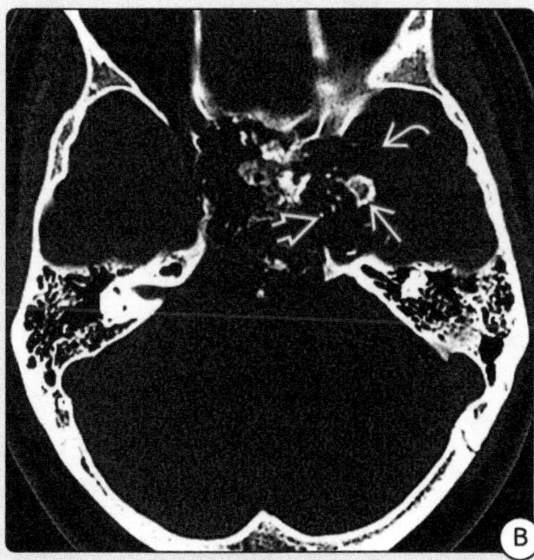

***(22-23A)** NECT in a 21-year-old man with blurred vision shows a hypodense central skull base mass ➡ with numerous matrix calcifications ➡. **(22-23B)** Bone CT in the same case shows erosion of the central skull base and anterior clinoid processes by the mass. Note matrix mineralization ➡, calcified arcs ➡, and dysplastic cortical bone ➡ within the mass.*

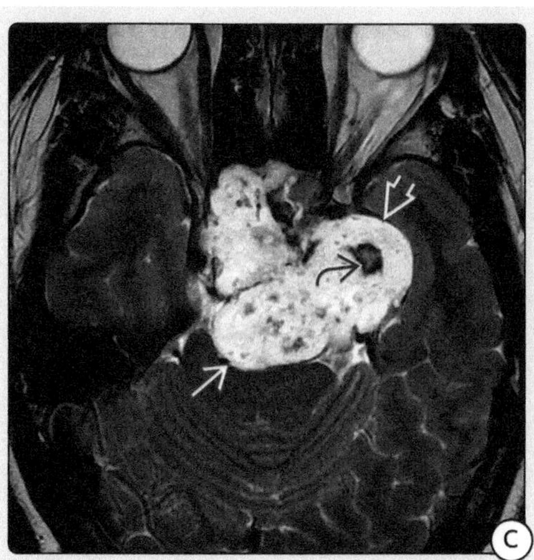

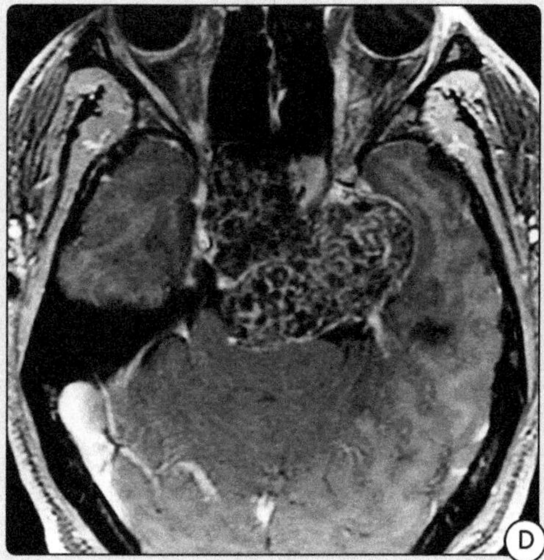

***(22-23C)** Axial T2 FS MR in the same case shows that the lobulated mass ➡ is well delineated and extremely hyperintense and compresses/displaces the pons posteriorly ➡. Dysplastic cortical bone ➡ within the mass is well seen. **(22-23D)** T1 C+ FS MR shows a "bubbly" enhancement pattern within the mass. Pathology showed enchondroma with foci of chondrosarcoma arising within the mass.*

Most BMTs occur as solitary nonsyndromic lesions. Multiple BMTs generally occur as part of inherited tumor syndromes. Multiple osteomas occur as part of **Gardner syndrome** (together with skin tumors and colon polyps). Multiple enchondromas or "enchondromatosis" are part of **Ollier disease**. Enchondromas associated with soft tissue hemangiomas are found in **Maffucci syndrome**.

Imaging findings vary with tumor type. Most BMTs are benign-appearing nonaggressive masses of the scalp, skull, or dura that resemble their counterparts found elsewhere in the body.

Hemangioma

Hemangiomas are benign nonmeningothelial mesenchymal tumors. They are common vascular neoplasms that closely resemble normal vessels and are found in all organs of the body. Hemangiomas are completely different from—and should not be confused with—cavernous angiomas, which are vascular malformations rather than neoplasms.

Intracranial hemangiomas occur in the calvarium **(22-24)**, dural venous sinuses, and dura. When they involve the calvarium, radiating spicules of lamellar bone are interspersed with vascular channels of varying sizes **(22-25)**. Hemangiomas of the venous sinuses and dura do not contain bone but otherwise resemble calvarial hemangiomas, consisting of large vascular channels in a soft, compressible mass. Hemangiomas are WHO grade I neoplasms, typically grow very slowly, and do not undergo malignant degeneration.

A calvarial hemangioma is seen as a sharply marginated, expansile diploic mass on NECT. Bone CT shows that the inner and outer tables are thinned but usually intact. A thin sclerotic margin may surround the lesion. "Spoke-wheel" or reticulated hyperdensities caused by fewer but thicker trabeculae are present within the hemangioma, giving it a "honeycomb" or "jail bars" appearance.

__(22-24)__ Coronal graphic depicts typical hemangioma of the calvarium ➡ as spicules of lamellar bone ➡ interspersed with vascular channels ➡. __(22-25)__ Photograph of resected calvarial hemangioma shows an unencapsulated, very vascular-appearing mass ➡ with radiating spicules of bone ➡.

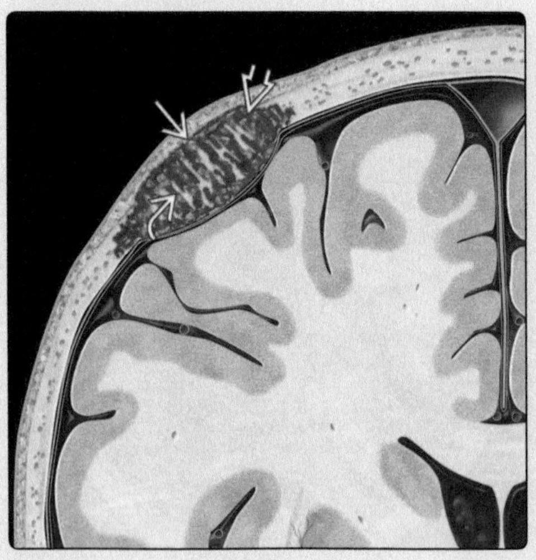

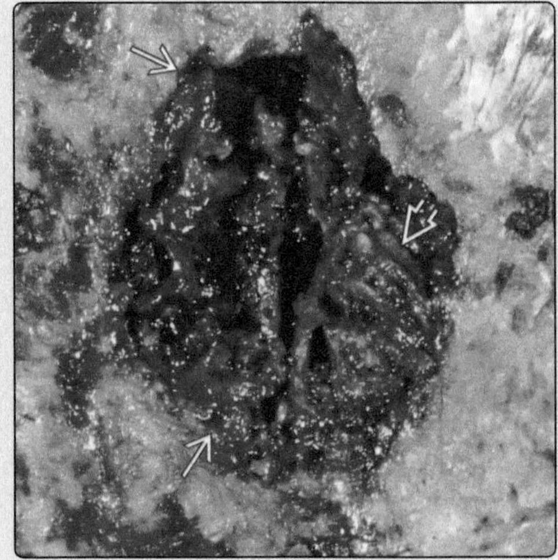

__(22-26A)__ Coronal T1 C+ FS MR shows a typical calvarial hemangioma ➡ that slightly expands the diploic space. The vascular channels enhance intensely, whereas the "dots" of bone spicules within the lesion ➡ do not. __(22-26B)__ Axial T2 MR of another calvarial hemangioma shows that the mass ➡ is mostly very hyperintense. The hypointense "dots" of radiating bone spicules give the lesion a striped appearance.

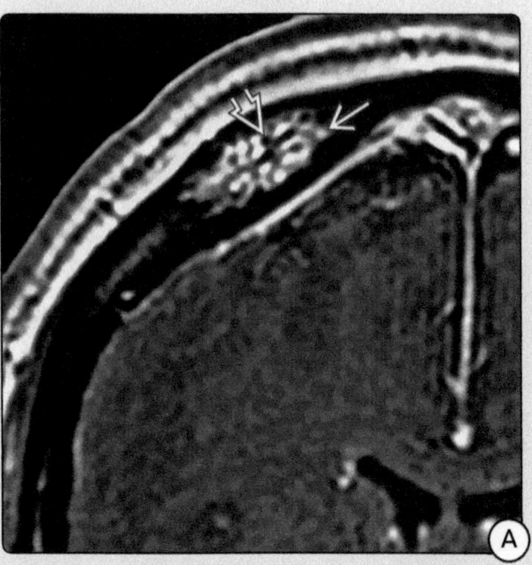

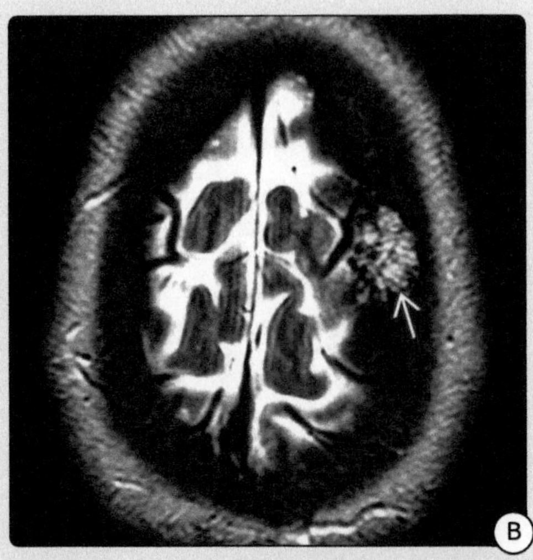

Mixed hypo- to isointensity is the dominant pattern on T1WI. Scattered hyperintensities are usually caused by fat—not hemorrhage—within the lesion. Most hemangiomas are markedly hyperintense on T2WI **(22-26)**. Contrast-enhanced scans show diffuse intense enhancement. Dynamic scans show slow centripetal "filling in" of the lesion **(22-27)**.

The major differential diagnosis for dural/venous sinus hemangioma is **meningioma**. Except for the microcystic variant, meningiomas do not display the marked hyperintensity on T2WI seen in most hemangiomas. Hemangiomas also exhibit the classic "filling in" from the periphery to the center of the lesion on rapid-sequence dynamic contrast-enhanced T1WIs.

CALVARIAL AND DURAL HEMANGIOMAS

Pathology
- Benign vasoformative neoplasm
  - Capillary-type growth pattern
- Calvarium > dura, dural venous sinuses

Clinical Features
- Any age, mostly small/asymptomatic

Imaging Findings
- CT: Radiating "spoke-wheel" bone spicules
- MR: T2 "honeycomb" hyperintensities
  - Dynamic T1 C+ shows "filling in" of lesion

Differential Diagnosis
- Calvarial = venous channels, arachnoid granulations, etc.
- Dura/venous sinus = meningioma

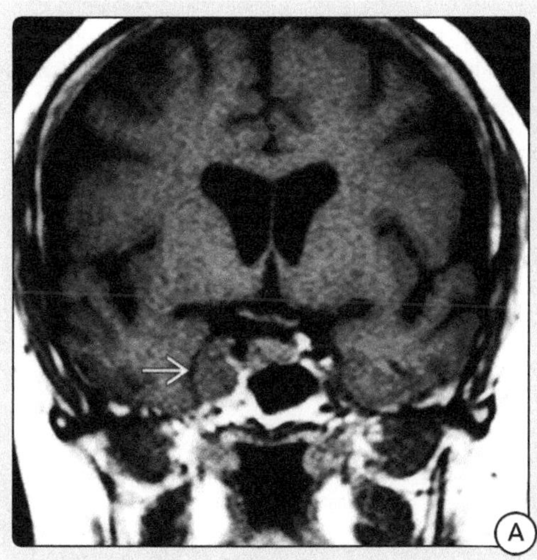

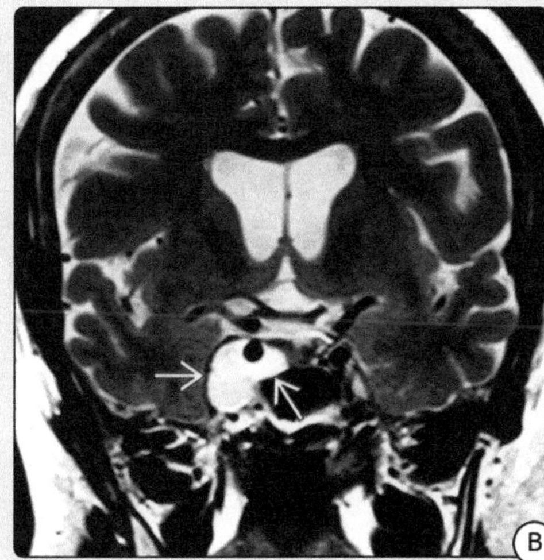

***(22-27A)** Coronal T1 MR in a 66-year-old woman with diagnosis of meningioma on outside MR shows a mass in the right cavernous sinus ➡ that is isointense with gray matter. **(22-27B)** Coronal T2 MR in the same case shows that the mass ➡ is extremely and uniformly hyperintense.*

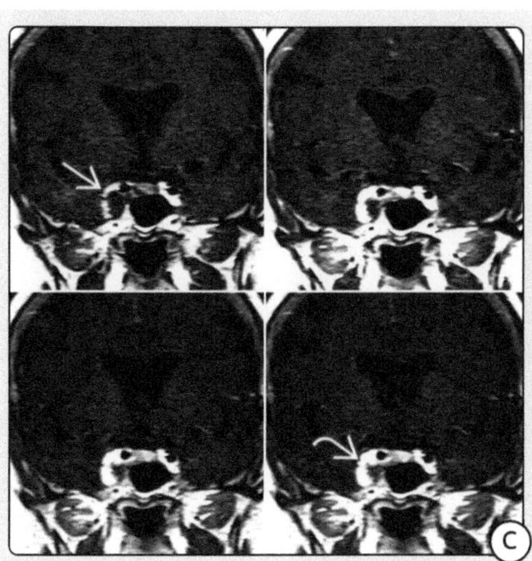

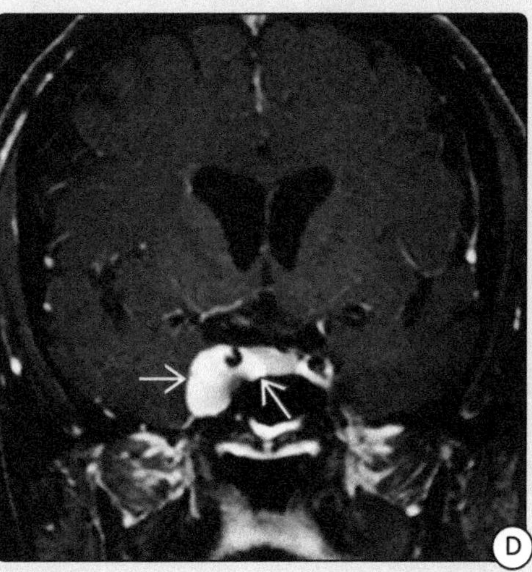

***(22-27C)** Dynamic contrast-enhanced fat-saturated T1 MRs show progressive "filling in" of mass by contrast with the periphery of the lesions filling first ➡ followed by centripetal (central) enhancement of the rest of the lesion with time ➡. **(22-27D)** T1 C+ FS MR 5 min after contrast injection for the dynamic sequence shows that the entire mass ➡ now enhances intensely and uniformly. This is cavernous sinus hemangioma. Surgery was cancelled.*

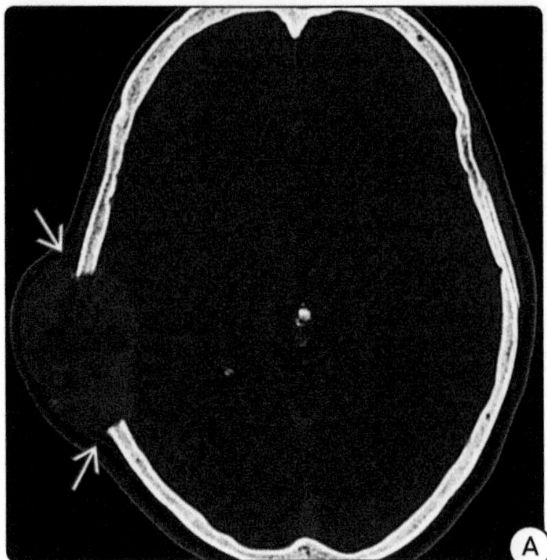

(22-28A) *Bone CT in 64y woman with a "lump" on her head shows a destructive soft tissue mass ➡ without intratumoral calcifications.*

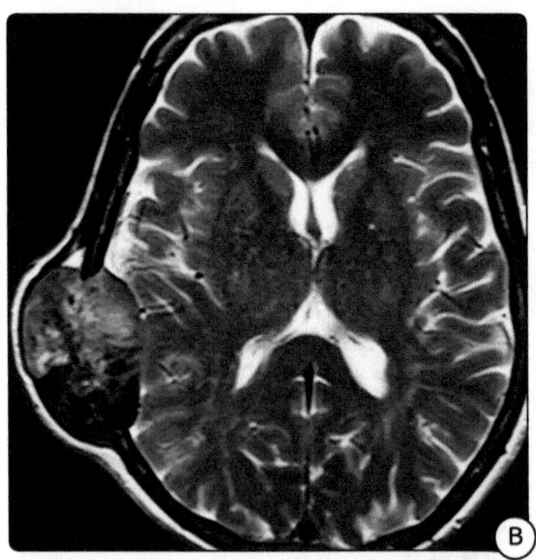

(22-28B) *Axial T2 MR in the same case shows that the mass is heterogeneously iso- and hypointense.*

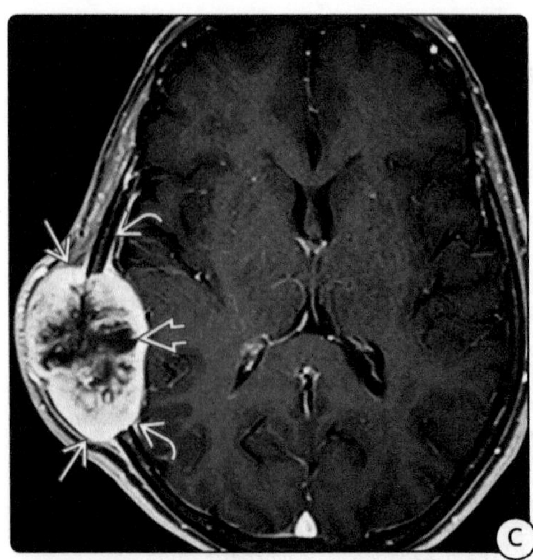

(22-28C) *The mass ➡ enhances intensely with a nonenhancing central necrotic core ➡, dural "tails" ➡. This is fibrosarcoma, WHO grade IV.*

Malignant Mesenchymal Tumors

MMTs are rare tumors. In the aggregate, they represent 0.5-2.0% of intracranial neoplasms. Most MMTs are **sarcomas** (of many histologic types) and other neoplasms, such as **undifferentiated pleomorphic sarcoma/malignant fibrous histiocytoma** (MFH). Most are WHO grade IV neoplasms.

Most intracranial MMTs arise in the dura or skull base. Some arise in the scalp or calvarium. Chondrosarcomas classically arise from the petrooccipital fissure.

Imaging findings of MMTs are those of highly aggressive dural, skull base, calvarial, or scalp lesions that invade adjacent structures **(22-28)**.

NECT scans show a mixed-density soft tissue mass that causes lysis of adjacent bone. Chondrosarcoma may have stippled calcifications or classic "rings and arcs." Sometimes "sunburst" calcifications can be seen in osteosarcomas. Periosteal reaction is generally absent with the exception of Ewing sarcoma.

Other than suggesting a highly aggressive mass, there are no MR findings specific for MMTs. Fibrous, chondroid, and osteoid tissue are often very hypointense on both T1- and T2WI. FLAIR is very helpful in demonstrating brain invasion. Most MMTs enhance strongly but heterogeneously. Foci of necrosis are common.

There are no characteristic radiologic findings that distinguish most MMTs from other aggressive neoplasms, such as **malignant meningioma** or **metastases**. Sarcoma subtypes are difficult to identify on the basis of imaging findings alone. For example, a histologically definite liposarcoma may demonstrate virtually no imaging features that would suggest the presence of fat.

Solitary Fibrous Tumor/Hemangiopericytoma

Terminology

Solitary fibrous tumor (SFT) represents a continuum of mesenchymal tumors with increasing cellularity. Because SFTs and hemangiopericytomas (HPCs) share the same molecular genetic profile, the 2016 WHO has created the combined term **solitary fibrous tumor/hemangiopericytoma (SFT/HPC)** to describe such lesions. Three grades of increasing malignancy are assigned to these tumors.

Although relatively rare, SFT/HPC is the most common primary intracranial nonmeningothelial mesenchymal neoplasm. These tumors are very cellular, highly vascular neoplasms known for their aggressive clinical behavior, high recurrence rates, and distant metastases even after gross total surgical resection.

Pathology

Location. Most SFT/HPCs are dura based, usually arising from the falx or tentorium. The most common site is the occipital region, where they often straddle the transverse sinus. Intraparenchymal SFT/HPCs occur in the cerebrum and spinal cord, often without a discernible dural attachment. The cerebral ventricles are another common site.

Size and Number. SFT/HPCs are almost always solitary lesions. They are relatively large tumors, reaching up to 10 cm in diameter. Lesions > 4-5 cm are not uncommon.

Gross Pathology. SFTs are solid, lobulated, relatively well-demarcated neoplasms **(22-29)**. HPCs contain abundant vascular spaces. Intratumoral hemorrhage and necrosis are common.

Microscopic Features. *STAT6* nuclear expression can be detected by immunohistochemistry and confirms the diagnosis of SFT/HPC. Most tumors with the SFT phenotype are low-grade lesions. Mitoses are rare. Anaplasia is uncommon.

Staging, Grading, and Classification. Three grades of SFT/HPC are recognized in the 2016 WHO. Grade I corresponds to the highly collagenous, low-cellularity spindle cell lesion previously diagnosed as **solitary fibrous tumor**. Grade II corresponds to the more cellular tumor with "staghorn" vasculature that was previously diagnosed as **hemangiopericytoma**.

Grade III SFT/HPC represents what was termed **anaplastic hemangiopericytoma**. More than five mitoses per ten high-power fields are present, and Ki-67 is usually 10% or more.

Clinical Issues

HPCs are rare tumors, accounting for < 1% of all primary intracranial neoplasms and 2-4% of all meningeal tumors. Mean age at diagnosis is 43 years.

Surgical resection with radiation therapy or radiosurgery is the treatment of choice. However, even with complete resection, local recurrence is the rule. The majority of meningeal HPCs eventually metastasize extracranially to bone, lung, and liver. There is no significant difference in survival between grade II and grade III HPCs.

Imaging

CT Findings. HPCs are hyperdense extraaxial masses that invade and destroy bone. Extracalvarial extension under the scalp is common. Calcification and reactive hyperostosis are absent.

Strong but heterogeneous enhancement is typical.

MR Findings. Low-grade intracranial SFTs are circumscribed masses that are usually dura based and resemble meningioma. Lesions are isointense with gray matter on T1WI and have variable signal intensity on T2WI. A mixed hyper- and hypointense pattern is common. Collagen-rich areas can be very hypointense **(22-30A)**. Avid enhancement following contrast administration is typical **(22-30B)**.

Most HPCs demonstrate mixed signal intensity on all sequences. They tend to be predominantly isointense to gray matter on T1 scans **(22-31A)** and iso- to hyperintense on T2 scans **(22-31)**. Prominent "flow voids" are almost always present **(22-31B)**.

Contrast enhancement is marked but heterogeneous. Nonenhancing necrotic foci are common. A "dural tail" sign is absent.

Angiography. HPCs may invade and occlude dural sinuses, so CTV or MRV are helpful noninvasive techniques for delineating patency.

DSA shows HPCs as hypervascular masses with prominent vascularity, "early draining" veins, and intense prolonged tumor "staining." HPCs usually recruit blood supply from both dural and pial vessels.

Differential Diagnosis

The major differential diagnosis of low-grade SFT is typical (WHO grade I) meningioma. The major differential of HPC is a highly vascular aggressive

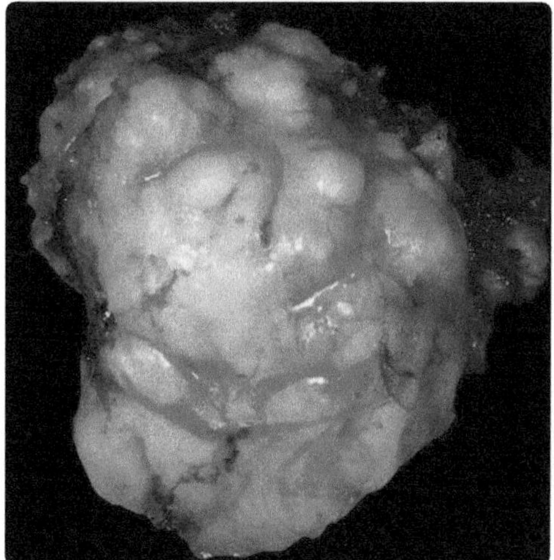

***(22-29)** Solitary fibrous tumors are firm, well-circumscribed masses that can appear identical to meningioma. (Courtesy E. Rushing, MD.)*

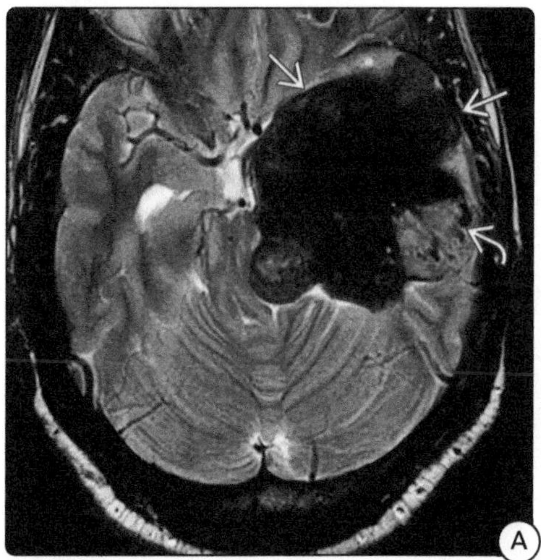

***(22-30A)** T2 MR shows well-delineated bosselated left hypointense middle cranial fossa mass ➡. Note prominent "flow voids" ➡.*

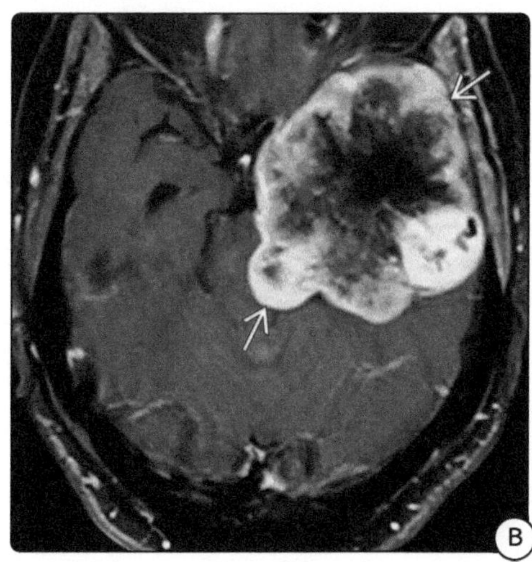

***(22-30B)** T1 C+ FS MR shows that the periphery of the mass ➡ enhances intensely & central part does not. Solitary fibrous tumor, WHO grade I.*

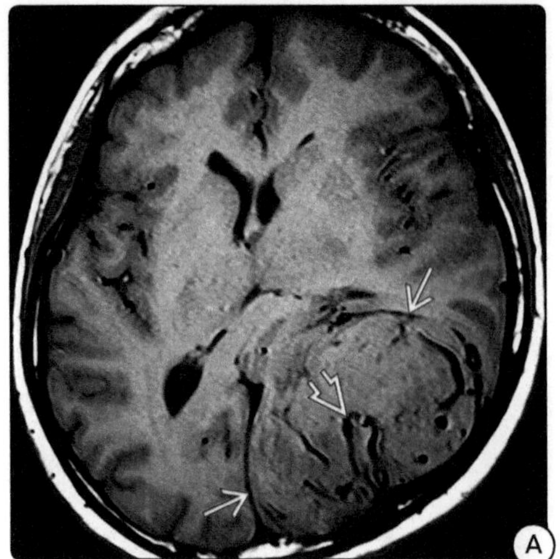

***(22-31A)** T1 MR in 21-year-old woman shows isointense left parietooccipital mass ➡. Note prominent "flow voids" ➡ within the mass.*

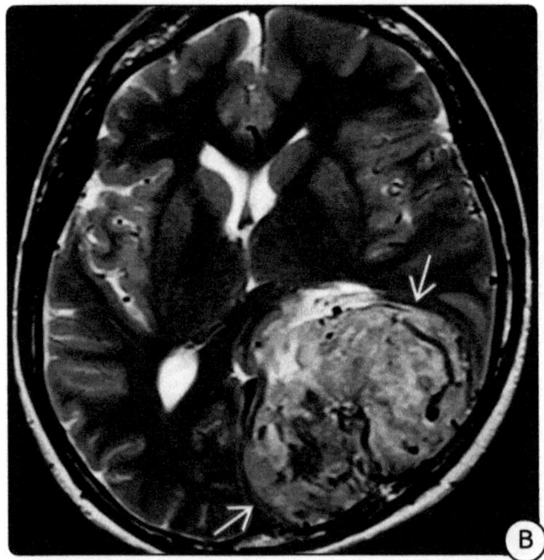

***(22-31B)** Axial T2 MR in the same case shows that the large mass is displacing brain around it ➡, suggesting that it is extraaxial in origin.*

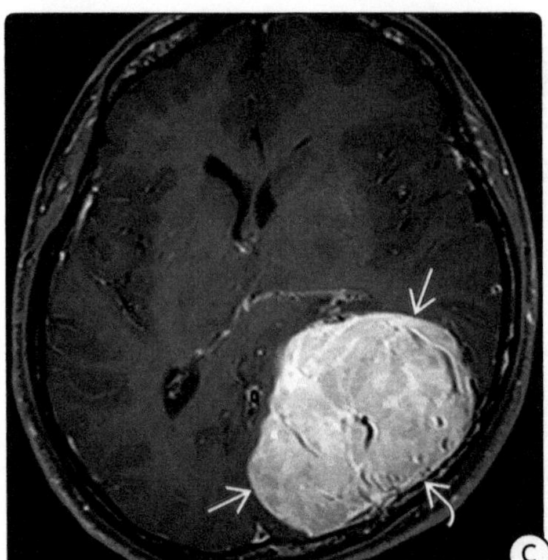

***(22-31C)** T1 C+ FS MR shows the intensely but heterogeneously enhancing mass ➡ has broad base ➡ abutting dura. SFT/HPC, WHO grade III.*

meningioma, particularly an **atypical** or **malignant meningioma**. HPCs rarely calcify or cause hyperostosis, and a "dural tail" sign is typically absent.

Dural metastases with skull invasion can be indistinguishable from HPC. Uncommon neoplasms that can resemble HPC include **gliosarcoma** and **malignant mesenchymal tumors**. Rarely, an intracranial SFT/HPC or malignant mesenchymal tumor can cause severe hypophosphatemia and metabolic bone disease not explained by any other metabolic or hereditary disease. These **osteomalacia-inducing tumors** (OITs) can be confused with aggressive meningioma.

SOLITARY FIBROUS TUMOR/HEMANGIOPERICYTOMA

Terminology, Etiology
- Solitary fibrous tumor (SFT)/hemangiopericytoma (HPC)
  - Spectrum of tumors sharing common molecular features
  - *NAB2* and *STAT6* fusion → *STAT6* nuclear expression (can be detected by IHC)

Pathology
- SFT/HPC WHO grade I
  - Collagenous, low-cellularity spindle cell lesion
  - Previously diagnosed as SFT
- SFT/HPC WHO grade II
  - More cellular, "staghorn" vasculature
  - Previously diagnosed in CNS as HPC
- SFT/HPC WHO grade III
  - ≥ 5 mitoses/HPF
  - Previously anaplastic HPC

Clinical Features
- Rare (< 1% of CNS primary neoplasms)
  - But are most common CNS nonmeningothelial mesenchymal tumor
  - SFT/HPC WHO grades II and III recur, metastasize

Imaging Findings
- SFT/HPC WHO grade I hypointense on T2WI
- SFT/HPC WHO grade II resembles aggressive meningioma
  - Calcification absent
  - Iso- to mildly hyperintense on T1WI
  - Iso- to heterogeneously hyperintense on T2WI
  - Very vascular, prominent "flow voids"
  - Enhances strongly but heterogeneously
  - "Dural tail" sign usually absent

Differential Diagnosis
- SFT/HPC WHO grade I = meningioma
- SFT/HPC WHO grade II, III
  - Atypical/malignant meningioma
  - Dural metastases
  - Gliosarcoma
  - Malignant mesenchymal tumor

Other Related Neoplasms

Hemangioblastoma

Terminology

Hemangioblastoma (HGBL) are benign, slow-growing, relatively indolent vascular neoplasms. HGBL occurs in both sporadic and multiple forms.

Multiple HGBLs are almost always associated with the autosomal dominant inherited cancer syndrome, **von Hippel-Lindau disease** (VHL). A rare non-VHL form of multiple disseminated HGBLs is termed **leptomeningeal hemangioblastomatosis**.

Etiology

VHL mutations (losses or inactivations) are present in 20-50% of sporadic HGBLs. Multiple key angiogenic pathways (including VEGF/VEGFR2 and Notch/Dll4) are massively activated in HGBL and contribute synergistically to the tumor's abundant vascularization.

Pathology

Location. HGBLs can occur in any part of the CNS, although the vast majority (90-95%) of intracranial HGBLs are located in the posterior fossa. The cerebellum is by far the most common site (80%) followed by the vermis (15%). Approximately 5% occur in the brainstem, usually the medulla. The nodule of an HGBL is superficially located and typically abuts a pial surface **(22-32)**.

Supratentorial tumors are rare, accounting for 5-10% of all HGBLs. Most are clustered around the optic pathways and occur in the setting of VHL.

Size and Number. Hemangiomas vary in size from tiny to large, especially when associated with a cyst. Unless they are syndromic, HGBLs are solitary lesions. If more than one HGBL is present, the patient, by definition, has VHL. Multiple HGBLs, positive family history, or presence of other VHL markers (such as visceral cysts, retinal angioma, renal cell carcinoma) should prompt genetic screening.

Gross Pathology. The common appearance is that of a beefy red, vascular-appearing nodule that abuts a pial surface **(22-33)**. A variably sized cyst is present in 50-60% of cases. Cyst fluid is typically yellowish, and the cyst wall is usually smooth. Approximately 40% of HGBLs are solid tumors.

Microscopic Features. The cyst wall of most HGBLs is nonneoplastic and composed of compressed brain. Cyst formation in HGBLs is a result of vascular leakage from tumor vessels, not tumor liquefaction, necrosis, or active secretion.

Mitoses in HGBLs are few or absent (MIB-1 usually < 1). HGBL is a WHO grade I neoplasm. There is no recognized atypical or anaplastic variant.

HEMANGIOBLASTOMA: PATHOLOGY AND CLINICAL ISSUES

Pathology

- Posterior fossa (90-95%)
  - Cerebellum most common site
- Cyst + nodule (60%), solid (40%)

Clinical Issues

- Epidemiology/demographics
  - Uncommon (1.0-2.5% of primary brain tumors)
  - 7% of all adult primary posterior fossa tumors
  - Peak age = 30-65 years (younger with VHL); rare < 15 years
- Presentation/natural history
  - May cause hydrocephalus
  - Dysmetria, ataxia
  - 5% have secondary polycythemia
  - Slow, "stuttering" growth
  - Metastasis rare

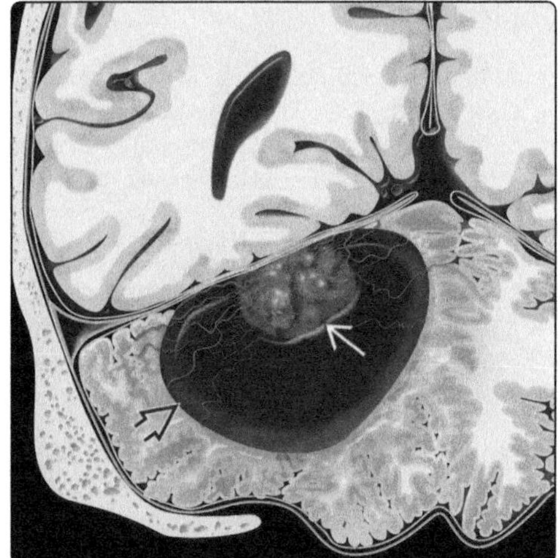

(22-32) Graphic depicts typical HGBL with cyst wall ⇨ composed of compressed cerebellum. Vascular tumor nodule ➡ abuts pial surface.

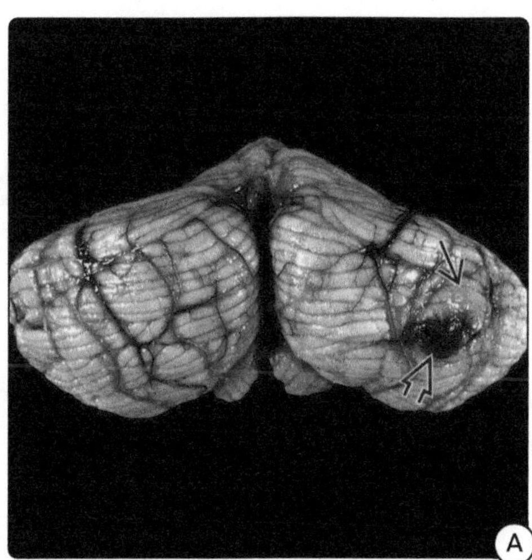

(22-33A) Autopsy specimen shows superficial nodule abutting the pia ⇨, hemorrhagic cyst ⇨ of a typical HGBL. (Courtesy E. Ross, MD.)

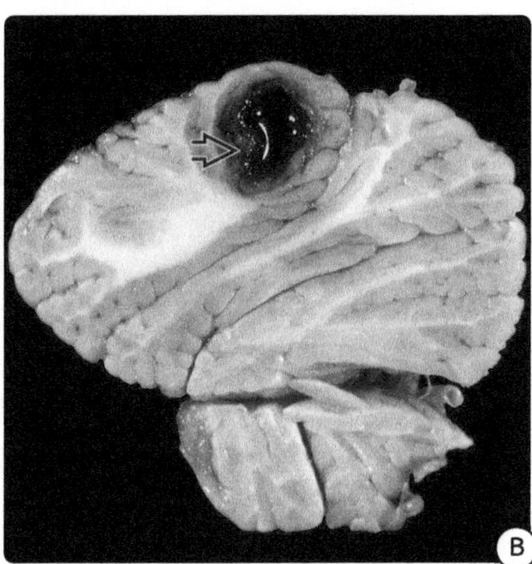

(22-33B) Sagittal section in the same case shows the hemorrhagic cyst ⇨. The tumor nodule is not visible. (Courtesy E. Ross, MD.)

Clinical Issues

Epidemiology. HGBL accounts for 1.0-2.5% of primary CNS neoplasms and ~ 7% of all primary posterior fossa tumors in adults. It is the second most common infratentorial parenchymal mass in adults (after metastasis).

Between 25-40% of HGBLs are associated with VHL.

Demographics. HGBL is generally a tumor of adults between the ages of 30 and 65 years. Pediatric HGBLs are rare. VHL-associated HGBLs tend to present at a significantly younger age but are still relatively rare in children under the age of 15.

Presentation. Most symptoms in patients with the cystic form of HGBL are caused by the cyst, not the neoplastic nodule. Headache is the presenting symptom in 85% of cases. HGBLs produce erythropoietin, which causes secondary polycythemia in ~ 5% of patients.

Natural History and Treatment Options. Because HGBLs exhibit a "stuttering" growth pattern, they are frequently stable lesions that can remain asymptomatic for long intervals. Imaging progression alone is not an indication for treatment, although tumor/cyst growth rates can be used to predict symptom formation and future need for treatment.

Although HGBLs show no intrinsic tendency to metastasize, there are sporadic reports of intraspinal dissemination. Complete en bloc resection is the procedure of choice. Total resection eliminates tumor recurrence, although new HGBLs may develop in the setting of VHL.

Imaging

General Features. HGBLs have four basic imaging patterns: (1) Solid HGBLs without associated cysts, (2) HGBLs with intratumoral cysts, (3) HGBLs with peritumoral cysts (nonneoplastic cyst with solid tumor nodule), and (4) HGBLs associated with both peri- and intratumoral cysts

(22-34A) Axial T1 MR in a 70-year-old woman with ataxia shows a cystic cerebellar mass ➲ with a mural nodule ➔. (22-34B) Axial T2 FS MR in the same case shows that the cyst fluid ➲ is very hyperintense, while the nodule is mostly isointense ➔ with adjacent brain.

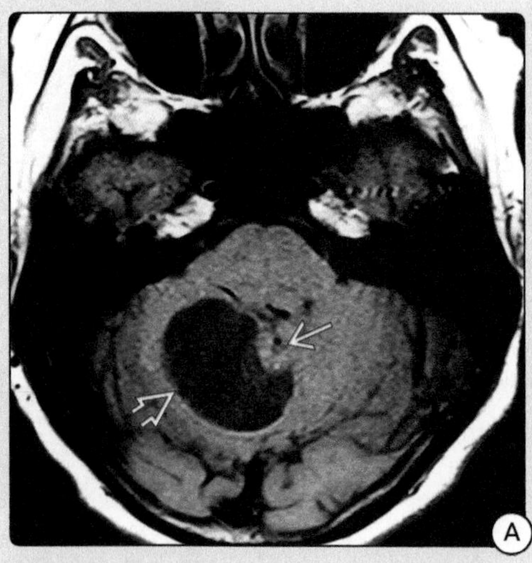

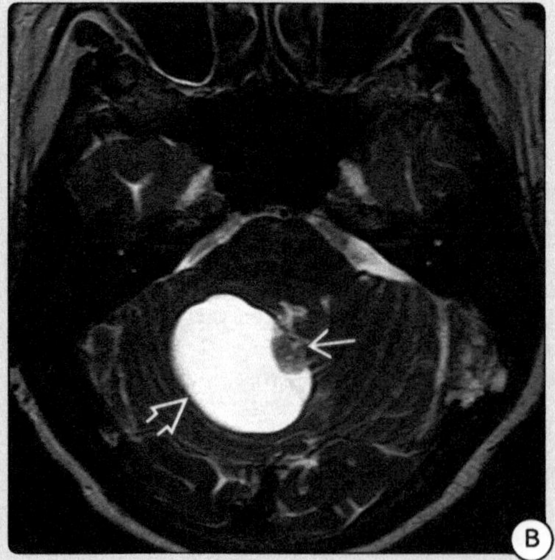

(22-34C) FLAIR MR shows that the fluid ➲ does not suppress, and the mural nodule ➔ is hyperintense to brain parenchyma. (22-34D) T1 C+ MR shows that the mural nodule enhances intensely ➔, while the cyst wall does not exhibit any contrast enhancement ➲. This is solitary hemangioblastoma, WHO grade I.

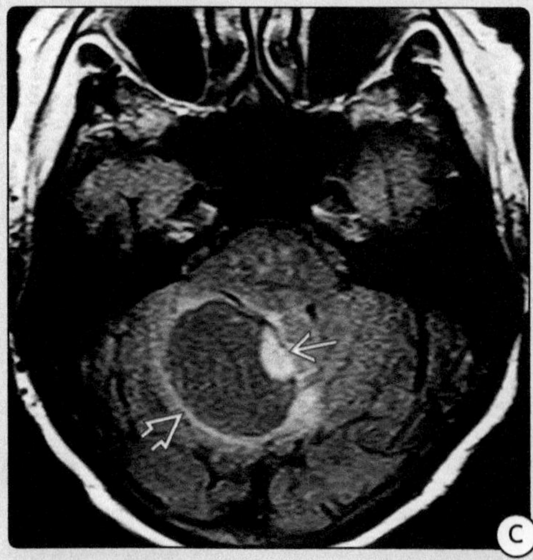

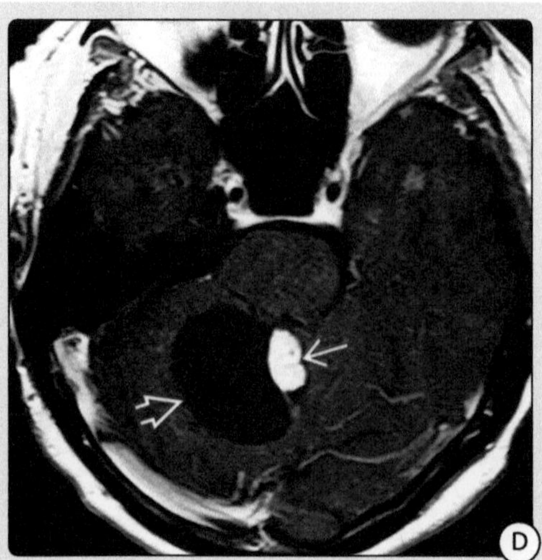

(nonneoplastic cyst with cysts in the tumor nodule). A nonneoplastic peritumoral cyst with solid nodule is the most common pattern, seen in 50-65% of cases. The second most common pattern is the solid form, seen in ~ 40% of cases.

CT Findings. The most common appearance is a well-delineated iso- to slightly hyperdense nodule associated with a hypodense cyst. Calcification and gross hemorrhage are absent. The nodule enhances strongly and uniformly following contrast administration.

MR Findings. An isointense nodule with prominent "flow voids" is seen on T1WI. If an associated peritumoral cyst is present, it is typically hypointense to parenchyma on T1WI but hyperintense compared with CSF **(22-34)**.

Compared with brain parenchyma, the tumor nodule of an HGBL is moderately hyperintense on T2WI and FLAIR. Intratumoral cysts and prominent "flow voids" are common. The cyst fluid is very hyperintense on T2WI and FLAIR **(22-34)**.

Occasionally, an HGBL hemorrhages. If present, blood products "bloom" on T2*. Intense enhancement of the nodule—but not the cyst itself—is typical. Cyst wall enhancement should raise the possibility of tumor involvement, as compressed, nonneoplastic brain does not enhance.

Noncystic HGBLs enhance strongly but often heterogeneously **(22-35)**. Multiple HGBLs are seen in VHL and vary from tiny punctate to large solid tumors (see Chapter 40).

Supratentorial HGBLs are rare. Most occur around the optic nerves or chiasm. HGBL occasionally occurs as a hemispheric mass with a "cyst + nodule" appearance **(22-37)**.

Angiography. The most common appearance is that of an intensely vascular tumor nodule that shows a prolonged vascular "blush" **(22-36)**. "Early draining" veins are common. If a tumor-associated cyst is present, vessels appear displaced and "draped" around an avascular mass.

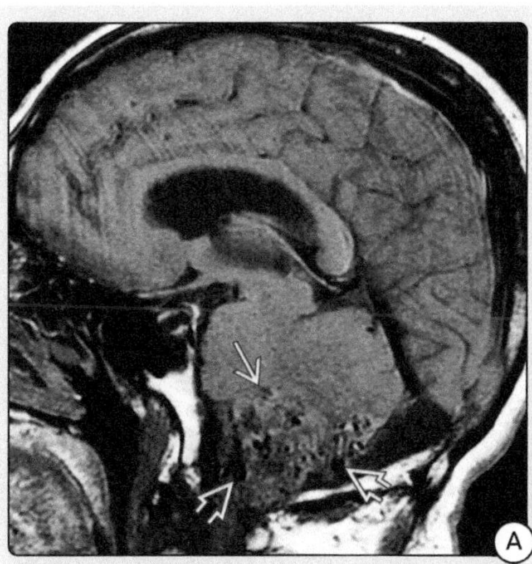

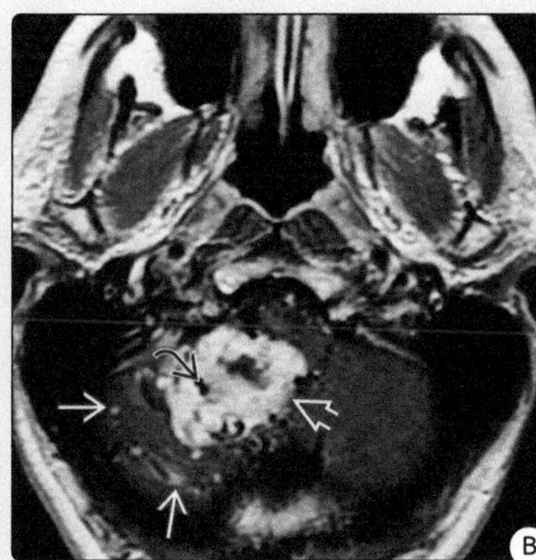

***(22-35A)** Sagittal T1 MR in a 63-year-old man with vertigo shows a posterior fossa mass ➡ with numerous prominent "flow voids" ➡. **(22-35B)** Axial T1 C+ MR shows that the mass ➡ enhances intensely but heterogeneously. Note the vascular "flow voids" ➡ and the enhancing, enlarged draining veins ➡.*

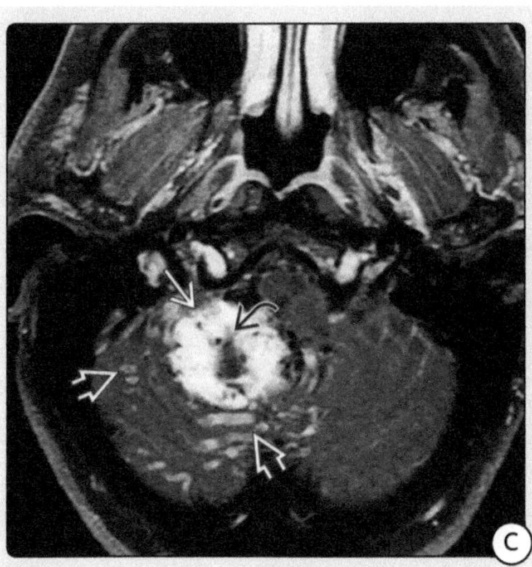

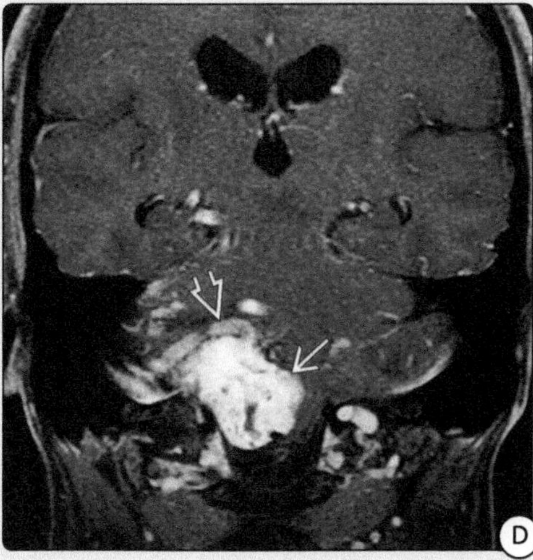

***(22-35C)** More cephalad axial T1 C+ FS MR in the same case shows that the mass ➡ enhances intensely, appears solid with an area of central necrosis ➡. Note numerous prominent serpentine enhancing vessels ➡ in the adjacent cerebellum. **(22-35D)** Coronal T1 C+ FS MR shows the solid mass ➡ and prominent draining vein ➡. This is hemangioblastoma, WHO grade I.*

Differential Diagnosis

The differential diagnosis of HGBL varies with age. In a middle-aged or older adult, the statistically most common cause of an enhancing posterior fossa intraaxial (parenchymal) mass is **metastasis**, not HGBL! DWI and DSC-PWI are helpful in the characterization and differentiation of HGBL from brain metastases. HGBL has higher minimum ADC values and relative ADC ratios compared with metastases.

A cerebellar mass with "cyst + nodule" in a child or young adult is most likely a **pilocytic astrocytoma**, not HGBL or metastasis. Occasionally, a **cavernous malformation** can mimic an HGBL with hemorrhage.

Selected References: The complete reference list is available on the Expert Consult™ eBook version included with purchase.

HEMANGIOBLASTOMA: IMAGING

General Features

- "Cyst + nodule" (60%); nodule abuts pial surface
- Solid (40%)

CT

- Low-density cyst
- Strongly enhancing nodule

MR

- Cyst
  - Fluid slightly hyperintense to CSF
  - Wall usually nonneoplastic
- Nodule
  - Isointense to brain
  - "Flow voids" common
  - Enhances intensely

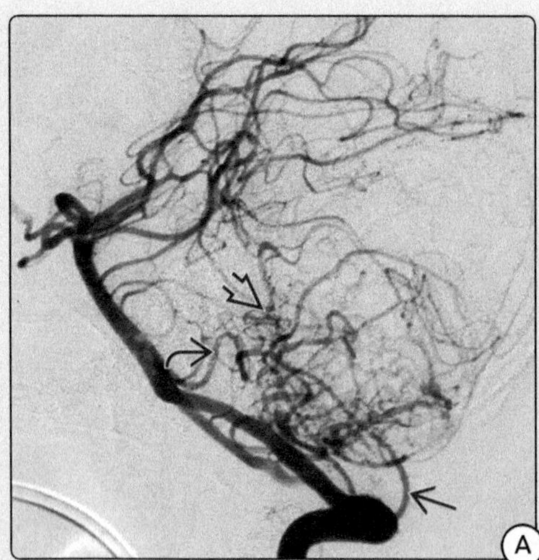

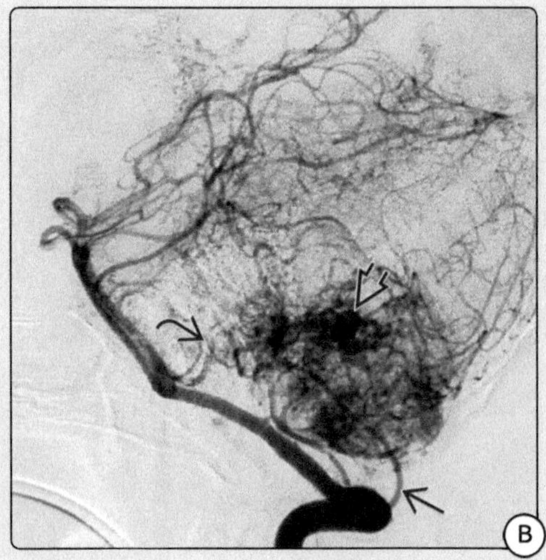

***(22-36A)** Early arterial phase, lateral view of a vertebrobasilar DSA shows a patient with cerebellar hemangioblastoma. Note vascular tumor mass ⇨ supplied primarily by enlarged branches of the anterior ⇨ and posterior inferior cerebellar arteries ⇨. **(22-36B)** Late arterial phase in the same case shows the characteristic prolonged tumor "blush" ⇨ coming from branches of enlarged PICA ⇨ and AICA ⇨.*

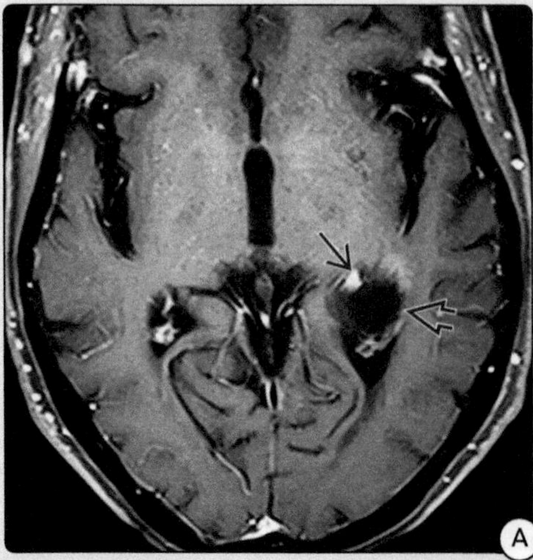

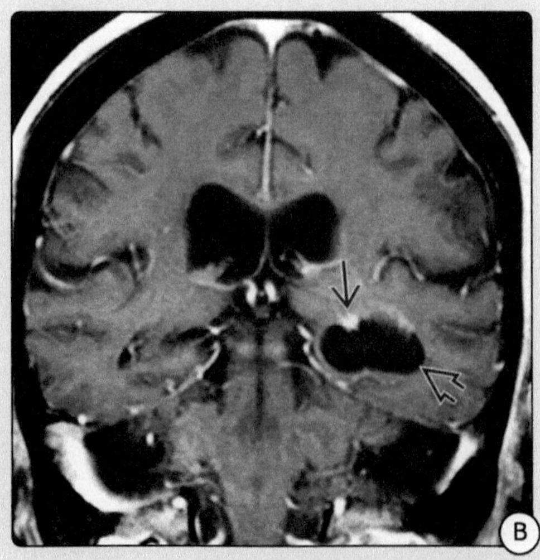

***(22-37A)** Axial T1 C+ FS MR in an 84-year-old woman with a positive family history of VHL shows a cystic lesion ⇨ with an enhancing nodule ⇨ in the left posteromedial temporal lobe. **(22-37B)** Coronal T1 C+ MR in the same case shows that the cyst wall ⇨ does not enhance, but the nodule enhances strongly, uniformly ⇨. The lesion has been stable for 5 years. This is presumed supratentorial hemangioblastoma in the setting of VHL.*

Nerve Sheath Tumors

The 2016 WHO made relatively few changes in the way tumors of the cranial and paraspinal nerves are classified. The four basic categories of ***schwannoma, neurofibroma, perineurioma,*** *and* ***malignant peripheral nerve sheath tumor*** *were retained.*

With the exception of vestibular schwannoma (VS), all intracranial nerve sheath tumors are rare. They occur ether sporadically or as part of tumor-associated familial tumor syndromes, such as neurofibromatosis types 1 and 2.

The vast majority of nerve sheath neoplasms are benign. The two major tumor types that are found intracranially and at or near the skull base are schwannomas and neurofibromas. Both are discussed in this chapter.

Schwannomas

Schwannoma Overview

Terminology

Schwannomas are benign slow-growing encapsulated tumors that are composed entirely of well-differentiated Schwann cells. Less common terms are neurinoma and neurilemmoma.

Etiology

General Concepts. Schwannomas originate from Schwann cells, which are derived from the embryonic neural crest. Schwannomas may arise along the course of any peripheral nerve or cranial nerves (CNs) III-XII. The olfactory and optic nerves do not contain Schwann cells so schwannomas do not arise from CNs I and II. "Olfactory groove schwannomas" are probably tumors that arise from olfactory ensheathing cells.

Schwann cells are also not a component of normal brain parenchyma. The exceptionally rare intraparenchymal schwannoma is thought to arise from neural crest remnants that later express aberrant Schwann cell differentiation.

Genetics. Biallelic inactivation (the classic "two-hit mechanism") of the *NF2* gene is detected in nearly all sporadic vestibular schwannomas and 50-70% of meningiomas.

Pathology

Location. Schwannomas arise at the glial-Schwann cell junction of CNs III-XII **(23-1)**. The distance from the brain to the interface where the glial covering

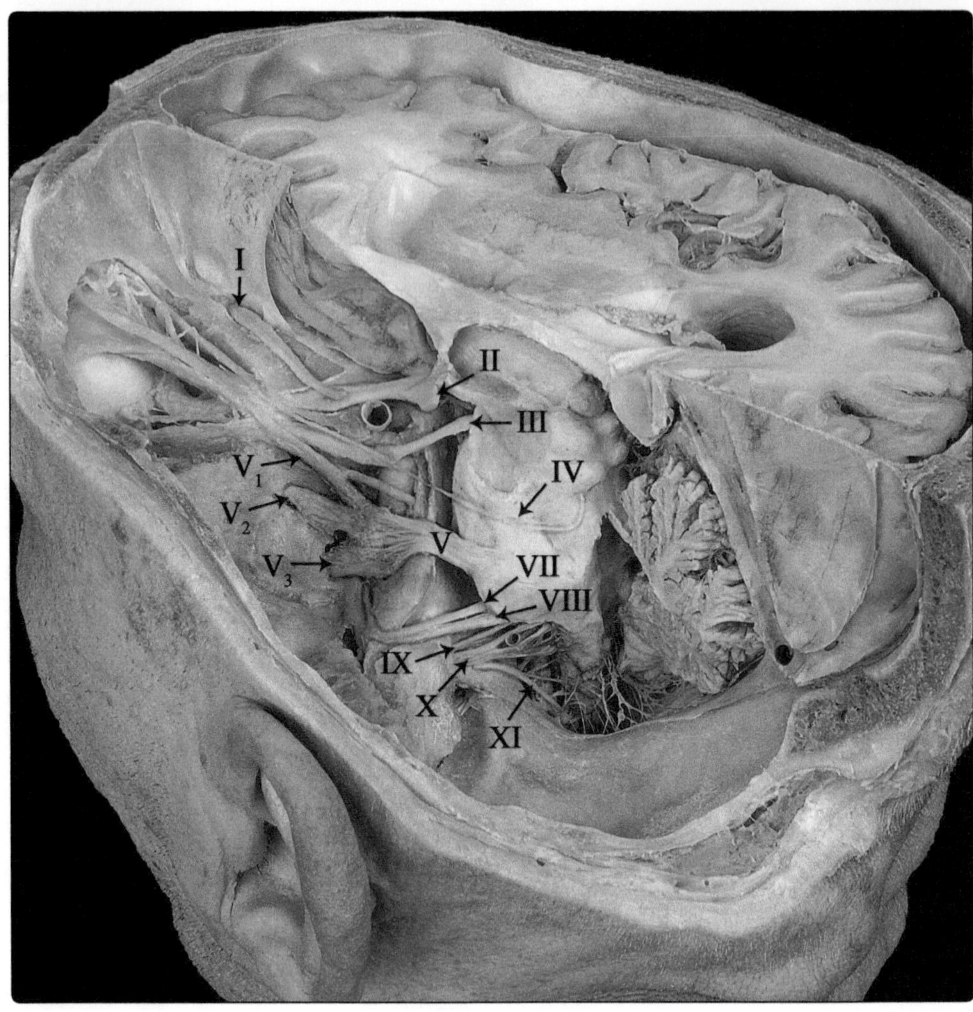

***(23-1)** Olfactory nerve (I), optic chiasm (II), oculomotor nerve (III), trochlear nerve (IV) coursing anteriorly in the ambient cistern, and the trigeminal nerve (V) with its ophthalmic (V1), maxillary (V2), and mandibular (V3) branches are shown. Abducens (VI) and hypoglossal (XII) nerves are not visualized. CPA segments of the facial (VII) and vestibulocochlear (VIII) nerves are shown. Glossopharyngeal (IX), vagus (X), and spinal accessory (XI) nerves course toward the jugular foramen. (Courtesy M. Nielsen, MS.)*

terminates and Schwann cell ensheathing begins varies with each cranial nerve. In some—such as the oculomotor nerve (CNIII)—the junction is in close proximity to the brain. Here, schwannomas arise close to the exit of the parent nerve from the brain. In others—such as the vestibulocochlear nerve (CNVIII)—the junction lies at some distance from the nerve exit or entrance into the brainstem.

Sensory nerves are much more commonly affected by schwannomas compared with pure motor cranial nerves. The vestibulocochlear nerve is by far the most common intracranial site (90%). The second most common site is the trigeminal nerve (CNV) (2-4%). Schwannomas of cranial nerves other than CNVIII and CNV (e.g., jugular foramen or hypoglossal tumors) are very rare, accounting for just 1-2% of cases.

Size and Number. Most intracranial schwannomas are small, especially those that arise from motor nerves. Some, especially trigeminal schwannomas, can attain a huge size and involve both intra- and extracranial compartments.

Most schwannomas are "sporadic" or "solitary." The presence of multiple schwannomas in the same individual suggests an underlying tumor predisposition syndrome (see Chapter 39).

Gross Pathology. Schwannomas arise eccentrically from their parent nerves and are smooth or nodular well-encapsulated lesions **(23-2)** **(23-3)**. Cystic change is common. Microhemorrhages occur, but gross macroscopic bleeds are rare.

INTRACRANIAL SCHWANNOMAS: PATHOLOGY

Location
- Vestibular (CNVIII) most common (90-95%)
  - All other sites combined (1-5%)
- Trigeminal (CNV) 2nd most common
- Jugular foramen (CNs IX, X, XI) 3rd most common
- Solitary > > multiple (NF2, schwannomatosis)

Pathology
- Arise at glial-Schwann cell junction
  - Distance from brain varies according to cranial nerve
- Benign encapsulated nerve sheath tumor
- Well-differentiated neoplastic Schwann cells
- Biphasic histology with 2 components
  - Compact, highly ordered cellularity ("Antoni A")
  - Less cellular, myxoid matrix ("Antoni B")

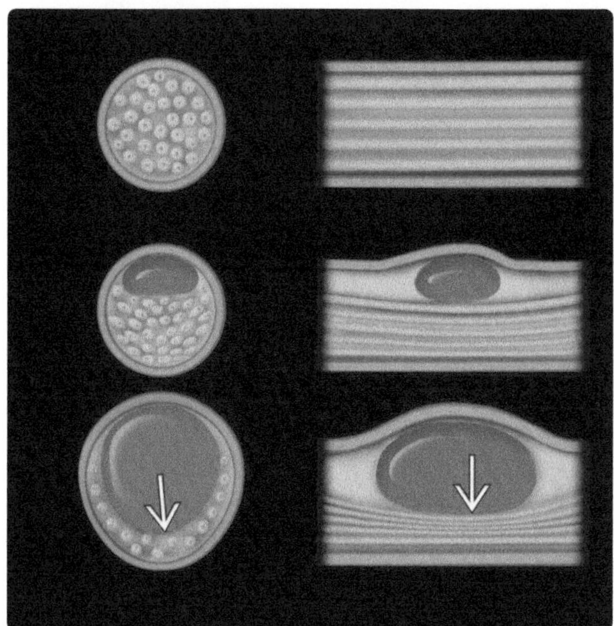

(23-2) Axial (L) and sagittal (R) graphics show a schwannoma arising within a unifascicular nerve. The tumor displaces other nerve fibers peripherally ➡.

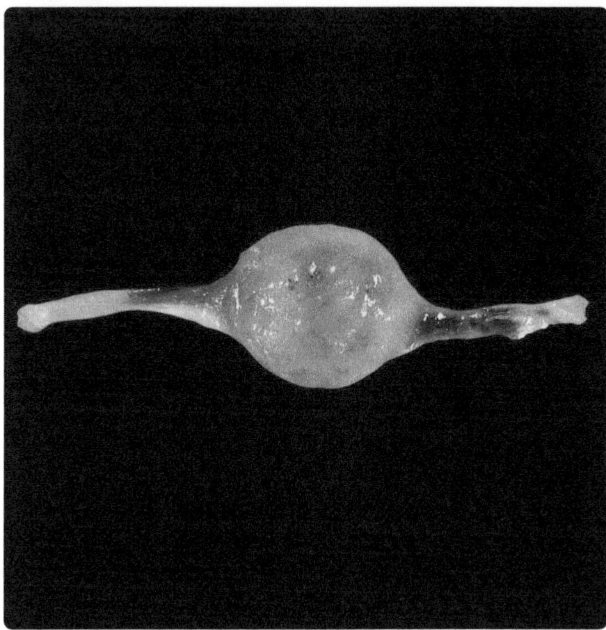

(23-3) Schwannomas are encapsulated by perineurium and epineural collagen and grow eccentrically to the nerve of origin. (From DP: Neuropathology, 2e.)

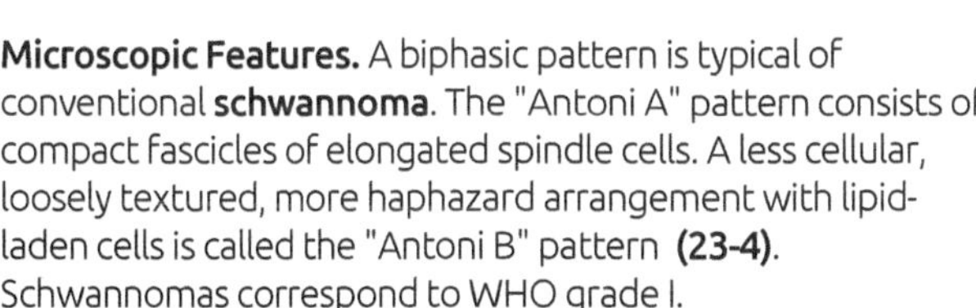

Microscopic Features. A biphasic pattern is typical of conventional **schwannoma**. The "Antoni A" pattern consists of compact fascicles of elongated spindle cells. A less cellular, loosely textured, more haphazard arrangement with lipid-laden cells is called the "Antoni B" pattern **(23-4)**. Schwannomas correspond to WHO grade I.

Clinical Issues

Intracranial schwannomas are relatively uncommon, constituting ~ 7% of all primary neoplasms. All ages are affected, but the peak incidence is in the 4th-6th decades. Schwannomas do occur in children but are uncommon unless associated with neurofibromatosis type 2 (NF2). Symptoms are location specific.

Schwannomas are benign tumors that tend to grow very slowly. The exception is VSs in young patients with NF2. These tumors have higher MIB-1 indices.

Imaging

General Features. Neuroimaging findings reflect their slow growth and benign biologic behavior. A well-circumscribed extraaxial mass that originates within or near a cranial nerve and displaces but does not invade adjacent structures is typical **(23-5)**.

CT Findings. Most schwannomas exhibit low to intermediate attenuation on NECT scans and show smooth expansion/remodeling of osseous foramina on bone CT. Cystic change is common. Gross intratumoral hemorrhage is uncommon, and calcification is rare. Strong, moderately heterogeneous enhancement after contrast administration is typical.

MR Findings. Schwannomas are generally isointense with cortex on T1WI and heterogeneously hyperintense on T2WI and FLAIR **(23-7A)**. Although macroscopic intratumoral hemorrhage is rare, T2* (GRE, SWI) scans often reveal "blooming" foci of microbleeds.

Secondary changes of muscle edema or denervation with atrophy and fatty infiltration can occur with motor nerve schwannomas. Vagal nerve schwannomas may cause vocal cord paralysis.

Virtually all schwannomas enhance intensely. Approximately 15% have nonenhancing intratumoral cysts. Nonneoplastic peritumoral cysts occur in 5-10% of cases, especially with larger lesions **(23-10)**.

Differential Diagnosis

The differential diagnosis of a **solitary enlarged enhancing cranial nerve** includes schwannoma, multiple sclerosis, viral and postviral neuritis, Lyme disease, sarcoid, ischemia, and malignant neoplasms (metastases, lymphoma, and leukemia).

The most common cause of **multiple enhancing cranial nerves** is metastasis. NF2, neuritis (especially Lyme disease), lymphoma, and leukemia are significantly less common than metastasis. Rare but important causes include multiple sclerosis and chronic inflammatory demyelinating polyneuropathy, a disorder that usually affects spinal nerves but may occasionally involve cranial nerves.

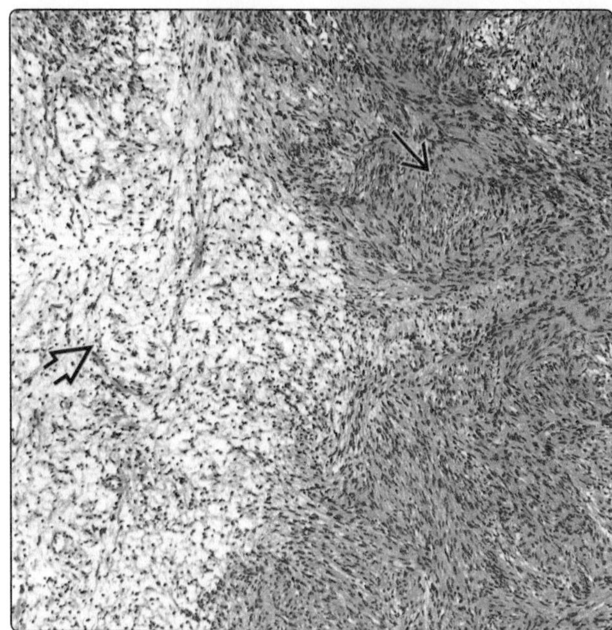

(23-4) The juxtaposition of the cellular "Antoni A" ➡ and loose "Antoni B" ➡ patterns is classic for conventional schwannoma. (From DP: Neuropathology, 2e.)

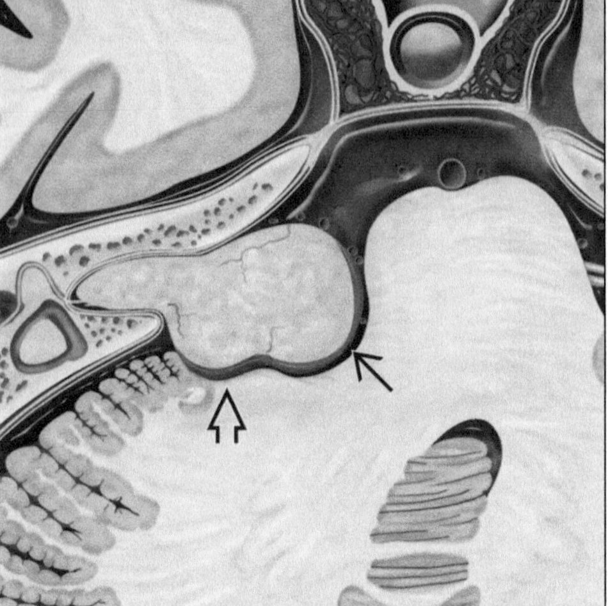

(23-5) Graphic of a large vestibular schwannoma shows the typical "ice cream on cone" morphology. Note the prominent CSF-vascular "cleft" between the middle cerebellar peduncle ➡ and the cerebellar hemisphere ➡.

Vestibular Schwannoma

Terminology

Vestibular schwannoma (VS) is the preferred term for a CNVIII schwannoma. VSs are also known as **acoustic schwannomas** and **acoustic neuromas**.

Etiology

VSs arise from the vestibular portion of CNVIII at the glial-Schwann cell junction, inside the IAC near the porus acusticus. Schwannomas rarely arise from the cochlear portion of CNVIII. The majority of sporadic VSs have inactivating mutations of *NF2*.

Pathology

VSs may occur at any location along the course of the nerve. Small VSs are often completely intracanalicular. Larger lesions frequently protrude medially through the porus acusticus into the cerebellopontine angle (CPA) cistern.

Small VSs are round or ovoid lesions that generally measure 2-10 mm in length. VSs that extend into the CPA cistern can become very large, up to 5 cm in diameter. Bilateral VSs are pathognomonic of NF2.

Clinical Issues

VS is by far the most common intracranial schwannoma. VS is also the most common cerebellopontine cistern mass, accounting for 85-90% of lesions in this location.

Peak presentation is 40-60 years of age. The most common presentation is an adult with slowly progressive unilateral sensorineural hearing loss (SNHL). Small VSs may present initially with tinnitus. Large lesions often present with trigeminal &/or facial neuropathy.

The growth rate of VSs varies. On average, they tend to enlarge between 1 mm or 2 mm per year. Approximately 60% grow very slowly (< 1 mm per year), whereas 10% of patients experience rapid enlargement of their lesions (> 3 mm per year).

Imaging

General Features. The classic imaging appearance of VS is an avidly enhancing mass that looks like "ice cream on a cone" **(23-6)**. Many VSs extend medially from their origin within the IAC. The intracanalicular part of the tumor represents the "cone." If a VS passes through the porus acusticus, it typically expands when it enters the CPA, forming the "ice cream" on the cone.

Precisely defining the size and extent of a VS is one of the most important goals of imaging. Some VSs remain as small slow-growing lesions that are entirely intracanalicular **(23-8)** **(23-9)**. Many intracanalicular VSs have a distinctive fundal "cap" of CSF interposed between the lesion and the modiolus **(23-9)**. Others grow laterally, extending deep into the IAC fundus, and may eventually pass through the cochlear aperture into the modiolus.

CT Findings. CT is generally negative unless lesions are large enough to expand the IAC or protrude into the CPA cistern.

MR Findings. VSs are generally iso-/hypointense with brain on T1WI **(23-7B)**. An intracanalicular VS appears as a hypointense filling defect within the bright CSF on CISS **(23-6A)**. Larger VSs are iso- to heterogeneously hyperintense on T2WI and may have associated cysts **(23-10)**. Microhemorrhage on T2* is common, although macroscopic hemorrhage is rare (0.4% of all newly diagnosed VSs but 5-6% of anticoagulated patients).

Virtually all VSs enhance strongly following contrast administration **(23-6B)**. A schwannoma-associated "dural tail" sign occurs but is rare compared with CPA meningiomas.

Differential Diagnosis

The major differential diagnosis of VS is **CPA meningioma**. Most meningiomas "cap" the IAC and do not extend deep to the porus. However, a reactive dural "tail" in the IAC may make distinction between VS and meningioma difficult unless other dural "tails" along the petrous ridge are also present.

A **facial nerve schwannoma** confined to the IAC may be difficult to distinguish from a VS. Facial nerve schwannomas are much less common and usually have a labyrinthine segment "tail." **Metastases** can coat the facial and vestibulocochlear nerves within the IAC. Metastases are usually bilateral with other lesions present.

Other CPA masses, such as **epidermoid cysts, arachnoid cysts**, and **aneurysms**, can usually be distinguished easily from VS. VSs occasionally have prominent intramural cysts, but a completely cystic schwannoma without an enhancing tumor rim is very rare.

Trigeminal Schwannoma

Although trigeminal schwannomas are the second most common intracranial schwannoma, they are rare tumors. They may involve any part of the CNV complex, including extracranial peripheral divisions of the nerve. Nearly 2/3 of all Meckel cave tumors are schwannomas.

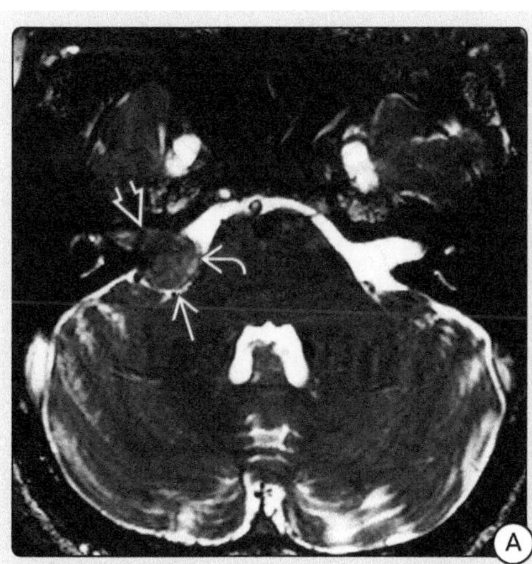

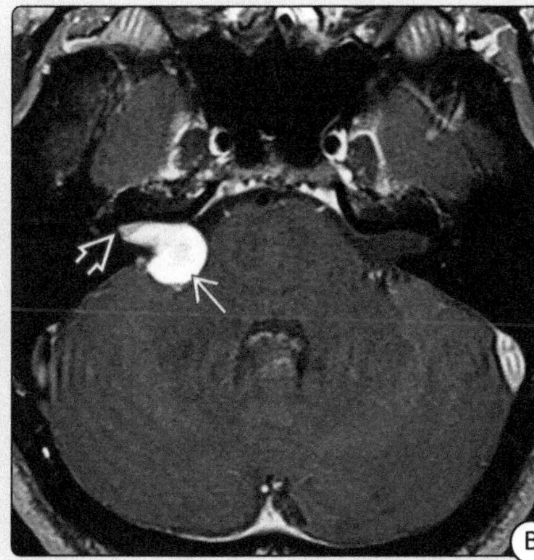

***(23-6A)** Thin-section CISS demonstrates a classic vestibular schwannoma (VS) with the "ice cream ➡ on a cone" ➡ appearance and thin CSF-vascular "cleft" ➡ where the tumor slightly indents the adjacent pons and middle cerebellar peduncle. **(23-6B)** Strong, relatively uniform enhancement ➡ is seen on T1 C+ FS MR. The tumor extends to the IAC fundus ➡.*

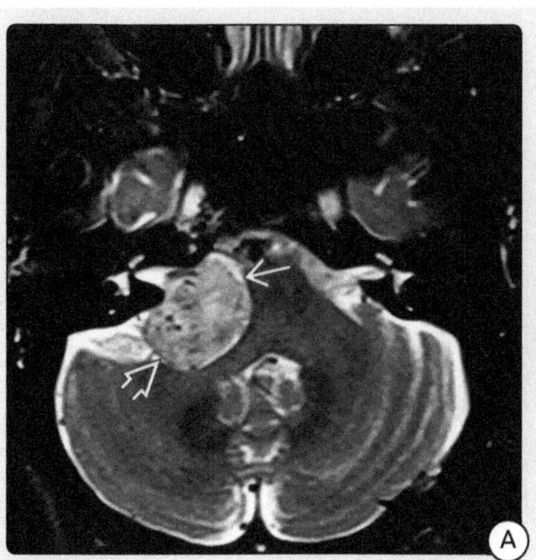

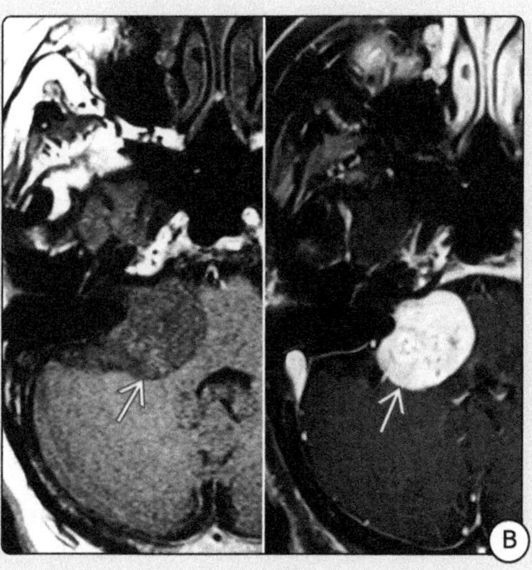

***(23-7A)** Axial T2 FS MR shows heterogeneously hyperintense signal of typical large VS ➡. The tumor indents the pons and cerebellar peduncle, deforming the 4th ventricle. Note CSF "cleft" ➡ between the tumor and brainstem. **(23-7B)** Precontrast T1 MR (L) and postcontrast T1 C+ FS MR (R) in the same case show that the tumor ➡ enhances intensely but somewhat heterogeneously. This is a VS with conventional histology.*

Imaging

Trigeminal schwannomas arise from the junction of the gasserian ganglion and the trigeminal nerve root **(23-11)**. Small lesions may be confined to Meckel cave. They have a very characteristic appearance on coronal T2WI, the "winking Meckel cave" sign. Because at least 90% of each Meckel cave is normally filled with CSF, any lesion that fills the cave with soft tissue contrasts sharply with the bright signal on the opposite normal side **(23-12)**.

Bicompartmental tumors are common. Schwannomas that originate in Meckel cave can extend into the posterior fossa (through the porus trigeminus). These tumors have a characteristic "dumbbell" configuration **(23-13)**. Tumors that involve all three locations are uncommon and termed "three-compartment" trigeminal schwannomas **(23-14)**.

Schwannomas that involve the mandibular division (CNV3) may cause denervation atrophy of the muscles of mastication.

Differential Diagnosis

The appearance of a bi- or tricompartmental CNV schwannoma is distinctive. The major differential diagnoses of a Meckel cave schwannoma are **meningioma** and **metastasis**.

Jugular Foramen Schwannoma

Although schwannomas account for ~ 40% of all jugular foramen (JF) neoplasms, JF schwannomas constitute only 2-4% of all intracranial schwannomas.

Glossopharyngeal schwannomas are the most common JF schwannoma, but they are still rare. The vast majority present with vestibulocochlear symptoms secondary to compression and displacement, not CNIX symptoms. Glossopharyngeal schwannomas can occur anywhere along the course of CNIX, but the majority of symptomatic cases are intracranial/intraosseous.

__(23-8)__ Graphic depicts an intracanalicular VS as round or fusiform enlargement of the nerve ➔. __(23-9)__ Small intracanalicular VS ➔ (top) is shown on axial T1 C+ MR. High-resolution axial T2 MR (bottom) in the same patient nicely shows the VS as a round isointense mass in the IAC ➔. Note the fundal "cap" of CSF ➔.

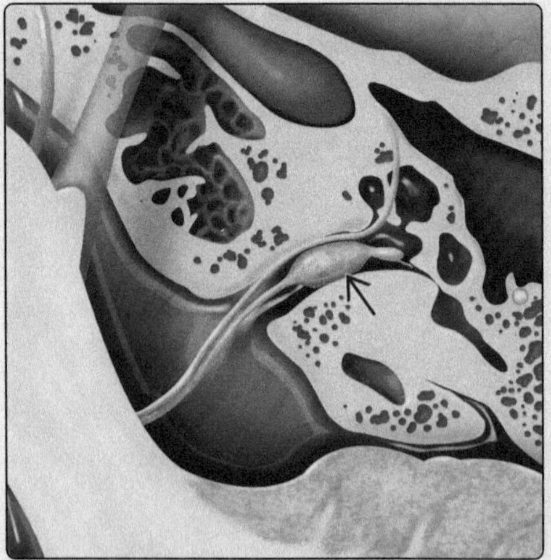

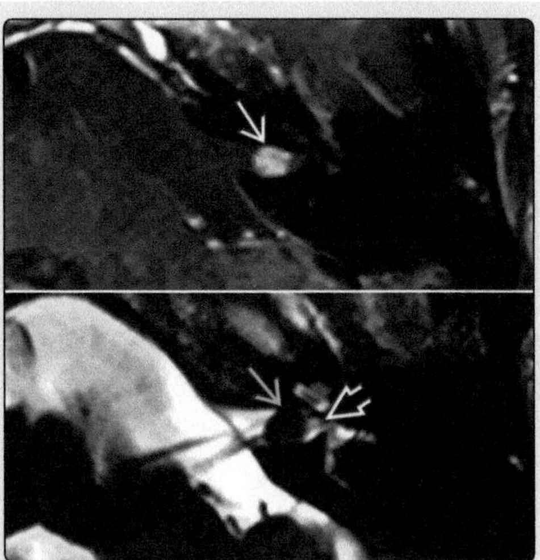

__(23-10A)__ Axial FIESTA MR in a 31-year-old man with headaches, left facial numbness shows large VS with intratumoral ➔ and marginal cysts with fluid-fluid level suggesting hemorrhage ➔. Peritumoral cysts ➔ are present, exhibit different signal from normal CSF in CPA cistern ➔. __(23-10B)__ T1 C+ FS shows nonenhancing intratumoral cysts ➔, rim enhancement along marginal ➔ and peritumoral cysts ➔. This is cystic VS with intracystic hemorrhage.

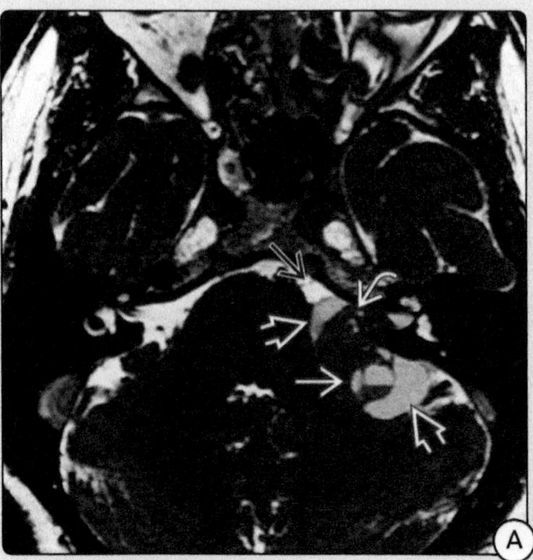

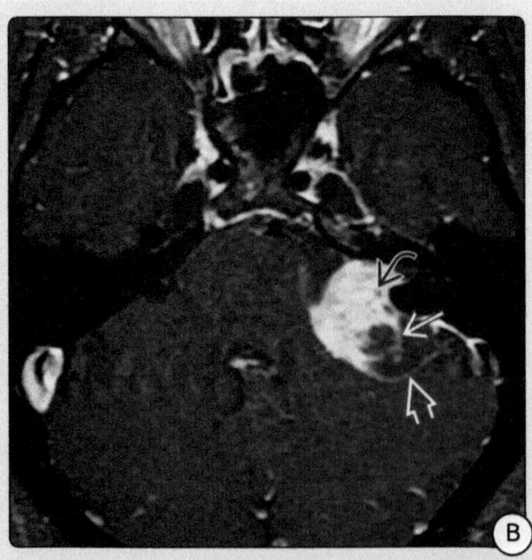

Most **vagal schwannomas** are "dumbbell" lesions that extend from the basal cistern through the JF into the high, deep carotid space **(23-15) (23-16)**.

The major differential diagnoses of JF schwannoma include **meningioma, glomus jugulare tumor**, and **metastasis**. Only a JF schwannoma smoothly enlarges and remodels the jugular fossa.

Facial Nerve Schwannoma

Facial nerve schwannomas (FNSs) are rare lesions that can arise anywhere along the course of the facial nerve, from its origin in the CPA to its extracranial ramifications in the parotid space **(23-17) (23-18)**.

CPA-IAC FNSs are radiologically indistinguishable from vestibular schwannomas if they do not demonstrate extension into the labyrinthine segment of the facial nerve canal. Lesions that traverse the labyrinthine segment often have a "dumbbell" appearance.

Almost 90% of FNSs involve more than one facial nerve segment **(23-19)**. The **geniculate fossa** is the most common site, involved in > 80% of all FNSs **(23-20)**. The **labyrinthine** and **tympanic segments** are each involved in slightly over 1/2 of FNSs. **Tympanic segment** FNSs often pedunculate into the middle ear cavity, losing their tubular configuration.

Schwannomas of Other Intracranial Nerves

Less than 1% of intracranial schwannomas arise from CNs other than VIII, V, VII, and IX/X. Most resemble their more common counterparts on imaging studies.

Olfactory nerve "schwannomas" actually arise from modified glial cells, not Schwann cells. Once termed "olfactory groove schwannoma" or "subfrontal schwannoma," these neoplasms

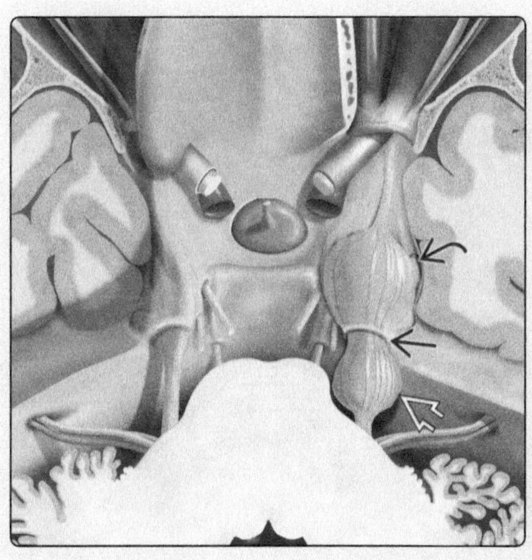

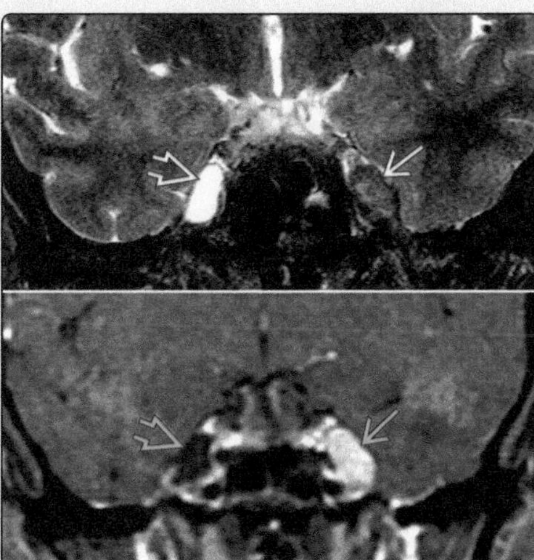

***(23-11)** "Dumbbell" trigeminal schwannoma shows that cisternal tumor segment ➡ is constricted as it passes through porus trigeminus ➡. Schwannoma then expands again ➡ when it enters Meckel cave. **(23-12)** Coronal T2 MR of left CNV schwannoma (top) shows "winking Meckel cave" sign. CSF-filled right side ➡ contrasts with tumor-filled left Meckel cave ➡. Schwannoma enhances ➡, while right side ➡ is normal (bottom).*

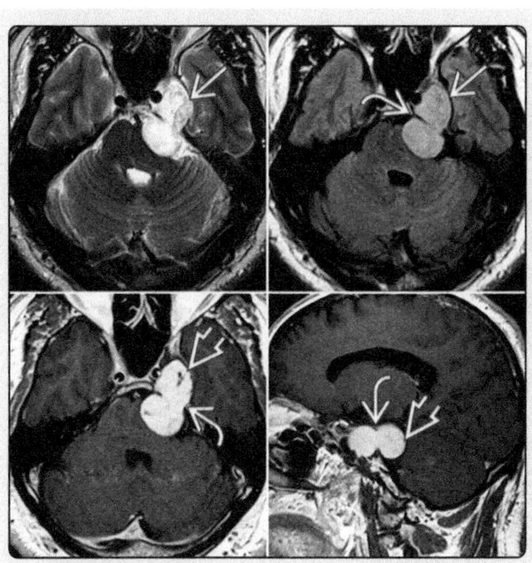

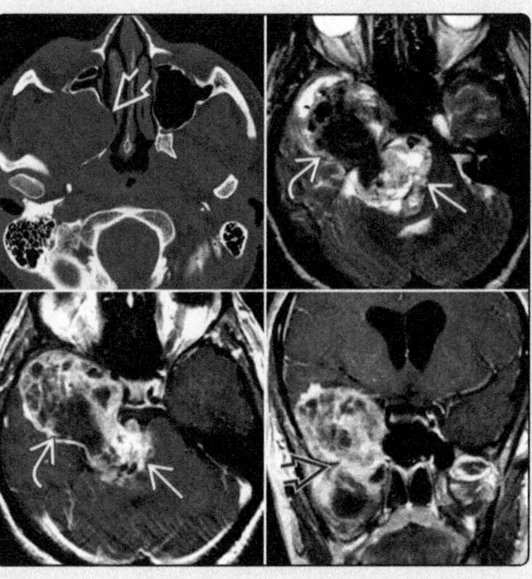

***(23-13)** This is a large "dumbbell" trigeminal schwannoma. Tumor is hyperintense on T2WI, and FLAIR ➡ enhances strongly on T1 C+ ➡. Note prominent constriction by dural ring of the porus trigeminus ➡. **(23-14)** Giant "tricompartmental" schwannoma of CNs V2 and V3 with cystic and hemorrhagic changes enlarges pterygopalatine fossa ➡, extends from posterior fossa ➡ into middle fossa ➡, through foramen ovale into masticator space ➡.*

are more accurately called **"olfactory ensheathing cell (OEC) tumors."** Many reach a large size **(23-21)**, causing frontal lobe signs, such as emotional lability and complex partial seizures.

Neoplasms of the optic nerve (a brain tract) are astrocytomas, not schwannomas. Intraorbital schwannomas arise from peripheral branches of CNs IV, V1, or VI or from sympathetic or parasympathetic fibers (not the optic nerve).

Oculomotor schwannomas are the most common of all the pure motor nerve schwannomas **(23-22)**. The most frequent location of a CNIII schwannoma is in the interpeduncular cistern near the nerve exit from the midbrain **(23-23)**. **Trochlear schwannomas** are uncommon **(23-24)**. They cause diplopia (isolated unilateral superior oblique palsy) and compensatory head tilt that may be misdiagnosed clinically as "wry neck." Most CNIV schwannomas are small and either simply watched or treated with prism spectacles.

Hypoglossal tumors are the rarest of the "other" schwannomas, accounting for only 5% of all nonvestibular intracranial schwannomas **(23-25)**. Over 90% present with denervation hemiatrophy of the tongue. Most originate intracranially **(23-26)** but can also extend extracranially as a "dumbbell" tumor that expands and remodels the hypoglossal canal **(23-27)**.

Parenchymal Schwannomas

Because the brain parenchyma does not normally contain Schwann cells, so-called "ectopic" schwannomas not associated with cranial nerves are very rare (< 1% of cases). Most intraparenchymal schwannomas are solitary and nonsyndromic.

On imaging studies, most intracranial parenchymal schwannomas appear well demarcated. The most common imaging pattern is that of a cyst with a mural nodule and peripheral enhancement. One-third are solid tumors with

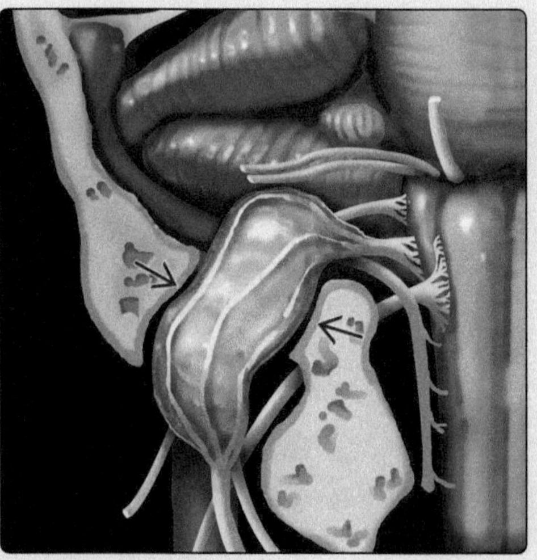

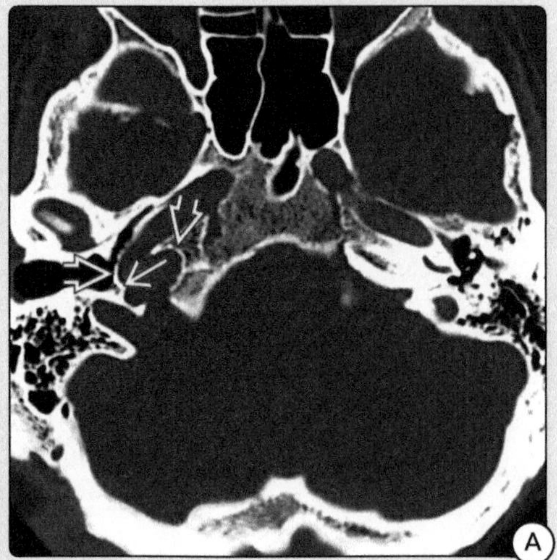

***(23-15)** Coronal graphic of a vagal schwannoma shows the tumor enlarging and remodeling the bony margins of the jugular foramen ➡. The "beak" of the "eagle" is eroded. **(23-16A)** NECT shows osseous remodeling of the right jugular foramen. The jugular spine ➡ is eroded, but the surrounding cortex ➡ appears intact (compare with Fig. 23-6).*

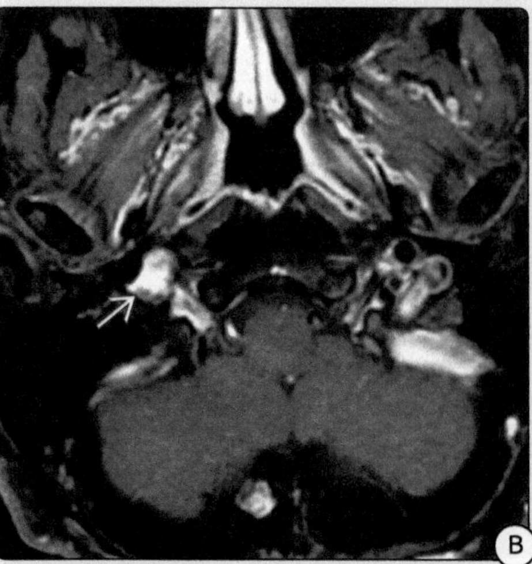

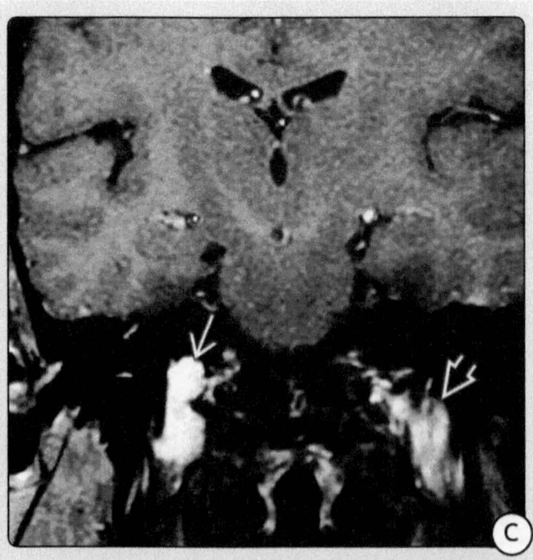

***(23-16B)** Axial T1 C+ FS MR shows an enhancing mass in the jugular foramen ➡. **(23-16C)** Coronal T1 C+ FS MR shows the intensely enhancing mass ➡. Contrast this with the normally enhancing left jugular bulb and vein ➡. At surgery, this jugular foramen schwannoma proved to be arising from the vagal nerve (CNX).*

strong homogeneous or heterogeneous enhancement. Peritumoral edema varies from none to moderate.

Melanotic Schwannoma

Melanotic schwannoma (MS) is a rare tumor composed of melanin-producing cells that have ultrastructural features resembling Schwann cells. Paraspinal and extraneural locations (e.g., skin, soft tissues, bone, and viscera) are the most common sites. Craniofacial and intracranial MSs are very rare.

Peak age at diagnosis is about a decade younger compared with conventional schwannoma. MSs can be sporadic or syndromic. Approximately 1/2 of all patients with psammomatous MS have **Carney complex**.

Because melanin causes T1 shortening, most MSs are hyperintense on T1WI and hypointense on T2WI. Enhancement varies from minimal to striking.

The main imaging differential diagnosis in MS is **metastatic melanoma** and **hemorrhagic conventional schwannoma**.

Schwannomatosis

Nonsyndromic schwannomas are almost always solitary lesions. Multiple schwannomas occur in the setting of two familial tumor syndromes, **neurofibromatosis type 2** (NF2) and **schwannomatosis**. Bilateral vestibular schwannomas are pathognomonic of NF2. Multiple, mostly nonvestibular schwannomas in the absence of other NF2 features are characteristic of schwannomatosis. Both of these syndromes are discussed in Chapter 39.

Neurofibromas

Intracranial neurofibromas (NFs) are much less common than schwannomas. In contrast to schwannomas, NFs consist of

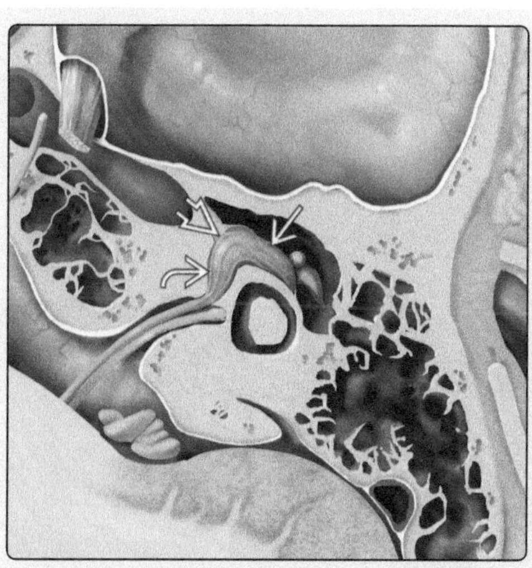

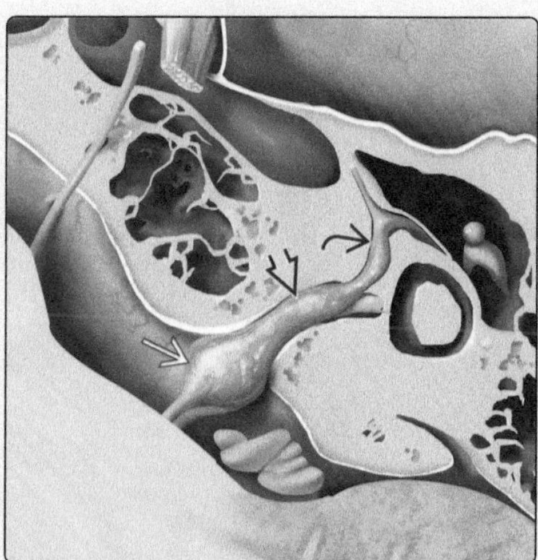

***(23-17)** Axial graphic depicts a small tubular facial nerve schwannoma involving the labyrinthine segment ➡, geniculate ganglion ➡, and anterior tympanic segment ➡ on CNVII. **(23-18)** Graphic depicts a larger facial nerve schwannoma with CPA ➡ and IAC ➡ segments. This can mimic a vestibular schwannoma ("ice cream on cone" appearance) except for the "tail" of tumor ➡ extending into the labyrinthine segment.*

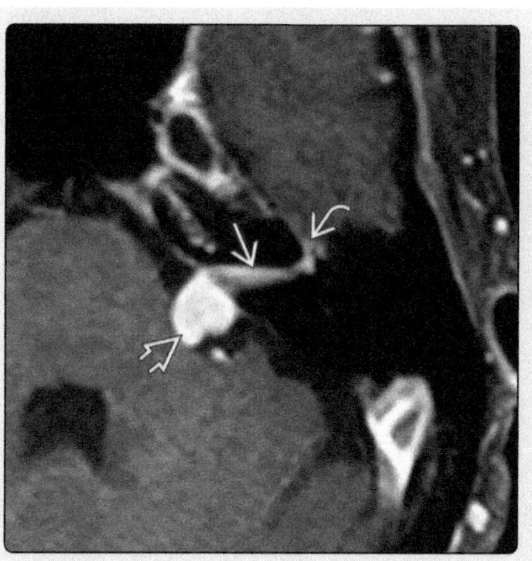

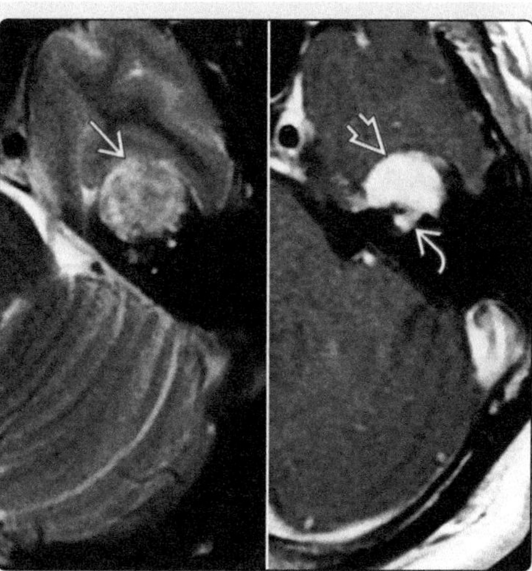

***(23-19)** Close-up view of T1 C+ FS MR shows a facial nerve schwannoma in the CPA ➡, extending into the IAC ➡ and geniculate ganglion ➡. **(23-20)** Geniculate fossa VII schwannoma is shown. T2WI (L) shows globular heterogeneously hyperintense mass ➡ tracking along the GSPN and extending extradurally into the middle cranial fossa. The labyrinthine ➡, geniculate ganglion ➡ segments (R) enhance intensely. (Courtesy P. Hildenbrand, MD.)*

(23-21A) Sagittal T1 C+ FS MR shows intensely enhancing, subfrontal, "dumbbell" mass ➡ extended through the eroded cribriform plate into the nasal cavity ⇨. (23-21B) Axial T1 C+ MR in the same patient shows well-circumscribed, intensely enhancing mass centered on cribriform plate. Diagnosis was olfactory nerve schwannoma. Most similar-appearing cases are likely olfactory ensheathing cell tumors, not schwannomas. (Courtesy G. Parker, MD.)

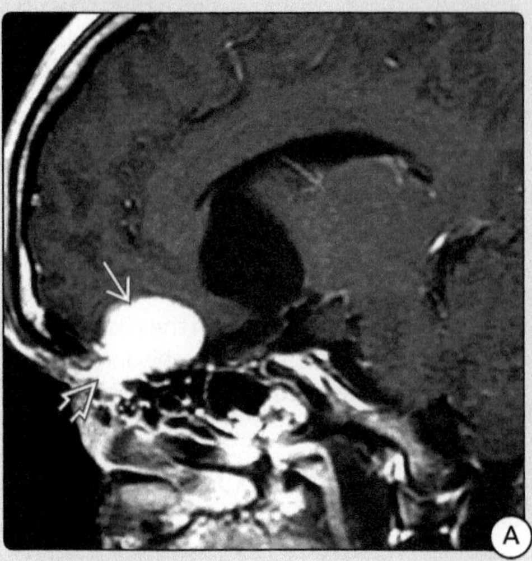

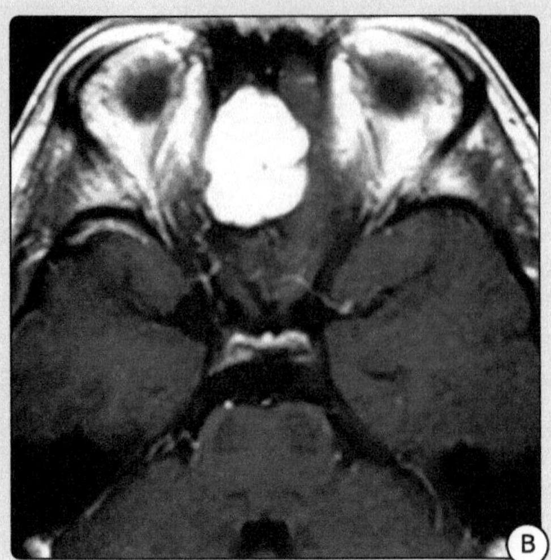

(23-22) Coronal autopsy case shows incidental left oculomotor schwannoma ➡ seen between the posterior cerebral artery above ⇨ and the superior cerebellar artery below ⇨. Contrast with the normal right CNIII ➡. (Courtesy E. T. Hedley-Whyte, MD.) (23-23A) Coronal T1 C+ MR demonstrates the enlarged, enhancing right oculomotor nerve ➡.

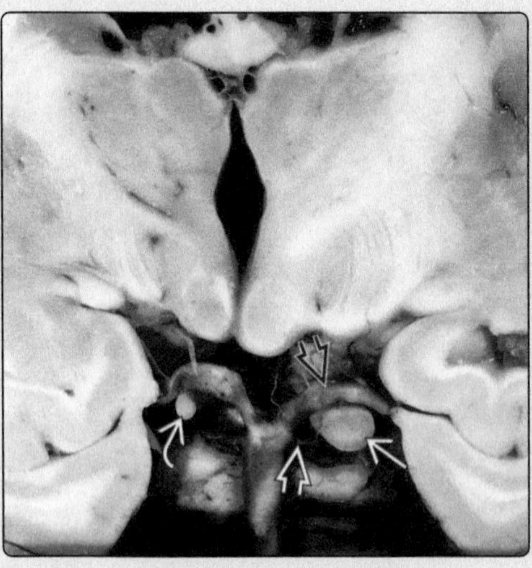

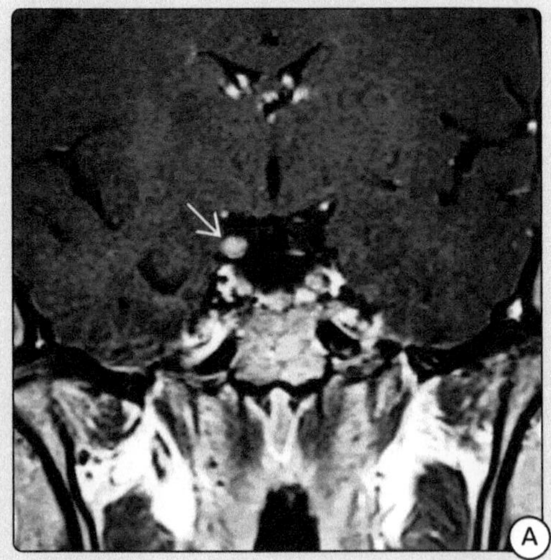

(23-23B) Sagittal T1 C+ MR in the same patient shows tubular enlargement of the oculomotor nerve ➡ extending from its midbrain exit to the cavernous sinus. (23-23C) Axial T1 C+ MR in the same patient shows the enlarged, intensely enhancing right oculomotor nerve ➡. The lesion was unchanged after 3 years. This was presumed schwannoma.

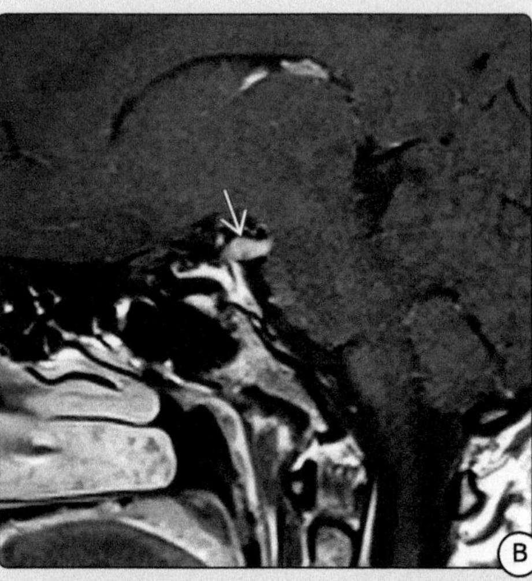

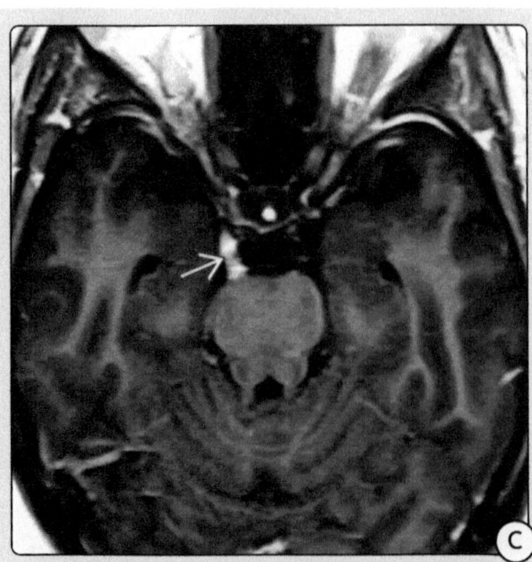

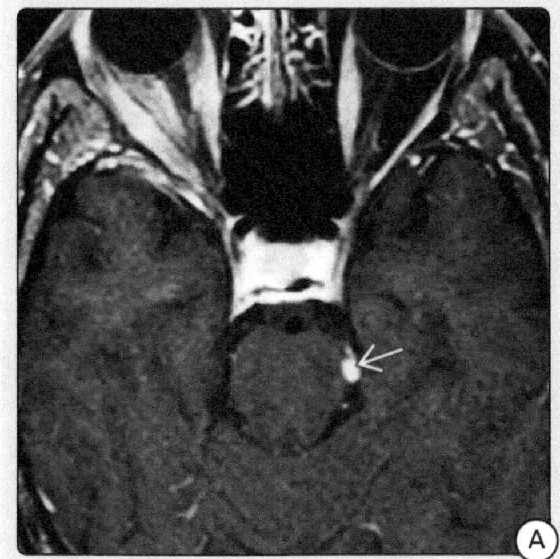

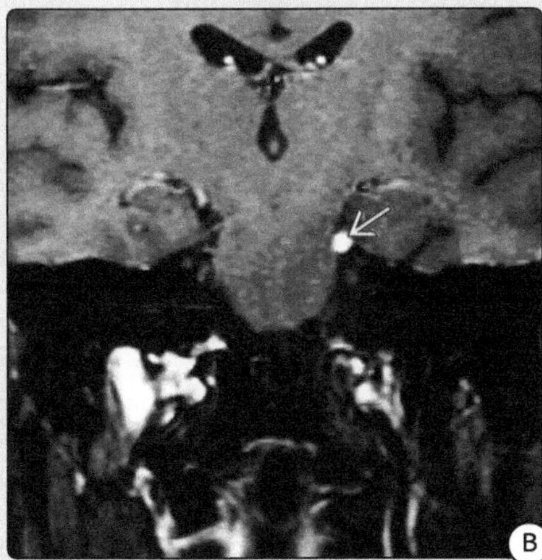

(23-24A) *Axial T1 C+ FS MR shows a small enhancing tumor in the left ambient cistern ➡.* ***(23-24B)*** *Coronal T1 C+ FS MR in the same patient shows that the tumor ➡ lies along the expected course of CNIV. This was probable trochlear schwannoma.*

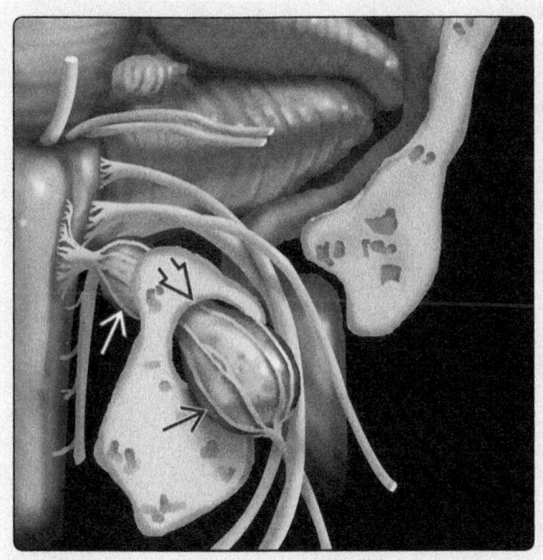

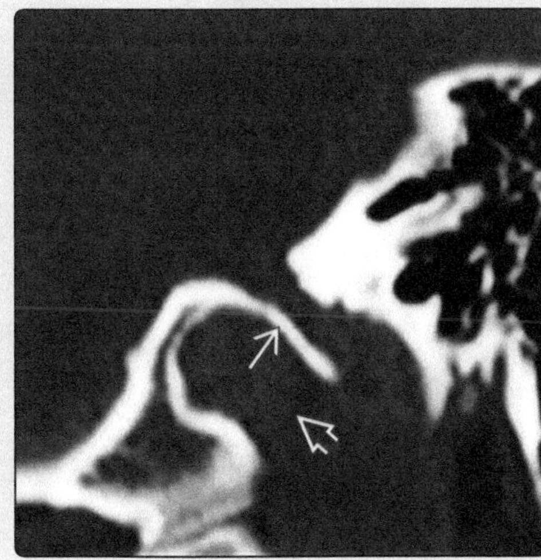

(23-25) *Graphic depicts hypoglossal schwannoma. CNXII schwannomas have a "dumbbell" shape with a cisternal segment ➡, relative constriction in the bony hypoglossal canal ➡, and a larger extracranial component ➡.* ***(23-26)*** *Coronal bone CT with hypoglossal schwannoma shows enlarged hypoglossal canal ➡ with thinning, remodeling of the jugular tubercle ➡ ("head" and "beak" of the "eagle").*

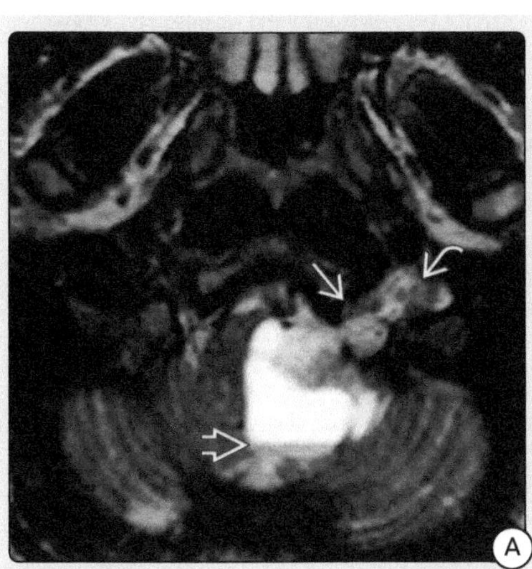

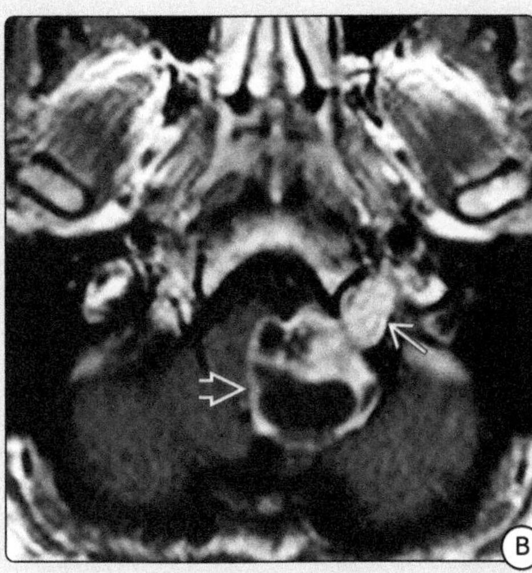

(23-27A) *Axial T2 FS MR in a patient with excruciating left arm pain shows a heterogeneously hyperintense posterior fossa mass with a large partially cystic intracranial component that exhibits a blood-fluid level ➡. Note extension through an enlarged hypoglossal canal ➡ into the high deep carotid space ➡.* ***(23-27B)*** *T1 C+ shows the partially cystic ➡, partially solid ➡ enhancing mass. This is "dumbbell" hypoglossal schwannoma.*

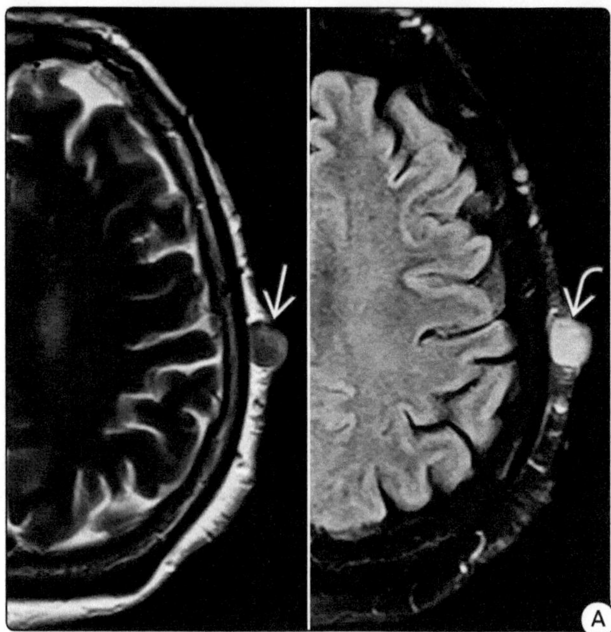

(23-28A) Axial T2 MR (L) in a 62-year-old woman with a solitary scalp neurofibroma ➡ shows that the well-demarcated mass extends from the calvarium to the skin surface. The neurofibroma is hyperintense on FLAIR ➡ (R).

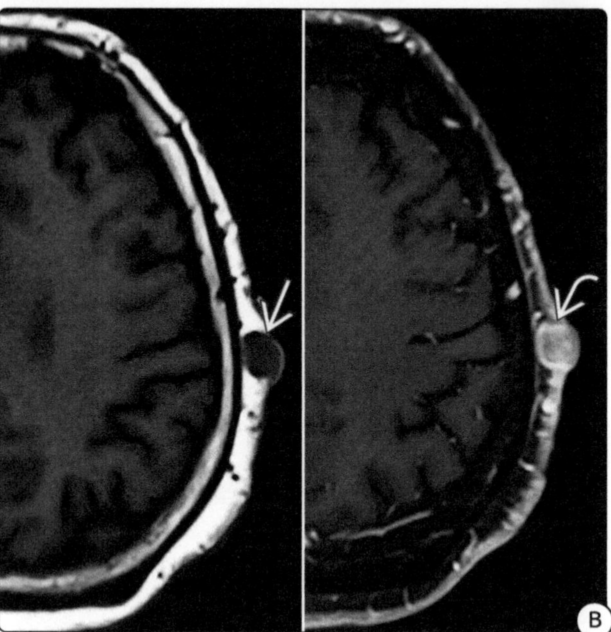

(23-28B) Axial precontrast T1 MR (L) compared to the postcontrast fat-saturated scan (R) shows that the lesion ➡ enhances strongly in a somewhat "target" fashion ➡.

both Schwann cells and fibroblasts. NFs can affect the scalp, skull, some cranial nerves (especially CNV1), or—rarely—the brain. They are found at all ages. Both sexes are affected equally.

The gross appearance of NFs is different from that of schwannomas. Schwannomas are well-delineated encapsulated lesions that arise eccentrically from their parent nerve. Schwannomas typically displace elements of the normal parent nerve to one side. In contrast, NFs generally present as more diffuse nerve expansions. They display single or multiple fascicles that enter and leave the affected nerve. Axons of the parent nerve pass through NFs and are intermixed with tumor cells, distinguishing them from schwannoma.

NFs can be solitary or multiple. Multiple NFs and plexiform NFs occur only in connection with neurofibromatosis type 1 (NF1).

Solitary Neurofibroma

A solitary NF in the head and neck rarely—if ever—involves cranial nerves. Solitary NFs affect patients of all ages and are usually sporadic (nonsyndromic). Most occur in the absence of NF1 and present as a painless scalp or skin mass.

Scalp solitary NFs are seen on imaging studies as well-delineated, focal, enhancing masses that abut but do not invade the calvarium **(23-28)**. Solitary NFs are WHO grade I neoplasms and do not undergo malignant degeneration.

Plexiform Neurofibroma

Terminology and Etiology

Plexiform NFs (PNFs) are infiltrative intra- and extraneural neoplasms that occur almost exclusively in patients with NF1 **(23-29)**. PNFs and NFs of major nerves are considered potential precursors of malignant peripheral nerve sheath tumors (MPNSTs).

Pathology

Cranial PNFs usually involve CNs V, IX, or X. The most typical locations are the scalp **(23-29)**, orbit, pterygopalatine fossa, and parotid gland. Scalp and orbital PNFs most commonly involve the ophthalmic branches of the trigeminal nerve. Parotid PNFs involve peripheral branches of the facial nerve.

PNFs are typically extensive, diffusely infiltrating lesions with a distinctive "bag of worms" appearance **(23-30)**. PNFs demonstrate a predominant intrafascicular growth pattern **(23-31)** with redundant loops of expanded nerve fascicles intermixed with collagen fibers and mucoid material. PNFs are WHO grade I neoplasms but 5% eventually degenerate into MPNSTs.

Imaging

PNFs are poorly delineated, worm-like masses that diffusely infiltrate and enlarge soft tissues, typically the scalp and periorbita. They are generally isodense with muscle on NECT. Calcification and hemorrhage are rare. CECT shows heterogeneous enhancement. Bone CT may show expansion of the superior orbital fissure and pterygopalatine fossa.

PNFs are isointense on T1WI and hyperintense on T2WI. Strong, sometimes heterogeneous enhancement is common **(23-32)**. A "target" sign of hypointensity within an enhancing tumor fascicle is seen in some PNFs but is not pathognomonic.

Differential Diagnosis

The major differential diagnosis of PNF is **malignant peripheral nerve sheath tumor (MPNST)**. If a previously quiescent PNF enlarges rapidly or becomes painful, malignant degeneration into MPNST should be suspected. Most MPNSTs are invasive as well as infiltrating lesions.

Schwannomas are well-circumscribed solitary lesions that involve CNs, especially CNVIII. In contrast to PNF, scalp and orbital schwannomas are uncommon. **Basal cell carcinoma** and infiltrating skin/scalp **metastases** without concomitant involvement of the underlying skull are rare.

NEUROFIBROMA

Solitary Neurofibroma
- Most are sporadic (nonsyndromic)
- All ages (children to adults)
- Nodular to polypoid
- Scalp, skin
- Rarely (if ever) involves cranial nerves

Plexiform Neurofibroma
- Pathology
  - Composed of Schwann cells + fibroblasts, mucoid material
  - Fusiform, infiltrates nerve
  - Often multicompartmental
  - Does not respect fascial boundaries
- Clinical issues
  - Usually diagnostic of NF1
  - "Sporadic" PNFs can occur without other signs of NF1, but most have *NF1* gene alterations
  - Risk of malignant degeneration in PNF = 5%
  - Rapid/painful enlargement, invasion? Suspect malignant peripheral nerve sheath tumor (MPNST)!
- Imaging
  - Multifocal scalp, orbit lesions most common
  - "Bag of worms" appearance
  - May enlarge superior orbital fissure, extend into CS
  - Intracranial involvement rare unless malignant degeneration
- Differential diagnosis
  - MPNST (invasive)
  - Schwannoma (usually solitary; skin/scalp lesions, plexiform schwannoma rare)
  - Metastases

Malignant Peripheral Nerve Sheath Tumor

Malignant Peripheral Nerve Sheath Tumor

A malignant peripheral nerve sheath tumor (MPNST) is any malignant tumor that arises from a peripheral nerve or shows nerve sheath differentiation.

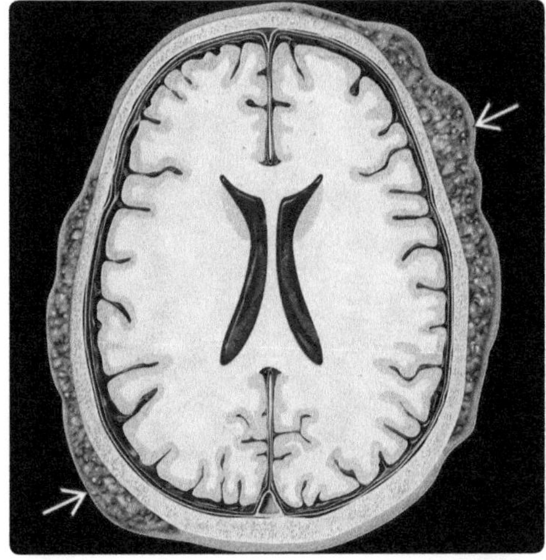

***(23-29)** Graphic depicts plexiform neurofibromas (PNFs) diffusely infiltrating and deforming the scalp ➡.*

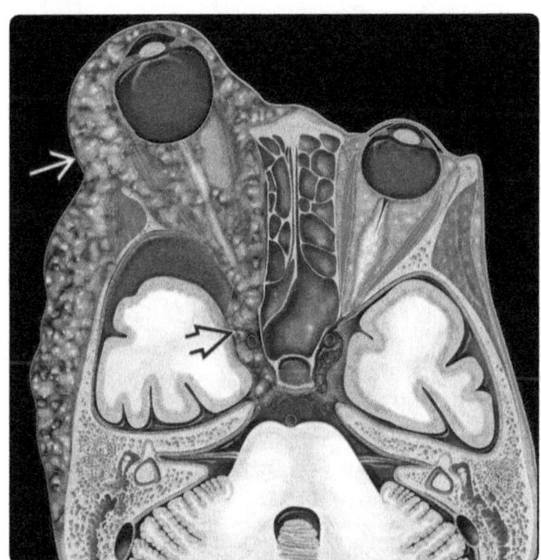

***(23-30)** Extensive PNF ➡ of the right face and orbit infiltrates cavernous sinus ⇨ in a patient with neurofibromatosis type 1 (NF1).*

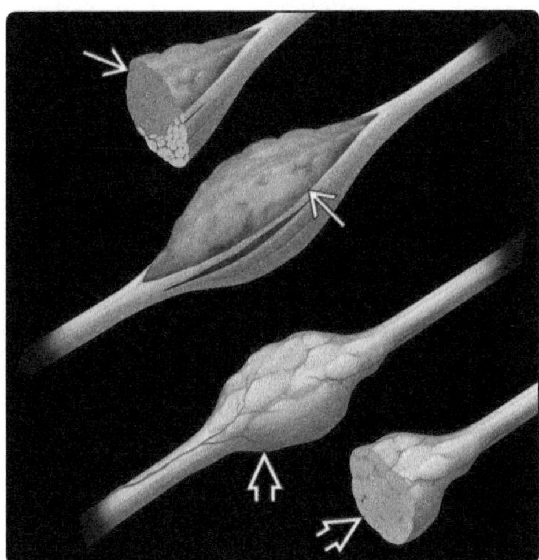

***(23-31)** Schwannomas ➡ displace nerve fascicles, whereas neurofibromas ⇨ infiltrate between fascicles.*

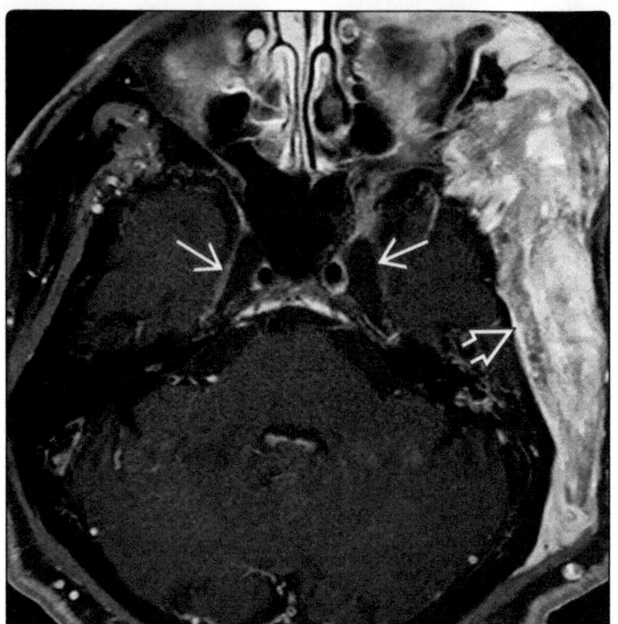

***(23-32)** T1 C+ FS MR in a patient with NF1 shows an extensively infiltrating plexiform neurofibroma of the scalp ➡ that enhances intensely but heterogeneously. Note patulous Meckel caves ➡, a finding of dural ectasia in some patients with NF1.*

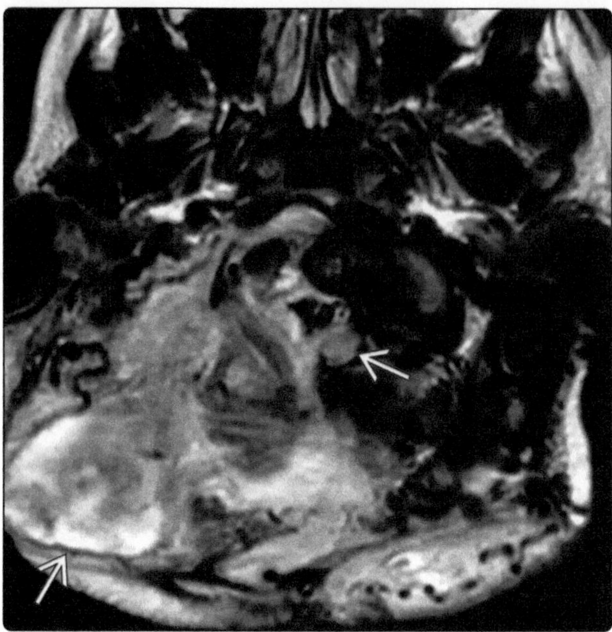

***(23-33)** T1 C+ in a patient with NF1 shows intensely but very heterogeneously enhancing mass ➡. Size, extent, and skull base invasion were significantly different from prior baseline studies. Malignant peripheral nerve sheath tumor was found at biopsy.*

Approximately 2/3 of *peripheral* MPNSTs are associated with malignant degeneration of tumors associated with NF1. The overall lifetime risk of developing an MPNST at any location in patients with NF1 is estimated at 8-13%.

MPNST is much more common in the peripheral or spinal nerves than in the cranial nerves. The most commonly affected cranial nerves are the vestibular, facial, and trigeminal nerves.

The 2016 WHO recognizes two histologic subtypes of MPNST: **Epithelioid MPNST** and **MPNST with perineurial differentiation**. There is no clinically validated and reproducible grading system for MPNSTs, so tumors are generally grouped into low-grade (15%) and high-grade lesions (85%).

There are no obvious characteristics that would differentiate MPNST from benign nerve sheath tumor on a single baseline imaging study. It is the behavior on *serial* imaging studies that helps distinguish MPNST from benign nerve sheath tumors. Aggressive growth with brain and bone invasion is typical **(23-33)**.

Other Nerve Sheath Tumors and Mimics

Intraneural **perineuriomas** account for just 1% of all nerve sheath tumors. Perineuriomas involving cranial nerves are very rare. **Neurofibrosarcomas** are more properly considered MPNSTs (either peripheral or intracranial).

Some nonneoplastic infiltrating disorders like **chronic interstitial demyelinating polyneuropathy (CIDP)** and **Charcot-Marie-Tooth disease** are benign conditions that rarely affect cranial nerves. When they do, diffuse enlargement and enhancement of one or more cranial nerves can be seen.

Selected References: The complete reference list is available on the Expert Consult™ eBook version included with purchase.

Lymphomas and Hematopoietic and Histiocytic Tumors

*This chapter focuses on hematopoietic tumors and tumor-like conditions. We begin with an increasingly common group of neoplasms, **lymphomas and related disorders**, then turn our attention briefly to **histiocytic tumors**, such as Langerhans cell histiocytosis.*

Plasma cell myeloma and **solitary plasmacytoma** affecting the skull and brain are usually secondary to extracranial disease, but they are a form of mature B-cell neoplasms and hence are included here rather than in Chapter 27 on metastases. We conclude the chapter with a brief discussion of **extramedullary hematopoiesis**—benign, nonneoplastic proliferations of blood-forming elements—which can appear virtually identical to malignant hematopoietic neoplasms.

Lymphomas and Related Disorders

The 2016 WHO divides primary CNS lymphoma into diffuse large B-cell lymphomas (DLBCLs) (> 95% of lesions), immunodeficiency-associated CNS lymphomas, intravascular large B-cell lymphoma, and a group of miscellaneous subtypes that includes T- and NK-/T-cell lymphomas as well as MALT lymphoma of the dura.

We begin this chapter by focusing on DLBCL. We then consider the fascinating spectrum of **immunodeficiency-associated CNS lymphomas** (including lymphomatoid granulomatosis and posttransplant lymphoproliferative disorder).

We follow with a discussion of **intravascular large B-cell lymphoma**, an uncommon but increasingly well-recognized cause of unexplained cognitive decline in elderly patients. Uncommon primary CNS lymphomas, such as MALT lymphoma of the dura, are then briefly discussed. We close the section with a brief review of CNS metastatic lymphoma.

Diffuse Large B-Cell Lymphoma of the CNS

Terminology

Diffuse large B-cell lymphoma (DLBCL) of the CNS is an extranodal B-cell lymphoma that arises exclusively inside the CNS. The vast majority of primary CNS lymphomas (PCNSLs) are DLBCLs. For purposes of discussion, in this text, the terms PCNSL and DLBCL are used interchangeably.

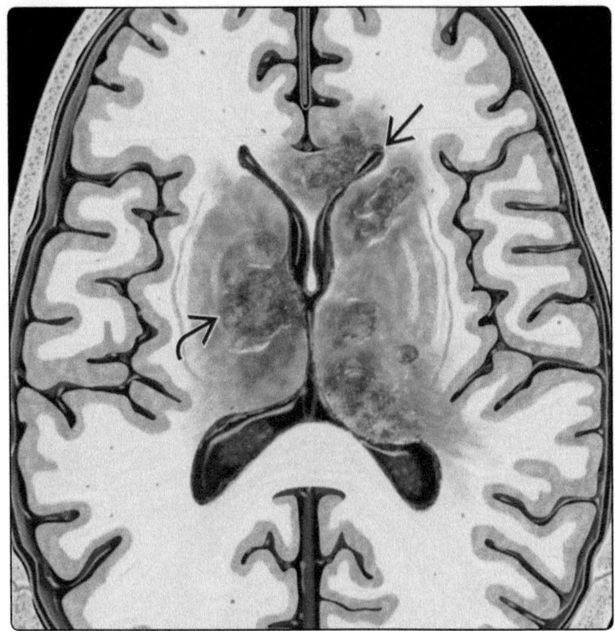

***(24-1)** This is primary CNS lymphoma (PCNSL). Periventricular lesions ➔ are in basal ganglia (BG), thalamus, corpus callosum with extensive subependymal spread of disease ➔.*

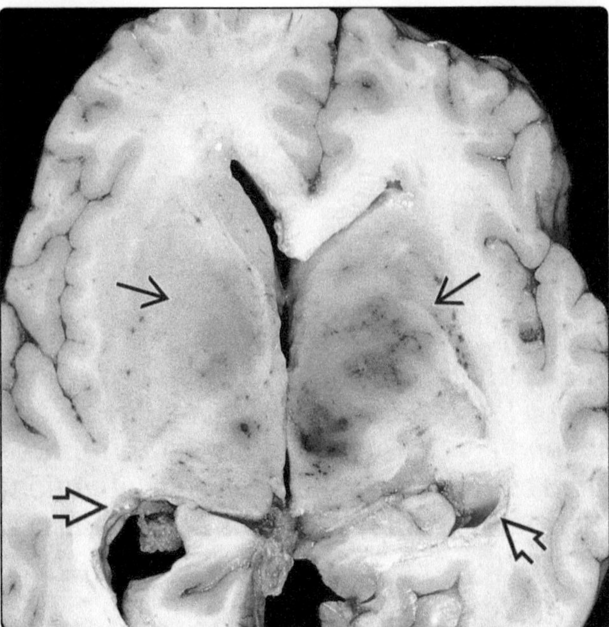

***(24-2)** Autopsy shows PCNSL with bilateral deep basal ganglionic, thalamic masses ➔, ependymal spread ➔. (Courtesy R. Hewlett, MD.)*

> **2016 WHO CLASSIFICATION OF PRIMARY CNS LYMPHOMAS**
>
> **Diffuse Large B-Cell Lymphoma of the CNS**
>
> **Immunodeficiency-Associated CNS Lymphomas**
> - AIDS-related diffuse large B-cell lymphoma
> - Epstein-Barr virus-positive diffuse large B-cell lymphoma, NOS
> - Lymphomatoid granulomatosis
> - Posttransplant lymphoproliferative disorder
>
> **Intravascular Large B-Cell Lymphoma**
>
> **Miscellaneous Rare CNS Lymphomas**
> - Low-grade B-cell lymphomas
> - T-cell and NK-/T-cell lymphoma
> - Anaplastic large cell lymphoma
>
> **MALT Lymphoma of Dura**

Etiology

The brain parenchyma normally contains very few lymphocytes. So how and why lymphomas arise as primary CNS neoplasms in immunocompetent individuals is unknown. To date, no genetic predispositions to PCNSL have been identified.

What is clear is that lymphoma cells—regardless of whether they originate within or outside the brain—exhibit a distinct, highly selective neurotropism for the CNS microenvironment and its vasculature. Intra- and perivascular tumor spread is common.

Pathology

Location. DLBCL can affect any part of the neuraxis. Up to 75% all PCNSLs contact a CSF surface, either the ventricular ependyma or pia **(24-1)**. Lesions are often deep seated with a predilection for the periventricular white matter, especially the corpus callosum **(24-4)**. The basal ganglia and thalami are the next most common locations **(24-2)**.

The hypothalamus, infundibulum, and pituitary gland are less common sites. Primary DLBCL may also develop in the leptomeninges, calvarial vault, and central skull base, although these areas are more commonly involved by metastatic spread from extracranial primary tumors.

Gross Pathology. DLBCL lesions vary in size from microscopic implants to large bulky masses. Up to 2/3 are solitary lesions.

Single or multiple hemispheric masses that appear relatively well demarcated rather than diffusely infiltrating lesions is typical. Large confluent areas of frank necrosis and gross intratumoral hemorrhage are more common in AIDS-related PCNSLs **(24-5)**.

Rarely, DLBCL diffusely infiltrates the brain, involving both gray and white matter structures. So-called "lymphomatosis cerebri," like "gliomatosis cerebri," is an anatomic pattern, not a distinct disease entity.

Microscopic Features. PCNSLs are highly cellular tumors. MIB-1 is high, often exceeding 50% (significantly higher than with glioblastoma). The WHO does not assign a grade to PCNSL.

PCNSL: ETIOLOGY AND PATHOLOGY

Etiology

- CNS lacks lymphatics, normally contains few lymphocytes
- Precise origin in immunocompetent individuals unknown

Pathology

- 3-6% of all primary CNS neoplasms
- Vast majority (90-95%) are DLBCLs
  - Large atypical cells
  - CD20(+), CD45(+)
  - MIB-1 > 50%
- Predilection for deep brain
  - Periventricular white matter, basal ganglia
  - Perivascular lymphoid clusters also common
- Solitary (2/3), multiple (1/3)
  - Multiple compartments may be involved
- Focal > > diffusely infiltrating lesions (lymphomatosis cerebri)
- Hemorrhage, necrosis rare in immunocompetent patients
- "Sentinel" demyelinating lesion indistinguishable from MS or ADEM can precede PCNSL!
- Corticosteroids → ↑ apoptosis, can obscure diagnosis of PCNSL!

Clinical Issues

Although PCNSLs account for only 3% of all malignant CNS neoplasms, worldwide prevalence is increasing as a result of the HIV/AIDS epidemic and the use of immunosuppressive therapies. PCNSLs are generally tumors of middle-aged and older adults. Peak age (in immunocompetent patients) is 60 years.

Most patients present with focal neurologic deficits, altered mental status, and neuropsychiatric disturbances. Seizures are less common than in patients with other primary brain tumors.

CNS DLBCL is an aggressive tumor with a median survival of only a few months in untreated patients. In general, immunocompetent patients younger than 60 years fare slightly better than older patients and patients with acquired immunodeficiency syndromes.

Early diagnosis is crucial for proper management of PCNSLs. Stereotactic biopsy is typically performed for diagnostic confirmation and histologic tumor typing. Treatment options include corticosteroids, high-dose methotrexate-based polychemotherapy, and radiation.

Approximately 70% of patients initially respond to treatment, but relapse is very common. Progression-free survival is approximately one year, and overall survival is approximately three years. Only 20-40% of patients experience prolonged progression-free survival.

Imaging

General Features. Contrast-enhanced cranial MR is the modality of choice in evaluating patients with suspected PCNSL. Contrast-enhanced CT of the chest, abdomen, and pelvis or PET/CT is generally recommended in patients with suspected PCNSL to look for an extracranial source of disease. Occult systemic lymphomas are found in 5-8% of patients with putative PCNSL.

CT Findings. All PCNSLs are highly cellular tumors. White matter or basal ganglia lesions in contact with a CSF surface are typical. Most lesions appear hyperdense compared with normal brain on NECT scans **(24-3A)**. Marked peritumoral edema is common, but gross necrosis, hemorrhage, and

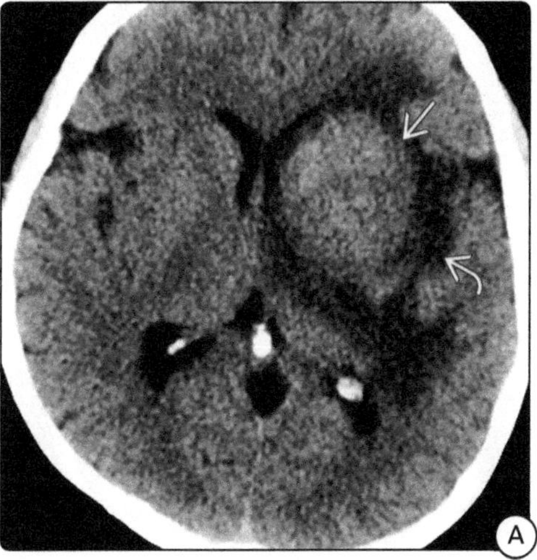

***(24-3A)** NECT in a 63-year-old woman with right-sided weakness shows a solitary hyperdense mass ➡ in the left BG with moderate edema ➡.*

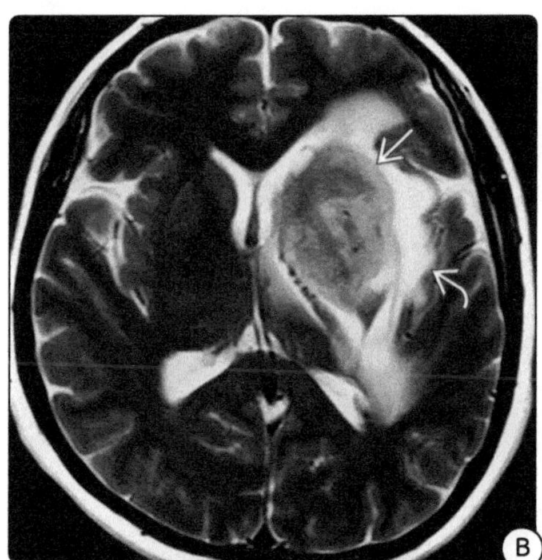

***(24-3B)** T2 MR shows mass ➡ is mixed iso- to hypointense relative to cortex. Moderate amount of hyperintense peripheral edema ➡ is present.*

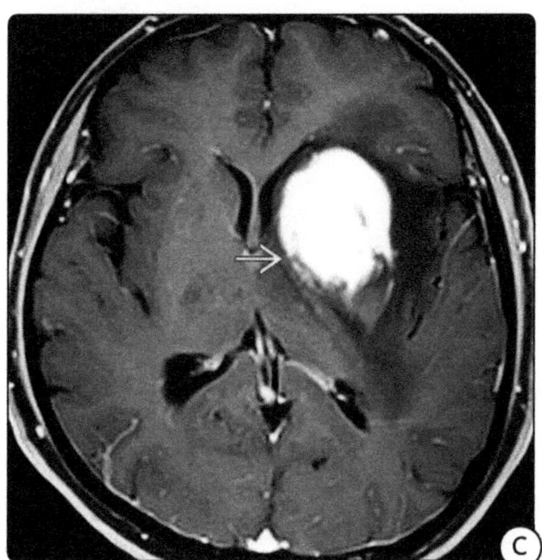

***(24-3C)** T1 C+ FS MR shows that the mass ➡ enhances intensely and uniformly. DLBCL was found at surgery.*

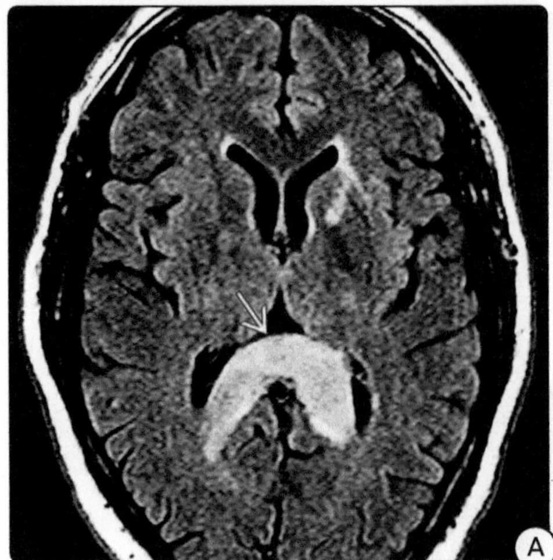

(24-4A) FLAIR MR in a patient with primary large B-cell lymphoma shows a hyperintense mass in the corpus callosum splenium ➡.

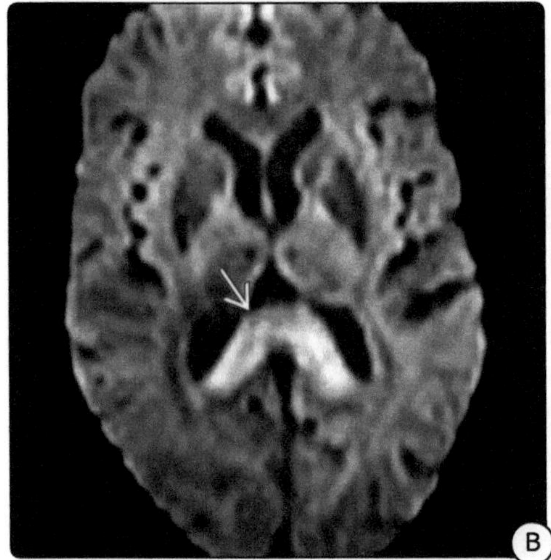

(24-4B) DWI MR shows diffusion restriction ➡ characteristic of a densely cellular mass.

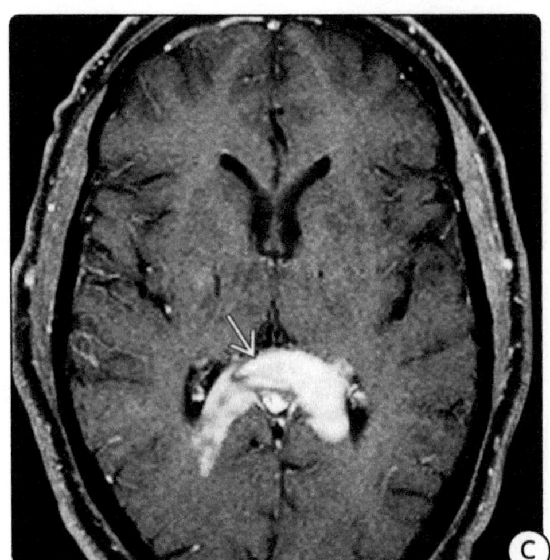

(24-4C) T1 C+ FS MR in the same patient shows that the mass ➡ enhances strongly, mostly uniformly.

calcification are rare (2-5%) unless the patient is immunocompromised **(24-6A)**.

DLBCLs in immunocompetent patients show mild to moderate, relatively homogeneous enhancement on CECT. Irregular ring enhancement is rare unless the patient is immunocompromised.

MR Findings. Over 3/4 of DLBCLs in **immunocompetent** patients are iso- or slightly hypointense compared with gray matter on T1WI and isointense on T2WI.

FLAIR signal is variable but usually iso- or hyperintense **(24-4A)**. Microhemorrhages with intratumoral "blooming" on T2* are present in 5-8% of cases, but gross hemorrhage is uncommon unless the patient is immunocompromised.

Nearly all PCNSLs in immunocompetent patients enhance **(24-4C)**. Solid homogeneous **(24-3C)** or mildly heterogeneous enhancement **(24-4C)** is common; ring enhancement is rare. MRS typically demonstrates elevated choline and high lipids.

Because of their high cellularity, over 95% of PCNSLs show mild to moderate diffusion restriction with low ADC values **(24-4B)**. MRS is nonspecific with elevated choline, reduced NAA and myoinositol, and prominent lipids. Tumor neovascularization is absent in PCNSLs; therefore, rCBV is relatively low, and permeability is not increased on DCE pMR even though the tumor is highly malignant.

Lymphomatosis cerebri mimics diffuse white matter disease with confluent T2/FLAIR hyperintensities. Enhancement can be subtle, patchy, or even absent.

Steroid administration significantly alters the imaging findings of PCNSLs. Cell lysis with tumor regression and normalization of the blood-brain barrier occurs in 40-85% of patients with **corticosteroid-treated PCNSLs**. Tumors typically diminish in size. Contrast enhancement also decreases or even disappears completely ("ghost tumor"), although some T2 and FLAIR signal abnormalities may persist.

Differential Diagnosis

The major differential diagnosis of PCNSL is **glioblastoma** (GBM). Although both tumors often cross the corpus callosum, hemorrhage and necrosis are rare in PCNSL. Enhancement in immunocompetent patients with PCNSL is strong and relatively homogeneous, whereas a peripheral ring pattern is more typical of GBM. Advanced MR techniques, such as DWI, MRS, and DCE pMR are helpful in distinguishing PCNSLs from other highly aggressive primary brain tumors.

The second most common differential diagnosis of PCNSL is **metastasis**. Dura-based PCNSLs may resemble **meningioma** or—due to their hyperdensity—even look like an acute epi- or subdural hematoma.

In the setting of solid organ or hematopoietic stem cell transplants, **lymphomatoid granulomatosis** and **posttransplant lymphoproliferative disorder** (PTLD) may closely resemble PCNSL. Biopsy is necessary for confirmation and patient management.

PCNSL: IMAGING AND DDx IN IMMUNOCOMPETENT PATIENTS

General Features
- Periventricular white matter, basal ganglia common sites
  - 95% contact a CSF surface
- Cautions
  - Findings vary with immune status
  - Steroids may mask/↓ imaging findings!

CT
- Hyperdense on NECT
- Hemorrhage, necrosis rare

MR
- Generally isointense with gray matter on T1-, T2WI
- Petechial hemorrhage in immunocompetent patients
- Gross hemorrhage, necrosis rare
- Strong, relatively uniform enhancement
- Often restricts on DWI
- Lymphomatosis cerebri
  - Mimics diffuse white matter disease with T2/FLAIR confluent hyperintensity
  - Enhancement can be subtle or patchy, occasionally absent

Differential Diagnosis
- Glioblastoma, metastasis
- Lymphomatosis cerebri
  - Microvascular disease
  - Encephalitis (infectious, inflammatory, autoimmune)
  - Toxic-metabolic disorders
  - Diffusely infiltrating glioma

Immunodeficiency-Associated CNS Lymphomas

Lymphomas associated with either inherited or acquired immunodeficiency are grouped together as immunodeficiency-associated CNS lymphomas. The immunodeficiency-associated CNS lymphomas include **AIDS-related diffuse large B-cell lymphoma, Epstein-Barr virus (EBV)-positive DLBCL** in elderly patients with no known immunodeficiency, **lymphomatoid granulomatosis**, and **posttransplant lymphoproliferative disorders**.

PCNSLs associated with **EBV** account for 10-15% of all cases. Congenital immunodeficiency syndromes increase the risk of lymphoma, as do severe acquired immunosuppression and autoimmune diseases.

AIDS-Related Diffuse Large B-Cell Lymphoma

Although HIV-associated PCNSL has become rarer with the introduction of highly active antiretroviral therapy (HAART), between 2% and 12% of HIV/AIDS patients eventually develop CNS lymphoma, generally during the later stages of their disease.

Pathology

Multiple lesions are common, as are larger, more confluent necrotic areas and intratumoral hemorrhages **(24-5)**.

Clinical Issues

Mean age at onset in HIV/AIDS patients is 40 years, two decades younger than immunocompetent patients. Lymphomas in transplant recipients occur

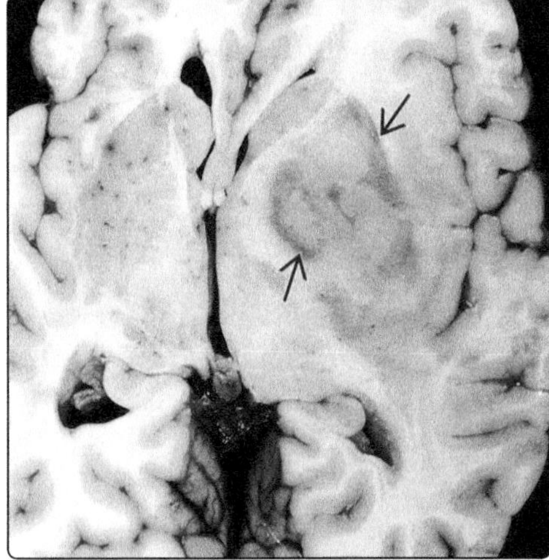

***(24-5)** Autopsy of PCNSL in HIV/AIDS shows hemorrhagic, necrotic left BG mass ➡. (Courtesy R. Hewlett, MD.)*

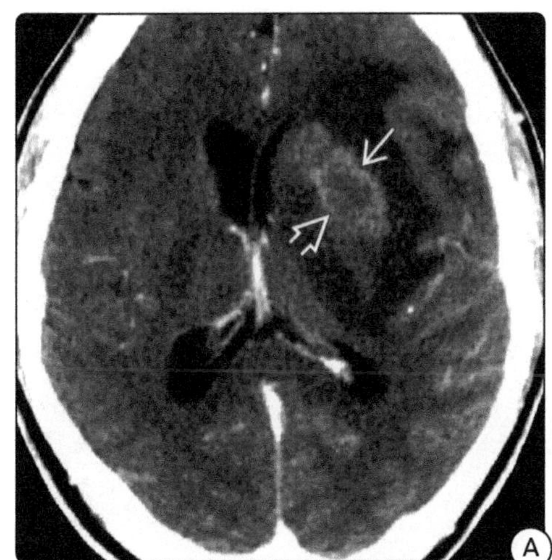

***(24-6A)** CECT scan shows necrosis ➡ and only faint rim enhancement ➡ in this HIV-positive patient with PCNSL.*

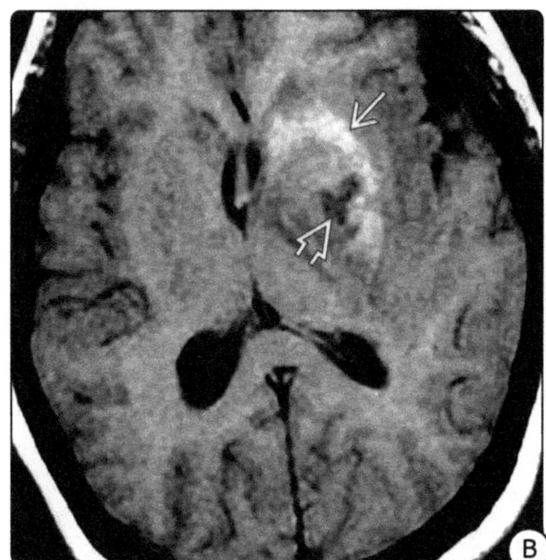

***(24-6B)** T1 MR shows T1 shortening due to subacute hemorrhage ➡ with more acute hemorrhage in the necrotic core of the lesion ➡.*

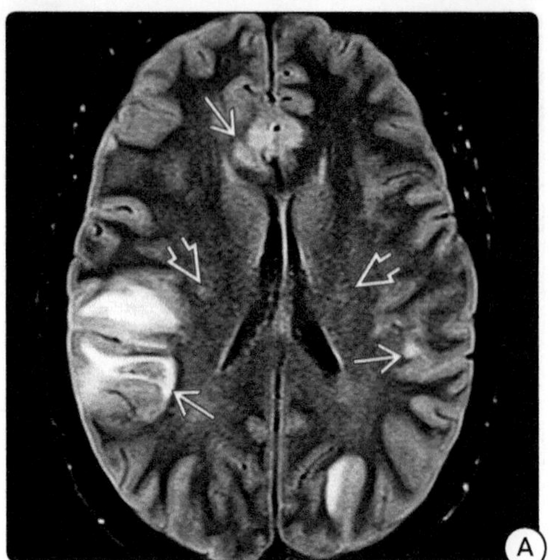

(24-7A) *FLAIR MR in a patient with confusion, altered mental status shows multiple subcortical ➡, deep ➡ white matter (WM) hyperintensities.*

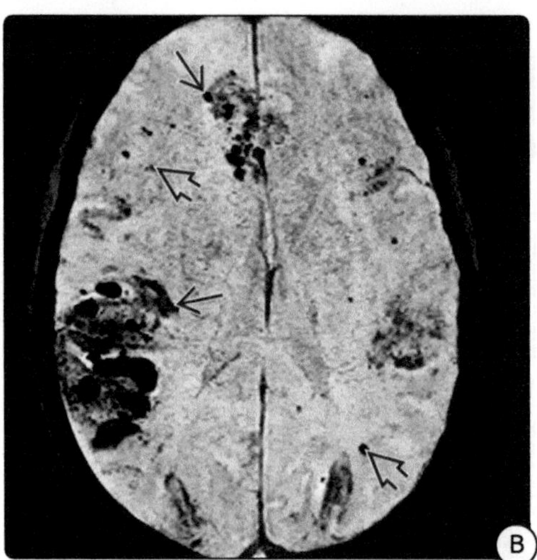

(24-7B) *T2* SWI MIP shows multifocal petechial WM ➡ confluent cortical/subcortical hemorrhages ➡. Biopsy disclosed IVL.*

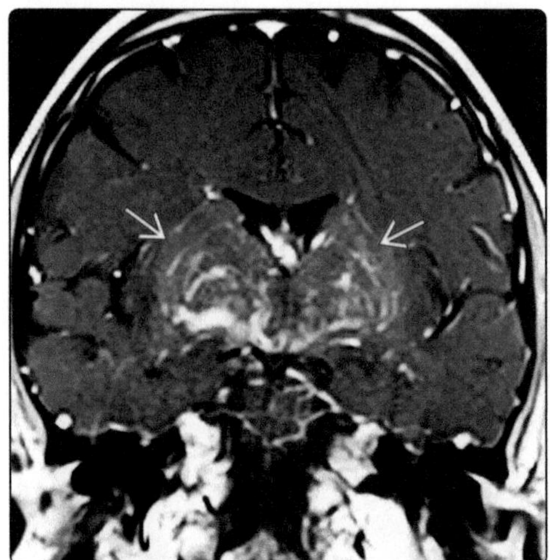
(24-8) *Coronal T1 C+ MR shows prominent curvilinear enhancement following penetrating arteries ➡. Intravascular DLBCL found at biopsy.*

even earlier, generally between the ages of 35 and 40 years. Mean age of onset in children with inherited immunodeficiencies is 10 years.

Imaging

Multiple lesions are common, as are more frequent and larger confluent areas of necrosis **(24-6A)**. Intratumor hemorrhage with T1 shortening **(24-6B)** and "blooming" on T2* scans is common. Enhancement is variable but often mild. Ring enhancement surrounding a nonenhancing core of necrotic tissue is typical.

Differential Diagnosis

In immunocompromised patients, the major differential diagnosis of PCNSL is **toxoplasmosis**. *A solitary ring-enhancing lesion in an HIV/AIDS patient is most often lymphoma,* whereas multiple lesions are more characteristic of toxoplasmosis. An "eccentric target" sign is suggestive of toxoplasmosis, although necrotic lymphomas occasionally show an enhancing "ring with a nodule" pattern.

Intravascular (Angiocentric) Lymphoma

Intravascular lymphoma (IVL) is a rare subtype of DLBCL characterized by proliferating malignant cells within small and medium-sized vessels. Although it can involve any organ, IVL typically affects the skin and the CNS.

Terminology

IVL is also called angiocentric or angioendotheliotropic lymphoma, angiotropic large cell lymphoma, endovascular lymphoma, and malignant angioendotheliomatosis.

Etiology

IVL is an aggressive malignant lymphoma that usually arises from B cells. T cells or NK cells may occasionally be the cell of origin. A possible association of IVL (especially the NK type) with EBV has been reported.

Pathology

The gross macroscopic appearance varies from normal to small multifocal infarcts of varying ages scattered throughout the cortex and subcortical white matter. Focal cerebral masses are rare. Petechial microhemorrhages may be present and are more common than confluent macroscopic bleeds.

At histologic examination, markedly atypical cells with large round nuclei and prominent nucleoli are found in small and medium-sized vessels. Extension into the adjacent perivascular spaces is minimal or absent. CD20 staining is helpful in identifying tumor cells, especially when they are sparse and widely scattered.

Clinical Issues

Epidemiology. IVL is rare. CNS involvement occurs in 75-85% of patients.

Demographics. IVL is typically a tumor of middle-aged and elderly patients. Mean age at presentation is 60-65 years.

Presentation. Sensory and motor deficits, neuropathies, and multiple stroke-like episodes are common symptoms. Some patients present with progressive neurologic deterioration and cognitive decline characterized by confusion and memory loss. Skin changes with elevated plaques or nodules are present in 1/2 of all cases.

Natural History. Outcome is generally poor. By the time of initial presentation, most patients have advanced disseminated disease. IVL is a relentless, rapidly progressive disease with a high mortality rate. Mean survival is 7-12 months.

Treatment Options. Because IVL is a widely disseminated disease, systemic chemotherapy is the recommended treatment. High-dose chemotherapy with autologous stem cell transplantation is often used in younger patients.

Imaging

There are no pathognomonic neuroimaging findings for IVL. Ischemic foci with infarct-like lesions are the most common imaging finding. CT may be normal or nonspecific, demonstrating only scattered white matter hypodensities. MR shows multiple T2/FLAIR hyperintensities **(24-7A)**. Both macro- and microhemorrhages are common, so "blooming" foci on T2* (GRE, SWI) are often present **(24-7B)**. Linear/punctate enhancement oriented along penetrating arteries and perivascular spaces is suggestive of IVL **(24-8)**. Multifocal areas of diffusion restriction may be present.

Differential Diagnosis

IVL is a "great imitator," both clinically and on imaging studies. Stereotactic biopsy is thus necessary to establish the definitive diagnosis. **Vasculitis** with punctate and linear enhancing foci may be virtually indistinguishable from IVL on imaging studies alone.

PCNSL, especially in the setting of immunodeficiency syndromes, may mimic IVL. IVL is most often multifocal, whereas 2/3 of PCNSLs are solitary lesions. Diffuse multifocal PCNSL, especially when it occurs in the form of **lymphomatosis cerebri**, may be difficult to distinguish from IVL. Lymphomatosis cerebri often shows little or no enhancement.

Rapidly progressive leukoencephalopathy with confluent nonenhancing white matter lesions is a rare presentation of diffusely infiltrating CNS IVL and may mimic a cerebral **demyelinating disorder**.

Diffuse **subacute viral encephalitis** can likewise mimic IVL, especially on biopsy. Parenchymal **neurosarcoid** with perivascular nodular spread may also resemble IVL on imaging studies.

INTRAVASCULAR (ANGIOCENTRIC) LYMPHOMA

Pathology
- Small/medium-sized vessels filled with tumor
- Little/no parenchymal tumor; focal masses rare
- Microhemorrhages common
- Multifocal infarcts

Clinical Issues
- Older patients with dementia, cognitive decline, TIAs
- Skin lesions (50%)

Imaging
- Multifocal T2/FLAIR hyperintensities
- Punctate hemorrhages on T2* (SWI > GRE)
- Foci of restricted diffusion
- Linear/punctate enhancement

Common Differential Diagnoses
- PCNSL
- Vasculitis

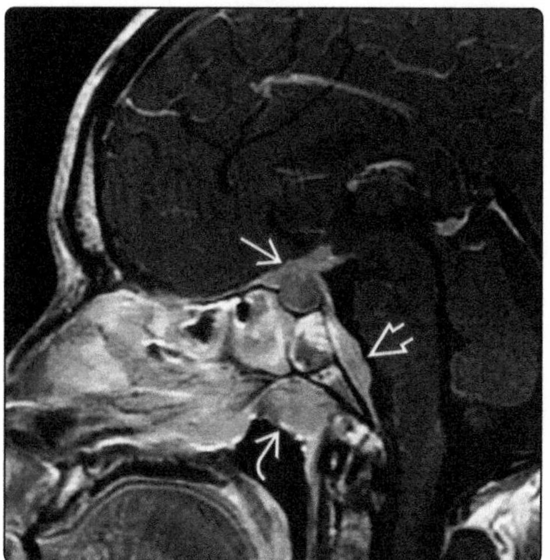

***(24-9)** T1 C+ MR of extranodal NK-/T-cell lymphoma shows nasopharyngeal ➡, clivus mass ➡ involving pituitary gland and stalk ➡.*

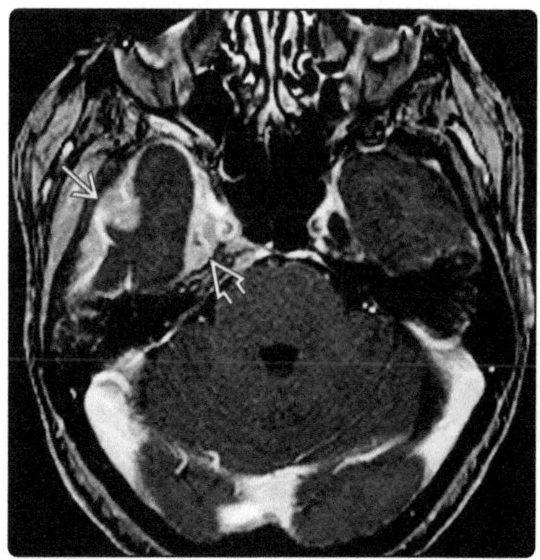

***(24-10)** T1 C+ FS in 67y woman with right CNVI palsy shows dural-based mass in right middle fossa ➡, cavernous sinus ➡. MALT lymphoma.*

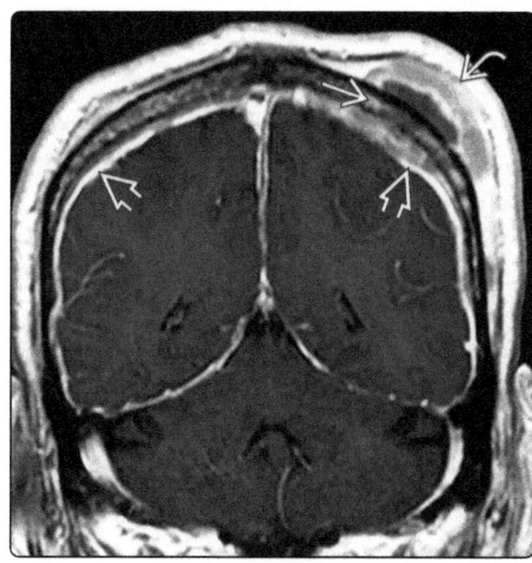

***(24-11)** T1 C+ MR shows systemic large B-cell lymphoma metastatic to skull ➡, scalp ➡, and dura ➡.*

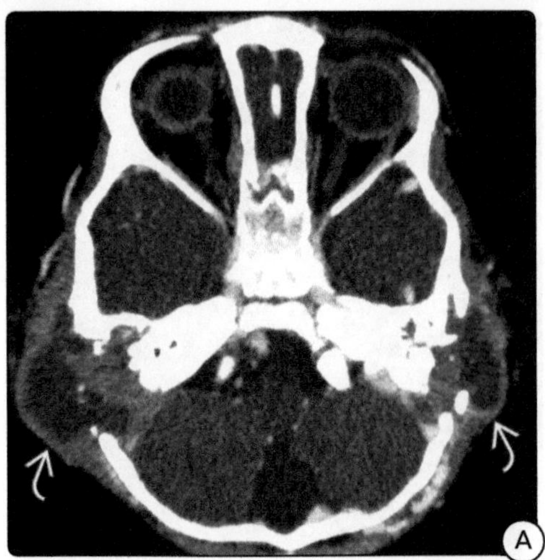

***(24-12A)** CECT in 15-month-old girl with mastoid region swelling, central DI, and ataxia shows bilateral destructive temporal bone masses ➡.*

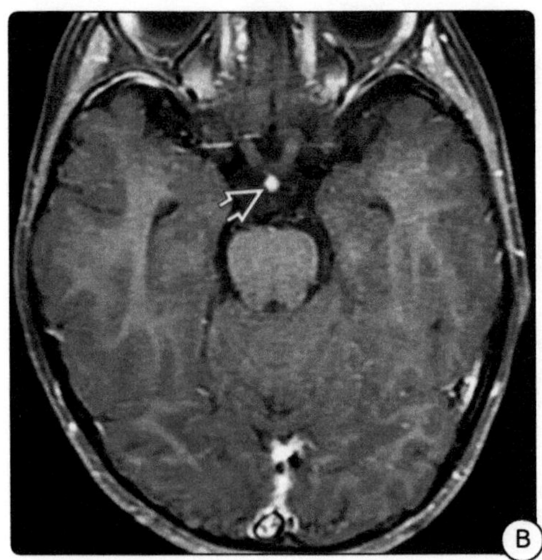

***(24-12B)** Axial T1 C+ FS MR in the same case demonstrates a thickened, enhancing infundibular stalk ➡.*

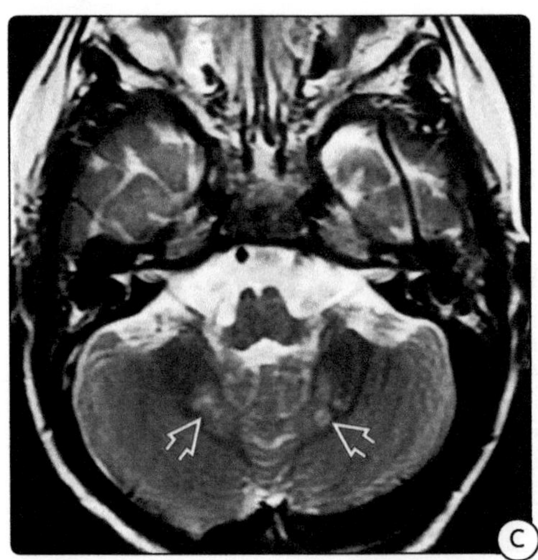

***(24-12C)** T2 MR shows dentate hyperintensities ➡ representing autoimmune-mediated demyelination. Langerhans cell histiocytosis.*

Miscellaneous Rare CNS Lymphomas

Other than DLBCL, primary CNS lymphomas are rare.

Low-grade lymphomas, most of which are B cell, account for ~ 3% of all CNS lymphomas and almost exclusively affect immunocompetent adults. **Primary CNS T-cell lymphomas (TCLs) and NKTCLs** are very rare, accounting for ~ 2% of all PCNSLs **(24-9)**. Most reported cases are associated with prior EBV infection. Imaging findings are generally indistinguishable from parenchymal DLBCL.

MALT Lymphoma of the Dura

Extranodal marginal zone lymphomas of mucosa-associated lymphoid tissue (MALT lymphomas) in the head and neck are most often ocular adnexal tumors, occurring in the conjunctiva, lacrimal glands, orbit, and eyelids. The cranial meninges, especially the dura, are occasional intracranial sites. Diffuse dura-arachnoid thickening with one or more meningioma-like masses is the most typical imaging finding **(24-10)**. Parenchymal lesions are rare. Prognosis is excellent with a 5-year survival rate of 85%.

Metastatic Intracranial Lymphoma

Metastatic intracranial lymphoma is also called secondary CNS lymphoma (SCNSL). Between 3-5% of patients with diffuse large B-cell systemic lymphomas eventually develop CNS involvement.

Metastatic lymphoma rarely presents as a parenchymal mass. In contrast with PCNSL, skull and dural involvement is much more frequent. Both calvarial vault and skull base metastases are common.

Calvarial lesions often involve the adjacent scalp and epidural space **(24-11)**. Dural "tails" are common. Involvement of the leptomeninges and underlying brain parenchyma may occur as late complications. Parenchymal lesions in the absence of skull and dural disease are uncommon. Leptomeningeal and CSF spread with cranial nerve, choroid plexus, and spine "drop" metastases occur but are rare.

Histiocytic Tumors

Histiocytic CNS neoplasms are a heterogeneous group of tumors that are histologically and immunologically identical to their extracranial counterparts.

The 2016 WHO classification recognizes five histiocytic tumors that affect the CNS: **Langerhans cell histiocytosis (LCH), Erdheim-Chester disease, Rosai-Dorfman disease (RDD), juvenile xanthogranuloma**, and **histiocytic sarcoma**. We discuss the most common of these, LCH and RDD, in this chapter.

Langerhans Cell Histiocytosis

LCH is a clonal neoplastic proliferation of immature, partially activated dendritic Langerhans cells. Between 50% and 60% of patients with LCH have *BRAF* V600E mutations, but the RAF-MEK-ERK pathway is activated in all patients. *MAP2K1*, which encodes MEK1, is mutated in 25% of cases.

LCH is now classified on the basis of disease extent as unifocal, multifocal (usually polyostotic), and disseminated disease. Most cases with isolated lesions present in young children under 2 years of age. Multifocal disease onset is generally between 2 and 5 years of age.

Geographic destructive bone lesions with "beveled edges" are the most common manifestation of LCH (80-95% of cases). The craniofacial bones and skull base are the most commonly affected sites (55%) **(24-12A)**. Half of LCH cases affect the hypothalamic-pituitary region, often with absence of the posterior pituitary "bright spot" and a thickened, enhancing nontapering infundibular stalk **(24-12B)**. Nearly 1/3 of cases involve the cranial meninges.

Approximately 1/3 of patients exhibit parenchymal lesions. A leukoencephalopathy-like pattern, often with degenerative changes in the dentate nuclei &/or basal ganglia, occurs in nearly 1/3 of all LCH cases **(24-12C)**.

LCH: IMAGING

CT
- > 50% have lytic craniofacial lesion(s)
- "Beveled" lesion > geographic destruction

MR
- Soft tissue mass adjacent to bone lesion
- Hypothalamus/pituitary stalk
  - Absent posterior pituitary "bright spot"
  - Thickened (> 3 mm), nontapering stalk
- Enhancing lesions
  - Dura-based mass(es)
  - Choroid plexus
  - Punctate/linear parenchymal enhancing foci
- Nontumorous degenerative changes
  - Symmetric T2/FLAIR hyperintensity in cerebellum/dentate nuclei, basal ganglia

Rosai-Dorfman Disease

Rosai-Dorfman disease (RDD), also called sinus histiocytosis with massive lymphadenopathy, is a rare benign histioproliferative disorder of unknown etiology. It is defined histopathologically by the accumulation of CD68-positive, S100-positive, and CDE1a-negative proliferating histiocytes with intact, mature hematolymphoid cells floating freely within their cytoplasm ("emperipolesis"). A prominent lymphoplasmacytic infiltrate is also frequently present within the tumor mass.

RDD can occur at any age, but almost 80% of patients are younger than 20 years old at the time of initial diagnosis. Bilateral massive but painless cervical lymphadenopathy is the most common presentation. CNS involvement is rare and generally occurs *without* cervical adenopathy or other extranodal involvement.

RDD has a protean imaging appearance but most frequently presents as bilateral cervical lymphadenopathy. Extranodal involvement is seen in 50% of cases. The skin, nose, sinuses, and orbit (especially the eyelids and lacrimal glands) are often affected.

Intracranial RDD occurs in 5% of cases. Solitary or multiple dura-based masses that are isointense with gray matter on T1WI **(24-13A)** and slightly hypointense on T2WI **(24-13B)** are typical. Intense homogeneous enhancement occurs following contrast administration **(24-13C)**. Less commonly, multiple cranial and peripheral enhancing nerves can be identified. Sellar/suprasellar and intraspinal lesions are even less common. They can be isolated or occur in concert with more typical dura-based &/or orbital lesions.

The major imaging differential diagnosis of *intra*cranial RDD is **meningioma**. **Neurosarcoid** with dura-based and sellar/suprasellar involvement can mimic

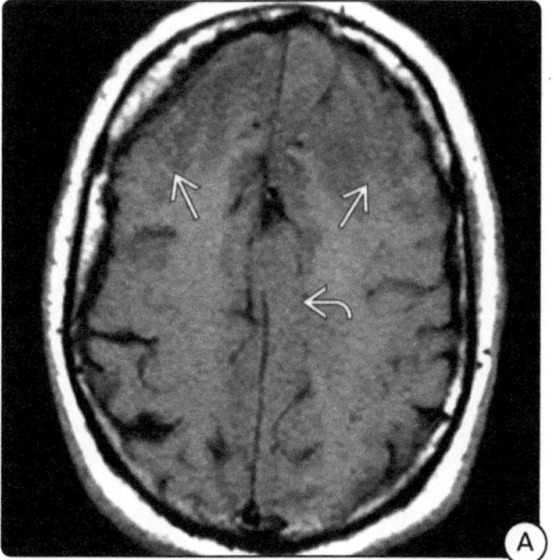

***(24-13A)** T1 MR shows effaced sulci and GM-WM interfaces in both frontal lobes ➡ and along the interhemispheric fissure ⮌.*

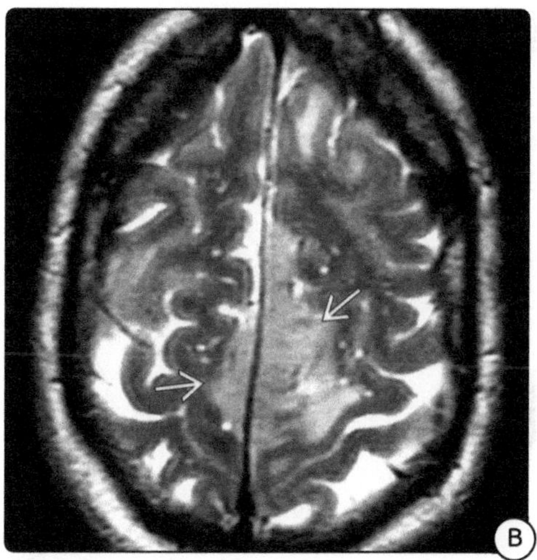

***(24-13B)** T2 MR shows lobulated parafalcine masses ➡ that are iso- to slightly hyperintense relative to cortex.*

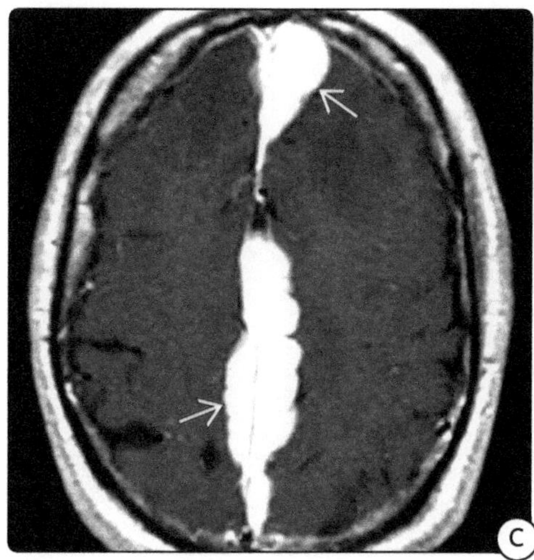

***(24-13C)** T1 C+ MR shows lobulated intensely enhancing parafalcine masses ➡. Rosai-Dorfman disease diagnosed by cervical lymph node biopsy.*

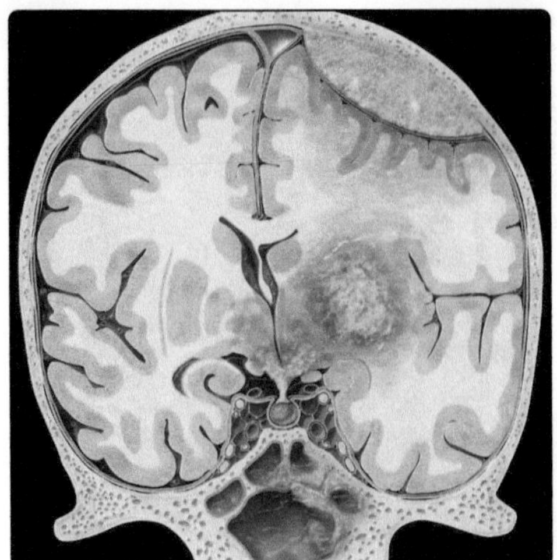

***(24-14)** Graphic depicts CNS leukemia with skull, dura, sinus, parenchymal, and juxtasellar disease.*

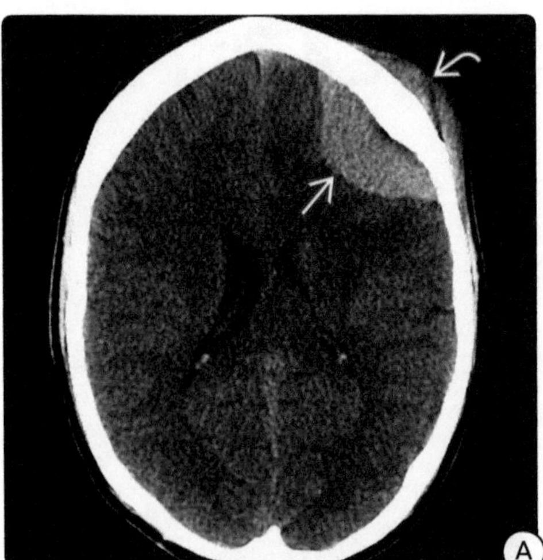

***(24-15A)** NECT in a 28-year-old man with AML and a scalp "lump" shows left frontal subgaleal ➡ and hyperdense extraaxial mass ➡.*

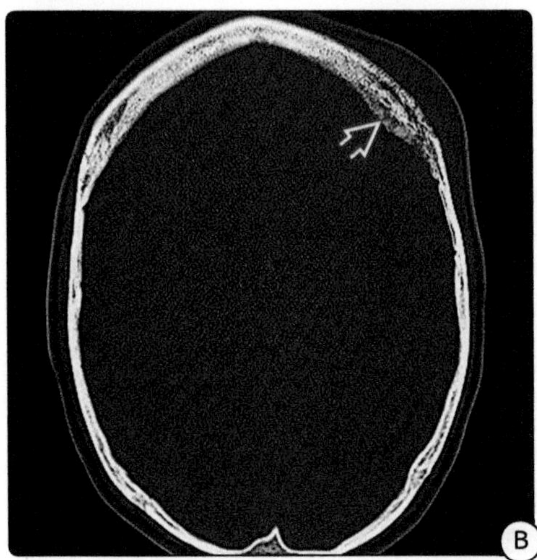

***(24-15B)** Bone CT with edge enhancement shows permeative, destructive changes in the adjacent calvarium ➡.*

RDD, as can other dural-based masses, such as **metastasis, plasma cell granuloma, infectious granuloma** (e.g., TB), **IgG4-related disease**, and **extramedullary hematopoiesis (24-15)**.

Hematopoietic Tumors and Tumor-Like Lesions

Leukemia

Leukemia is the most common form of childhood cancer, representing ~ 1/3 of all cases. Acute lymphoblastic leukemia (ALL) accounts for 80% and acute myeloid leukemia (AML) for most of the remaining 15-20%. Chronic myelocytic leukemia (CML) and lymphocytic leukemia are much more common in adults. Regardless of specific type, the general clinical features of leukemias are similar.

Leukemic masses were initially called **chloromas** (for the greenish discoloration caused by high levels of myeloperoxidase in immature cells). These tumors have been renamed **granulocytic sarcomas**.

Overt CNS leukemia presents in three forms: (1) Meningeal disease ("carcinomatous meningitis"), (2) intravascular tumor aggregates with diffuse brain disease ("carcinomatous encephalitis"), and (3) focal tumor masses (granulocytic sarcoma) **(24-14)**.

Most intracranial lesions are located adjacent to malignant deposits in the orbits, paranasal sinuses, skull base, or calvarium. Multifocal involvement is typical. Extraaxial lesions are generally large and seen as extensive bony infiltrates and dura-based masses **(24-15)**. Intraaxial granulocytic sarcomas occur but are less common and usually smaller, ranging from a few millimeters to 1 or 2 cm.

Imaging is key to the diagnosis of CNS involvement, as CSF studies may be negative.

Granulocytic sarcomas typically present as one or more iso- or hyperdense dura-based masses on NECT. Strong uniform enhancement is typical. Bone CT often shows infiltrating, permeative, destructive lucent lesions. An adjacent soft tissue mass may be present.

Nearly 75% of patients with leukemia and positive CSF cytology have abnormal findings on MR. Pachymeningeal (30%), leptomeningeal (25%), cranial nerve (30%), and spinal meningeal (70%) types of enhancement are typical. Parenchymal lesions ("chloroma") are much less common than meningeal disease. Chloromas are hypo- to isointense on T1WI and heterogeneously iso- to hypointense on T2/FLAIR. Enhancement of parenchymal and focal dural chloromas is typically strong and relatively homogeneous.

Differential diagnosis depends on location. Dura-based granulocytic sarcomas may resemble **extraaxial hematoma, lymphoma**, or **meningioma**. In younger children, **metastatic neuroblastoma** and **Langerhans cell histiocytosis** can mimic granulocytic sarcoma. **Extramedullary hematopoiesis** is a diagnostic consideration but is typically more hypointense than granulocytic sarcoma on T2WI.

Plasma Cell Tumors

Three major forms of neoplastic plasma cell proliferations are recognized: (1) Solitary bone plasmacytoma (SBP), (2) solitary extramedullary plasmacytoma (EMP), and (3) multiple myeloma (MM).

SBPs are sometimes simply called plasmacytoma or solitary plasmacytoma (SP). SPs are characterized by a mass of neoplastic monoclonal plasma cells in either bone or soft tissue without evidence of systemic disease. SPs are rare (5-10% of all plasma cell neoplasms) and are most commonly found in the vertebrae and skull.

EMP is usually seen in the head and neck, typically in the nasal cavity or nasopharynx.

Multifocal disease is **MM (24-16)**. **Plasmablastic lymphoma** is an uncommon, aggressive lymphoma that most frequently arises in the oral cavity of HIV-infected patients. Rarely, **atypical monoclonal plasma cell hyperplasia** occurs as an intracranial inflammatory pseudotumor (discussed in Chapter 28).

MM shows numerous lytic lesions on bone CT **(24-17)**, usually centered in the spine, skull base **(24-18)**, calvarial vault, or facial bones. A variegated "salt and pepper" pattern is typical.

Osseous lesions replace normal hyperintense fatty marrow and are typically hypointense on T1WI. T2 and fat-saturated sequences, such as T2-weighted STIR imaging, also highlight the extent of marrow infiltration. Focal and diffuse lesions appear hyperintense. Both SBPs and MM enhance strongly following contrast administration. Leptomeningeal and parenchymal disease occurs but is uncommon.

Multiple "punched-out" destructive myeloma lesions can appear virtually identical to lytic **metastases**. Spine and skull base MM can resemble **leukemia** or non-Hodgkin **lymphoma. Invasive pituitary macroadenoma** may be difficult to distinguish from MM, as both are isointense with gray matter. An elevated prolactin is often present with macroadenoma, and the pituitary gland cannot be separated from the mass.

Extramedullary Hematopoiesis

Extramedullary hematopoiesis (EMH) is the compensatory formation of blood elements due to decreased medullary hematopoiesis. Various anemias (thalassemia, sickle cell disease, hereditary spherocytosis, etc.) are the most common etiologies, accounting for 45% of cases. Myelofibrosis/myelodysplastic syndromes (35%) are the next most common underlying causes associated with EMH.

Multiple smooth, juxtaosseous, circumscribed, hypercellular masses are typical **(24-19)**. The most common site is along the axial skeleton. The face and skull are the most common head and neck sites. The subdural space is the most common intracranial location.

EMH is hyperdense on NECT **(24-20A)**, enhances strongly and homogeneously on CECT, and may show findings of underlying disease on bone CT (e.g., "hair on end" pattern in thalassemia, dense bone obliterating the diploic space in osteopetrosis).

Round or lobulated subdural masses that are iso- to slightly hyperintense relative to gray matter on T1WI and hypointense on T2WI are typical **(24-20B)**. EMH enhances strongly and uniformly on postcontrast T1WI **(24-20C)**.

The major differential diagnoses of intracranial EMH are **dural metastases** and **meningioma**. **Neurosarcoid** and **lymphoma** are other considerations. **Rosai-Dorfman disease** and other histiocytoses can cause multiple dural-based masses.

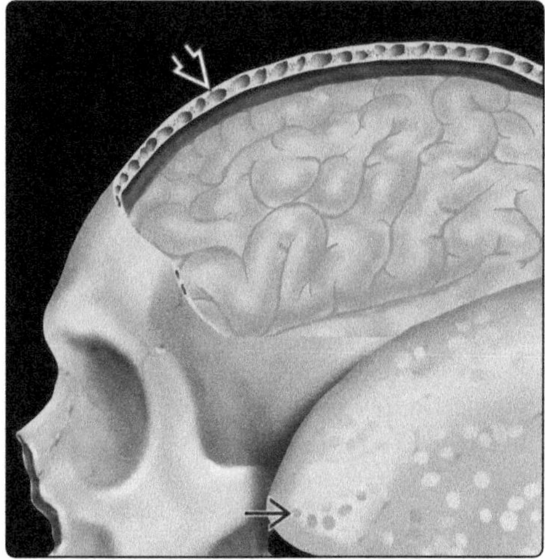

***(24-16)** Graphic shows multiple lytic foci ⇒ characteristic of MM. Sagittal section shows the "punched-out" lesions in the diploic space ➡.*

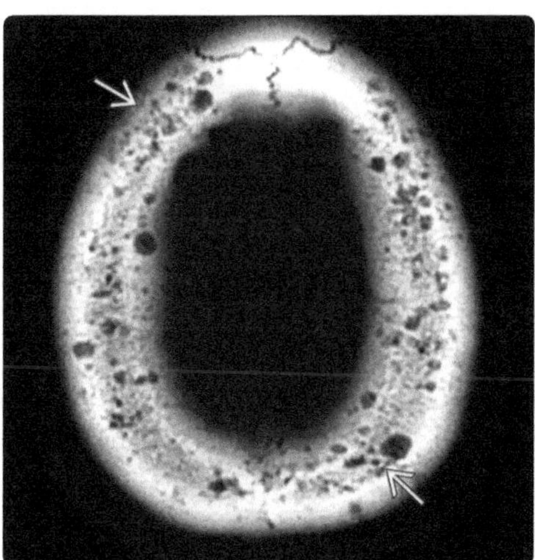

***(24-17)** Bone CT shows MM. Innumerable lytic "punched-out" lesions ➡ give the calvarium the characteristic "salt and pepper" appearance.*

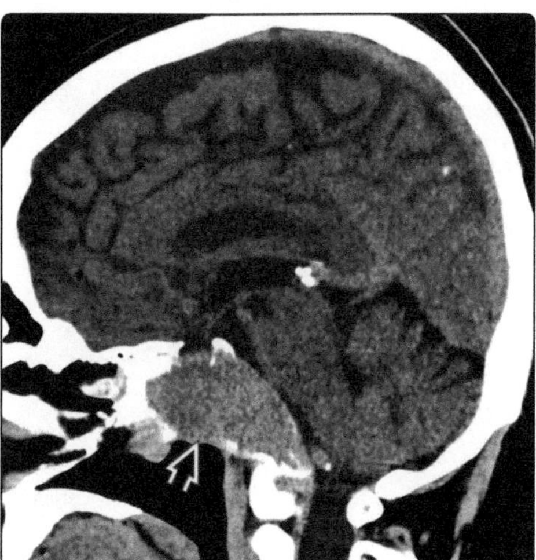

***(24-18)** Sagittal NECT in a 67-year-old man with multiple cranial neuropathies shows hyperdense, destructive central skull base mass ➡.*

EXTRAMEDULLARY HEMATOPOIESIS

Etiology

- Decreased medullary hematopoiesis
- Compensatory formation of blood elements
- Anemias (45%), myelofibrosis/myelodysplasia (35%)

Imaging

- Multiple smooth juxtaosseous masses
  - Spine, face, skull, dura
- Hyperdense on NECT
- T1 iso-/hypo-, T2 hypointense
- Enhances strongly

Differential Diagnosis

- Dural metastases
- Meningioma
- Neurosarcoid
- Lymphoma

Selected References: The complete reference list is available on the Expert Consult™ eBook version included with purchase.

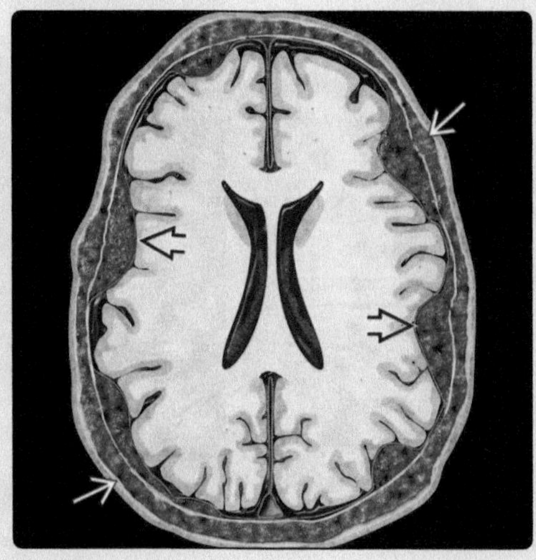

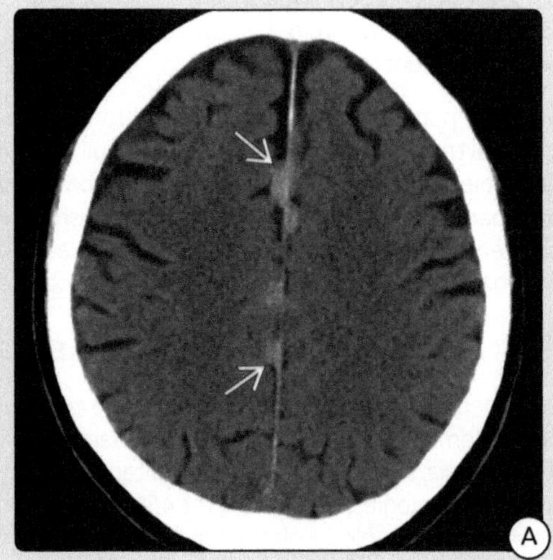

(24-19) Graphic shows extramedullary hematopoiesis (EMH), hematopoietic calvarial marrow ➡, and lobulated extraaxial masses ⇨. (24-20A) NECT of EMH shows several hyperdense nodules ➡ along the falx cerebri.

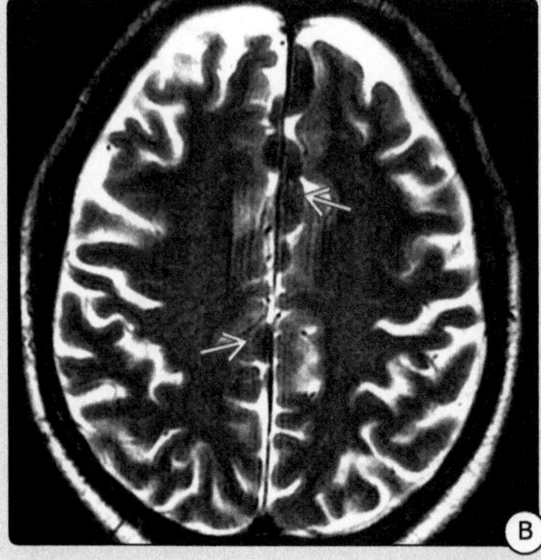

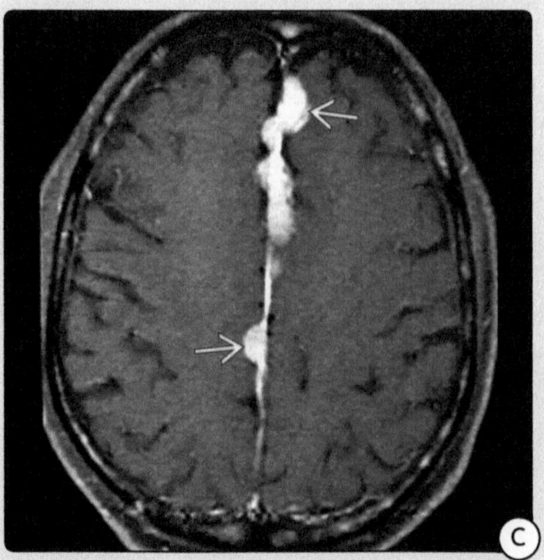

(24-20B) The lobulated lesions are very hypointense on T2WI ➡. (24-20C) EMH enhances strongly and uniformly ➡ as shown on this T1 C+ FS MR in the same patient.

Sellar Neoplasms and Tumor-Like Lesions

The sellar region is one of the most anatomically complex areas in the brain. It encompasses the bony sella turcica and pituitary gland plus all the normal structures that surround it ***(25-1)****. Virtually any of these can give rise to pathology that ranges from incidental and innocuous to serious, potentially life-threatening disease.*

At least 30 different lesions occur in or around the pituitary gland, arising from either the pituitary gland itself **(25-2)** or the structures that surround it. These include the cavernous sinus and its contents, arteries (the circle of Willis), cranial nerves, meninges, CSF spaces (the suprasellar cistern and third ventricle), central skull base, and brain parenchyma (the hypothalamus).

Despite the overwhelming variety of lesions that can occur in this region, at least 75-80% of all sellar/juxtasellar masses are due to one of the **"Big Five": Macroadenoma, meningioma, aneurysm, craniopharyngioma**, and **astrocytoma**. All other lesions combined account for < 1/4 of sellar region masses.

We begin the chapter with normal variants, such as physiologic hypertrophy, that can mimic pituitary pathology. Congenital lesions (such as tuber cinereum hamartoma) that can be mistaken for more ominous pathology are also delineated. Pituitary gland and infundibular stalk neoplasms are then discussed. A brief consideration of miscellaneous lesions, such as lymphocytic hypophysitis, pituitary apoplexy, and the postoperative sella, follows.

The goal of imaging is to determine precisely the location and characteristics of a sellar mass, delineate its relationship to—and involvement with—surrounding structures, and construct a reasonable, limited differential diagnosis to help direct patient management. We then conclude the chapter with a summary of—and approach to—a differential diagnosis of sellar masses.

Diagnostic Considerations

Anatomic sublocation is the single most important key to establishing an appropriate differential diagnosis of a sellar region mass. The first step is assigning a lesion to one of three anatomic compartments, identifying it as an (1) intrasellar, (2) suprasellar, or (3) infundibular stalk lesion.

The key to determining anatomic sublocation accurately is the question: "Can I find the pituitary gland separate from the mass?" If you can't, and the gland *is* the mass, the most likely diagnosis is macroadenoma.

If the mass is clearly *separate* from the pituitary gland, it is extrapituitary and therefore not a macroadenoma. Other pathologies, such as meningioma in

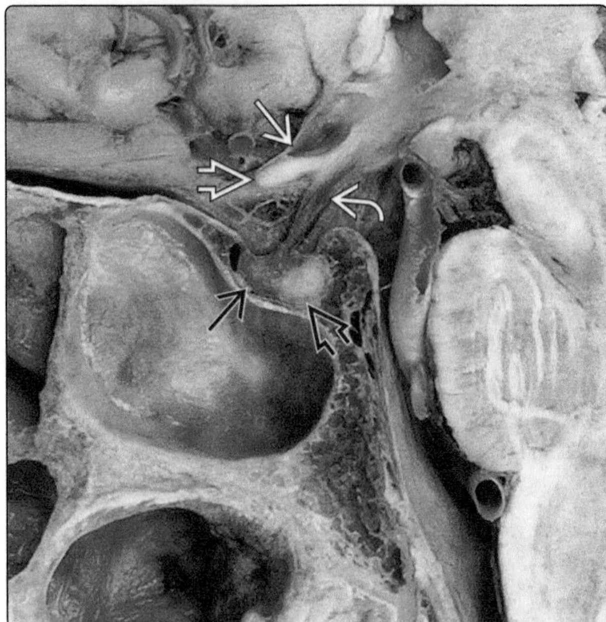

(25-1) *Midline anatomic section depicts sella and surrounding structures. Adenohypophysis ⇒, neurohypophysis ⇒ are shown, along with the optic chiasm ➡ and optic ➡ and infundibular ➡ recesses of the third ventricle. (Courtesy M. Nielsen, MS.)*

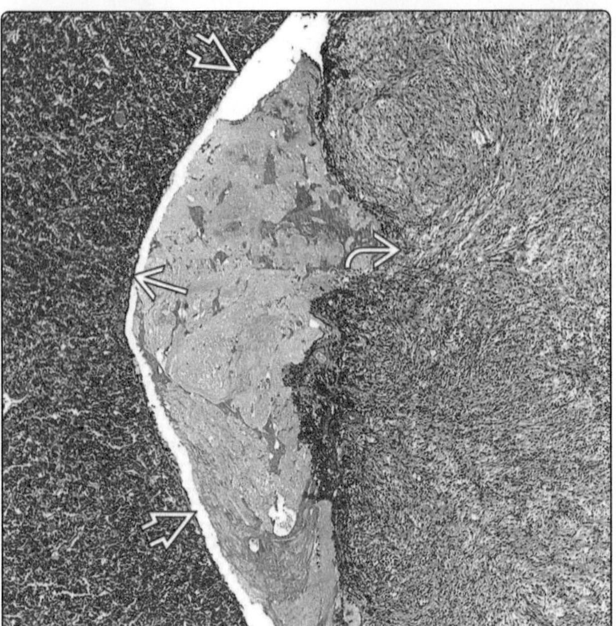

(25-2) *Photomicrograph of a sectioned normal pituitary gland shows Rathke pouch remnant as a "cleft" ➡ between the anterior ➡ and posterior ➡ lobes of the pituitary gland. (Courtesy A. Ersen, MD, B. Scheithauer, MD.)*

an adult or craniopharyngioma, should be considered in such cases.

Clinical Considerations

The single most important clinical feature in establishing an appropriate differential diagnosis for a sellar region mass is **patient age**. Lesions that are common in adults (macroadenoma, meningioma, and aneurysm) are generally rare in children. A lesion in a prepubescent child—especially a boy—that looks like a macroadenoma is almost never a neoplasm. Nonneoplastic pituitary gland enlargement in children is much more common than tumors. Therefore, an enlarged pituitary gland in a child is almost always either normal physiologic hypertrophy or nonphysiologic nonneoplastic hyperplasia secondary to end-organ failure (most commonly hypothyroidism).

Some lesions that are common in children (e.g., opticochiasmatic/hypothalamic pilocytic astrocytoma and craniopharyngioma) are relatively uncommon in adults.

Sex is also important. Imaging studies of young menstruating female patients and postpartum women often demonstrate plump-appearing pituitary glands due to temporary physiologic hyperplasia.

Imaging Considerations

Imaging appearance is very helpful in evaluating a lesion of the sellar region. After establishing the anatomic sublocation of a lesion, look for imaging clues. Are other lesions present? Is the lesion calcified? Does it appear cystic? Does it contain blood products? Is it focal or infiltrating? Does it enhance? Does it enlarge or invade the sella turcica?

Normal Imaging Variants

A number of variants occur in the pituitary gland and around the sella turcica; these should not be mistaken for disease on imaging studies. Pituitary hyperplasia can be abnormal, but it can also be physiologic and normal. An empty sella is a common normal variant but can be a manifestation of idiopathic intracranial hypertension (pseudotumor cerebri).

Pituitary Hyperplasia

Physiologic increase in pituitary volume is common and normal in many circumstances **(25-3)**. Physiologic hypertrophy of puberty and enlarged pituitary glands in young menstruating female patients is very common **(25-4)**. Pituitary gland enlargement also occurs during pregnancy and lactation or in response to exogenous estrogen treatment.

Pathologic hyperplasia most commonly occurs in response to **end-organ failure**. Primary hypothyroidism, usually in the setting of longstanding primary hypothyroidism, is the most common cause of pathologic pituitary hyperplasia **(25-5)**.

NECT scans show that the superior margin of the gland is convex upward, measuring 10-15 mm in height. There is no evidence of erosion of the bony sella turcica. Enhancement is strong and generally uniform on CECT.

MR demonstrates an enlarged gland that bulges upward and may even contact the optic chiasm. The enlarged pituitary is isointense with cortex on both T1- and T2WI. Dynamic contrast-enhanced MR scans with 2- to 3-mm slice thickness and small field of view show that the gland enhances homogeneously.

Pituitary hyperplasia must be distinguished from **macroadenoma**. Age, sex, and endocrine status are helpful. Primary neoplasms of the pituitary gland are rare in children, whereas physiologic enlargement is common. **Remember**: *An enlarged pituitary gland in a prepubescent male patient is almost always hyperplasia, not adenoma!*

Other important causes of a diffusely enlarged pituitary gland include **lymphocytic hypophysitis**. Lymphocytic hypophysitis is most common in pregnant and postpartum female patients and may be difficult to distinguish from physiologic hyperplasia on imaging studies alone. If stalk enlargement is present, hypophysitis is more likely than hyperplasia.

Intracranial hypotension results in pituitary enlargement above the sella turcica in 50% of patients. These patients typically present with headaches related to decreased intracranial CSF pressure. The classic imaging appearance of intracranial hypotension includes diffuse dural thickening and enhancement, downward displacement of the brain through the incisura ("slumping midbrain"), and distension of the venous structures and dural sinuses.

Empty Sella

An **empty sella** (ES) is an arachnoid-lined, CSF-filled protrusion that extends from the suprasellar cistern through the diaphragma sellae into the sella turcica **(25-6)**. An ES is rarely completely "empty"; a small remnant of flattened pituitary gland is almost always present at the bottom of the bony sella **(25-7)**, even if it is inapparent on imaging studies.

The major differential diagnosis of an ES is a **suprasellar arachnoid cyst** that may herniate into the sella turcica. The bony sella is often not simply enlarged but eroded and flattened. Sagittal T2WI often shows an elevated, compressed third ventricle draped over the suprasellar arachnoid cyst.

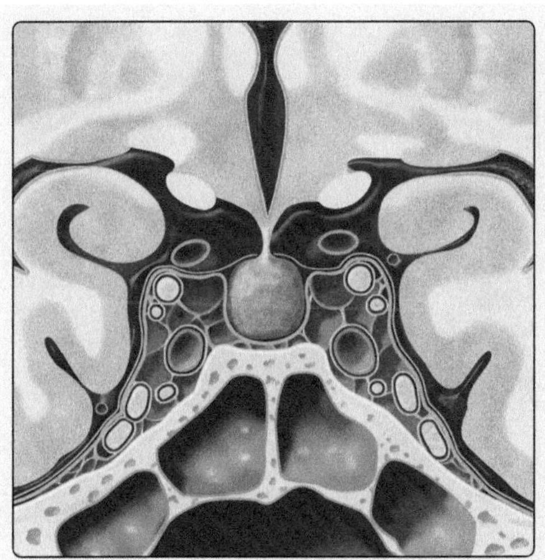

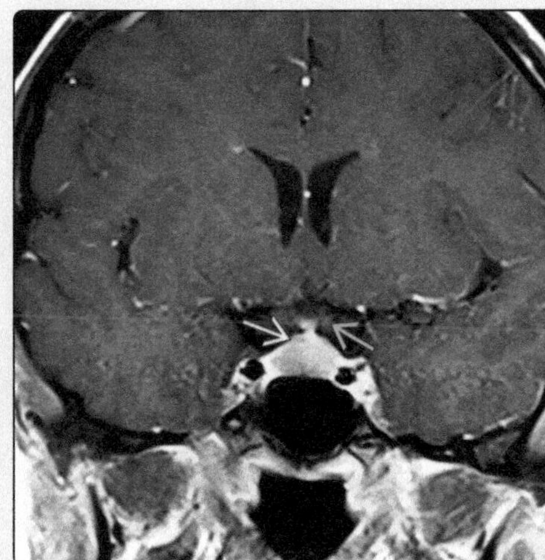

***(25-3)** Coronal graphic shows physiologic pituitary hyperplasia. The gland is uniformly enlarged and has a mildly convex superior margin. **(25-4)** Coronal T1 C+ MR in the same patient shows the upwardly convex gland ➡ almost touching the optic chiasm ➡. The overall volume of the pituitary gland is almost 2x the size of one in a postmenopausal woman.*

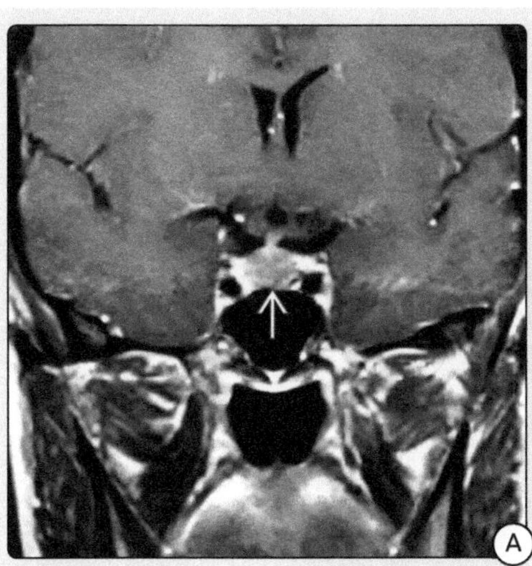

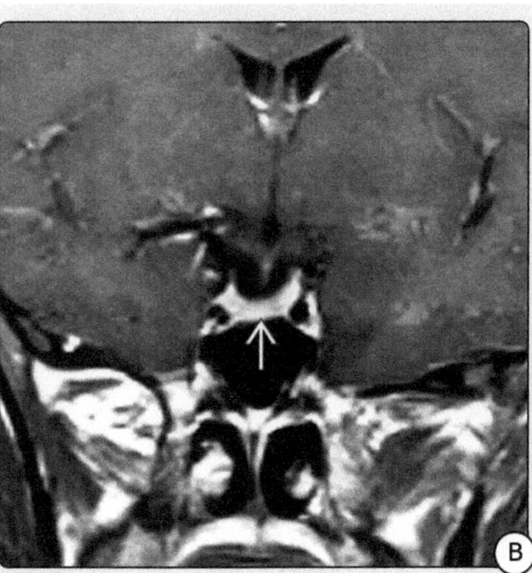

***(25-5A)** Coronal T1 C+ MR in a prepubescent male patient with hypothyroidism shows pituitary hyperplasia ➡ with an upwardly bulging gland that mimics macroadenoma. **(25-5B)** Repeat scan obtained a few weeks following initiation of thyroid hormone replacement shows that the pituitary gland returns to a normal size ➡.*

The other major consideration of patients with an ES is **idiopathic intracranial hypertension** (IIH) a.k.a. "pseudotumor cerebri." Both incidental ES and patients with IIH have an increased prevalence in obese females. Imaging findings also show some overlap, as both conditions often demonstrate an empty sella. In IIH, the optic nerve sheaths are often dilated, and the ventricles and CSF cisterns often appear smaller than normal. Patients with IIH will also typically have papilledema, which can be seen on MR as protrusion of the optic nerve papilla into the posterior globes.

Increased intracranial pressure (↑ ICP) caused by obstructive hydrocephalus usually results in displacement of the enlarged anterior third ventricle recesses—not the suprasellar cistern—toward or into the bony sella. Transependymal CSF migration is common in ↑ ICP but absent in ES.

Congenital Lesions

Pituitary Anomalies

A **hypoplastic pituitary gland** is the most frequent abnormality in children with *isolated* growth hormone deficiency, whereas **stalk abnormalities** are more common in children with *multiple* hormone deficiencies. Nearly 75% of children with hypopituitarism are male.

Imaging abnormalities include a small sella and anterior pituitary lobe, hypoplasia or absence of the stalk, and an "ectopic" posterior pituitary "bright spot" seen as displacement of the T1-hyperintense posterior lobe into the infundibulum or median eminence of the hypothalamus **(25-8)** **(25-9)**.

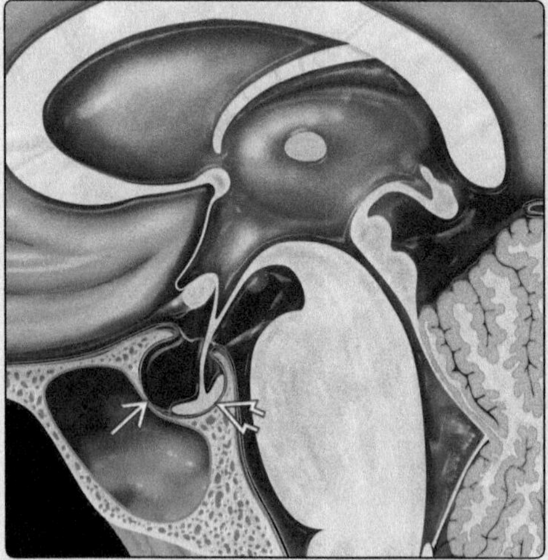

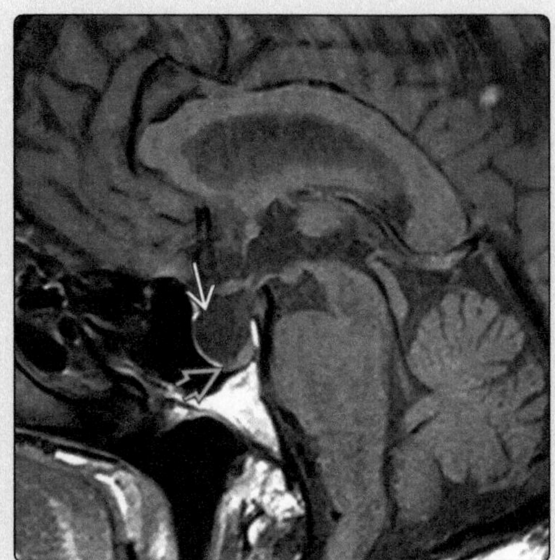

(25-6) *Graphic depicts primary empty sella ➡ with CSF-filled arachnoid cistern protruding inferiorly into the enlarged sella turcica, flattening the pituitary gland posteroinferiorly against the sellar floor ➡.* ***(25-7)*** *Sagittal T1 MR shows a classic empty sella ➡ with an enlarged sella turcica in this 58-year-old woman with Cushing syndrome. The pituitary gland is thinned and flattened against the sellar floor ⇨.*

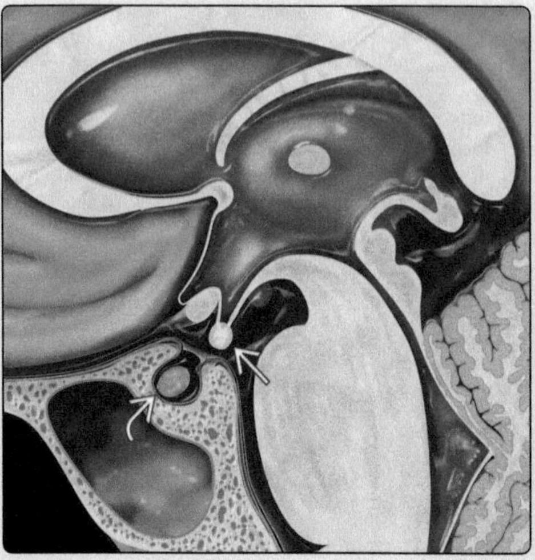

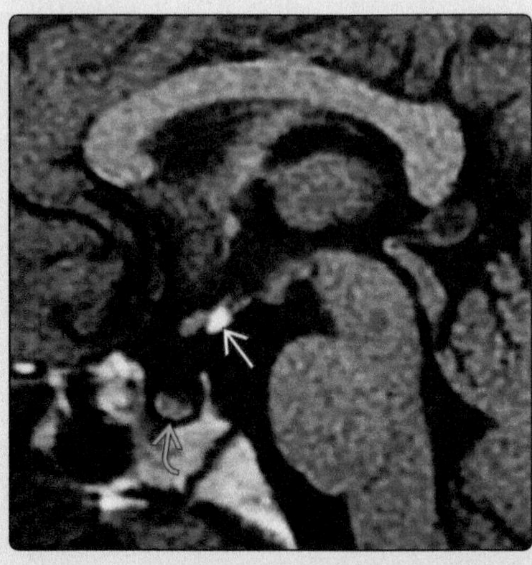

(25-8) *Sagittal graphic demonstrates ectopia of the posterior pituitary gland ➡, located at the distal end of a truncated pituitary stalk. The sella turcica and adenohypophysis ➡ are both small.* ***(25-9)*** *Sagittal T1 MR shows an ectopic posterior pituitary gland at the hypothalamic median eminence ➡. The infundibulum is absent, and the anterior pituitary gland ⇨ is small. The normal posterior pituitary "bright spot" is not in its typical location.*

Hypothalamic Hamartoma

Hypothalamic hamartoma (HH), a.k.a. diencephalic or **tuber cinereum hamartoma**, is a nonneoplastic congenital malformation associated with precocious puberty, behavioral disturbances, and gelastic seizures.

The majority of HHs are located in the tuber cinereum, i.e., between the infundibular stalk in front and the mammillary bodies behind. They can be pedunculated or sessile. Pedunculated lesions extend inferiorly from the hypothalamus into the suprasellar cistern, whereas sessile HHs project from the floor of the third ventricle into its lumen. HHs are solitary lesions that vary in size from a few millimeters to huge mixed solid-cystic lesions measuring several centimeters in diameter.

Most HHs present between 1 and 3 years of age. Three-quarters of patients with histologically verified HHs have precocious puberty, and 50% have seizures, often "gelastic" (ictal laughing fits). Gelastic seizures are more common with sessile tumors, whereas precocious puberty is more often present in patients with small pedunculated lesions.

NECT scan shows a homogeneous suprasellar mass that is isodense to slightly hypodense compared with brain. HHs do not enhance on CECT.

Pedunculated HHs are shaped like a collar button on sagittal T1WI, extending inferiorly into the suprasellar cistern. Signal intensity is usually isointense to normal gray matter on T1WI and iso- to slightly hyperintense on T2/FLAIR **(25-12A)**. Intralesional cysts may be present in larger HHs. HHs do not enhance with contrast **(25-12B)**.

The differential diagnoses of HH are craniopharyngioma and chiasmatic/hypothalamic astrocytoma. **Craniopharyngioma** is the most common suprasellar mass in children. Over 90% of craniopharyngiomas are cystic, 90% calcify, and 90% show nodular and rim enhancement. **Optic pathway/hypothalamic**

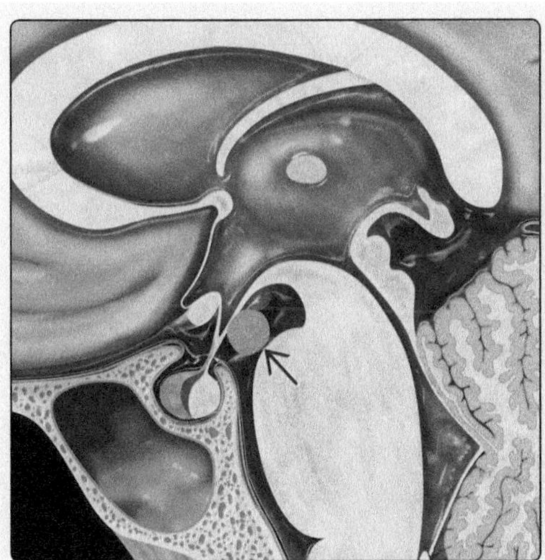

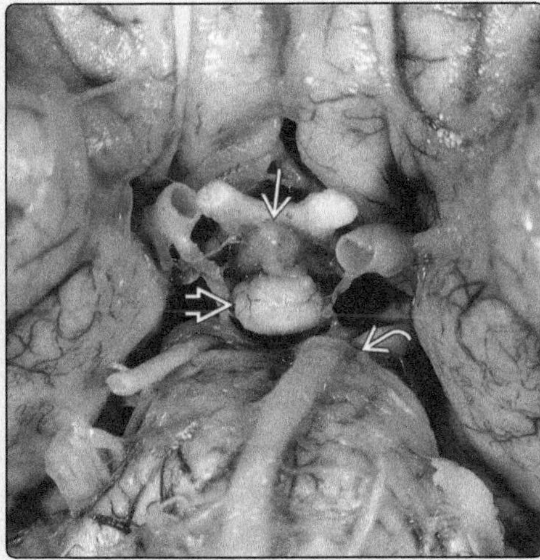

***(25-10)** Sagittal graphic shows a pedunculated hypothalamic hamartoma ➡ interposed between the infundibulum anteriorly and the mammillary bodies posteriorly. The mass resembles gray matter. **(25-11)** Submentovertex view shows a classic "collar button" pedunculated HH ➡ positioned between the infundibular stalk ➡ in front, mammillary bodies (not visible), and pons ➡ behind. (Courtesy R. Hewlett, MD.)*

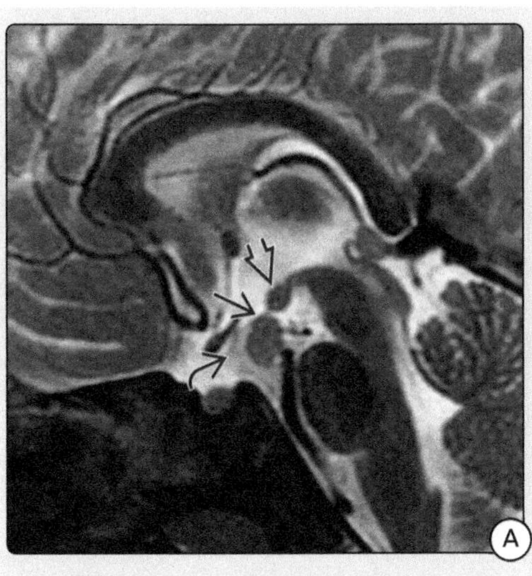

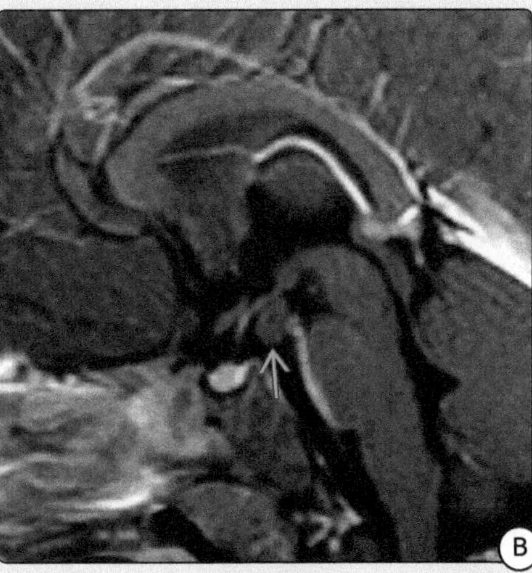

***(25-12A)** Sagittal T2 MR in a 12-month-old child with central precocious puberty shows a classic "collar button" hypothalamic hamartoma ➡ between the infundibular stalk ➡ and the mammillary bodies ➡. The mass is isointense with gray matter. **(25-12B)** Sagittal T1 C+ MR in the same patient shows that the hypothalamic hamartoma ➡ does not enhance. If the mass enhanced, a glioma should be considered.*

pilocytic astrocytoma is the second most common pediatric suprasellar mass. Astrocytomas are hyperintense on T2/FLAIR and often enhance on T1 C+.

Rathke Cleft Cyst

Rathke cleft cyst (RCC) is a benign endodermal cyst of the sellar region, thought to arise from remnants of the fetal Rathke pouch. Approximately 40% are completely intrasellar and 60% are either suprasellar or combined intra- and suprasellar **(25-13)**.

Most RCCs are asymptomatic and discovered incidentally at imaging. Symptomatic RCCs cause pituitary dysfunction, visual disturbances, and headache. Mean age at presentation is 45 years.

NECT scans show a well-delineated round or ovoid mass within or just above the sella. Three-quarters of RCCs are hypodense, 20% are of mixed density, and 5-10% are hyperdense. Calcification is rare.

Signal intensity varies with cyst contents; 1/2 of RCCs are hypointense on T1WI and 1/2 are hyperintense **(25-14)**. The majority are hyperintense on T2WI **(25-15)**, whereas 25-30% are iso- to hypointense. A hypointense intracystic nodule occurs in 40-75% of cases **(25-15)**. RCCs are almost always hyperintense on FLAIR. An enhancing rim ("claw" sign) of compressed pituitary gland can often be seen surrounding the nonenhancing cyst on T1 C+ **(25-16)**.

The major differential diagnosis of RCC is **craniopharyngioma**. Calcifications are common in craniopharyngioma. The rim or nodular enhancement in craniopharyngioma is generally thicker and more irregular than the "claw" of enhancing pituitary gland that surrounds the nonenhancing RCC. A cystic pituitary adenoma—especially a **nonfunctioning cystic microadenoma**—can be difficult to distinguish from a small intrasellar RCC.

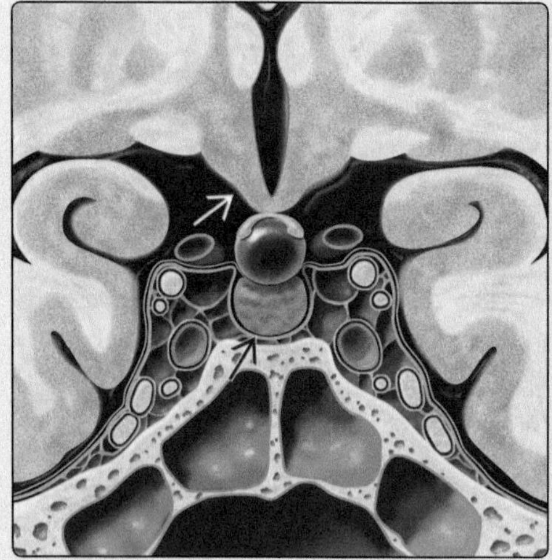

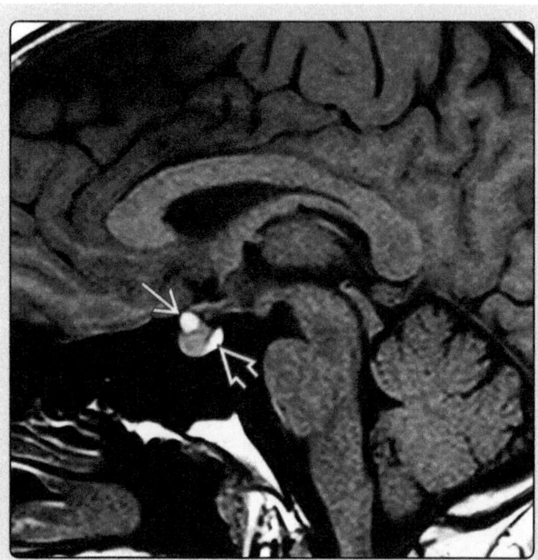

***(25-13)** Coronal graphic shows a typical suprasellar Rathke cleft cyst interposed between the pituitary gland ⇨ and the optic chiasm ➡. **(25-14)** Sagittal T1 MR in an asymptomatic patient shows a tiny hyperintense suprasellar mass ➡ that appears separate from the pituitary gland "bright spot" of the neurohypophysis ➡. This is presumed Rathke cleft cyst.*

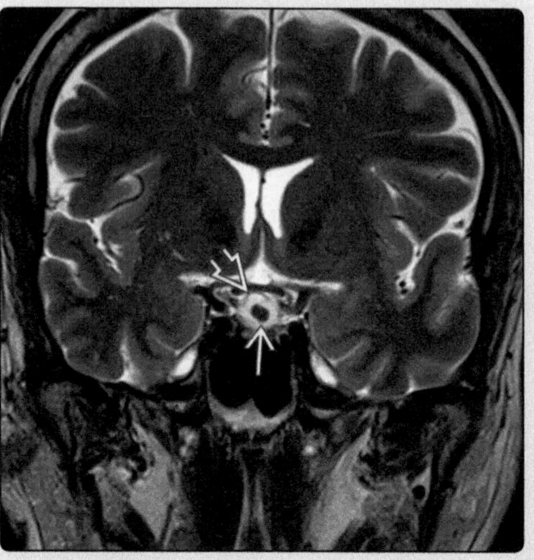

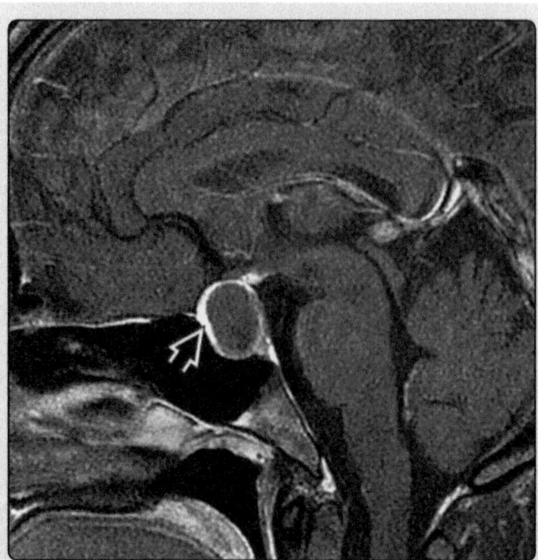

***(25-15)** Coronal T2 MR in a 62-year-old woman with headaches shows a hyperintense intra- and suprasellar cyst ➡ with a hypointense intracystic nodule ➡. This is RCC. **(25-16)** Sagittal T1 C+ MR in a 42-year-old patient with a Rathke cleft cyst shows the classic "claw" sign ➡ of compressed pituitary gland wrapping around the anterior aspect of the cyst.*

Other nonneoplastic cysts that can occur in the sellar region are dermoid (fat, calcification common) and epidermoid cysts (rarely midline, usually CSF-like, DWI hyperintense), arachnoid cysts (larger, CSF-like, lacking an intracystic nodule), and inflammatory cysts (e.g., neurocysticercosis; multiple far more prevalent than solitary cysts).

Neoplasms

Pituitary Adenomas

Terminology

Pituitary adenomas are adenohypophysial tumors composed of secretory cells that produce pituitary hormones. **Microadenomas** are defined as tumors ≤ 10 mm in diameter, whereas larger adenomas are designated **macroadenomas (25-17) (25-18) (25-19)**.

Pathology

Location. Adenomas arise from the adenohypophysis. Specific sublocation follows the normal distribution of peptide-containing cells. Prolactinomas and growth-hormone-secreting tumors—the two most common pituitary adenomas—tend to arise laterally within the adenohypophysis, whereas thyroid-stimulating hormone (TSH)- and ACTH-secreting tumors are more often midline.

Size and Number. Adenomas vary in size from microscopic lesions to giant tumors that invade the skull base and extend into multiple cranial fossae.

Gross Pathology. Macroadenomas are red-brown, lobulated masses that often bulge upward through the opening of diaphragma sella **(25-18)** or, less commonly, extend laterally toward the cavernous sinus. Approximately 1/2 of macroadenomas contain cysts &/or hemorrhagic foci. Pituitary adenomas are WHO grade I tumors.

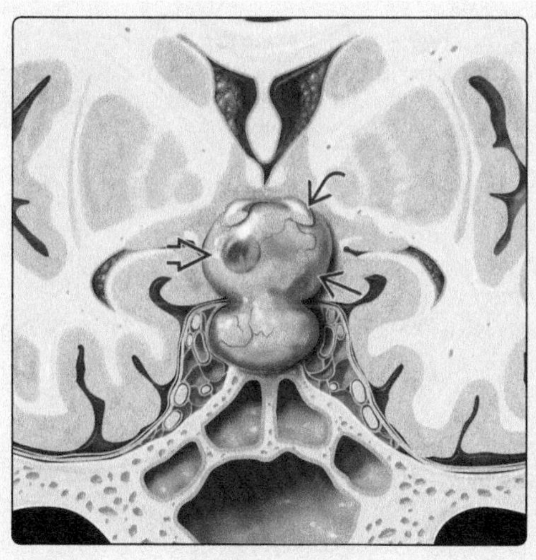

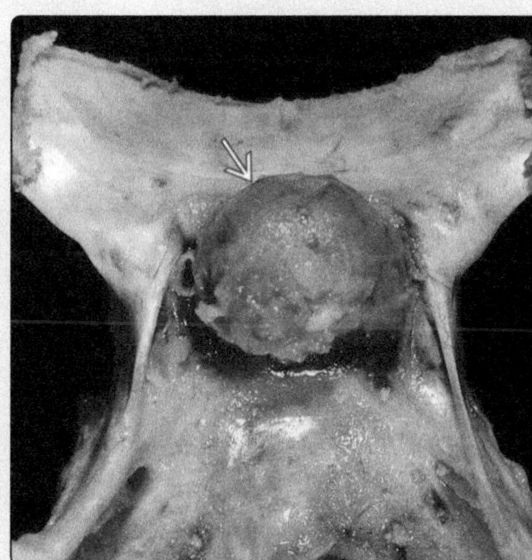

***(25-17)** Coronal graphic shows a snowman-shaped or "figure 8" sellar and suprasellar mass ➙. Small foci of hemorrhage ➙ and cystic change ➙ are present within the lesion. The pituitary gland cannot be identified separately from the mass; indeed, the gland is the mass. **(25-18)** Autopsy specimen shows a macroadenoma ➙ protruding superiorly into the suprasellar cistern. (Courtesy R. Hewlett, MD.)*

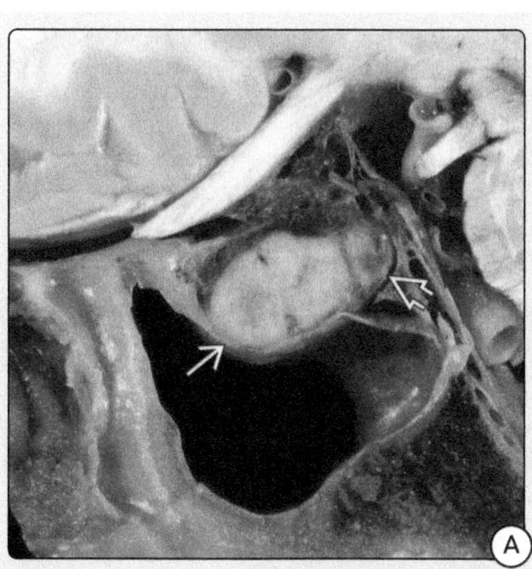

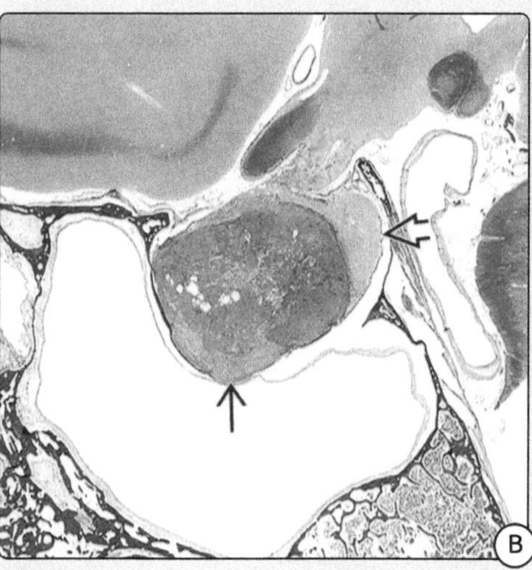

***(25-19A)** Pituitary adenomas ➙ are well-circumscribed masses that compress and displace the normal pituitary gland ➙. (Courtesy A. Ersen, MD, B. Scheithauer, MD.) **(25-19B)** Sagittal low-power photomicrograph shows a prolactinoma eroding the sellar floor ➙, compressing and displacing the normal pituitary gland posteriorly ➙. (Courtesy A. Ersen, MD, B. Scheithauer, MD.)*

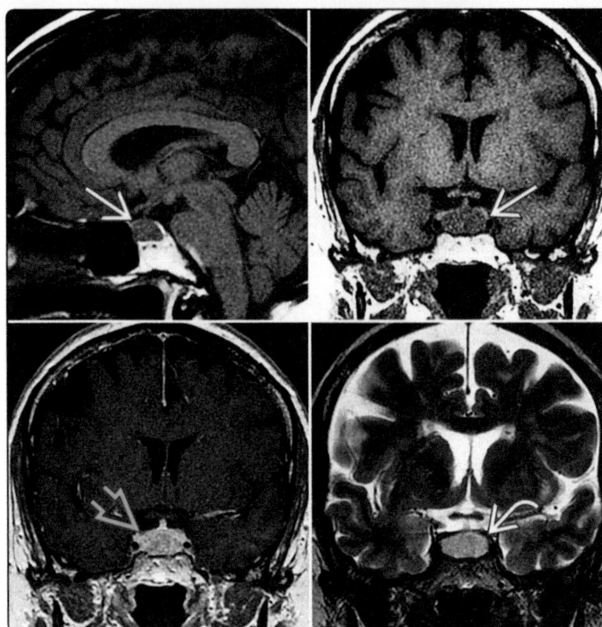

(25-20) Series of MRs shows a small macroadenoma that measured 12 mm in height. The mass is isointense with GM ➡ on T1- and T2WI ➡ and enhances strongly and uniformly ⇨.

(25-21) Sagittal T1WI ➡, T2WI ⇨, FLAIR ➡, and T1 C+ ⇨ show a very large "snowman" or "figure 8" sellar and suprasellar mass. The pituitary gland cannot be identified as separate from the mass (macroadenoma).

Clinical Issues

Epidemiology. Pituitary adenomas are among the most common of all CNS neoplasms, accounting for 10-15% of primary intracranial neoplasms. Microadenomas are much more common than macroadenomas; clinically silent incidental microadenomas are identified in 15-25% of autopsies.

Peak age of presentation is between the fourth and seventh decades. Only 2% of pituitary adenomas are found in children. Most of these occur in adolescent girls. Pituitary adenomas in prepubescent boys are very rare.

Presentation. Almost 2/3 of pituitary adenomas secrete a hormone (~ 40-50% prolactin, 10% growth hormone, 6% corticotropin, 1% thyrotropin) and cause typical hypersecretory syndromes. One-third do not produce hormones and are referred to as "nonfunctioning" or "null cell" adenomas.

Macroadenomas generally present with mass effect. Headache and visual disturbances are common. Diabetes insipidus is rarely associated with pituitary adenoma, so its presence should prompt consideration of an alternative diagnosis.

Although pituitary adenoma growth rates are quite variable, most enlarge slowly over a period of years. Malignant degeneration into pituitary carcinoma is exceptionally rare. Treatment options are numerous and range from medical treatment to surgical resection.

Imaging

General Features. A sellar or combined intra- and suprasellar mass that cannot be identified separately from the pituitary gland (the mass *is* the gland) is the most characteristic imaging finding.

CT Findings. Pituitary adenomas demonstrate variable attenuation on NECT scans. Macroadenomas are usually isodense with gray matter, but cysts (15-20%) and hemorrhage (10%) are common. Calcification is rare (< 2%). Moderate but heterogeneous enhancement of macroadenomas is typical on CECT.

Bone CT may show an enlarged, remodeled sella turcica. "Giant" pituitary adenomas may erode and extensively invade the skull base **(25-23)**.

MR Findings

Macroadenomas. Macroadenomas are usually isointense with cortex on T1WIs **(25-20)** **(25-21)**. Small cysts and hemorrhagic foci are common. Fluid-fluid levels can be present but are more common in patients with pituitary apoplexy.

Adenomas are generally isointense with gray matter on T2WI but can also demonstrate heterogeneous signal intensity **(25-22)**. Hemorrhagic adenomas "bloom" on T2*.

Most macroadenomas enhance strongly but heterogeneously on T1 C+ **(25-21)**. Subtle dural thickening (a dural "tail") is present in 5-10% of cases.

Microadenomas. Unless they hemorrhage, small microadenomas may be inapparent on standard nonenhanced sequences **(25-24)**. Many microadenomas appear slightly

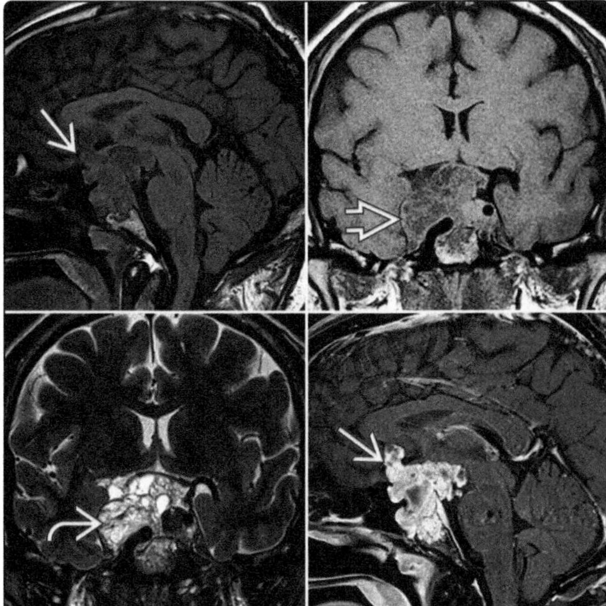

(25-22) Lobulated, invasive sellar/suprasellar mass ➡ has multiple medium/small-sized T2-hyperintense cysts ➡. Macroadenoma also invades the right cavernous sinus ➡.

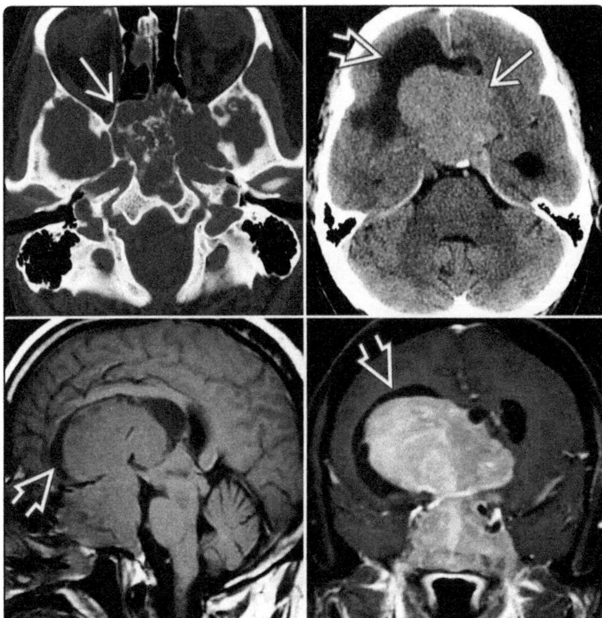

(25-23) Bone CT (top left), CECT (top right) show a huge invasive pituitary macroadenoma ➡. CECT, sagittal T1WI, coronal T1 C+ FS all show trapped pools of CSF ➡ adjacent to the tumor. These are nonneoplastic peritumoral cysts.

hypointense on T1 C+ **(25-25)** **(25-26)**. Others enhance more strongly and may become isointense with the enhancing pituitary gland, rendering them virtually invisible.

Microadenomas enhance more slowly than the normal pituitary tissue. This discrepancy in enhancement timing can be exploited by using thin-section coronal dynamic contrast-enhanced scans. Fast image acquisition during contrast administration can often discriminate between the slowly enhancing microadenoma and rapidly enhancing normal gland. Between 10-30% of microadenomas are seen only on dynamic T1 C+ imaging.

Differential Diagnosis

The major differential diagnosis of pituitary *macro*adenoma is **pituitary hyperplasia**. Tumors that can resemble pituitary adenoma include meningioma, metastasis, and craniopharyngioma. **Meningioma** of the diaphragma sellae can usually be identified as clearly separate from the pituitary gland below.

Metastasis to the stalk &/or pituitary gland from an extracranial primary neoplasm is uncommon. Lung, breast, and systemic **lymphoma** are the most common sources.

Craniopharyngioma is the most common suprasellar tumor of childhood, whereas pituitary adenomas in children are rare. Craniopharyngiomas in middle-aged adults are typically solid papillary tumors that infrequently calcify. In adults with craniopharyngioma, the pituitary gland can usually be identified as anatomically separate from the mass.

Nonneoplastic entities that can mimic macroadenoma include **hypophysitis** (and, rarely, aneurysm).

Pituitary *micro*adenoma may be difficult to distinguish from incidental nonneoplastic intrapituitary cysts, such as **Rathke cleft cyst** or **pars intermedia cyst**. Microadenomas enhance; cysts are seen as nonenhancing foci within the intensely enhancing pituitary gland.

PITUITARY MACROADENOMA: IMAGING AND DDx

CT

- Sella usually enlarged, remodeled, cortex intact
- Invasive adenomas erode, destroy bone
- Majority are isodense with brain
  - Cysts (15-20%), hemorrhage (10%)
  - Ca^{++} rare (1-2%)

MR

- Usually isointense with cortex
- Heterogeneous signal intensity common (cysts, hemorrhage)
- Strong, heterogeneous enhancement
- Microadenomas sometimes seen only with dynamic T1 C+

Differential Diagnosis

- Pituitary hyperplasia (know patient age, sex, endocrine status!)
- Other tumors
  - Meningioma, craniopharyngioma, metastasis, lymphoma
  - Aggressive-looking adenoma is almost never malignant!
- Nonneoplastic lesions
  - Hypophysitis
  - Aneurysm (usually eccentric, "flow void")

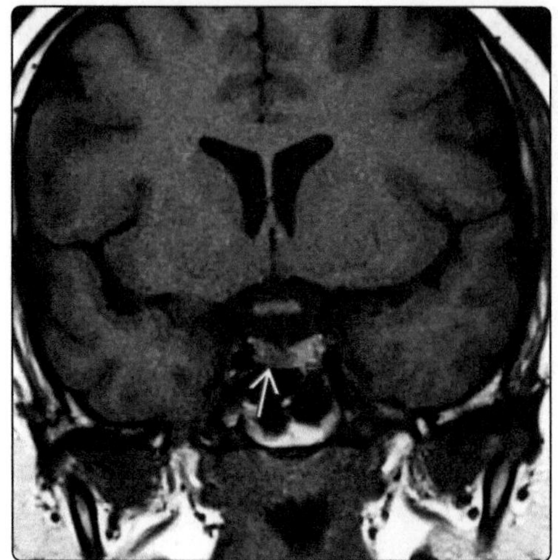

(25-24) T1WI in a patient with amenorrhea, elevated prolactin demonstrates a hypointense mass ➡ in the right lateral pituitary gland.

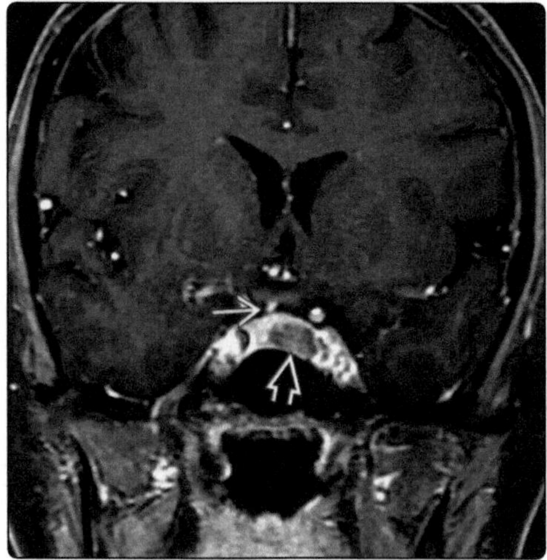

(25-25) T1 C+ shows small macroadenoma ➡ displacing infundibulum ➡. Mass enhances more slowly than gland, appearing hypointense.

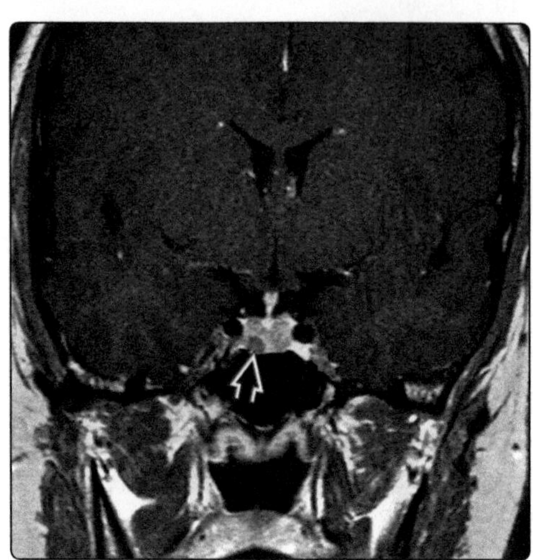

(25-26) T1 C+ MR shows pituitary microadenoma ➡. Microadenoma enhances but less than intensely enhancing normal gland.

Germinoma

Germinomas are discussed in detail in Chapter 20. Germinomas of the suprasellar region are classically hyperdense on CT, similar to lymphoma. When involving the pituitary axis, a germinoma involves the infundibulum &/or neurohypophysis and often presents in a child with an absent posterior pituitary "bright spot." T2 hypointensity and diffuse enhancement of an enlarged infundibulum/anterior third ventricle is the typical MR appearance. Diffusion restriction on DWI is typical.

Craniopharyngioma

Terminology and Etiology

Craniopharyngioma (CP) is a benign, often partly cystic sellar/suprasellar mass that probably arises from epithelial remnants of Rathke pouch.

Pathology

Completely intrasellar CPs are rare. CPs are primarily suprasellar tumors (75%). A small intrasellar component is present in 20-25% of cases. Occasionally, CPs (especially the papillary type) arise mostly or entirely within the third ventricle.

Lesions > 5 cm are common. Giant CPs may extend into both anterior and middle cranial fossae. Posteroinferior extension between the clivus and pons down to the foramen magnum can be seen in exceptionally large lesions.

Two types of CPs are recognized: Adamantinomatous (90%) and papillary (10%). The typical gross appearance of an **adamantinomatous CP** is that of a multilobulated, partially solid but mostly cystic suprasellar mass **(25-27)**. Multiple loculated cysts are common. The cysts often contain dark, viscous, "machinery oil" fluid rich in cholesterol crystals **(25-28)**. Adamantinomatous CPs often adhere to adjacent structures, such as the hypothalamus.

Papillary CP is usually a discrete encapsulated mass with a smooth surface that does not adhere to adjacent brain. Papillary CPs are often solid with a cauliflower-like configuration **(25-32)**. When they contain cysts, the fluid is clear (unlike the "machinery oil" cholesterol-rich contents of adamantinomatous CPs).

Both adamantinomatous and papillary CPs are WHO grade I neoplasms. MIB-1 is low.

CRANIOPHARYNGIOMA: ETIOLOGY AND PATHOLOGY

Etiology
- Epithelial remnants of Rathke pouch

Pathology
- 2 types
  - Adamantinomatous (90%)
  - Papillary (10%)
  - Both are WHO grade I
- Adamantinomatous
  - Multiple cysts
  - Squamous epithelium, "wet" keratin
  - Cholesterol-rich "machinery oil" fluid
- Papillary
  - Solid > > cystic (clear fluid)
  - Almost always adults (40-55 years old)

Clinical Issues

CP is the most common nonglial neoplasm in children, accounting for 6-10% of all pediatric brain tumors and slightly > 1/2 of suprasellar neoplasms.

CPs occur nearly equally in children and adults. Adamantinomatous CPs have a bimodal age distribution with a large peak between 5 and 15 years and a second, smaller peak at 45-60 years. CPs are rare in newborns and infants; only 5% arise in patients between birth and 5 years of age. Papillary CPs almost always occur in adults with a peak incidence between 40 and 55 years.

Patients most commonly present with visual disturbances, either with or without accompanying headache. Endocrine deficiencies including growth failure, delayed puberty, and diabetes insipidus are common.

CPs are slow-growing neoplasms with a propensity to recur following surgery. More than 85% of patients survive at least three years following diagnosis. However, the recurrence rate at 10 years approaches 20-30%, even in patients with gross total resection.

Imaging

General Features. A partially calcified, mixed solid and cystic extraaxial suprasellar mass in a child is the classic appearance. A compressed, displaced pituitary gland can sometimes be identified as separate from the mass.

CT Findings. Adamantinomatous CPs follow a "rule of ninety," i.e., 90% are mixed cystic/solid, 90% are calcified, and 90% enhance **(25-29)**. Papillary CPs rarely calcify. They are often solid or mostly solid.

MR Findings. Signal intensity varies with cyst contents **(25-30)**. Multiple cysts are common, and intracystic fluid within each cyst varies from hypo- to hyperintense compared with brain on T1WI **(25-30B)**.

CP cysts are variably hyperintense on T2WI and FLAIR. The solid nodule is often calcified and moderately hypointense. Hyperintensity extending along the optic tracts is common and usually represents edema, not tumor invasion. Cyst walls **(25-31)** and solid nodules typically enhance following contrast administration **(25-30D)**.

MRS shows a large lipid-lactate peak, characteristic of the cholesterol and lipid constituents of a CP. pMR shows low rCBV.

CRANIOPHARYNGIOMA: CLINICAL ISSUES, IMAGING, AND DDx

Clinical Issues
- Occurs equally in children, adults
  - Peak in children = 5-15 years (usually adamantinomatous)
  - Peak in adults = 40-55 years (papillary more common)

Imaging
- CT
  - Adamantinomatous: 90% cystic, 90% calcify, 90% enhance
  - Papillary: Solid > cystic
- MR
  - Variable signal on T1WI
  - Usually hyperintense on T2/FLAIR
  - Enhancement (nodular or rim) 90%
  - MRS: Large lipid-lactate peak
  - Main differential diagnosis = Rathke cleft cyst

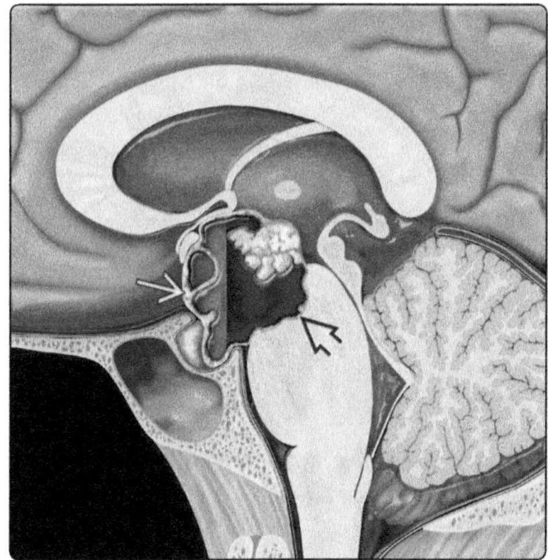

***(25-27)** Graphic shows craniopharyngioma as predominantly cystic, partially solid suprasellar mass with rim Ca^{++} ➡, dark viscous fluid ⇨.*

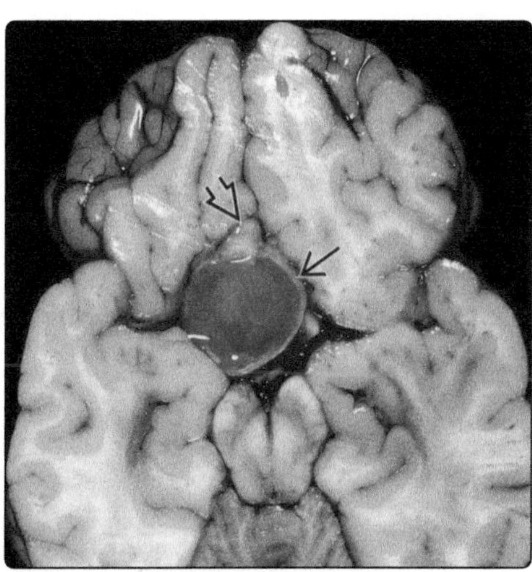

***(25-28)** Specimen shows mostly cystic craniopharyngioma ⇨ with small tumor nodule present ⇨. (Courtesy R. Hewlett, MD.)*

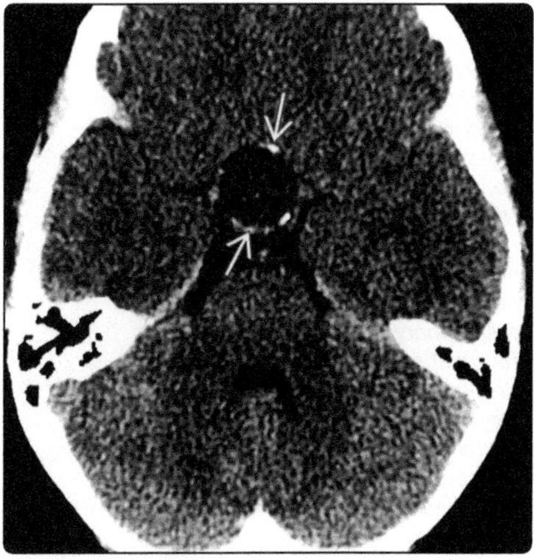

***(25-29)** (L) NECT shows cystic suprasellar mass with rim Ca^{++} ➡. (R) Rim enhances on CECT. This is adamantinomatous craniopharyngioma.*

Differential Diagnosis

The major differential diagnosis of CP is **Rathke cleft cyst** (RCC). RCCs do not calcify, appear to be much less heterogeneous, and do not show nodular enhancement. The ADC of RCC is significantly increased compared with that of cystic CPs. Immunohistochemistry is helpful, as RCCs express specific cytokeratins that CPs do not.

Hypothalamic/chiasmatic astrocytoma is usually a solid suprasellar mass that is clearly intraparenchymal. Calcifications and cysts are uncommon. These tumors are T2 hyperintense and have variable enhancement.

Pituitary adenoma is rare in prepubescent children (peak age period for CP). A **dermoid cyst** can be hyperintense on T1WI and may demonstrate calcification. An **epidermoid cyst** (EC) is usually off-midline with DWI restriction. Suprasellar ECs are uncommon. Neither dermoid nor epidermoid cysts enhance.

Nonadenomatous Pituitary Tumors

The 2016 WHO recognizes three rare, histologically distinct pituitary region neoplasms: Pituicytoma, spindle cell oncocytoma (SCO), and granular cell tumor. All are WHO grade I tumors. All rarely present with diabetes insipidus, typically having visual disturbances or panhypopituitarism.

Pituicytoma arises from modified glial cells ("pituicytes") that reside in the infundibular stalk and neurohypophysis. The majority of pituicytomas are isointense with brain on T1WI and hyperintense on T2WI. They usually arise along the infundibulum or neurohypophysis and enhance homogeneously following contrast enhancement.

Spindle cell oncocytoma has imaging findings that are similar to—and cannot be distinguished from—those of pituitary adenoma or lymphocytic hypophysis.

(25-30A) Sagittal T1 MR in the same patient as Fig. 25-29 shows a lobulated sellar and suprasellar mass ➡ that is nearly isointense with white matter in the corpus callosum. (25-30B) The mass ➡ is very hyperintense on sagittal T2WI. Some hypointense debris ⇨ is present at the bottom of the mostly cystic mass. There is mild expansion of the sella turcica.

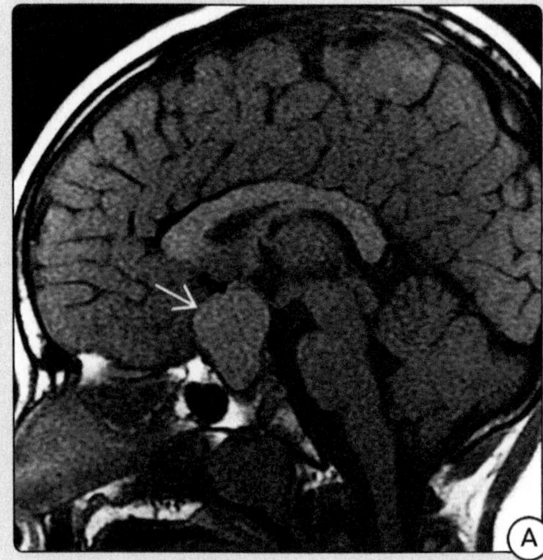

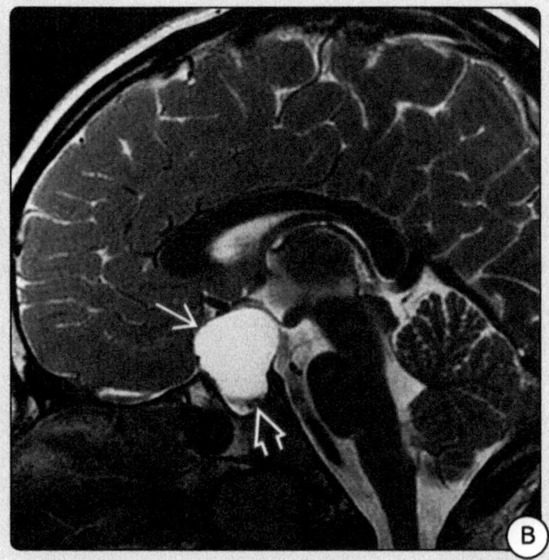

(25-30C) Sagittal T1 C+ MR shows thin rim enhancement around the mass ➡. (25-30D) Coronal T1 C+ MR shows the thin enhancing tumor rim ➡ with a small tumor nodule ⇨. Adamantinomatous craniopharyngioma was found at surgery. Craniopharyngioma is the most common nonglial tumor in children. The enhancing nodule helps differentiate this tumor from a Rathke cleft cyst.

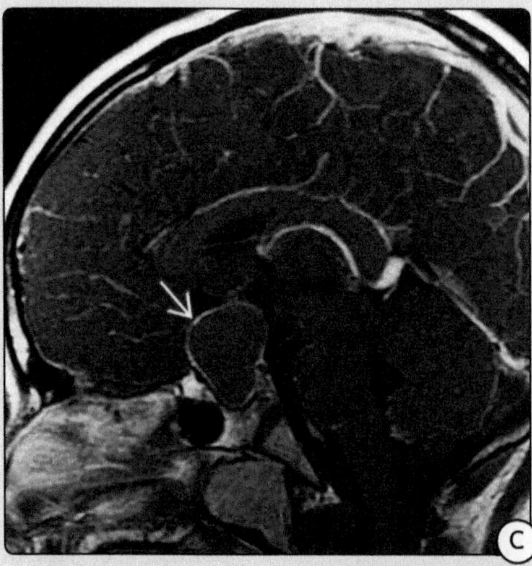

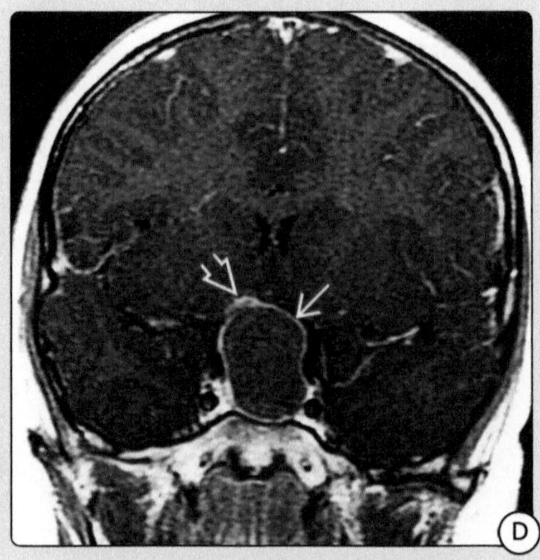

Like pituicytoma, **granular cell tumor** is a suprasellar tumor of the neurohypophysis. Granular cell tumors are typically suprasellar masses. They are hyperdense on NECT and isointense with brain on both T1- and T2WI. Granular cell tumors enhance strongly and homogeneously following contrast administration.

Miscellaneous Lesions

Hypophysitis

Hypophysitis is an inflammation of the pituitary gland. There are two main histologic forms of hypophysitis: Lymphocytic hypophysitis (LH) **(25-34)** and nonlymphocytic hypophysitis. We focus on LH, the most common form. We then briefly discuss nonlymphocytic hypophysitis, including granulomatous hypophysitis and some of the newly described entities that are often characterized by plasma cell infiltrates.

Lymphocytic Hypophysitis

LH is also called lymphocytic adenohypophysitis, primary hypophysitis, and stalkitis. LH is an uncommon autoimmune inflammatory disorder of the pituitary gland. Between 80% and 90% of patients with LH are female; 30-60% of cases occur in the peripartum period.

The most common presenting symptoms are headache and multiple endocrine deficiencies with partial or total hypopituitarism. Diabetes insipidus is common. Adrenocorticotrophic hormone deficits often appear first. Hyperprolactinemia occurs in 1/3 of all patients, probably secondary to stalk compression.

Imaging shows a combined intra- and suprasellar mass with a thickened, nontapering infundibular stalk **(25-35)**. A rounded, symmetrically enlarged pituitary gland is common. The sellar floor is intact, not expanded or eroded. The posterior pituitary

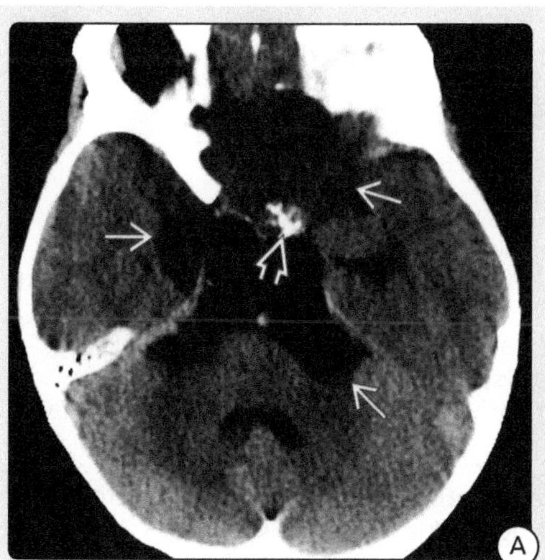

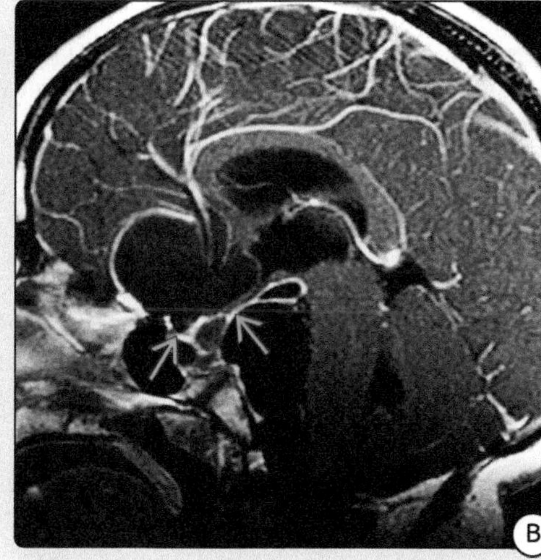

***(25-31A)** Axial NECT in a 9-year-old boy shows an extensive hypodense mass involving the anterior, middle, and posterior cranial fossae ➡. A small focus of calcification ➡ is present inside the mass. **(25-31B)** Sagittal T1 C+ MR in the same patient demonstrates some thin rim enhancement ⇨ around parts of the sellar and suprasellar mass. This is adamantinomatous craniopharyngioma.*

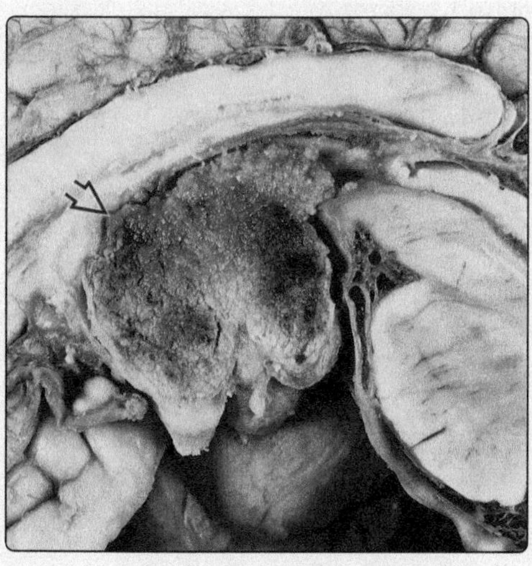

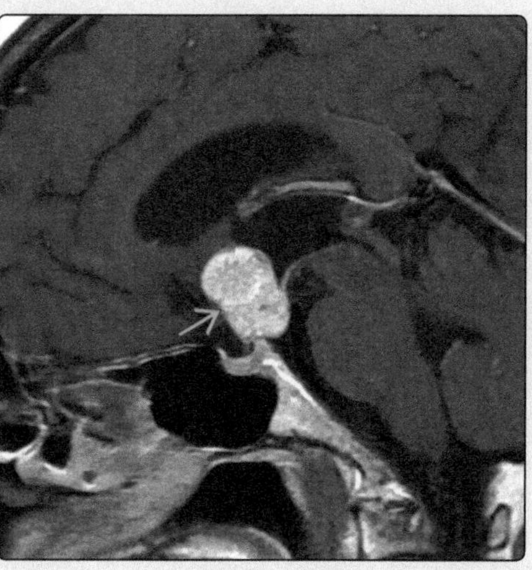

***(25-32)** Midline sagittal autopsy section shows a solid mass filling the 3rd ventricle ⇨. This was papillary craniopharyngioma. (Courtesy B. Scheithauer, MD.) **(25-33)** Sagittal T1 C+ MR in a 60-year-old man shows a solidly enhancing mass in the anterior 3rd ventricle ⇨. Note that the pituitary gland is separate from the mass. Imaging is typical of a papillary craniopharyngioma.*

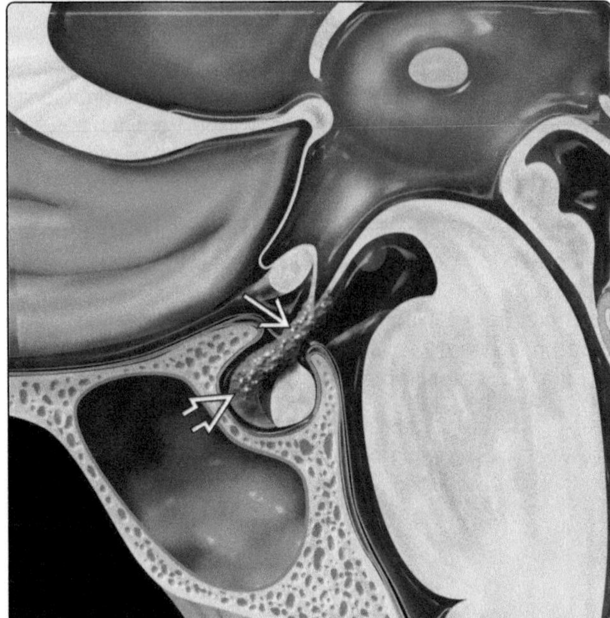

(25-34) Sagittal graphic shows lymphocytic hypophysitis. Note thickening of the infundibulum ➡ and infiltration into the anterior lobe of the pituitary gland ⇨.

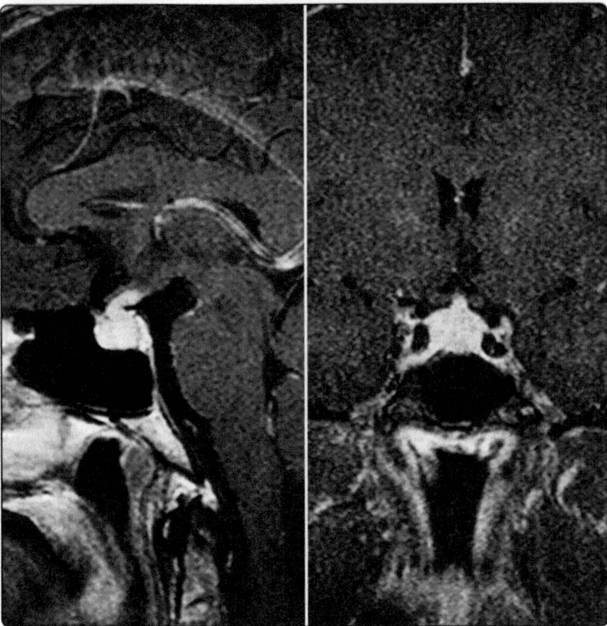

(25-35) Patient on ipilimumab for metastatic melanoma developed drug-induced hypophysitis with infiltration of the stalk and pituitary gland.

"bright spot" (PPBS) is absent in 75% of cases. LH enhances intensely and uniformly.

The major differential diagnosis for LH is nonsecreting **pituitary macroadenoma**. The distinction is important, as treatment differs significantly. LH is treated medically, whereas surgical resection is the primary treatment for pituitary macroadenoma. Macroadenomas can be giant, but LH only occasionally exceeds 3 cm in diameter. Clinical findings are also helpful, as LH commonly presents with diabetes insipidus.

The stalk is usually normal in **pituitary hyperplasia**, although patient age and sex are similar. **Metastasis** usually occurs in older patients with known systemic primary tumor.

Granulomatous hypophysitis may occur secondary to infection, sarcoidosis, or Langerhans cell histiocytosis. Granulomatous hypophysitis is less common than LH, has a different epidemiologic profile, and tends to enhance more heterogeneously. **IgG4-** and **drug-related hypophysitis** is very rare.

Granulomatous Hypophysitis

Granulomatous hypophysitis has different epidemiologic characteristics than LH does. Granulomatous hypophysitis is equally common in both sexes, and there is no association with pregnancy.

Granulomatous hypophysitis can be primary (idiopathic) or secondary. **Secondary granulomatous hypophysitis** is far more common than primary granulomatous hypophysitis and typically results from necrotizing granulomatous inflammation. Infectious/inflammatory secondary granulomatous hypophysitis can be caused by TB, sarcoid, fungal infection, syphilis, Langerhans cell histiocytosis, Wegener granulomatosis, Erdheim-Chester disease, granulomatous autoimmune hypophysitis, ruptured Rathke cleft cyst, or craniopharyngioma. Secondary granulomatous hypophysitis may also occur as a reaction to systemic inflammatory disorders, such as Crohn disease. Imaging findings are nonspecific, resembling those of LH or pituitary adenoma.

Primary granulomatous hypophysitis is a rare inflammatory disease without identifiable infectious organisms. The precise etiology of primary granulomatous hypophysitis is unknown. Nonnecrotizing granulomas with multinucleated giant cells, histiocytes, and various numbers of plasma cells and lymphocytes are typical. Primary granulomatous hypophysitis usually presents with diabetes insipidus. A symmetric sellar mass that enhances strongly but heterogeneously is seen on imaging studies.

Other Hypophysitis Variants

A number of new hypophysitis variants have been recently described. **IgG4-related hypophysitis** has a marked mononuclear infiltrate mainly characterized by increased numbers of IgG4-positive plasma cells. Imaging findings resemble those of lymphocytic infundibuloneurohypophysitis. The pituitary stalk and posterior pituitary lobe are enlarged and enhance intensely following contrast administration.

Drug-related hypophysitis has been reported in cases of cancer immunotherapy with antibodies that stimulate T-cell responses (e.g., ipilimumab) **(25-35)**. Clinicians and radiologists should be aware of autoimmune-induced hypophysitis as a complication of new treatments. Imaging of

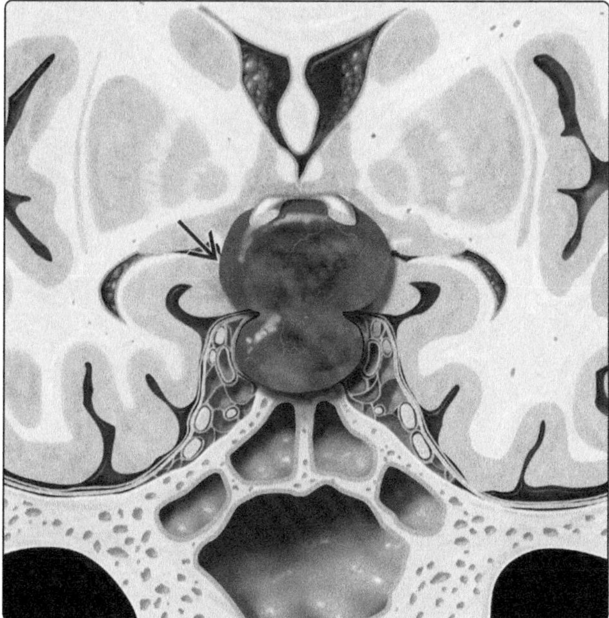

(25-36) Coronal graphic shows a macroadenoma with acute hemorrhage ➾ causing pituitary apoplexy.

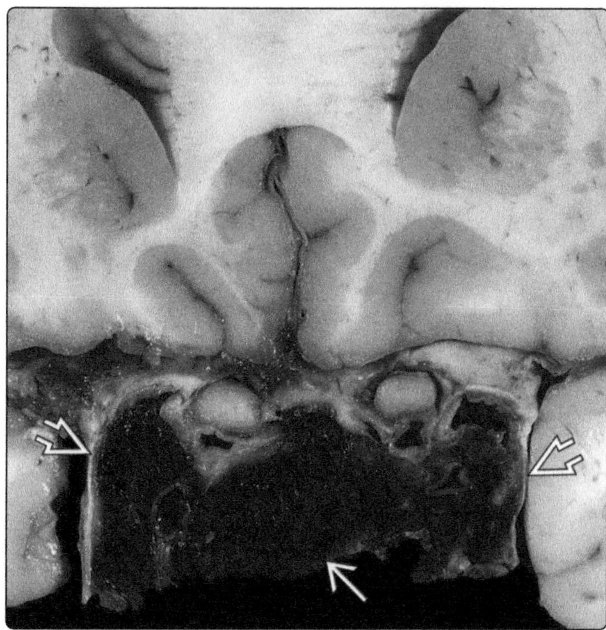

(25-37) Autopsy specimen of pituitary apoplexy shows hemorrhagic macroadenoma ➡ extending into both cavernous sinuses ➡. (Courtesy R. Hewlett, MD.)

drug-related hypophysitis usually shows enlargement of the pituitary gland with or without infundibulum.

Langerhans Cell Histiocytosis

Langerhans cell histiocytosis (LCH) is discussed in detail in Chapter 24. LCH typically presents with diabetes insipidus. The typical patient is < 2 years of age.

The classic imaging of LCH of the pituitary axis is an absent posterior bright spot with a thickened, enhancing pituitary infundibulum. LCH may also present as a sellar and suprasellar mass. The major differential diagnosis of LCH in a child is **germinoma**. In an adult, the major differential diagnosis of LCH affecting the pituitary axis is **neurosarcoid** or **hypophysitis**.

Neurosarcoid

Neurosarcoid is a multisystem inflammatory disease characterized by noncaseating epithelioid-cell granulomas. Neurosarcoid is discussed in more detail in Chapter 15. Neurosarcoid may present as diffuse or focal dural (pachymeningeal) &/or leptomeningeal thickening and enhancement, pituitary infundibulum &/or hypothalamic thickening and enhancement, cranial nerve enhancement, brain parenchymal lesions, or, less commonly, choroid plexus lesions.

The main differential diagnoses for pituitary axis neurosarcoid are lymphocytic hypophysitis, lymphoma, and metastatic disease.

INFUNDIBULAR STALK MASSES

Adults
- Neurosarcoid (isolated stalk lesion rare)
- Hypophysitis ("stalkitis")
- Metastasis
- Lymphoma
- Pituicytoma
- IgG4-related disease

Children
- Germinoma
- Langerhans cell histiocytosis (look for other lesions)
- Ectopic neurohypophysis (displaced PPBS)
- Leukemia

Pituitary Apoplexy

Pituitary apoplexy (PAP) is a well-described acute clinical syndrome with headache, visual defects, and variable endocrine deficiencies. In some cases, profound pituitary insufficiency develops and may become life threatening.

Etiology

PAP is caused by hemorrhage into—or ischemic necrosis of—the pituitary gland **(25-36)**. A preexisting macroadenoma is present in 65-90% of cases **(25-37)**, but PAP can also occur in microadenomas or histologically normal pituitary glands. What precipitates the hemorrhage or necrosis is unknown.

In rare cases, patients undergoing treatment with bromocriptine or cabergoline for pituitary adenoma have

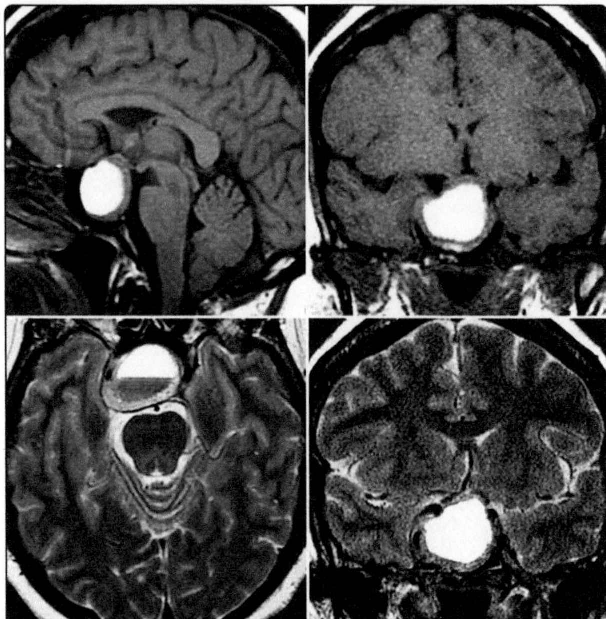

(25-38) Pituitary apoplexy in a 50-year-old woman with 4 days of visual changes shows subacute hemorrhage in the pituitary gland with a blood-fluid level.

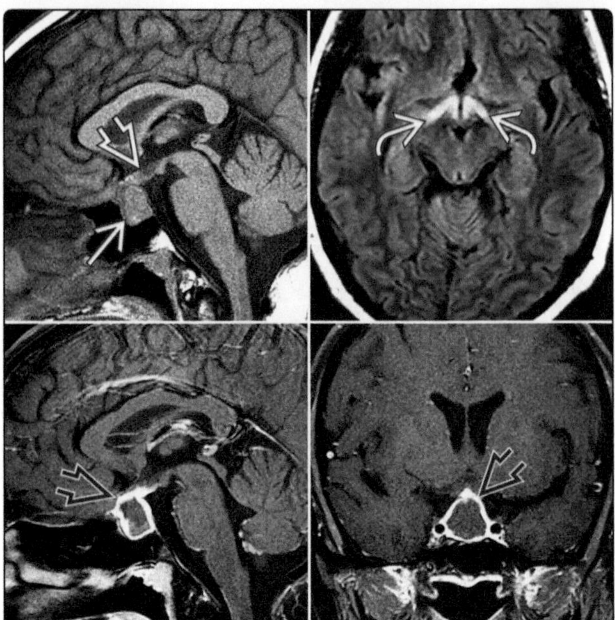

(25-39) (Top left) T1WI shows an enlarged pituitary gland ➡, thick hypothalamus ➡. (Top right) FLAIR hyperintensity is along both optic tracts ➡. (Bottom) Rim enhancement ➡ is shown. This is nonhemorrhagic pituitary apoplexy.

developed life-threatening PAP. More often, this medical therapy results in a subclinical hemorrhage into the adenoma.

Pathology

The most common gross appearance of PAP is that of a large intrasellar or combined intra- and suprasellar mass **(25-36)**. Between 85% and 90% of cases demonstrate gross hemorrhagic infarction **(25-37)**. Nonhemorrhagic ("bland") pituitary infarction causes an enlarged, edematous-appearing pituitary gland. Microscopic features are nonspecific and generally unremarkable.

Clinical Issues

PAP is rare, occurring in ~ 1% of all patients with pituitary macroadenomas. Peak age is 55-60 years. PAP is rare in patients under the age of 15 years. The M:F ratio is 2:1.

Headache is almost universal in patients with PAP and is the most common presenting symptom followed by nausea (80%) and visual field disturbance (70%). Hemorrhagic tumors that extend into the cavernous sinus may compress cranial nerves III, IV, V, and VI. Almost 80% of patients with PAP have panhypopituitarism.

PAP varies from a clinically benign event to catastrophic presentation with permanent neurologic deficits. Coma or even death may ensue in severe cases.

Imaging

An enlarged pituitary gland with peripheral rim enhancement is typical of pituitary apoplexy. Gross intraglandular hemorrhage is common but not invariably present.

NECT scans are often normal. Hemorrhage into the pituitary gland with a hyperdense sellar/suprasellar mass can be identified in 20-25% of cases.

MR is the procedure of choice to evaluate suspected PAP. Signal intensity depends on whether the PAP is hemorrhagic or nonhemorrhagic. Hemorrhage can be identified in 85-90% of cases **(25-38)**.

Signal intensity depends on clot age. Acute PAP is heterogeneously iso- to hypointense to brain on T1WI. Initially iso- to mildly hyperintense on T2WI, PAP rapidly becomes hypointense on T2WI. Acute compression of the hypothalamus and optic chiasm may cause visible edema along the optic tracts on T2/FLAIR scans.

"Blooming"/susceptibility artifact on T2* is common if blood products are present but may be obscured by artifact from the adjacent paranasal sinuses. T1 C+ shows rim enhancement **(25-39)**. Dural thickening and enhancement is seen in 50%, and mucosal thickening in the adjacent sphenoid sinus occurs in 80% of all patients. PAP usually restricts on DWI.

Differential Diagnosis

The major differential diagnosis of PAP is **hemorrhagic macroadenoma**. Focal hemorrhages in adenomas are common, but, in contrast to PAP, the clinical course is typically subacute or chronic. Most adenomas enhance strongly but heterogeneously, whereas PAP demonstrates rim enhancement around a predominantly nonenhancing, expanded pituitary gland.

PITUITARY APOPLEXY

Etiology
- Hemorrhagic or nonhemorrhagic pituitary necrosis
- Preexisting macroadenoma (65-90%)

Clinical Issues
- Sudden onset
- Headache, visual defects
- Hypopituitarism (80%)
- Can be life threatening
- Can result in permanent pituitary insufficiency
- Sheehan syndrome = postpartum pituitary necrosis

Imaging
- Enlarged pituitary
  - ± hemorrhage (85-90%)
- Rim enhancement around nonenhancing gland
- May cause hypothalamic, optic tract edema

Differential Diagnosis
- Hemorrhagic macroadenoma without apoplexy
- Rathke cleft cyst apoplexy
- Pituitary abscess
- Acute thrombosed aneurysm

Pre- and Postoperative Sella

Preoperative Evaluation

Most surgical approaches (transethmoid, transnasal, or transseptal) pass through the sphenoid sinus to reach the sella. Regardless of which operative technique—microscopic or endoscopic—is used, delineating sphenoid sinus anatomy and identifying anatomic variants that might impact surgery are important to successful patient outcome.

CT and MR each has a unique contribution to the full preoperative evaluation of sellar lesions. Multiplanar MR is the procedure of choice to characterize the lesion and define its extent. In concert with MR, preoperative CT helps define relevant bony anatomy.

Location and extent of sphenoid sinus pneumatization as well as the presence and location of bony septa are the major concern. Pneumatization of the planum sphenoidale and dorsum sellae should also be noted. The specific type of pneumatization is generally determined from sagittal MRs.

Postoperative Evaluation

To evaluate the postoperative sella, thin-section, small field-of-view imaging in both the sagittal and coronal planes is mandatory. Precontrast T1- and T2WI images plus postcontrast fat-saturated sequences are standard.

The appearance on postoperative MR scans is complicated by hemorrhage, use of hemostatic agents, packing materials (muscle, fat, fascia lata), and residual tumor. Typical findings include a bony defect in the anterior sphenoid sinus wall, fluid and mucosal thickening in the sinus, fat packing within the sella turcica, hemorrhage, and varying amounts of residual mass effect **(25-40)**.

The first postoperative scan provides the baseline against with which subsequent imaging is compared. With time, hemorrhage evolves and resorbs, fat packing fibroses and retracts, and mass effect decreases. A partially empty sella with or without traction on the infundibular stalk and optic chiasm is typical in the months and years following the initial surgery.

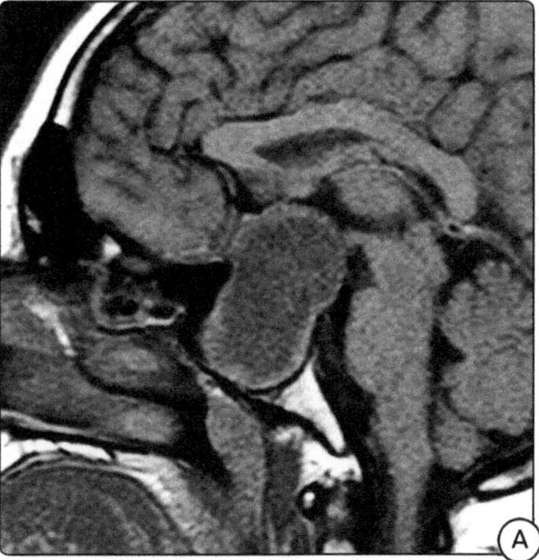

***(25-40A)** Preoperative sagittal T1 MR shows a large sellar/suprasellar solid and cystic mass that expands, erodes, and deepens the sella turcica.*

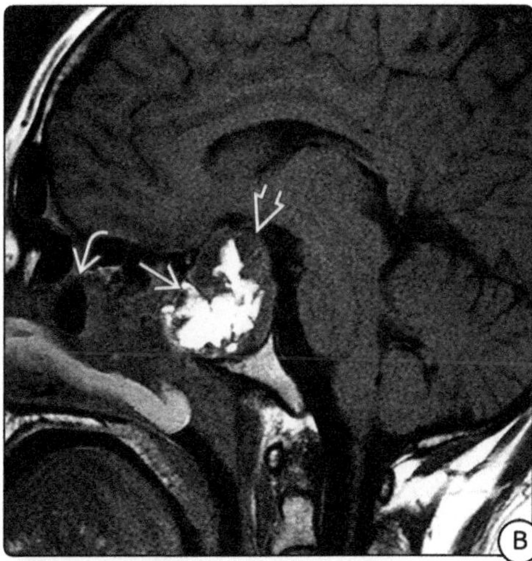

***(25-40B)** Postoperative T1 C+ MR after tumor debulking shows fat packing ➡, residual tumor ➡, and sphenoid air-fluid level ➡.*

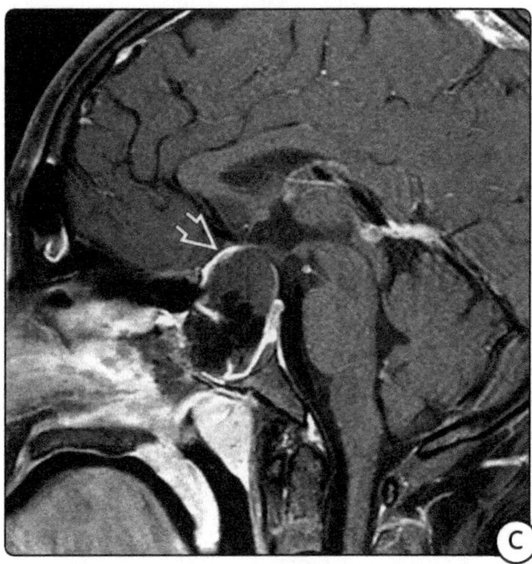

***(25-40C)** T1 C+ FS MR shows suppressed fat and a thin rim of enhancing tissue ➡.*

Complications such as diabetes insipidus, stalk transection, and electrolyte disturbances are usually temporary. Long-term complications include CSF leaks and cranial neuropathy.

Differential Diagnosis of a Sellar Region Mass

In establishing a helpful differential diagnosis of a sellar mass, determining anatomic sublocation is the first, most important step. Is the lesion (1) intrasellar, (2) suprasellar, or (3) in the infundibular stalk? Or is it a combination of these locations?

Whether a sellar/suprasellar mass *is* the pituitary gland itself or is separate from the mass is the most important imaging task and the most helpful finding **(25-41)** **(25-42)** **(25-43)** **(25-44)**. Masses that can be clearly distinguished as separate from the pituitary gland are rarely—if ever—macroadenomas.

The most helpful clinical feature is patient age. Some lesions are common in adults but rarely occur in children. Sex and endocrine status are helpful ancillary clues. For example, pituitary macroadenomas rarely cause diabetes insipidus, but it is one of the most common presenting symptoms of hypophysitis.

Lastly, consider some specific imaging findings. Is the mass cystic? Is it calcified? What is the MR signal intensity? Does the lesion enhance?

Intrasellar Lesions

Intrasellar lesions can be mass-like or non-mass-like. Keep two concepts in mind: (1) Not all "enlarged pituitary glands" are abnormal. Pituitary size and height vary with sex and age. A "fat" pituitary can also occur with intracranial hypotension. (2) Pituitary "incidentalomas" are common (identified in 15-20% of normal MR scans), often cystic microadenomas or Rathke cleft cysts **(25-47)**.

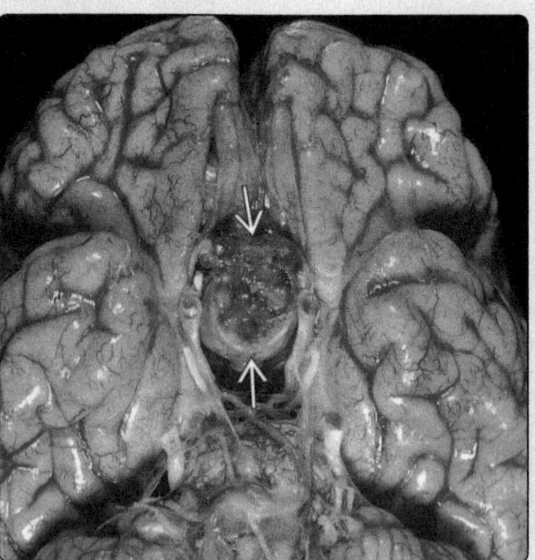

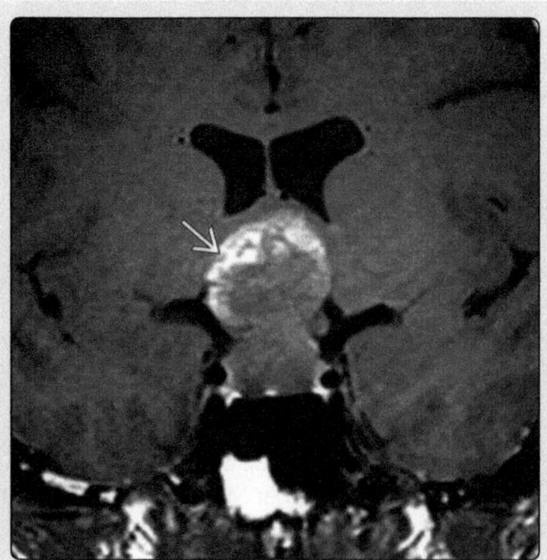

***(25-41)** Submentovertex view of autopsied brain shows large intra- and suprasellar mass ➡. The pituitary gland cannot be separated from the mass and indeed is the mass. (Courtesy R. Hewlett, MD.) **(25-42)** Coronal T1 MR shows the classic "snowman" or "figure 8" shape of a macroadenoma ➡. The mass and pituitary gland are indistinguishable from each other.*

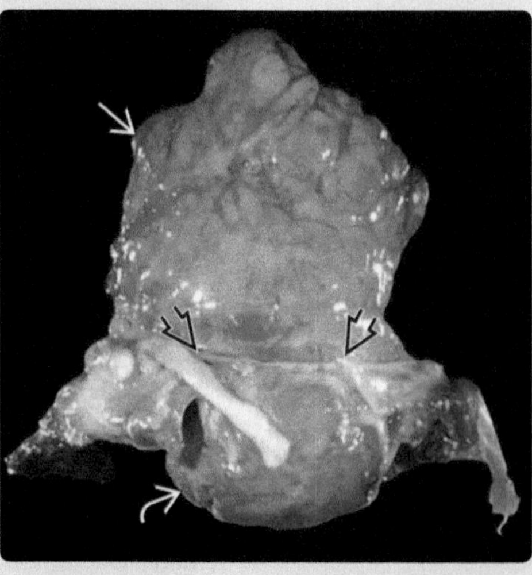

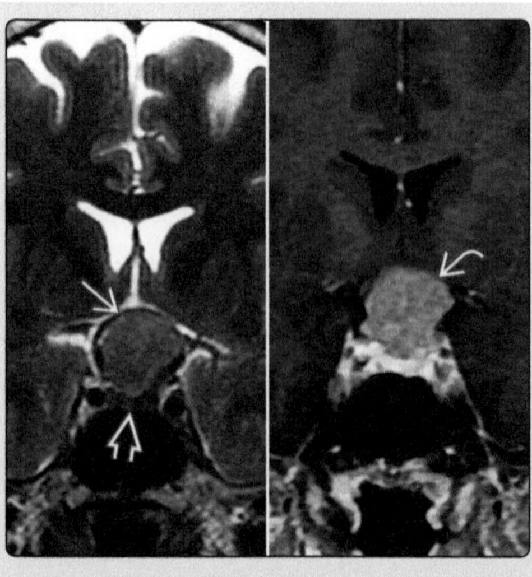

***(25-43)** Coronal view shows autopsied suprasellar meningioma. The tumor ➡ is separated from the pituitary gland below ➡ by the diaphragma sellae ➡ from which the meningioma arose. (Courtesy J. Paltan, MD.) **(25-44)** (L) T2 of meningioma ➡ arising from diaphragma sellae shows the signal intensity is different from underlying normal pituitary gland ➡. (R) T1 C+ FS MR shows the meningioma ➡ does not enhance as strongly as the gland below.*

WHEN THE MASS *CANNOT* BE SEPARATED FROM THE PITUITARY GLAND

Common
- Pituitary macroadenoma
- Pituitary hyperplasia (physiologic, pathologic)

Less Common
- Neurosarcoid
- Langerhans cell histiocytosis
- Hypophysitis

Rare but Important
- Metastasis
- Lymphoma
- Germinoma

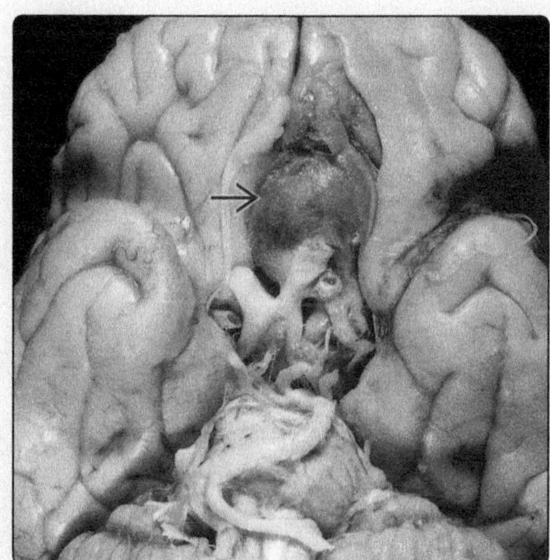

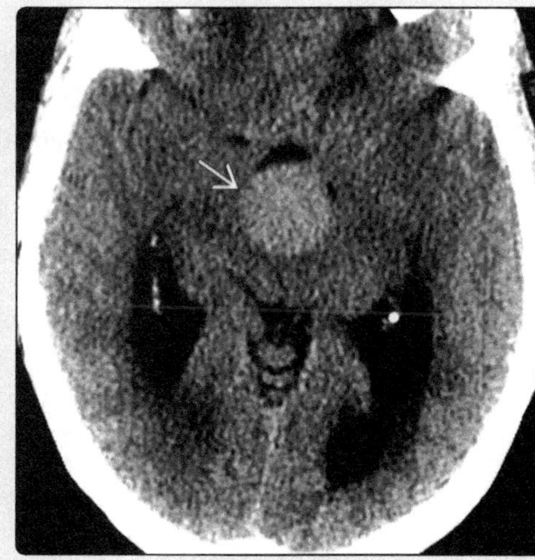

***(25-45)** Autopsy specimen demonstrates an unruptured suprasellar aneurysm ➡. (Courtesy R. Hewlett, MD.) **(25-46)** NECT in a 55-year-old man with headaches shows hyperdense noncalcified mass ➡ in the suprasellar cistern. Considerations in an adult include macroadenoma, meningioma, and aneurysm. This is large basilar tip aneurysm.*

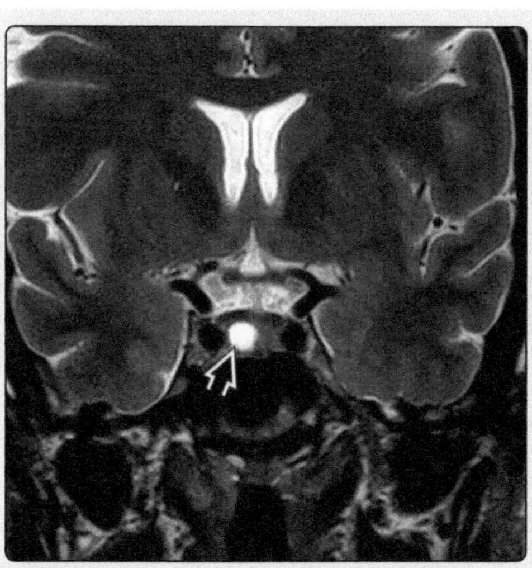

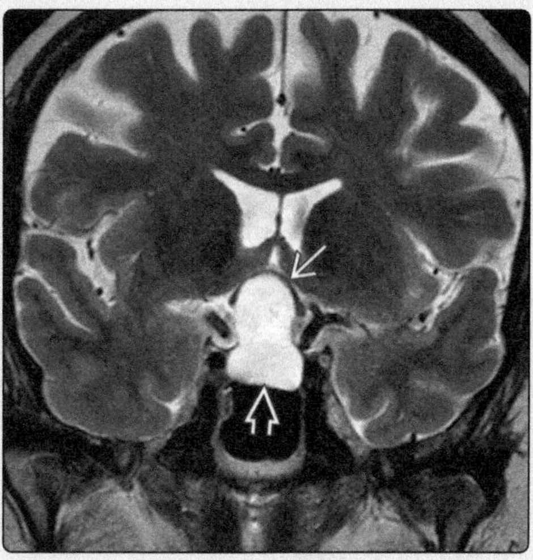

***(25-47)** Coronal T2 MR shows a cystic intrasellar mass ➡ in a young adult with elevated prolactin. Cystic microadenoma was found at resection. Imaging mimics a Rathke cleft cyst. **(25-48)** Coronal T2 MR shows a cystic intra- and suprasellar mass ➡. The optic chiasm ➡ is elevated and draped over the cyst. Arachnoid cyst was found at surgery. ACs follow CSF signal intensity on all MR sequences.*

INTRASELLAR LESION

Common
- Pituitary hyperplasia (physiologic, pathologic)
- Pituitary microadenoma
- Empty sella

Less Common
- Pituitary macroadenoma
- Rathke cleft (or other) cyst
- Craniopharyngioma
- Neurosarcoid

Rare but Important
- Lymphocytic hypophysitis
- Intracranial hypotension (venous congestion)
- Vascular ("kissing" carotids, aneurysm)
- Meningioma
- Metastasis
- Lymphoma

Common Suprasellar Masses

The five most common overall suprasellar masses, i.e., the "Big Five," are pituitary macroadenoma, meningioma, aneurysm, craniopharyngioma, and astrocytoma. Together, they account for 75-80% of all sellar region masses. Three of the "Big Five" (the "Big Three")—adenoma, meningioma, aneurysm—are common in adults but rare in children **(25-45)** **(25-46)**.

COMMON SUPRASELLAR MASSES

Adults
- Pituitary adenoma (mass = gland)
- Meningioma (mass separate from gland)
- Aneurysm ("flow void," pulsation artifact)

Children
- Craniopharyngioma (90% cystic, 90% calcify, 90% enhance)
- Hypothalamic/optic chiasm astrocytoma (solid, no calcification)

Less Common Suprasellar Masses

The presence of some less common lesions can often be inferred from imaging studies **(25-48)**.

LESS COMMON SUPRASELLAR MASSES

- Rathke cleft cyst (well delineated, separate from pituitary)
- Arachnoid cyst (behaves just like CSF)
- Dermoid cyst (looks like fat)
- Neurocysticercosis (usually multiple)

Rare Suprasellar Masses

Keep these lesions in mind—they can mimic more common lesions, but the appropriate treatment differs sharply.

RARE BUT IMPORTANT SUPRASELLAR MASSES

- Hypophysitis (may look like adenoma)
- Hypothalamic hamartoma ("collar button" between stalk, mammillary bodies)
- Metastasis (systemic cancer; look for other lesions)
- Lymphoma (often infiltrates adjacent structures)

Cystic Intra-/Suprasellar Mass

If an intra- or suprasellar mass is primarily or exclusively cystic, the differential diagnosis considerations change. The key issue is to distinguish a cystic mass that originates *within* the sella vs. intrasellar extension *from* a suprasellar lesion **(25-47)**. Other than Rathke cleft cyst, completely intrasellar nonneoplastic cysts are rare, as is a totally intrasellar craniopharyngioma without suprasellar extension.

In a **child** with a suprasellar cystic mass, consider an enlarged third ventricle, craniopharyngioma, neurocysticercosis, and astrocytoma. In an **adult**, consider arachnoid cyst, neurocysticercosis, RCC, adenoma, and aneurysm **(25-48)**.

CYSTIC *INTRA*SELLAR MASS

Common
- Empty sella
- Idiopathic intracranial hypertension

Less Common
- Cystic pituitary adenoma
- Rathke cleft cyst
- Neurocysticercosis cyst

Rare but Important
- Craniopharyngioma
- Epidermoid cyst, arachnoid cyst
- Pituitary apoplexy
- Thrombosed aneurysm

CYSTIC *SUPRA*SELLAR MASS

Common
- Enlarged 3rd ventricle
- Arachnoid cyst
- Craniopharyngioma
- Neurocysticercosis cyst

Less Common
- Rathke cleft cyst
- Dermoid cyst
- Epidermoid cyst

Rare but Important
- Pituitary macroadenoma, apoplexy
- Astrocytoma (usually solid)
- Ependymal cyst
- Aneurysm (patent or thrombosed)

Selected References: The complete reference list is available on the Expert Consult™ eBook version included with purchase.

Miscellaneous Tumors and Tumor-Like Conditions

Some important neoplasms that affect the calvarium, skull base, and cranial meninges are not included in the most recent standardized WHO classification of CNS tumors. This chapter covers several of these intriguing tumors as well as tumor-like lesions that do not easily fit into other sections of this text.

Extracranial Tumors and Tumor-Like Conditions

Fibrous Dysplasia

Fibrous dysplasia (FD) is a benign dysplastic fibroosseous lesion. Abnormal differentiation of osteoblasts results in replacement of normal marrow and cancellous bone by immature "woven" bone and fibrous stroma.

Virtually any bone in the head and neck can be affected by FD. The skull and facial bones are the location of 10-25% of all monostotic FD lesions. The frontal bone is the most common calvarial site followed by the temporal bone, sphenoid, and parietal bones. Involvement of the clivus is rare. The orbit, zygoma, maxilla, and mandible are the most frequent sites in the face.

Pathology

FD lesions range in size from relatively small (< 1 cm) to massive lesions that involve virtually an entire bone. Altered osteogenesis may occur within a single bone ("monostotic FD") or multiple bones ("polyostotic FD"). **Monostotic FD** accounts for ~ 60-80% of all lesions; **polyostotic FD** occurs in 20-40% of cases. Polyostotic FD with endocrinopathy is known as **McCune-Albright syndrome** (MAS) and occurs in 3-5% of cases.

FD is tan to whitish gray **(26-1)**. Fibrous and osseous tissues are admixed in varying proportions. Different stromal patterns can be admixed with the usual fibroblastic elements. These include focal fatty metamorphosis (20-25%), myxoid stroma (15%), and calcifications (12%). Cystic degeneration occurs but is uncommon.

Clinical Issues

Although FD can present at virtually any age, most patients are younger than 30 years at the time of initial diagnosis. Polyostotic FD presents earlier; the mean age is 8 years. FD is rare, representing ~ 1% of all biopsied primary bone tumors.

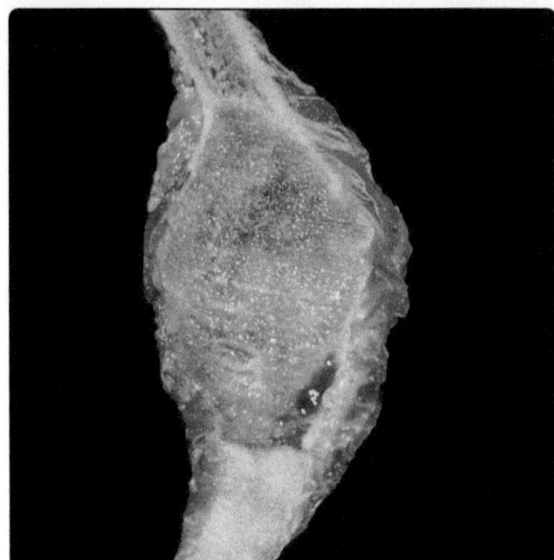

***(26-1)** FD in a rib is a solid tan tumor that expands bone & has ground-glass appearance. (Courtesy A. Rosenberg, MD, G. P. Nielsen, MD.)*

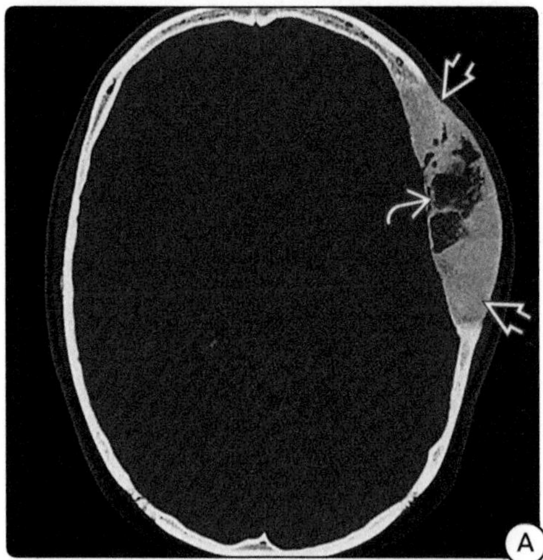

***(26-2A)** Bone CT in a 26y woman shows classic monostotic FD with ground-glass appearance ➡, central noncalcified fibrous stroma ➡.*

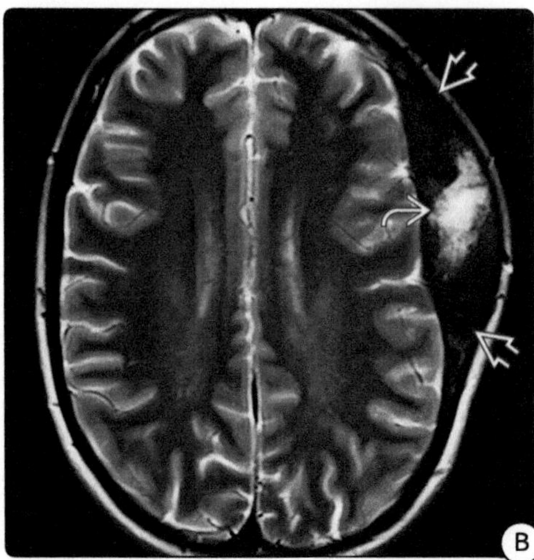

***(26-2B)** T2 MR shows that dense, ossified bone is hypointense ➡, but a central area of active disease is hyperintense ➡.*

Imaging findings depend on disease stage. In general, very early lesions are radiolucent and then undergo progressive calcification, resulting in a ground-glass appearance on bone CT. Mixed patterns are common.

Nonaggressive osseous remodeling and thickening of the affected bone are typical. NECT shows a geographic expansile lesion centered in the medullary cavity. Abrupt transition between the lesion and adjacent normal bone is typical.

Imaging

CT appearance varies with the relative content of fibrous vs. osseous tissue. FD can be sclerotic, cystic, or mixed (sometimes called "pagetoid"). A pattern with mixed areas of radiopacity and radiolucency is found in ~ 1/2 of all cases **(26-2A)**. The classic, relatively homogeneous ground-glass appearance occurs in 25%. Densely sclerotic lesions are common in the skull base. Almost 1/4 of all FD cases have some cystic changes seen as central lucent areas with thinned but sclerotic borders.

FD is usually homogeneously hypointense on T1WI. Signal intensity on T2WI is variable. Moderate hypointensity is characteristic of ossified &/or fibrous portions of the lesion **(26-2B)**. Active lesions may be heterogeneous and may have hyperintense areas on T2 or FLAIR. Cysts appear as rounded high-signal foci.

Signal intensity following contrast administration varies depending on the lesion stage and ranges from no enhancement to diffuse, avid enhancement in active lesions.

Differential Diagnosis

The major differential diagnoses for craniofacial FD are Paget disease and ossifying fibroma (OF).

Paget disease typically occurs in elderly patients and usually involves the calvarium and temporal bone. A cotton wool appearance is typical on digital skull radiographs and bone CT.

Intraosseous meningioma is another differential consideration. Intraosseous meningiomas are more common in the calvarium than in the skull base and facial bones. A strongly enhancing en plaque soft tissue mass is often associated with the bony lesion. A mixed sclerotic-destructive skull base **metastasis** may mimic FD. In most cases, an extracranial primary site is known.

FIBROUS DYSPLASIA: IMAGING AND DDx

Imaging

- CT
  - Bone remodeled, expanded
  - Ground-glass appearance is classic
  - Sclerotic, cystic, mixed ("pagetoid") changes
- MR
  - T1 hypointense, T2 variable (usually hypointense)
  - Enhancement varies from none to intense

Differential Diagnosis

- Paget disease (older patients)
- Ossifying fibroma, other benign fibroosseous lesions
- Intraosseous meningioma
- Renal osteodystrophy

Paget Disease

Paget disease (PaD) of bone, also called osteitis deformans, is the most exaggerated example of abnormal osseous remodeling. PaD is characterized by rapid bone turnover within one or more discrete skeletal lesions.

Pathology

The skull (both calvarium and skull base) is affected in 25-65% of patients **(26-3)**. In contrast to FD, PaD is more commonly polyostotic (65-90% of cases).

The pagetoid skull shows diffuse thickening **(26-4)**. Patches of fibrovascular tissue initially replace fatty marrow.

In the early lytic stage, active PaD is characterized by cellular fibroosseous lesions with minimally calcified osteoid trabeculae. Increased vascularity is common. Osteoblastic rimming is present together with osteoclastic resorptive lacunae.

Malignant transformation to **osteosarcoma** occurs in 0.5-1.0% of cases and is generally seen in patients with widespread disease. Most osteosarcomas are high grade and have already metastasized at the time of diagnosis. Only 15% of patients survive beyond two or three years.

Clinical Issues

Classic PaD is a disease of the elderly. Most patients are 55-85 years of age with < 5% of cases occurring in patients under the age of 40. There is a moderate male predominance.

Presentation varies with location, and all bones of the craniofacial complex can be affected. Patients with calvarial PaD may experience increasing hat size. Cranial neuropathy is common with skull base lesions, most commonly affecting CNVIII. Patients may present with either conductive (ossicular involvement) or sensorineural hearing loss (cochlear involvement or bony compression). Markedly elevated serum alkaline phosphatase is a constant feature, whereas calcium and phosphate levels remain within normal range.

Imaging

Imaging findings in PaD vary with disease stage. In early PaD, radiolucent lesions develop in the calvarium, a condition termed **osteoporosis circumscripta**. Enlarged bone with mixed lytic and sclerotic foci and confluent nodular calcifications follows (the **cotton wool** appearance) in the mixed active stage **(26-5)**. The final inactive or quiescent stage is seen as **dense bony sclerosis**.

Multifocal T1-hypointense lesions replace fatty marrow **(26-6A)**. Signal intensity on T2WI is often heterogeneous **(26-6B)**. Patchy enhancement on T1 C+ can occur in the advancing hypervascular zone of active PaD **(26-6C)**.

Differential Diagnosis

FD may appear very similar to craniofacial PaD. However, PaD occurs mostly in the elderly and does not have the typical ground-glass appearance that often characterizes FD.

Sclerotic metastases may resemble PaD, but no trabecular coarsening or bony enlargement is present. The early lytic phase of PaD may resemble lytic metastases or multiple myeloma; neither enlarges the affected bone.

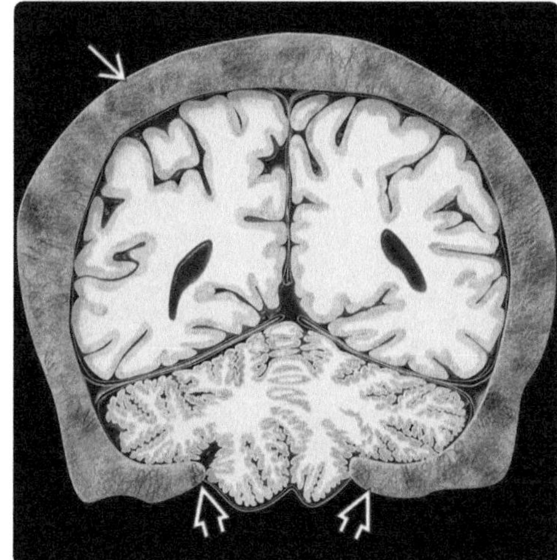

***(26-3)** Graphic shows diffuse Paget disease of the skull with severe diploic widening ➡ and basilar invagination ➡.*

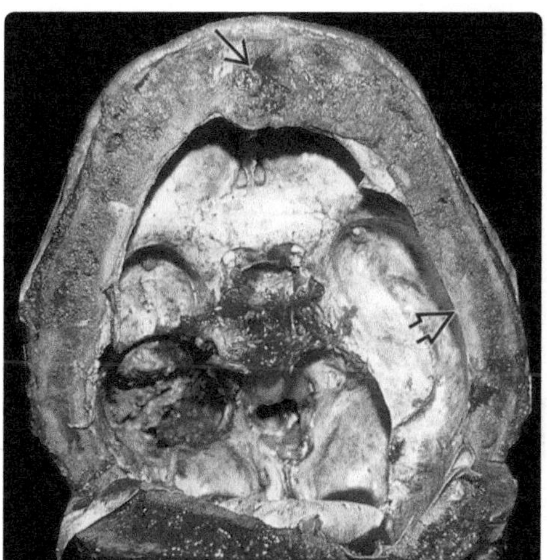

***(26-4)** Autopsied Paget disease shows calvarial thickening with sclerotic bone ➡, patches of fibrovascular tissue ➡. (From Dorfman, 2016.)*

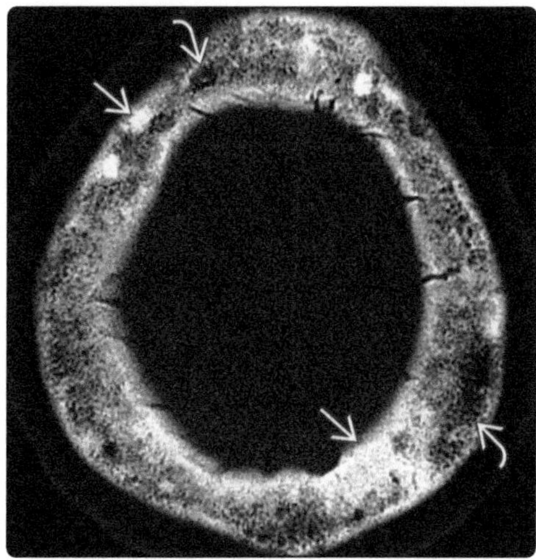

***(26-5)** Bone CT in a 63-year-old woman with Paget disease shows thick calvarium with mixed sclerotic ➡ and lucent areas ➡.*

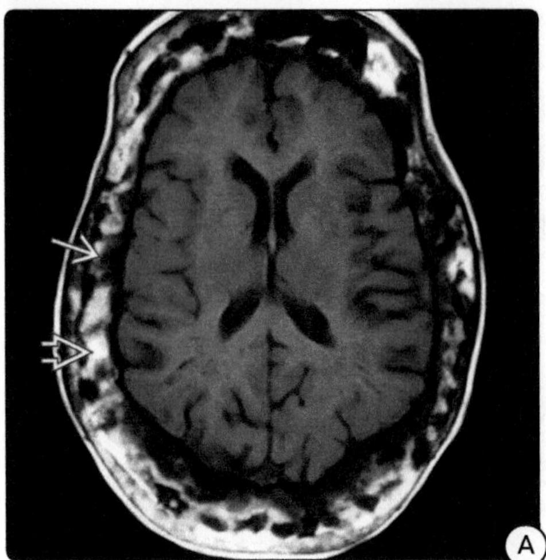

(26-6A) T1 MR shows mixed hyper- ➡, hypointense ➡ diploic lesions in a calvarium massively expanded by Paget disease.

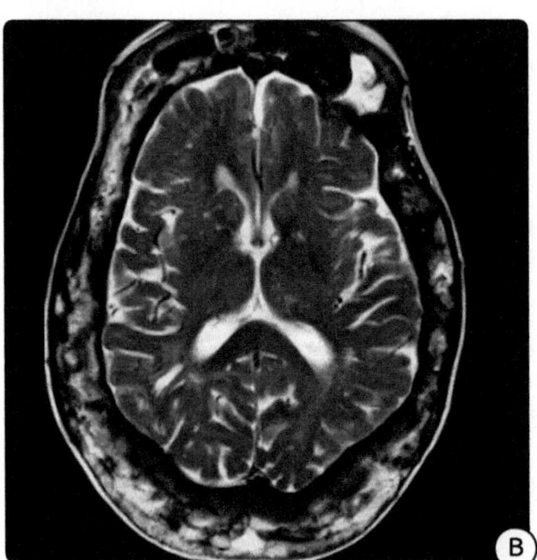

(26-6B) T2 MR in the same case shows the extremely "mottled" heterogeneous appearance of calvarial Paget disease.

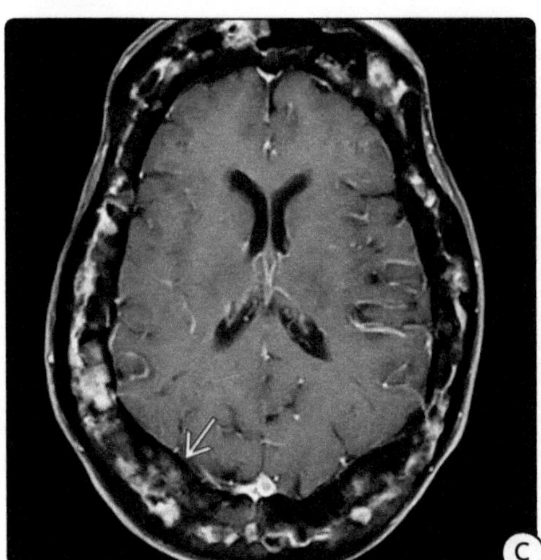

(26-6C) Patchy enhancement ➡ is seen on T1 C+ FS MR, indicating that some active disease is present in this longstanding case.

PAGET DISEASE

Pathology
- Monostotic (65-90%)
- Calvarium, skull base affected (25-60%)
- Fibroosseous tissue replaces fatty marrow

Clinical Issues
- Affects up to 10% of patients > 80 years
- Enlarging skull, CNVIII neuropathy common
- Malignant transformation (0.5-1.0%)
  - Sarcoma > giant cell tumor

Imaging
- Early: Lytic ("osteoporosis circumscripta")
- Mid: Mixed lytic, sclerotic ("cotton wool")
- Late: Dense bony sclerosis

Differential Diagnosis
- Fibrous dysplasia (younger patients)
- Metastases, myeloma

Chordoma

Chordomas are rare, locally aggressive primary malignant neoplasms with a phenotype that recapitulates the notochord.

Etiology

Skull base (clival) chordomas probably arise from the cranial end of primitive notochordal remnants. Subpopulations of cancer stem-like cells have been identified in some chordomas.

Pathology

Chordomas are midline tumors that may arise anywhere along the primitive notochord. The sacrum is the most common site (50% of all chordomas) followed by the sphenooccipital (clival) region (35%) and spine (15%).

Most sphenooccipital chordomas are midline lesions **(26-7)**. Occasionally, a chordoma is predominantly extraosseous and arises off-midline, usually in the nasopharynx or cavernous sinus.

Three major histologic forms of chordoma are recognized: Conventional ("classic"), chondroid, and dedifferentiated. Conventional chordoma is the most common type and consists of physaliphorous cells that contain mucin and glycogen vacuoles, giving a characteristic bubbly appearance to its cytoplasm.

Chondroid chordomas have stromal elements that resemble hyaline cartilage with neoplastic cells nestled within lacunae. Dedifferentiated chordoma represents < 5% of chordomas and typically occurs in the sacrococcygeal region, not the clivus, and is associated with dismal prognosis.

Clinical Issues

Chordomas account for 2-5% of all primary bone tumors but cause almost 40% of sacral tumors. Although chordomas may occur at any age, peak prevalence is between the fourth and sixth decades. There is a moderate male predominance.

Clival chordomas (CCh) typically present with headaches and diplopia secondary to CNVI compression. Large chordomas may cause multiple cranial neuropathies, including visual loss and facial pain. Although they grow slowly, chordomas are eventually lethal unless treated with aggressive resection and proton beam irradiation. The overall 5-year survival rate of patients following radical resection is 75%.

Imaging

NECT shows a relatively well-circumscribed, moderately hyperdense midline or paramedian clival mass with permeative lytic bony changes **(26-8A)**. Intratumoral calcifications generally represent sequestrations from destroyed bone **(26-9A)**.

Chordomas exhibit substantial heterogeneity on MR. Most conventional chordomas are typically intermediate to low signal intensity on T1WI. On sagittal images, a "thumb" of tumor tissue is often seen extending posteriorly through the cortex of the clivus and indenting the pons **(26-9B)**.

Conventional chordomas are very hyperintense on T2WI **(26-9C)**, reflecting high fluid content within the physaliphorous cells. Intratumoral calcifications and hemorrhage may cause foci of decreased signal within the overall hyperintense mass. Moderate to marked but heterogeneous enhancement is typical after contrast administration **(26-8B)**.

Differential Diagnosis

A large **invasive pituitary macroadenoma** can mimic CCh. CChs typically displace but do not invade the pituitary gland, whereas macroadenomas cannot be identified separate from the gland.

Signal intensity of a **skull base chondrosarcoma** is very similar to that of CCh. Chondrosarcomas typically arise off-midline, along the petrooccipital fissure. **Ecchordosis physaliphora (EP)** is a rare nonneoplastic notochordal remnant that may arise anywhere from the skull base to the sacrum. Most are small and found incidentally at autopsy or imaging. They usually lie just in front of the pons and have a thin stalk-like connection to a smaller intraclival component.

Skull base **metastases** and **plasmacytoma** are destructive lesions that are usually isointense with brain on all sequences. Predominantly intraosseous **meningioma** is rare in the skull base. It usually causes sclerosis and hyperostosis rather than a permeative destructive pattern.

EP is a small (usually < 1 cm) gelatinous soft tissue mass that represents an ectopic notochordal remnant. Best demonstrated on MR, EPs are hypointense to brain on T1WI and hyperintense relative to CSF on T2WI. The key imaging feature of EP that distinguishes it from chordoma and other similar-appearing lesions is the presence of a small pedicle or stalk that connects the clival lesion to an intradural component in the prepontine cistern.

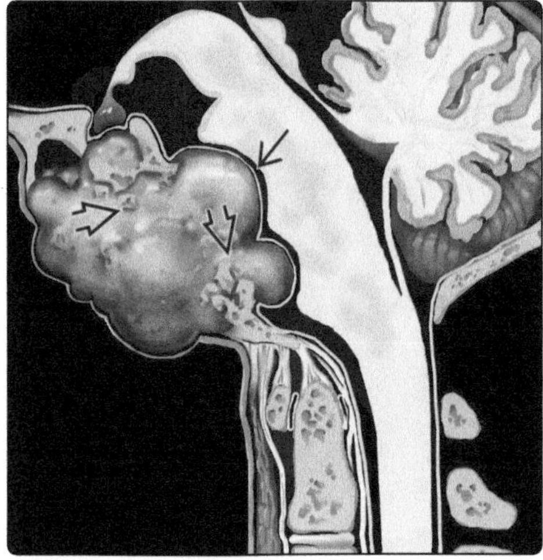

***(26-7)** Destructive, lobulated clival mass has a "thumb" of tumor ➙ indenting pons. Note the bone fragments ➙ "floating" in the chordoma.*

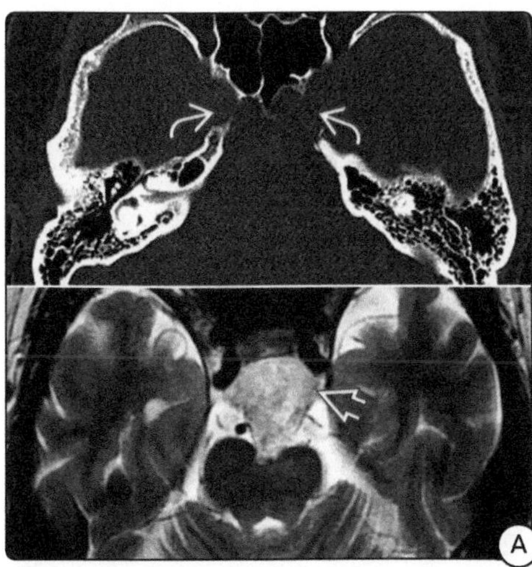

***(26-8A)** (Top) Bone CT shows destructive central skull base lesion ➙. (Bottom) Lesion ➙ is T2 hyperintense.*

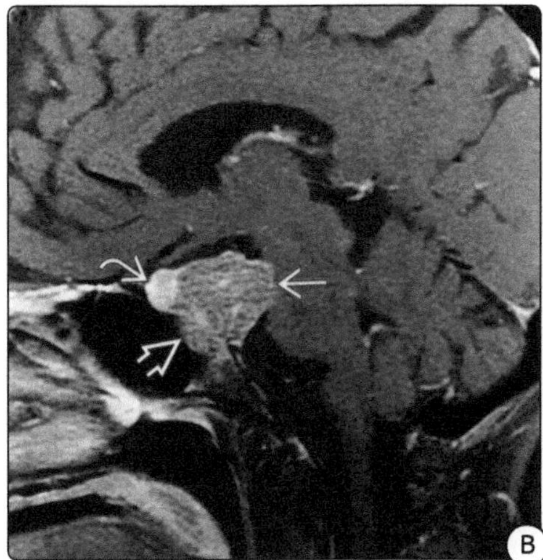

***(26-8B)** T1 C+ FS shows destructive enhancing mass ➙ displaces pituitary gland anteriorly ➙, indents the pons posteriorly ➙. This is chordoma.*

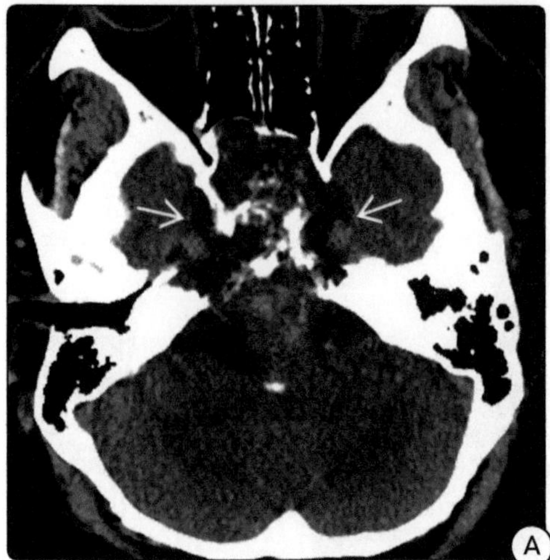

(26-9A) NECT in 39y man with multiple cranial nerve palsies shows destructive, heterogeneous-appearing central skull base mass ➡.

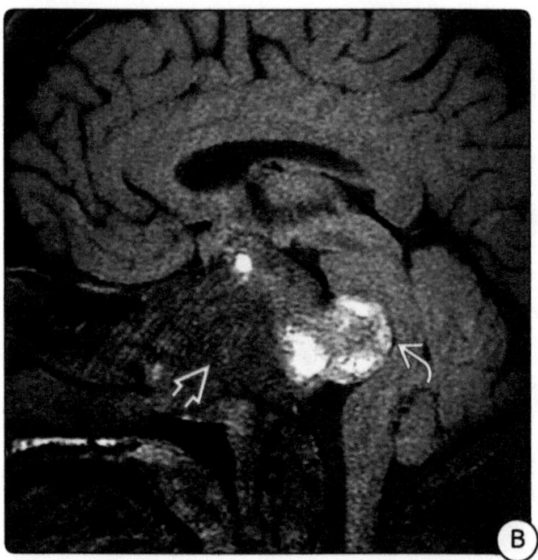

(26-9B) Sagittal T1 FS shows that the mass has destroyed almost the entire sphenoid bone ➡ with "thumb" of tumor ➡ indenting the pons.

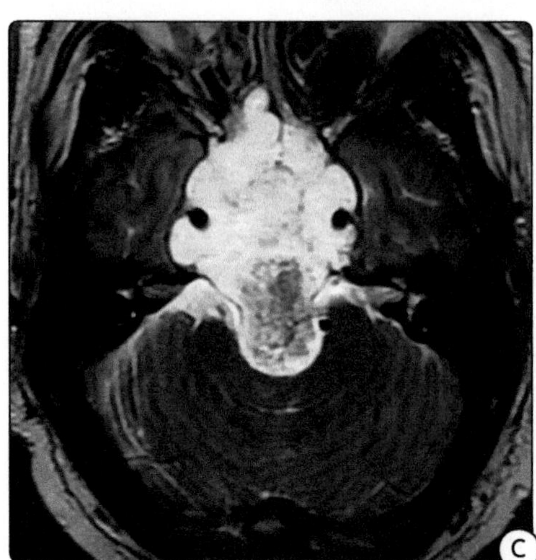

(26-9C) The lobulated mass is very hyperintense and displaces both carotid arteries and the basilar artery. This is conventional chordoma.

CHORDOMA

Etiology
- Arises from cranial end of primitive notochordal remnants

Pathology
- Typically midline
  - 50% sacrum
  - 35% sphenooccipital (clivus)
  - 15% vertebral body
- 3 types
  - Typical ("classic") with physaliphorous cells
  - Chondroid
  - Dedifferentiated (< 5%, usually sacral)

Clinical Features
- Any age but peak = 4th-6th decades
- Cranial neuropathies

Imaging Findings
- CT
  - Permeative destructive central skull base lesion
  - Often contains sequestered bony fragments
- MR
  - T1 hypointense
  - T2 hyperintense
  - "Thumb" of tumor extends posteriorly, indents pons
  - Usually moderate enhancement
  - Variable

Differential Diagnosis
- Invasive pituitary macroadenoma
  - Look for displaced but intact gland
- Chondrosarcoma
  - Typically off-midline
  - Petrooccipital fissure
- Ecchordosis physaliphora

Intracranial Pseudoneoplasms

Textiloma

Terminology

Textiloma refers to a mass created by a retained surgical element (inadvertently or deliberately left behind) and its associated foreign body inflammatory reaction. The terms "gossypiboma," "gauzoma," and "muslinoma" refer specifically to retained nonresorbable cotton or woven materials.

Etiology

Hemostatic agents can be resorbable or nonresorbable. All classes of resorbable and nonresorbable agents may produce textilomas as an allergic response.

Resorbable agents include gelatin sponge, oxidized cellulose, and microfibrillar collagen. Nonresorbable agents include various forms of cotton pledgets, cloth (i.e., muslin), and synthetic rayon. Although bioabsorbable hemostats are often left in place, nonresorbable agents are typically removed prior to surgical closure. Any of these materials may induce an inflammatory reaction, creating a textiloma.

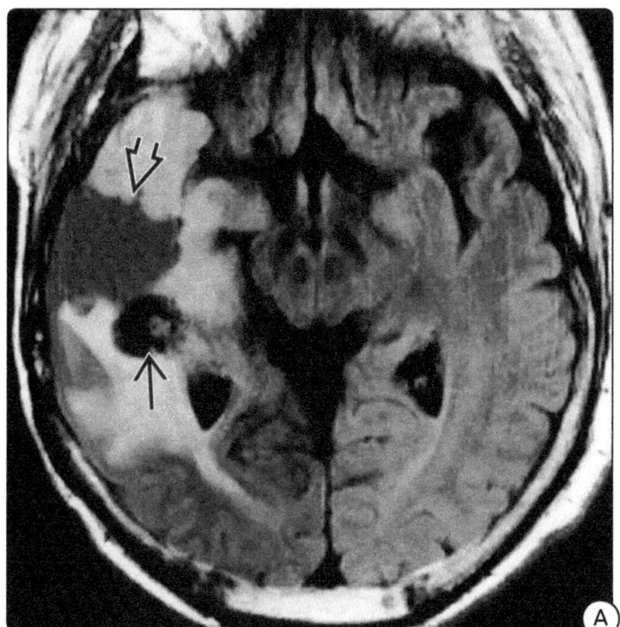

(26-10A) Axial FLAIR MR shows a hypointense mass ➡ adjacent to the tumor resection cavity ⇨.

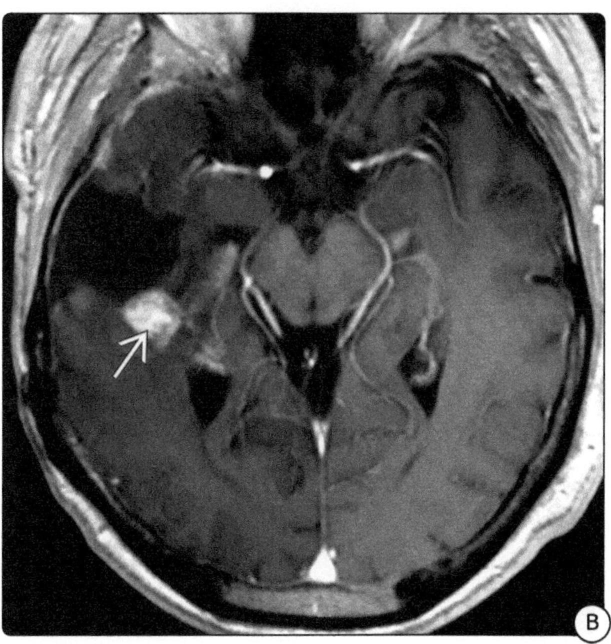

(26-10B) The lesion ➡ demonstrates solid but heterogeneous enhancement on T1 C+ FS MR.

Textilomas are uncommon. The highest reported prevalence is following abdominal and orthopedic surgery. Intracranial textilomas are rare with < 75 reported cases.

Pathology

Hemostatic elements that are introduced into the CNS occasionally induce an excessive inflammatory reaction. Most textilomas occur within surgical resection sites or around muslin-reinforced aneurysms.

Histologic examination typically shows a core of degenerating inert hemostatic agent surrounded by inflammatory reaction. Foreign body giant cells and histiocytes are often present. Each agent exhibits distinctive histologic features, often permitting specific identification.

Imaging

Intracranial textilomas are almost always iso- or hypointense on T1WI. Approximately 45% are iso- and 40% are hypointense on T2/FLAIR **(26-10A)**. Some "blooming" on T2* may be present. All reported cases of textiloma enhance on postcontrast scans. Ring and heterogeneous solid enhancement patterns occur almost equally **(26-10B)**.

Differential Diagnosis

The major differential diagnosis is **recurrent neoplasm** or **radiation necrosis**. Residual or recurrent tumor can coexist with textiloma. If present, T2 hypointensity helps distinguish textiloma from neoplasm or **abscess**. Definitive diagnosis typically requires biopsy and histologic examination with both routine stains and polarized light.

Calcifying Pseudoneoplasm of the Neuraxis

Terminology

Calcifying pseudoneoplasm of the neuraxis (CAPNON) is a rare but distinctive nonneoplastic lesion of the CNS. Calcifying pseudoneoplasms are also known as fibroosseous lesions, cerebral calculi, "brain stones," and "brain rocks."

Etiology

CAPNONs have been characterized as foreign body reactions with giant cells, tissue ossification, and the formation of lamellar bone or scattered psammoma bodies. The surrounding brain often exhibits inflammatory changes with gliosis and edema leading to mass effect.

Pathology

CAPNONs are nonneoplastic, noninflammatory lesions. They are discrete intra- or extraaxial masses that contain various combinations of chondromyxoid and fibrovascular stroma, metaplastic calcification, and ossification.

Positive immunoreactivity to vimentin and epithelial membrane antigen (EMA) are typical. GFAP and S100 protein are typically negative, helping distinguish CAPNON from astrocytic neoplasms and meningioma.

Clinical Issues

Intracranial CAPNONs are usually asymptomatic and discovered incidentally on imaging studies, although seizures and headache have been reported. A few cases have been

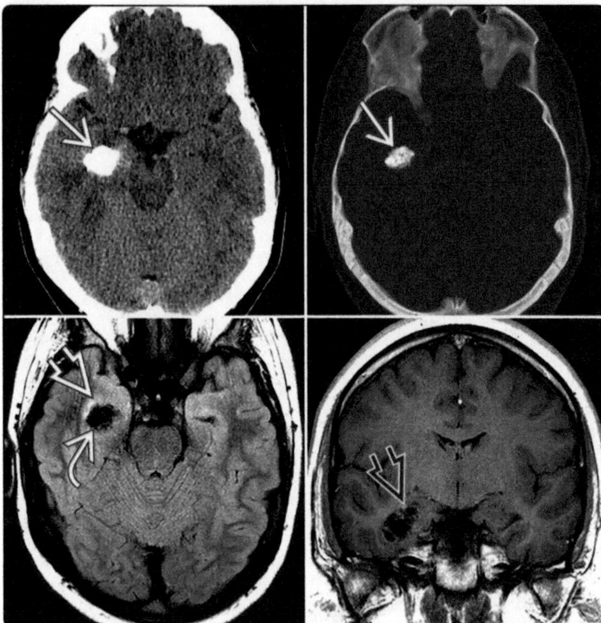

***(26-11)** NECT (upper L) and bone CT (upper R) show densely calcified mass ➡. FLAIR (lower L) shows that hypointense mass ➡ is surrounded by edema ➡ and does not enhance ➡ (lower R). This is CAPNON. (Courtesy S. Blaser, MD.)*

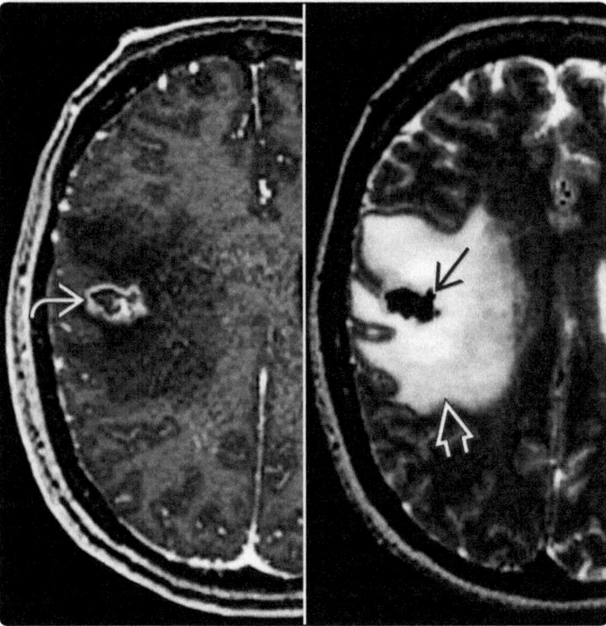

***(26-12)** Sometimes surgically proven CAPNONs are extremely hypointense on T2WI ➡, incite intense edema ➡, and exhibit rim enhancement ➡. (Courtesy B. K. Kleinschmidt-DeMasters, MD.)*

reported in association with meningioangiomatosis and neurofibromatosis type 2.

Imaging

NECT scans demonstrate a densely calcified leptomeningeal, deep intrasulcal, or brain parenchymal "rock." The temporal lobe is the most common site **(26-11)**.

On MR, CAPNONs demonstrate little mass effect, are isointense on T1WI, and are uniformly hypointense on T2WI and FLAIR. Mild "blooming" is seen on T2* GRE. Perilesional edema varies from none to extensive. Enhancement varies from none to moderate. Solid, linear, serpiginous, and peripheral rim-like enhancement patterns have all been reported **(26-12)**.

Differential Diagnosis

The differential diagnosis of CAPNON includes an ossified vascular lesion—most often a **cavernous malformation**—and densely calcified neoplasm, such as **oligodendroglioma, meningioma**, and **choroid plexus papilloma** with osseous metaplasia. Although cavernous malformations can often be distinguished by their "popcorn" mixed hyperintensity on T2WI, biopsy is usually necessary for definitive diagnosis.

INTRACRANIAL PSEUDOTUMORS

Textiloma
- Foreign body reaction
  - Usually to hemostatic elements
  - Other = introduced embolic materials
- Iso-/hypointense on T2WI
- Ring, heterogeneous enhancement on T1 C+

Calcifying Pseudoneoplasm of the Neuraxis (CAPNON)
- Chondrocalcific or ossified mass
  - Usually in sulcus
- Very hypointense on T2/FLAIR
- Enhancement varies (none to rim-like)

Selected References: The complete reference list is available on the Expert Consult™ eBook version included with purchase.

Metastases and Paraneoplastic Syndromes

Up to 40% of all patients with advanced cancers (particularly lung and breast) will eventually develop CNS involvement. Brain metastases are often ultimately responsible for patient mortality, even in the face of controlled systemic disease.

We begin the chapter with a brief overview of CNS metastases, then follow with a discussion of cranial metastases by anatomic location, beginning with the brain parenchyma (the most common overall CNS location). We conclude with remote effects of cancer on the CNS, so-called paraneoplastic syndromes.

Metastatic Lesions

Metastases are secondary tumors that arise from primary neoplasms at another site. As a group, metastases are now the most common CNS neoplasm in adults.

Overview

Etiology

Routes of Spread. CNS metastases can arise from both extra- and intracranial primary tumors. Metastases from **extracranial primary neoplasms** ("body-to-brain metastases") most commonly spread via **hematogeneous dissemination**.

Direct geographic extension from a lesion in an adjacent structure (such as squamous cell carcinoma in the nasopharynx) also occurs but is much less common than hematogeneous spread. Invasion is usually through natural foramina and fissures where bone is thin or absent. **Perineural** and **perivascular spread** are less common but important direct geographic routes by which head and neck tumors gain access to the CNS.

Primary intracranial neoplasms sometimes spread from one CNS site to another, causing brain-to-brain or brain-to-spine metastases. Spread occurs preferentially along compact white matter tracts, such as the corpus callosum and internal capsule, but can also involve the ventricular ependyma, pia, and perivascular spaces.

CSF dissemination with "carcinomatous meningitis" occurs with both extra- and intracranial primary neoplasms.

Origin of CNS Metastases. Both the source and location of metastases vary significantly with patient age. Approximately 10% of all brain metastases originate from an unknown primary neoplasm at the time of initial diagnosis.

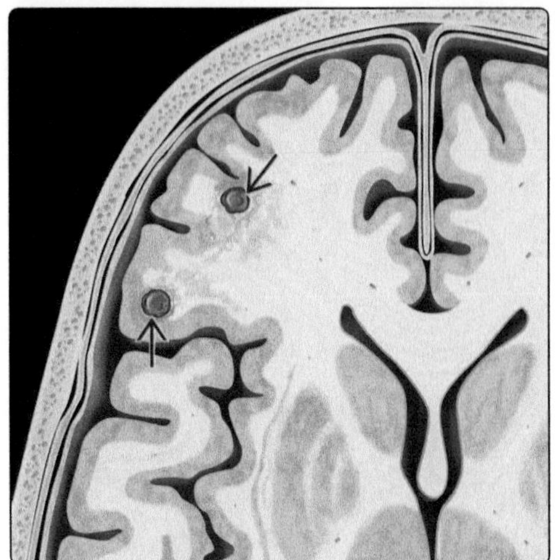

***(27-1)** Graphic shows parenchymal metastases ➡ at GM-WM junction, the most common site. Most metastases are round, not infiltrating.*

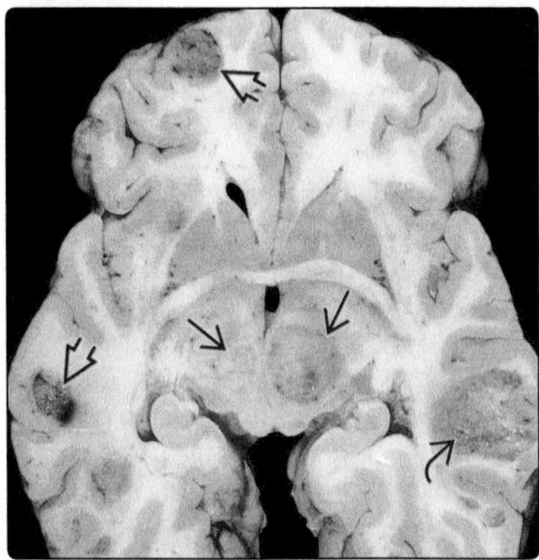

***(27-2)** Multiple metastases shown, some with hemorrhage ➡ or necrosis ➡. Midbrain lesions are gray-tan ➡. (Courtesy R. Hewlett, MD.)*

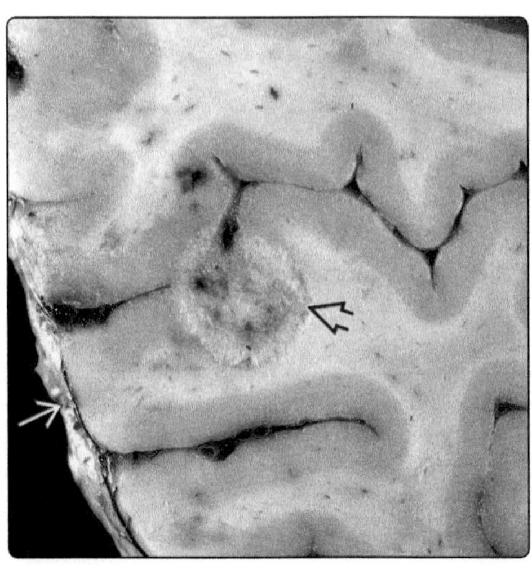

***(27-3)** Metastases are often at depths of sulci ➡. This specimen also has pial metastases ➡.*

Children. The most common sources of cranial metastases in children are hematologic malignancies, such as leukemia and lymphoma. The preferential locations are the skull and dura. Parenchymal metastases are much less common in children compared with adults.

Adults. Lung, breast, and melanoma account for at least 2/3 of all brain metastases in adults. The most common primary tumor that metastasizes to the brain is lung cancer. Breast is the second most common primary tumor source followed by melanoma, renal carcinoma, and colorectal cancer.

Skull, dura, and spine metastases are typically caused by prostate, breast, or lung cancer followed by hematologic malignancies and renal cancers.

CNS METASTASES: EPIDEMIOLOGY AND ETIOLOGY

Epidemiology

- Adults > > children
  - Metastases = most common CNS neoplasm in adults
  - 5x increase in past 50 years
  - Brain metastases occur in > 30-40% of cancer patients

Routes of Spread

- Most common = extracranial primary to CNS via
  - Hematogeneous dissemination
  - Direct geographic extension (nasopharynx, sinuses)
  - Perineural, perivascular spread
- Less common
  - Brain to brain from CNS primary
  - Brain to CSF from CNS primary
- Least common
  - Tumor-to-tumor metastasis
  - Sometimes called "collision tumor"
  - Most common "donor" tumor = breast, lung
  - Most common "recipient" tumor = meningioma

Origin

- 10% unknown primary at initial diagnosis
  - Children: Leukemia, lymphoma, sarcoma
  - Adults: Lung, breast cancer, melanoma, renal carcinoma, colorectal cancer

Pathology

Location. The brain parenchyma is the most common site (80%) followed by the skull and dura (15%). Diffuse leptomeningeal (pial) and subarachnoid space infiltration is relatively uncommon, accounting for just 5% of all cases.

The vast majority of parenchymal metastases are located in the cerebral hemispheres, especially at the junction between the cortex and subcortical white matter **(27-1) (27-2)**. Only 15% of metastases are found in the cerebellum.

Uncommon sites include the pons and midbrain, choroid plexus, ventricular ependyma, pituitary gland/stalk, and retinal choroid. Rarely, tumor cells diffusely infiltrate the brain perivascular spaces, a process termed "carcinomatous encephalitis."

Size and Number. Most parenchymal metastases are between a few millimeters and 1.5 cm. Large hemispheric metastases are rare. In contrast, skull and dural metastases can become very large.

Approximately 50% of metastases are solitary while 50% are multiple. About 20% of patients have two lesions, 30% have three or more, and only 5% have more than five lesions.

Gross Pathology

Parenchymal Metastases. Parenchymal metastases are focal round, relatively circumscribed lesions that exhibit sharp borders with the adjacent brain **(27-3)**. Diffusely infiltrating parenchymal metastases are rare. Peritumoral edema, necrosis, hemorrhage, and mass effect range from none to striking.

Skull/Dural Metastases. Calvarial and skull base metastases are typically destructive, poorly marginated lesions **(27-4)** **(27-5)**.

Dural metastases usually occur in combination with adjacent skull lesions, appearing as focal nodules **(27-6)** or more diffuse, plaque-like sheets of tumor. Dural metastasis without skull involvement is much less common.

Leptomeningeal Metastases. The term "leptomeningeal metastases" actually describes metastases to the subarachnoid spaces and pia **(27-7)**. Diffuse sugar-like coating of the pia is typical **(27-8)**. Multiple nodular deposits and infiltration of the perivascular (Virchow-Robin) spaces with extension into the adjacent cortex may occur **(27-9)**.

Microscopic Features. Although metastases may display more marked mitoses and elevated labeling indices compared with their primary systemic source, they generally preserve the same cellular features.

CNS METASTASES: PATHOLOGY

Location
- Adults
  - Brain (80%, cerebral hemispheres > > cerebellum)
  - Skull/dura (15%)
  - Pia ("leptomeningeal"), CSF (5%)
  - Other (1%)
- Children
  - Skull/dura > > brain parenchyma

Size
- Parenchymal metastases
  - Microscopic to a few centimeters (most 0.5-1.5 cm)
- Skull/dura metastases
  - Variable; can become very large

Number
- Solitary (50%)
- 2 lesions (20%)
- ≥ 3 lesions (30%)
  - Only 5% have > 5 lesions

Gross Pathology
- Round, well circumscribed > > > infiltrating
- Variable edema, necrosis, hemorrhage

Microscopic Features
- Preserves general features of primary tumor
- May have more mitoses, elevated labeling indices

Clinical Issues

Demographics. Up to 40% of patients with treated systemic cancers eventually develop brain metastases. Peak prevalence is in patients over 65 years of age. Only 6-10% of children with extracranial malignancies develop brain metastases.

Presentation. Seizure and focal neurologic deficit are the most common presenting symptoms of parenchymal metastases. Half of all patients with

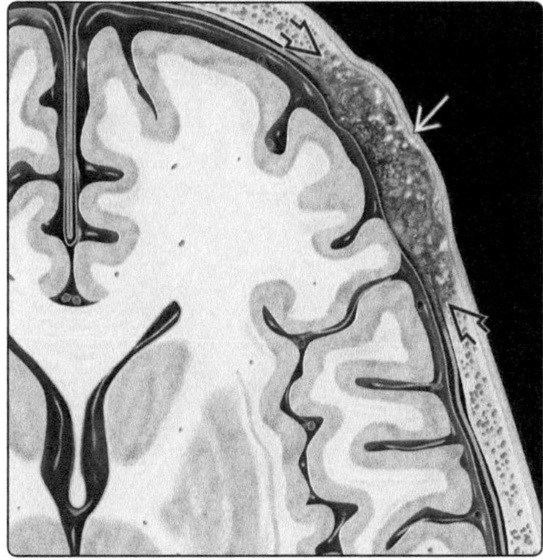

***(27-4)** Graphic shows skull metastasis ➡ expanding diploic space, invading/thickening the underlying dura (light blue linear structure) ⇨.*

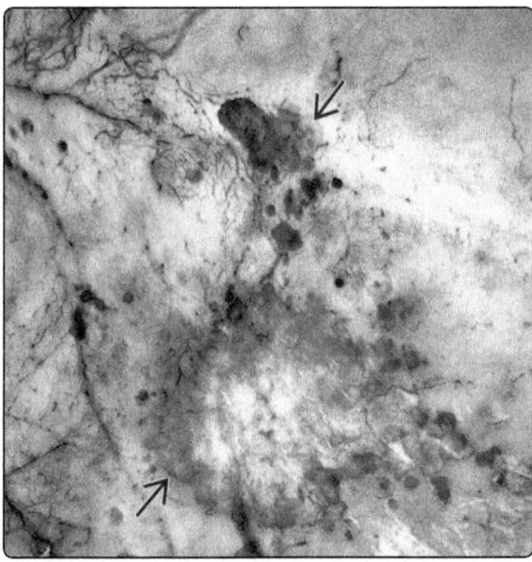

***(27-5)** Skull metastases are seen here as permeative, lytic, and destructive lesions ⇨.*

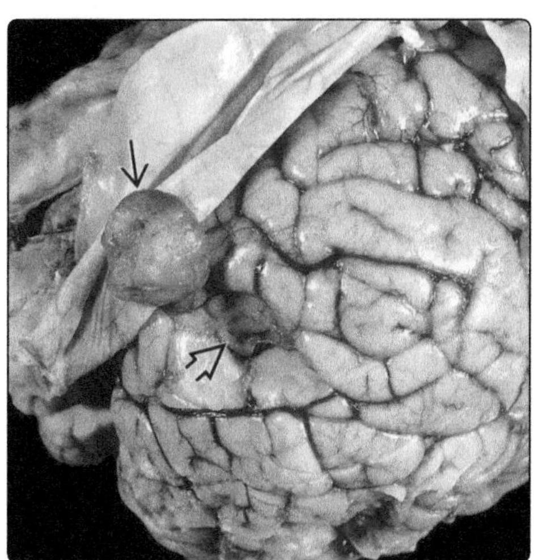

***(27-6)** Solitary dural metastasis ⇨ indents the brain ⇨ and appears identical to a meningioma. (Courtesy R. Hewlett, MD.)*

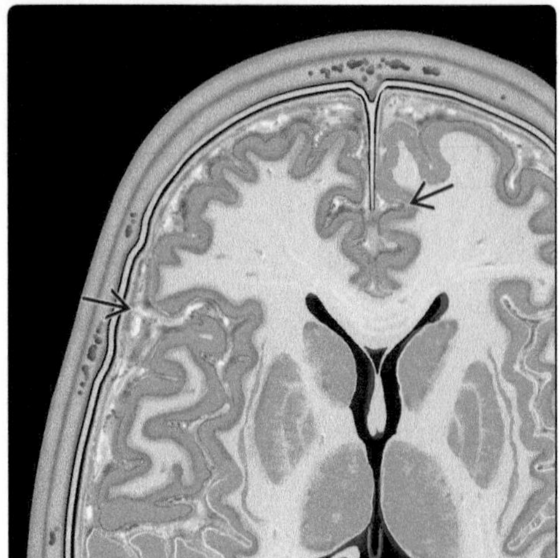

(27-7) Graphic depicts "sugar icing" appearance of leptomeningeal metastases ➡ covering the brain and extending into the sulci.

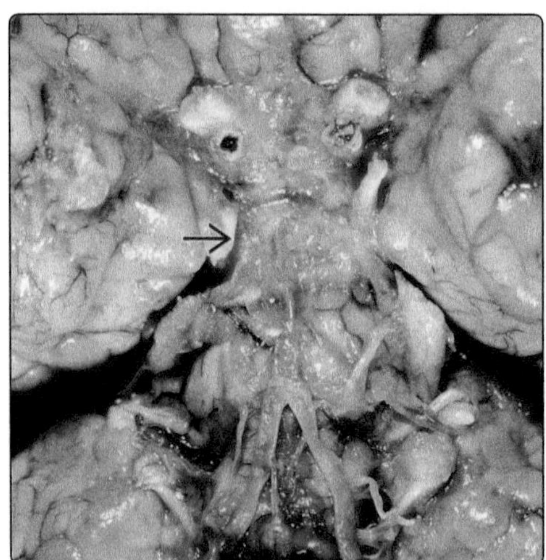

(27-8) Pia-subarachnoid ("leptomeningeal") metastases coat the brain, fill the subarachnoid cisterns ➡. (Courtesy R. Hewlett, MD.)

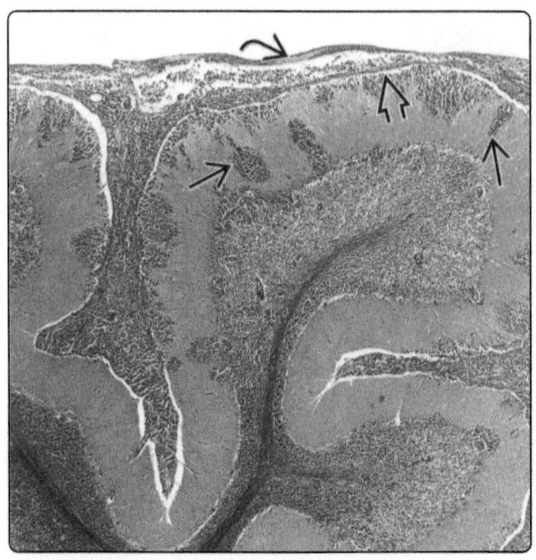

(27-9) Mets fill space between the arachnoid ➡ and pia ➡ and extend along perivascular spaces into cortex ➡. (Courtesy P. Burger, MD.)

skull/dural metastases present with headache. Seizure, sensory or motor deficit, cranial neuropathy, or a palpable mass under the scalp are other common symptoms.

Natural History. The natural history of parenchymal metastases is grim. Relentless progressive increase in both number and size of metastases is typical. Median survival after diagnosis is short, generally averaging between 3 and 6 months.

Imaging

Imaging findings and differential diagnosis vary with metastasis location. Each anatomic site has special features; each is discussed separately in this chapter.

Parenchymal Metastases

Imaging

CT Findings. Most metastases are iso- to slightly hypodense relative to gray matter on NECT **(27-10A)**. With the exception of treated metastases, calcification is rare. Occasionally, the first manifestation of an intracranial metastasis is a brain bleed **(27-11)**.

The vast majority of parenchymal metastases enhance strongly following contrast administration **(27-10B)**. Double-dose delayed scans may increase lesion conspicuity. Solid, punctate, nodular, or ring patterns can be seen.

MR Findings

T1WI. Most metastases are iso- to mildly hypointense on T1WI. The exception is melanoma metastasis, which has intrinsic T1 shortening and thus appears moderately hyperintense **(27-13)**. Subacute hemorrhagic metastases show disordered, heterogeneous signal intensity, often with bizarre-appearing intermixed foci of T1 hyper- and hypointensities.

T2/FLAIR. Signal intensity on T2WI varies widely depending on tumor type, lesion cellularity, presence of hemorrhagic residua, and amount of peritumoral edema. Many metastases are hypointense on T2WI and FLAIR **(27-12A)**. Exceptions are mucinous tumors, cystic metastases, and tumors with large amounts of central necrosis, all of which can appear moderately hyperintense.

Some hyperintense metastases show little or no surrounding edema. Multiple small hyperintense metastases ("miliary metastases") can be mistaken for small vessel vascular disease unless contrast is administered.

T2*. Both subacute hemorrhage and melanin cause prominent signal intensity loss ("blooming") on T2* (GRE, SWI) images **(27-13B)**.

T1 C+. Virtually all nonhemorrhagic metastases enhance following contrast administration **(27-12B)**. Patterns vary from solid, uniform enhancement to nodular, "cyst + nodule," and ring-like lesions. Multiple metastases in the same patient may exhibit different patterns.

DWI, MRS. DWI is variable but metastases generally do not exhibit restricted diffusion. Some highly cellular tumors show low ADC values. MRS may show a prominent lipid peak.

Differential Diagnosis

The major differential diagnosis for punctate and ring-enhancing metastases is abscess. **Abscesses** and **septic emboli** typically restrict on DWI. Primary neoplasms like **glioblastoma** tend to be infiltrating, whereas metastases are almost always round and relatively well demarcated.

Both metastases and **multiple embolic infarcts** share a predilection for arterial "border zones" and the gray matter-white matter interfaces. Most acute infarcts restrict strongly on DWI and rarely demonstrate a ring-enhancing pattern on T1 C+ scans. Chronic infarcts and age-related microvascular disease are hyperintense on T2WI and do not enhance following contrast administration.

Multiple cavernous malformations can mimic hemorrhagic metastases but are typically surrounded by a complete hemosiderin rim. **Multiple sclerosis** occurs in younger patients and is preferentially located in the deep periventricular white matter, not the gray matter-white matter interface.

Primary infratentorial parenchymal brain tumors in adults are rare. No matter what the imaging findings are, *a solitary cerebellar mass in a middle-aged or older adult should be considered a metastasis until proven otherwise!*

PARENCHYMAL METASTASES: IMAGING AND DDx

CT
- Variable density (most iso-, hypodense)
- Most enhance on CECT
- Perform bone CT for calvarial, skull base metastases

T1WI
- Most metastases: Iso- to slightly hypointense
- Melanoma metastases: Hyperintense
- Hemorrhagic metastases: Heterogeneously hyperintense

T2/FLAIR
- Varies with tumor type, cellularity, hemorrhage
- Most common: Iso- to mildly hyperintense
- Can resemble small vessel vascular disease

T2*
- Subacute blood, melanin "bloom"

T1 C+
- Almost all nonhemorrhagic metastases enhance strongly
- Solid, punctate, ring, "cyst + nodule"

DWI
- Variable; most common: No restriction
- Highly cellular metastases may restrict

MRS
- Most prominent feature: Lipid peak
- Elevated Cho, depressed/absent Cr

Differential Diagnosis
- Most common
  - Abscess
  - Septic emboli
- Less common
  - Glioblastoma
  - Multiple embolic infarcts
  - Small vessel (microvascular) disease
  - Demyelinating disease
  - Multiple cavernous malformations

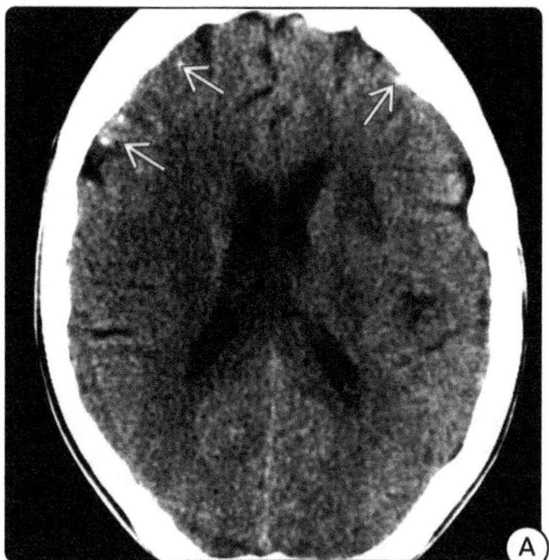

***(27-10A)** Axial NECT in a 63-year-old woman with known breast carcinoma shows a few scattered bifrontal hyperdensities ➡.*

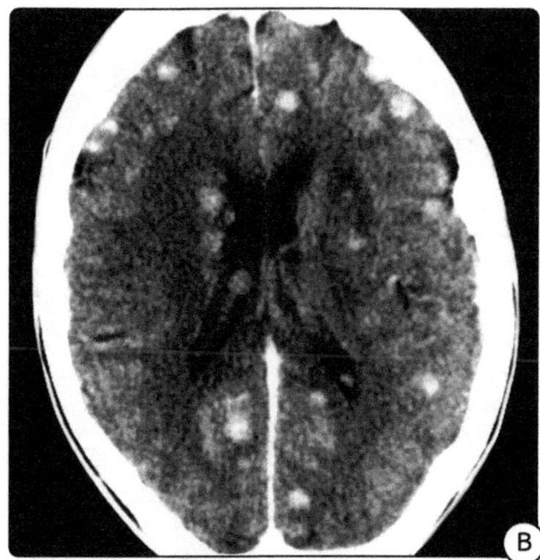

***(27-10B)** CECT shows "too numerous to count" enhancing metastases, most of which were invisible on the precontrast study.*

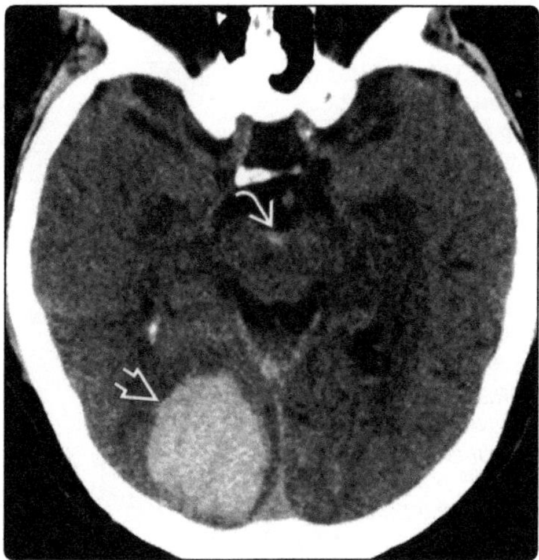

***(27-11)** NECT in 74yF with headache shows hematoma ➡, subarachnoid hemorrhage ➡. Renal cell carcinoma met, unknown at diagnosis.*

Skull and Dural Metastases

Terminology

The term "skull" refers both to the calvarium and to the skull base. As one cannot distinguish neoplastic involvement of the periosteal vs. meningeal dural layers, we refer to these layers collectively as the "dura." In actuality, the arachnoid—the outermost layer of the leptomeninges—adheres to the dura, so it too is almost always involved any time tumor invades the dura.

Overview

The skull and dura are the second most common sites of CNS metastases from extracranial primary tumors. Calvarial and skull base metastases can occur either with or without dural involvement.

In contrast, dural metastases without coexisting calvarial lesions are less common. Between 8-10% of patients with advanced systemic cancer have dural metastases. Breast (35%) and prostate (15-20%) cancers are the most frequent sources. Single lesions are slightly more common than multiple dural metastases.

Imaging

General Features. Solitary or multiple focal lesions involve the skull, dura (and underlying arachnoid), or both. A less common pattern is diffuse neoplastic dura-arachnoid thickening, seen as a curvilinear layer of tumor that follows the inner table of the calvarium.

CT Findings. Complete evaluation requires *both* soft tissue and bone algorithm reconstructions of the imaging data **(27-14)**. Scans with soft tissue reconstruction obscure skull lesions, which may be invisible unless bone algorithms are utilized.

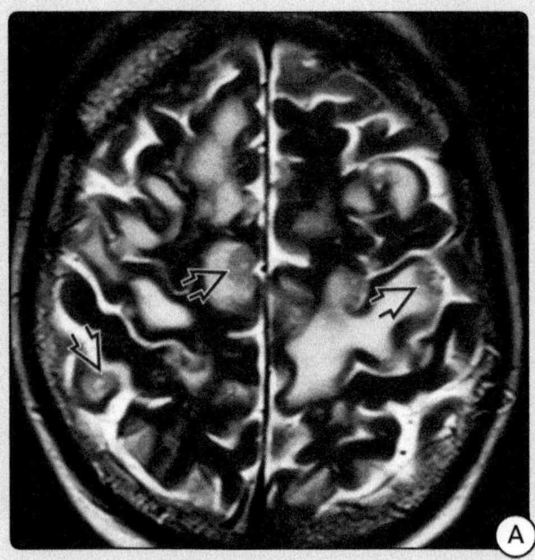

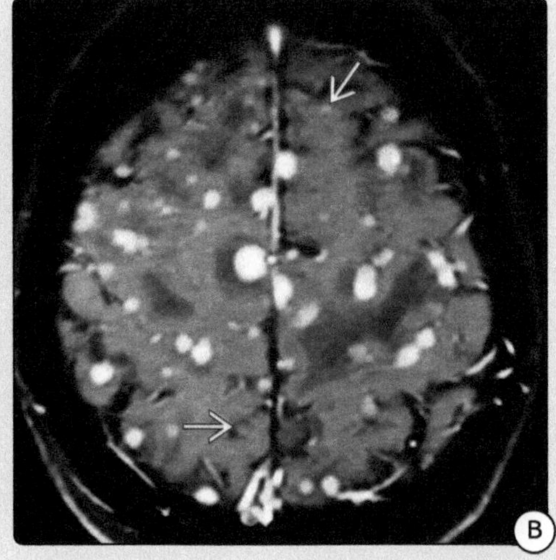

***(27-12A)** A 63-year-old man with a urogenital primary carcinoma presented with seizure. T2 MR shows multiple iso- to slightly hyperintense nodules at the GM-WM interfaces ⇨ surrounded by edema. **(27-12B)** The lesions enhance intensely on T1 C+ FS. A number of tiny enhancing foci ➡ that were not seen on T2 or FLAIR are identified.*

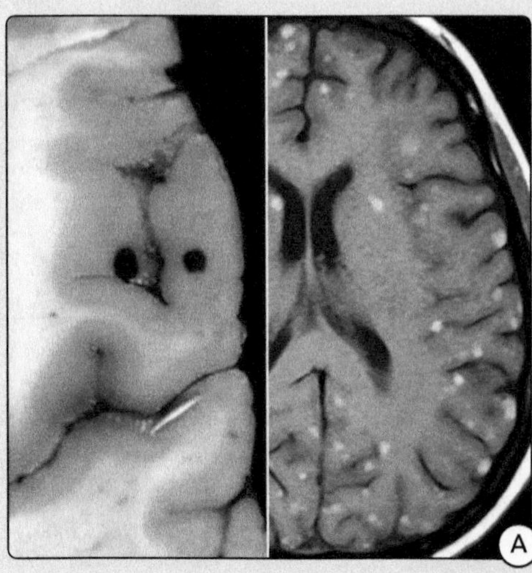

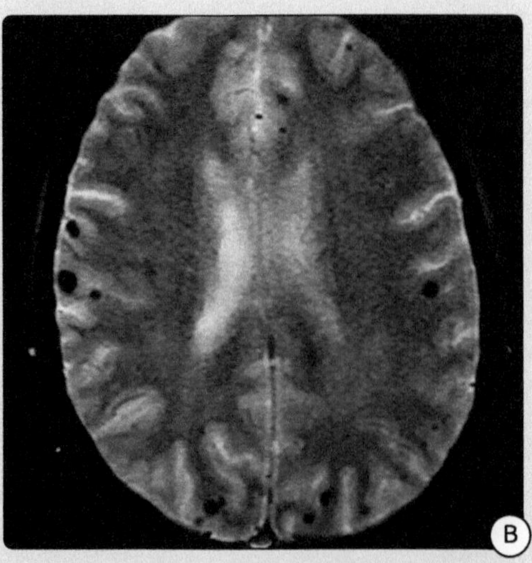

***(27-13A)** (L) Autopsy shows round black nodules in the cortex, GM-WM interface. This is melanoma metastasis. (Courtesy R. Hewlett, MD.) (R) T1 MR in a patient with metastatic melanoma shows innumerable hyperintense metastases. **(27-13B)** T2* GRE in same patient shows that only a few of the metastases visible on the T1 MR "bloom," indicating that most of the T1 shortening was secondary to melanin, not subacute hemorrhage.*

Soft tissue scans viewed with bone windows do not provide sufficient detail for adequate assessment.

NECT. Large dural metastases displace the brain inward, buckling the gray matter-white matter interface medially **(27-15)**. Hypodensities in the underlying brain suggest parenchymal invasion or venous ischemia.

Bone CT usually demonstrates one or more relatively circumscribed intraosseous lesions. Permeative, diffusely destructive lesions are the second most common pattern **(27-14)**. A few osseous metastases—mostly those from prostate and treated breast cancer—can be blastic and sclerotic.

CECT. The most common finding is a focal soft tissue mass centered on the diploic space. A biconvex shape with both subgaleal and dural extension is typical **(27-14)**. Most dural metastases enhance strongly.

MR Findings

T1WI. Hyperintense fat in the diploic space provides excellent, naturally occurring demarcation from skull metastases. Metastases replace hyperintense yellow marrow and appear as hypointense infiltrating foci **(27-15)**. Dural metastases thicken the dura-arachnoid and are typically iso- or hypointense to underlying cortex **(27-16)** **(27-17)**.

T2/FLAIR. Most skull metastases are hyperintense to marrow on T2WI, but the signal intensity of dural metastases varies. FLAIR hyperintensity in the underlying sulci suggests pia-subarachnoid tumor spread. Hyperintensity in the underlying brain is present in 1/2 of all cases and suggests either tumor invasion along the perivascular spaces or compromise of venous drainage.

T1 C+. Nearly 70% of dural metastases are accompanied by metastases in the overlying skull **(27-16)**. Involvement of the adjacent scalp is also common. Contrast-enhanced T1WI

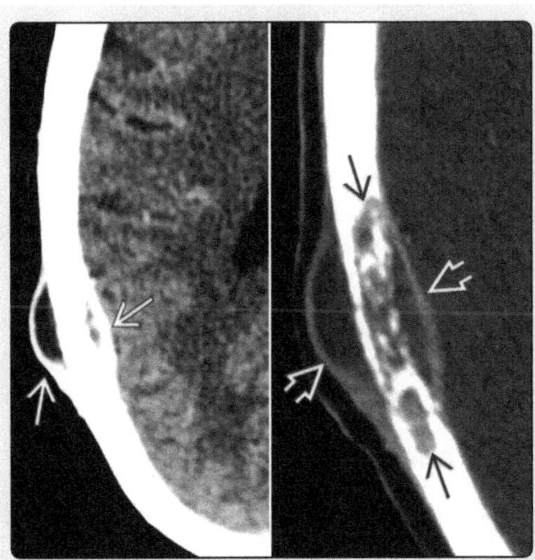

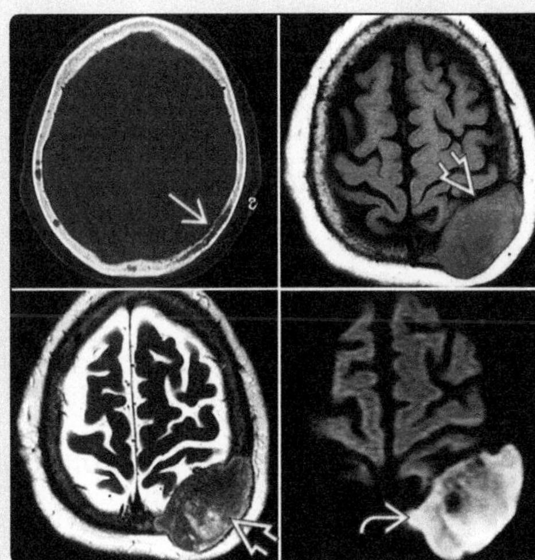

(27-14) (L) CECT with soft tissue windows shows a lesion ➡ centered on diploic space of calvarium. (R) Intermediate windows show extent of the lytic, destructive metastasis ➡, better delineate the subgaleal and extradural components ➡. (27-15) Metastatic breast carcinoma to the skull, dura is seen as a permeative destructive lesion in the left parietal diploë ➡. Lesion is mostly isointense to brain on T1-, T2WI ➡ and restricts on DWI ➡.

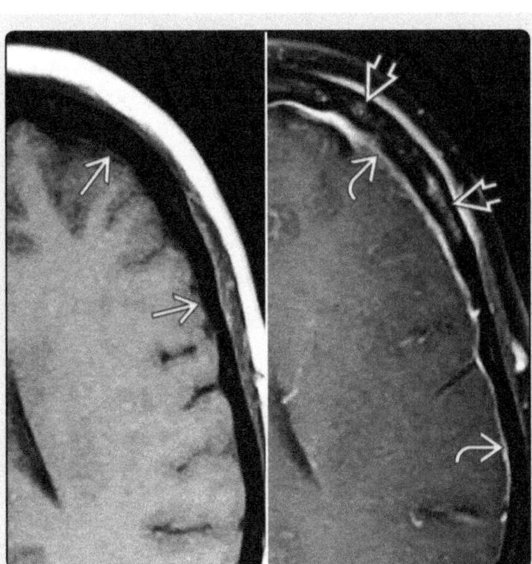

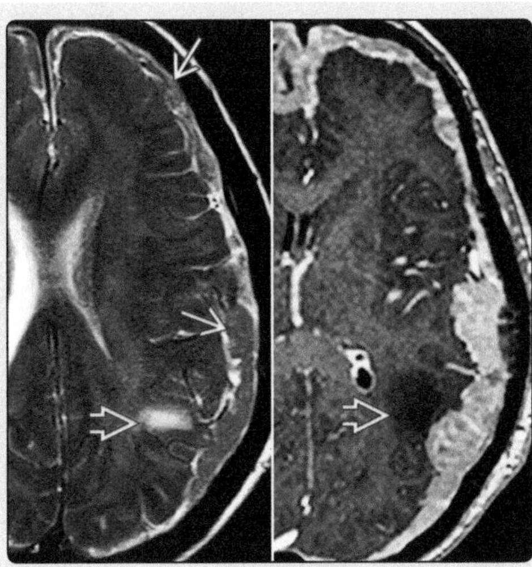

(27-16) (L) Subtle dura-arachnoid metastasis is seen as mild thickening ➡. (R) Thickened dura ➡ enhances on T1 C+ FS MR. Enhancing lesions in the diploic space can now be identified ➡. (27-17) Metastases from prostate cancer thicken the dura, fill the subarachnoid space ➡. Edema ➡ indicates infiltration along the perivascular spaces into the brain parenchyma. (Courtesy N. Agarwal, MD.)

should be performed with fat saturation (T1 C+ FS) for optimal delineation, as some calvarial lesions may enhance just enough to become isointense with fat.

Most dural metastases enhance strongly, appearing as biconvex masses centered along the adjacent diploic space **(27-15)**. Dural "tails" are present in ~ 1/2 of all cases. Frank tumor invasion into the underlying brain is seen in 1/3 of cases **(27-17)**. Dural thickening can be smooth and diffuse or nodular and mass-like.

DWI. Hypercellular metastases with enlarged nuclei and reduced extracellular matrix may show diffusion restriction (hyperintense) and decreased ADC values (hypointense).

SKULL/DURA METASTASES

General Features
- 2nd most common site of CNS metastases
- Skull alone or skull + dura > > isolated dural metastases
- "Dural" metastases: Usually dura *plus* arachnoid!

CT
- Use both soft tissue, bone reconstructions
- Skull: Permeative lytic lesion(s)
- Scalp, dura: Biconvex mass centered on skull

MR
- T1WI: Metastases replace hyperintense fat
- T2WI: Most skull metastases are hyperintense
- FLAIR: Look for
  - Underlying sulcal hyperintensity (suggests pia-subarachnoid space tumor)
  - Parenchymal hyperintensity (suggests brain invasion along perivascular spaces)
- T1 C+
  - Use fat-saturation sequence
  - Skull/scalp/dural lesion(s) can be focal or diffuse, enhance strongly
  - "Dural tail" sign (50%)
  - Less common: Diffuse dura-arachnoid thickening ("lumpy-bumpy" or smooth)
- DWI: Hypercellular metastases may restrict

Differential Diagnosis
- Skull metastases
  - Surgical defect, venous lakes/arachnoid granulations
  - Myeloma
  - Osteomyelitis
- Dural metastases
  - Meningioma (solitary or multiple)

Differential Diagnosis

The major differential diagnoses for skull metastases are surgical defects and normal structures. A **surgical defect**, such as a burr hole or craniotomy, can be distinguished from a metastasis by clinical history and the presence of defects in the overlying scalp. **Venous lakes, vascular grooves, arachnoid granulations**, and sometimes even **sutures** can mimic calvarial metastases. Normal structures are typically well corticated, and the underlying dura is normal.

Myeloma can be indistinguishable from multiple lytic skull metastases. Skull base **osteomyelitis** is a rare but life-threatening infection that can resemble diffuse skull base metastases. ADC values are generally higher in infection than in malignant neoplasms.

The major differential diagnosis for solitary or multifocal dura-arachnoid metastases is **meningioma**. Metastases, especially from breast cancer, can be virtually indistinguishable from solitary or multiple meningiomas on the basis of imaging studies alone.

The differential diagnosis of diffuse dura-arachnoid thickening is much broader. Nonneoplastic pachymeningopathies, such as meningitis, chronic subdural hematoma, and intracranial hypotension, can all cause diffuse dura-arachnoid thickening. Metastatic dural thickening is generally—although not invariably—more "lumpy-bumpy" **(27-16)** **(27-17)**.

Leptomeningeal Metastases

Terminology

The anatomic term "leptomeninges" refers to both the arachnoid *and* the pia. The widely used term "leptomeningeal metastases" (LM) is technically incorrect, as it is employed to designate the imaging pattern seen when tumor involves the subarachnoid spaces and pia **(27-9)**.

Synonyms for leptomeningeal metastases include meningeal carcinomatosis, neoplastic meningitis, and carcinomatous meningitis.

Epidemiology and Etiology

LMs from **systemic cancers** **(27-8)** are rare, occurring in 5% of cases. The most common sources are breast and small cell lung cancers.

Intracranial primary tumors more commonly cause LM. In adults, the two most common are glioblastoma and lymphoma. The most common intracranial sources of childhood LM are medulloblastoma and other embryonal tumors, such as embryonal tumors with multilayered rosettes C19MC-altered, ependymoma, and germinoma.

Imaging

General Features. LMs follow the brain surfaces, curving along gyri and dipping into the sulci. The general appearance on contrast-enhanced scans is as though the CSF "turns white" **(27-7)**.

CT Findings. NECT scans may be normal or show only mild hydrocephalus. Sulcal-cisternal enhancement, especially at the base of the brain, can sometimes be seen on CECT.

CECT scans may also be normal.

MR Findings. T1 scans may be normal or show only "dirty" CSF. Most LMs are hyperintense on T2WI and may be indistinguishable from normal CSF. Sulcal-cisternal hyperintensity on FLAIR is common **(27-18A)**. If tumor has extended from the pia into the perivascular spaces, underlying brain parenchyma may show hyperintense vasogenic edema.

Postcontrast T1 scans show meningitis-like findings **(27-18B)**. Smooth or nodular enhancement seems to coat the brain surface, filling the sulci **(27-18C)** and sometimes almost the entire subarachnoid space, including the thecal sac. Cranial nerve thickening with linear, nodular, or focal mass-like enhancement may occur with or without disseminated disease.

Tiny enhancing miliary nodules or linear enhancing foci in the cortex and subcortical white matter indicate extension along the penetrating perivascular spaces.

Differential Diagnosis

The major differential diagnosis of leptomeningeal metastases is **infectious meningitis**. It may be difficult or impossible to distinguish between carcinomatous and infectious meningitis on the basis of imaging findings alone. Other diagnostic considerations include **neurosarcoid**. Clinical history and laboratory features are essential elements in establishing the correct diagnosis.

LEPTOMENINGEAL METASTASES

General Features
- Pia + subarachnoid space metastases
- Uncommon
  - 5% of systemic cancers
  - More common with primary tumors (e.g., GBM, medulloblastoma, germinoma)

CT
- NECT: May be normal ± mild hydrocephalus
- CECT: Sulcal-cisternal enhancement (looks like pyogenic meningitis)

MR
- T1WI: Normal or "dirty" CSF
- T2WI: Usually normal
- FLAIR: Sulcal-cisternal hyperintensity (nonspecific)
- T1 C+: Sulcal-cisternal enhancement (nonspecific)

Differential Diagnosis
- Meningitis
- Neurosarcoid

Miscellaneous Metastases

Several "secret" sites may also harbor metastases. The ventricles and choroid plexus, pituitary gland/infundibular stalk, pineal gland, and eye are less obvious places where intracranial metastases occur and may escape detection.

CSF Metastases

Both extra- and intracranial metastases can seed the CSF. Intracranial CSF metastases are usually seen as "dirty" CSF on T1WI and FLAIR **(27-18A)**, often occurring together with diffuse pial spread. "Drop metastases" into the spinal subarachnoid space are a manifestation of generalized CSF spread.

Ependymal spread around the ventricular walls occurs with primary CNS tumors much more often than with extracranial sources.

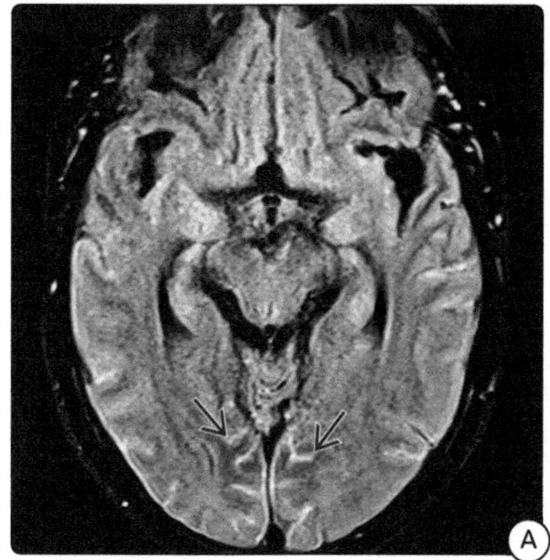

***(27-18A)** FLAIR MR in a 61-year-old woman with remote history of breast cancer shows diffuse symmetric sulcal hyperintensity ➙.*

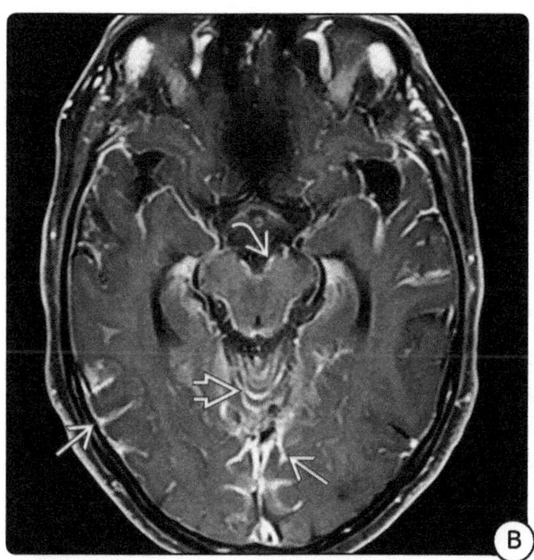

***(27-18B)** T1 C+ FS MR shows diffuse pia-subarachnoid enhancement over hemispheres ➙, midbrain ➙, and cerebellum ➙.*

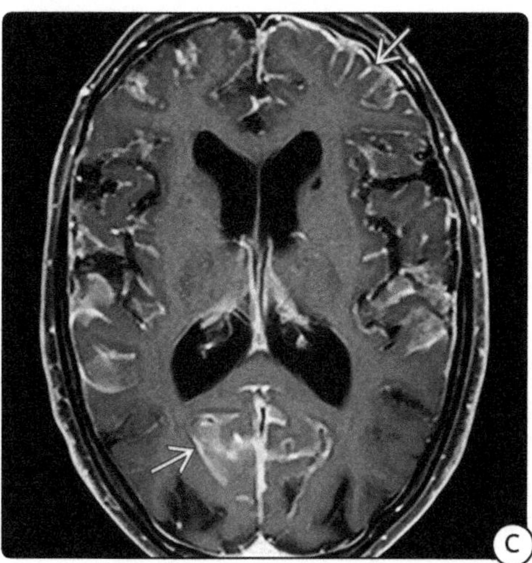

***(27-18C)** More cephalad T1 C+ FS MR through the ventricles shows diffuse enhancing leptomeningeal metastases ➙.*

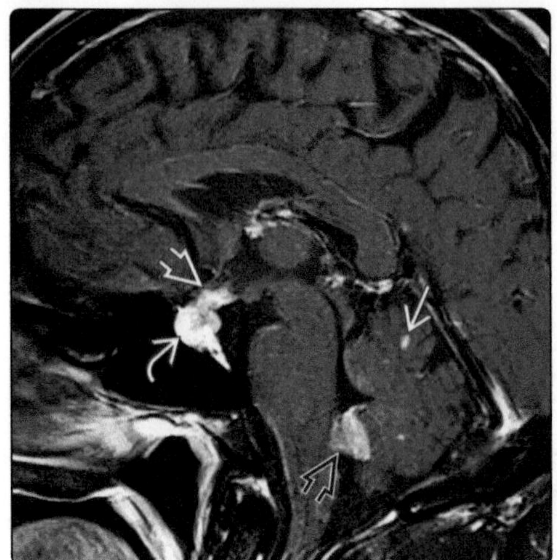

(27-19) T1 C+ FS MR shows metastases to pituitary gland/stalk ➡, 3rd ventricle ➡, 4th ventricle choroid plexus ➡, and vermian folia ➡.

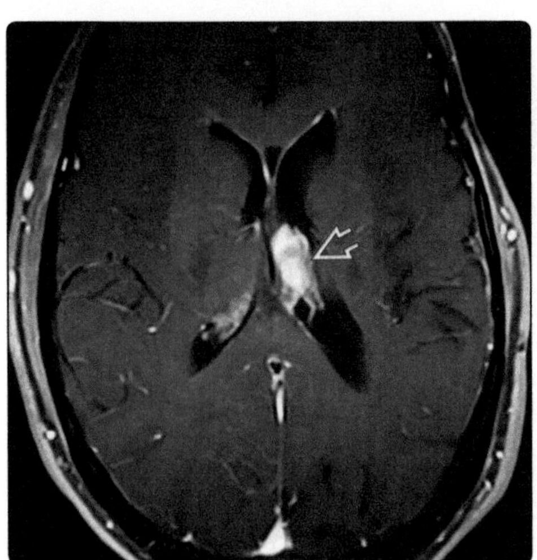

(27-20) T1 C+ MR shows large choroid plexus metastasis ➡.

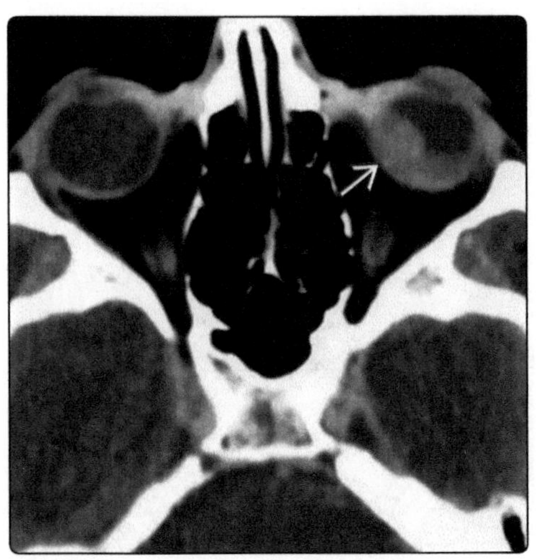

(27-21) CECT shows a lobulated enhancing mass in the posterior segment of the left globe ➡. This was metastatic breast carcinoma.

Ventricles/Choroid Plexus Metastases

The lateral ventricle choroid plexus is the most common site for ventricular metastases followed by the third ventricle. Only 0.5% of ventricular metastases occur in the fourth ventricle. Solitary choroid plexus metastases are more common than multiple lesions.

Choroid plexus metastases enlarge the choroid plexus **(27-20)** and are iso- to hyperdense compared with normal choroid plexus on NECT scans. They enhance strongly but heterogeneously on CECT and T1 C+ **(27-19)**.

Most nonhemorrhagic choroid plexus metastases are hypointense to brain on T1WI and hyperintense on T2/FLAIR. Intense enhancement following contrast administration is typical.

In an older patient (especially one with known systemic cancer, such as renal cell carcinoma), the differential diagnosis of a choroid plexus mass should always include metastasis. Other common choroid plexus lesions in older patients are **meningioma** and **choroid plexus xanthogranuloma**. Choroid plexus meningiomas enhance strongly and generally uniformly. Choroid plexus cysts (xanthogranulomas) are usually bilateral, multicystic-appearing lesions.

Pituitary Gland/Infundibular Stalk Metastases

Metastasis causes ~ 1% of all pituitary tumors and is found in 1-2% of autopsies. Breast and lung primaries account for 2/3 of cases.

Most pituitary metastases involve the posterior lobe, probably because of its direct systemic arterial supply via the hypophyseal arteries. Coexisting brain metastases are common, but solitary lesions do occur.

A sellar mass with or without bone erosion, stalk thickening, loss of posterior pituitary "bright spot," and cavernous sinus invasion is typical but nonspecific. An infiltrating, enhancing pituitary &/or stalk mass is the most common finding **(27-19)**.

The major differential diagnosis of pituitary metastasis is **macroadenoma**. Macroadenomas rarely present with diabetes insipidus. In the setting of a known systemic cancer, rapid growth of a pituitary mass with onset of clinical diabetes insipidus is highly suggestive but certainly not diagnostic of metastasis. **Lymphocytic hypophysitis** can also resemble pituitary metastasis on imaging studies.

Pineal Gland Metastases

Although the pineal gland is a relatively common source of primary CNS tumors that seed the CSF, it is one of the rarest sites to harbor a metastasis. Only 0.3% of intracranial metastases involve the pineal gland. Lung, breast, skin (melanoma), and kidney are the most frequent sources. When pineal metastases do occur, they are usually solitary lesions without evidence of metastatic deposits elsewhere and are indistinguishable on imaging studies from primary pineal neoplasms.

Ocular Metastases

Metastases to the eye are rare. The highly vascular choroid is by far the most commonly affected site, accounting for nearly 90% of all ocular metastases. Breast cancer is the most common cause of ocular metastases followed by lung cancer.

CT and MR findings are nonspecific, demonstrating a posterior segment mass that often enhances strongly after contrast administration **(27-21)**.

Whole-brain imaging is recommended, as 20-25% of patients with choroidal metastases have concurrent CNS lesions.

The differential diagnosis of choroidal metastasis includes other hyperdense posterior segment masses. Primary **choroidal melanoma** and **hemangioma** may appear similar on both CT and MR. Melanoma and metastases may also incite **hemorrhagic choroidal** or **retinal detachment**.

Perineural Metastases

Perineural tumor (PNT) spread is defined as extension of malignant tumor along neural sheaths. Squamous cell carcinoma (SCCa) and major/minor salivary gland malignancies, such as adenoid cystic carcinoma, are all prone to PNT spread. Other tumors, such as non-Hodgkin lymphoma, also frequently spread along major nerve sheaths. Perineural invasion occurs in 2-6% of cutaneous head and neck basal carcinomas and SCCas.

The most common nerves to be affected by PNT are the maxillary division of the trigeminal nerve (CNV2) **(27-22)** and the facial nerve (CNVII).

Tubular enlargement and enhancement of the affected nerve together with widening of its bony canal or foramen is typical. If the nerve passes through a structure such as the PTPF that is normally filled with fat, the fat becomes "dirty" or effaced. *Look for denervation atrophy*—common with CNV3 lesions—seen as small, shrunken muscles of mastication with fatty infiltration **(27-22B)**.

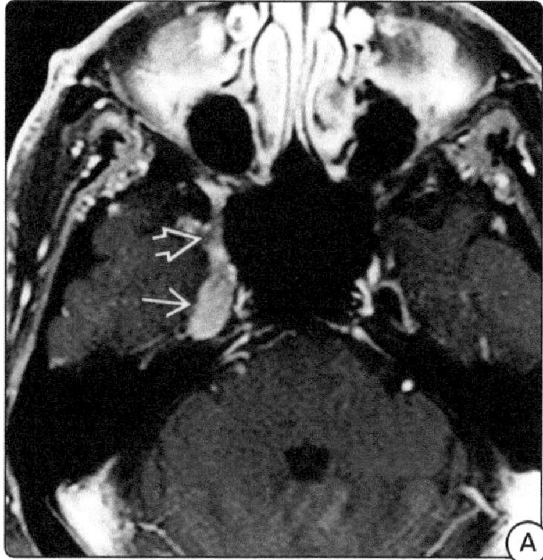

***(27-22A)** Enhancing metastasis fills right Meckel cave ➡, infiltrates and thickens CNV2 ➡. Tumor also involved CNV3 (not shown).*

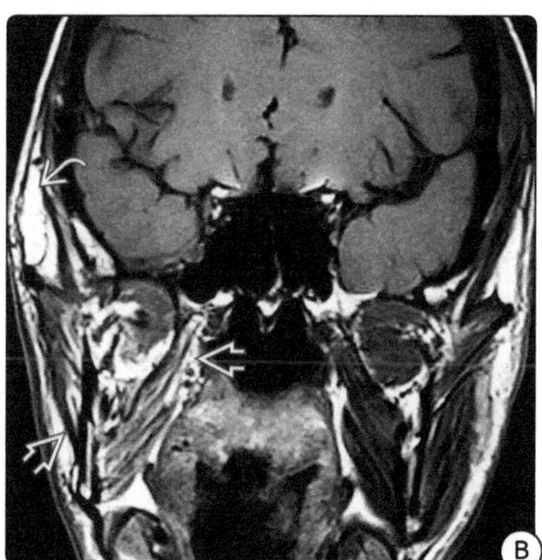

***(27-22B)** Coronal T1 C+ MR shows muscles of mastication ➡, temporalis ➡ are atrophic, fatty infiltrated. This was denervation atrophy.*

Paraneoplastic Syndromes

We close this chapter with a brief discussion of cancer-induced remote neurologic effects, collectively called **paraneoplastic syndromes** or **paraneoplastic neurologic disorders** (PNDs). By definition, PNDs are not related to direct (local or metastatic) tumor invasion, adverse effects of chemotherapy, malnutrition, or infection. In a paraneoplastic syndrome, extra-CNS tumors exert their adverse influence on the brain, not via metastasis but indirectly.

Paraneoplastic neurologic syndromes are rare, affecting < 1% of all patients with systemic cancer. In most cases, a paraneoplastic syndrome is diagnosed only after other etiologies—primarily metastatic disease—have been excluded. However, in 70% of patients with PND, neurologic symptoms are the *first* manifestation of a tumor.

Most PNDs are mediated by antibodies against known neural antigens ("onconeuronal antibodies"). Several types of PND have been recognized. These include **paraneoplastic limbic encephalitis, paraneoplastic encephalomyelitis, paraneoplastic cerebellar degeneration, paraneoplastic opsoclonus-myoclonus, paraneoplastic sensorimotor neuropathy, retinopathy, stiff-person syndrome**, and **Lambert-Eaton myasthenic syndrome**.

PNDs may involve any part of the CNS (brain, spinal cord) or peripheral nervous system, although the temporal lobes seem to be the most favored site and paraneoplastic limbic encephalitis is the most common PND.

Paraneoplastic Encephalomyelitis

The most common form of paraneoplastic encephalomyelitis is paraneoplastic limbic encephalitis (PLE). Note that limbic encephalitis is a heterogeneous group of immune-mediated disorders that also includes *non*paraneoplastic autoimmune encephalitides, such as anti-GAD and LGI1

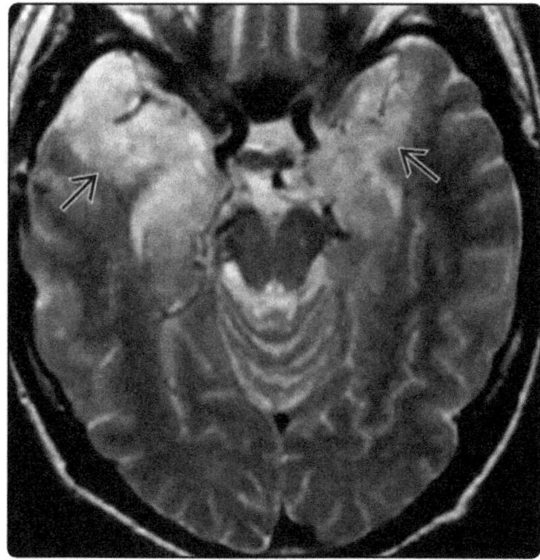

***(27-23)** T2 MR in a 75y man with small cell lung cancer shows paraneoplastic limbic encephalitis in both anteromedial temporal lobes ➡.*

encephalitis. The nonparaneoplastic autoimmune encephalitides were discussed in Chapter 15.

Terminology

By definition, paraneoplastic limbic encephalitis is a limbic system disorder. The medial temporal lobes are preferentially involved, but the inferior frontal region, insular cortex, and cingulate gyrus can also be affected.

Etiology

The most frequent neoplasm associated with PLE is small cell lung cancer identified in ~ 1/2 of all cases. Other associated tumors include testicular neoplasms (20%), breast carcinoma (8%), thymoma, and lymphoma.

Antineuronal antibodies are frequently but not invariably found in the CSF or serum of patients with PLE. The most common is the anti-Hu antibody, which is present in ~ 1/2 of the patients with small cell lung cancer-associated PLE. Anti-Ma2 PLE is associated with testicular germ cell tumors.

Other neuronal autoantibodies include anti-Ri (breast, small cell lung cancer), anti-Yo (ovarian, breast), and anti-Ma2 (testicular germ cell cancer). These often affect the brainstem (midbrain, pons, medulla) either in isolation or as part of a more widespread autoantibody-mediated encephalitis.

Clinical Issues

Neurologic symptoms often precede identification of the inciting tumor by weeks or months. Confusion and short-term memory loss with relative preservation of other cognitive functions—with or without mood and behavioral changes—are typical. Complex partial seizures are common.

Imaging

MR is the procedure of choice in diagnosing PLE. T2/FLAIR shows hyperintensity in one or both medial temporal lobes **(27-23)**.

Differential Diagnosis

The major differential diagnosis of PLE is **herpes encephalitis**. Other causes of limbic encephalitis that can mimic PLE include **glutamic acid decarboxylase 65 (GAD65) autoantibody-associated LE**, **posttransplant acute limbic encephalitis** (PALE) syndrome, and **human herpesvirus 6 (HHV-6) encephalitis**.

HHV-6 encephalitis is associated with hematologic malignancies, such as Hodgkin and angioimmunoblastic T-cell lymphoma and leukemia.

PARANEOPLASTIC NEUROLOGIC DISORDERS AND ANTINEURONAL ANTIBODIES

Paraneoplastic Limbic Encephalitis
- Primary autoantibody = anti-Hu (small cell lung)
- Other = anti-Ma2 (testicular germ cell)

Paraneoplastic Brainstem Encephalitis
- Anti-Hu, Anti-Ri (breast)
- Anti-NMDA (ovarian teratoma)

Paraneoplastic Cerebellar Degeneration
- Primary autoantibody = anti-Yo (ovarian, breast)
- Anti-Hu, anti-Ri, anti-Tr, or pmGLuR1 (Hodgkin lymphoma)
- Anti-VGCC (small cell lung)

Stiff-Person Syndrome
- Primary antineuronal antibody = anti-GAD65
- Other = antiamphiphysin

Opsoclonus-Myoclonus Syndrome
- Primary antineuronal antibody = anti-Ri
- Other = anti-Yo, anti-Hu, anti-amphiphysin, anti-Nova 1/2

IMAGING OF MAJOR PARANEOPLASTIC NEUROLOGIC DISORDERS

Paraneoplastic Encephalomyelitis
- Limbic encephalitis is most common form
- T2/FLAIR hyperintensity in one or both medial temporal lobes
- No enhancement on T1 C+

Paraneoplastic Cerebellar Degeneration
- Usually normal
- Subacute/chronic may show cerebellar atrophy

Stiff-Person Syndrome
- Usually normal
- SPS with limbic encephalitis may exhibit T2/FLAIR hyperintensity in medial temporal lobes
- F-FDG-PET may show hypermetabolism in medial temporal lobes

LGI1 (Voltage-Gated Potassium Channel-Complex Disorders)
- Only 25% associated with systemic malignancy
- T2/FLAIR hyperintensity in medial temporal lobes, basal ganglia
- PET/CT intense uptake in basal ganglia

Selected References: The complete reference list is available on the Expert Consult™ eBook version included with purchase.

Nonneoplastic Cysts

There are many types of intracranial cysts. Some are incidental and of no significance. Others may cause serious—even life-threatening—symptoms.

In this chapter, we consider a number of different intracranial cysts: Cystic-appearing anatomic variants that can be mistaken for disease, congenital/developmental cysts, and a variety of miscellaneous cysts. Parasitic cysts, cystic brain malformations, and cystic neoplasms are excluded as they are discussed in their respective chapters.

While there are many different ways to classify cysts, an *imaging-based* approach to classification of intracranial cysts is the most practical as most of these lesions are discovered on CT or MR examination.

An imaging-based approach takes into account three easily defined features: (1) Anatomic location, (2) imaging characteristics (i.e., density/signal intensity of the contents, presence/absence of calcification &/or enhancement), and (3) patient age. Of these three, anatomic location is the most helpful.

While many types of intracranial cysts occur in more than one location, some sites are "preferred" by certain cysts. In this chapter, we discuss cysts by location from the outside in, beginning with intracranial extraaxial cysts before turning our attention to intraaxial (parenchymal and intraventricular) cysts.

There are four key anatomy-based questions to consider about a cystic-appearing intracranial lesion (see below). A summary chart based on these simple questions, together with the cysts discussed throughout the text, is included on the next page **(Table 28-1)**.

4 KEY ANATOMY-BASED QUESTIONS

- Is the cyst extra- or intraaxial?
- Is the cyst supra- or infratentorial?
- If the cyst is extraaxial, is it midline or off-midline?
- If the cyst is intraaxial, is it in the brain parenchyma or inside the ventricles?

Extraaxial Cysts

Extraaxial cysts lie between the skull and brain. With few exceptions, most are contained within the arachnoid membrane or in the subarachnoid space.

Determining sublocation of an extraaxial cyst (supra- vs. infratentorial, midline vs. off-midline) is helpful in establishing a meaningful differential diagnosis **(Table 28-1)**. For example, an arachnoid cyst is the only type that commonly occurs in the posterior fossa. Some extraaxial cysts are usually

Intracranial Cystic-Appearing Lesions

	Supratentorial	Infratentorial
Extraaxial		
Midline	Pineal cyst Dermoid cyst Rathke cleft cyst Arachnoid cyst (suprasellar)	Neurenteric cyst Arachnoid cyst (retrocerebellar)
Off-midline	Arachnoid cyst (middle cranial fossa, convexity) Epidermoid cyst Tumor-associated cyst Trichilemmal ("sebaceous") cyst (scalp) Leptomeningeal cyst ("growing fracture")	Epidermoid cyst (CPA) Arachnoid cyst (CPA) Tumor-associated cyst
Intraaxial		
Parenchymal	Enlarged perivascular spaces Neuroglial cyst Porencephalic cyst Hippocampal sulcus remnants	Enlarged perivascular spaces (dentate nuclei)
Intraventricular	Choroid plexus cyst Colloid cyst Choroid fissure cyst Ependymal cyst	Epidermoid cyst (4th ventricle, cisterna magna) Cystic ("trapped") 4th ventricle

(Table 28-1) *CPA = cerebellopontine angle. Leptomeningeal cyst, Rathke cleft cyst, and cystic/trapped 4th ventricle are discussed in chapters 2, 25, and 34, respectively. All other entities listed in the table are considered here.*

(although not invariably) off-midline. Others—pineal and Rathke cleft cysts—occur only in the midline.

Arachnoid Cyst

An arachnoid cyst (AC) is a CSF-containing cyst that arises as an anomaly of meningeal development. The embryonic endomeninges fail to merge and remain separated, forming a "duplicated" arachnoid. CSF is secreted by cells in the cyst wall and accumulates between the layers.

Pathology

ACs are well-marginated cysts filled with clear, colorless fluid that resembles CSF **(28-1)**. They are devoid of internal septations and are completely encased by a delicate translucent membrane lined by a single layer of mature, histologically normal arachnoid cells **(28-2)**.

Most ACs are supratentorial. They are usually off-midline and are the most common off-midline extraaxial supratentorial cyst. Nearly 2/3 are found in the middle cranial fossa, anteromedial to the temporal lobe. 15% of ACs are found over the cerebral convexities, predominantly over the frontal lobes. Between 10-15% of ACs are found in the posterior fossa, predominately the cerebellopontine angle cistern.

ARACHNOID CYST: PATHOLOGY

Location
- Supratentorial (90%)
  - Middle fossa (67%)
  - Convexities (15%)
  - Other (5-10%): Suprasellar, quadrigeminal cisterns
- Infratentorial (10-12%)
  - Mostly CPA cistern (2nd most common cystic CPA mass)
  - Less common = cisterna magna

Gross Pathology
- Thin translucent cyst wall bulging with clear fluid
- Lined by mature arachnoid cells

Clinical Issues

ACs are the most common of all congenital intracranial cysts. They account for ~ 1% of all space-occupying intracranial lesions and are identified on imaging studies in 1-2% of patients. ACs can be seen at any age. Most (nearly 75%) are found in children and young adults.

Most ACs are asymptomatic and found incidentally, remaining stable over many years. Enlargement—if any—is very gradual.

Symptoms vary with size and location. Headaches are common. Some suprasellar ACs become very large and cause obstructive hydrocephalus.

Hemorrhage—either traumatic or spontaneous—into an intracranial AC is rare but may cause sudden enlargement. ACs carry a slightly increased risk of subdural hematoma.

Imaging

ACs vary in size, ranging from small incidental cysts to large space-occupying lesions. Uncomplicated ACs behave *exactly* like CSF on CT and MR **(28-3)**. FLAIR and DWI are the best sequences to distinguish cystic-appearing intracranial masses from one another.

There is a relationship between subdural hematomas (SDHs) and ACs, although whether this is causative or coincidental is unclear. Traumatic SDHs can rupture into ACs. The converse—AC rupture causing a spontaneous SDH—occurs but is rare.

CT Findings. Uncomplicated ACs are CSF density **(28-4)**. If intracystic hemorrhage has occurred, the cyst fluid may be moderately hyperdense compared with CSF. Large middle cranial fossa ACs expand the fossa and cause temporal lobe hypoplasia or displacement **(28-2)**.

With moderately large ACs, bone CT may show pressure remodeling of the adjacent calvarium. ACs do not cause frank bone invasion. ACs do not enhance.

MR Findings. ACs are sharply marginated, somewhat scalloped-appearing lesions that parallel CSF signal intensity on all sequences. They are therefore isointense with CSF on T1- and T2-weighted images. ACs cause moderate focal mass effect, *displacing but not engulfing adjacent brain, vessels, and cranial nerves* **(28-4)**.

The internal appearance of an AC is intrinsically featureless, containing neither septations, vessels, nor cranial nerves.

ACs suppress completely with FLAIR. Occasionally, CSF pulsations within large lesions may cause spin dephasing, producing heterogeneous signal intensity and significant propagation of phase artifact across the scan. ACs do not restrict on DWI and do not enhance.

CSF flow imaging, such as 2D cine PC, may demonstrate communication between cyst and adjacent subarachnoid space.

Differential Diagnosis

The major differential diagnosis of AC is **epidermoid cyst** (EC). ECs are often almost—but not quite—exactly like CSF. They have a cauliflower-like, lobulated configuration instead of the sharply marginated borders of an AC. ECs engulf vessels and nerves, insinuating themselves along CSF cisterns. ECs do not suppress completely on FLAIR and typically show moderate to marked hyperintensity on DWI.

Enlarged subarachnoid spaces caused by brain volume loss are usually more diffuse CSF collections and do not cause mass effect on adjacent structures.

A **subdural hygroma** or **chronic subdural hematoma** (cSDH) is not precisely like CSF and is usually crescentic, not round or scalloped. cSDHs usually show evidence of prior hemorrhage, especially on T2* sequences, and may have enhancing encasing membranes.

A **porencephalic cyst** looks just like CSF, but it is intraaxial and lined by gliotic white matter that is often hyperintense on FLAIR.

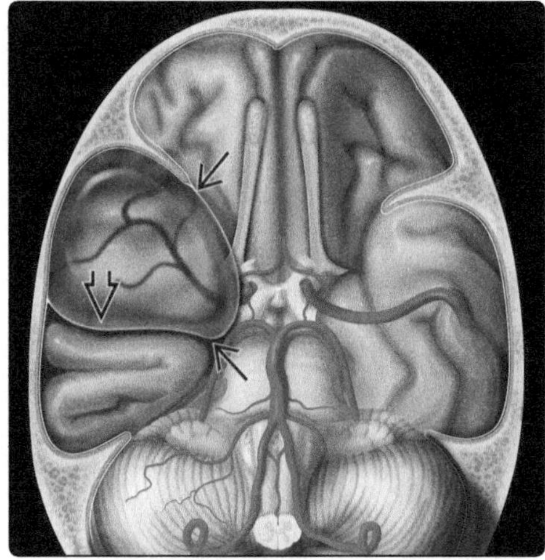

***(28-1)** Graphic shows the arachnoid ➡ splitting, enclosing CSF. Middle fossa is expanded; temporal lobe ➡ is displaced posteriorly.*

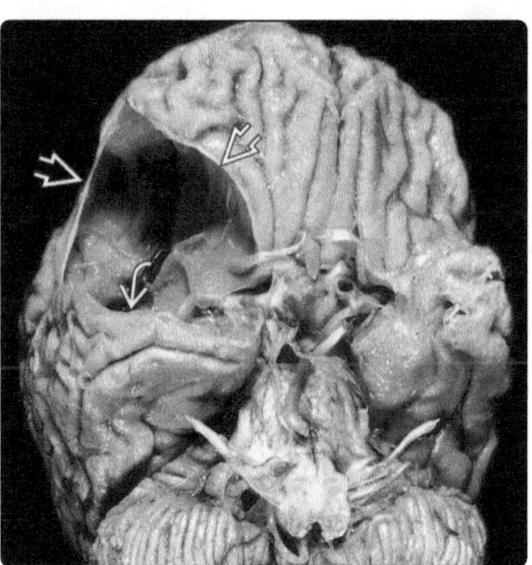

***(28-2)** Middle fossa AC is contained between layers of "duplicated" arachnoid ➡. Temporal lobe ➡ is displaced. (Courtesy J. Townsend, MD.)*

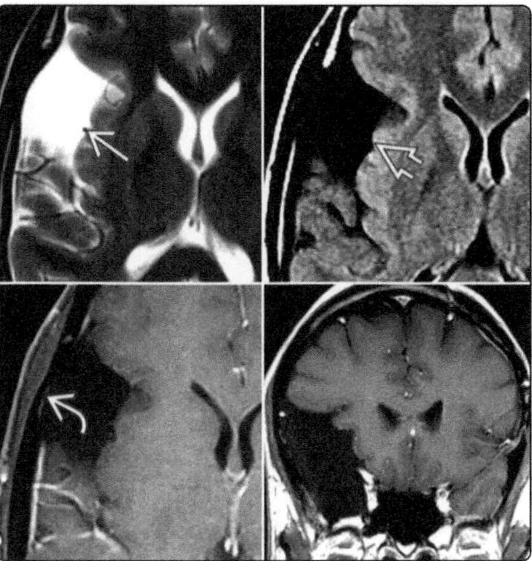

***(28-3)** ACs often have scalloped margins and are CSF-like on T2WI ➡. They suppress on FLAIR ➡, remodel the skull ➡, and do not enhance.*

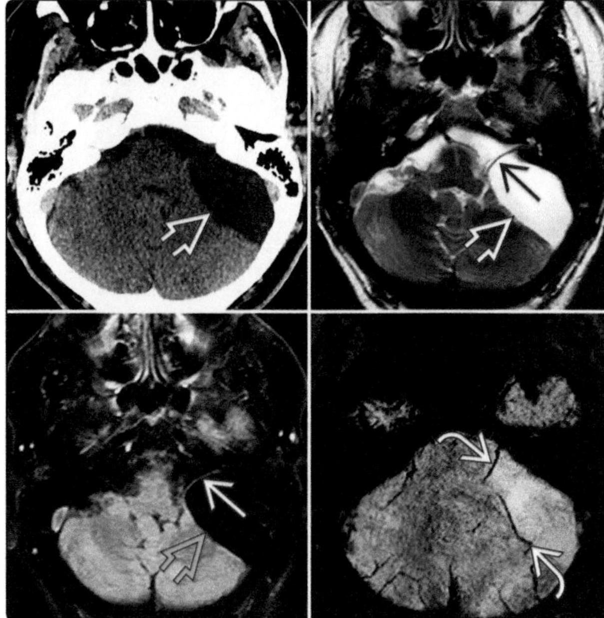

(28-4) (Upper L) AC ➡ is CSF-like on NECT, hyperintense-like on T2WI (upper R). CNs VII, VIII are displaced ➡ by AC. (Lower L) Cyst ➡ suppresses completely on FLAIR, displaces nerves ➡. (Lower R) T2 SWI shows vessels ➡ displaced around AC.*

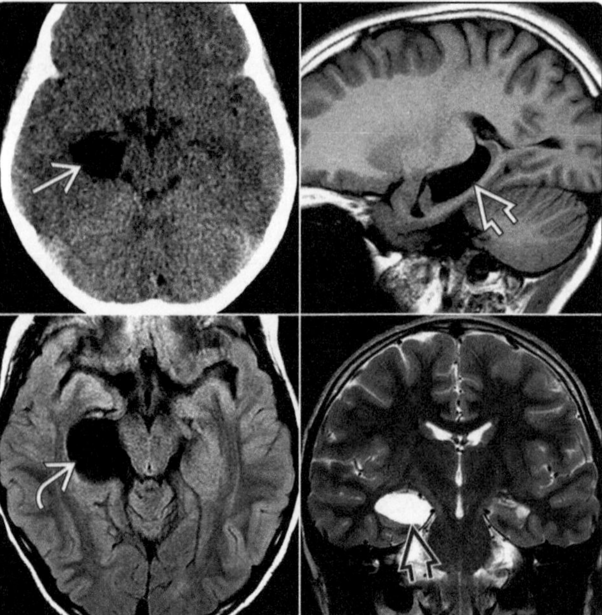

(28-5) Choroid fissure cyst is isodense with CSF on NECT ➡. Sagittal T1WI shows classic elongated "spindle" shape of cyst ➡. The lesion suppresses completely on FLAIR ➡ and is isointense with CSF on T2WI ➡.

ARACHNOID CYST: CLINICAL ISSUES, IMAGING, AND DDx

Clinical Issues
- Most common nonneoplastic intracranial cyst
  - 1% of all intracranial masses
  - All ages; children + young adults (75%)
  - Prevalence = 2% on imaging studies
- Most do not communicate freely with subarachnoid space

Imaging
- Behaves *exactly* like CSF
- FLAIR/DWI best to distinguish from other cysts

Differential Diagnosis
- Most common = epidermoid cyst
- Less common
  - Enlarged subarachnoid spaces
  - Loculated subdural hygroma/hematoma
  - Porencephalic cyst
  - Neoplasm-associated cyst
- Rare = neurenteric cyst

Choroid Fissure Cyst

The choroid fissure is an infolding of CSF between the fornix and thalamus. It is normally a shallow, inconspicuous, C-shaped cleft that curves posterosuperiorly from the anterior temporal lobe all the way to the atrium of the lateral ventricle. The choroidal arteries and choroid plexus lie just medial to the choroid fissure.

A CSF-containing cyst can form anywhere along the choroid fissure. These "choroid fissure cysts" are probably caused by maldevelopment of the embryonic tela choroidea, a double layer of pia that invaginates through the choroid fissure to reach the lateral ventricles.

Imaging

Most choroid fissure cysts are discovered incidentally on imaging studies. They lie just medial to the temporal horn of the lateral ventricle between the hippocampus and diencephalon. Choroid fissure cysts follow CSF density/signal intensity on all sequences **(28-5)**. On axial and coronal images, they are round to oval, but on sagittal images, they have a distinctive, somewhat elongated "spindle" shape **(28-5)**.

Epidermoid Cyst

Terminology

An intracranial epidermoid cyst (EC) is a developmental, nonneoplastic inclusion cyst that is derived from embryonic ectodermal elements.

Pathology

Location. ECs are extraaxial masses that have a predilection for the basilar cisterns. The CPA cistern is the single most common site, accounting for nearly 1/2 of all intracranial ECs. ECs insinuate themselves around cranial nerves and vessels **(28-6)**.

Gross Pathology. The outer surface of an EC is often shiny, resembling mother of pearl **(28-7)**. Multiple "cauliflower" excrescences are typical. The cyst wall consists of stratified squamous epithelium. The cyst itself is filled with soft, waxy, creamy, or flaky material with keratinaceous debris and solid

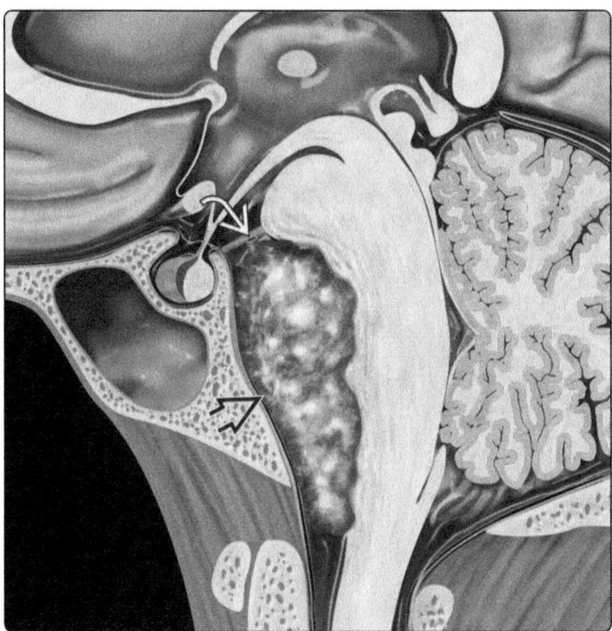

(28-6) ***Graphic shows a multilobulated epidermoid cyst ➡ within prepontine cistern encasing the basilar artery ➡, displacing pons.***

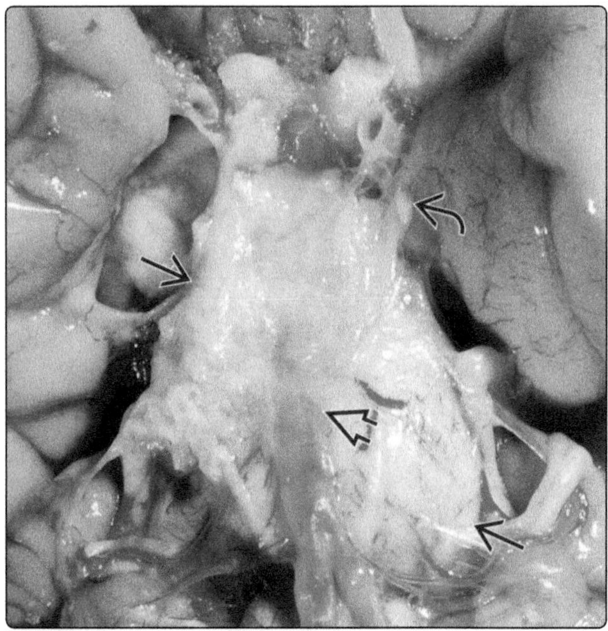

(28-7) ***Autopsy shows epidermoid cyst as a whitish, "pearly" tumor ➡. Note the encased basilar artery ➡, oculomotor nerves ➡.***

crystalline cholesterol. *Dermal appendages, such as hair follicles (a characteristic of dermoid cysts), are absent.*

Clinical Issues

ECs may remain clinically silent for many years. They grow very slowly via progressive accumulation of epidermal cells and accretions of desquamated keratin. ECs often reach considerable size before becoming symptomatic. Symptoms vary according to location; peak age at presentation is 20-60 years.

EPIDERMOID CYST: ETIOLOGY, PATHOLOGY, AND EPIDEMIOLOGY

Etiology
- Congenital inclusion cyst

Pathology
- Gross pathology
  - Insinuates in/around CSF cisterns
  - Encases vessels/cranial nerves
  - "Cauliflower-like" excrescences
  - "Pearly" whitish surface
  - Waxy, creamy, or flaky contents
- Microscopic pathology
  - Squamous epithelium + keratin debris, solid cholesterol
  - *No* dermal appendages!

Epidemiology
- 4-9x more common than dermoid cysts
- Peak age: 20-60 years (rare in children)

Imaging

Epidermoid cysts resemble CSF on imaging. Irregular frond-like excrescences and an insinuating growth pattern within CSF cisterns are characteristic.

CT Findings. Over 95% of ECs are hypodense and appear almost identical to CSF on NECT scans. Calcification is present in 10-25%. Hemorrhage is very rare. Hyperdense "white" epidermoids are uncommon, representing 3% of reported lesions. Enhancement is rare.

MR Findings. ECs are iso- or slightly hyperintense compared with CSF on both T1- **(28-8A)** and T2-weighted sequences **(28-8B)**. Slight heterogeneity in signal intensity is often present.

ECs either do not suppress at all or suppress incompletely on FLAIR **(28-8C)**. They restrict on DWI **(28-8D)** and are therefore moderately to strikingly hyperintense. Enhancement is generally absent, although mild peripheral enhancement can be seen in 25% of cases.

Differential Diagnosis

The major differential diagnosis is **arachnoid cyst (AC)**. ACs are smoothly marginated, behave *exactly* like CSF on all sequences, suppress completely on FLAIR, and do not restrict on DWI. ACs displace nerves and vessels while ECs surround and engulf them. **Dermoid cysts** should not be confused with ECs. Dermoid cysts contain fat and dermal appendages and do not resemble CSF on imaging studies.

EPIDERMOID CYST: FEATURES, IMAGING, AND DDx

General Features
- Resembles CSF (vs. fat-like dermoid)
- Insinuates around/along CSF cisterns
- Encases, displaces vessels and cranial nerves

Imaging
- Hypodense (> 95%)
- Slightly hyperintense to CSF on T1WI
- Does not suppress on FLAIR
- Restricts ("bright") on DWI

Differential Diagnosis
- Arachnoid cyst
  - Suppresses on FLAIR, restricts on DWI
- Other
  - Inflammatory cyst (e.g., neurocysticercosis)
  - Neurenteric cyst (not exactly like CSF)

Dermoid Cyst

Pathology

Dermoid cysts (DCs) are congenital inclusion cysts. The cyst wall contains mature squamous epithelium, keratinous material, and adnexal structures (hair follicles and sebaceous and sweat glands). DCs typically contain a thick, greasy sebaceous material with lipid and cholesterol elements.

DCs are usually extraaxial lesions that are most often found in the midline. The suprasellar cistern is the most common site **(28-9)** followed by the posterior fossa and frontonasal region.

Clinical Issues

DCs are much less common (4-10x) than epidermoid cysts. DCs grow slowly secondary to the production of hair and oils from the internal dermal elements.

*(**28-8A**) Sagittal T1 MR shows a scalloped posterior fossa mass ➡ that encases the basilar artery ➡, wraps around the midbrain, elevates the 3rd ventricle, and deforms the pons. Mass is slightly hyperintense compared to CSF in the 3rd ventricle ➡. (**28-8B**) T2 MR in the same case shows a lobulated, irregular hyperintense mass in the right CPA ➡ and basilar ➡ cisterns encasing the basilar artery ➡. The CSF looks "dirty."*

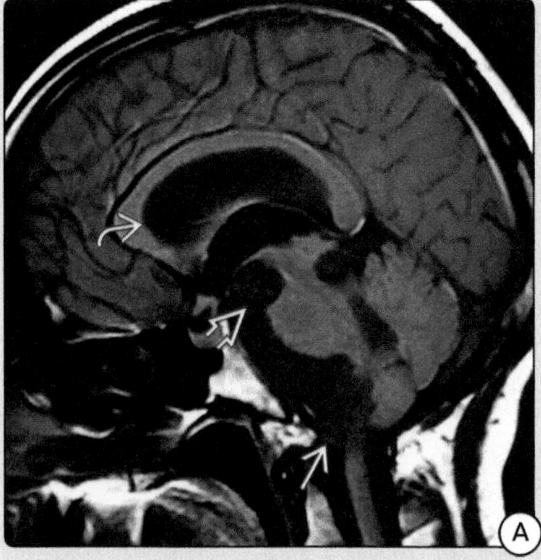

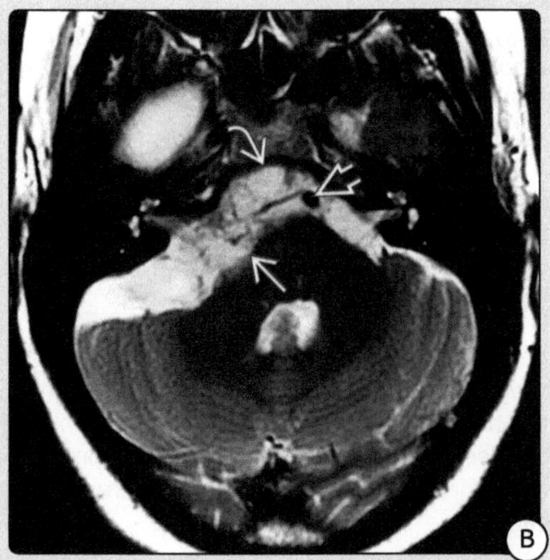

*(**28-8C**) FLAIR MR demonstrates that the lobulated, cauliflower-like mass ➡ does not suppress. (**28-8D**) The mass ➡ restricts on DWI MR. This is a classic epidermoid cyst.*

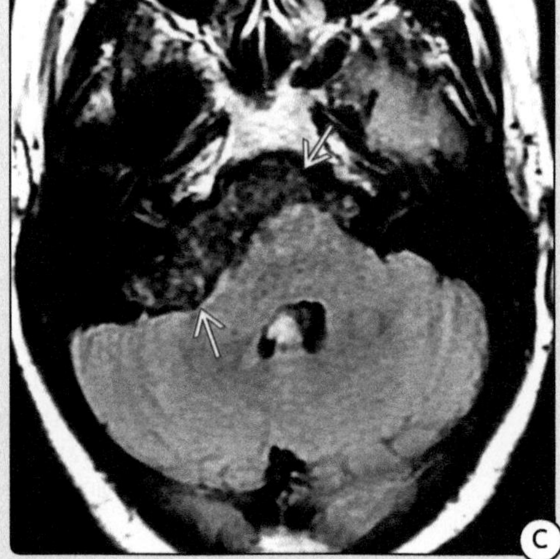

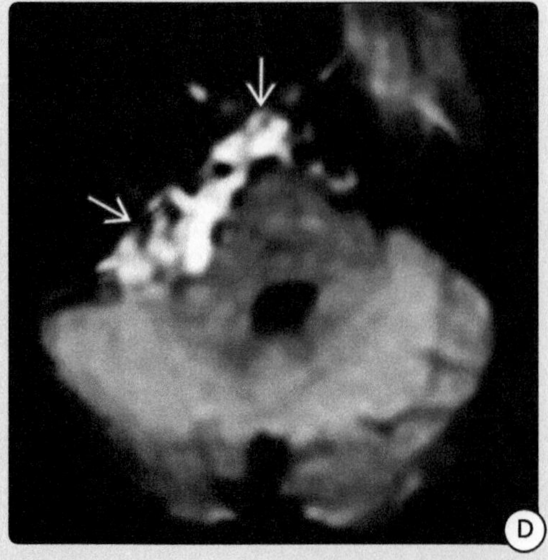

Presentation occurs at significantly younger ages compared with epidermoids, peaking in the second to third decades. DCs often remain asymptomatic until they rupture. Chemical meningitis with seizure, coma, vasospasm, infarction, and even death may ensue as a consequence.

Imaging

DCs resemble fat. A round, well-circumscribed, lipid-containing mass is the usual appearance.

CT Findings. DCs are quite hypodense on NECT scans. With rupture, hypodense fatty "droplets" disseminate in the CSF cisterns **(28-10A)** and may cause discernible fat-fluid levels in the ventricles.

MR Findings. Signal intensity varies with fat content in the cyst. Most DCs are heterogeneously hyperintense on T1WI **(28-10B)**. T1WI is also the most sensitive sequence to detect disseminated fat "droplets" in the subarachnoid space, diagnostic of ruptured dermoid **(28-10C)**. Fat suppression is helpful to confirm the presence of lipid elements.

Standard PD and T2 scans show increasingly more pronounced "chemical shift" artifact in the frequency-encoding direction as the time of repetition is lengthened. Fat is very hypointense on standard T2WI but is "bright" (hyperintense) on fast spin-echo T2-weighted sequences. DCs demonstrate heterogeneous hyperintensity with linear or striated laminations if hair is present within the cyst.

Uncomplicated DCs are heterogeneously hyperintense on FLAIR. Ruptured DCs demonstrate subtle FLAIR sulcal hyperintensity and "bloom" on T2* GRE or SWI.

Most DCs do not enhance, although ruptured DCs may cause significant chemical meningitis with extensive leptomeningeal reaction and enhancement.

Spectroscopy may show an elevated lipid peak at 0.9-1.3 ppm.

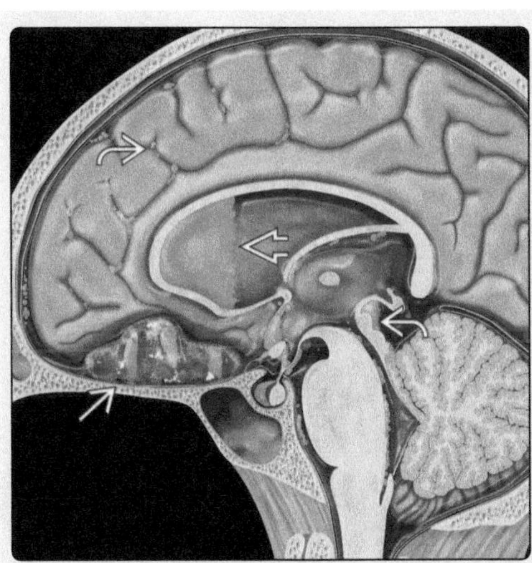

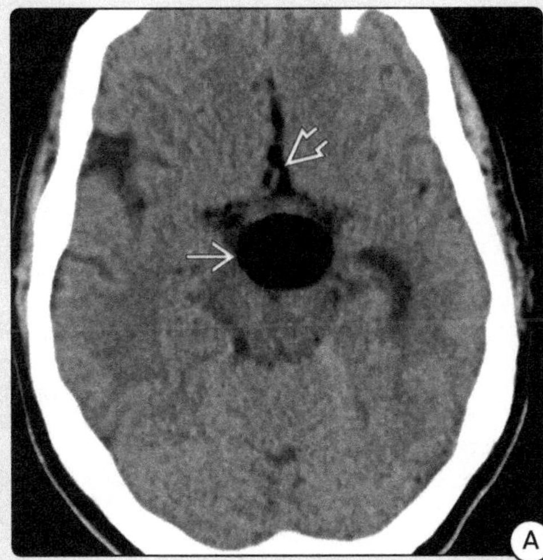

(28-9) Ruptured DC ➡ is a heterogeneous fat-containing midline mass with ventricular fat-fluid level ➡ and fat droplets in SASs ➡. (28-10A) Axial NECT of a ruptured dermoid cyst shows a hypodense suprasellar mass ➡ and fat droplets in the interhemispheric fissure ➡.

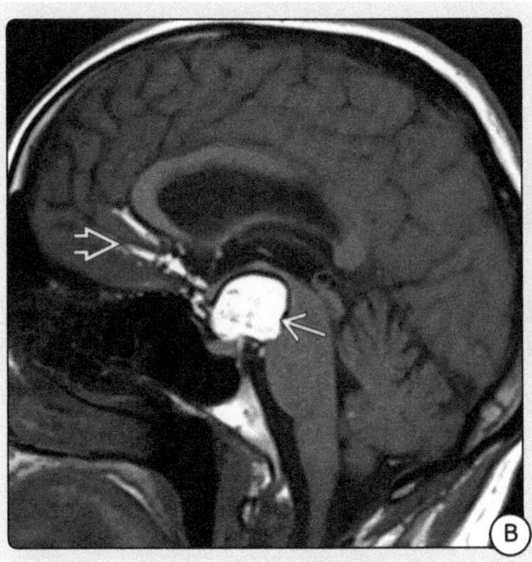

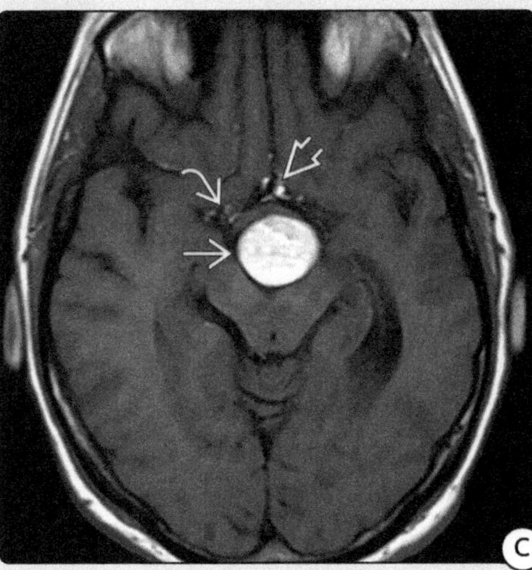

(28-10B) The cyst contents ➡ and subarachnoid fatty droplets ➡ are hyperintense on sagittal T1 MR. (28-10C) Axial T1 MR shows the midline heterogeneously hyperintense dermoid ➡. Rupture has spilled fatty droplets into the suprasellar cistern ➡ and interhemispheric fissure ➡.

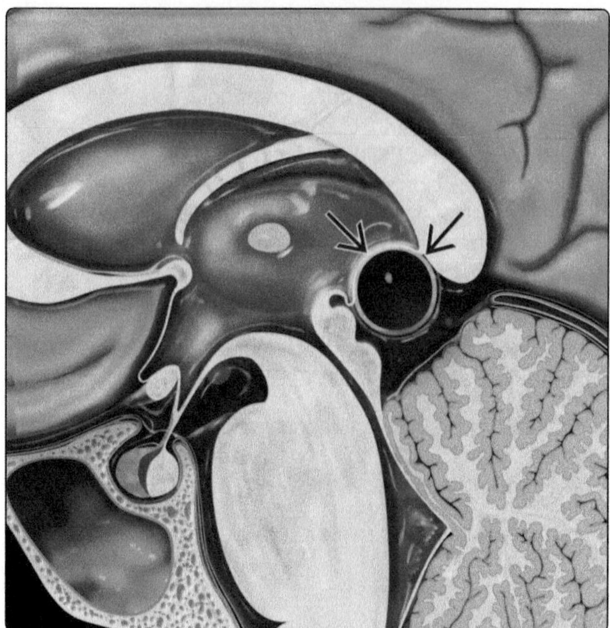

(28-11) Sagittal graphic shows a small cystic lesion within the pineal gland ➡. Small benign pineal cysts are often found incidentally at autopsy or imaging.

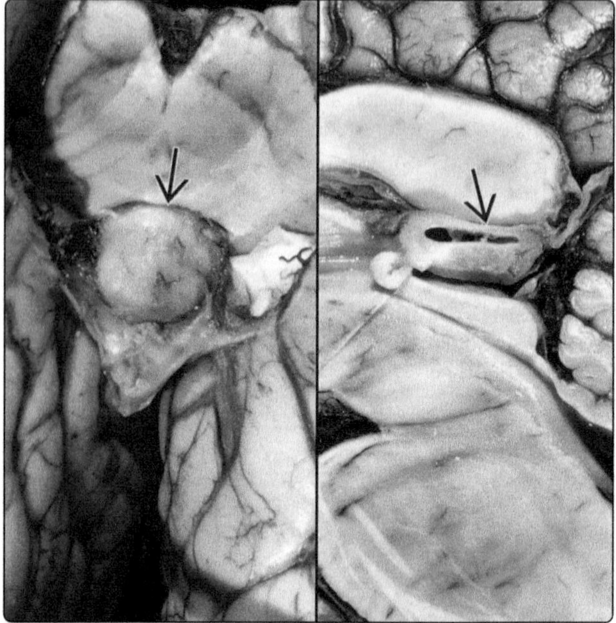

(28-12) Axial (L), sagittal (R) autopsy views of pineal cyst ➡ show the typical location behind the tectal plate. (Courtesy E. T. Hedley-Whyte, MD.)

DERMOID CYST

Pathology
- Location
  - Usually extraaxial
  - Midline > off-midline
  - Suprasellar > posterior fossa > frontonasal
- Wall of squamous epithelium
  - Cyst contains fatty sebaceous material, keratin, skin adnexa

Clinical Findings
- Grow slowly
- Usually asymptomatic until rupture

Imaging
- NECT
  - Hypodense, Ca^{++} in 20%
  - "Fatty" droplets in cisterns if ruptured
- MR
  - Heterogeneously hyperintense on T1WI/FSE T2
  - Heterogeneously hyperintense on FLAIR
  - Ruptured DCs "bloom" on T2*GRE

Differential Diagnosis

The major differential diagnosis of DC is **epidermoid cyst**. Epidermoid cysts behave more like CSF on both CT and MR, whereas DCs resemble fat on imaging studies. Dermoids often rupture, spilling fatty droplets into the subarachnoid space. Epidermoid cyst rupture does occur but is much less common and may demonstrate high serum carbohydrate antigen, CA 199.

Lipoma may resemble a DC but is generally much more homogeneous on MR and is often associated with other congenital malformations, such as callosal dysgenesis.

Craniopharyngioma is often multicystic, extends into the sella, calcifies, and enhances. **Teratoma** may resemble a DC but most commonly occurs in the pineal gland and is much more heterogeneous on imaging than the typical DC.

DERMOID vs. EPIDERMOID CYST

Pathology
- *Both* dermoid, epidermoid contain squamous epithelium + keratin debris
- *Only* dermoid also contains fat, dermal appendages

Clinical Issues
- Dermoid cysts *less* common than epidermoids
- Dermoid cysts more common in children/young adults
- Dermoid cysts commonly rupture

Imaging
- DC behaves mostly like fat
  - Most often midline, supra- or juxtasellar
- Epidermoid cyst more like CSF
  - Most often midline
  - Most common site = posterior fossa (cerebellopontine angle cistern)

Pineal Cyst

Cystic-appearing lesions in the pineal gland are common incidental findings on MR scans, seen in 1/2 of children and over 1/4 of healthy adults with only vague complaints and no symptoms referable to the pineal region.

Pathology

Between 25-40% of autopsied pineal glands contain cysts. PCs are well-demarcated, round or ovoid expansions within an otherwise normal-appearing pineal gland **(28-11)**. Most are < 10 mm in diameter. The largest reported PC is 4.5 cm. PCs are usually unilocular, but lesions containing multiple smaller cysts do occur.

Gross Pathology. The general appearance is that of a smooth, soft, tan-yellow pineal gland that contains a uni- or multilocular cyst **(28-12)**. PCs do not have ependymal or epithelial lining so the cyst "wall" is actually compressed pineal parenchyma. The inner surface of the cyst cavity is often hemosiderin stained as the result of intralesional hemorrhage. Cyst fluid is clear to yellowish.

There are no gross pathologic or histologic features that distinguish symptomatic from asymptomatic PCs.

Clinical Issues

Demographics. PCs can occur at *any* age, although they are more often discovered in middle-aged and older adults.

The overall F:M ratio is 2:1. The incidence among women ages 21-30 years is significantly higher than in any other group.

Presentation. Most PCs are clinically benign and asymptomatic, discovered incidentally at imaging or autopsy. Large PCs may obstruct the cerebral aqueduct, resulting in hydrocephalus and headache. Parinaud syndrome (tectal compression) is less common.

Pineal "apoplexy" occurs with sudden intracystic hemorrhage. Acute worsening of headaches combined with visual symptoms can occur. A "thunderclap" headache may mimic symptoms of aneurysmal subarachnoid hemorrhage. Pineal "apoplexy" can result in acute intraventricular obstructive hydrocephalus.

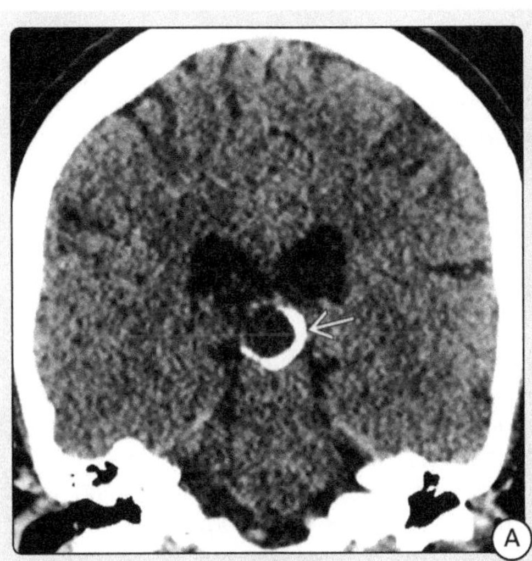

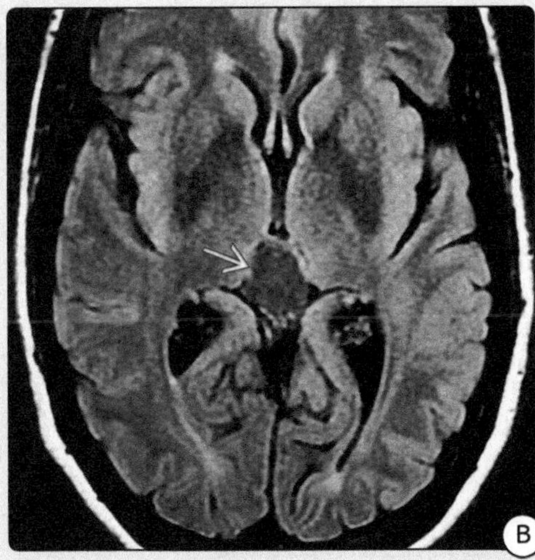

***(28-13A)** Coronal NECT in a 49-year-old woman with chronic headaches shows a large cystic pineal gland with thick rim calcification ➡. **(28-13B)** Axial FLAIR MR in the same case shows that the fluid in the pineal cyst ➡ does not compress completely.*

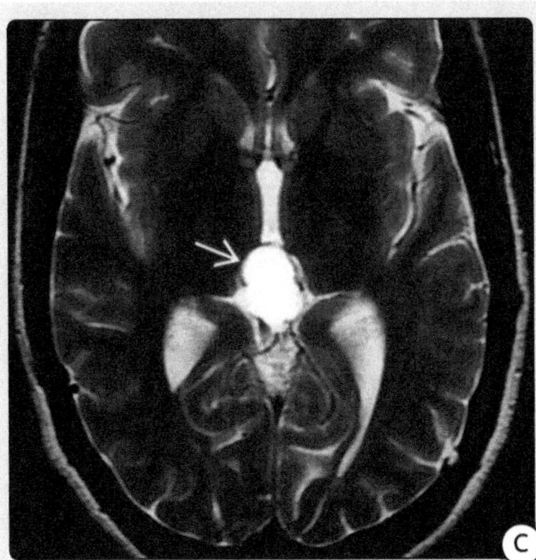

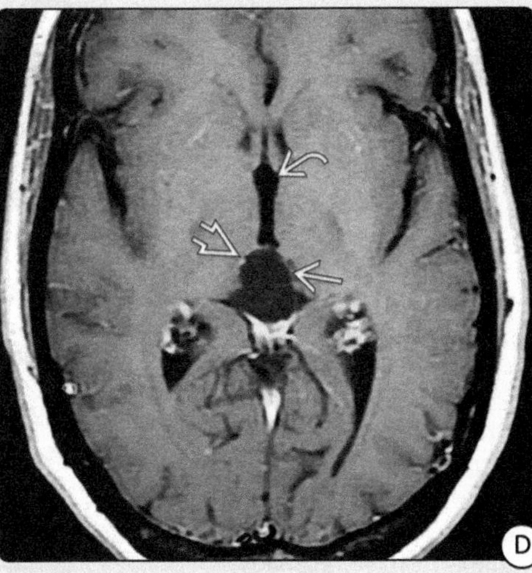

***(28-13C)** T2 MR in the same case shows that the cyst fluid ➡ appears slightly hyperintense compared with CSF in the ventricles. **(28-13D)** T1 C+ MR shows that the cyst fluid ➡ is slightly hyperintense compared with CSF in the adjacent 3rd ventricle ➡. Minimal enhancement of the cyst wall ➡ is present. This is a nonneoplastic pineal cyst.*

Natural History. Most PCs are "leave me alone" lesions. Follow-up of indeterminate cystic lesions of the pineal region usually shows no significant change over time intervals from months to years. Most investigators recommend that incidentally identified PCs be followed clinically and do not require serial imaging. Patients with growing lesions, atypical contrast enhancement, or hemorrhage on MR are more likely to develop hydrocephalus and have malignant pathology, so follow-up serial MRs are recommended.

Imaging

CT Findings. At least 25% of PCs show calcification within the cyst wall **(28-13A)**. The cyst fluid is iso- to slightly hyperdense compared with CSF. A very hyperdense PC in a patient with severe headache should raise suspicion of hemorrhage with cyst "apoplexy." Rim, crescentic, or nodular enhancement patterns have all been described with PCs.

The ventricles are usually normal. Large ventricles with "blurred" margins indicate acute obstructive hydrocephalus.

MR Findings. As with other cysts, PC signal intensity varies with imaging sequence and cyst contents. Between 50% and 60% of PCs are slightly hyperintense compared with CSF on T1WI. Approximately 40% are isointense with CSF. Approximately 1-2% are very hyperintense, which may indicate intracystic hemorrhage. A blood-fluid level may be present.

Most PCs are small and cause minimal or no mass effect. Large cysts may cause obstructive hydrocephalus. In such cases, PD and T2/FLAIR scans show "fingers" of hyperintensity extending into the periventricular white matter due to subependymal accumulation of brain interstitial fluid. These are especially well demonstrated on sagittal scans.

The vast majority of PCs are iso- to slightly hyperintense on T2WI **(28-13C)** and do not suppress completely on FLAIR **(28-13B)**. Internal septations are visible in 20-25% of cases, and 10% are multicystic. If acute hemorrhage has occurred, intracystic blood may appear very hypointense on T2WIs and "bloom" on T2* (GRE, SWI). PCs typically do not restrict on DWI.

Between 1/3 and 2/3 of PCs enhance. The most common pattern is a thin circumferential rim of enhancement **(28-13D)**. Less common patterns include nodular, crescentic, or irregular enhancement.

Differential Diagnosis

The most common differential diagnosis is **normal pineal gland**. Normal pineal glands often contain one or more small cysts and can have nodular, crescentic, or ring-like enhancement.

The most important pathologic entity to be differentiated from a PC is **pineocytoma**. Pineocytoma is a WHO grade I pineal parenchymal tumor that is usually solid or at least partially solid/cystic. Purely cystic pineocytomas are much less common and can be indistinguishable from PC on imaging. Pineocytomas can remain stable for many years without significant change on serial imaging.

Atypical imaging findings, focal invasion, or significant interval change in a presumed PC or pineocytoma should raise suspicion for the more aggressive **pineal parenchymal tumor of intermediate differentiation** (PPTID), which is a WHO grade II or III lesion.

PINEAL CYST

Pathology
- Usually < 1 cm; unilocular > multicystic
- Wall consists of compressed pineal parenchyma
- Fluid clear to yellowish

Clinical Issues
- Common
    - 23% of normal MRs; 25-40% of autopsies
- Occurs at any age; more common in adults
- Usually asymptomatic, found incidentally

Imaging
- Ca^{++} (25%)
- Fluid slightly hyperintense to CSF on MR
- Rim, nodular, or crescentic enhancement

Differential Diagnosis
- Normal pineal gland, pineocytoma

Parenchymal Cysts

Parenchymal (intraaxial) cysts are much more common than either their extraaxial or intraventricular counterparts. Once a cyst has been identified as lying within the brain itself, the differential diagnosis is limited. The most common parenchymal cysts—prominent perivascular spaces and hippocampal sulcus remnants—are anatomic variants. Neuroglial cysts and porencephalic cysts are relatively uncommon. All other nonneoplastic, noninfectious brain cysts are rare.

Enlarged Perivascular Spaces

By far, the most common parenchymal brain "cysts" are enlarged perivascular spaces (PVSs). They vary from solitary, small, inconspicuous, and unremarkable to multiple, large, bizarre, alarming-looking collections of CSF-like fluid. They are often asymmetric, may cause mass effect, and have frequently been mistaken for multicystic brain tumors.

Terminology

PVSs are also known as Virchow-Robin spaces. PVSs are pia-lined spaces that accompany penetrating arteries and arterioles into the brain parenchyma **(28-14)**. The PVSs do not communicate directly with the subarachnoid space.

Etiology

General Concepts. The brain PVSs form a complicated intraparenchymal network that is distributed throughout the cerebral hemispheres, midbrain, and cerebellum. They are filled with interstitial fluid (ISF), not CSF, and are thought to be a major pathway for ISF and cerebral metabolites to exit the brain. Recent evidence suggests the PVSs also perform an essential role in maintaining intracranial pressure homeostasis.

Precisely why some PVSs become enlarged is unknown. Most investigators believe ISF egress is blocked, causing cystic enlargement of the PVSs.

Genetics. Sporadic PVS enlargement has no known genetic predilection. Patients with Hurler, Hunter, or Sanfilippo disease accumulate undegraded mucopolysaccharides within enlarged PVSs. A few congenital muscular dystrophies have also been associated with cystic PVSs.

Pathology

Location. Although PVSs can be found virtually anywhere in the brain, they have a striking predilection for the inferior 1/3 of the basal ganglia, especially near the anterior commissure **(28-14)**. They are also common in the subcortical and deep white matter as well as the midbrain and dentate nuclei of the cerebellum.

Size and Number. Enlarged PVSs tend to occur in clusters. Collections of multiple variably sized PVSs are much more common than solitary unilocular lesions.

Most PVSs are smaller than 2 mm. PVSs increase in size and prevalence with age **(28-16)**. Giant so-called tumefactive PVSs measuring up to 9 cm in diameter have been reported.

Gross Pathology. Enlarged PVSs appear as collections of smoothly demarcated cysts filled with clear colorless fluid **(28-17)**.

Microscopic Features. PVSs are bounded by a single or double layer of invaginated pia. Cortical PVSs are lined by a single layer of pia, whereas two layers accompany lenticulostriate and midbrain arteries.

As a PVS penetrates into the subcortical white matter, it becomes fenestrated and discontinuous. The pial layer disappears completely at the capillary level.

The brain parenchyma surrounding enlarged PVSs is typically normal without gliosis, inflammation, hemorrhage, or discernible amyloid deposition.

Clinical Issues

Epidemiology. PVSs are the most common nonneoplastic parenchymal brain "cysts." With high-resolution 3T MR, small PVSs are seen in nearly all patients **(28-15)**, in virtually every location, and at all ages. Between 25-30% of children have identifiable PVSs on high-resolution MR scans.

Demographics. Enlarged PVSs are more common in middle-aged and older patients and increase in both size and number with age **(28-16)**. Recent studies have linked enlarged PVSs with age, lacunar stroke subtype, and white matter lesions and consider them as an MR marker of cerebral small vessel disease.

Presentation. Most enlarged PVSs do not cause symptoms and are discovered incidentally on imaging studies or at autopsy. Neuropsychological evaluation is typically normal. Nonspecific symptoms, such as headache, dizziness, memory impairment, and Parkinson-like symptoms, have been reported in some cases, but their relationship to enlarged PVSs is unclear. Large PVSs in the midbrain may cause obstructive hydrocephalus and present with headache.

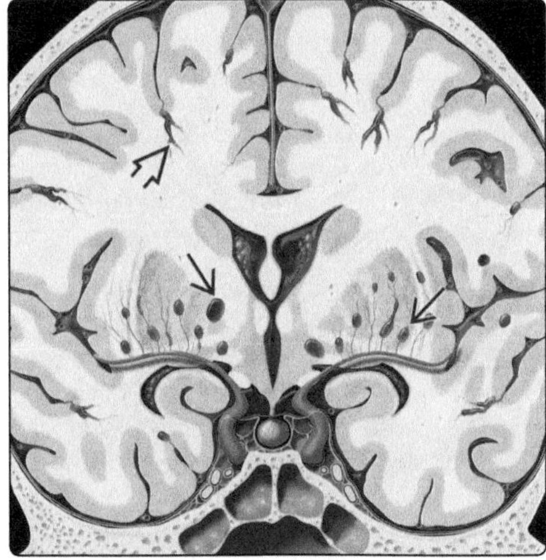

***(28-14)** Graphic shows normal PVSs along penetrating arteries in the basal ganglia ➔ and subcortical white matter ⇨.*

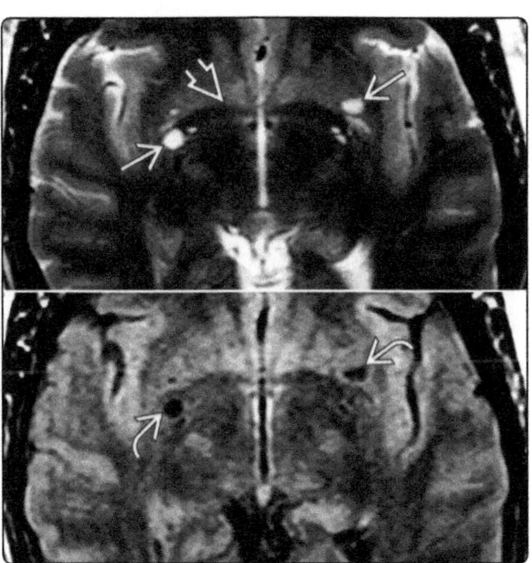

***(28-15)** (Top) T2 MR shows perivascular spaces ➔ clustered around the anterior commissure ⇨. ISF-filled VRSs suppress on FLAIR ↪ (bottom).*

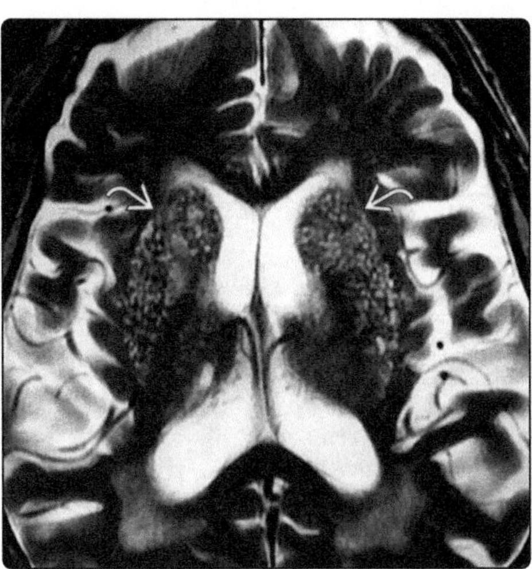

***(28-16)** Basal ganglia PVSs can become very prominent in older patients ↪, a condition termed "état criblé" or cribriform state.*

Natural History. Enlarged PVSs tend to be stable in size and remain unchanged over many years, although a few cases of progressively enlarging PVSs have been reported.

Treatment Options. Enlarged PVSs are "leave me alone" lesions that should not be mistaken for serious disease. If midbrain PVSs cause obstructive hydrocephalus, the generally accepted treatment is to shunt the ventricles, not the cysts.

Imaging

General Features. The common pattern of enlarged PVSs is one or more clusters of variably sized CSF-like cysts. They commonly cause focal mass effect. For example, if they occur in the subcortical white matter, the overlying gyri are enlarged with concomitant compression of adjacent sulci **(28-19)**.

CT Findings. Enlarged PVSs are groups of round/ovoid/linear/punctate CSF-like lesions that do not demonstrate calcification or hemorrhage. PVSs do not enhance following contrast administration.

MR Findings. Even though they are filled with ISF, PVSs closely parallel CSF signal intensity on all imaging sequences. Focal mass effect is common. Enlarged PVSs in the subcortical white matter expand overlying gyri **(28-19)** **(28-20)**. Enlarged "tumefactive" PVSs in the midbrain may compress the aqueduct and third ventricle, resulting in intraventricular obstructive hydrocephalus **(28-17)**.

PVSs are isointense with CSF on T1-, PD, and T2WI. They suppress completely on FLAIR **(28-15)**. Edema in the adjacent brain is absent, although 25% of "tumefactive" PVSs have minimal increased signal intensity around the cysts.

PVSs do not hemorrhage, enhance, or demonstrate restricted diffusion.

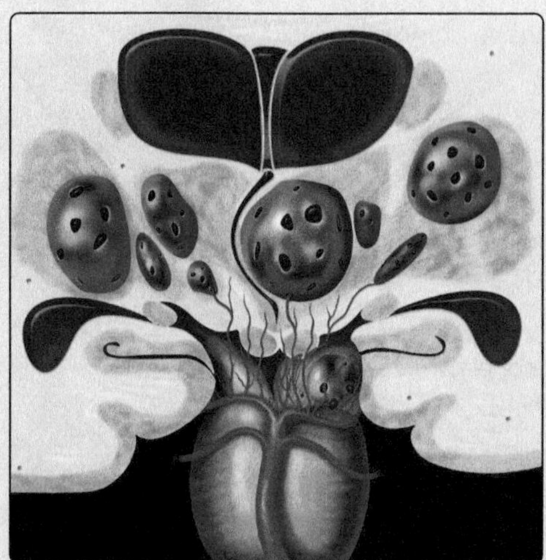

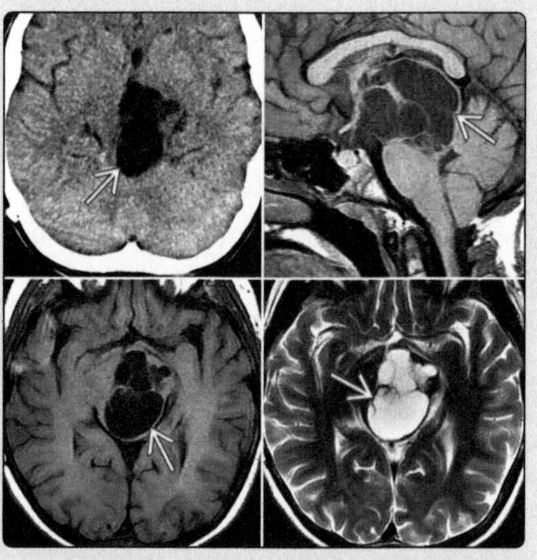

***(28-17)** Coronal graphic shows enlarged perivascular spaces in the midbrain and thalami that cause mass effect on the 3rd ventricle and aqueduct with resulting hydrocephalus. **(28-18)** NECT and MR scans show a cluster of variably sized CSF-like cysts ➡ grossly expanding the midbrain. These are giant "tumefactive" perivascular spaces.*

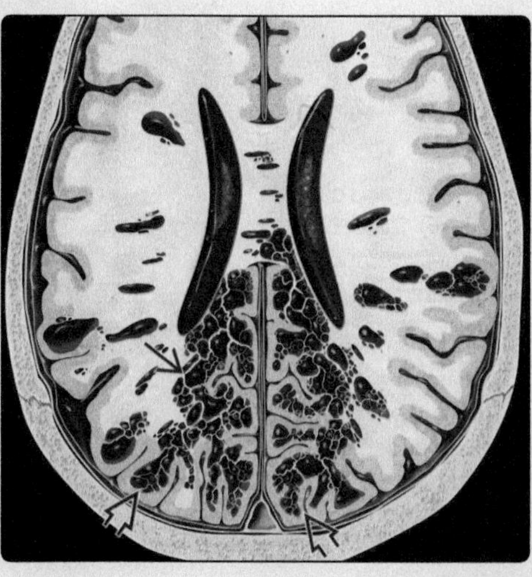

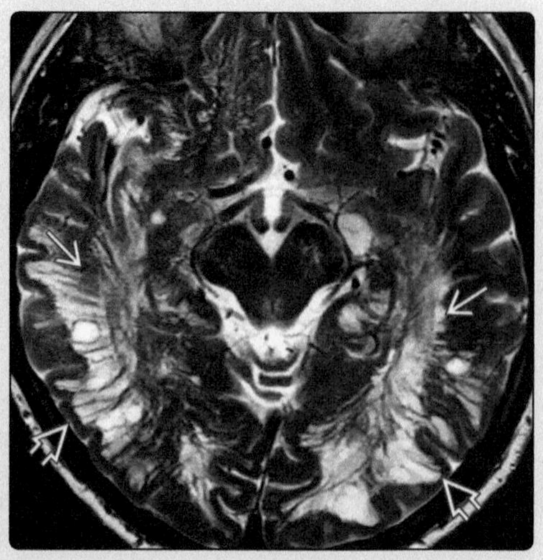

***(28-19)** Graphic depicts innumerable hemispheric enlarged PVSs ➡ in subcortical, deep white matter. Note that the overlying gyri ➡ are expanded but otherwise normal. **(28-20)** Axial T2 MR in a 69-year-old moderately demented man shows innumerable enlarged PVSs ➡. Note sparing of overlying cortex, which appears expanded ➡. (Courtesy M. Warmuth-Metz, MD.)*

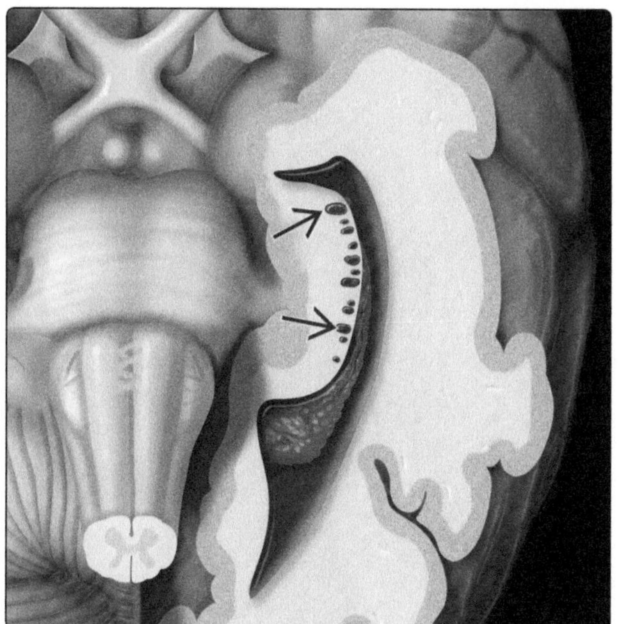

***(28-21)** Graphic of normal temporal lobe shows a string of cysts within the lateral hippocampus, along the residual cavity of the primitive hippocampal sulcus ⇨. Hippocampal sulcus remnant cysts are incidental, a normal finding.*

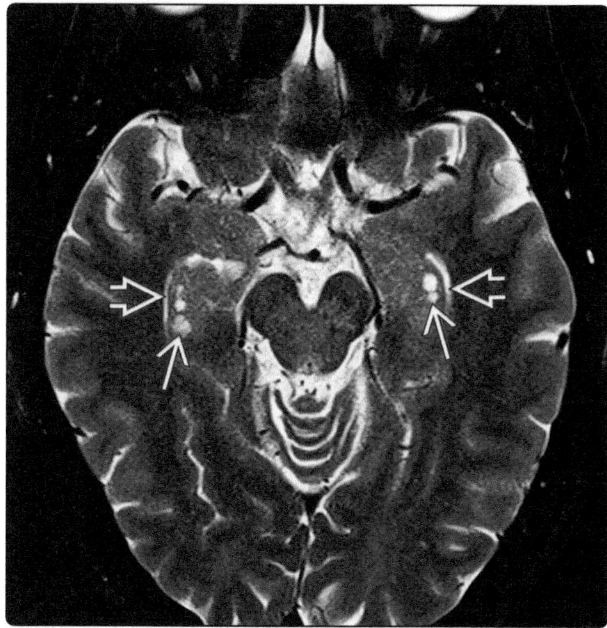

***(28-22)** Axial T2 MR shows bilateral hippocampal sulcus remnants ➡ located just medial to the temporal horns of the lateral ventricles ➡. The cysts suppressed completely on FLAIR (not shown).*

Differential Diagnosis

The major differential diagnosis is chronic **lacunar infarction**. Although they often affect the basal ganglia and suppress on FLAIR, lacunar infarcts do not cluster around the anterior commissure, are often irregular in shape, and frequently exhibit hyperintensity in the adjacent brain.

In some older patients, very prominent PVSs in the basal ganglia are present. This condition, called **"état criblé"** (cribriform state), should not be mistaken for multiple lacunar infarcts. PVSs are round/ovoid and regular in configuration, and the adjacent brain parenchyma is usually normal without gliosis or edema.

Infectious cysts (especially parenchymal neurocysticercosis cysts) are usually small. Although often multiple or multilocular, they typically do not occur in clusters of variably sized cysts as is typical for enlarged PVSs.

ENLARGED PERIVASCULAR SPACES (PVSs)

Terminology
- a.k.a. Virchow-Robin spaces
- Found around penetrating blood vessels
- Lined by pia; filled with interstitial fluid
- Do not communicate directly with subarachnoid space

Pathology
- Normal PVSs common; < 2 cm
- Giant "tumefactive" PVSs up to 9 cm reported
- Basal ganglia, subcortical white matter most common

Imaging
- Often bizarre-looking
- Occur in clusters
- Variably sized cysts
- Follow CSF

Hippocampal Sulcus Remnants

Etiology

At 15 fetal weeks, the hippocampus normally surrounds an "open" shallow fissure—the hippocampal sulcus—along the medial surface of the temporal lobe. The walls of the hippocampal sulcus gradually fuse, and the sulcus is eventually obliterated. One or more residual cystic cavities may remain and persist into adult life **(28-21)**. These remnant cavities—hippocampal remnant cysts—are normal anatomic variants and are of no clinical significance.

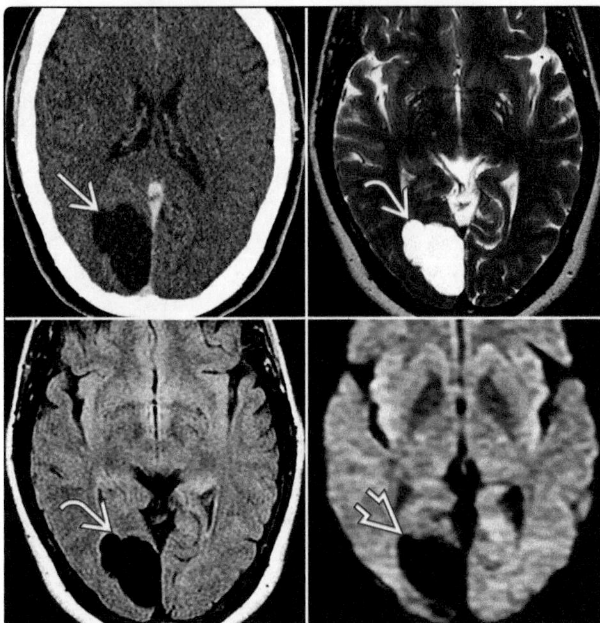

(28-23) Proven neuroglial cyst in the right occipital lobe does not enhance on CECT ➡, follows CSF on T2/FLAIR ➡, and does not restrict ➡.

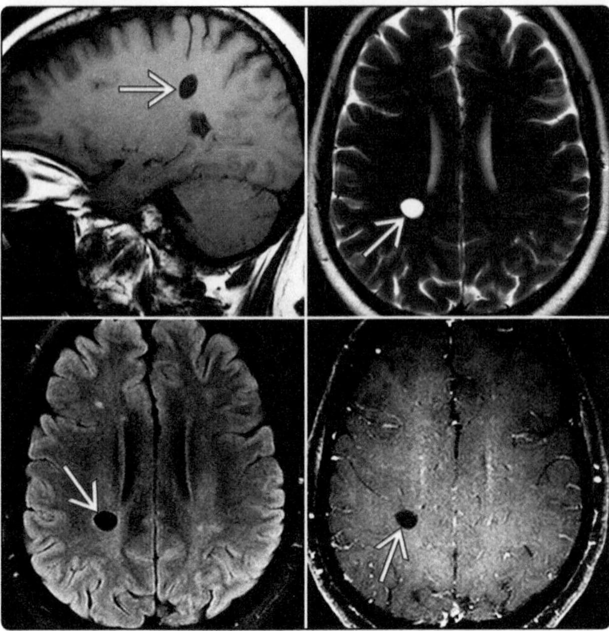

(28-24) MR shows a small presumed right parietal neuroglial cyst ➡. The cyst follows CSF on all sequences and has been stable for 9 years.

Imaging

HCSRs are seen in 10-15% of normal high-resolution MR scans. They appear as a "string of beads" with multiple small round or ovoid cysts curving along the hippocampus between the dentate gyrus and subiculum, just medial to the temporal horn of the lateral ventricle **(28-22)**. HCSRs follow CSF in signal intensity on all sequences. They suppress completely on FLAIR, do not enhance, and do not restrict on DWI.

Differential Diagnosis

The major differential diagnosis is **enlarged perivascular spaces**. When they occur in the temporal lobe, enlarged perivascular spaces are found in the subcortical white matter of the insula and anterior tip of the temporal lobe, not medial to the temporal horn of the lateral ventricle.

Neuroglial Cyst

Terminology

Neuroglial cysts (NGCs) are sometimes called **glioependymal cysts** or **neuroepithelial cysts**. They are benign fluid-containing cavities buried within the cerebral white matter.

Pathology

The frontal lobe is the most common site. NGCs often lie adjacent to—but do not communicate directly with—the cerebral ventricles. Most are solitary, unilocular cysts that vary in size from a few millimeters up to several centimeters in diameter.

Grossly, NGCs are rounded, smooth, unilocular cysts that contain clear CSF-like fluid. Most NGCs are lined with a simple, nonstratified, low columnar/cuboidal epithelium.

Clinical Issues

Parenchymal NGCs are uncommon, representing < 1% of all intracranial cysts. NGCs occur in all age groups but are generally more common in adults. There is no sex predilection.

NGCs are often asymptomatic and found incidentally at imaging or autopsy. Many—if not most—NGCs remain stable over many years. Serial observation with imaging studies is the usual course, although some large NGCs have been fenestrated or drained.

Imaging

NGCs are fluid density, typically resemble CSF on NECT, do not contain calcifications, and do not hemorrhage.

MR signal intensity varies with cyst content. Most NGCs are iso- or slightly hyperintense to CSF **(28-23)**. They usually suppress on FLAIR, do not restrict, and do not enhance **(28-24)**. The parenchyma surrounding an NGC is usually normal or may show minimal gliosis.

Differential Diagnosis

The diagnosis of NGC is mostly a process of elimination, excluding other, sometimes more ominous possibilities.

The major differential diagnosis of NGC is a solitary **enlarged perivascular space**. Most enlarged PVSs are multiple (not solitary) and occur as clusters of variably sized cysts. A **porencephalic cyst** is a result of an insult to the brain

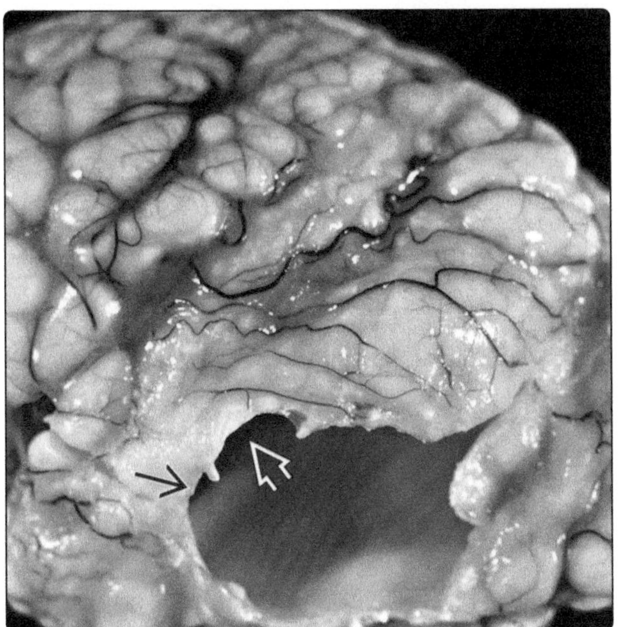

(28-25) Autopsy specimen shows a typical porencephalic cyst as a CSF-filled cavity that extends from the brain surface ⇒ to the ventricular ependyma ⇒. (Courtesy J. Townsend, MD.)

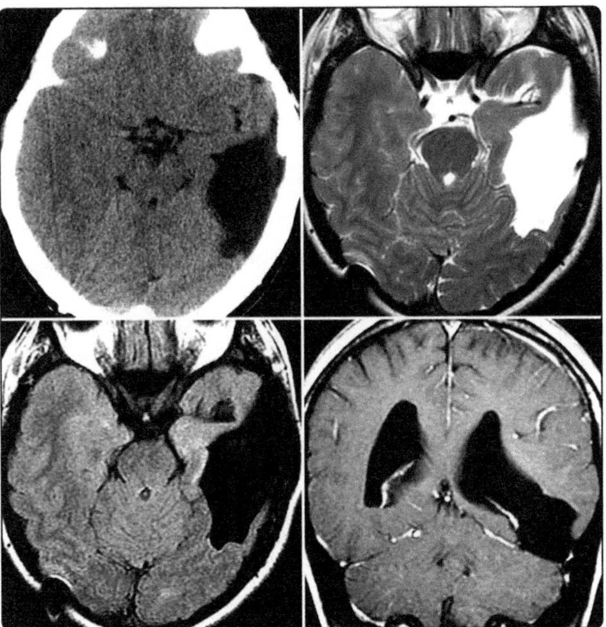

(28-26) NECT, MR scans show a posttraumatic porencephalic cyst extending from the surface of the temporal lobe to the temporal horn of the lateral ventricle. The cyst contains CSF.

parenchyma. Porencephalic cysts communicate with the ventricle and are lined by gliotic or spongiotic white matter.

Arachnoid cysts are extraaxial, not intraaxial, and are lined with flattened arachnoid cells. **Epidermoid cysts** are almost always extraaxial, do not suppress on FLAIR, and restrict on DWI. **Ependymal cysts** are intraventricular. **Neoplastic** and **inflammatory cysts** generally do not follow CSF, often demonstrate wall enhancement or calcification, and are frequently surrounded by edema.

Porencephalic Cyst

Terminology

"Porencephaly" literally means a hole in the brain. Porencephalic cysts are congenital or acquired CSF-filled parenchymal cavities that usually—but not invariably—communicate with the ventricular system.

Pathology

Porencephalic cysts are encephaloclastic lesions, the end result of a destructive process (e.g., trauma, infection, vascular insult, surgery) that compromises brain parenchyma. They range in size from a few centimeters to cysts that involve virtually an entire cerebral hemisphere.

Porencephalic cysts are typically deep, uni- or bilateral, smooth-walled cavities or excavations within the brain parenchyma. They are often "full-thickness" lesions, extending from the ventricle to the cortex **(28-25)**. Occasionally, a thin rim of ependyma or subependymal white matter may separate the cyst from the ventricle.

Clinical Issues

Porencephalic cysts are relatively common, especially in children, in whom they represent 2.5% of congenital brain lesions. Spastic hemiplegia, medically refractory epilepsy, and psychomotor retardation are the most common symptoms.

Most porencephalic cysts remain stable for many years. Occasionally, a porencephalic cyst will continue to sequester fluid and expand, causing mass effect.

Imaging

CT Findings. Porencephalic cysts are sharply marginated, smooth-walled, CSF-filled cavities that usually communicate directly with an adjacent ventricle **(28-26)**. The ipsilateral ventricle is often enlarged secondary to volume loss in the adjacent parenchyma.

Calcification is rare. Bone CT may show skull thinning and remodeling caused by chronic CSF pulsations. Porencephalic cysts do not enhance.

MR Findings. Porencephalic cysts follow CSF signal intensity on all sequences **(28-26)**. Large cysts may show internal inhomogeneities secondary to spin dephasing. These cysts suppress completely on FLAIR, although there is often a rim of hyperintense gliotic or spongiotic white matter around the cyst. No restriction on DWI is present.

Differential Diagnosis

The major differential diagnosis is **cystic encephalomalacia**. An encephalomalacic cavity is often more irregular and does not communicate with the adjacent ventricle.

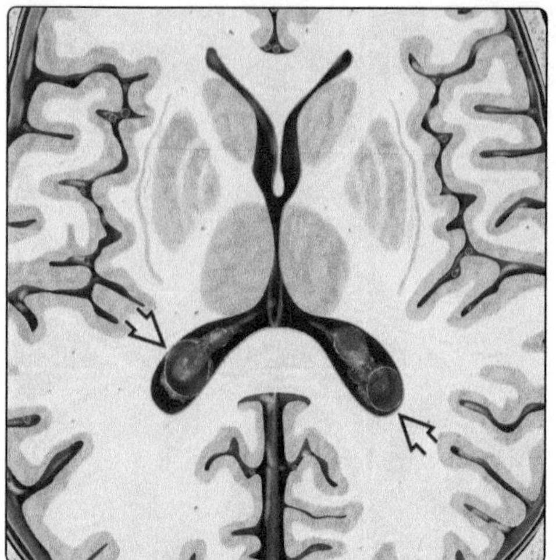

***(28-27)** Multiple cystic masses are in choroid plexus glomi ⇒; in adults, it increases with age. Most are degenerative xanthogranulomas.*

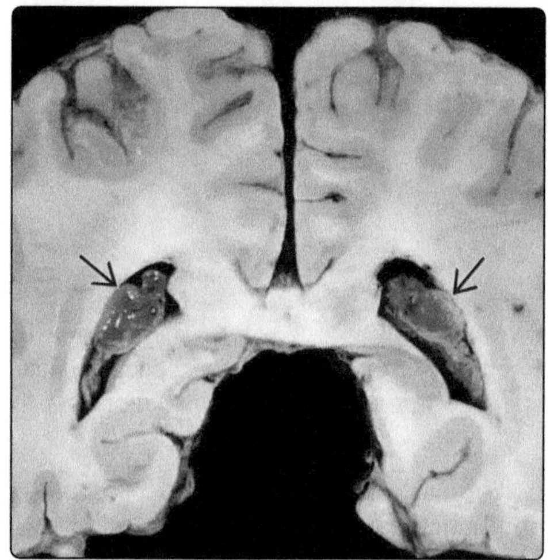

***(28-28)** Autopsy specimen shows multiple cysts in the choroid plexus glomi of both lateral ventricles ⇒. (Courtesy N. Nakase, MD.)*

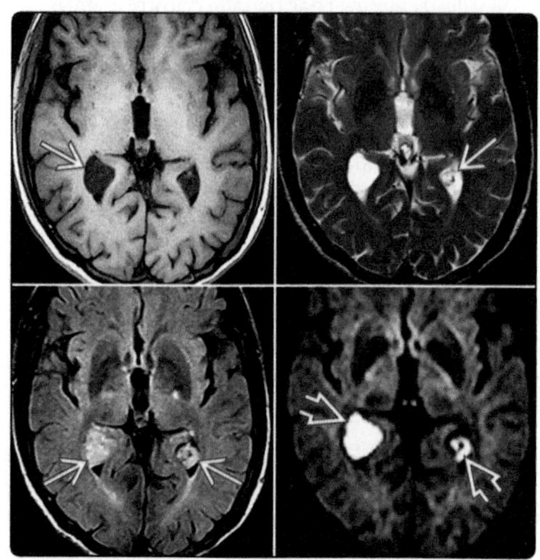

***(28-29)** Choroid plexus cysts are usually bilateral and hyperintense compared with CSF ➡ and are often very bright on DWI ➡.*

Porencephalic cysts are lined by reactive gliosis (glial "scar"), which occurs when histologically benign astrocytes proliferate in and around damaged brain parenchyma. A porencephalic cyst with surrounding **reactive gliosis** must be distinguished from **spongiosis**, a process that represents tissue loss (not astrocytic proliferation) with formation of empty (spongiform) areas ("holes") in the brain. Gliosis is a low to medium cellularity lesion that is hyperintense on T2WI and does not suppress on FLAIR. Spongiosis is T2 hyperintense but suppresses on FLAIR.

An **arachnoid cyst** is extraaxial and does not communicate with the ventricle. **Schizencephaly** (literally "split brain") is a congenital lesion that can be either "open" or "closed lip." An "open lip" schizencephalic cleft can look very much like a porencephalic cyst but is lined with dysplastic gray matter, not gliotic white matter.

Intraventricular Cysts

Intraventricular cysts include choroid plexus cysts, colloid cysts, and ependymal cysts.

Choroid Plexus Cysts

Choroid plexus cysts (CPCs), also called choroid plexus xanthogranulomas, are one of the most common types of intracranial cyst. Most are small and unremarkable. Occasionally, large cysts may appear somewhat atypical and cause diagnostic concern.

Terminology

A CPC is also often called a choroid plexus xanthogranuloma. CPCs are nonneoplastic noninflammatory cysts of the choroid plexus **(28-27)**.

Etiology

General Concepts. CPCs can be either congenital or acquired. Acquired lesions are much more common; lipid that accumulates from desquamating, degenerating choroid plexus epithelium coalesces into macrocysts and provokes a xanthomatous response.

Genetics. Large (> 10 mm), congenital CPCs can be associated with aneuploidy, particularly trisomy 18. CPCs, together with choroid plexus papillomas, also occur as part of Aicardi syndrome.

Pathology

Most CPCs are found in the atrium of the lateral ventricle, within the choroid plexus glomus **(28-28)**. Most are small, ranging from a few millimeters up to 1 cm, although occasionally larger cysts exceed 2 cm in diameter. Multiple bilateral lesions are significantly more common than solitary unilateral CPCs.

CPCs are nodular, partly cystic, yellowish-gray masses that are most often found in the choroid plexus glomus. They are highly proteinaceous and often gelatinous. Gross hemorrhage is rare.

CHOROID PLEXUS CYSTS: ETIOLOGY, PATHOLOGY, AND CLINICAL ISSUES

Etiology

- Congenital
  - Aicardi syndrome
  - Trisomy 18
- Acquired
  - Desquamated, degenerated epithelium
  - Xanthomatous response

Pathology

- Bilateral, usually multiloculated
- Most common in glomi of choroid plexus
- Proteinaceous, gelatinous contents

Clinical Issues

- Most common intracranial cyst
- Most found incidentally
- Most common in fetus/infants, older adults

Clinical Issues

CPCs are the most common of all intracranial cysts, occurring in up to 50% of autopsies. CPCs are found at both ends of the age spectrum. In adults, their prevalence increases with age, whereas fetal CPCs decrease with gestational age. There is no sex predilection.

Most adult CPCs are found incidentally and are asymptomatic, remaining stable for many years. Congenital CPCs are detected on prenatal ultrasound in 1% of fetuses during the second trimester and generally resolve during the third trimester. When detected postnatally, CPCs are of no clinical significance in otherwise normal neonates.

Imaging

CT Findings. CPCs are iso- to slightly hyperdense compared with intraventricular CSF. Irregular clumps of calcification around the margins are common findings. Enhancement varies from none to a complete rim surrounding each cyst.

MR Findings. CPCs do not precisely follow CSF signal intensity. They are iso- to slightly hyperintense compared with CSF on T1WI and are hyperintense on PD and T2WI. FLAIR signal is variable **(28-29)**.

Enhancement following contrast administration varies from none to striking. Solid, ring, and nodular patterns occur **(28-30)**.

Between 60-80% of CPCs appear quite bright on DWI but often remain isointense with parenchyma on ADC. This may therefore represent pseudorestriction rather than true restricted diffusion.

Differential Diagnosis

The major differential diagnosis of a CPC is an **ependymal cyst**. Ependymal cysts generally displace and compress the choroid plexus rather than arise from it. Ependymal cysts usually behave much more like CSF than CPCs do. **Neurocysticercosis cysts** are relatively uncommon and are not associated with the choroid plexus.

Choroid plexus papilloma of the lateral ventricle is a tumor of children younger than 5 years old. An enhancing, enlarged choroid plexus without frank cyst formation can also be seen with **Sturge-Weber malformation, collateral venous drainage**, and **diffuse villous hyperplasia**.

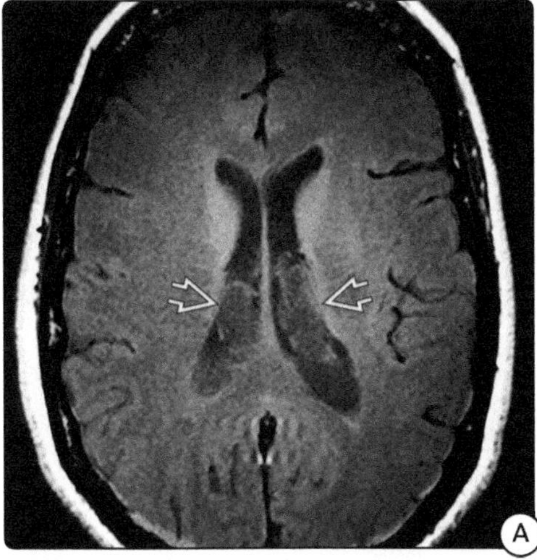

***(28-30A)** Variant choroid plexus cysts are in the body of the lateral ventricle. Cyst contents ➡ are slightly hyperintense compared with CSF.*

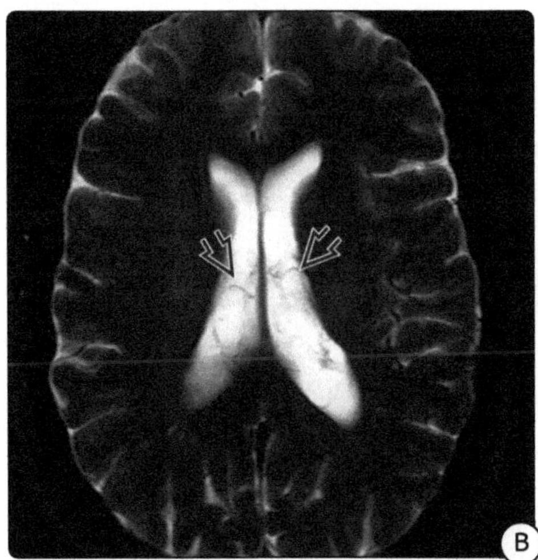

***(28-30B)** The cysts are so hyperintense on T2WI that the thin cyst walls are barely visible ➡.*

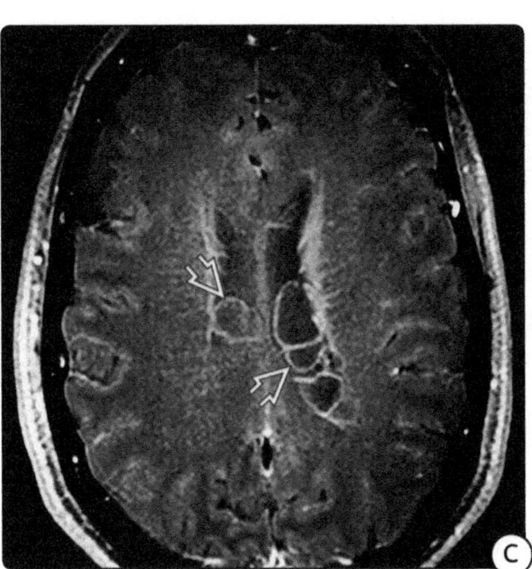

***(28-30C)** T1 C+ FS MR shows that the thin walls of these multiloculated choroid plexus cysts enhance moderately ➡.*

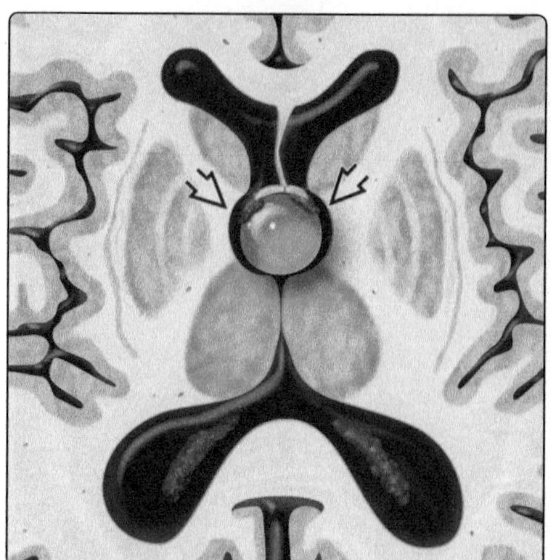

***(28-31)** Graphic shows colloid cyst ➪ at the foramen of Monro causing mild/moderate obstructive hydrocephalus.*

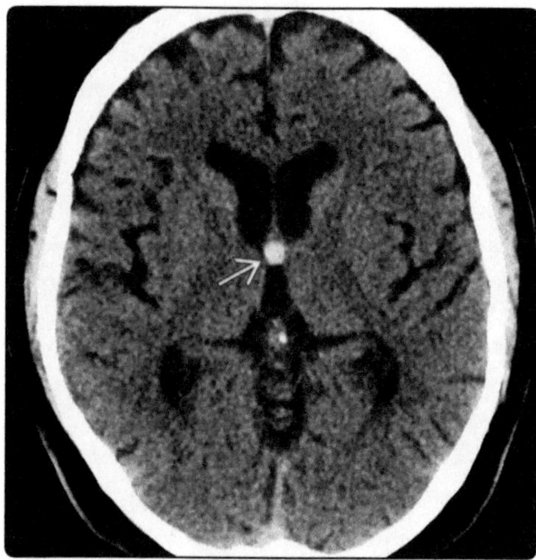

***(28-32)** NECT reveals a classic colloid cyst as a well-circumscribed hyperdense mass ➡ in the foramen of Monro.*

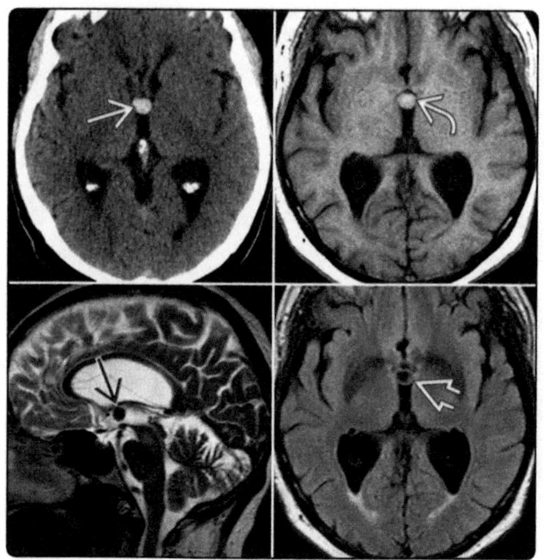

***(28-33)** NECT shows hyperdense colloid cyst ➡ that is hyperintense on T1WI ➡, hypointense on T2WI ➡, with mixed signal intensity on FLAIR ➪.*

CHOROID PLEXUS CYST: IMAGING AND DDx

CT

- Iso-/mildly hyperdense
- Ca^{++} common

MR

- Iso-/mildly hyperintense to CSF on T1WI
- Hyperintense on PD/T2WI, FLAIR variable
- Variable enhancement (usually thin rim)
- Bright on DWI but isointense on ADC

Differential Diagnosis

- Most common = ependymal cyst
- Uncommon/rare
  - Epidermoid cyst (rarely intraventricular)
  - Cystic metastasis

Colloid Cyst

Terminology

Colloid cysts (CCs) are also called paraphyseal cysts. They are unilocular, mucin-containing endodermal cysts. They are almost always found wedged into the top of the third ventricle at the foramen of Monro **(28-31)**.

Pathology

CCs are virtually always solitary lesions. Size varies from tiny (a few millimeters) up to 3 cm. Mean diameter is 1.5 cm. CCs are smooth-walled, well-demarcated, spherical or ovoid cysts that have a thin fibrous capsule and gelatinous center of variable viscosity. They are lined with simple or pseudostratified columnar epithelium with variable mucin-secreting goblet cells interspersed throughout the cyst lining.

Clinical Issues

CCs represent ~ 1% of all intracranial tumors but 15-20% of all intraventricular tumors.

Most symptomatic CCs present between the third and fifth decades. The peak age is 40 years. Pediatric CCs are rare; < 8% of all patients are younger than 15 years old at the time of initial diagnosis.

The clinical presentation of CCs is diverse, ranging from asymptomatic, incidentally discovered cysts (nearly 1/2 of all patients) to acute deterioration, coma, and death. CCs cause symptoms when they obstruct CSF flow at the foramina of Monro. Headache is the presenting symptom in 50-60% of symptomatic patients.

Over 90% of CCs—especially small cysts found in older patients—are stable and do not enlarge. The roughly 10% that *do* enlarge tend to be larger lesions, often causing hydrocephalus, and are found in younger patients. Incidental lesions rarely cause acute obstructive hydrocephalus or sudden neurological deterioration. Cyst "apoplexy" with intracystic hemorrhage and sudden enlargement occurs but is rare.

COLLOID CYST: PATHOETIOLOGY AND CLINICAL ISSUES

Etiology

- Endodermal cyst
- Probably derived from ectopic elements in diencephalic roof

Pathology

- Foramen of Monro (> 99%)
- Size varies from a few millimeters up to 3 cm
- Fibrous capsule
- Cyst lining
  - Columnar epithelium
  - Mucin-secreting goblet cells
- Gelatinous center (variable viscosity)

Clinical Issues

- Epidemiology
  - 1% of all intracranial tumors
  - 15-20% of intraventricular masses
- Peak age = 40 years (rare in children)
- Asymptomatic, found incidentally (50%)
- Headache most common symptom
- Sudden obstruction can cause coma, death
- Stable, do not enlarge (90%)

Treatment Options. Small asymptomatic CCs that are discovered incidentally and followed with serial imaging rarely grow or cause obstructive hydrocephalus. However, their treatment is debated. Neuroendoscopic management has emerged as a safe, effective alternative.

Imaging

CCs are well-delineated round or ovoid masses. Imaging appearance depends on their viscosity &/or cholesterol content. The relative amounts of mucous material, cholesterol, protein, and water content all affect density/signal intensity. Desiccated, inspissated cysts appear very different from water-rich lesions.

CT Findings. Density on NECT correlates directly with the hydration state of the cyst contents. Nearly 2/3 of all CCs are hyperdense compared with brain **(28-32)**, whereas 1/3 are iso- to hypodense. Hydrocephalus is variable. Intracystic hemorrhage and calcification are very rare.

Most CCs show no enhancement. Occasionally, a thin enhancing rim surrounds the cyst. Solid or nodular enhancement almost never occurs.

MR Findings. Signal intensity varies with cyst content.

Signal intensity on T1WI reflects cholesterol concentration. Most CCs are hyperintense compared with brain **(28-33)**, but 1/3 are isointense. Small isointense CCs may be very difficult to identify on T1WI.

Signal on PD and T2WI is more variable, as it is more reflective of water content. Most CCs are minimally hyperintense to brain on PD and usually isointense on T2WI **(28-33)**. A few CCs with inspissated contents are hypointense. Approximately 25% demonstrate mixed hypo- and hyperintensity (the "black hole" effect). Fluid-fluid levels are rare.

CCs do not suppress on FLAIR nor do they restrict on DWI.

CCs generally do not enhance. A thin peripheral rim of enhancement can be seen in some cases.

Differential Diagnosis

A well-delineated focal hyperdense lesion at the foramen of Monro on NECT scan is virtually pathognomonic of a CC. On MR, the most common "lesion" that mimics a CC is artifact caused by **pulsatile CSF flow**.

Neoplasms, such as **metastasis** and **subependymoma** (usually in the frontal horn or foramen of Monro, not anterosuperior third ventricle), can be hyperdense on NECT scans. Large **craniopharyngiomas** and pituitary **macroadenomas** occasionally extend superiorly almost to the foramen of Monro.

COLLOID CYST: IMAGING AND DDx

Imaging

- CT
  - 2/3 hyperdense
  - 1/3 iso- to hypodense
  - Usually do not enhance
- MR
  - Signal intensity varies with sequence, cyst contents
  - Typical: T1 hyper-, T2 hypointense
  - Inspissated: T2 hypointense
  - "Black hole" effect (25%)
  - Do not suppress on FLAIR
  - Generally do not enhance
  - Thin peripheral rim enhancement may occur
  - No restriction on DWI

Differential Diagnosis

- Most common
  - Ectatic basilar artery (NECT)
  - CSF flow artifact (MR)
- Less common
  - Metastasis
  - Subependymoma
  - Pituitary macroadenoma
  - Craniopharyngioma
- Rare but important
  - Low-grade astrocytoma
  - Lymphoma
  - Choroid plexus papilloma
  - Choroid plexus cyst
  - Xanthogranuloma

Ependymal Cyst

Ependymal cysts are also called glioependymal cysts. Some authors consider ependymal cysts a subtype of neuroepithelial cyst.

Ependymal cysts are solitary lesions, thin-walled, usually unilocular cysts that are filled with clear, CSF-like liquid. They

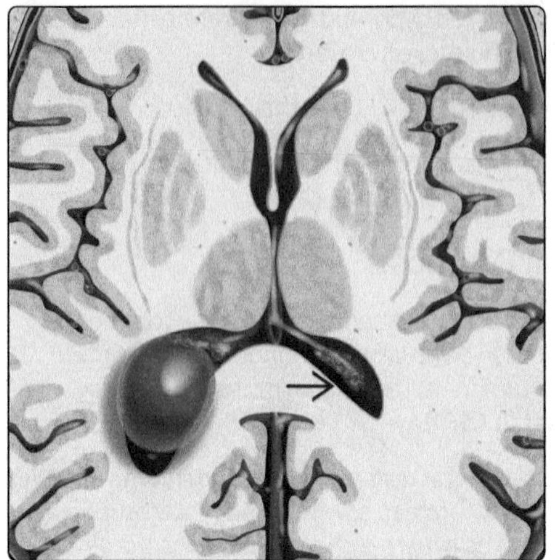

(28-34) Graphic depicts ependymal cyst of the lateral ventricle ⇒ as a CSF-containing simple cyst that displaces the choroid plexus around it.

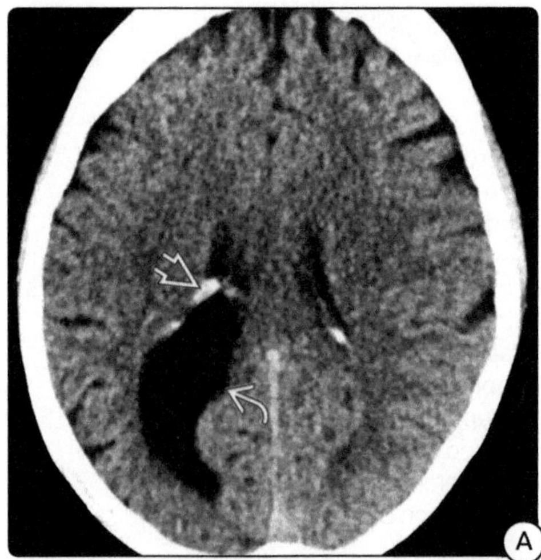

(28-35A) Axial NECT of ependymal cyst shows a CSF-containing mass ⇒ displacing the calcified choroid plexus around it ⇒.

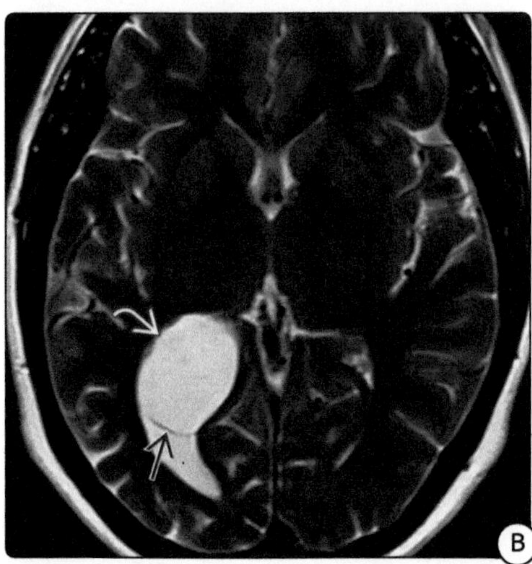

(28-35B) T2 MR in the same case shows that the unilocular ependymal cyst ⇒ is exactly like CSF. Note the distinct cyst wall ⇒.

are most often found in the atrium of the lateral ventricles, where they may cause significant ventricular asymmetry **(28-34)**. Less commonly, they occur in the brain parenchyma.

Clinical Issues

Ependymal cysts are typically asymptomatic and discovered incidentally at imaging or autopsy. Most patients present as young adults (under 40 years of age). Nonspecific symptoms, such as headache and cognitive dysfunction, are common. Large ependymal cysts occasionally cause obstructive hydrocephalus and increased intracranial pressure.

Imaging

Ependymal cysts parallel CSF in density/signal intensity **(28-35)**. They suppress completely on FLAIR, do not enhance, and do not demonstrate diffusion restriction. Thin-section heavily T2-weighted sequences, such as constructive interference in a steady state (CISS), may be necessary to delineate the cyst wall.

Differential Diagnosis

The major intraventricular mass that can mimic ependymal cyst is a **choroid plexus cyst**. Choroid plexus cysts are typically bilateral, often multilocular, and located within the choroid plexus glomi. Ependymal cysts arise *outside* the choroid plexus and usually displace it superolaterally.

Epidermoid cysts are rare in the lateral ventricle. They do not suppress completely on FLAIR and demonstrate diffusion restriction on DWI. **Arachnoid cysts** are identical to ependymal cysts in density and signal intensity but are rarely intraventricular. **Cystic metastases** to the choroid plexus are rare; nodular or irregular rim enhancement is typical.

EPENDYMAL CYST

Terminology
- Also called glioependymal or neuroepithelial cyst

Pathology
- 1% of intracranial cysts
- Solitary, usually unilocular
- Lined by columnar epithelium
- Contain CSF

Clinical Issues
- Most asymptomatic, discovered incidentally
- All ages, but usually < 40 years

Imaging
- Density, signal intensity = CSF
- No enhancement, no restriction

Differential Diagnosis
- Most common
  - Choroid plexus cyst
- Uncommon/rare
  - Epidermoid cyst
  - Arachnoid cyst
  - Cystic metastasis

Selected References: The complete reference list is available on the Expert Consult™ eBook version included with purchase.

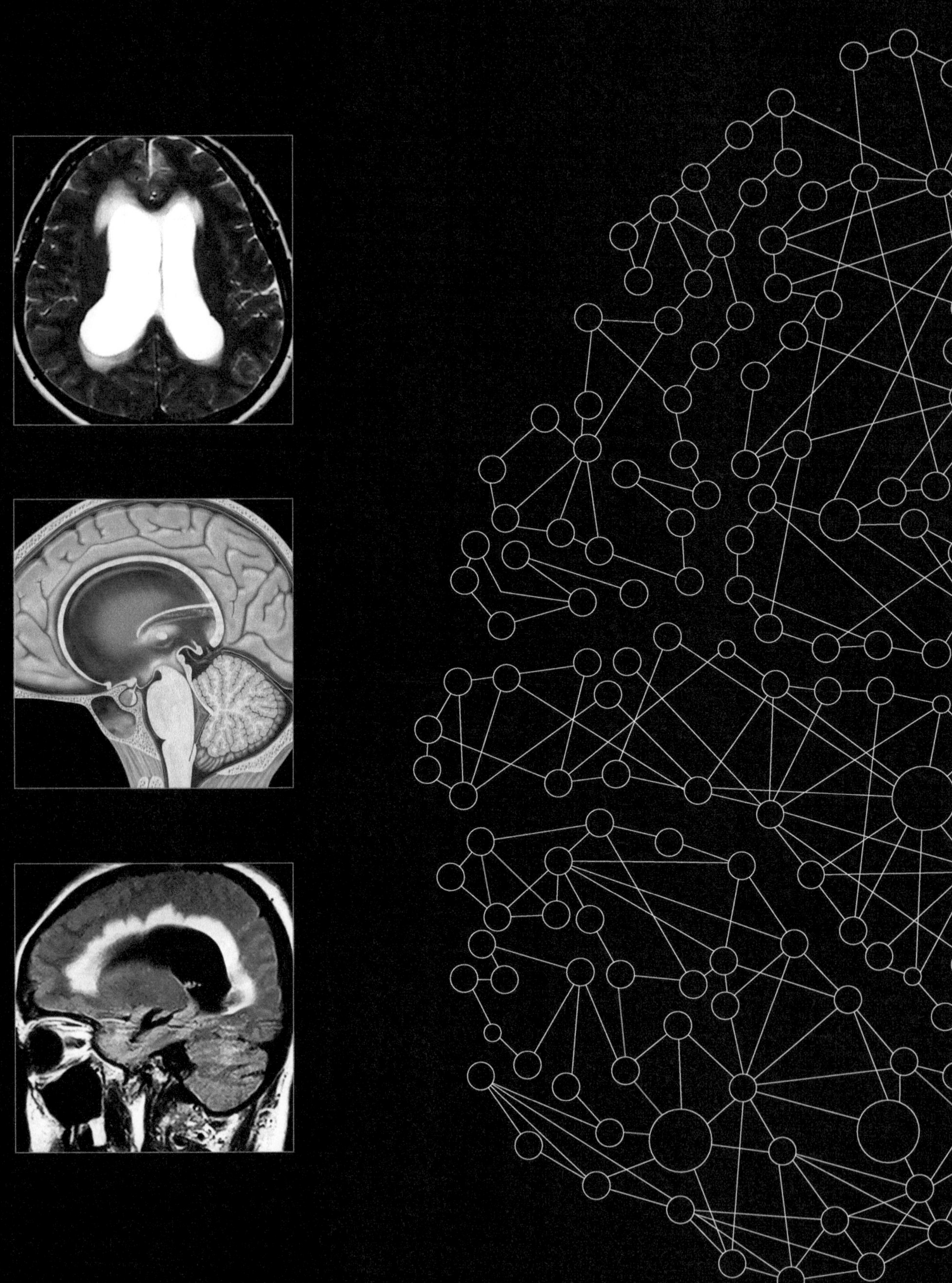

Section 5

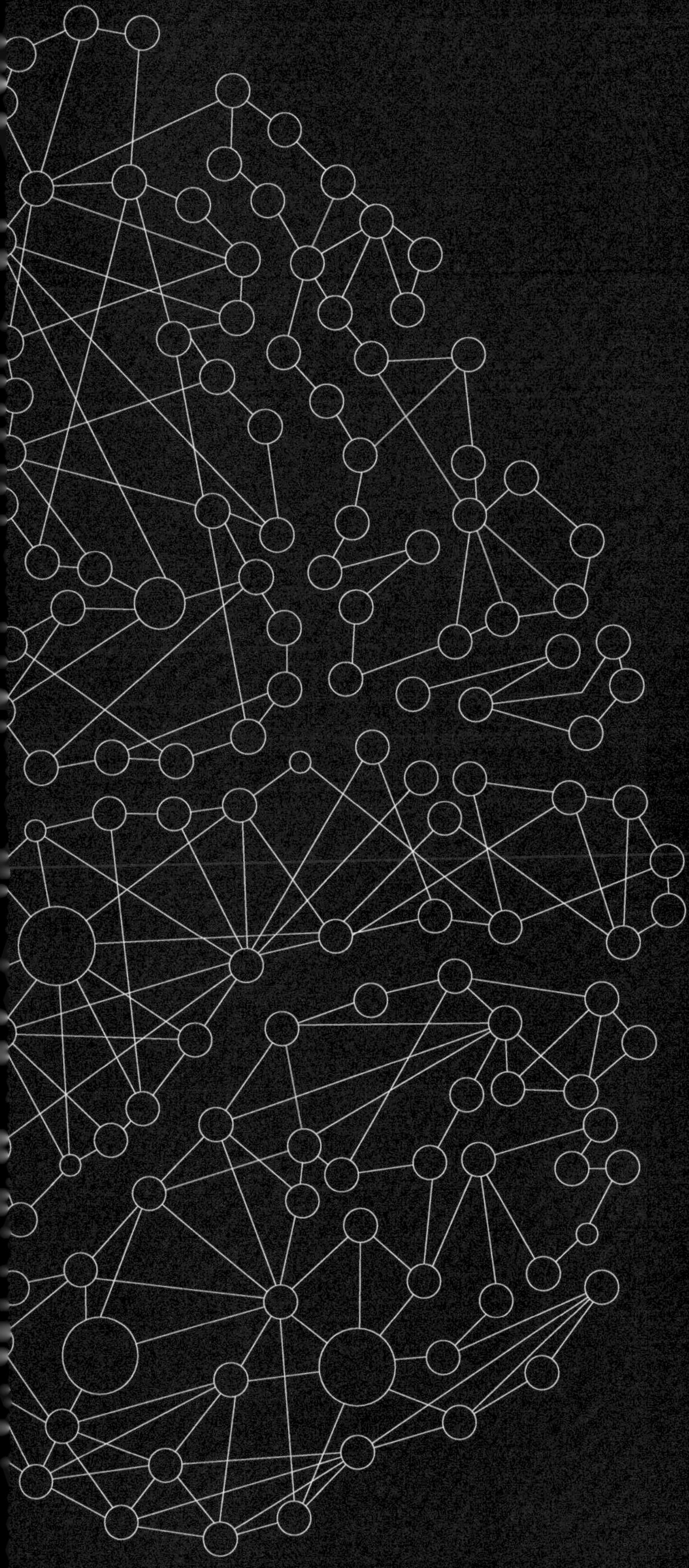

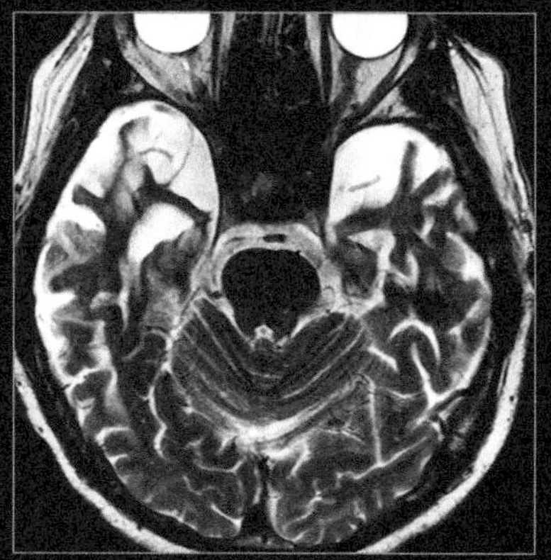

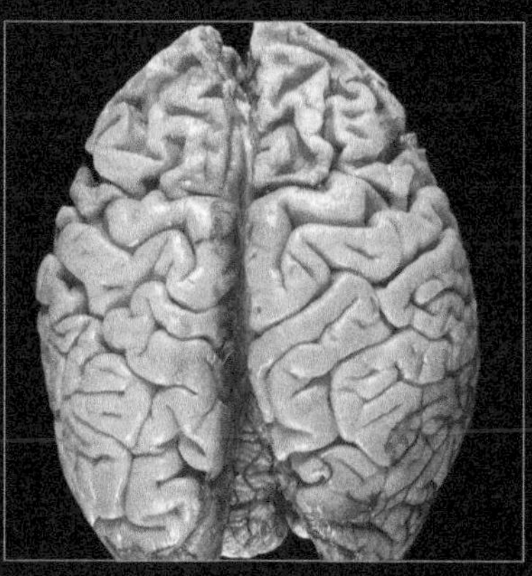

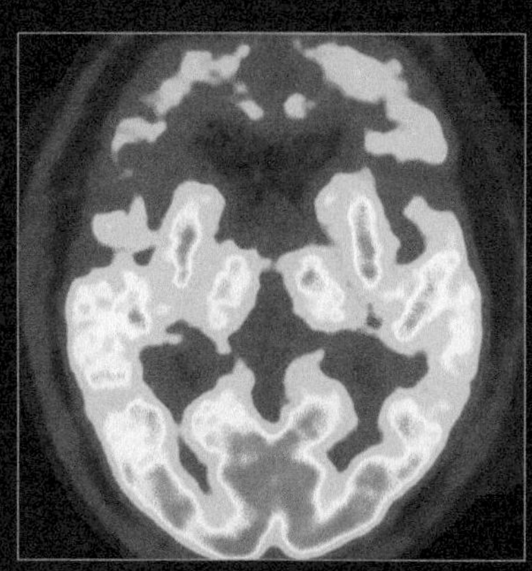

Section 5

Toxic, Metabolic, Degenerative, and CSF Disorders

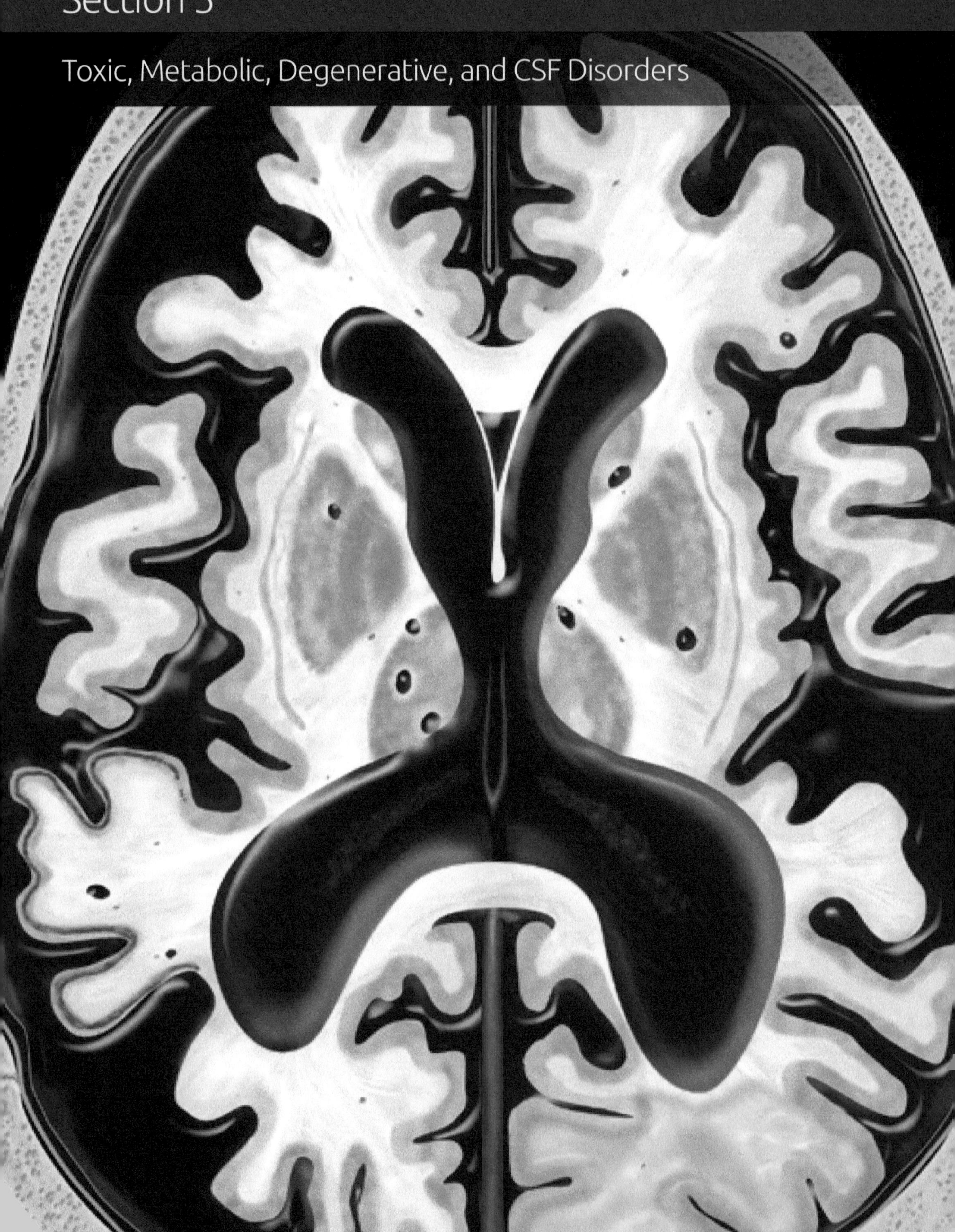

Approach to Toxic, Metabolic, Degenerative, and CSF Disorders

Metabolic disorders are relatively uncommon but important diseases in which imaging can play a key role in early diagnosis and appropriate patient management. Drug and alcohol abuse are increasing around the world, and the list of environmental toxins that can affect the CNS continues to increase. Recognizing toxic and metabolic-induced encephalopathies has become a clinical and imaging imperative. The two etiologies are often linked because many toxins induce metabolic derangements and some systemic metabolic diseases have a direct toxic effect on the brain.

With rapidly increasing numbers of aging people, the prevalence of dementia and brain degeneration is also becoming a global concern. Brain scans in elderly patients with mental status changes are now some of the most frequently requested imaging examinations, so normal and pathologic age-related CNS changes are discussed in this section.

Anatomy and Physiology of the Basal Ganglia and Thalami

Physiologic Considerations

By weight and volume, the brain is a small structure. However, relative to its size, the brain is one of the most metabolically active of all organs. It normally receives ~ 15% of total cardiac output, consumes ~ 20% of blood oxygen, and metabolizes up to 20% of blood glucose.

Because of its high intrinsic metabolic demands, the brain is exquisitely sensitive to processes that decrease delivery or utilization of blood, oxygen, and glucose. A variety of toxic substances do exactly that.

Two areas of the brain are especially susceptible to toxic and metabolic damage: The deep gray nuclei and the cerebral white matter (WM). The basal ganglia (BG) are highly vascular, rich in mitochondria, and loaded with neurotransmitters. The BG—especially the putamen and globus pallidus (GP)—are particularly susceptible to hypoxia or anoxia and are also commonly affected by toxins and metabolic derangements. The cerebral WM is particularly vulnerable to lipophilic toxic substances.

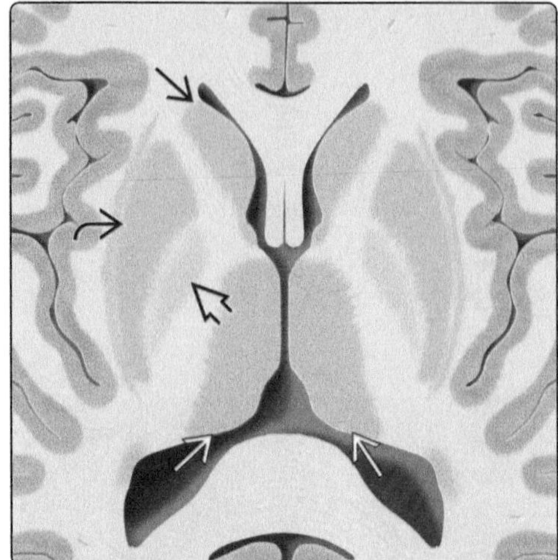

(29-1) Graphic depicts basal ganglia, caudate nucleus ➡, putamen ➡, and globus pallidus (GP) ➡. Thalami ➡ form borders of the 3rd ventricle.

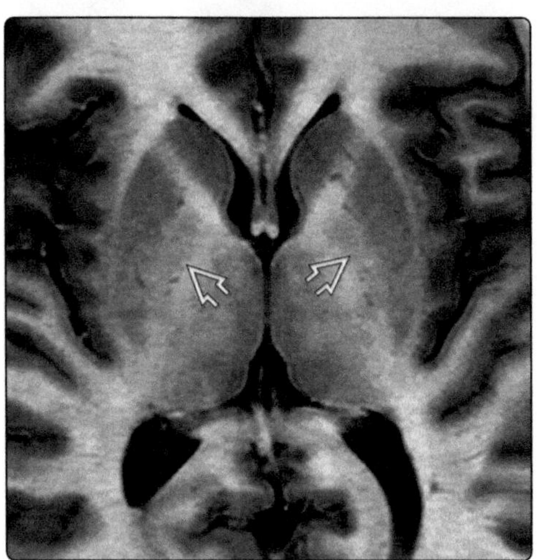

(29-2) Axial T1WI shows basal ganglia, thalami as isointense with gray matter. GP ➡ are slightly hyperintense to the caudate and putamen.

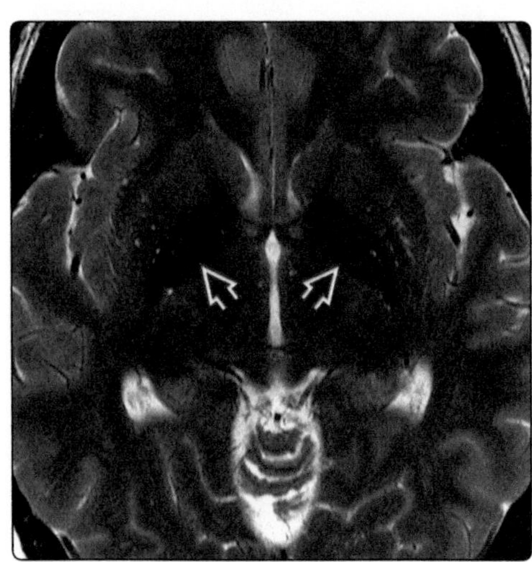

(29-3) On T2WI, the GP ➡ are more hypointense than putamen, caudate. Putamen reaches same hypointensity in 7th or 8th decade.

Normal Gross Anatomy

The **BG** are symmetric paired subcortical (deep gray matter) nuclei that form the core of the extrapyramidal system and control motor activity. The BG consist of (1) the caudate nucleus (CNuc), (2) the putamen, and (3) the GP **(29-1)**.

The thalami are the largest and most prominent of the deep gray matter nuclei but are generally not included in the term "basal ganglia."

Normal Imaging Anatomy

NECT

The BG and thalami are symmetrically hyperdense compared to normal WM. Physiologic calcifications in the globi pallidi are common in adults **(29-4)**.

T1WI

The CNuc, putamina, and thalami are isointense with cortex on T1 scans **(29-2)**. As the site of both physiologic calcification and age-related iron deposition, the GP segments vary in signal intensity **(29-3)**. Calcification may cause T1 shortening and mild hyperintensity in the medial segment.

T2WI

The CNuc, putamina, and thalami are isointense with cortical gray matter on T2 scans **(29-3)**. Increasing iron deposition occurs with aging, and the putamen becomes progressively more hypointense. A "dark" putamen is normal by the seventh or eighth decade of life.

T2*

The GP is hypointense relative to cortex on GRE or SWI imaging. By the seventh or eighth decade of life, iron deposition in the putamen "blooms," and the lateral putamen appears hypointense relative to the thalami but not as intensely hypointense as the GP.

Toxic and Metabolic Disorders

Many toxic, metabolic, systemic, and degenerative diseases affect the BG and thalami in a strikingly symmetric fashion **(29-5)** **(29-6)**. Lesions are most often secondary to diffuse systemic or metabolic derangements. Patchy, discrete, focal, and asymmetric lesions are more commonly infectious, postinfectious, traumatic, or neoplastic in origin.

Differential Diagnoses of Bilateral Basal Ganglia Lesions

The most common bilateral BG lesions are normal variants (e.g., physiologic Ca^{++} and prominent perivascular spaces). Vascular disease, hypoxic-ischemic insults, and common metabolic disorders, such as chronic liver failure, are the most frequent causes **(29-10)**. Infection, toxins, drug abuse, or metabolic disorders, such as osmotic demyelination and Wernicke encephalopathy, are less common causes of bilateral BG lesions.

COMMON BILATERAL BASAL GANGLIA LESIONS

Normal Variants
- Physiologic mineralization
  - Medial globus pallidus (GP) > > caudate, putamen
- Prominent perivascular spaces
  - Follow CSF, suppress on FLAIR

Vascular Disease
- Lacunar infarcts
  - Multiple bilateral, scattered, asymmetric
- Diffuse axonal/vascular injury
  - Hemorrhage, other lesions

Hypoxic-Ischemic Injury
- Hypoxic-ischemic encephalopathy (HIE)
  - BG ± cortex/watershed, hippocampi, thalami

Metabolic Disorders
- Chronic liver disease
  - GP, substantia nigra hyperintensity

LESS COMMON BILATERAL BASAL GANGLIA LESIONS

Infection/Post Infection
- Viral
  - Especially flaviviral encephalitides (West Nile virus, Japanese encephalitis, etc.)
- Post virus, post vaccination
  - Acute disseminated encephalomyelitis (ADEM): Patchy > confluent; WM, thalami, cord often involved
  - Acute striatal necrosis

Toxic Poisoning and Drug Abuse
- Carbon monoxide
  - GP (WM may show delayed involvement)
- Heroin
  - BG, WM ("chasing the dragon")
- Methanol
  - Putamen, WM
- Cyanide
  - Putamen (often hemorrhagic)
- Nitroimidazole
  - Dentate nuclei, inferior colliculi, splenium, BG

Metabolic Disorders
- Osmotic ("extrapontine") demyelination
  - BG, ± pons, WM
- Wernicke encephalopathy
  - Medial thalami, midbrain (periaqueductal), mammillary bodies

Vascular Disease
- Internal cerebral vein/vein of Galen/straight sinus thrombosis
  - BG, deep WM
- Artery of Percheron infarct
  - Bilateral thalami, midbrain ("V" sign)

Neoplasm
- Primary CNS lymphoma
  - Periventricular (WM, BG)
- Astrocytoma
  - Bithalamic "glioma"

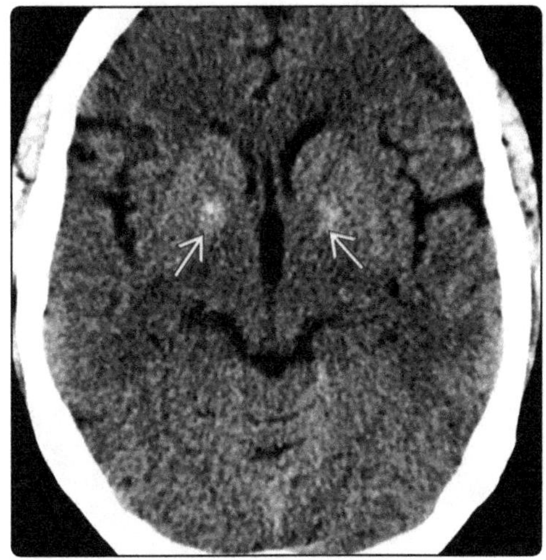

***(29-4)** NECT in a 34-year-old woman with headaches shows normal bilateral symmetric physiologic calcifications in the medial GP ➡.*

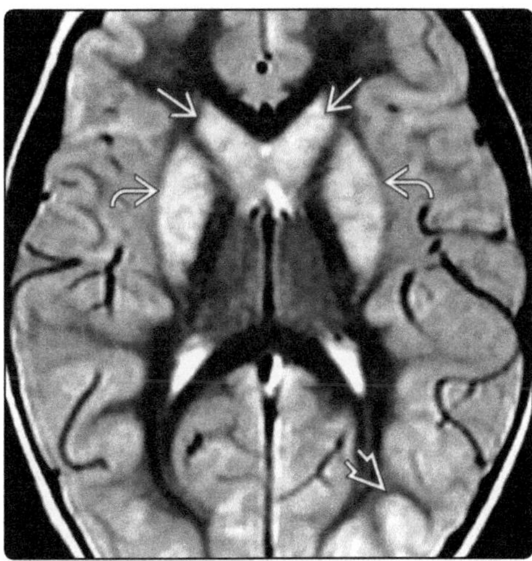

***(29-5)** T2 MR in anoxia shows bilateral hyperintensity in caudates ➡, putamina, GP ➡, and cortex ➡. Thalamus is relatively spared.*

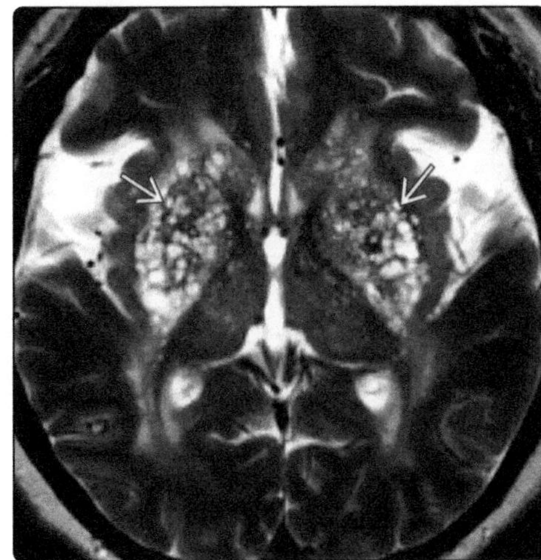

***(29-6)** T2 MR shows CSF-like basal ganglia cysts ➡ representing enlarged perivascular spaces ("état criblé" or "cribriform state").*

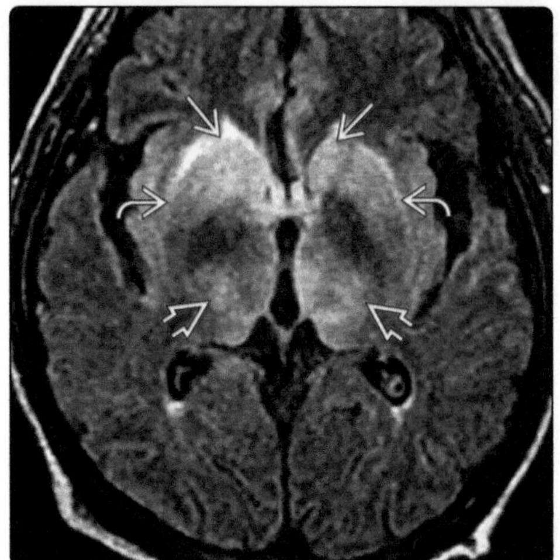

(29-7) FLAIR MR shows bilateral CNuc ➡, putamina ➡, thalamic hyperintensity ➡; West Nile encephalitis. (Courtesy M. Colombo, MD.)

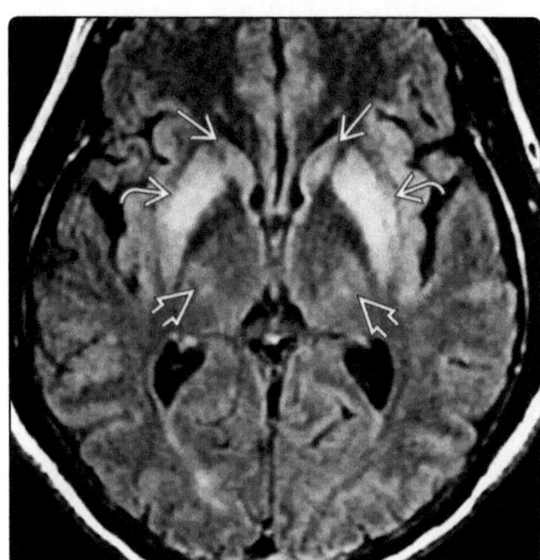

(29-8) Axial FLAIR shows CNuc ➡, putamina ➡, thalamic ➡ symmetric hyperintensity. This is extrapontine osmotic myelinolysis.

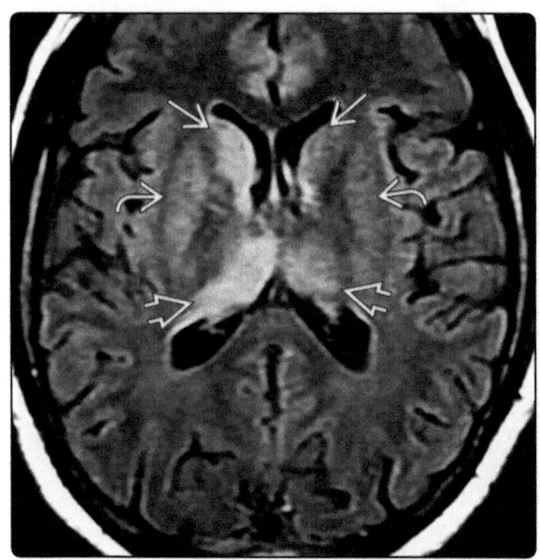

(29-9) Axial FLAIR MR shows bilateral but asymmetric CNuc ➡, putamen ➡, thalamic ➡ hyperintensity. This is deep vein occlusion.

RARE BUT IMPORTANT BILATERAL BASAL GANGLIA LESIONS

Metabolic Disorders

- Acute diabetic uremia
  - GP, putamen, caudate
- Acute hyperammonemia
  - Acute liver failure
  - Ornithine transcarbamylase deficiency, etc.
- Acute hyperglycemia
  - GP, caudate
- Severe hypoglycemia
  - Occipital cortex, hippocampi, ± WM

Infection and Inflammation

- Toxoplasmosis
  - Often HIV-positive, other ring-enhancing lesions
- Behçet disease
  - Midbrain often involved
  - Orogenital aphthous ulcers
- Chronic longstanding multiple sclerosis (MS)
  - BG become very hypointense
  - Putamina, thalami > GP, caudate nucleus (CNuc)
  - Extensive WM disease, volume loss
- Creutzfeldt-Jakob disease (CJD)
  - Anterior BG (caudate, putamen)
  - Posteromedial thalami (T2-/FLAIR-hyperintense "hockey stick" sign)
  - Variable cortical (occipital = Heidenhain variant)

Inherited Disorders

- Neurofibromatosis type 1 (NF1)
  - GP T1 hyperintensity, T2-hyperintense foci
- Mitochondrial encephalopathies
  - Mitochondrial encephalopathy with lactic acidosis and stroke-like episodes (MELAS), myoclonic epilepsy with ragged red fibers (MERRF)
  - Leigh disease (putamen, periaqueductal region, cerebral peduncles)
- Wilson disease
  - Putamina, CNuc, ventrolateral thalami
- Pantothenate kinase-associated neurodegeneration (PKAN)
  - GP ("eye of the tiger")
- Huntington disease
  - Atrophic CNuc, putamina
- Fahr disease
  - Dense symmetric BG, thalami, dentate nuclei, subcortical WM Ca^{++}
- Iron storage disorders
  - Symmetric BG "blooming" hypointensity

Putamen Lesions

Toxic, metabolic, and hypoxic-ischemic events and degenerative disorders account for the vast majority of symmetric putamen lesions. In general, the putamina are less commonly affected than either the globi pallidi or thalami. The most common lesion to affect the putamen is hypertensive hemorrhage. Acute hypertensive bleeds are usually unilateral, although T2* scans often disclose evidence of prior hemorrhages.

COMMON PUTAMEN LESIONS
Metabolic Disorders • Hypertensive hemorrhage   o Lateral putamen/external capsule **Hypoxic-Ischemic Encephalopathy** • HIE in term infants • Hypotensive infarction

Bilateral symmetric putamen lesions usually occur with more generalized BG involvement. However, there are some lesions that predominantly or almost exclusively involve the putamina **(29-17)**.

LESS COMMON PUTAMEN LESIONS

Toxic Disorders
• Methanol toxicity*
  o Often hemorrhagic
  o ± subcortical WM
• Osmotic demyelination
  o Extrapontine myelinolysis
Inherited Disorders
• Leigh disease
• Neuroferritinopathy
  o Putamina, GP, dentate
** Predominantly or almost exclusively involves the putamina*

RARE BUT IMPORTANT PUTAMEN LESIONS

Degenerative Diseases
• Huntington disease
  o CNuc, putamina
• Parkinson disease
  o Putamen hypointensity
• Multiple system atrophy
  o Parkinsonian type* (hyperintense putaminal rim)
Miscellaneous
• Creutzfeldt-Jakob disease*
  o Anterior putamina, CNuc
  o Posteromedial thalami
  o Variable cortex (± predominant or exclusive involvement)
** Predominantly or almost exclusively involves the putamina*

Globus Pallidus Lesions

The globus pallidus (GP) is the part of the BG that is most sensitive to hypoxia. The vast majority of symmetric GP lesions are secondary to hypoxic, toxic, or metabolic processes. Most cause bilateral symmetric abnormalities on imaging studies **(29-10)** **(29-11)** **(29-12)**.

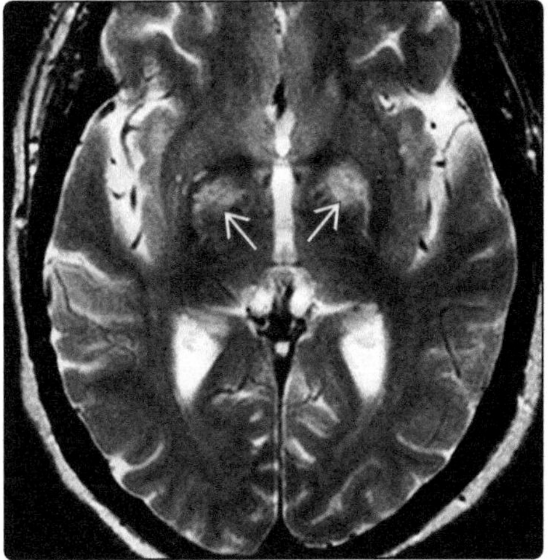

***(29-10)** T2 MR in a patient with hypotensive infarct following narcotic overdose shows bilateral GP hyperintensities ➡.*

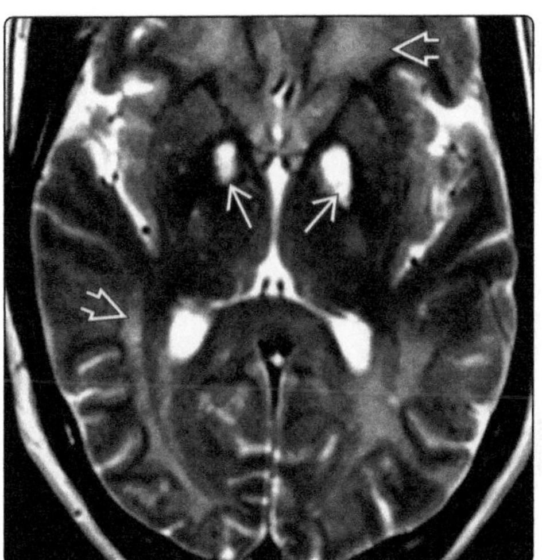

***(29-11)** T2 MR shows bilateral medial GP hyperintensities ➡, confluent WM hyperintensity ⇨; this is carbon monoxide poisoning.*

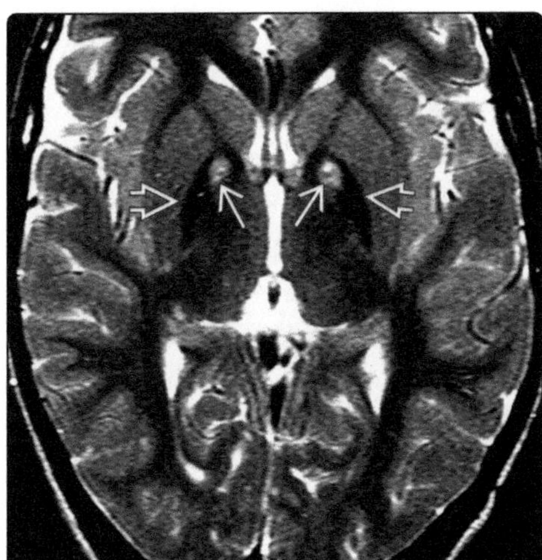

***(29-12)** T2 MR shows classic "eye of the tiger" with medial GP hyperintensities ➡ surrounded by well-defined hypointensity ⇨. This is PKAN.*

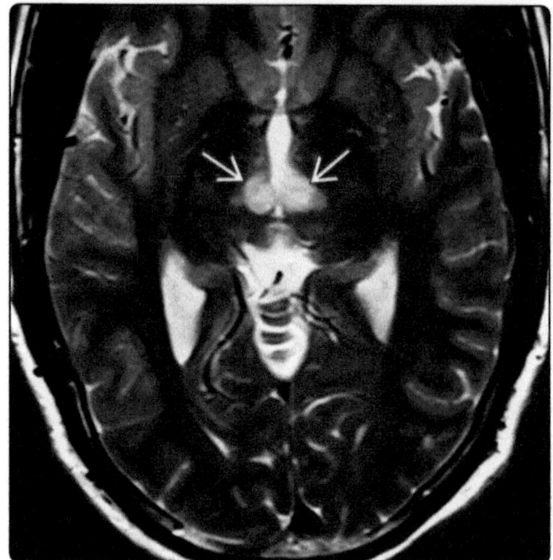

***(29-13)** Axial T2 MR shows bilateral medial thalamic infarcts ➡ caused by artery of Percheron occlusion.*

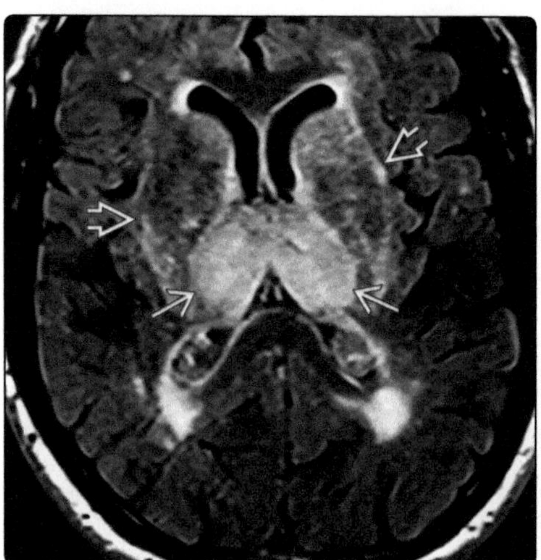

***(29-14)** Axial FLAIR shows bithalamic lesions ➡ with less extensive involvement of putamina ⇨ and GP. This is internal cerebral vein occlusion.*

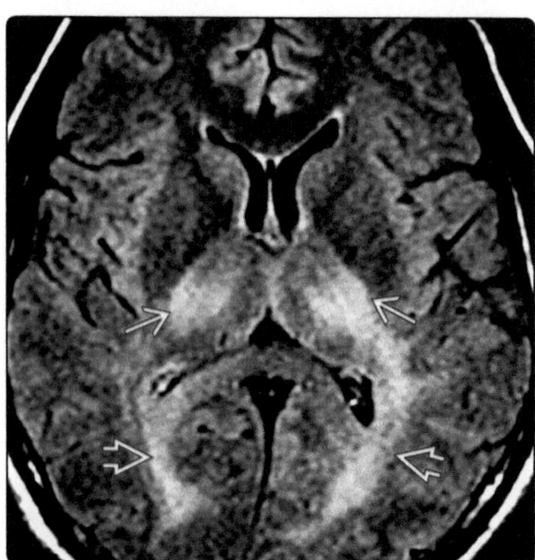

***(29-15)** FLAIR MR in a patient with Epstein-Barr virus encephalitis shows bithalamic ➡ and occipital WM involvement ⇨.*

COMMON GLOBUS PALLIDUS LESIONS

Normal Variant

- Physiologic calcification
  - Medial GP

Hypoxic-Ischemic Encephalopathy

- Anoxia, hypoxia (near-drowning, cerebral hypoperfusion)
- Neonatal HIE (profound acute)

Toxic/Metabolic Disorders

- Chronic liver disease
  - T1 hyperintensity, T2* hypointensity
- Carbon monoxide
  - T2-hyperintense medial GP

LESS COMMON GLOBUS PALLIDUS LESIONS

Toxic/Metabolic Disorders

- Postopioid toxic encephalopathy
  - Often combined with HIE
- Hyperalimentation
  - Manganese deposition, short T1
- Chronic hypothyroidism
  - Punctate calcification
  - T1 hyperintensity, T2 hypointensity

Inherited Disorders

- NF1
- Leigh disease

RARE BUT IMPORTANT GLOBUS PALLIDUS LESIONS

Toxic/Metabolic Disorders

- Kernicterus
  - T1 shortening
- Cyanide poisoning
  - Hemorrhagic GP, laminar cortical necrosis

Inherited Disorders

- Fahr disease
  - Dense symmetric confluent calcification
- Wilson disease
  - T2 hyperintensity in GP, putamen
  - "Face of giant panda" sign in midbrain
- PKAN
  - "Eye of the tiger" (central T2 hyperintensity, peripheral hypointensity)
  - Not always present!
- Neurodegeneration with brain iron accumulation (NBIA)
  - GP, substantia nigra hypointensity ± putamen
- Maple syrup urine disease (MSUD)
  - Edema (GP, brainstem, thalami, cerebellar WM)
- Methylmalonic acidemia (MMA)
  - Symmetric GP T2 hyperintensity ± WM

Degenerative Diseases

- Hepatocerebral degeneration
  - 1% of patients with cirrhosis, portosystemic shunts
  - T1 shortening
- Progressive supranuclear palsy
  - Also affects subthalamic nucleus, substantia nigra

Globus Pallidus Lesions by Appearance

Some GP lesions can be distinguished by their typical attenuation on CT or signal intensity on MR.

GLOBUS PALLIDUS LESIONS BY CHARACTERISTIC APPEARANCE

NECT Hypodensity
- HIE
- Carbon monoxide poisoning

NECT Hyperdensity
- Physiologic Ca^{++}
- Hypothyroidism
- Fahr disease

T1 Hyperintensity
- Chronic hepatic encephalopathy
- Hyperalimentation (manganese deposition)
- NF1
- Hypothyroidism
- Kernicterus (acute)
- Wilson disease

T2 Hyperintensity
- HIE
- Drug abuse
- Carbon monoxide poisoning
- NF1
- Leigh disease
- Kernicterus (chronic)
- Wilson disease
- PKAN, MSUD, MMA

Thalamic Lesions

Because lacunar infarcts and hypertensive bleeds are so common, *unilateral* thalamic lesions are much more common than bilateral symmetric abnormalities.

UNILATERAL THALAMIC LESIONS

Common
- Lacunar infarction
- Hypertensive intracranial hemorrhage

Less Common
- NF1
- Diffuse astrocytoma (low-grade fibrillary)
- Glioblastoma multiforme
- Anaplastic astrocytoma
- ADEM

Rare but Important
- MS
- Unilateral internal cerebral vein thrombosis
- Germinoma

In contrast, *bilateral* symmetric thalamic lesions are relatively uncommon and have a somewhat limited differential diagnosis. As with the symmetric BG lesions discussed previously, bilateral thalamic lesions tend to be toxic, metabolic, vascular, infectious, or hypoxic-ischemic **(29-13) (29-14) (29-15) (29-16) (29-17) (29-18)**.

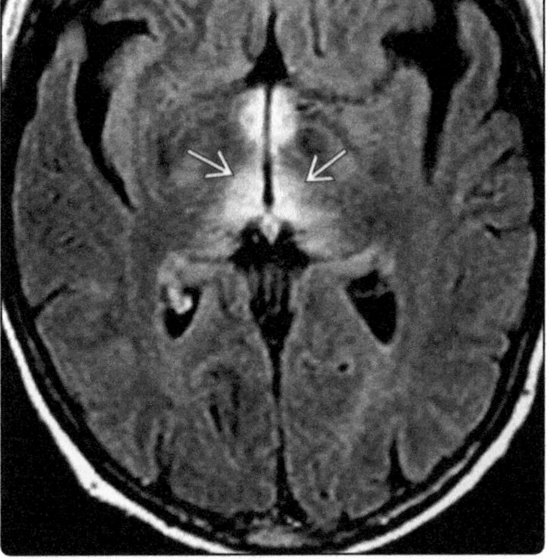

***(29-16)** FLAIR MR in a patient with Wernicke encephalopathy shows symmetric lesions in both medial thalami ➡.*

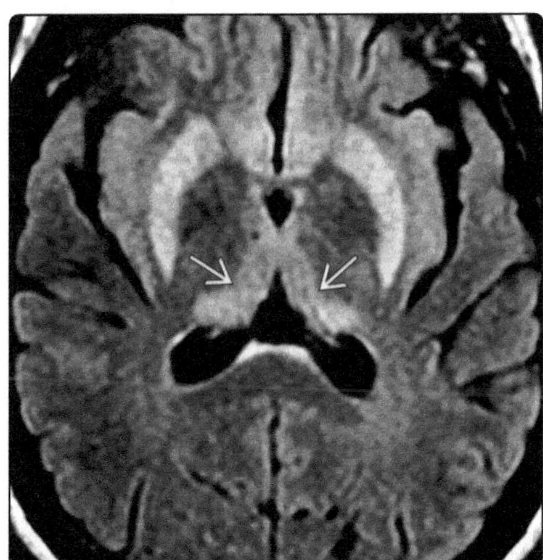

***(29-17)** FLAIR MR in a patient with CJD shows classic "hockey stick" sign ➡ as well as anterior caudate and putamen hyperintensity.*

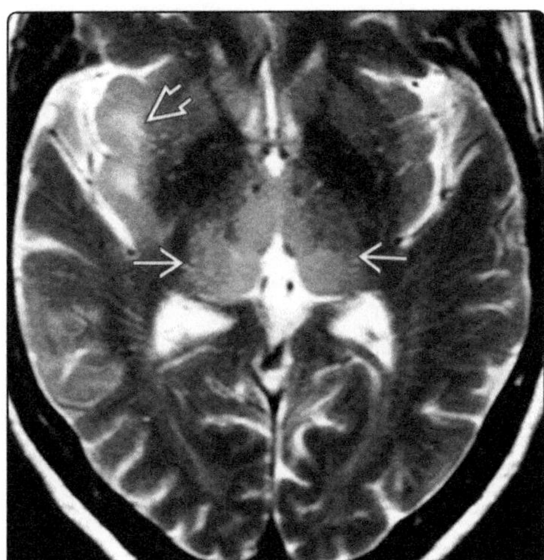

***(29-18)** T2 MR shows bithalamic ➡ and right insular ➡ hyperintensity in a patient with gliomatosis cerebri, WHO grade II astrocytoma.*

COMMON BITHALAMIC LESIONS

Vascular Lesions
- Deep venous occlusion
  - Thalami > GP, putamina
  - CNuc ± deep WM
- Arterial ischemia
  - Artery of Percheron infarct
  - "Top of the basilar" thrombosis
- Vasculitis

Hypoxic-Ischemic Encephalopathy
- Profound hypoperfusion
  - BG, hippocampi, cortex
- Usually occurs in full-term neonates

LESS COMMON BITHALAMIC LESIONS

Infection/Postinfection/Inflammatory Disorders
- ADEM
  - Usually with WM lesions
- Viral encephalitis
  - *Many* agents affect thalami
  - Epstein-Barr virus, West Nile virus, Japanese encephalitis, etc.
- CJD
  - "Hockey stick" sign
  - Pulvinar, medial thalami

Toxic/Metabolic Disorders
- Osmotic myelinolysis
  - Extrapontine involvement variable
  - Thalami
  - External capsules, putamina, CNuc
- Wernicke encephalopathy
  - Medial thalami (around 3rd ventricle)
  - Pulvinar
  - Midbrain (periaqueductal)
  - Mammillary bodies
  - Cortex variable
- Solvent inhalation
  - Toluene
  - Glue
  - Ethylene glycol
- Acute hypertensive encephalopathy (PRES)
  - Occipital lobes, watershed zones
  - "Atypical" PRES may involve BG, thalami
- Status epilepticus
  - Pulvinar
  - Corpus callosum splenium (usually transient excitotoxic)
  - Often hippocampi ± cortex

Neoplasms
- Bithalamic low-grade astrocytoma
- Germinoma
- Lymphoma

RARE BUT IMPORTANT BITHALAMIC LESIONS

Infection/Postinfection/Inflammatory Disorders
- MS (severe, chronic)
  - Hypointense BG on T2*
- Acute necrotizing encephalopathy of childhood
- Flavivirus encephalitis
- Neuro-Behçet

Inherited Disorders
- Mitochondrial disorders
- Krabbe disease
  - Hyperdense on CT, hypointense on T2
- Wilson disease
  - Putamina, CNuc > thalami
- Fahr disease
  - GP > thalami
- Fabry disease
  - T1-hyperintense posterior thalamus ("pulvinar")
  - M > > F
  - Strokes (territorial, lacunar)
  - Renal, cardiac disease

Neoplasm
- Glioblastoma
- Anaplastic astrocytoma

Paraneoplastic Syndromes
- Paraneoplastic can mimic prion disease (variant of Creutzfeldt-Jakob disease)
- Limbic involvement not always present

Selected References: The complete reference list is available on the Expert Consult™ eBook version included with purchase.

Toxic Encephalopathy

The list of toxins and poisons that affect the CNS is long and continues to grow. Some agents are deliberately injected, inhaled, or ingested, whereas others are accidentally encountered or administered in a controlled medical setting. Some toxins accumulate slowly, so their clinical manifestations are subtle and onset insidious. Others cause profound, virtually immediate CNS toxicity with rapid onset of coma and death. Still others—such as ethanol—have both acute and chronic effects.

Use of "street" drugs, opioids, synthetic "designer" drugs and the emergence of fentanyl are fueling a worldwide epidemic. Overdoses (ODs) are increasingly common. An accurate history is often difficult to obtain in patients with suspected OD and clinical symptoms are frequently nonspecific. Presentation may also be confounded by "polydrug" abuse and secondary effects, such as hypoxia, that mask the underlying pathology.

In this chapter, we focus on the most common types of toxic encephalopathies, beginning with the acute and long-term effects of alcohol on the brain followed by a discussion of drug abuse and various poisons that affect the CNS. We conclude with a brief discussion of treatment-related disorders.

Alcohol and Related Disorders

We begin our discussion of alcohol and the brain by briefly considering the acute effects of alcohol poisoning. We then consider chronic alcoholic encephalopathy before turning to other complications of alcohol abuse, including alcohol-induced demyelination syndromes and Wernicke encephalopathy.

Acute Alcohol Poisoning

Etiology

The acute effects of binge drinking—and its complication, acute alcohol poisoning—are striking. Life-threatening cytotoxic cerebral edema and nonconvulsive status epilepticus may ensue **(30-1)**. A blood alcohol concentration of 0.40% typically results in unconsciousness, and a level exceeding 0.50% is usually lethal.

Imaging

Imaging findings in patients with acute alcohol poisoning include diffuse brain swelling and confluent hyperintensity in the supratentorial subcortical and deep white matter on T2/FLAIR **(30-2)**. Seizure-induced changes in the cortex, with gyral hyperintensity and diffusion restriction, may also be associated.

Chronic Alcoholic Encephalopathy

Imaging

General Features. Progressive brain volume loss is seen with chronic alcoholic encephalopathy. Initially, the superior vermis atrophies and the cerebellar fissures become prominent **(30-3)**. In later stages, the frontal white matter becomes involved, reflected by widened sulci and enlarged lateral ventricles **(30-5B)**. In the final stages, global volume loss is present **(30-3)**.

CT Findings. NECT scans show generalized ventricular and sulcal enlargement **(30-5A)**. The great horizontal fissure of the cerebellum and the superior vermian folia are unusually prominent relative to the patient's age **(30-5)**.

MR Findings. Brain volume loss, especially in the prefrontal cortex, is common as is more focal atrophy of the superior vermis. Focal and confluent cerebral white matter hyperintensities on T2/FLAIR sequences are frequently present.

Chronic liver failure secondary to cirrhosis may cause basal ganglia hyperintensity on T1WI, probably secondary to manganese accumulation. Increased iron deposition in the basal ganglia and dentate nuclei may occur.

(30-1) EtOH poisoning shows brain swelling with white matter (WM) necrosis ➡, especially marked in the corpus callosum ➡. Basal ganglia/thalami are swollen, pale, infarcted ➡. (Courtesy R. Hewlett, MD.) (30-2) T2 MR in a comatose patient who drank 1 gallon of vodka or whisky daily for a full week shows diffuse brain swelling, hyperintense WM ➡, bithalamic lesions ➡. This is acute alcohol poisoning.

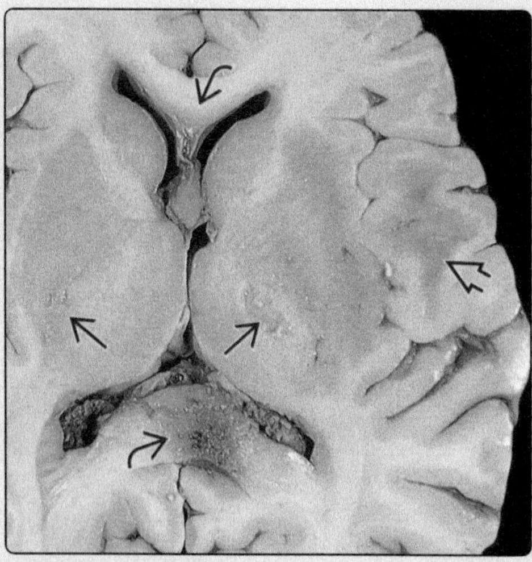

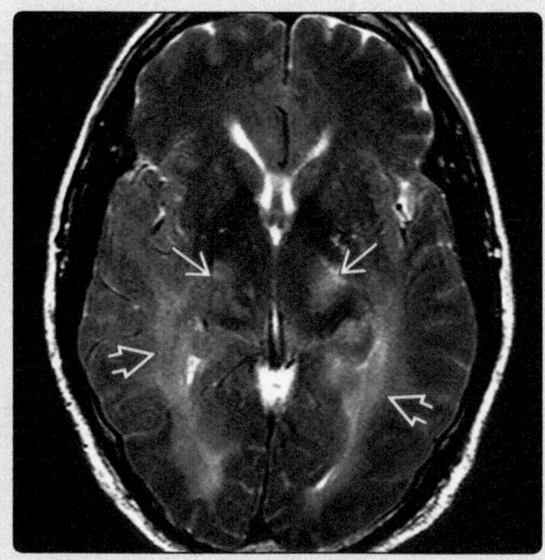

(30-3) Graphic shows cortical, superior vermian atrophy, corpus callosum necrosis ➡ from EtOH abuse. Mammillary ➡, periaqueductal gray necrosis ➡ characterize Wernicke encephalopathy (WE). (30-4) Sagittal T1 MR in chronic alcoholic encephalopathy and Marchiafava-Bignami disease shows hypointensity in the entire middle corpus callosum ➡. Mammillary bodies ➡ and superior vermis ➡ are atrophic. (Courtesy A. Datir, MD.)

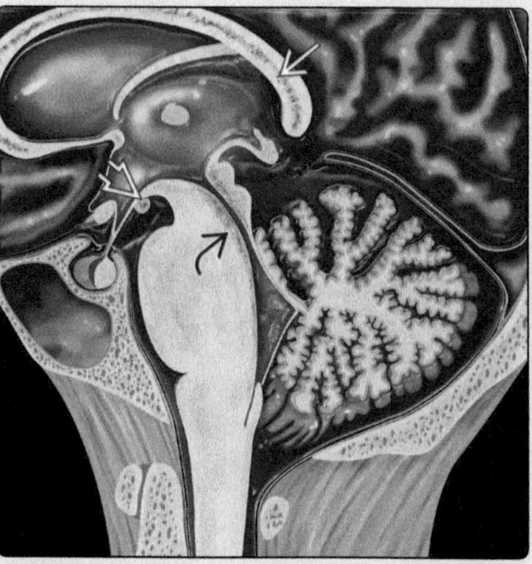

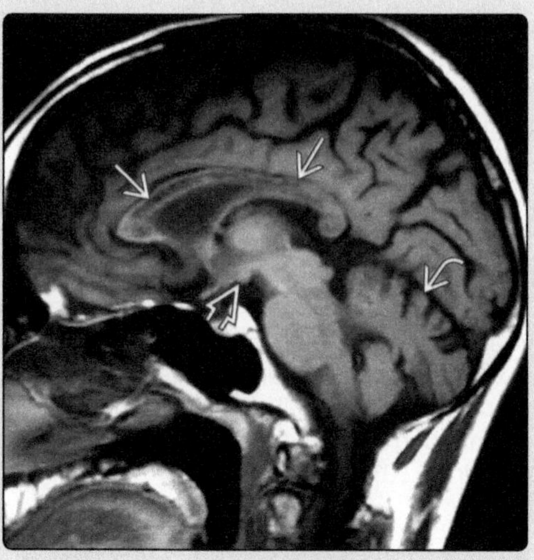

ACUTE/CHRONIC ALCOHOLIC ENCEPHALOPATHY

Acute Alcohol Poisoning

- Rare; caused by binge drinking
- Imaging
  - Diffuse cerebral edema
  - Acute demyelination

Chronic Alcoholic Encephalopathy

- Primary toxic effect on neurons
- Secondary effects related to liver, GI disease
  - Hepatic encephalopathy
  - Malnutrition, malabsorption, electrolyte imbalance
- Imaging
  - Atrophy (superior vermis, cerebellum, generalized)
  - White matter myelinolysis

Wernicke Encephalopathy

Pathology

The mammillary bodies, hypothalamus, medial thalamic nuclei (adjacent to the third ventricle), tectal plate, and periaqueductal gray matter are most commonly affected **(30-6)**. Less commonly involved areas include the cerebellum (especially the dentate nuclei), red nuclei, corpus callosum splenium, and cerebral cortex.

Demyelination and petechial hemorrhages are common in the acute stage of Wernicke encephalopathy (WE). Callosal necrosis, white matter rarefaction with brain volume loss, and mammillary body atrophy can be seen in chronic WE.

Clinical Issues

Alcohol abuse is the most common cause of WE. However, *almost 1/2 of all WE cases occur in nonalcoholics.* Although

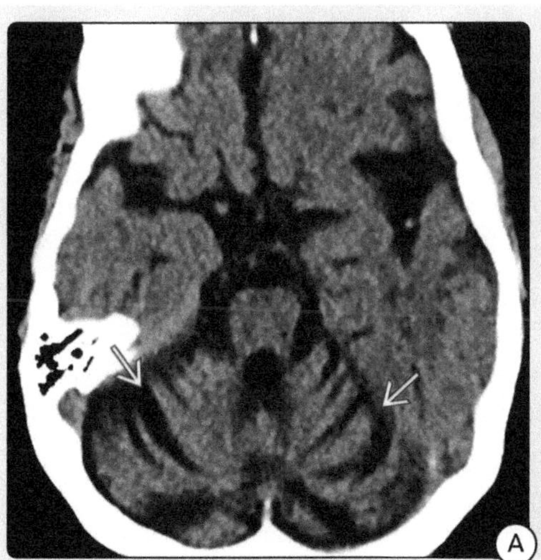

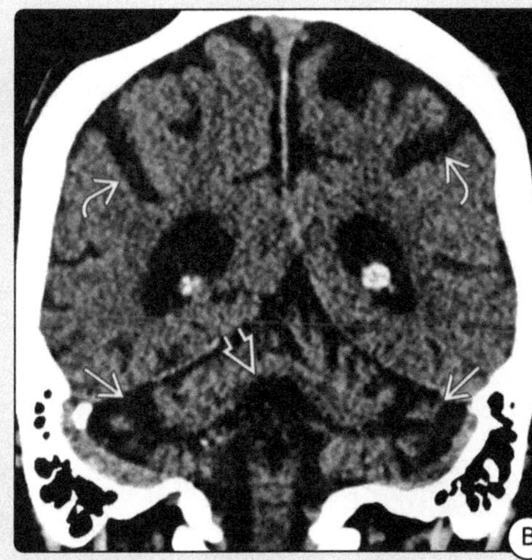

***(30-5A)** NECT in a 56-year-old woman with chronic alcoholism and multiple falls shows severe cerebellar atrophy with grossly enlarged sulci ➡. **(30-5B)** Coronal NECT in the same case shows the striking cerebellar volume loss ➡. Note enlarged 4th ventricle ➡. The cerebral hemispheres also appear moderately atrophic with prominent superficial sulci ➡.*

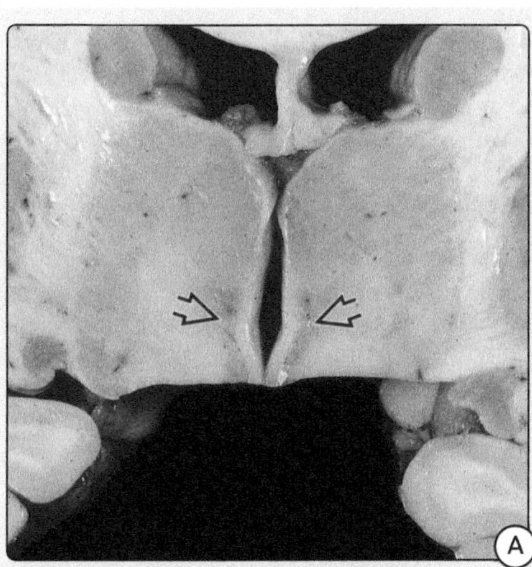

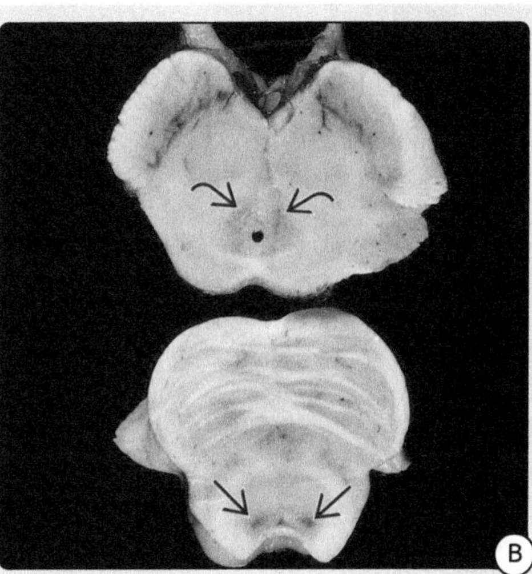

***(30-6A)** Coronal autopsy of WE shows bithalamic necrosis around the walls of the 3rd ventricle ➡. **(30-6B)** Axial section through the midbrain (above) and upper pons (below) in the same case show hemorrhagic necrosis in the periaqueductal gray matter ➡ and tectum ➡.*

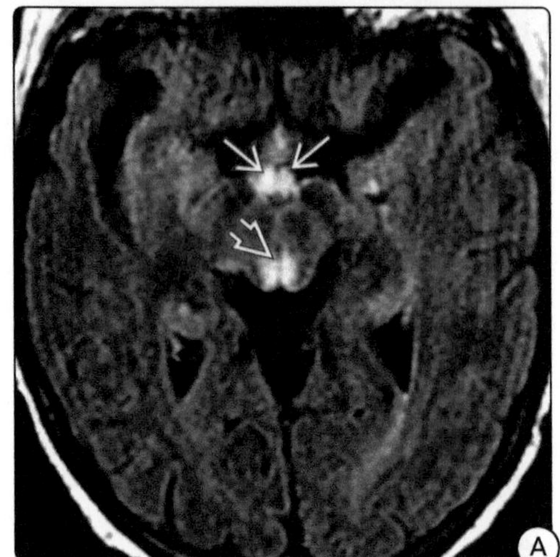
(30-7A) FLAIR MR in acute WE shows periaqueductal gray matter ➡ and mammillary body hyperintensity ➡.

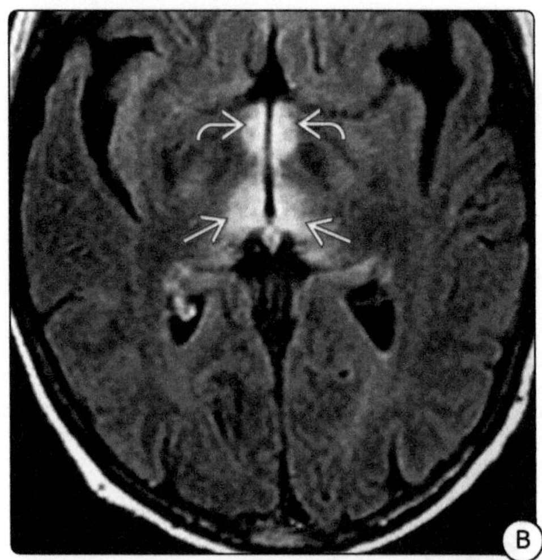
(30-7B) Hyperintensity in the medial thalami around the walls of the 3rd ventricle ➡ is shown. The hypothalamus ➡ is also involved.

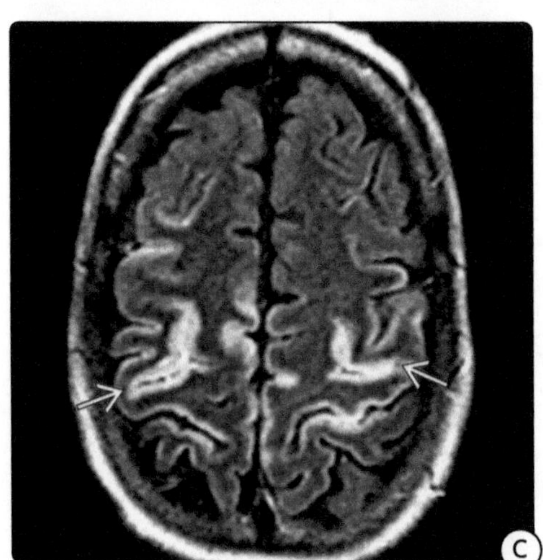
(30-7C) FLAIR MR through the cerebral convexities shows bilateral, relatively symmetric cortical hyperintensities ➡.

nonalcoholic WE is generally more common in adults, it *can and does occur in children!*

The underlying pathophysiology of *nonalcoholic* WE is identical to that of alcoholic WE, but the etiology is different. Malnutrition secondary to hyperemesis gravidarum (pregnancy-related vomiting), eating disorders, or bariatric surgery with drastically reduced thiamine intake is typical. Hyperemesis (e.g., pregnancy, chemotherapy) and prolonged hyperalimentation are other common causes of nonalcoholic WE.

Only 30% of patients demonstrate the classic WE clinical triad of (1) ocular dysfunction (e.g., nystagmus, conjugate gaze palsies, ophthalmoplegia), (2) ataxia, and (3) altered mental status. Mortality of untreated WE is high. Rapid intravenous thiamine replacement is imperative to prevent the most severe sequelae of WE.

Imaging

MR is the procedure of choice in evaluating patients with possible WE. T1WI may show hypointensity around the third ventricle and cerebral aqueduct. In severe cases, petechial hemorrhages are present and may cause T1 hyperintensities in the medial thalami and mammillary bodies. T2* SWI sequences may be helpful in detecting microhemorrhages in the affected areas.

During the acute phase, T2/FLAIR hyperintensity can be seen in the affected areas **(30-7)**. Bilateral symmetric lesions in the putamina and medial thalami around the third ventricle are present in 85% of cases **(30-8)**. The tectal plate and periaqueductal gray matter are involved in nearly 2/3 of cases. T2/FLAIR hyperintensity in the mammillary bodies is seen in 50-60% of cases.

Less commonly, the dorsal medulla is affected **(30-8)**. Bilateral but asymmetric cortical hyperintensities can be present **(30-7C)**.

DWI shows corresponding restricted diffusion in the affected areas. Some cases show an isolated focus of diffusion restriction in the corpus callosum splenium **(30-8C)**.

In ~ 1/2 of all alcoholic WE cases, postcontrast scans demonstrate enhancement of the periventricular and periaqueductal lesions. Strong uniform enhancement of the mammillary bodies is seen in up to 80% of acute cases and is considered pathognomonic of WE. With chronic WE, mammillary body atrophy ensues.

Differential Diagnosis

The medial thalami and midbrain can be symmetrically involved in **artery of Percheron (AOP) infarct** and **deep cerebral vein thrombosis (CVT)**. **Viral infections**, such as influenza A and West Nile virus meningoencephalitis, cause symmetric medial thalamic and midbrain lesions that may mimic WE. Mammillary bodies are usually not involved.

A rare but reported imaging differential diagnosis is demyelination in **neuromyelitis optica spectrum disorder (NMOSD)**. Therefore, measurement of aquaporin 4 antibodies should be considered if no obvious cause for thiamine deficiency is present.

WERNICKE ENCEPHALOPATHY

Etiology
- Thiamine (vitamin B1) deficiency
- Alcohol related (50%), nonalcoholic (50%)

Pathology
- Acute = petechial hemorrhages (especially mammillary bodies), demyelination
- Chronic = callosal necrosis, mammillary atrophy

Clinical Issues
- Classic triad = ocular dysfunction, ataxia, altered mental status
- Can occur in children!
- Intravenous thiamine imperative

Imaging
- MR > > CT (usually unhelpful)
- T2/FLAIR hyperintensity, DWI restriction
    - Common = medial thalami (85%), periaqueductal gray matter (65%), mammillary bodies (60%), tectum (30%)
    - Less common = dorsal medulla (8%), cerebellum/cranial nerve nuclei (1%), corpus callosum splenium
- SWI may show microhemorrhages
- Enhancement varies
    - More common in alcoholic WE
    - Mammillary body enhancement pathognomonic

Differential Diagnosis
- Artery of Percheron infarct, deep cerebral vein thrombosis
- Viral infection (e.g., influenza A, West Nile virus)
- Neuromyelitis optica

Amphetamines and Derivatives

CNS stimulants include cocaine, amphetamine, methamphetamine, methylenedioxymethamphetamine (MDMA), and methylphenidate. Although not a classic CNS stimulant, nicotine is a prototypic drug that is avidly self-administered and has some stimulating properties. All of these drugs have a high human abuse liability.

Most addictive drugs are excitotoxic and cause two major types of pathologies: Vascular events (e.g., ischemia, hemorrhage) and leukoencephalopathy.

Methamphetamine

Methamphetamine (MA or "meth") is a highly addictive psychostimulant drug. "Crystal" methamphetamine abuse has been steadily increasing over the past decade. Even a single acute exposure to MA can result in profound changes in cerebral blood flow. Both hemorrhagic and ischemic strokes occur **(30-9)**.

MR in chronic adult MA users demonstrates lower gray matter volumes on T1WI, especially in the frontal lobes, and more white matter hyperintensities on T2/FLAIR scans than are appropriate for the patient's age. MRS shows increased choline and myoinositol levels in the frontal lobes. DTI shows lower fractional anisotropy in the frontal lobes and higher ADC values in the basal ganglia.

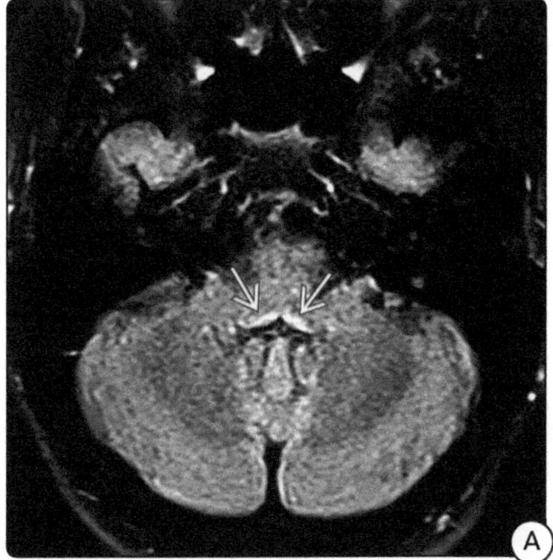

***(30-8A)** FLAIR MR in an anorexic woman after vomiting for several days shows symmetric hyperintensities in the dorsal medulla ➡.*

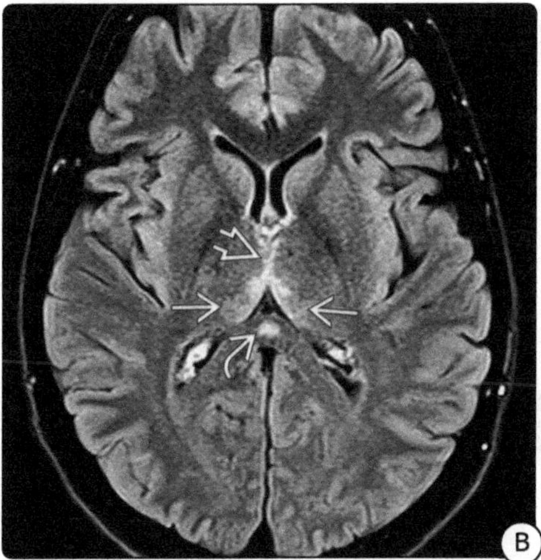

***(30-8B)** Symmetric FLAIR hyperintensity is seen in the pulvinars ➡, around the 3rd ventricle walls ➡, and corpus callosum splenium ➡.*

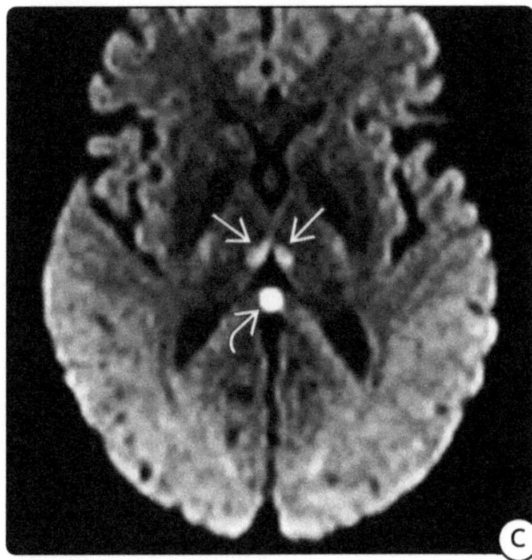

***(30-8C)** DWI MR shows restricted diffusion in medial thalami ➡, corpus callosum splenium ➡. Intractable vomiting caused nonalcoholic WE.*

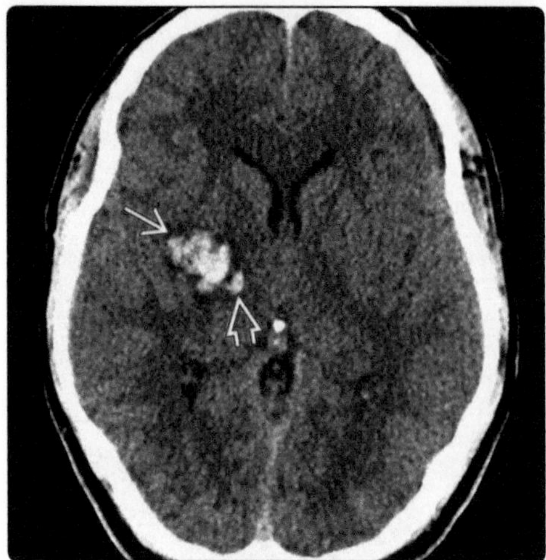

(30-9) NECT in amphetamine abuse shows focal acute hemorrhage in the right basal ganglia ➡ and posterior limb of the internal capsule ⇨.

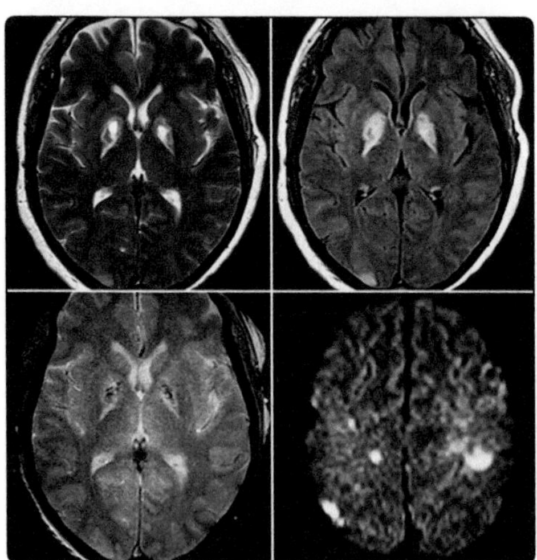

(30-10) MR scans in opiate, benzodiazepine OD show globi pallidi (GP), cortical infarcts. She also had hemorrhagic cerebellar infarcts (not shown).

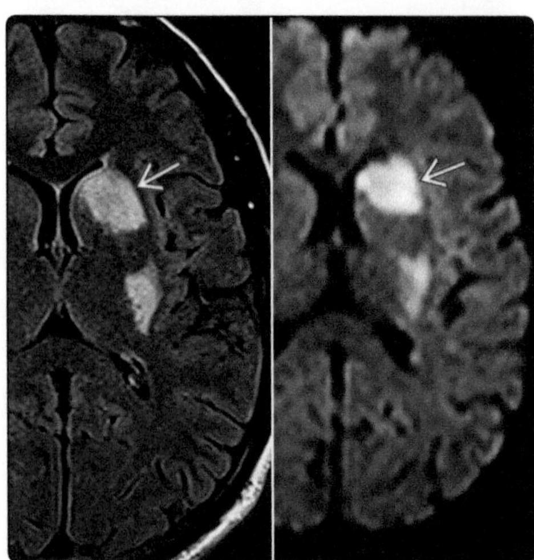

(30-11) FLAIR (left) and DWI (right) show acute cocaine-induced basal ganglia infarcts ➡.

MDMA ("Ecstasy")

3-,4-Methylenedioxymethamphetamine is also known as **MDMA** or **ecstasy**. MDMA can cause arterial constriction, vasculitis, or prolonged vasospasm with acute ischemic infarcts. MDMA-induced ischemia is most pronounced in serotonin-rich brain areas, such as the globus pallidus and occipital cortex, which are especially vulnerable.

Benzodiazepines

Benzodiazepines, sometimes called "**benzo**," are psychoactive drugs used to treat anxiety, insomnia, seizures, muscle spasms, and alcohol withdrawal. Benzodiazepines, such as temazepam and midazolam, act selectively on GABA-A receptors in the brain, inhibiting or reducing the activity of neurons.

Benzodiazepine overdose has been associated with hypoxic-ischemic encephalopathy **(30-10)**, hemorrhagic ischemic strokes, and delayed toxic leukoencephalopathy.

Cocaine

Cocaine can be sniffed/snorted, smoked, or injected. In its most common form (cocaine hydrochloride), it is ingested via the nasal mucosa. "Crack," the alkaloidal freebase form of cocaine hydrochloride, can also be smoked.

Regardless of the route of administration, the adverse impact of cocaine on the brain is largely related to its vascular effects. Systemic hypertension can be extreme, causing spontaneous hemorrhagic strokes.

Etiology

Nearly 1/3 of strokes in patients younger than 45 years old are drug related with 80-90% occurring in the fourth and fifth decades. Stroke risk is highest within the first six hours after drug use.

Rupture of a preexisting aneurysm or underlying vascular malformation accounts for nearly 1/2 of all cocaine-related hemorrhagic strokes. Cocaine also facilitates platelet aggregation and may lead to thrombotic vascular occlusion.

Acute cerebral vasoconstriction &/or cocaine-induced vasculopathy may lead to ischemic strokes. Snorted cocaine causes severe vasoconstriction in the vascular plexus of the nasal septal mucosa (Kiesselbach plexus). Chronic abuse may lead to septal necrosis and perforation.

Imaging

Strokes—both ischemic and hemorrhagic—are the major manifestations of cocaine-induced brain damage **(30-11)**. The hemorrhages can be parenchymal (secondary to hypertension or vascular malformation) or subarachnoid (aneurysm rupture). Hypertensive bleeds are usually centered in the external capsule/putamen or in the thalamus.

Ischemic strokes can be caused by vasospasm, cocaine-induced vasoconstriction, vasculitis, or thrombosis. Bilateral globus pallidus infarction has also been reported as a stroke subtype in cocaine abuse.

Acute cocaine-induced strokes are positive on DWI. MRA, CTA, or DSA may show focal areas of arterial narrowing and irregularity.

Acute hypertensive encephalopathy with posterior reversible encephalopathy (PRES-like syndrome) can also occur. Vasogenic edema in the occipital lobes is the most common finding.

Differential Diagnosis

Unexplained parenchymal hemorrhage in young and middle-aged adults should prompt evaluation for possible drug abuse. **Embolic infarcts** as well as **vasculitis** may appear identical to cocaine vasculopathy.

COCAINE AND AMPHETAMINE EFFECTS ON THE BRAIN

Amphetamines
- Methamphetamine
  - Hemorrhagic, ischemic strokes
- MDMA ("ecstasy")
  - Vasospasm, infarcts
  - Location: Occipital cortex, globus pallidus
- Benzodiazepines
  - Delayed toxic leukoencephalopathy

Cocaine
- Intracranial hemorrhage
  - Hypertensive intracranial hemorrhage (50%)
  - "Unmasked" aneurysm or arteriovenous malformation (50%)
- Ischemic stroke
  - Vasospasm, vasculitis
- Acute hypertensive encephalopathy
  - Posterior reversible encephalopathy syndrome (PRES)
  - Vasogenic edema (typically bioccipital)

Opioids and Derivatives

The ten drugs most frequently involved in overdose deaths include several opioids: **Heroin, oxycodone, methadone, morphine, hydrocodone**, and **fentanyl**. Of these, heroin is the most commonly abused opioid.

Heroin

Heroin is usually injected intravenously. The most common acute complication of *injected* heroin is stroke. Globus pallidus ischemia, very similar to that seen in carbon monoxide poisoning, is common.

The most dramatic acute effects occur with *inhaled* heroin. The freebase form is heated over aluminum foil and the vapors inhaled (**"chasing the dragon"**). Heroin vapor inhalation causes a striking toxic leukoencephalopathy.

Acute CNS toxicity from inhaled heroin ("chasing the dragon") is characterized by symmetric hypodensities in the cerebellar white matter, sometimes described as a "butterfly wing" pattern **(30-12)**. The cerebral white matter, posterior limb of the internal capsule, and globi pallidi are also commonly affected. The anterior limb of the internal capsule is typically spared.

T2 and FLAIR scans in patients with early heroin-related leukoencephalopathy show symmetric hyperintensity in the cerebellar white matter with relative sparing of the dentate nuclei **(30-12)**. There is often selective symmetric involvement of the posterior limb of the internal capsule, the corticospinal tract, the medial lemniscus, and the tractus solitarius **(30-12)**.

Confluent hyperintensity in the cerebral white matter, including the corpus callosum, is common in severe cases of heroin vapor encephalopathy **(30-13)**. DWI shows acute diffusion restriction in the affected areas; MRS shows a lactate peak in the cerebral white matter.

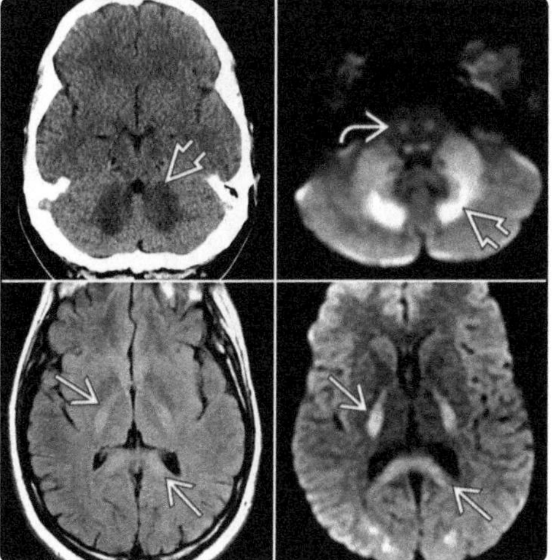

***(30-12)** Inhaled heroin results in abnormalities in pons ➡, cerebellum ➡, corpus callosum, and internal capsules ➡. (Courtesy K. Nelson, MD.)*

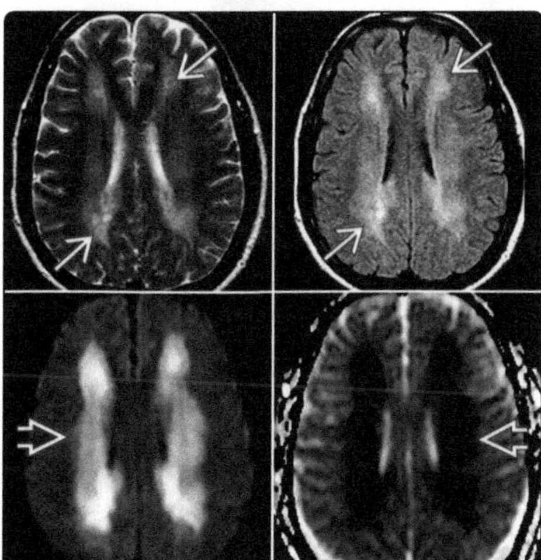

***(30-13)** "Chasing the dragon" shows hyperintensity ➡ and restricted diffusion ➡ in periventricular WM. (Courtesy M. Michel, MD.)*

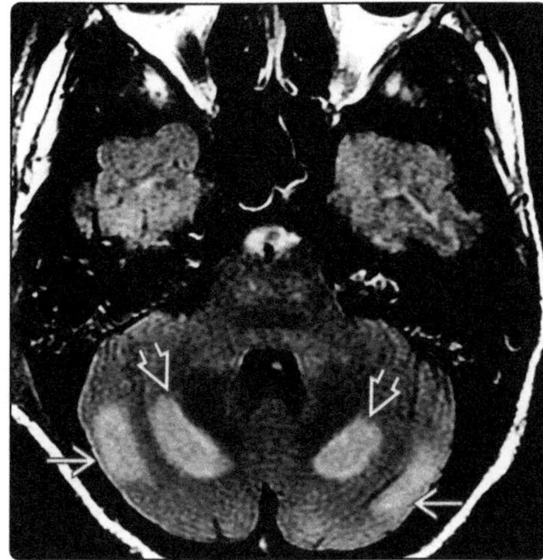

***(30-14)** FLAIR MR shows symmetric cerebellar ➡ and WM lesions ➡ in oxycodone overdose.*

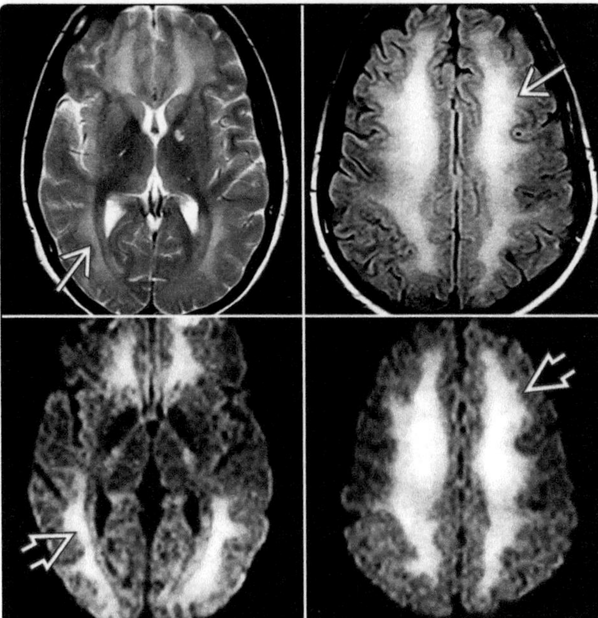

***(30-15)** MR scans in a 33-year-old woman who overdosed on methadone show striking symmetric confluent hyperintensity (leukoencephalopathy) on FLAIR and restricted diffusion on DWI.*

***(30-16)** Accidental methadone poisoning in a child shows bilateral cerebellar hypodensity on NECT, T2/FLAIR hyperintensity, and restricted diffusion.*

Methadone

So-called substitute drugs, such as the synthetic opioid methadone, are used in the medication-assisted therapy for drug abuse/dependence as well as in the management of intractable pain. With increasing use and availability, methadone overdose is likewise growing.

A postopioid delayed toxic leukoencephalopathy similar to that caused by inhaled heroin has been reported with methadone. Diffuse, symmetric, confluent hyperintensity in the cerebral white matter on T2/FLAIR is seen **(30-15)**. Sparing of the subcortical U-fibers is typical. In contrast to heroin toxicity, cerebellar and brainstem changes are subtle or absent in adults. MRS shows elevated choline, decreased NAA, and increased lactate.

Oxycodone

Imaging in the few reported cases of oxycodone and OxyContin overdose shows restricted diffusion in the cerebellar hemispheres and globi pallidi **(30-14)**.

Fentanyl

Accidental or intentional fentanyl and fentanyl analogue overdoses are skyrocketing worldwide and have become a major case of OD-related deaths. Many occur because fentanyl is illicitly manufactured, often mixed with heroin and other opioids. Toxic spongiform leukoencephalopathy similar to heroin overdose has been reported as having changes associated with delayed hypoxic-ischemic encephalopathy.

OPIOID DRUGS

Heroin
- Injected
  - Most common = ischemic strokes
  - Globi pallidi, white matter (resembles carbon monoxide poisoning)
- Inhaled
  - "Chasing the dragon"
  - Most common = leukoencephalopathy
  - Cerebellum, cerebral white matter

Methadone
- Adults
  - Toxic leukoencephalopathy
- Children
  - Usually accidental ingestion
  - Cerebellar edema

Oxycodone
- Cerebellar, globus pallidus ischemia
- Less common = toxic leukoencephalopathy

Fentanyl
- Leukoencephalopathy (like "chasing the dragon")
- Hypoxic-ischemic changes basal ganglia, white matter

Inhaled Gases and Toxins

Carbon monoxide and nitrous oxide are purely inhaled toxins. Some toxins such as cyanide can be inhaled, ingested, or absorbed transdermally. Inhaled vapors from volatile, intrinsically liquid agents include amyl nitrite ("poppers") and industrial solvents (e.g., toluene).

Carbon Monoxide Poisoning

Carbon monoxide (CO) is a colorless, odorless, tasteless gas that is produced by the incomplete combustion of various fuels. CO poisoning is caused by deliberate (suicide) or accidental inhalation (inadequate ventilation).

Etiology

CO combines reversibly with hemoglobin (Hgb) with over 200x higher the affinity than that of oxygen. If carboxyhemoglobin (CO-Hgb) levels exceed 20%, brain and cardiac damage are common.

Pathology

Because the globi pallidi are exquisitely sensitive to hypoxia, the hallmark of acute CO poisoning is symmetric globus pallidi necrosis **(30-18)**. The cerebral white matter is the second most commonly affected and often shows delayed demyelination and necrosis that may appear several weeks after the initial insult **(30-17)**.

In addition to bilateral globi pallidi and cerebral white matter, various sites, such as the cerebral cortex, cerebellum, hippocampus, amygdala, corpus callosum splenium, and insula, are often involved.

Clinical Issues

Acute CO poisoning initially causes nausea, vomiting, headache, and impaired consciousness. Outcome depends on both duration and intensity of exposure. Seizures, coma, and death may ensue.

Patients who survive CO poisoning often develop delayed encephalopathy. Parkinson-like symptoms, memory deficits, and cognitive disturbances are common.

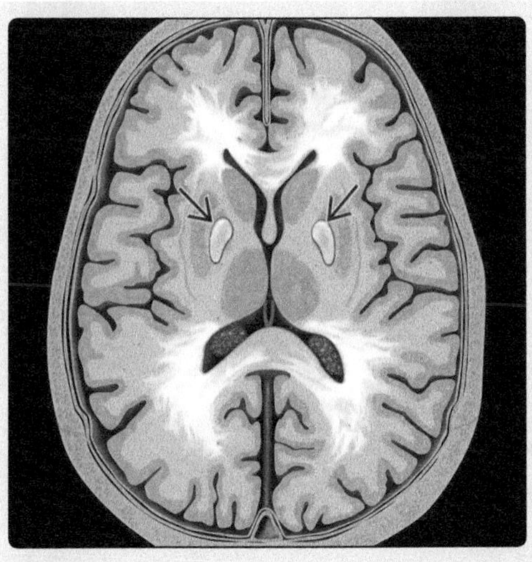

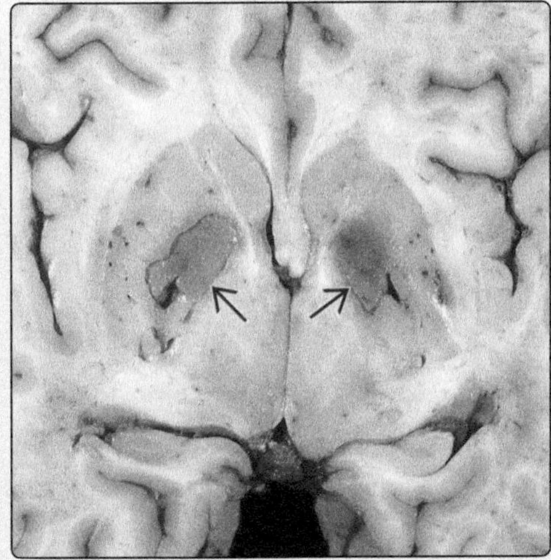

***(30-17)** Axial graphic shows the typical involvement of the brain by CO poisoning. The GP ⇨ are most affected followed by the cerebral WM. Pathologically, there is necrosis of the GP with variable areas of necrosis and demyelination in the WM. **(30-18)** Autopsy of CO poisoning shows symmetric coagulative (nonhemorrhagic) necrosis of both medial GP ⇨. (Courtesy R. Hewlett, MD.)*

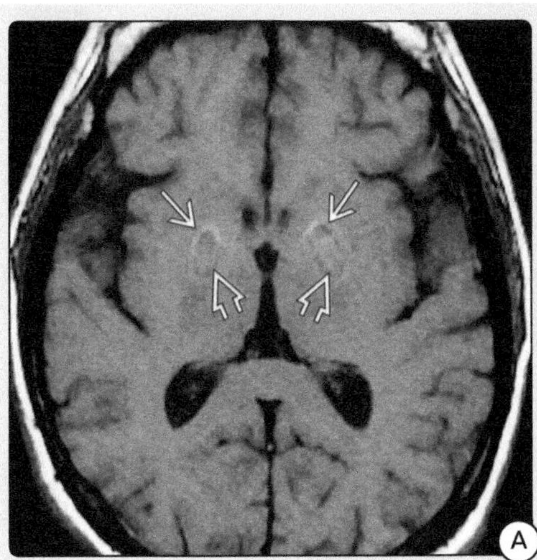

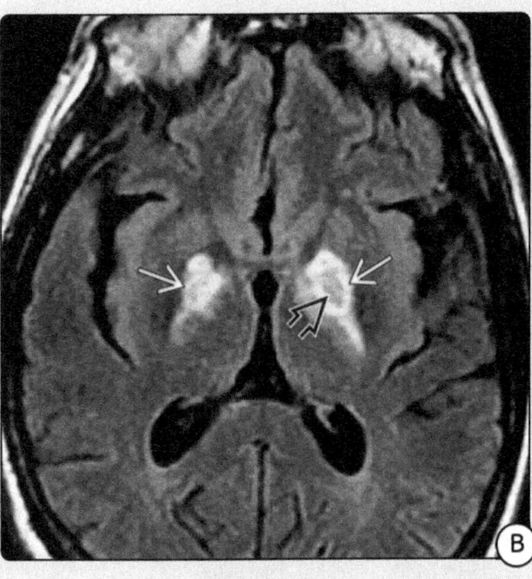

***(30-19A)** T1 MR in a 49-year-old man with CO poisoning shows symmetric lesions in both medial GP. Note faint hyperintense rim ➡, thin hypointense underlying rim, and central coagulative necrosis seen as mildly hyperintense lesions ➡. **(30-19B)** FLAIR MR in the same patient shows that the lesion is mostly hyperintense ➡ with central isointense core ⇨. The isointense parts of the lesions enhanced on T1 C+ (not shown).*

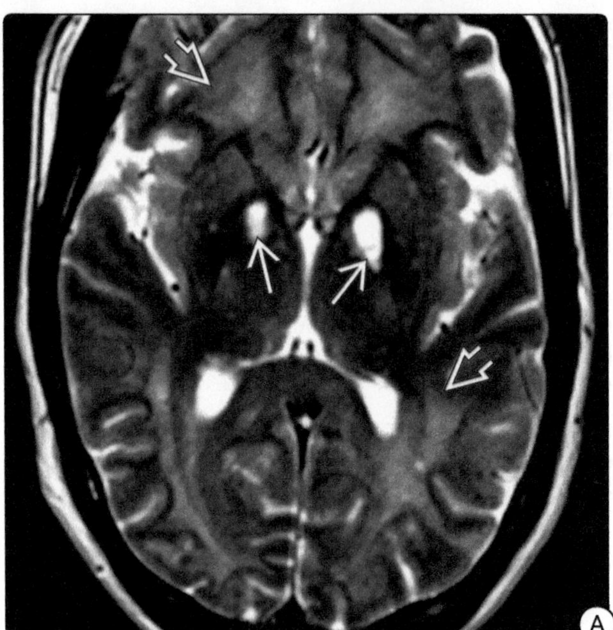

(30-20A) *Axial T2 MR in a patient with CO poisoning 2 weeks prior shows characteristic bilateral hyperintensities in GP ➡. Confluent hyperintensity now involves virtually all of the cerebral WM ➡ except the subcortical U-fibers.*

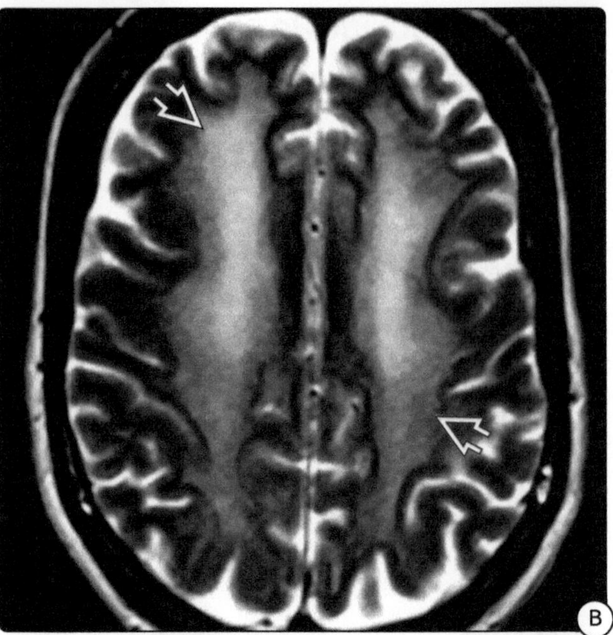

(30-20B) *More cephalad T2 MR shows that the hyperintensity involves most of the corona radiata ➡, mostly spares subcortical WM. This was the "interval" (subacute) form of CO poisoning with toxic demyelination.*

Imaging

CT Findings. Early NECT scans may be normal. Symmetric hypodensity in both globi pallidi develops within a few hours. Gross hemorrhage is rare. Variable diffuse hypodensity in the hemispheric white matter can be seen in severe cases.

MR Findings. Multiplanar MR (e.g., FLAIR, T2WI, and DWI) is the most sensitive technique for early detection of changes caused by CO poisoning. T1WI shows subtle hypointensity in the globi pallidi. A faint rim of hyperintensity caused by hemorrhage or coagulative necrosis may be present **(30-19A)**.

T2/FLAIR shows bilateral hyperintensities in the medial globi pallidi **(30-19B)** with the putamina and caudate nuclei less commonly affected. A thin hypointense rim around the lesion may be present.

In addition to the hyperintense areas seen on T2WI, FLAIR imaging may disclose subtle involvement of the caudate nuclei, thalami, hippocampi, corpus callosum, fornices, and cerebral cortex.

DWI/ADC maps show restricted diffusion in the affected areas. Bilateral globi pallidi hyperintensities as well as foci of restricted diffusion in the subcortical white matter are typical. ADC in the cerebral white matter increases significantly, reflecting extensive microstructural tissue damage. DTI shows fractional anisotropy decline in associated cortical areas.

T2* GRE or SWI may show hypointensity in the globi pallidi suggestive of petechial hemorrhage.

Within a week after exposure, MRS shows elevated Cho:Cr and lowered NAA:Cr ratios, indicating increased membrane metabolism and decreased neuroaxonal viability.

Up to 1/3 of CO patients develop a **delayed leukoencephalopathy** with progressive white matter demyelination, the "interval" (subacute) form of CO poisoning. Extensive bilateral symmetric confluent areas of hyperintensity on T2/FLAIR are characteristic findings **(30-20)**.

Differential Diagnosis

The major differential diagnoses of CO poisoning are **hypoxic-ischemic encephalopathy** (HIE) and **drug abuse**. As they share some common pathophysiology, imaging findings often overlap. HIE generally affects the entire basal ganglia and hippocampi, and less often affects the white matter or only the globi pallidi.

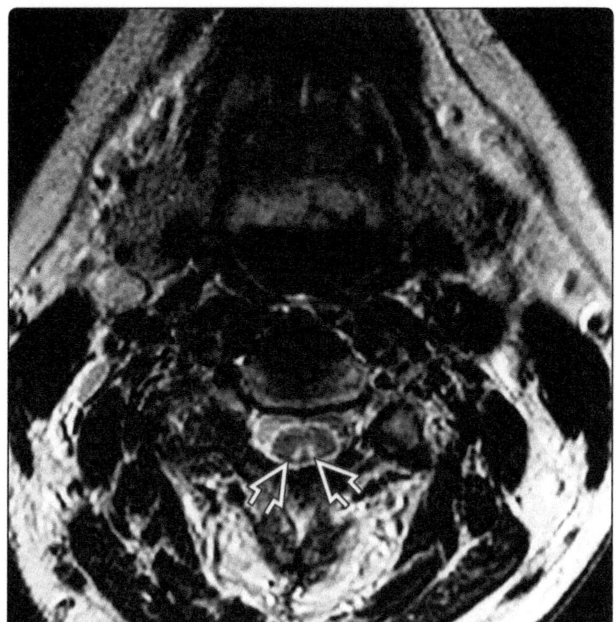

(30-21) *Axial T2 MR in a patient with nitrous oxide abuse shows selective symmetric demyelination of the posterior columns ➡, characteristic of subacute combined degeneration. (Courtesy C. Glastonbury, MBBS.)*

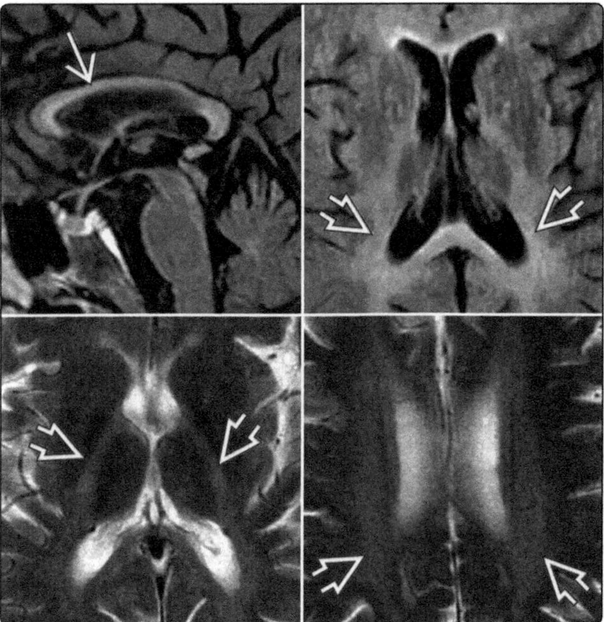

(30-22) *Sagittal T1 MR shows thinned corpus callosum ➡, and T2/FLAIR demonstrates confluent WM hyperintensity ➡. This was toluene toxicity due to chronic glue sniffing. (Courtesy S. Lincoff, MD.)*

INHALED GASES AND TOXINS

Carbon Monoxide Poisoning
- Acute: Symmetric globi pallidi necrosis
- Subacute ("interval"): Confluent leukoencephalopathy

Nitrous Oxide Abuse
- Brain lesions rare
- Subacute combined degeneration of spinal cord
  - Hyperintensity in dorsal columns

Toluene (Solvent) Abuse
- Chronic, repeated use
  - Atrophy
  - White matter lesions
  - Thalami, substantia nigra, red nuclei, dentate lesions

Organophosphate (Pesticide) Poisoning
- Basal ganglia hemorrhage, necrosis
- "Eye of the tiger" sign

Cyanide Poisoning
- Suicide, smoke inhalation
- Basal ganglia hemorrhage, necrosis
- Laminar cortical necrosis

Nitrous Oxide

Anesthetic gases, including N_2O, are sometimes inhaled for the putative euphoria. Excess N_2O irreversibly oxidizes the cobalt ion of vitamin B12, which is necessary for methylation of myelin sheath phospholipids. Long-term nitrous oxide abuse causes progressive myelopathy and a peripheral polyneuropathy. The end result is **subacute combined degeneration of the spinal cord**. The dorsal columns and corticospinal tracts are preferentially affected **(30-21)**. Brain lesions are rare.

Toluene Abuse

Toluene is a colorless liquid found in glues, paint thinners, inks, and other industrial products. Because it is lipid soluble, it is rapidly absorbed by the CNS.

The common methods of solvent abuse are "sniffing" (direct inhalation from a container), "huffing" (inhalation from a soaked rag held over the nose and mouth), and "bagging" (inhalation from a plastic bag). Solvent abuse is particularly prevalent among adolescents and young adults.

Imaging in patients with acute toluene abuse is usually normal. Abnormalities are typically seen only after several years of chronic inhalant abuse. Diffuse white matter lesions are seen in nearly 1/2 of all patients, initially seen as T2/FLAIR hyperintensity in the deep periventricular white matter with subsequent spread into the centrum semiovale and subcortical areas. The internal capsule, cerebellum, and pons are often affected **(30-22)**.

Cyanide Poisoning

Cyanide (CN) is one of the most potent and deadly of all poisons. Cyanogenic compounds may be found in household or workplace substances and deliberately or accidentally ingested.

CN exists in gas, solid, and liquid form. CN poisoning can occur by inhalation, ingestion, or transdermal absorption. Combustion of many common materials, such as some fabrics and plastics, may release CN and cyanogenic compounds.

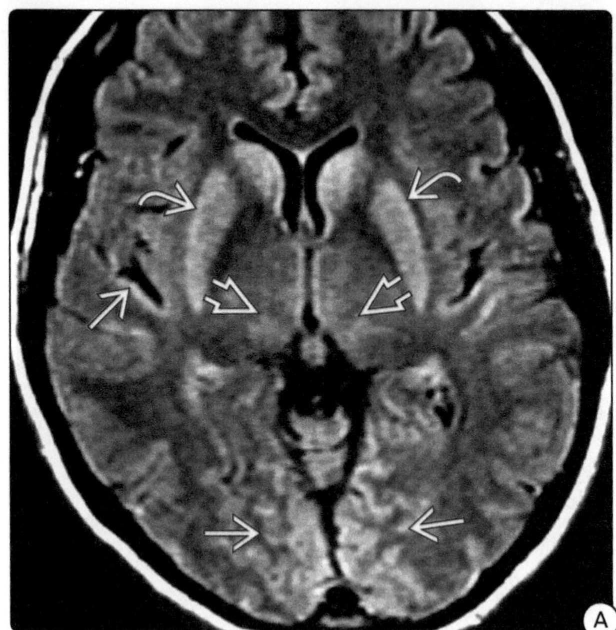

(30-23A) *FLAIR MR in smoke inhalation with CN poisoning from burning plastic shows symmetric hyperintensity in caudate nuclei and putamina ➡, more subtle lesions in posteromedial thalami ➡, and curvilinear cortical hyperintensities ➡.*

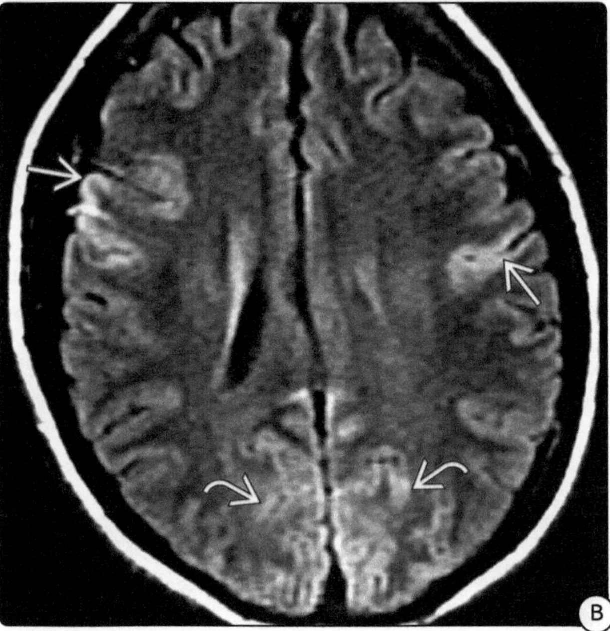

(30-23B) *More cephalad scan in the same patient shows the cortical hyperintensities ➡, which are especially prominent in both occipital lobes ➡.*

Cyanogenic compounds are also found in some foods, including almonds, the pits of stone fruits, lima beans, and cassava root.

Patients who survive the initial insult show symmetric hyperintensity in the basal ganglia and linear cortical hyperintensity on T2WI and FLAIR **(30-23)**.

The most important differential diagnosis of CN poisoning is **hypoxic-ischemic encephalopathy**. It may complicate CN poisoning. CN poisoning usually spares the hippocampi, but other features often overlap because the basal ganglia are affected in both disorders.

Metal Poisoning and Toxicity

A variety of metals can cause serious neurologic dysfunction when deposited in excess amounts in the CNS. **Manganese** accumulation is most common in the setting of chronic liver failure (see Chapter 32). Other environmental toxins, such as **lead** and **mercury**, are rare causes of neurotoxicity.

Gadolinium-based contrast agents (GBCAs) have been used routinely in clinical neuroimaging for nearly 30 years. **Gadolinium** brain deposition is now an increasingly common cause of heavy metal toxicity.

Gadolinium Deposition

Gadolinium Physiology

Gadolinium is a rare earth heavy metal in the lanthanide series. Its seven unpaired electrons induce a strong paramagnetic effect, reflected in its widespread use for contrast-enhanced MR sequences. Free gadolinium is extremely toxic so various chelating ligands are used to avoid the adverse effects of free gadolinium. Gadolinium in the blood must remain in chelated form until it is excreted by the kidneys. GBCAs are drained from the CSF through olfactory nerves via the "glymphatic" system.

Gadolinium-Based Contrast Agents (GBCAs)

GBCAs are divided into two categories: Linear and macrocyclic. In macrocyclic molecules, free gadolinium is isolated within the cage-like structure of the ligand agent. Ionic agents are chemically more stable than nonionic agents because the donor chelates are stronger in ionic agents. Laboratory evidence has shown that retained gadolinium from linear GBCAs is 10x higher than with macrocyclic GBCAs.

Life-threatening adverse reactions to GBCA are very rare. Potentially lethal nephrogenic systemic fibrosis (NSF) due to GBCA use in patients with renal failure were first described in 2006.

GBCA Brain Deposition

Dechelation of free gadolinium from an intact GBCA is the initial step in the mechanism of gadolinium deposition in the brain. GBCA brain deposition was first reported in 2014 and investigators have confirmed the association of repeated administration of GBCAs and high T1 signal intensity in the dentate nucleus and globi pallidi **(30-24)**. These iron-rich areas are the same sites specifically affected by neurodegenerative disorders with iron and manganese accumulation, viz., dentate nucleus, globus pallidus interna, and pulvinar of the thalamus. Signal intensity change seems to be significantly and exclusively related to the use of linear agents, although very low levels of deposition can also occur with macrocyclic agents.

To date, there is no strong evidence for harmful CNS effects of retained GBCAs. While the United States FDA has so far declined to restrict use of some GBCAs, European agencies have recommended suspension of marketing authorization for four linear GBCAs. Many clinical practices have subsequently switched to using macrocyclic GBCAs except in rare cases (e.g., prior allergic reaction).

Treatment-Related Disorders

A comprehensive treatment of all iatrogenic abnormalities in the brain is far beyond the scope of this text. Here, we discuss the most common disorders with a focus on treatment effects that must be recognized on imaging studies, namely radiation and chemotherapy.

Radiation Injury

Many investigators divide radiation-induced injury (RII) into three phases: Acute injury, early delayed injury, and late delayed injury. Pathologically, radiation injury varies from mild transient vasogenic edema to frank necrosis. The damage that results from XRT depends on a number of variables, including total dose, field size, number/frequency/fractionation of

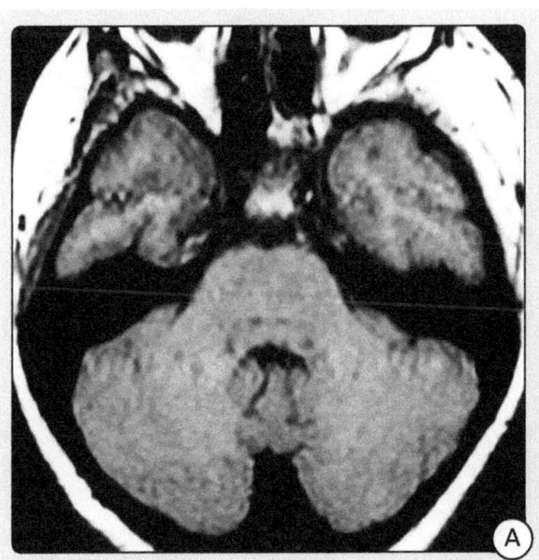

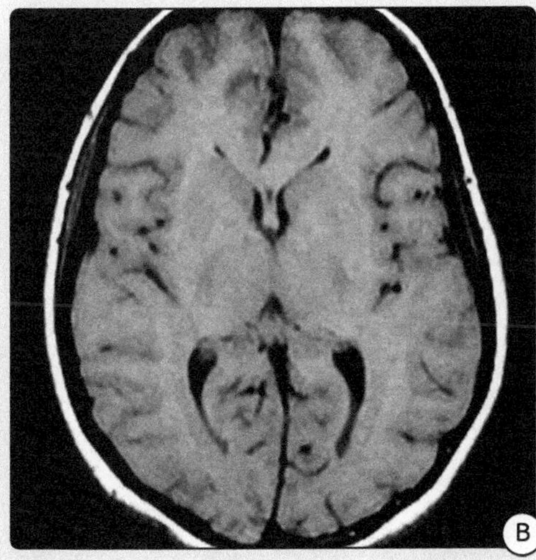

(30-24A) Baseline axial T1 MR through the 4th ventricle in a patient with multiple meningiomatosis shows no abnormalities. (30-24B) More cephalad T1 MR in the same patient shows no abnormalities.

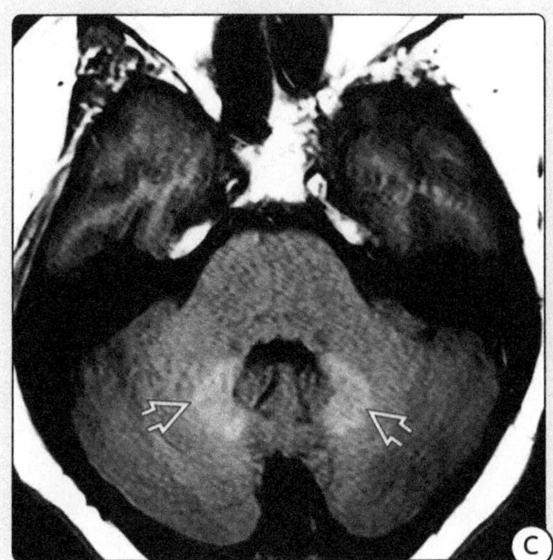

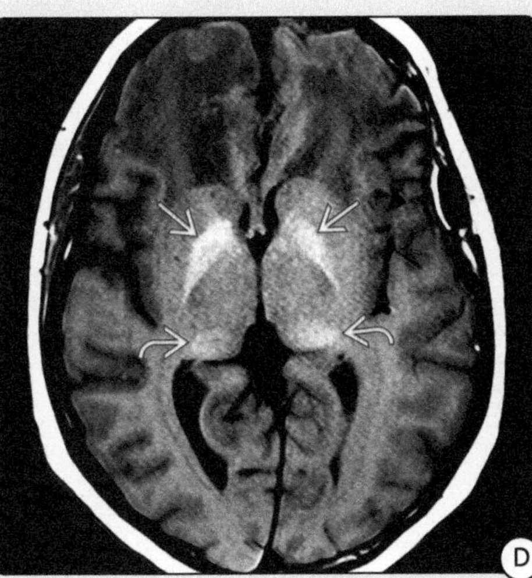

(30-24C) Fifteen years and 30+ contrast-enhanced MRs performed for follow-up, axial T1 MR through the 4th ventricle shows symmetric hyperintensity in both dentate nuclei ⇨. (30-24D) More cephalad T1 MR shows symmetric hyperintensity in both GP ➡ and pulvinars of both thalami ↪. Gadolinium deposition is from repeated use of GBCAs.

doses, and whether chemotherapy is used in conjunction with XRT.

Vascular endothelial cells, oligodendrocytes, astrocytes, microglia, and neurons probably all interact in the brain's response to radiation injury. Oligodendrocytes are especially vulnerable.

Acute Radiation Injury

Acute RII occurs days to weeks after irradiation and is very rarely encountered with modern XRT regimens. Standard imaging studies are usually normal, although MRS, DTI, and fMRI may detect changes before neurocognitive symptoms or anatomic alterations emerge. Occasionally, transient white matter edema can be seen on T2/FLAIR sequences.

Early Delayed Radiation Injury

In early delayed RII, imaging abnormalities can be detected as early as 1-6 months after XRT is completed. Early delayed RII is characterized pathologically by transient demyelination and clinically by somnolence, attention deficits, and short-term memory loss.

Confluent hypodense areas on NECT and periventricular white matter hyperintensity on T2/FLAIR are typical abnormalities. At this stage, RII changes are generally mild and reversible, often resolving spontaneously.

Late Delayed Radiation Injury

Late delayed RII is usually not observed until at least 6 months post irradiation. These late delayed injuries are viewed as progressive and largely irreversible, resulting from loss of glial and vascular endothelial cells.

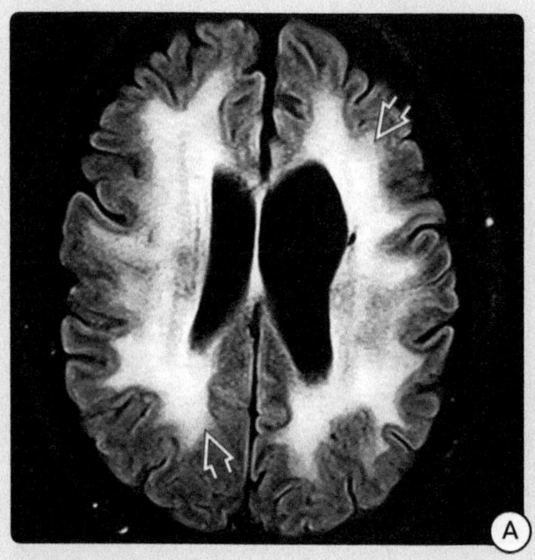

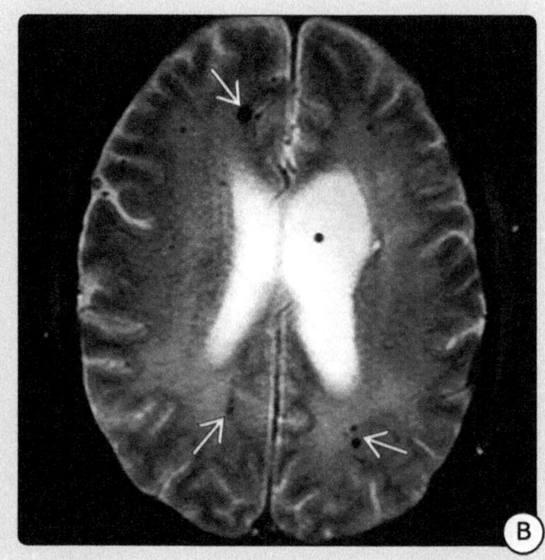

(30-25A) FLAIR MR in a patient with cognitive decline 3 years after whole-brain XRT for leukemia shows confluent WM hyperintensity ➔. (30-25B) T2 MR shows multiple foci of gradient blooming ➔, necrotizing leukoencephalopathy with XRT-induced vascular malformations.*

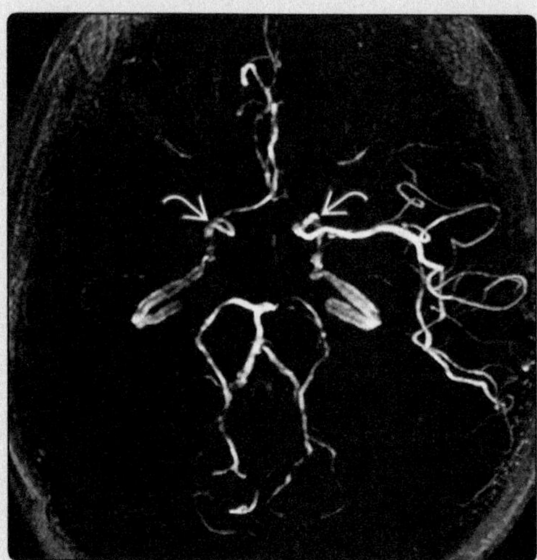

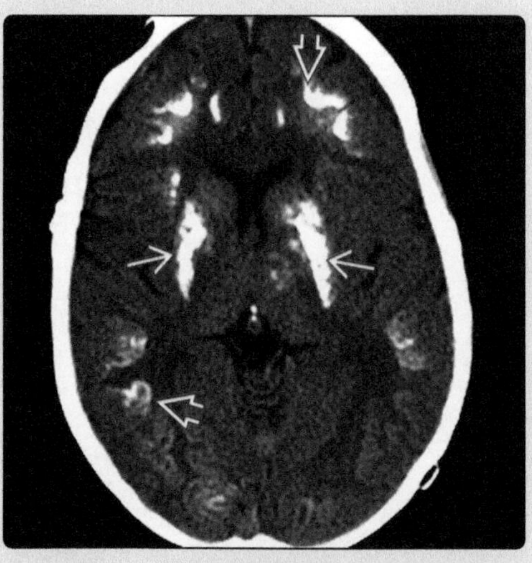

(30-26) MRA in a case with right MCA stroke years after XRT shows moyamoya and postradiation vasculopathy. Stenosis of both supraclinoid ICAs ➔ is present; right MCA is occluded. (Courtesy P. Hildenbrand, MD.) (30-27) NECT of 20-year-old man with XRT and chemo at age 8 for medulloblastoma shows BG ➔, subcortical WM calcifications ➔ are characteristic of mineralizing microangiopathy. (Courtesy P. Chapman, MD.)

Coagulative necrosis in a "mosaic" pattern with coalescing foci produces a necrotizing leukoencephalopathy in the deep cerebral white matter. The subcortical association or U-fibers and corpus callosum are typically spared. Vascular changes include fibrinoid necrosis, hyalinization, and sclerosis with thrombosis. Late delayed radiation necrosis is initially expansile and mass-like with necrosis largely confined to white matter.

Initially, late delayed RII shows mass effect and variable enhancement on imaging studies. Later, volume loss, white matter spongiosis with confluent hyperintensity, and calcifications can be seen **(30-25)**.

Long-Term Sequelae of Radiation Injury

In addition to **necrotizing leukoencephalopathy**, long-term complications of XRT include vasculopathy, mineralizing microangiopathy, telangiectasis (XRT-induced vascular malformations), and radiation-induced neoplasms.

Radiation-induced vasculopathy with endothelial hyperplasia results in diffusely narrowed large and medium-sized arteries. Ischemic strokes and moyamoya-like disease may result **(30-26)**.

Mineralizing microangiopathy is usually seen in patients treated with combination XRT and chemotherapy and generally does not appear until at least two years following treatment. Calcifications in the basal ganglia and subcortical white matter are typical findings **(30-27)**.

Radiation-induced vascular malformations (RIVMs) are primarily capillary telangiectasias or cavernous malformations most commonly seen in children who have received whole-brain radiotherapy for acute lymphoblastic leukemia. T2* (GRE, SWI) sequences demonstrate "blooming" microhemorrhages in the majority of patients **(30-25B)**. RIVMs rarely occur more than three years following XRT. Children under 10 years of age at the time of irradiation are at higher risk.

Radiation-induced neoplasms are rare but often devastating. XRT is the single most important risk factor for developing a new primary CNS neoplasm. Approximately 70% are meningiomas, 20% are malignant astrocytomas or medulloblastomas, and 10% are sarcomas. Meningiomas occur an average of 17-20 years after treatment, whereas gliomas occur at a mean of nine years. Sarcomas have a mean latency of seven or eight years following XRT.

RADIATION-INDUCED BRAIN INJURY

Pathology
- Microglial activation; proinflammatory cytokines

3 Phases of RII
- Acute radiation injury
  - Rare
  - T2/FLAIR may show white matter edema
  - TSPO-PET may show neuroinflammation
- Early delayed injury (at least 6 months)
  - Necrotizing leukoencephalopathy
  - Confluent hyperintensity
- Long-term sequelae
  - Necrotizing leukoencephalopathy
  - Vasculopathy, mineralizing microangiopathy
  - Vascular malformations (T2* "black dots")
  - Radiation-induced neoplasms

Chemotherapy Effects

Currently, the most common chemotherapy agents implicated in CNS toxicity are methotrexate, cytarabine, vincristine, asparaginase, and corticosteroids. Unlike radiation injury, chemotherapy-associated acute toxic CNS injury is common. The two most frequent abnormalities are posterior reversible encephalopathy syndrome and treatment-induced leukoencephalopathy.

Posterior reversible encephalopathy syndrome (PRES) is addressed in detail in Chapter 32. In chemotherapy-related PRES, imaging findings are often atypical. The occipital lobes are frequently spared, whereas the cerebellum, brainstem, and basal ganglia are frequently involved. Hemorrhage, contrast enhancement, and diffusion restriction—all relatively rare in "typical" PRES—are common.

Treatment-induced leukoencephalopathy is especially common in patients treated with methotrexate. Acute neurotoxicity occurs in 5-18% of children treated for acute lymphoblastic leukemia. Bilateral, relatively symmetric, confluent areas of T2/FLAIR hyperintensity in the periventricular white matter are typical. Imaging abnormalities typically resolve after treatment.

CHEMOTHERAPY EFFECTS ON THE BRAIN

Clinical Issues
- Acute effects common; often reversible

Imaging
- PRES common
  - Atypical > typical imaging findings
  - Occipital lobes often spared
  - Hemorrhage, enhancement, restricted diffusion common
- Acute leukoencephalopathy
  - Reflects acute neurotoxicity
  - Transient T2/FLAIR periventricular hyperintensity

Selected References: The complete reference list is available on the Expert Consult™ eBook version included with purchase.

Inherited Metabolic Disorders

***Inherited metabolic disorders (IMDs)**—a.k.a. **inborn errors of metabolism**—represent conditions in which a genetic defect leads to a deficiency of a protein (e.g., enzyme or nonenzyme protein) that subsequently affects mechanisms of synthesis, degradation, transport, &/or storage of molecules in the body. IMDs can present at virtually any age from infancy well into the fifth and sixth decades, although infantile and childhood presentation is most common.*

IMDs are relatively uncommon diseases. The informed radiologist can merge his or her understanding of the pathogenetic and pathomorphologic underpinnings of the various IMDs with imaging observations. Specifically, we observe *what part of the brain is involved* (e.g., gray matter vs. white matter), *what kind of involvement is present* (e.g., cortex, basal ganglia, white matter—subcortical, deep, or periventricular), and *what locations are most affected* (e.g., frontal lobes). Additional information, such as the presence of cysts, calcifications, diffusion restriction, and pathologic enhancement, aids in crystallizing the imaging differential diagnosis.

Because white matter abnormalities form a constant part of many, if not most, **inborn metabolic diseases**, familiarization with the normal progression of white matter myelination is a prerequisite for detecting and understanding IMDs. We therefore begin this chapter with a brief review of how normal myelination progresses from birth through 2 years of life.

Once we have reviewed the patterns of normal myelination as assessed with MR, we continue with an overview and introduction of the IMDs. A discussion of classification systems and a practical approach to analyzing imaging is delineated. A detailed discussion of the leukodystrophies and nonleukodystrophic white matter disorders is beyond the scope of this text, but selected IMDs representative of their groupings will be presented.

Normal Myelination and White Matter Development

General Considerations

Myelination

Myelination is an orderly, highly regulated, multistep process that begins during the fifth fetal month and is largely complete by 18-24 postnatal months. Some structures (e.g., cranial nerves) myelinate relatively early in

Selected Myelination Milestones

Age	T1 Hyperintensity	T2 Hypointensity
Birth		
	Dorsal brainstem	Dorsal brainstem
	Posterior limb IC	Partial posterior limb IC
	Perirolandic gyri	Perirolandic gyri
	Corticospinal tracts	Corticospinal tracts
3-4 Months		
	Ventral brainstem	Posterior limb IC
	Anterior limb IC	
	CC splenium	
	Central, posterior corona radiata	
6 Months		
	Cerebellar WM	Ventral brainstem
	CC genu	Anterior limb IC
	Parietal, occipital WM	CC splenium, genu by 8-9 months
	Frontal WM by 9 months	
12 Months		
	Posterior fossa (≈ adult)	Most of corona radiata
	Most of corona radiata	Posterior subcortical WM
	Posterior subcortical WM	Occipital WM
18 Months		
	All WM except temporal, frontal U-fibers	All WM except temporal, frontal U-fibers, occipital radiations
24 Months		
	Anterior temporal, frontal U-fibers	Anterior temporal, orbital frontal U-fibers

(Table 31-1) *CC = corpus callosum; IC = internal capsule; WM = white matter. WM maturation is seen earlier on T1WI.*

fetal development, whereas others (e.g., optic radiations and fibers to/from association areas) often do not completely myelinate until the third or even the fourth decade of life.

Brain myelination follows a typical topographical pattern, progressing from **inferior to superior, central to peripheral**, and **posterior to anterior**. For example, the brainstem myelinates before the peripheral cerebellar hemispheres, the posterior limbs of the internal capsules myelinate before the anterior limbs, and the deep periventricular white matter (WM) myelinates before the subcortical U-fibers. The dorsal brainstem myelinates before the anterior brainstem, and—with the exception of the parietooccipital association tracts—occipital WM myelinates earlier than WM in the anterior temporal and frontal lobes.

CT

At birth, the WM is largely unmyelinated, so it appears symmetrically hypoattenuating compared with regional gray matter (GM) due to the comparatively high water content of unmyelinated WM.

MR

The MR appearance of WM maturation varies with two important factors, i.e., **patient age** and the **imaging sequence** employed. Unmyelinated WM is hypointense relative to GM on T1WI and hyperintense to GM on T2WI.

As WM matures, it becomes more hyperintense on T1WI. Progressive T2 shortening (hypointensity) occurs in the first 2 years of life as myelin matures and proton density decreases.

During the first 6-8 months, T1 hyperintensity occurs earlier and is more conspicuous than T2 hypointensity, so T1WIs are best both to evaluate WM maturation and brain morphology **(31-1)** **(31-2)**. Heavily weighted T2 sequences are sensitive to follow WM maturation between 6 and 18 months. Fully myelinated WM has high T1 signal and low T2 signal.

Selected major milestones of normal myelination on T1- and T2-weighted images are summarized in the accompanying table **(Table 31-1)**.

Classification of Inherited Metabolic Disorders

Overview

An exhaustive discussion of IMDs is far beyond the scope of this book. The interested reader is referred to the superb definitive texts by A. James Barkovich. In this chapter, we consider the major inherited neurometabolic diseases, summarizing the pathoetiology, genetics, demographics, clinical presentation, and key imaging findings of each.

There are several strategies that can be used to conceptually frame IMDs. One way is to divide IMDs according to which cellular organelle (e.g., mitochondria, lysosomes) is predominantly affected. Another characterizes them by defects in a specific metabolic pathway (e.g., disorders of carbohydrate metabolism). However, these methods lack the pragmatic approach needed by the radiologist to be a contributing member of the clinical care team. We therefore emphasize—and advocate the use of—an approach to imaging analysis pioneered by A. James Barkovich that is primarily based on anatomic location and specific imaging features with an emphasis on MR—the **imaging-based approach.**

Organelle-Based Approach

Three cellular organelles are primarily affected in IMDs, i.e., the lysosomes, peroxisomes, and mitochondria. Classifying IMDs according to the affected organelle has the benefit of conceptual simplicity, but many IMDs do not arise from disordered organelle formation or function, making this classification scheme less than comprehensive. The organelle-based approach to IMDs is summarized in the box below.

ORGANELLE-BASED CLASSIFICATION OF IMDs

Lysosomal Disorders
- Mucopolysaccharidoses
- Gangliosidoses
- Metachromatic leukodystrophy
- Krabbe disease
- Fabry disease

Peroxisomal Disorders
- Abnormal peroxisomal formation
  - Zellweger syndrome
  - Neonatal adrenoleukodystrophy
  - Infantile Refsum disease
- Abnormal peroxisomal function
  - X-linked adrenoleukodystrophy
  - Classic Refsum disease

Mitochondrial Disorders
- Leigh syndrome
- **M**itochondrial **e**ncephalomyopathy with **l**actic **a**cidosis and **s**troke-like episodes (MELAS)
- Myoclonic epilepsy with ragged red fibers (MERRF)
- Kearns-Sayre
- Glutaric aciduria types 1 and 2

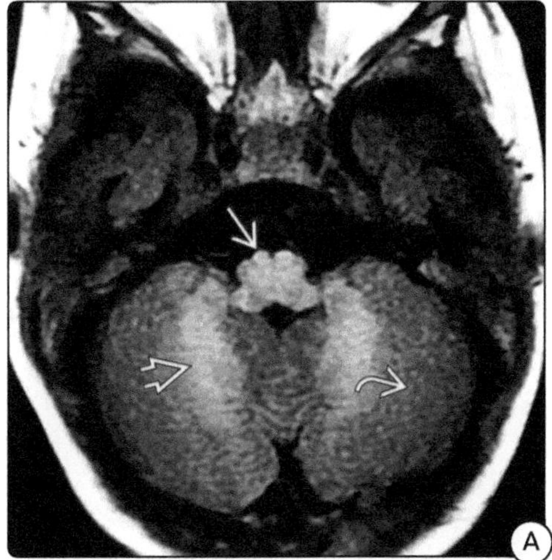

***(31-1A)** T1WI at 4m shows hyperintense medulla ➡, medial cerebellar hemispheres ➡ while peripheral unmyelinated WM is hypointense ➡.*

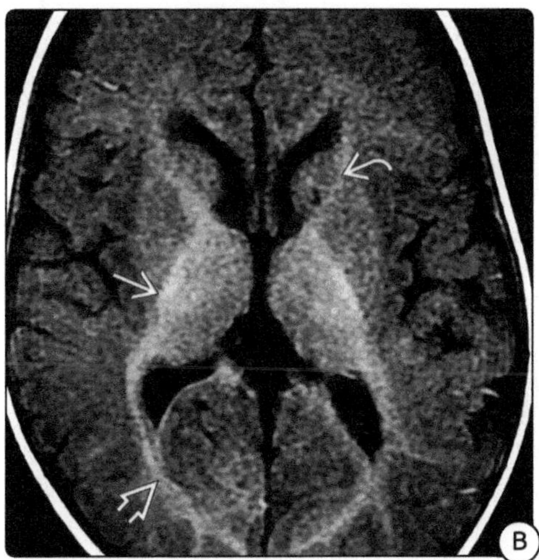

***(31-1B)** T1 MR shows normal T1 shortening in PLIC ➡, subtle in ALIC ➡. The optic radiation WM is beginning to myelinate ➡.*

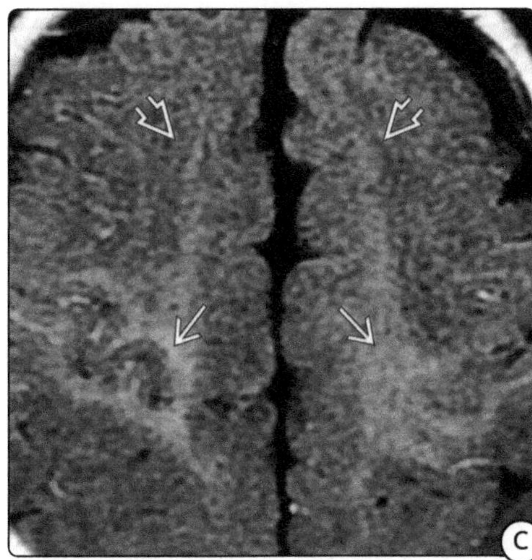

***(31-1C)** T1 MR shows corona radiata is unmyelinated ➡, although some myelination in WM of the perirolandic regions ➡ is present.*

(31-2A) T1 MR at 6m shows pons, peduncles completely myelinated. Hyperintensity extends further into cerebellar hemispheres.

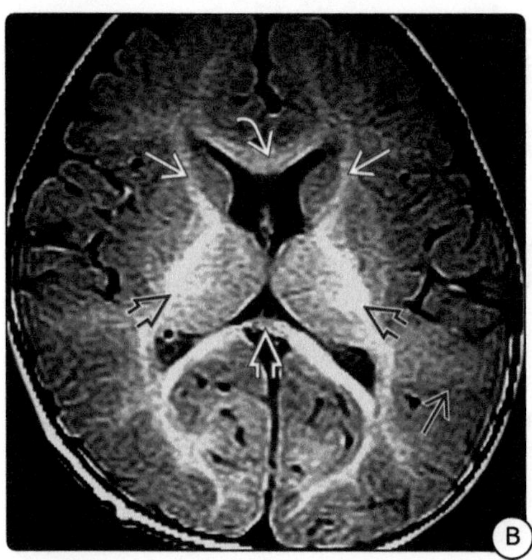

(31-2B) T1 MR shows myelinated WM in PLIC, ALIC, corpus callosum splenium, genu. Subcortical WM is unmyelinated.

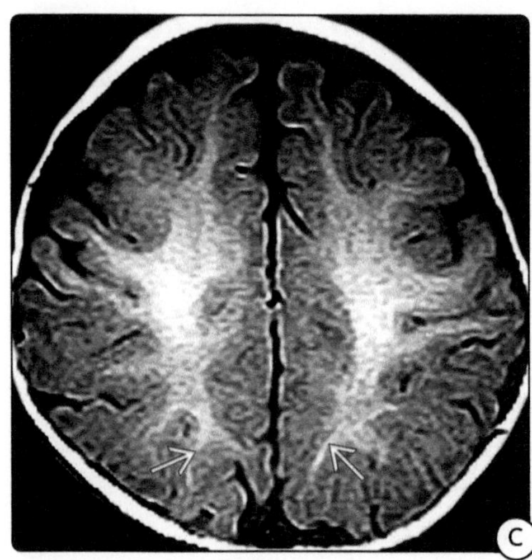

(31-2C) T1 MR shows hyperintensity extends to subcortical WM, especially parietal, occipital lobes. Change compared to 4m is striking.

Imaging-Based Approach

Barkovich et al have elaborated a practical imaging-based approach to the diagnosis of IMDs derived from the seminal work of van der Knaap and Valk. This approach is based on determining whether the disease involves primarily or exclusively (1) WM, (2) mostly GM, or (3) both. Furthermore, a heightened awareness of the region of the brain most heavily involved (e.g., periventricular WM vs. subcortical WM or frontal lobe vs. parietal occipital lobes) and the presence of miscellaneous findings (e.g., cysts &/or calcifications) leads to greater specificity.

In this text, we follow the **imaging-based approach**, the clinically practical classification based on three categories of predominant imaging features (e.g., WM, GM, or both being involved). We then discuss the major diagnostic entities in each imaging-based group.

IMDs Predominantly Affecting White Matter

Historically, nearly all abnormalities of the white matter (WM) have been described as "leukodystrophies." *"Leukodystrophies"* have been divided into three categories: (1) *Dys*myelinating disorders (i.e., normal myelination does not occur), (2) *de*myelinating disease (i.e., myelin forms normally, is deposited around axons, but later breaks down or is destroyed), and (3) *hypo*myelinating diseases (i.e., here, the WM may partially myelinate but never myelinates completely). Hypomyelinating leukoencephalopathies represent an important yet uncommon group of genetic disorders that cause delayed myelin maturation or undermyelination.

From an imaging perspective, it can be difficult to determine whether a disorder is *dys*myelinating, *de*myelinating, or *hypo*myelinating. In structuring a differential diagnosis, it is important to determine whether the disorder primarily affects *deep* (periventricular) WM or the *subcortical* short association WM fibers (U-fibers). In a few diseases, both the deep and peripheral WM are affected.

Examples of leukodystrophies that exhibit early *deep* WM predominance include metachromatic leukodystrophy and X-linked adrenoleukodystrophy. Leukodystrophies that involve the *subcortical* U-fibers early in the disease course include megaloencephalic leukoencephalopathy with cysts and infantile Alexander disease. The latter two diagnoses also present with a large head.

Diseases in which virtually *all* the WM (both periventricular *and* subcortical) remains unmyelinated are rare. The imaging appearance in these disorders resembles that of a normal newborn brain with immature, almost completely unmyelinated WM. Here, the entire WM—including the subcortical U-fibers—appears uniformly hyperintense on T2WI.

Periventricular White Matter Predominance

The prototypical disorder that typically begins with symmetric deep WM involvement and spares the subcortical U-fibers until late in the disease course is metachromatic leukodystrophy (MLD). Others with a similar pattern of periventricular predominance include Krabbe disease (globoid cell leukodystrophy), X-linked adrenoleukodystrophy, and vanishing WM disease (VWMD).

MAJOR IMDs WITH PERIVENTRICULAR WM PREDOMINANCE

Common
- Metachromatic leukodystrophy
- Classic X-linked adrenoleukodystrophy

Less Common
- Globoid cell leukodystrophy (Krabbe disease)
- Vanishing WM disease

Rare but Important
- Phenylketonuria
- Maple syrup urine disease
- Merosin-deficient congenital muscular dystrophy

Metachromatic Leukodystrophy (MLD)

Etiology. MLD is a devastating lysosomal storage disease caused by a reduction in or complete absence of arylsulfatase A (ARSA). Reduced or absent ARSA leads to increased lysosomal storage of sulfatide and eventually lethal demyelination.

Pathology. Sulfatide deposition occurs within glial cells, plasma membranes, inner layer of myelin sheath, neurons, Schwann cells, and macrophages. A brain affected by MLD may initially be normal but exhibits progressive volume loss. The periventricular WM shows a grayish discoloration (e.g., "tigroid" or "leopard" pattern) with relatively normal-appearing subcortical U-fibers.

Clinical Issues. MLD is one of the most common of all inherited WM disorders. Three distinct clinical forms are currently recognized: Late infantile (onset earlier than 3 years), juvenile (onset earlier than 16 years), and adult MLD. The *late infantile form* is the most common and typically presents in the second year of life with visuomotor impairment, gait disorder, and abdominal pain. Progressive decline and death within 4 years are expected. The *juvenile form* presents between 5-10 years, often with deteriorating school performance. Survival beyond 20 years is rare. The *adult form* may present with early-onset dementia, MS-like symptoms, and progressive cerebellar signs.

Imaging

CT Findings. Early NECT shows symmetric diminished attenuation involving the central hemispheric WM **(31-3A)**. CECT shows no enhancement.

MR Findings. The typical MR features of early MLD are confluent, symmetric, "butterfly-shaped" T2/FLAIR hyperintensities involving the periventricular WM **(31-3)**. The subcortical U-fibers and cerebellum are typically spared until late in the disease.

With disease progression, centrifugal spread of demyelination involves the corpus callosum (i.e., splenium), parietooccipital WM, and the frontal and then the temporal WM. Islands of normal myelin around medullary veins in the WM may produce a striking "tiger," "tigroid," or "leopard" pattern with linear hypointensities in a sea of confluent hyperintensity **(31-4)**. No enhancement is seen on T1 C+.

Miscellaneous Imaging. Reduction of diffusivity in zones of active demyelination is seen. Regions of "burned-out," aging or chronic demyelination demonstrate increased diffusivity. MRS is nonspecific; choline and myoinositol may be elevated in early and active disease.

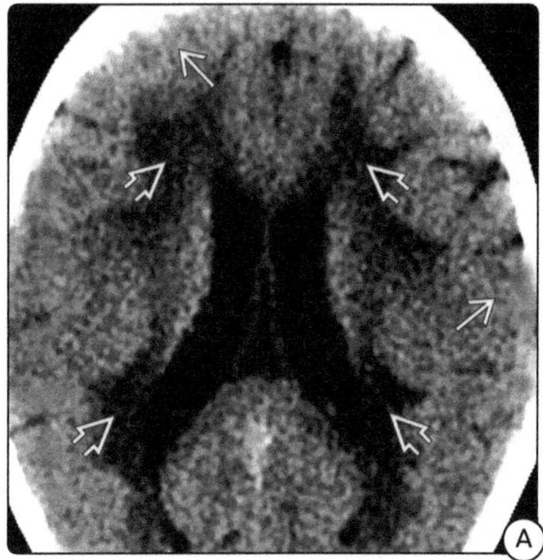

(31-3A) Axial NECT in a 6-year-old boy with MLD shows periventricular WM hypoattenuation ➡. The subcortical U-fibers are spared ➡.

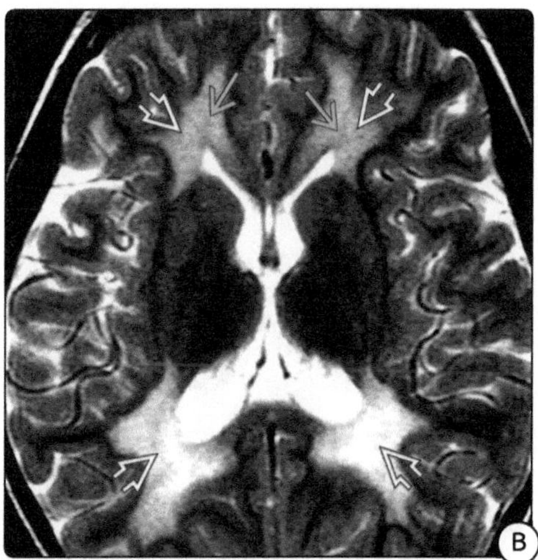

(31-3B) Axial T2 MR shows WM demyelination (hyperintensity) ➡. Note "granular" hypointense frontal perivenular myelin sparing ➡.

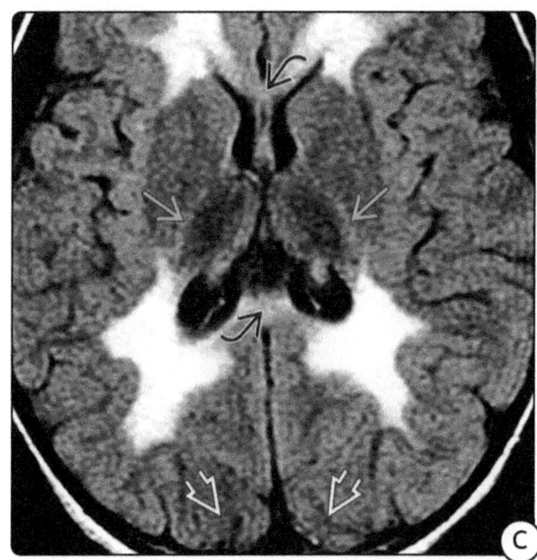

(31-3C) Axial FLAIR MR shows the "butterfly" pattern of MLD. U-fibers appear normal ➡. CC ➡ and PLIC ➡ are involved.

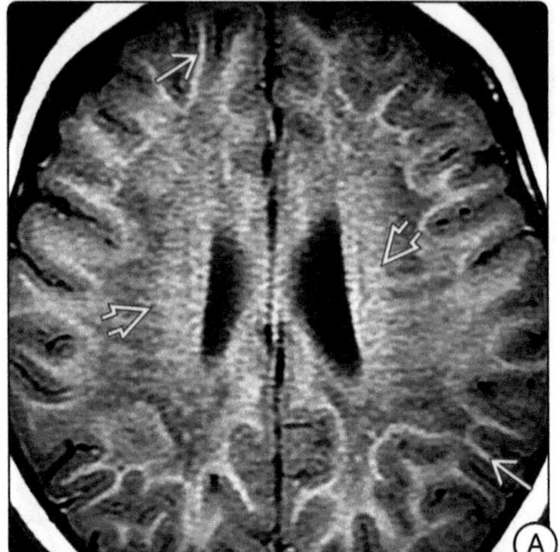

(31-4A) Axial T1 MR shows MLD in a 2-year-old boy with sparing of U-fibers ➡, preserved striate myelin surrounding venules (tigroid pattern) ➡.

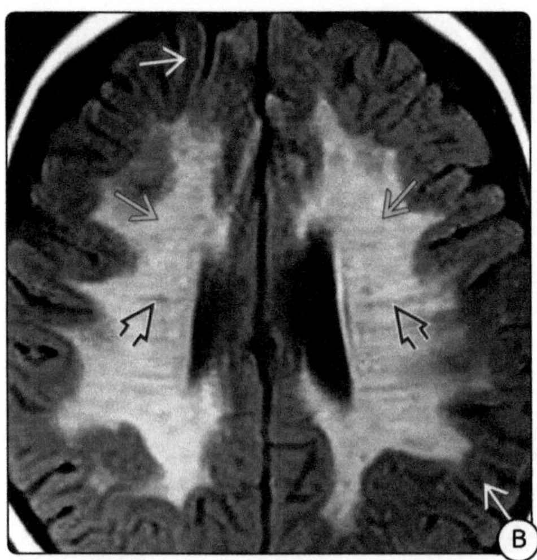

(31-4B) Axial FLAIR MR shows hyperintense demyelination ➡, preserved perivenule myelin ➡ (tigroid pattern), sparing of U-fibers ➡.

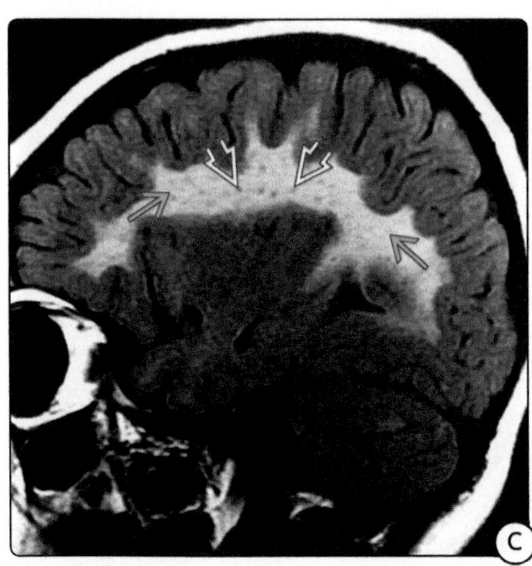

(31-4C) Sagittal FLAIR MR shows hypointense dots (leopard pattern) of preserved myelin ➡ within demyelinated WM ➡, sparing U-fibers.

Differential Diagnosis. The major differential diagnosis of MLD includes other IMDs that primarily affect the periventricular WM. Globoid cell leukoencephalopathy (**Krabbe disease**) shows bithalamic hyperattenuation on NECT, involves the cerebellum early, and often demonstrates enlarged optic nerves and optic chiasm.

Pelizaeus-Merzbacher disease usually presents in neonates and shows almost a total lack of myelination that does not show interval improvement on serial MRs. The cerebellum may be markedly atrophic.

Periventricular white matter injury (PVL) is associated with a history of low-birth-weight/preterm deliveries and clinical static spastic di- or quadriparesis and shows nonprogressive periventricular volume loss and T2/FLAIR hyperintensity.

Vanishing white matter disease (VWMD) begins in the periventricular WM but eventually involves all of the hemispheric WM. VWMD often cavitates and does not enhance.

METACHROMATIC LEUKODYSTROPHY (MLD)

Etiology and Pathology
- Lysosomal storage disorder
- Decreased ARSA → sphingolipid accumulation
- Periventricular demyelination

Clinical Issues
- Most common inherited leukodystrophy
- 3 forms
  - Late infantile (most common)
  - Juvenile
  - Adult (late onset)

Imaging
- Centrifugal spread of demyelination
  - Starts in corpus callosum splenium, deep parietooccipital WM
  - Frontal, temporal WM affected later
  - Spares subcortical U-fibers, cerebellum
- Classic = butterfly pattern
  - Symmetric hyperintensities around frontal horns, atria
- Tiger pattern
  - "Stripes" of perivenular myelin sparing in WM

Differential Diagnosis
- Other disorders that predominantly affect periventricular WM
  - Globoid cell leukodystrophy (Krabbe disease)
  - Pelizaeus-Merzbacher disease
  - Vanishing WM disease
- Destructive disorders
  - Periventricular leukomalacia

X-Linked Adrenoleukodystrophy (X-ALD)

Etiology. X-ALD is an inherited disorder of peroxisomal metabolism. Absent or deficient acyl-CoA synthetase leading to impaired oxidation of very-long-chain fatty acids (VLCFAs). VLCFAs accumulate in the WM, causing severe inflammatory demyelination ("brittle" myelin). Axonal degeneration in the posterior fossa and spinal cord are also typical of the disease. The definitive diagnosis of X-ALD is established by tissue assays for increased amounts of VLCFAs.

Pathology. Three distinct zones of myelin loss are seen in ALD **(31-5)**. The *innermost zone* consists of a necrotic core of demyelination with astrogliosis, ± Ca^{++}. An *intermediate zone* of active demyelination and perivascular inflammation lies just outside the necrotic, "burned-out" core of the lesion. The most *peripheral zone* represents the advanced edge of ongoing demyelination without inflammatory changes.

Clinical Issues. X-ALD is the most common single protein or enzyme deficiency disease to present in childhood. Several clinical forms of ALD and related disorders have been described. **Classic X-linked ALD** is the most common form (45%) and is seen almost exclusively in boys 5-12 years of age. Behavioral difficulties and deteriorating school performance are common. Approximately 10% of affected patients present acutely with seizures, adrenal crisis, acute encephalopathy, or coma.

Adrenomyeloneuropathy (AMN) is the second most common type (35%). It is another X-linked disorder that occurs primarily in male patients. It presents between 14 and 60 years, thus presenting later than classic X-ALD. AMN is characterized by axonal degeneration in the spinal cord more than the brain and peripheral nerves.

ADRENOLEUKODYSTROPHY (ALD): ETIOLOGY, PATHOLOGY, AND CLINICAL ISSUES

Etiology
- Peroxisomal disorder
- Impaired oxidation of VLCFAs

Pathology
- Severe inflammatory demyelination
- 3 zones
  - Necrotic "burned-out" core
  - Intermediate zone of active demyelination + inflammation
  - Peripheral demyelination without inflammation

Clinical Issues
- Classic X-linked ALD
  - Most common form (45%)
  - Preteen boys
  - Deteriorating cognition, school performance
- Adrenomyeloneuropathy (AMN)
  - 2nd most common form (35%)
  - Most common in male patients
- Addison disease without CNS involvement (20%)

Imaging. Although CT scans are sometimes obtained as an initial screening study in children with encephalopathy of unknown origin, MR without and with IV contrast is the procedure of choice.

CT Findings. NECT scans demonstrate hypoattenuation involving the corpus callosum splenium and WM around the atria and occipital horns. Calcification in the affected WM may be seen. CECT typically shows enhancement around the central hypoattenuating WM.

MR Findings. A *posterior-predominant* pattern is seen in 80% of patients with X-ALD **(31-6)**. The earliest finding is T2/FLAIR hyperintensity in the middle of the corpus callosum splenium. As the disease progresses, hyperintensity spreads from posterior to anterior and from the center to the periphery. The peritrigonal WM, corticospinal tracts, fornix, commissural fibers, plus the visual and auditory pathways can all eventually become involved.

The leading edge of demyelination appears hyperintense on T1WI but does not enhance. The intermediate zone of active inflammatory demyelination typically enhances T1 C+ **(31-6B)**.

X-ALD may present at an atypical age, demonstrate atypical sites of involvement, and lack enhancement. Approximately 10-15% of all patients

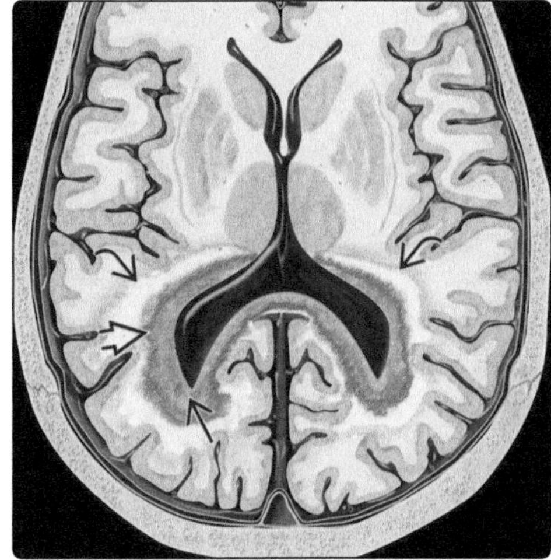

(31-5) X-ALD with burned-out deep zone ➡; intermediate zone of active demyelination ➡, advancing demyelinating edge ➡ are shown.

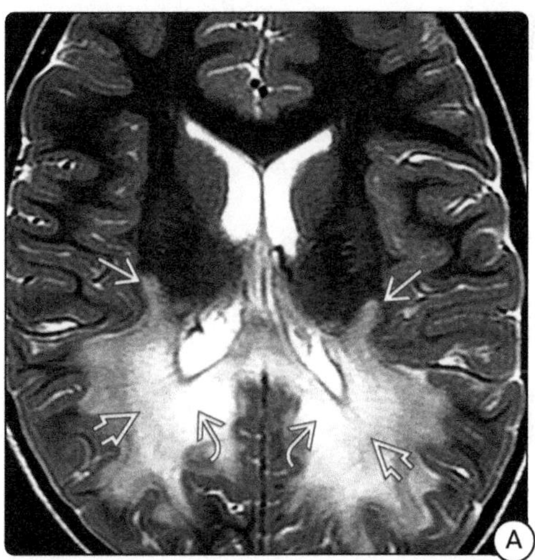

(31-6A) T2 MR of X-ALD shows burned-out WM ➡, demyelination/inflammation ➡, advancing edge without inflammation ➡.

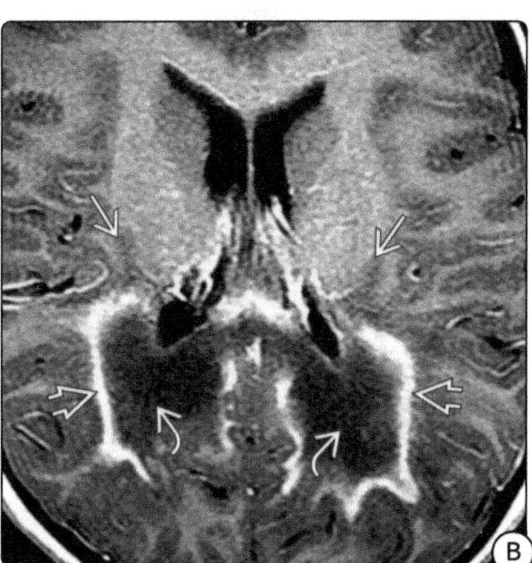

(31-6B) T1 C+ FS MR in X-ALD shows zone of active demyelination enhances ➡, while leading edge ➡ and central burned-out cores ➡ do not.

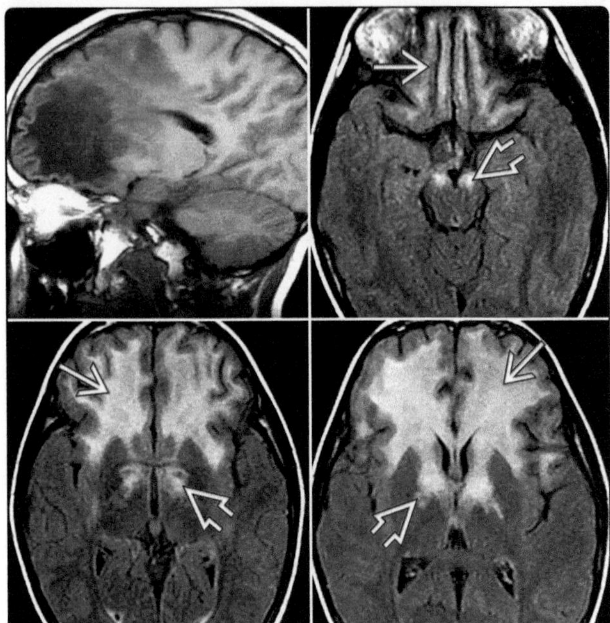

***(31-7)** MR multiplanar images of an atypical variant of ALD show symmetric confluent frontal lesions ➡ with sparing of parietooccipital WM. Note the involvement of internal capsules and cerebral peduncles ⇨.*

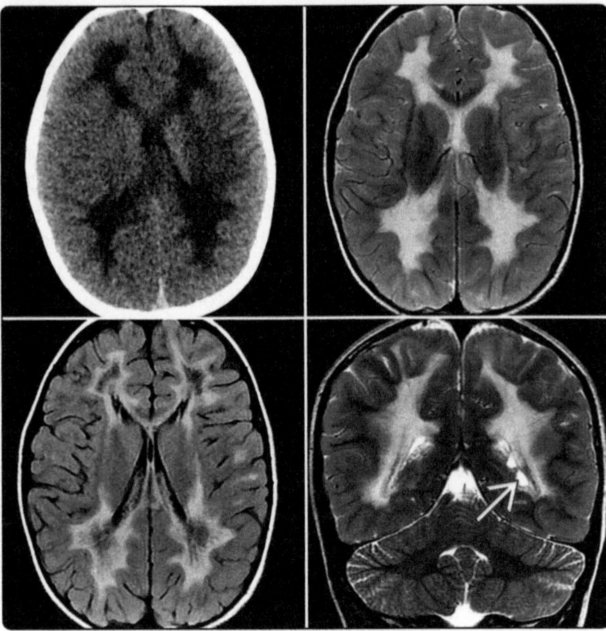

***(31-8)** Images show vanishing white matter disease in a 5-year-old boy originally diagnosed with MLD. Note the symmetric periventricular disease, spared U-fibers, and early cyst formation ➡. (Courtesy S. Harder, MD.)*

with classic X-ALD have an *anterior predominant* demyelination; T2/FLAIR hyperintensity initially appears in the corpus callosum genu (not the splenium) and spreads into the frontal lobe WM **(31-7)**.

In patients with AMN, the cerebral hemispheres are relatively spared with predominant involvement of the cerebellum, corticospinal tracts, and spinal cord. Enhancement is typically absent.

DWI/DTI shows reduced diffusivity in active zones of demyelination and increased diffusivity in regions of "burned-out" demyelination. DTI shows reduced connectivity (i.e., loss of fractional anisotropy) in WM that MR demonstrates as abnormal and in "normal" WM.

MRS shows, at TE of 35 ms, peaks at 0.8-1.4 (i.e., cytosolic amino acids and VLCFA macromolecules). Reduced *N*-acetyl-L-aspartate (NAA) may be detected prior to observed MR abnormality and predicts progression. Increased myoinositol, CHO, and lactate doublet are typical findings.

Differential Diagnosis. When X-ALD presents in patients of classic age and sex (i.e., 5- to 12-year-old boys) and with typical posterior predominance on imaging studies, the differential diagnosis is very limited.

ALD: IMAGING AND DIFFERENTIAL DIAGNOSIS

Imaging

- X-linked ALD posterior predominance in 80%
  - Earliest finding: Corpus callosum splenium hyperintensity
  - Spreads posterior to anterior, center to periphery
  - Intermediate zone often enhances, restricts
- Variant patterns
  - X-linked ALD with anterior predominance (10-15%)
  - AMN involves corticospinal tracts, cerebellum, cord more than hemispheric WM

Differential Diagnosis

- X-linked ALD pathognomonic if sex, age, imaging findings classic

Vanishing White Matter Disease

Vanishing white matter disease (VWMD) has become recognized as one of the most prevalent inherited leukoencephalopathies. VWMD is characterized by diffusely abnormal cerebral WM that literally "vanishes" over time. VWMD is an autosomal recessive disorder caused by point mutation of genes responsible for encoding any of the five subunits of the eukaryotic translation inhibiting factor 2B (*EIF2B*).

Pathology. VWMD is a slowly progressive, eventually cavitating WM disease that predominately involves the deep frontoparietal with lesser involvement of the temporal lobes. The basal ganglia, corpus callosum, anterior commissure, internal capsules, and cortex are characteristically spared. The

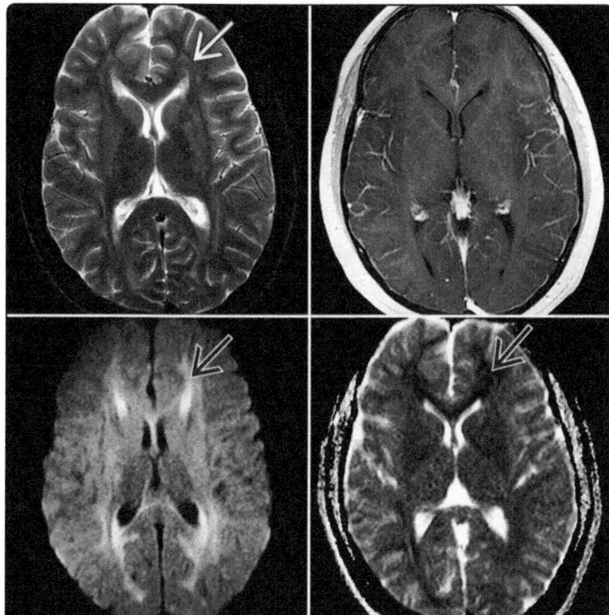

***(31-9)** Axial MR scans in a 13-year-old girl with PKU, mild cognitive impairment show subtle periventricular hyperintensity ➡, no enhancement, and restriction on DWI ➡.*

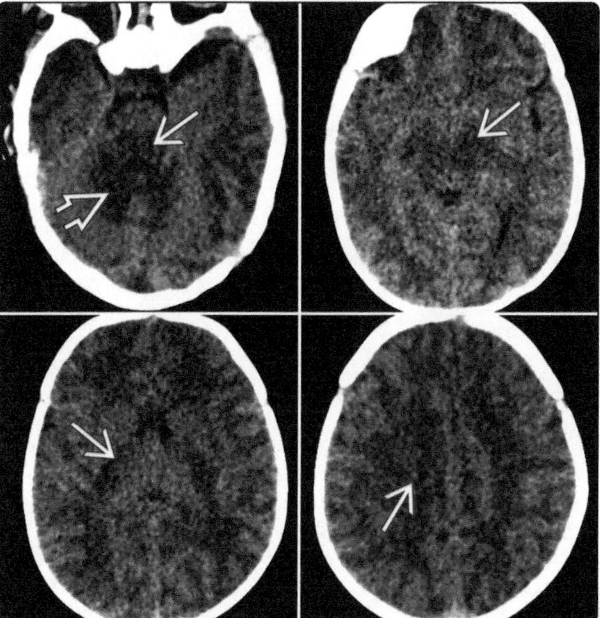

***(31-10)** Axial NECT in a 13-day-old boy with MSUD shows edema (low attenuation) ➡ in the dorsal midbrain and central cerebellar WM ➡, cerebral peduncles (upper R), internal capsules (lower L), and centrum semiovale.*

eventual appearance is areas of cystic degeneration with frank WM cavitation.

Clinical Issues. Classic VWMD presents in children 2-5 years of age. Development is initially normal, but progressive motor and cognitive impairment with cerebellar and pyramidal signs follows. Progression is typically slow. Death by adolescence is typical.

Approximately 15% of VWMD cases occur in adolescents and adults. Mean age of late-onset VWMD is 30 years.

Imaging. WM hypoattenuation without calcifications is typical in the early stages of VWMD. Eventually, profound WM volume loss is seen.

Extensive confluent WM T1 hypointensity with T2/FLAIR hyperintensity is typical. The disease is initially periventricular **(31-8)** but later spreads to involve the subcortical arcuate fibers. Over time, the affected WM undergoes rarefaction. Cavitary foci of CSF-like signal intensity eventually develop **(31-8)**. Diffuse volume loss with enlarged ventricles and sulci is seen on serial studies. VWMD does not enhance.

Differential Diagnosis. VWMD is not the only leukoencephalopathy that causes "melting away" or "vanishing" of the cerebral WM. Alexander disease and mitochondrial encephalopathies can be associated with WM rarefaction and cystic degeneration. **Alexander disease** presents with macrocephaly and is not associated with the episodic neurologic deterioration characteristic of VWMD; it demonstrates a frontoparietal gradient of disease. Frontal WM cysts can occur in end-stage disease. Approximately 10% of **mitochondrial encephalopathies** predominantly affect the WM and may form cavitations.

Phenylketonuria

Phenylketonuria (PKU) is the most common inborn error of amino acid metabolism. Phenylalanine (Phe) accumulates and is toxic to the developing brain. Newborns are usually asymptomatic and most cases are diagnosed with newborn metabolic disease-screening programs. With adherence to dietary protein restriction, mitigation of the ravages of this disease occurs. Early treatment is key to minimizing cognitive impairment.

Initial imaging in PKU can appear normal! When abnormality is detected, T2/FLAIR imaging shows hyperintensity in the periventricular WM, particularly frontal and peritrigonal regions **(31-9)**. The subcortical arcuate fibers are spared. There is no enhancement following contrast administration. *Centrifugal* progression eventually leads to end-stage disease. MRS shows a Phe peak resonating at 7.37 ppm (which is missed on routine clinical MRS that only displays to 4 ppm).

The differential diagnosis includes **periventricular WM injury (PVL)** (at-risk population of low-birth-weight, premature neonates who eventually manifest signs and symptoms of cerebral palsy, **metachromatic leukodystrophy** (demonstrating more confluent zones of deep WM T2/FLAIR hyperintensity), and **Krabbe disease** (optic and cranial nerve enlargement, thalamic hyperattenuation on NECT, MR showing T2/FLAIR hyperintensity in corticospinal tracts, deep cerebral WM, and early cerebellar involvement) are differential diagnoses for PKU.

Maple Syrup Urine Disease

Maple syrup urine disease (MSUD) is an autosomal recessive disorder of branched-chain amino acid (leucine, isoleucine,

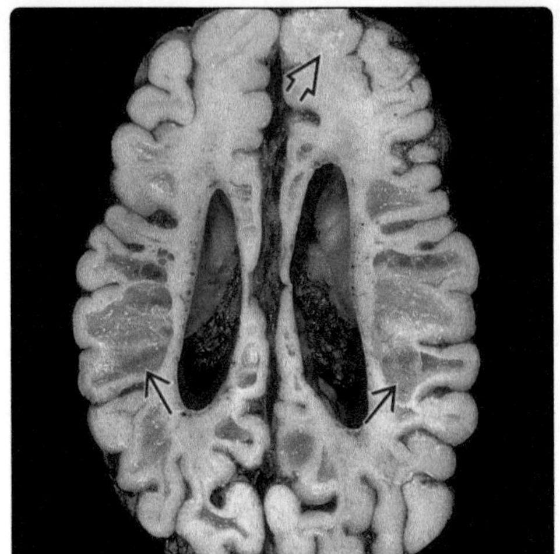

(31-11) MLC autopsy shows multiple subcortical cysts ➡ and WM rarefaction ➡ in frontal subcortical WM. (Courtesy R. Hewlett, MD.)

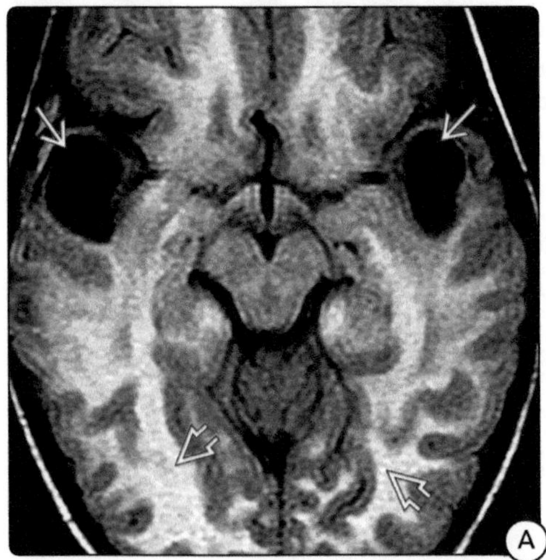

(31-12A) Axial FLAIR in a 22-month-old child with MLC shows swollen, hyperintense, "watery" WM ➡ and CSF-like temporal subcortical cysts ➡.

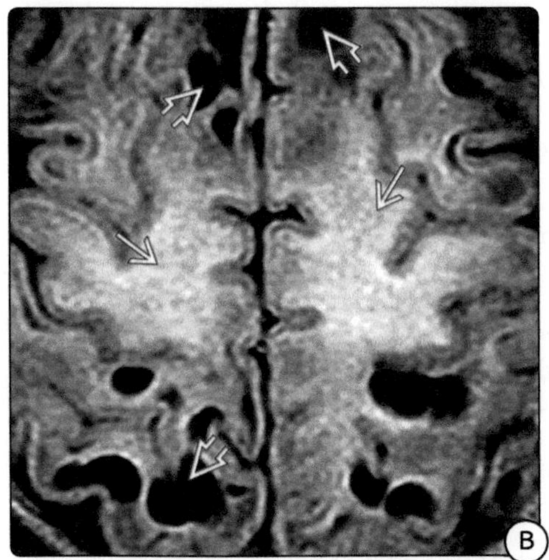

(31-12B) Axial FLAIR MR in a 2y child with MLC shows swollen, hyperintense subcortical WM ➡. Note fluid-filled subcortical hypointense cysts ➡.

valine) metabolism. Elevated levels of leucine and other leukotoxic metabolites induce cytotoxic or intramyelinic edema and spongiform degeneration.

Infants with classic MSUD are initially normal. Within days after birth, poor feeding, lethargy, vomiting, seizures, and encephalopathy may occur. In severe cases, the urine smells of maple syrup or burned sugar.

NECT scans show profound hypoattenuation within the myelinated WM as well as within the dorsal brainstem, cerebellum, cerebral peduncles, and posterior limb of the internal capsule **(31-10)**. MR shows striking T2/FLAIR hyperintensity involving the cerebellar WM, dorsal brainstem, cerebral peduncles, thalami, globi pallidi, posterior limbs of internal capsule, internal medullary lamina, and pyramidal and tegmental tracts.

MRS shows a peak at 0.9 ppm caused by accumulation of branched-chain α-keto amino acids. This peak is present at short (35 ms), intermediate (144 ms), and long (288 ms) PRESS MRS aquisitions, distinguishing them from the broad cytosolic amino acid peaks that only resonate at a short TE (35 ms).

The differential diagnosis includes **sepsis** (brain MR expected to be normal), **Alexander disease** (T2 hyperintensity of the frontal WM and enhancement), **hypoxic-ischemic injury** (with history of periparturitional distress, no significant symptom-free period), and **mitochondrial cytopathy** (episodic stroke-like clinical events of varied severity depending on the genotype of the disorder).

Subcortical White Matter Predominance

IMDs that initially or predominantly affect the subcortical WM are much less common than those that begin with deep periventricular involvement. The most striking IMD with preferential involvement of the subcortical WM is megaloencephalic leukoencephaly with subcortical cysts (MLC).

Megaloencephalic Leukodystrophy With Subcortical Cysts (MLC)

MLC, a.k.a. vacuolating megaloencephalic leukoencephalopathy, is a rare autosomal recessive disorder with characteristic MR features.

Pathology, Clinical Features. Gross pathology shows a swollen cerebral hemispheric WM, relative occipital sparing, variable involvement of the subcortical arcuate fibers, frequent involvement of the external capsules, and sparing of the internal capsules. Multiple variably sized subcortical cysts, initially involving the temporal lobes, are typical **(31-11)** **(31-12)**.

MLC is distinguished clinically from other leukoencephalopathies by its remarkably slow course of neurologic deterioration. Infantile-onset macrocephaly is characteristic, but neurologic deterioration is often delayed. Age at symptom onset varies widely, ranging from birth to 25 years. Slow cognitive decline is observed as the disease progresses.

Imaging. Cranial US in symptomatic infants shows unexplained hyperechogenicity of affected WM. NECT will demonstrate hypoattenuation of the cerebral hemispheric WM.

The diagnosis of MLC is typically established by MR. Macrocephaly with diffuse confluent WM T2/FLAIR hyperintensity in the subcortical WM is typical. The affected subcortical WM appears "watery" and swollen. The overlying gyri seemingly stretch over the swollen WM. The optic radiations, occipital subcortical WM, corpus callosum as well as the basal ganglia and internal capsule are usually spared.

Characteristic CSF-like subcortical cysts develop in the anterior temporal lobes followed in frequency by frontoparietal cysts. Unlike the "watery" WM, which exhibits T2/FLAIR hyperintensity, the cysts approximate the signal intensity of CSF on FLAIR. The number and size of the cysts may increase over time. The abnormal WM and cysts do not enhance on T1 C+.

Differential Diagnosis. MLC must be distinguished from other IMDs with macrocrania. The two major considerations are **Canavan disease** and **Alexander disease**, both of which are characterized by much greater clinical disability.

Canavan disease almost always involves the basal ganglia, lacks the development of subcortical cysts, and demonstrates a large NAA peak on MRS. Canavan disease also shows very early involvement of the subcortical U-fibers, which may appear uninvolved in the early presentation of MLC.

Alexander disease demonstrates a *frontal* WM gradient, involves the basal ganglia, and often enhances following contrast administration.

IMDs Predominantly Affecting Gray Matter

Inherited metabolic disorders (IMDs) that involve the gray matter (GM) without affecting the white matter (WM) can be subdivided into those that involve the cortex and those that mostly affect the deep gray nuclei. Inherited GM disorders that involve the deep gray nuclei are significantly more common than those that primarily affect the cortex.

IMDs Primarily Affecting Deep Gray Nuclei

A number of inherited disorders affect mostly the basal ganglia and thalami. Three inborn errors of metabolism with specific predilection for the deep gray nuclei include (1) *pantothenate kinase-associated neurodegeneration* (PKAN), (2) *creatine deficiency syndromes*, and (3) a cytosine-adenine-guanine (CAG) repeat disorder called *Huntington disease.*

We begin this section with an overview of brain iron accumulation disorders before turning our attention specifically to **PKAN** and **Huntington disease**. We close the section with a discussion of the most important inherited disorder with abnormal copper metabolism, **Wilson disease**.

Brain Iron Accumulation Disorders

Some iron accumulation within the basal ganglia and dentate nuclei occurs as part of normal aging (see Chapter 33). Neurodegeneration with brain iron accumulation (NBIA) represents a clinically and genetically heterogeneous group of conditions characterized by progressive neurodegeneration and abnormally elevated brain iron. We focus our discussion on PKAN, the most common type of NBIA, and Huntington disease.

MR is especially useful in diagnosing NBIAs. All feature iron deposition in the globus pallidus (GP) but differ in other associated findings. The distribution of T2 or T2* hypointensity can help distinguish between the different NBIA subtypes (see next box).

PKAN

Terminology and Etiology. PKAN, formerly known as Hallervorden-Spatz disease, is a rare familial autosomal recessive disorder characterized by excessive iron deposition in the GP and substantia nigra (SN).

Pathology. Grossly, PKAN is characterized by shrinkage and rust-brown discoloration of the medial GP, the reticular zone of the SN, and, sometimes, the dentate nuclei. The red nuclei are generally spared. Microscopically, increased iron content is found in the GP interna and pars reticulata SN. Iron deposition is found within astrocytes, microglial cells, neurons, and around vessels. The "eye of the tiger" corresponds to regions of reactive astrocytes, dystrophic axons, and vacuoles in the anteromedial GP.

Clinical Issues. PKAN or NBIA type 1 can develop at any age. Most cases are diagnosed late in the first decade or during early adolescence. The disorder classically begins with slowly progressive gait disturbances and delayed psychomotor development. Progressive mental deterioration finally leads to dementia.

Imaging. Imaging findings reflect the anatomic distribution of the excessive iron accumulation. T2WI demonstrates marked hypointensity in the GP and SN. A small focus of central hyperintensity in the medial aspect of the very hypointense GP (the classic "eye of the tiger" sign) is caused by tissue gliosis and vacuolization **(31-13)**. Note that *not all cases of PKAN demonstrate the "eye of the tiger"* **(31-14)**.

PKAN does not enhance on T1 C+ nor does it demonstrate restricted diffusion.

Differential Diagnosis. Abnormal iron deposition in the basal ganglia occurs with PKAN as well as other NBIAs. **Aceruloplasminemia** and **neuroferritinopathy** are both adult-onset disorders. Both involve the cortex, which is spared in PKAN.

Disorders with increased T2 signal within the GP can be grouped within *metabolic* derangements and *toxic/ischemic* insults. These entities lack pallidal GRE and SWI "blooming."

Inherited metabolic disorders to consider in the differential diagnosis of basal ganglia T2 hyperintensity include **neuroferritinopathy** (variable GP T2 hyperintensity), **Wilson disease, Leigh syndrome, infantile bilateral striatal necrosis**, and **mitochondrial encephalopathies**, which show striatal hyperintensity (not hypointensity or blooming). These disorders predominantly involve the caudate and putamen, not the medial GP.

Toxic/ischemic insults include hypoxic-ischemic injury (positive health history, T2 hyperintensity involving striatum, GP, thalami, corticospinal tracts, with or without cortical involvement), *CO poisoning* (increased T2 signal involving GP,

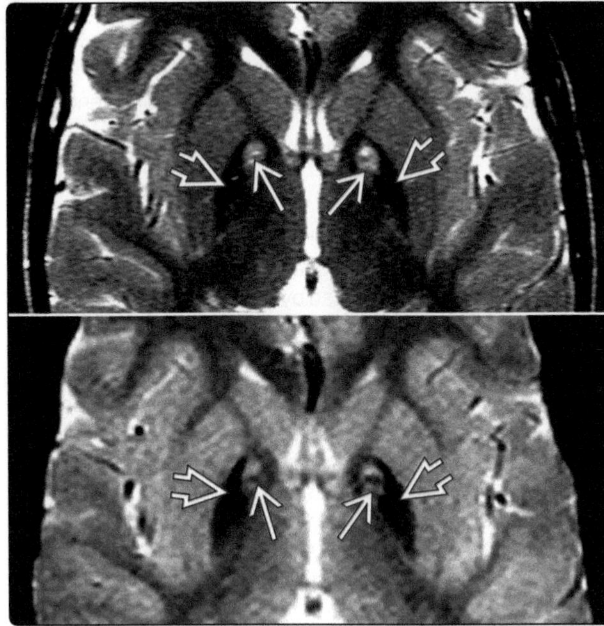

(31-13) T2 MR (top), GRE (bottom) in a patient with PKAN show classic "eye of the tiger" sign with bilateral hyperintense central foci ➡ in the medial globi pallidi surrounded by striking hypointensity ➡.

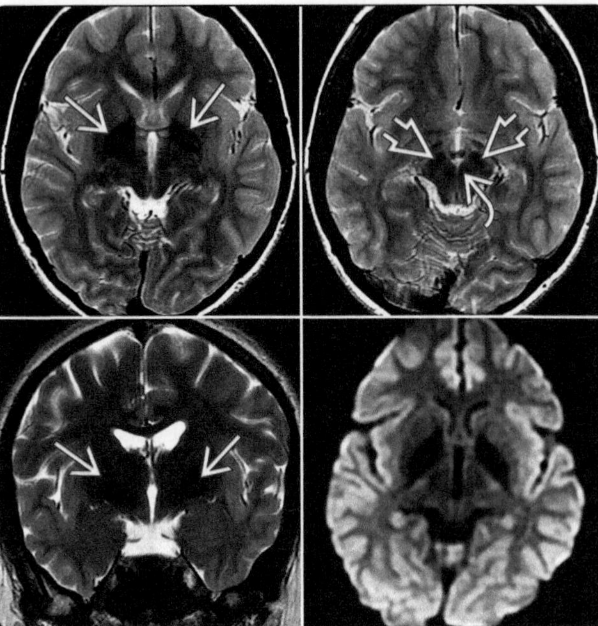

(31-14) Multiplanar MR shows a 19-year-old woman with documented PKAN. Note the profound hypointensity in the GP ➡, SN ➡, red nuclei ➡, and the lack of an "eye of the tiger" sign. DWI is normal (bottom right).

other deep nuclei, cortex, and WM), **cyanide toxicity** (T2 increased within basal ganglia with or without hemorrhagic necrosis), and **kernicterus** (neonate) (increased T1/T2 GP).

NBIA T2* HYPOINTENSITY

PKAN
- GP, SN, dentate nuclei
- "Eye of the tiger" sign variable
- *Spares* cortex

Infantile Neuroaxonal Dystrophy
- Cerebellar atrophy (95%)
- T2* hypointensity in GP, SN (50%)
- *Spares* cortex

Neuroferritinopathy
- T2* hypointensity in GP, SN
- Then dentate/caudate nuclei, thalami
- *Affects* cortex

Aceruloplasminemia
- GP, caudate nuclei, putamen, thalamus
- Red nucleus, SN, dentate nuclei
- *Affects* cerebral, cerebellar cortices

Huntington Disease

Terminology and Etiology. HD is a.k.a. Huntington chorea. HD is an autosomal dominant chronic hereditary neurodegenerative disorder with complete penetrance. The huntingtin gene includes a repeating CAG trinucleotide segment of variable length. The presence of > 38 repeats confirms the diagnosis of HD.

Pathology. The most characteristic gross abnormality is volume loss with rarefaction of the caudate nucleus, putamen, and GP **(31-15) (31-16)**. The cerebellum is also atrophic in juvenile-onset HD.

Clinical Issues. Mean age at symptom onset is 35-45 years. Only 5-10% of patients present before the age of 20 years (juvenile-onset HD). CAG repeat length and age influence both the expression and the progression of HD.

Adult-onset HD is characterized by progressive loss of normal motor function, development of stereotypic choreiform movements, and deteriorating cognition. Once symptoms appear, the disease progresses relentlessly and results in death within 10-20 years.

Imaging. NECT scans show caudate atrophy with enlarged, outwardly convex frontal horns and variable generalized diffuse atrophy **(31-17)** with or without cerebellar atrophy.

MR shows diffuse volume loss in the frontal lobes with T2/FLAIR hyperintensity in shrunken caudate heads. Putaminal hyperintensity is also common **(31-18)**. MR volumetric studies may demonstrate decreased basal ganglia volumes years before the onset of motor disturbances.

Differential Diagnosis. *Adult* HD mimics include **multiple system atrophy** (MSA), **corticobasal degeneration**, and **frontotemporal lobar dementia**. These disorders are often accompanied by basal ganglia atrophy. Unlike HD, the caudate nuclei are not disproportionately affected.

HUNTINGTON DISEASE

Etiology
- Autosomal dominant, complete penetrance
- CAG trinucleotide repeat disorder

Pathology
- Caudate nuclei, putamina, GP
  - Huntingtin protein nuclear inclusions
  - Neuronal loss, gliosis, iron accumulation

Clinical
- Adult-onset HD (35-45 years): 90%
- Juvenile-onset HD (< 20 years): 10%

Imaging
- Caudate nuclei, putamina T2/FLAIR hyperintense
- Frontal horns outwardly convex

Disorders of Copper Metabolism

Copper homeostasis is a delicate balance that requires both adequate dietary intake and proper excretion. Excess copper is neurotoxic. The most common disorder of copper metabolism—Wilson disease (WD)—has striking CNS manifestations. The major manifestations of WD are found in the basal ganglia, midbrain, and dentate nucleus of the cerebellum.

Wilson Disease

Etiology. WD is an uncommon autosomal recessive disorder of copper trafficking. The mutation causes defective incorporation of copper into ceruloplasmin and impaired biliary copper excretion. There is excessive accumulation of Cu in hepatocytes, which later spills into the circulation. Copper deposition results in oxidative damage primarily to the liver, brain, kidney, skeletal system, and eye **(31-19)**.

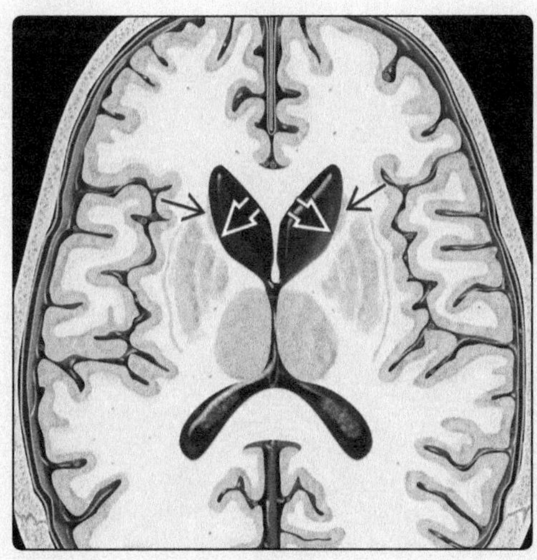

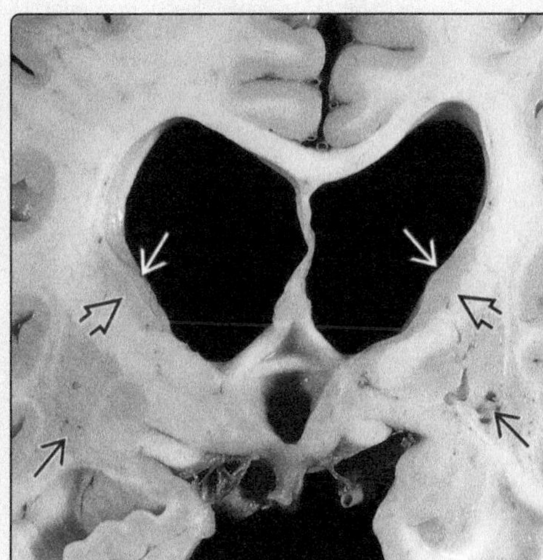

***(31-15)** Axial graphic shows shrunken, atrophic caudate nuclei ⇨ with the outwardly convex frontal horns ➡ that are typical of Huntington disease (HD). **(31-16)** Coronal autopsy of HD shows outwardly convex frontal horns ➡, severely shrunken caudate nuclei ⇨, and atrophic putamina ⇨. (Courtesy R. Hewlett, MD.)*

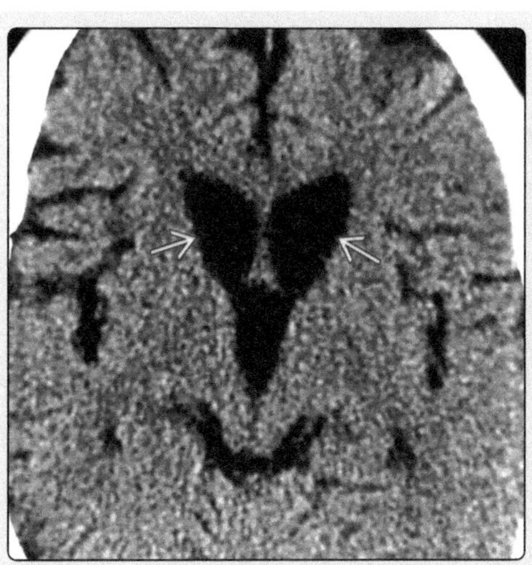

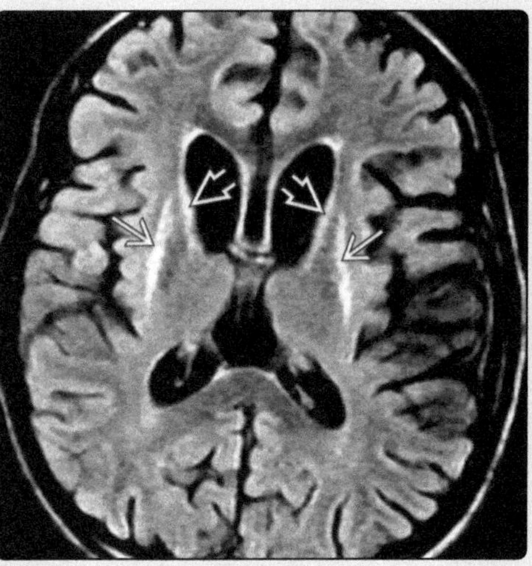

***(31-17)** Axial NECT of a patient with HD shows moderate generalized, severe caudate atrophy seen as outwardly convex frontal horns ➡. (Courtesy M. Huckman, MD.) **(31-18)** Axial FLAIR MR in a patient with HD shows almost nonexistent caudate heads ➡, basal ganglia atrophy, and thinned atrophic hyperintense putamina ➡.*

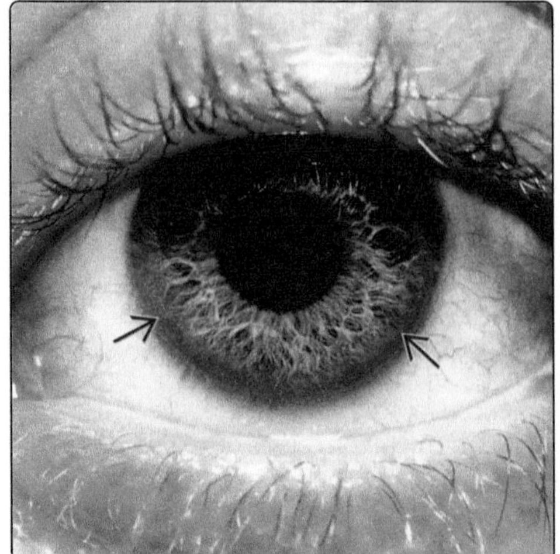

(31-19) Wilson disease (WD) is shown with classic peripheral greenish yellow Kayser-Fleischer ring ➡. (Courtesy AFIP Archives.)

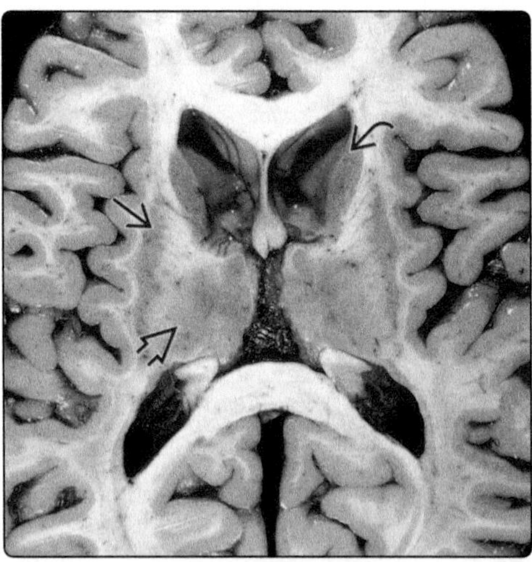

(31-20) Autopsy in WD shows atrophic putamina ➡, caudate ➡, and basal ganglia ➡ characteristic of WD. (Courtesy R. Hewlett, MD.)

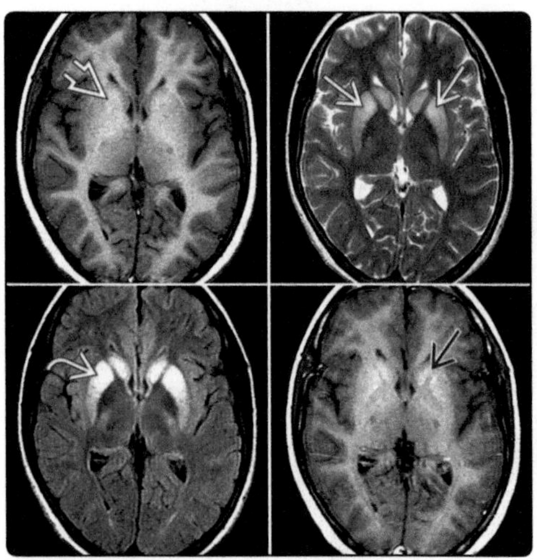

(31-21) Acute WD shows hyperintensity on T1 ➡ and T2 ➡, DWI restriction ➡, and no enhancement ➡. (Courtesy M. Ayadi, MD.)

Pathology. Selective vulnerability of the corpus striatum to mitochondrial dysfunction accounts for the predominant basal ganglia volume loss seen in WD **(31-20)**. Gross pathologic features are nonspecific with ventricular enlargement and widened sulci seen at autopsy in severe cases.

Clinical Issues. WD most commonly affects children and young adults. Symptoms of early-onset WD (8-16 years of age) are usually related to liver failure. Later-onset WD symptoms are primarily neurologic and are generally recognized in the second or third decade. Dysarthria, dystonia, tremors, ataxia, Parkinson-like symptoms, and behavioral disturbances are common. Copper deposition in the cornea causes the characteristic greenish yellow Kayser-Fleischer rings seen on slit-lamp examination **(31-19)**.

WILSON DISEASE

Etiology
- Abnormal copper metabolism
- Autosomal recessive
- *ATP7B* gene mutations

Pathology
- Copper accumulates in hepatocytes, brain, eye
- Mitochondrial dysfunction damages basal ganglia

Clinical Issues
- Childhood WD: Liver disease
- Young adults: Parkinson-like
- Kayser-Fleischer rings

Imaging
- T2/FLAIR hyperintensity
  - Putamina, caudate, thalami, midbrain
- T2* "blooming"

Differential Diagnosis
- Leigh syndrome
- PKAN

Imaging. NECT scans may be normal, especially early in the disease course. Signal intensity on T1WI is variable. Some cases demonstrate T1 shortening similar to that seen in chronic hepatic encephalopathy (see Chapter 32). Basal ganglia T2 signal reflects paramagnetic effects of Cu.

The most common imaging finding of WD on MR is bilaterally symmetric T2/FLAIR hyperintensity (sometimes heterogeneous) in the putamina (70%), caudate nuclei (60%), ventrolateral thalami (55-60%), and midbrain (50%) **(31-21)**. Hyperintensity can sometimes be seen in the pons (20%), medulla (10-15%), and cerebellum (10%). The cerebral (25%) and cerebellar WM (10%) can show focal or diffuse confluent hyperintensities.

In 10-12% of cases, diffuse tegmental (midbrain) hyperintensity with sparing of the red nuclei gives an appearance that has been termed the **"face of a giant panda."**

T2* (GRE, SWI) sequences show blooming in the putamina, caudate nuclei, ventrolateral thalami, and often the dentate nuclei. Contrast enhancement is typically absent. Restricted diffusion in the corpus striatum can be seen in the early stages of WD.

PET shows markedly reduced glucose metabolism and diminished dopa-decarboxylase activity indicative of striatonigral dopaminergic pathway dysfunction.

Differential Diagnosis. The differential diagnoses of WD includes other inherited metabolic disorders that affect the basal ganglia, such as Leigh syndrome, NBIAs, the organic acidurias, and Japanese encephalitis (JE). **Leigh syndrome** (subacute necrotizing encephalomyelopathy) shows bilateral, symmetric, spongiform, and hyperintense lesions, particularly in the *putamen* and brainstem. The WM is often affected in Leigh syndrome, whereas the caudate and thalamus are less commonly involved. MRS demonstrates elevated lactate levels in the basal ganglia.

PKAN can also resemble WD. WD predominantly affects the putamina and caudate nuclei rather than the medial GP and lacks the "eye of the tiger" sign often seen in PKAN.

Disorders Affecting Both Gray and White Matter

In the last section of this chapter, we discuss inherited metabolic disorders (IMDs) that affect *both* GM and WM.

Mucopolysaccharidoses

Terminology and Etiology

The mucopolysaccharidoses (MPSs) are lysosomal storage disorders characterized by incomplete degradation and progressive accumulation of toxic glycosaminoglycan (GAG) in various organs. In the brain, this accumulation includes GAG deposits in the perivascular spaces (PVSs), leptomeninges, and craniocervical junction ligamentous structures.

The MPSs have a classification of 1-9. Each has a specific enzyme deficiency and gene defect that leads to the inability to break down GAG. For example, MPS 1H (Hurler) has an α-L-iduronidase (4p16.3) deficiency while MPS 2 (Hunter disease) is characterized by iduronate 2-sulfatase deficiency (Xq28).

Pathology

The two distinctive gross features of the MPSs are thickened meninges and dilated PVSs packed with undegraded GAG **(31-23)**. The enlarged PVSs give a cribriform appearance to the brain on both pathology and imaging **(31-22)**.

Clinical Issues

Each MPS subtype has different clinical phenotypes. Age at presentation varies, as do sex predilection and prognosis based on the inherited MPS type.

Hurler (MPS 1H) and Hunter (MPS 2) diseases are two of the most common "prototypical" MPSs. Hurler patients appear normal at birth but soon develop CNS symptoms, including delayed development and mental retardation. Untreated Hurler disease typically results in death by age 10.

MPS 2 (Hunter disease) is an X-linked disorder and is seen only in male patients. Hunter disease is characterized by progressive multisystem involvement in the CNS, joints, bones, heart, skin, liver, eyes, and other organs. Patients often survive into their mid teens but usually expire from cardiac disease.

Imaging

The prototypical imaging findings in MPSs are illustrated by Hurler (MPS 1H) and Hunter (MPS 2) diseases.

Macrocephaly. NECT and MR scans show an enlarged head, often with metopic "beaking" and scaphocephalic configuration. Sagittal MR scans also

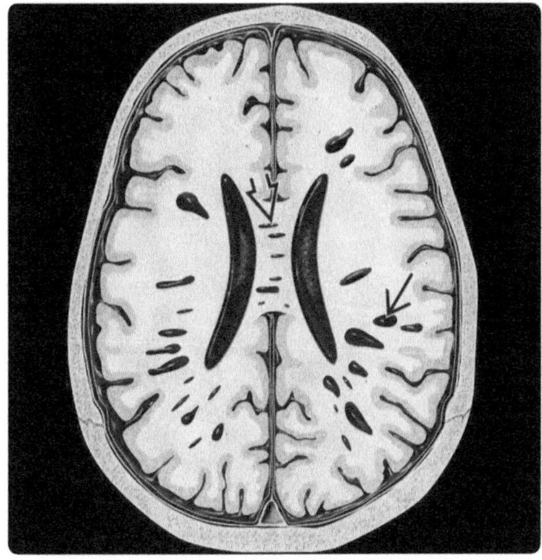

(31-22) MPS with dilated PVSs ➙ is radially oriented in the WM. Posterior predominance and involvement of the corpus callosum ➙ are seen.

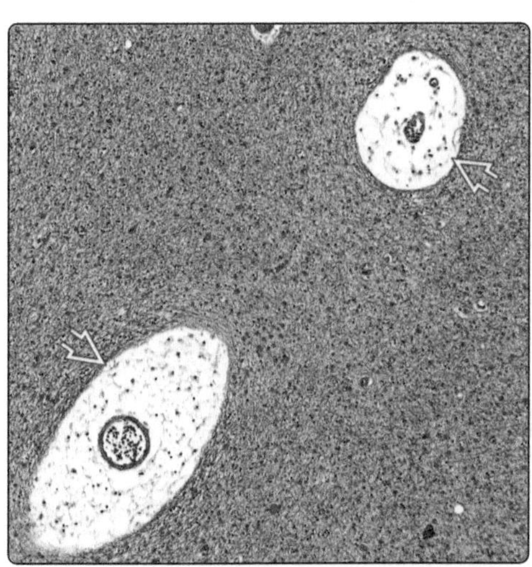

(31-23) MPS 1HS (Hurler-Scheie) myelin stain shows large PVSs ➙ packed with undegraded mucopolysaccharides. (Courtesy P. Shannon, MD.)

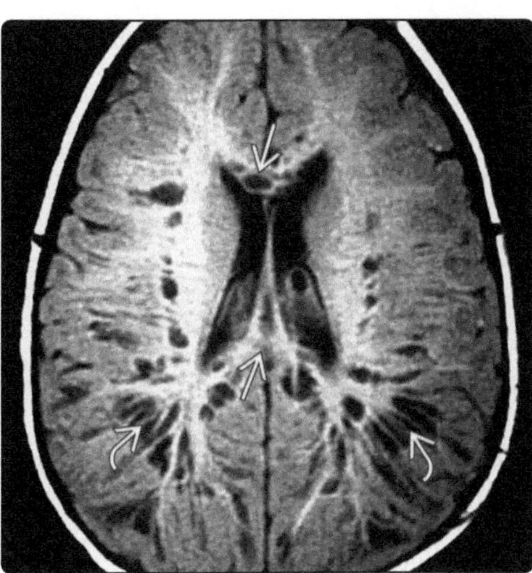

(31-24) T1 MR in a toddler with MPS 1H (Hurler disease) shows markedly enlarged WM ➙ PVSs, including the corpus callosum ➙.

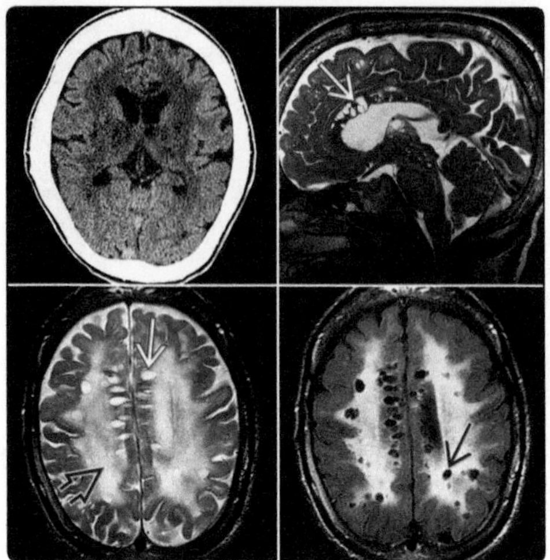

(31-25) *MPS 2 (Hunter) shows enlarged PVSs in corpus callosum, confluent WM disease. PVSs suppress on FLAIR; WM disease does not.*

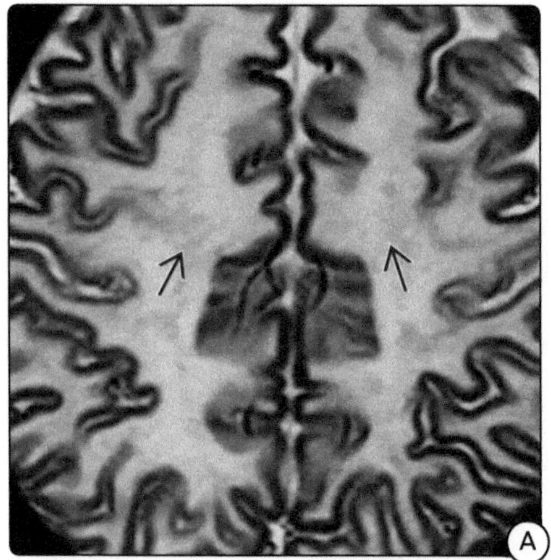

(31-26A) *T2 MR through corona radiata in 2y boy with Canavan disease shows hyperintense WM, virtually complete absence of myelination.*

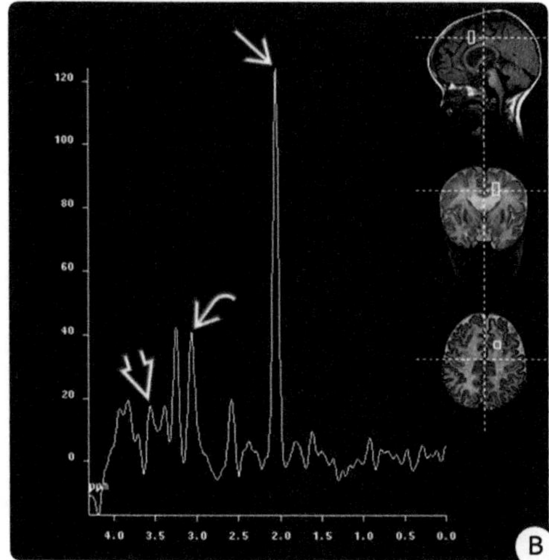

(31-26B) *MRS with TE = 135 ms shows elevated NAA peak at 2.0 ppm. Cr is significantly reduced. A small myoinositol peak is present.*

demonstrate a large head with craniofacial disproportion. Pannus of ligaments at craniocervical junction can be seen.

Enlarged Perivascular Spaces and WM Abnormalities. A striking sieve-like cribriform appearance in the posterior cerebral WM and corpus callosum is characteristic and caused by numerous dilated PVSs **(31-24) (31-25)**. Although sometimes called "Hurler holes," these enlarged PVSs are typical of both Hurler and Hunter diseases. They are much less common in the other MPSs.

T2 scans show CSF-like hyperintensity in the enlarged PVSs. The PVSs themselves suppress completely on FLAIR. The enlarged PVSs do not "bloom" on T2* and do not enhance following contrast administration.

Pachymeningopathy. The meninges, especially around the craniovertebral junction, are often thickened and appear very hypointense on T2-weighted images. In severe cases, the thickened meninges can compress the medulla or upper cervical cord. Odontoid dysplasia and a short C1 posterior arch—common in the MPSs—can exacerbate the craniovertebral junction stenosis, causing progressive myelopathy.

Differential Diagnosis

The differential diagnosis of MPS is limited. **Prominent PVSs** can be normal findings in patients of any age but are more common in middle-aged and older patients. No macrocephaly is present with this normal variant.

Canavan Disease (CD)

Canavan disease is a fatal autosomal recessive neurodegenerative disorder and the only identified genetic disorder caused by a defect in a metabolite—*N*-acetyl-L-aspartate (NAA)—that is produced exclusively in the brain. Mutations in the *ASPA* gene, located on the long arm of chromosome 17, cause abnormal NAA accumulation in the brain and result in CD.

Pathology

The brain in CD appears grossly swollen. Microscopic analysis shows spongiform WM degeneration with swollen astrocytes in the globi pallidi and thalami.

Clinical Issues

Three clinical variants of CD are recognized. The *congenital form* presents within the first few days of life and leads to profound hypotonia with poor head control. Death rapidly ensues. The most common form by far is *infantile CD*. Infantile CD presents between 3 and 6 months and is characterized by hypotonia, macrocephaly, and seizures. Death between 1 and 2 years is typical. *Juvenile-onset CD* begins between 4 and 5 years of age and is the most slowly progressive form.

Imaging

NECT shows a large head with diffuse WM hypoattenuation in the cerebral hemispheres and cerebellum. The globi pallidi also appear hypoattenuating.

MR eventually shows virtually complete absence of myelination with confluent T2/FLAIR hyperintensity throughout the WM and globi pallidi. The gyri may appear swollen and the subcortical U-fibers are involved early in the disease course **(31-26A)**. As the disease progresses, widespread volume loss with ventricular and sulcal enlargement ensues.

DWI reveals bright DWI signal with normal to reduced ADC values in the involved areas. CD does not enhance.

MRS is the key to the definitive imaging diagnosis of CD. Markedly elevated NAA is seen in virtually all cases **(31-26)**. Cr is reduced. An elevated myoinositol peak is sometimes present. The choline:creatine (Ch:Cr) ratio is reduced.

Differential Diagnosis

The major differential diagnosis of CD is **Alexander disease**. Both CD and Alexander disease cause macrocephaly, but an elevated NAA peak on MRS and enhancement on T1 C+ distinguish the two disorders.

Megalencephaly with leukoencephalopathy and cysts involves the subcortical arcuate fibers, as does CD; however, the basal ganglia are not affected. **Pelizaeus-Merzbacher disease** demonstrates virtually complete lack of myelination but does not cause macrocephaly and does not affect the basal ganglia.

Alexander Disease (AxD)

Etiology

More than 95% of AxD patients have de novo heterozygous dominant mutations in the *GFAP* gene (17q21). *GFAP* encodes for glial fibrillary acidic protein, a protein that is expressed only in astrocytes. *GFAP* mutations cause accumulation of mutant GFAP aggregates, which begins during fetal development.

Pathology

The brains of infants with AxD have markedly increased astrocytic density and are grossly enlarged. Dramatic myelin loss makes the WM—especially in the frontal lobes—appear very pale. In severe cases, the WM appears partially or almost entirely cystic. In contrast to CD, the subcortical arcuate fibers are relatively spared.

The hallmark histopathologic feature of AxD is the presence of enormous numbers of Rosenthal fibers (RFs) in astrocytes. The striking lack of nearly all myelin in AxD is considered a secondary phenomenon that arises from severely disrupted astrocyte-derived myelination signaling.

Clinical Issues

Three clinical forms are recognized: Infantile, juvenile, and adult. In the infantile form, which is the most common, patients younger than 2 years old present with megalencephaly, progressive psychomotor retardation, and seizures. Spasticity and eventually quadriplegia often develop. All forms eventually lead to death. Care is supportive.

Imaging

NECT scans of infants with AxD show a large head with symmetric WM hypoattenuation in the frontal lobes that extends posteriorly into the caudate nuclei and internal/external capsules. Intense bifrontal periventricular enhancement can be seen on CECT scans early in the disease course.

MR shows macrocephaly, T1 hypointensity, and T2/FLAIR hyperintensity involving the frontal WM, caudate nuclei, and anterior putamina. Although infantile AxD involves the subcortical U-fibers early in the disease course, the periventricular WM is more severely affected in the juvenile and adults forms **(31-27)**. A classic finding is a T1-hyperintense, T2-hypointense rim around the frontal horns. FLAIR scans may demonstrate cystic encephalomalacia in the frontal WM in more severe, protracted cases.

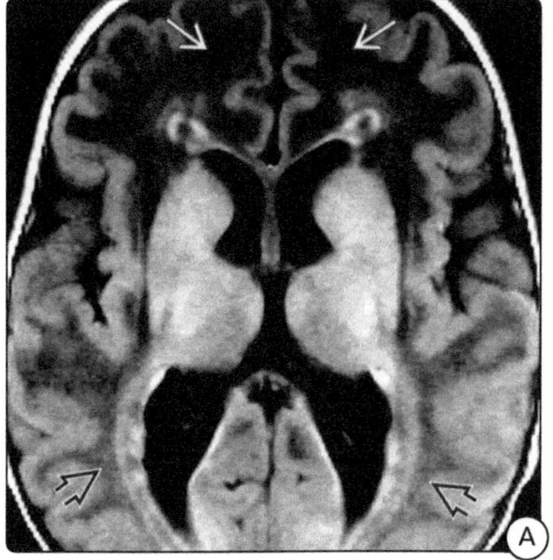

***(31-27A)** T1 MR in 6m boy with AxD shows exceptionally hypointense frontal WM ➡ with more normal-appearing parietooccipital WM ⇨.*

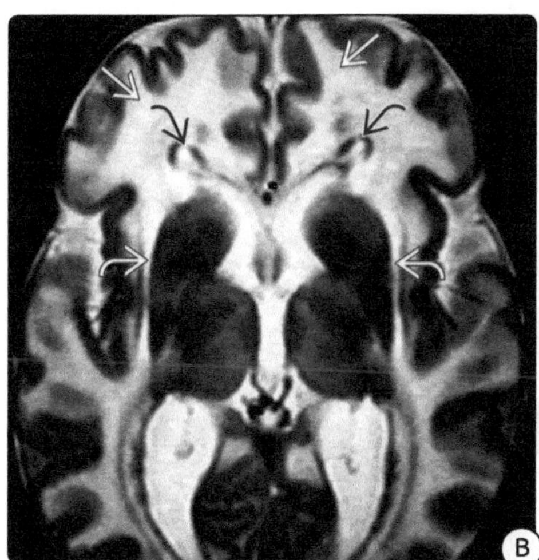

***(31-27B)** T2 MR shows hyperintense frontal WM ➡, external capsule ↪. Hypointense rim around the frontal horns ↪ is characteristic.*

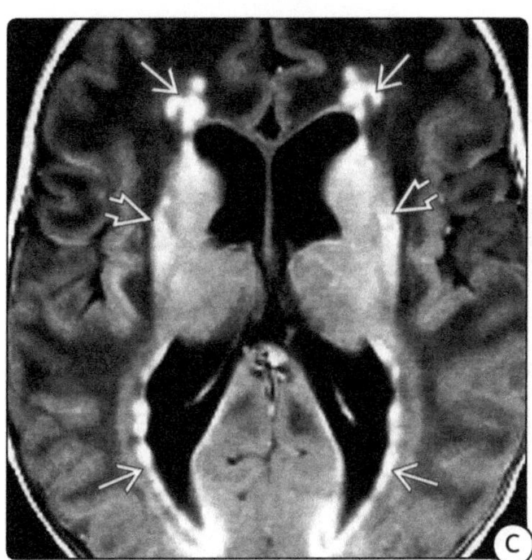

***(31-27C)** Axial T1 C+ MR shows enhancement in the periventricular WM ➡ and basal ganglia ⇨.*

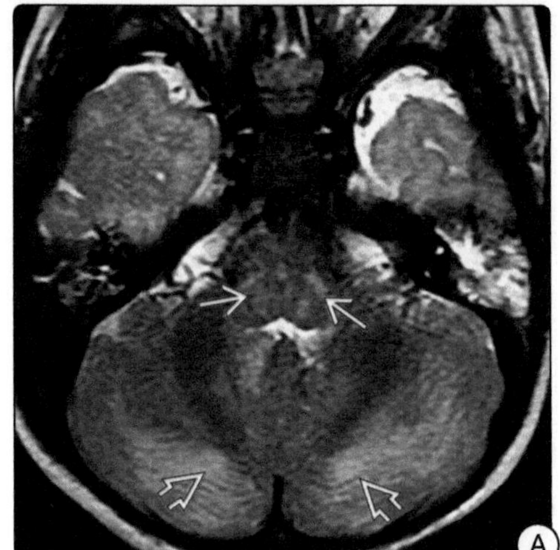

***(31-28A)** T2 MR in Leigh syndrome shows symmetric hyperintensities in the white matter of both cerebellar hemispheres ➩ and medulla ➩.*

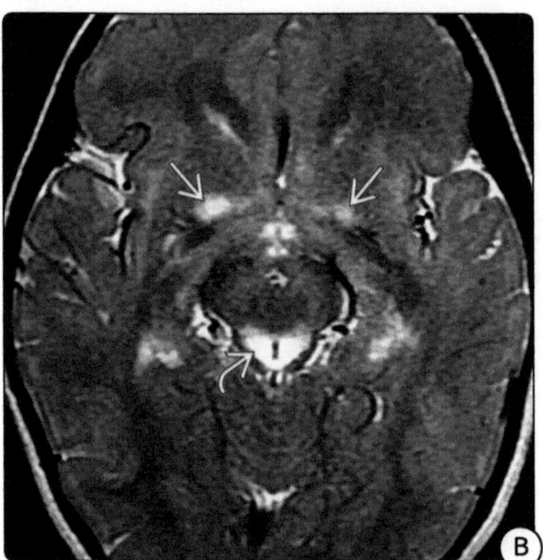

***(31-28B)** More cephalad T2 MR shows striking hyperintensity in the periaqueductal gray matter ➩. Note the globi pallidi hyperintensities ➩.*

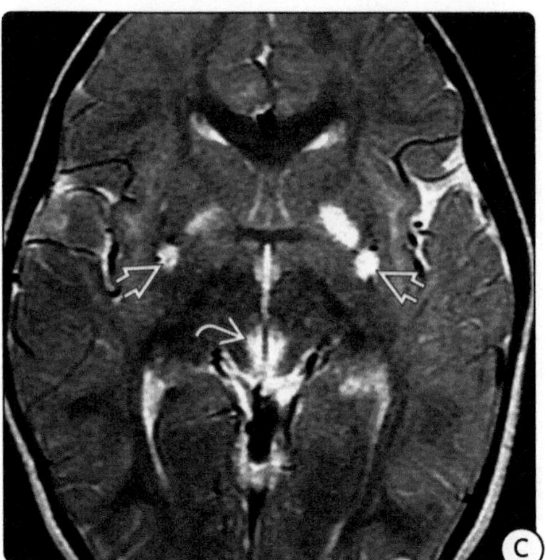

***(31-28C)** Axial T2 MR in the same patient shows symmetric hyperintensity in the upper midbrain ➩ and basal ganglia ➩.*

A unique finding in AxD is enlargement of the caudate heads and fornices, which appear swollen and hyperintense. The thalami, globi pallidi, brainstem, and cerebellum are less commonly affected.

AxD is one of the few IMDs that demonstrates enhancement on T1 C+. Rims of intense enhancement can be seen around the surfaces of the swollen caudate nuclei and affected frontal lobe WM **(31-27C)**. In the juvenile and adult forms, brainstem and cerebellar involvement can be striking and may even mimic a neoplasm.

Differential Diagnosis

The major differential diagnoses of AxD are other inherited leukodystrophies with macrocephaly. These primarily include **Canavan disease (CD)** and the **mucopolysaccharidoses**. Although both AxD and CD show almost complete lack of myelination with T2/FLAIR WM hyperintensity, the predilection of AxD for the frontal lobes, caudate heads, and enhancement help distinguish it from CD.

The mucopolysaccharidoses, especially Hurler and Hunter diseases, display a striking "cribriform" appearance of the WM and corpus callosum caused by enlarged perivascular spaces. Deep gray involvement is absent, and the lesions do not enhance. Dural thickening is also absent in AxD.

DIFFERENTIAL DIAGNOSIS: CHILD WITH A LARGE HEAD

Common

- Normal variant
- Benign familial macrocrania
- Benign macrocrania of infancy

Less Common

- Nonaccidental trauma with subdural hematomas

Rare but Important

- Inherited metabolic disorder
  - Canavan disease
  - Alexander disease
  - Mucopolysaccharidoses
  - Megalencephaly with leukoencephalopathy and cysts
  - Glutaric aciduria type 1

Mitochondrial Diseases (Respiratory Chain Disorders)

The mitochondria are cellular organelles that are the "power plants" responsible for energy production. Mitochondrial disorders are caused by mitochondrial DNA (mtDNA) mutations and are among the most common of all IMDs. Although virtually every organ or tissue of the body can be affected, the nervous system and skeletal muscle are especially vulnerable because of their high energy demands.

Four major encephalomyopathic syndromes have been described: *Leigh syndrome*, *Kearns-Sayre syndrome*, *MELAS*, and *MERRF*. Two other less common disorders, glutaric aciduria types 1 and 2, are also caused by mtDNA-mediated enzyme abnormalities.

Mitochondrial disorders have significant clinical and imaging overlap and are challenging to distinguish from each other. We focus on Leigh syndrome, MELAS, and type 1 glutaric aciduria.

Leigh Syndrome

Terminology and Pathology. Leigh syndrome (LS) is also known as subacute necrotizing encephalopathy. LS demonstrates brownish gray gelatinous or cavitary foci within the basal ganglia, brainstem, dentate nuclei, thalami, and spinal cord with variable WM spongiform degeneration and demyelination.

Clinical Issues. Clinical manifestations of LS are variable. Most patients with LS present in infancy or childhood with failure to thrive, central hypotonia, developmental regression, ataxia, bulbar dysfunction, and ophthalmoplegia. Serum &/or CSF lactate levels are increased.

Imaging. MR in LS shows bilaterally symmetric areas of T2/FLAIR hyperintensity (often *speckled*) in the basal ganglia **(31-28)**. The putamina (especially the posterior segments) are consistently affected, as are the caudate heads. The dorsomedial thalami can also be involved, whereas the globi pallidi are less commonly affected. Acute lesions show swelling of the basal ganglia.

Mid and lower brainstem (pons/medulla) lesions are typical in LS and, in a few cases, can be the *only* finding. Symmetric lesions in the cerebral peduncles are common, and the periaqueductal GM is frequently affected. Brainstem lesions are especially common in cytochrome-C oxidase deficiency.

Acute lesions restrict on DWI but do not enhance. MRS of the brain and CSF typically shows a lactate doublet at 1.3 ppm. Lactate resonates above baseline at short (35 ms) and long (288 ms) TEs and inverts at an intermediate TE (144 ms).

Differential Diagnosis. As their imaging findings often overlap, the differential diagnosis of LS includes the other mitochondrial encephalomyopathies. **MELAS** typically shows stroke-like abnormalities in the cortical GM in a nonvascular distribution in the hemispheres, peripheral in location and often crossing vascular territories and sparing underlying WM.

MELAS

Terminology and Etiology. Mitochondrial **e**ncephalomyopathy with **l**actic **a**cidosis and **s**troke-like episodes (MELAS) is caused by several different point mitochondrial tRNA mutations.

Clinical Issues. MELAS is an uncommon but important cause of childhood stroke. The diagnosis of MELAS should always be considered when encountering a child or young adult with atypical stroke and encephalitis presenting with seizures.

The clinical triad of lactic acidosis, seizures, and stroke-like episodes is the classic presentation. Other common symptoms include progressive sensorineural hearing loss, migraines, episodic vomiting, alternating hemiplegia, and progressive brain injury. Cardiac abnormalities, renal dysfunction, GI motility disorders, and generalized muscle weakness are also common.

Mean age at symptom onset is 15 years, although some patients may not become symptomatic until 40-50 years of age.

Imaging. Imaging findings vary with disease acuity **(31-29)**. *Acute* MELAS often shows swollen T2-/FLAIR-hyperintense gyri. The underlying WM is normal, and the cortical abnormalities cross arterial territories, distinguishing MELAS from acute cerebral infarction **(31-30)**. The parietal and occipital lobes are most commonly affected **(31-30B)**.

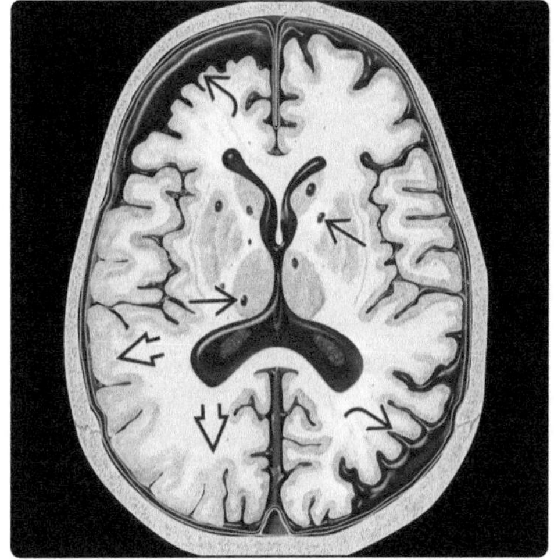

***(31-29)** MELAS with acute gyral edema crossing vascular territories ⇨ spares underlying WM. Old lacunar infarcts ➡, cortical atrophy ⇨.*

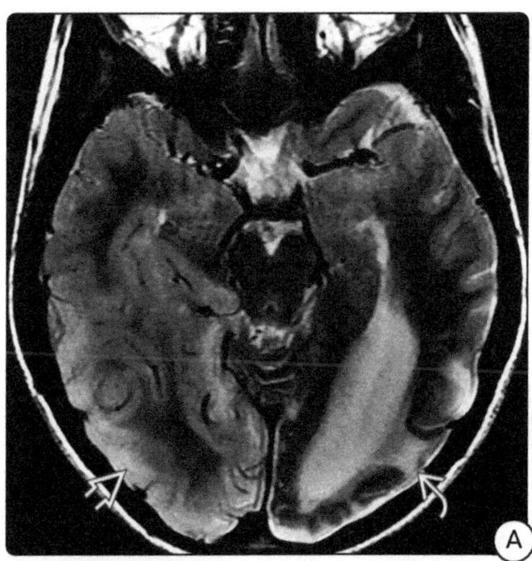

***(31-30A)** T2 MR in 10y girl with MELAS shows old left parietooccipital infarct ⇨, acute right gyral swelling ⇨ that spares underlying WM.*

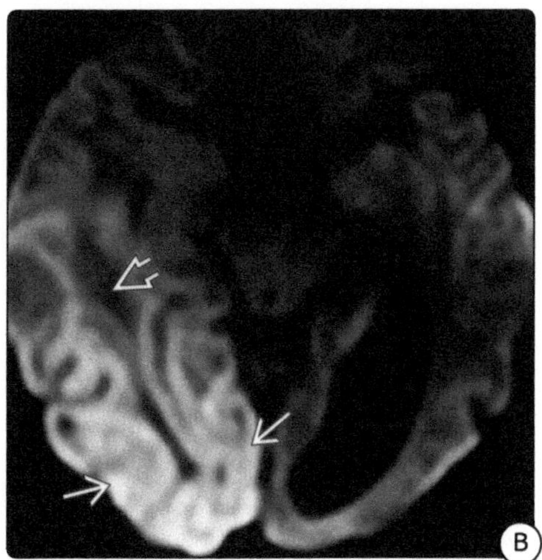

***(31-30B)** DWI MR shows restricted diffusion ➡ in acutely swollen edematous cortex spares the underlying WM ⇨. Lactate on MRS is not shown.*

The appearance of *strokes of differing ages* is often a clue to the diagnosis of MELAS. Gyral enhancement on T1 C+ is typical. MRA in MELAS shows no evidence of major vessel occlusion.

Chronic MELAS shows multifocal lacunar-type infarcts, symmetric basal ganglia calcifications, WM volume loss, and progressive atrophy of the parietooccipital cortex.

MRS is extremely helpful in the diagnosis of most mitochondrial encephalopathies. Nearly 2/3 of cases with MELAS show a prominent lactate "doublet" at 1.3 ppm in otherwise normal-appearing brain. **Caution**: 1/3 of cases show no evidence for elevated lactate levels in the brain parenchyma but may demonstrate a lactate peak in the ventricular CSF.

Differential Diagnosis. The differential diagnosis of acute MELAS includes territorial **arterial infarction**. MELAS spares the subcortical and deep WM and *crosses vascular distributions* (often the middle and posterior cerebral territories). **Prolonged seizures** can cause gyral swelling, hyperintensity, and enhancement that appears identical to MELAS. MRS shows no evidence of elevated lactate levels in the CSF and normal-appearing brain.

LS often involves the brainstem, which is less commonly involved in MELAS. **MERRF** shows a propensity to involve the basal ganglia, caudate nuclei, and vascular watershed zones.

Glutaric Aciduria Type 1

Etiology and Pathology. Glutaric aciduria type 1 (GA1) is an autosomal recessive IMD caused by deficiency of the mitochondrial enzyme, *GCDH*. The accumulation of excess glutaric acid is neurotoxic. Cells in the basal ganglia and WM are especially vulnerable. Spongiform changes with neuronal loss, myelin splitting and vacuolation, and intramyelinic fluid accumulation are typical pathologic features of GA1.

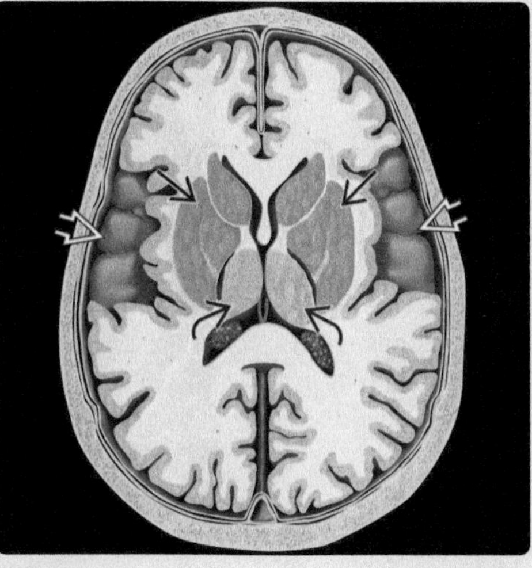

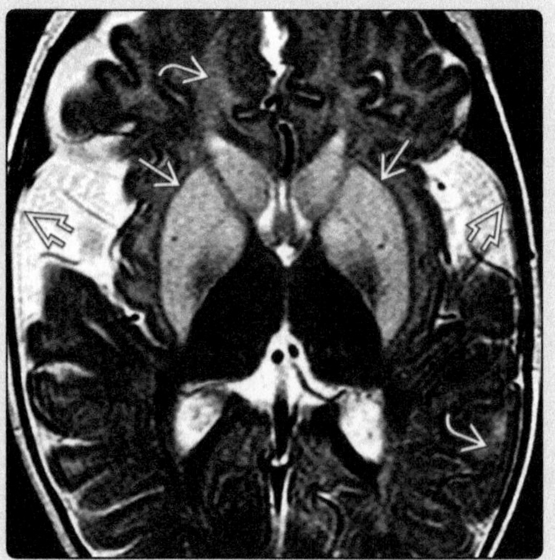

***(31-31)** Graphic depicts typical findings of GA type 1. Note the symmetrically enlarged ➡ basal ganglia and the bilateral "open" sylvian or lateral cerebral fissures ➡. The thalami ➡ appear normal. **(31-32)** Axial T2 MR in a 7m child with GA1 shows enlarged, hyperintense caudate nuclei, putamina, and globi pallidi ➡ with thalamic sparing. The sylvian fissures ➡ are enlarged. The hemispheric WM myelination ➡ is grossly delayed.*

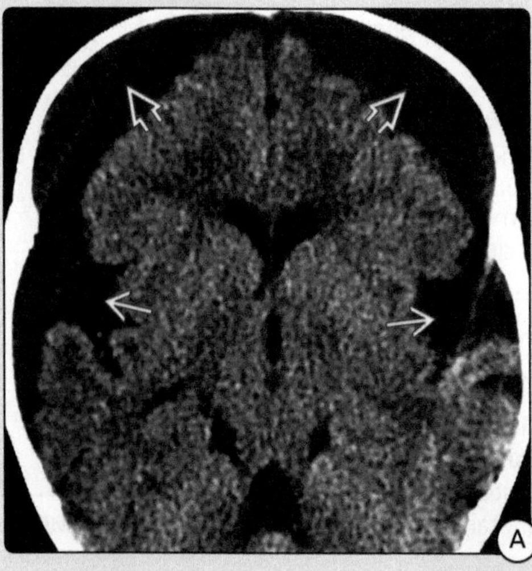

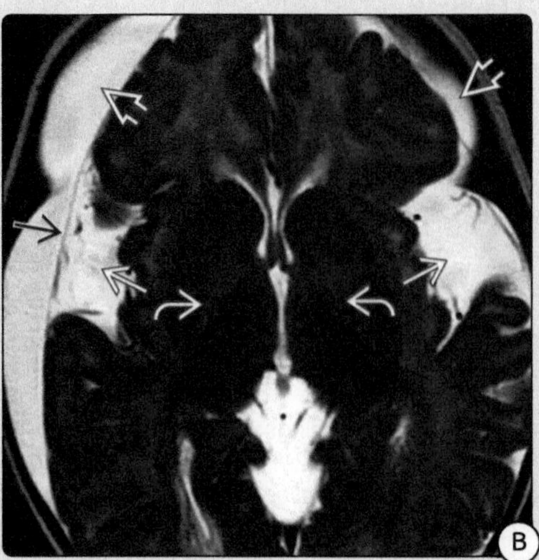

***(31-33A)** NECT of GA1 in a 7m infant with a large head and delayed development shows "open" sylvian (lateral cerebral) fissures ➡ and large bifrontal hypoattenuating chronic subdural hematomas (cSDH) ➡. **(31-33B)** Axial T2 MR in the same patient shows the "open" sylvian fissures ➡, membrane-bound ➡ subdural fluid collections ➡, and significantly delayed myelination for a child 7 months of age. GP shows T2 hyperintensity ➡.*

Clinical Issues. The majority of infants with GA1 exhibit macrocephaly at birth. More than 85% of GA1 patients present during the first year of life, usually with acute encephalopathy, seizures, dystonia, choreoathetosis, vomiting, &/or opisthotonus. These episodic crises are often triggered by febrile illness or immunization. Patients may also develop an acute Reye-like encephalopathy with ketoacidosis and vomiting.

Imaging. The three "signature" imaging findings of classic GA1 are (1) macrocrania, (2) bilateral widened ("open") lateral cerebral (sylvian) fissures, and (3) bilaterally symmetric basal ganglia lesions **(31-31)**. Severe GA1 may also cause diffuse hemispheric WM abnormalities (i.e., central and periventricular).

GA1 infants in metabolic crisis often present with acute striatal necrosis. Bilateral diffusely swollen basal ganglia that are T2/FLAIR hyperintense **(31-32)** and that restrict on DWI are typical.

Chronic GA1 causes enlarged CSF spaces and cerebral atrophy. Volume loss leads to tearing of cortical dural bridging veins, resulting in recurrent subdural hematomas **(31-33)**.

GA1 does not enhance on T1 C+ scans. DWI in the acute phase or during crises shows restricted diffusion within the globi pallidi. MRS is nonspecific.

Differential Diagnosis. The major differential diagnosis of GA1 is **subdural hemorrhage** in **abusive head trauma**. However, GA1 is not associated with fractures, exhibits basal ganglia lesions, and the associated subdural hematomas do not occur in the absence of enlarged CSF spaces.

Urea Cycle/Ammonia Disorders

Urea cycle disorders result in elevated serum ammonia, which readily crosses the blood-brain barrier and causes diffuse cerebral edema. The two most common disorders are ornithine transcarbamylase deficiency (**OTCD**) and **citrullinemia**.

Both OTCD and citrullinemia are characterized by diffuse brain swelling. MR shows basal ganglia and cortical swelling with T2/FLAIR hyperintensity. The periinsular cortex is usually affected first (cortical T2/FLAIR hyperintensity and restricted diffusion) **(31-34)**. Involvement progresses into the frontal, parietal, temporal, and (finally) the occipital lobes. The globi pallidi, putamina, and thalami are affected with prolonged hyperammonemia and may show restricted diffusion.

The major imaging differential diagnosis of acute hyperammonemia is **hypoxic-ischemic encephalopathy** (HIE). Infants with HIE typically have more thalamic and perirolandic cortical abnormalities.

Fabry Disease

Fabry disease is a rare but important cause of strokes in young children and adult men with cryptogenic stroke.

Etiology and Pathology

Fabry disease is an X-linked lysosomal storage disorder of glycosphingolipid metabolism. Mutation in α-galactosidase leads to glycosphingolipid deposition in the vascular endothelium and smooth muscle cells. Impaired endothelial function results in progressive multisystem vasculopathy. The renal, cardiac, and cerebral vessels are severely affected. Cardiac emboli, large vessel arteriopathy, and microvascular disease all occur.

Clinical Issues

Late-onset Fabry disease is difficult to diagnose. Although mean onset of first stroke is 39 years in men and 45 years in women, nearly 22% of patients are younger than 30 years at initial presentation. Over 85% of strokes in Fabry disease are ischemic strokes. Hemorrhagic strokes are less common and usually occur secondary to renovascular hypertension.

Imaging

NECT scans show bilateral, often symmetric calcifications in the basal ganglia and thalami **(31-35A)**. Multifocal deep WM hypodensities consistent with lacunar infarcts can be identified in some cases. Patients with long-standing Fabry disease show volume loss with enlarged ventricles and sulci.

MR may show T1 shortening in the basal ganglia and posterior thalami ("pulvinar" sign) **(31-35B)**, a rare but typical finding of Fabry disease. Between 45% and 50% of adult patients with Fabry disease have patchy multifocal T2/FLAIR hyperintensities in the basal ganglia, thalami, and cerebral WM **(31-36)**. 10% demonstrate "blooming" hypointensities on T2* (GRE, SWI) due to microbleeds.

Differential Diagnosis

Other disorders marked by basal ganglia calcifications include **Fahr disease**, which causes bilateral, dense, thick calcifications in the basal ganglia and thalami. The cerebellum and GM-WM interfaces are usually not involved in Fabry disease. Hyperparathyroidism, hypoparathyroidism, and hypothyroidism may have similar calcifications but lack the multifocal infarcts typical of Fabry disease. A pulvinar sign can be seen in variant Creutzfeldt-Jakob disease.

Selected References: The complete reference list is available on the Expert Consult™ eBook version included with purchase.

(31-34A) Axial T2 MR in a patient with ornithine OTCD shows BG ➲ and cortical hyperintensity, most striking in the periinsular and frontal cortices ➔. Note that the occipital lobes ➲ are relatively spared. (31-34B) Axial DWI MR in the same patient shows diffusion hyperintensity in the periinsular and frontal cortices ➔ and left thalamus with less striking involvement of the corpus callosum ➲. The occipital lobes ➲ show no evidence of restricted diffusion.

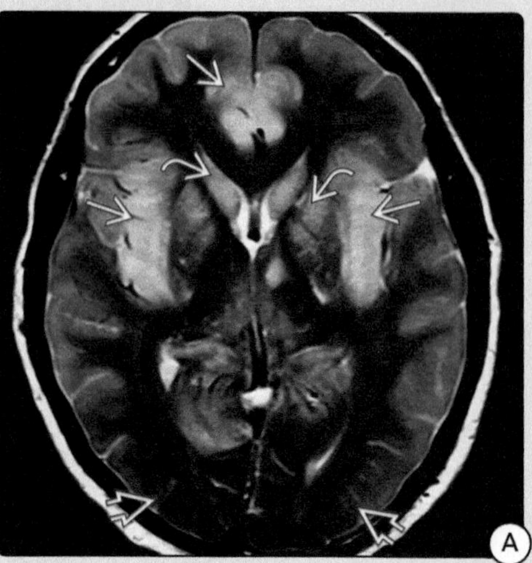

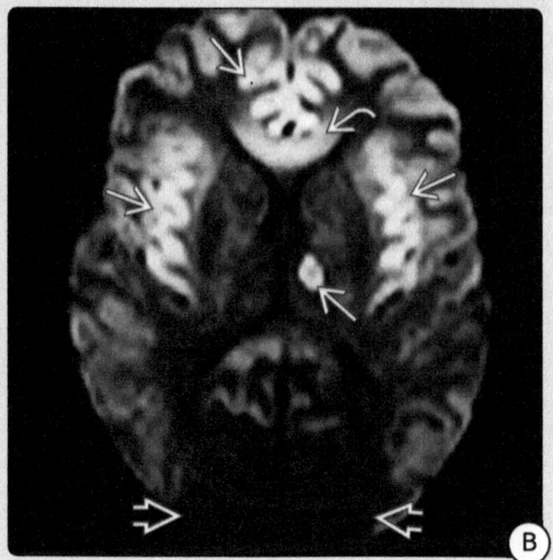

(31-35A) NECT in a patient with Fabry disease shows symmetric calcifications in the basal ganglia ➔, posterior thalami (pulvinars) ➲. (31-35B) T1 MR in the same case shows symmetric T1 shortening in the basal ganglia ➔. The T1 shortening in the pulvinars of both thalami ➲ is particularly striking.

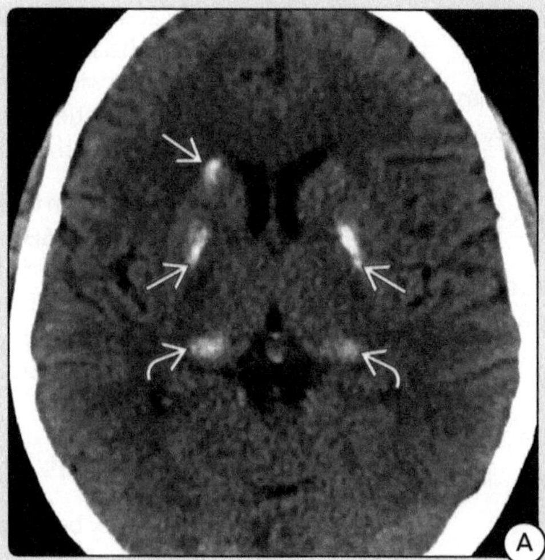

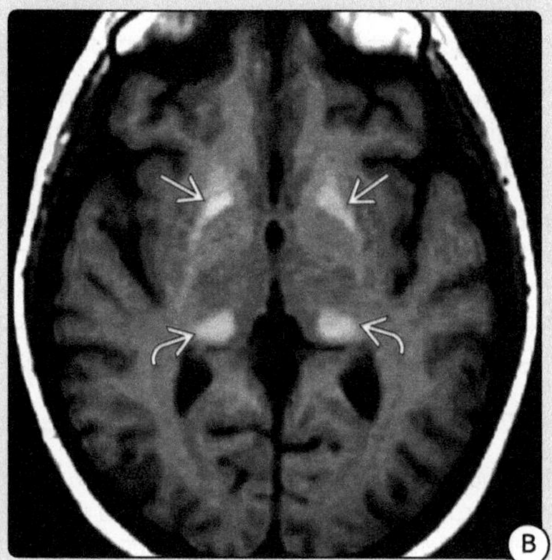

(31-36A) T2 MR in a 50-year-old man with multiple cryptogenic lacunar infarcts shows hyperintense foci in the basal ganglia ➔, thalami ➲, and deep periventricular WM ➲. (31-36B) More cephalad T2 MR in the same case shows multiple subcortical ➲, deep periventricular ➔ lacunar infarcts. This is Fabry disease.

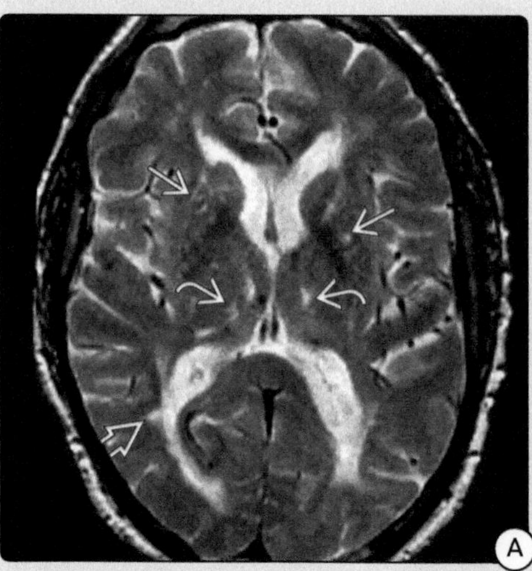

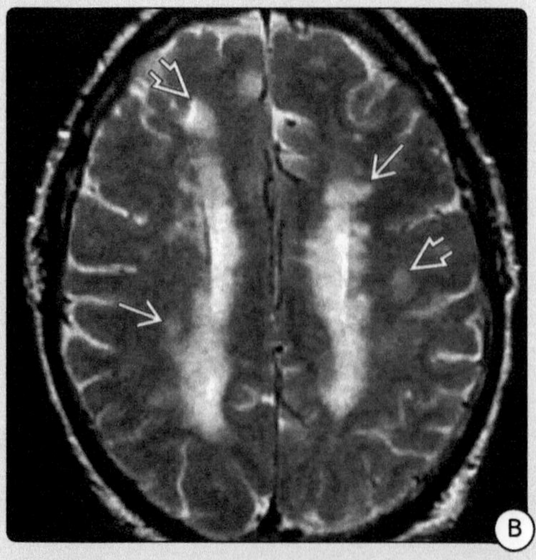

Acquired Metabolic and Systemic Disorders

In this chapter, we focus on acquired metabolic and systemic disorders that involve the CNS. We begin with the most common—hypertension—before turning our attention to abnormalities of glucose metabolism and thyroid/parathyroid function.

We then discuss seizure disorders, as sustained ictal activity with hypermetabolism can have profound effects on the brain. We finish the section by exploring cytotoxic corpus callosum injury and transient global amnesia.

We close with miscellaneous but important acquired metabolic diseases, such as hepatic encephalopathy (both acute and chronic) and the osmotic demyelination syndromes.

Hypertensive Encephalopathies

If not recognized and treated, the effects of both acutely elevated blood pressure and chronic hypertension (HTN) on the brain can be devastating. We begin this section with a discussion of acute hypertensive encephalopathy, then delve into the CNS damage caused by chronic HTN.

Acute Hypertensive Encephalopathy

Terminology

The most common manifestation of acute hypertensive encephalopathy is **p**osterior **r**eversible **e**ncephalopathy **s**yndrome (**PRES**). Despite the syndrome's name, lesions are rarely limited to the "posterior" (parietooccipital) aspects of the brain, and atypical is more common than "classic" PRES.

Etiology

General Concepts. The pathogenesis of PRES is not yet completely understood. The most common explanation is that severe HTN leads to failed cerebral autoregulation and breakthrough hyperperfusion with *vasodilatation*. However, between 15-20% of patients with PRES are normotensive or even hypotensive, whereas < 1/2 have a mean arterial pressure above 140-150 mm Hg.

Alternative theories for the development of PRES invoke vasculopathy with vascular endothelial injury and dysfunction.

Associated Conditions. PRES is associated with a multitude of diverse clinical entities, the most common of which are **eclampsia**, **HTN**, and **immunosuppressive treatment**.

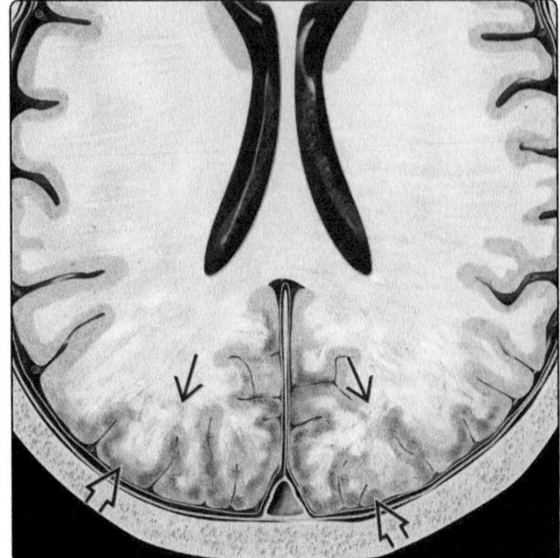

(32-1) PRES with cortical/subcortical vasogenic edema ➡ in the posterior circulation with some petechial hemorrhage ⇨ is shown.

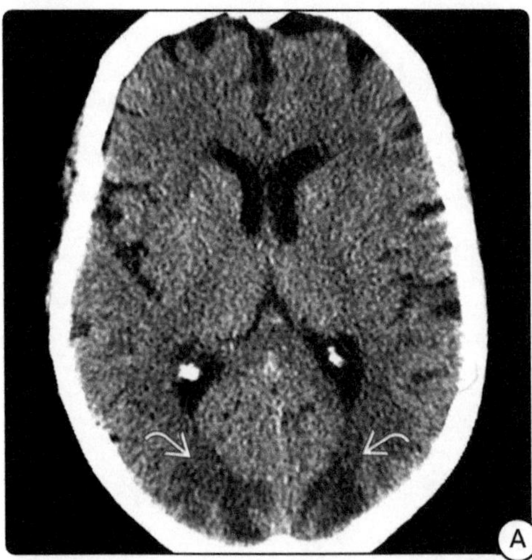

(32-2A) NECT in severe hypertension shows bioccipital hypodensities in the subcortical white matter ➡.

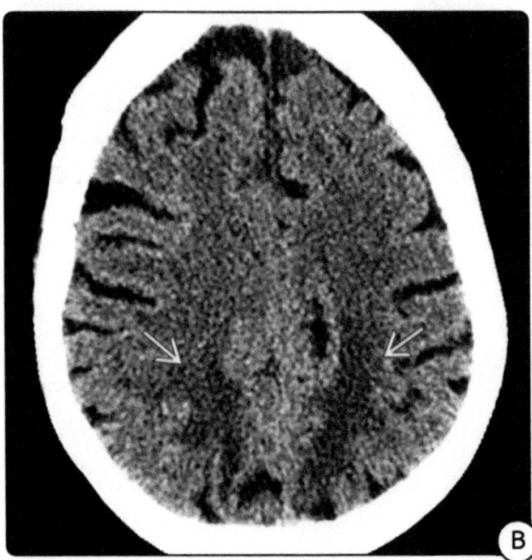

(32-2B) More cephalad NECT shows symmetric hypodensity in the posterior parietal and high occipital white matter ➡. This is classic PRES.

Other conditions associated with PRES include renal failure with hemolytic-uremic syndrome (HUS), thrombotic thrombocytopenic purpura (TTP), autoimmune disorders (e.g., lupus nephropathy and acute glomerulonephritis), shock/sepsis syndrome, postcarotid endarterectomy with reperfusion syndrome, endocrine disorders, stimulant drugs, such as ephedrine and pseudoephedrine, and ingestion of some food products (e.g., licorice).

Pathology

Autopsied brains from patients with complicated PRES show diffuse cerebral edema. Intracranial hemorrhage complicates 15-25% of PRES cases. The most common finding is multiple bilateral petechial microhemorrhages in the occipital lobes **(32-1)**.

Microvascular pathology includes fibrinoid arteriolar necrosis with petechial hemorrhages, proteinaceous exudates, and macrophage infiltration along the perivascular spaces.

Pathologic evidence of partial irreversible damage has been documented in PRES despite radiographic resolution of abnormalities. Scattered microinfarcts, white matter (WM) rarefaction with subpial gliosis, and hemosiderin deposition—especially in the posterior cerebrum—have been reported.

PRES: TERMINOLOGY, ETIOLOGY, AND CLINICAL ISSUES

Terminology

- **P**osterior **r**eversible **e**ncephalopathy **s**yndrome (PRES)
- *Lesions often not* just *posterior, not always reversible!*

Etiology

- HTN-induced dysautoregulation vs. vasospasm, ↓ perfusion
- ↑ ↑ BP → failed autoregulation → hyperperfusion
  - Vasogenic (not cytotoxic) edema
  - Endothelial dysfunction ± excessive circulating cytokines → "leaky" blood-brain barrier
  - Fluid, macromolecules ± blood extravasate
- Causes (HTN typical but not invariable)
  - Preeclampsia/eclampsia
  - Chemotherapy, immunosuppressive drugs
  - Thrombotic microangiopathies (e.g., HUS/TTP)
  - Renal failure
  - Shock/sepsis
  - Tumor lysis syndrome
  - Food/drug-induced mineralocorticoid excess

Clinical Issues

- All ages (peak = 20-40 years)
- F >> M
- BP usually ↑ ↑ *but*
  - < 50% have *mean* arterial pressure > 140-50 mm Hg
  - 15-20% normotensive or hypotensive
- Usually resolves completely with BP normalization

Clinical Issues

Epidemiology and Demographics. Although the peak age of onset is 20-40 years, PRES can affect patients of all ages from infants to the elderly. There is a moderate female predominance, largely because of the strong association of PRES and preeclampsia.

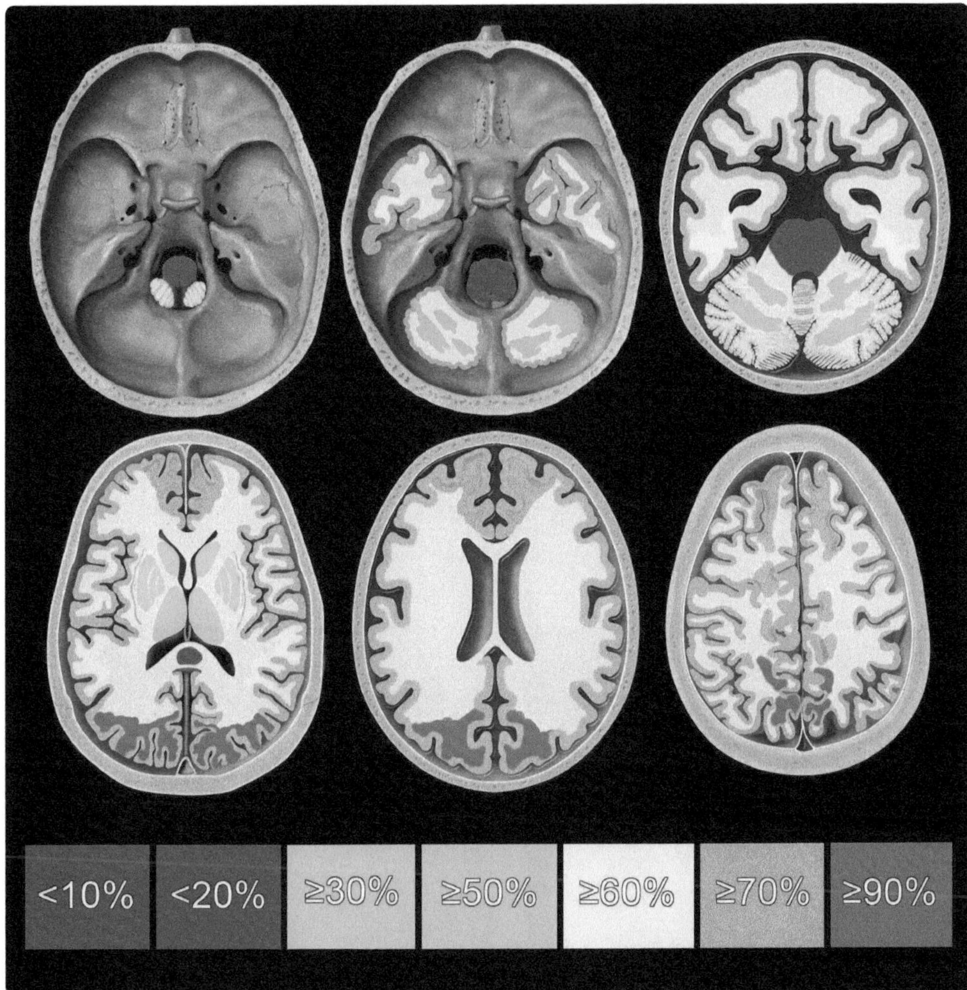

(32-3) Diagrams show location, relative frequency of PRES lesions. Although > 90% have lesions in the parietooccipital subcortical WM (classic PRES, shown in red), note that multifocality is the rule, not the exception. Most cases of PRES also have lesions in areas other than the classic parietooccipital location. Both classic PRES (red) and the superior frontal sulcus pattern (orange) are frequently combined with additional lesions distributed along the hemispheric cortical (superficial) watershed zones (depicted in the lower right image). The cerebellum is affected in nearly 1/2 of PRES cases, whereas about 1/3 have basal ganglionic lesions (light blue). The pons, medulla, cervical spinal cord, and corpus callosum splenium are less common sites involved by PRES, although in some cases, only the posterior fossa is affected. Remember: Atypical PRES is actually more common than the classic isolated parietooccipital involvement! (Adapted from Ollivier et al.)

Preeclampsia is the most common overall cause of PRES. HTN (blood pressure exceeding 140/90 mm Hg) and proteinuria are typical. Progression from preeclampsia to **eclampsia** (mean systolic ≥ 160 mm Hg) occurs in 0.5% of patients with mild and 2-3% of patients with severe preeclampsia.

Presentation. Although 92% of patients with PRES have acutely elevated blood pressure, *PRES can also occur in the absence of hypertension.* The most common clinical symptoms and signs in patients with PRES are encephalopathy (50-80%), seizure (60-75%), headache (50%), visual disturbances (33%), and focal neurological deficit (10-15%).

Natural History and Treatment Options. Reversibility is a typical feature of PRES and is associated with good prognosis. If the inciting substances or precipitating conditions are eliminated and any existing HTN is promptly treated, PRES often resolves with minimal or no residual abnormalities.

Extensive vasogenic edema, hemorrhage, and restricted diffusion on initial imaging are associated with worse clinical outcomes. Severe PRES can be life threatening. In rare cases, lesions are irreversible and permanent damage occurs, typically hemorrhagic cortical/subcortical or basal ganglionic infarcts.

Imaging

General Features. Three distinct imaging patterns of PRES have been described. The most common is a dominant **parietal-occipital pattern** (classic or typical PRES). Two less common (atypical) patterns are a **superior frontal sulcus pattern** (involvement of the mid and posterior aspects of the superior frontal sulcus) and a **holohemispheric watershed pattern** (involvement of the frontal, parietal, and occipital lobes along the internal watershed zones). Combinations of these three patterns as well as involvement of other anatomic areas are also common **(32-3)**.

The parietooccipital lobes are involved in > 90% of PRES cases **(32-2)**. The frontal lobes are involved in 75-77% of cases with the temporal lobes (65%) and cerebellum (50-55%) also commonly affected. Other atypical distributions include the basal ganglia and thalami, deep WM, corpus callosum splenium, brainstem, and cervical spinal cord.

CT Findings. NECT scans are commonly obtained as an initial screening study **(32-4A)**. It is therefore extremely important to identify even subtle abnormalities that may be suggestive of PRES. **If the screening NECT is normal and PRES is suspected on clinical grounds, an MR scan with DWI and T2***

in addition to the routine sequences (T1 and T2/FLAIR) should be obtained.

Screening NECTs are normal in ~ 1/4 of all PRES cases **(32-4)**. Subtle, patchy cortical/subcortical hypodensities—usually in the parietooccipital lobes, watershed zones, &/or cerebellum—may be the only visible abnormalities on NECT **(32-2)**. PRES-associated intracranial hemorrhage is uncommon.

MR Findings. PRES has both classic and atypical (i.e., variant) MR features. Keep in mind that (1) atypical PRES is actually more common than classic (i.e., purely parietal-occipital) PRES; (2) PRES is rarely *just* posterior; and (3) PRES is *not always reversible.*

Classic PRES demonstrates bilateral parietooccipital cortical/subcortical hypointensities that are hypointense on T1WI and hyperintense on T2/FLAIR **(32-4)**. T2* (GRE or SWI) sequences may demonstrate hemorrhagic foci. Transient patchy cortical-subcortical enhancement on T1 C+ may occur **(32-4C)**.

Imaging findings in *atypical* PRES include involvement of the frontal lobes, watershed zones, basal ganglia &/or thalami, brainstem, cerebellum, and even the spinal cord **(32-5)**. Findings of both classic and atypical PRES very commonly occur together.

In unusual cases, brainstem &/or cerebellar lesions may be the *only* abnormality present. The spinal cord has been reported as a rare site of isolated PRES involvement.

Frank infarction is quite rare in PRES. Because most cases of PRES are caused by vasogenic—not cytotoxic—edema, DWI is usually negative. However, PRES with restricted diffusion occurs in 15-30% of cases and is usually seen as small foci of restricted diffusion within larger regions of nonrestricting vasogenic edema.

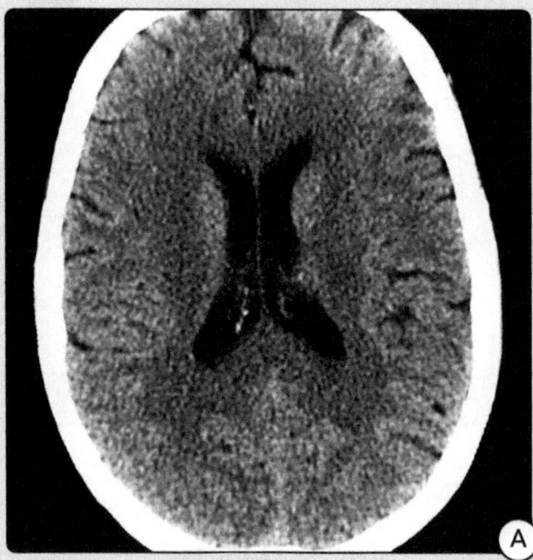

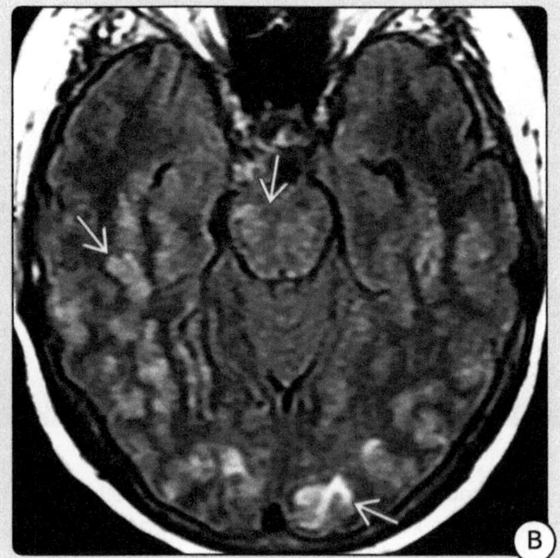

***(32-4A)** A 63y woman with end-stage renal disease had a seizure, then fell. Blood pressure on admission was 220/140. NECT performed to evaluate for intracranial hemorrhage shows normal findings. **(32-4B)** MR was obtained because of suspected PRES. FLAIR MR obtained 1 hour after the NECT shows multifocal patchy hyperintensities in the midbrain, posteroinferior temporal lobes, and parietooccipital cortex ➡.*

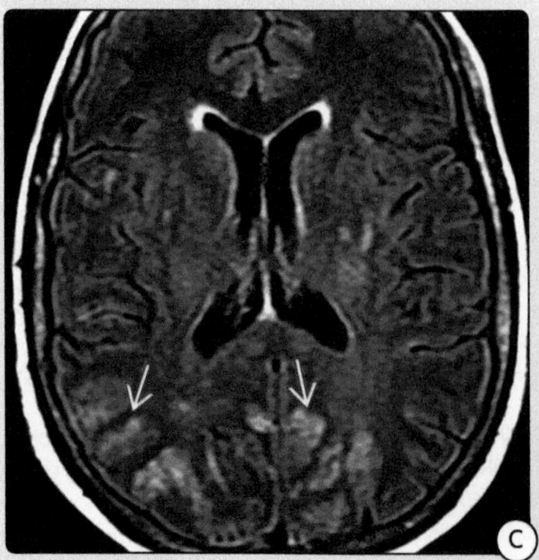

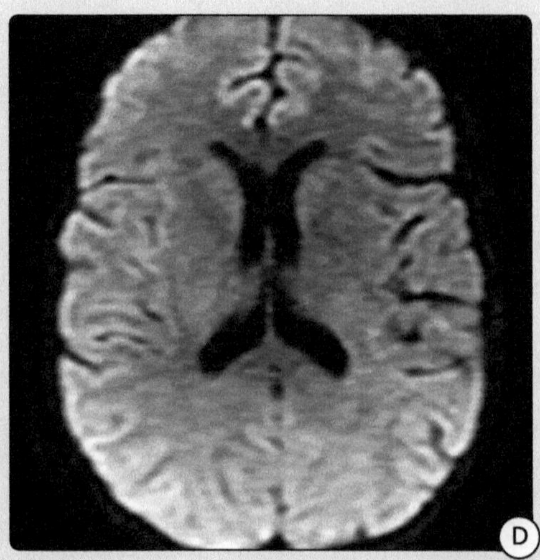

***(32-4C)** FLAIR MR through the lateral ventricles shows bilateral, relatively symmetric lesions in the parietooccipital cortex ➡. **(32-4D)** DWI MR in the same patient shows no evidence for diffusion restriction. DWI scans are usually (although not invariably) normal in PRES because the edema is mostly vasogenic, not cytotoxic.*

Following blood pressure normalization, imaging findings in most cases of PRES resolve completely. Irreversible lesions are relatively uncommon, occurring in ~ 15% of cases.

Differential Diagnosis

The major differential diagnoses of PRES include acute cerebral ischemia-infarction, vasculitis, hypoglycemia, status epilepticus, sinovenous thrombosis, reversible cerebral vasoconstriction syndrome (RCVS), and the thrombotic microangiopathies.

PRES rarely involves *just* the posterior circulation, so **acute cerebral ischemia-infarction** is often easily distinguished. **Vasculitis** can resemble PRES-induced vasculopathy on CTA or DSA.

The distribution of lesions in vasculitis is much more random and less symmetric, usually does not demonstrate the parietooccipital predominance seen in PRES, and more often enhances following contrast administration. In contrast to vasculitis, high-resolution vessel wall imaging is usually negative in PRES.

Hypoglycemia typically affects the parietooccipital cortex and subcortical WM, so the clinical laboratory findings (i.e., low serum glucose, lack of systemic HTN) are important differentiating features. **Status epilepticus** can cause transient gyral edema but is rarely bilateral and can affect any part of the cortex.

Less common entities that can mimic PRES include **RCVS**. RCVS shares some features (e.g., convexal subarachnoid hemorrhage) with PRES but is typically limited to a solitary sulcus or just a few adjacent sulci.

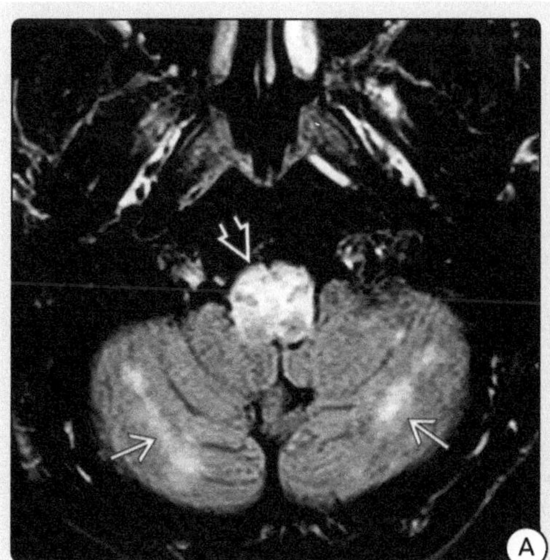

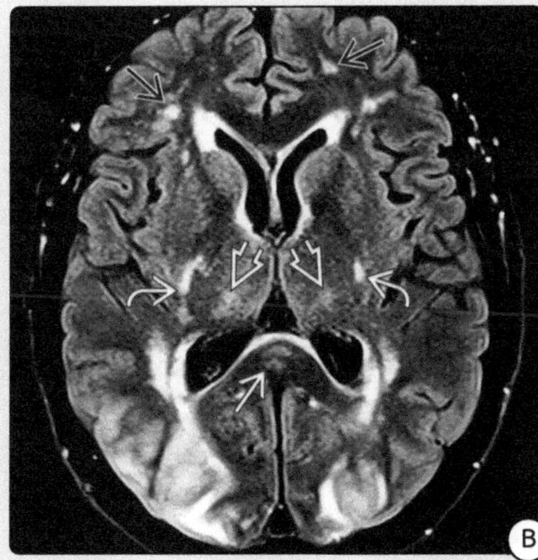

***(32-5A)** Axial FLAIR MR in a 50-year-old man with severe hypertension (BP = 200/120) shows confluent hyperintensity involving the entire medulla ➡. Note patchy hyperintensities in the white matter of both cerebellar hemispheres ➡. **(32-5B)** Additional lesions are present in the thalami ➡, internal capsules ➡, corpus callosum splenium ➡, and frontal WM ➡.*

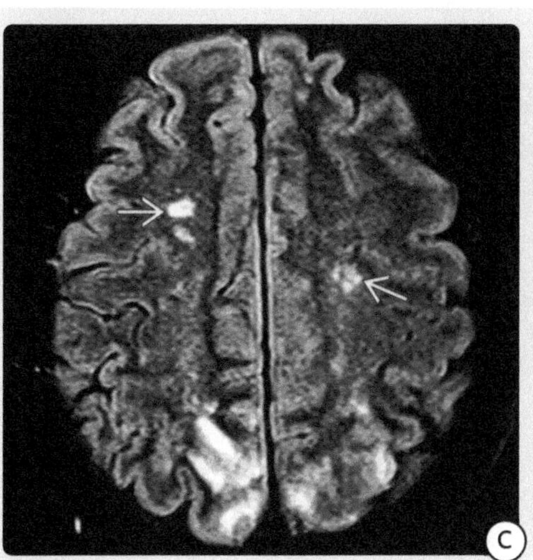

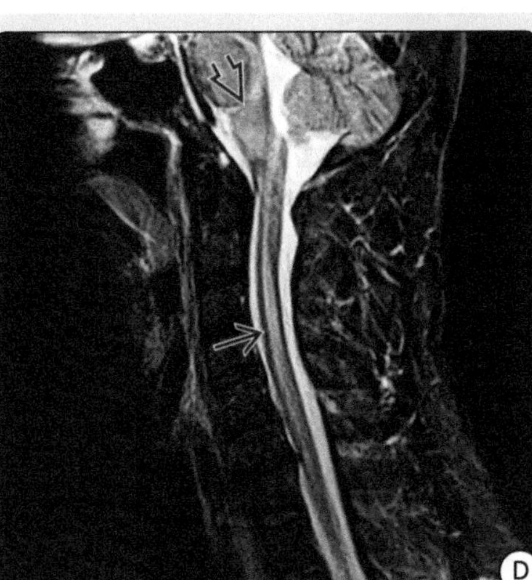

***(32-5C)** More cephalad FLAIR shows lesions along the watershed zones ➡. **(32-5D)** Sagittal STIR of the cervical spine shows confluent hyperintensity extending from the medulla ➡ inferiorly throughout the entire cervical spinal cord ➡. This is atypical PRES. Remember: "Atypical" PRES is more common than "classic" PRES!*

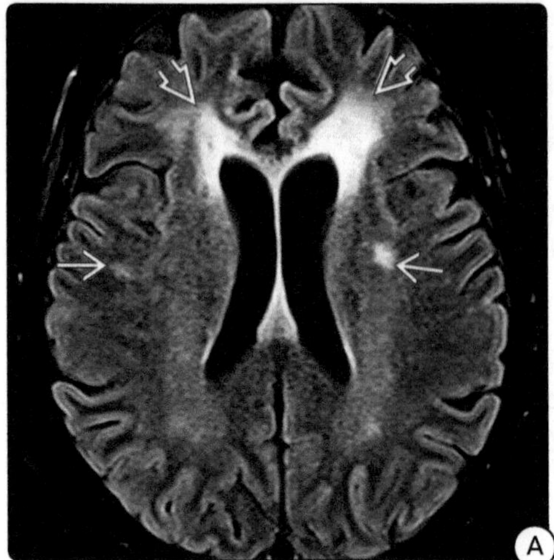

***(32-6A)** FLAIR in 54y woman with chronic renal failure, TTP, confusion shows bifrontal confluent ➡ and scattered WM ➡ hyperintensities.*

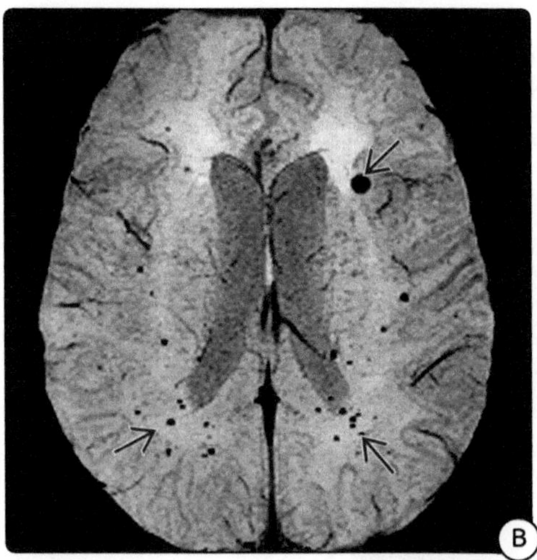

***(32-6B)** T2* SWI shows multiple "blooming" foci ➡ throughout the white matter. The cortex is spared.*

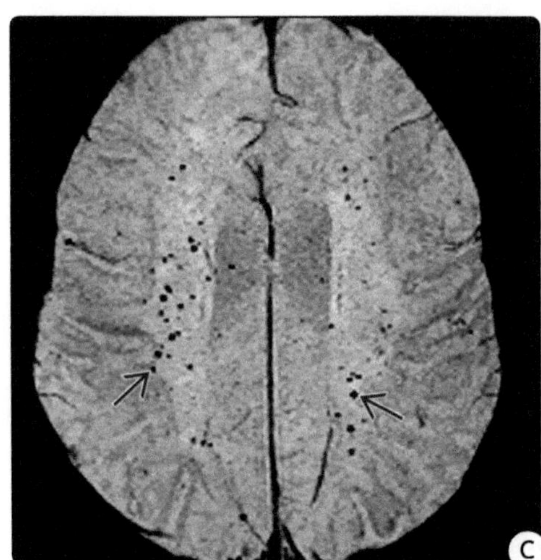

***(32-6C)** More cephalad T2* SWI demonstrates more blooming WM hypointensities ➡.*

PRES: IMAGING AND DDx

3 Anatomic Patterns
- Classic PRES
  - **Parietooccipital pattern** (> 90%)
- Variant PRES
  - **Superior frontal sulcus pattern** (70%)
  - **Holohemispheric watershed pattern** (50%)
  - Other: Cerebellum (50%), basal ganglia (30%), brainstem (20%), spinal cord (< 10%)
- Combinations *very* common (> 90%)

CT
- Can be normal or only subtly abnormal
  - If PRES suspected and CT normal, get MR!
- Posterior cortical/subcortical hypodensities
- Gross hemorrhage rare (parenchymal > convexal subarachnoid hemorrhage)

MR
- T2/FLAIR hyperintensity (parietooccipital most common)
- T2* (GRE/SWI) shows hemorrhage in 15-25%
- DWI usually but not invariably negative
- Enhancement none/mild (unless severe PRES)

Differential Diagnosis
- Posterior circulation ischemia-infarction
  - Top of basilar syndrome
- Vasculitis
- Status epilepticus
- Hypoglycemia
- Thrombotic microangiopathy
  - Primary (ADAMTS13-mediated TMA/TTP, Shiga toxin-mediated HUS)
  - Secondary (malignant HTN, HELLP syndrome, autoimmune disorders, DIC)
- Sinovenous thrombosis
  - Internal cerebral veins, vein of Galen/straight sinus
- Reversible cerebral vasoconstriction syndrome

Malignant Hypertension

Terminology and Etiology

Malignant hypertension (mHTN) is characterized clinically by extreme blood pressure elevation and papilledema. Diastolic levels often exceed 130-140 mm Hg. **The abruptness of blood pressure elevation seems to be more important than the absolute level of either systolic or mean arterial blood pressure.**

Pathology

Macroscopically, the brain appears swollen and edematous. Gross parenchymal hematomas and perivascular petechial microhemorrhages may be present. Acute microinfarcts, especially in the basal ganglia and pons, are common.

Imaging

Imaging findings in mHTN range from classic PRES to "atypical" features. "Atypical" features are more common in mHTN. Brainstem-dominant hypertensive encephalopathy and basal ganglia &/or watershed lesions are common cerebral manifestations of mHTN.

Lobar &/or multifocal parenchymal microhemorrhages in the cortex, basal ganglia, pons, and cerebellum are common in mHTN and are best seen as "blooming" foci on T2* sequences (GRE, SWI) **(32-6)**. Convexal subarachnoid hemorrhage has been reported in a few cases of mHTN.

ACUTE HYPERTENSIVE ENCEPHALOPATHY

Terminology
- a.k.a. malignant hypertension, hypertensive crisis

Etiology
- Abrupt rise in BP > absolute value of BP
- Many causes (uncontrolled HTN, drug abuse, etc.)

Imaging
- Brainstem, basal ganglia > > cortex, watershed
- Microbleeds on T2* (GRE, SWI) common

Differential Diagnosis
- Major differential diagnosis is PRES (can, often does overlap)

Chronic Hypertensive Encephalopathy

Although the clinical and imaging manifestations of posterior reversible encephalopathy syndrome (PRES) and malignant hypertension (mHTN) can be dramatic and life threatening, the effects of longstanding untreated or poorly treated HTN on end-organ function can be equally devastating and are far more common.

Pathology

The most consistent histopathologic feature of chronic hypertensive encephalopathy (CHtnE) is a microvasculopathy characterized by arteriolosclerosis and lipohyalinosis (see Chapter 10). The microvasculopathy is accompanied by myelin pallor, gliosis, and spongiform WM volume loss. Multiple lacunar infarcts are common.

Clinical Issues

CHtnE is most common in middle-aged and elderly patients. In addition to age and chronically elevated blood pressure, smoking is an independent risk factor as is metabolic syndrome (impaired glucose metabolism, elevated blood pressure, central obesity, and dyslipidemia).

Imaging

The two cardinal imaging features of CHtnE are (1) diffuse patchy &/or confluent WM lesions and (2) multifocal microbleeds. The WM lesions are concentrated in the corona radiata and deep periventricular WM—especially around the atria of the lateral ventricles. The damaged WM appears hypodense on NECT scans and hyperintense on T2/FLAIR imaging.

Multiple petechial bleeds ("microhemorrhages") are the second most common manifestation of CHtnE. These are not usually identifiable on NECT and may be invisible on standard MR sequences (FSE T2WI and FLAIR). T2* (GRE, SWI) scans show multiple "blooming" hypointensities ("black dots") that tend to be concentrated in the basal ganglia and cerebellum **(32-7)**.

Differential Diagnosis

The major differential diagnosis of CHtnE is **cerebral amyloid angiopathy** (CAA). The WM lesions in both diseases often appear similar, and both disorders can cause hemorrhagic microangiopathy. The microbleeds of CAA are more often peripheral (e.g., cortex, siderosis of the leptomeninges) and

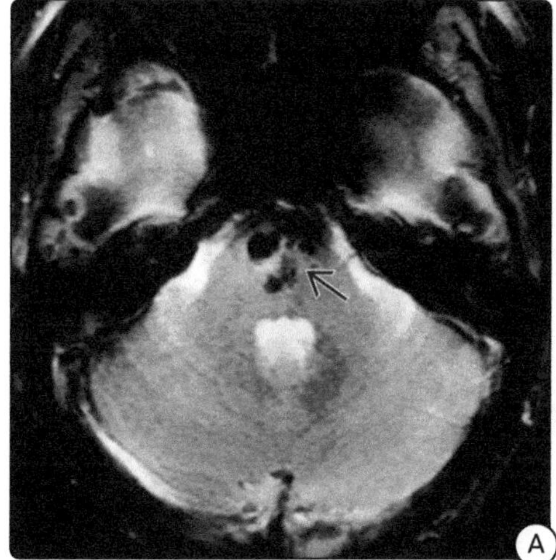

***(32-7A)** T2* GRE in a 37y woman with longstanding, poorly treated hypertensions shows multiple "blooming" foci in the pons ⇨.*

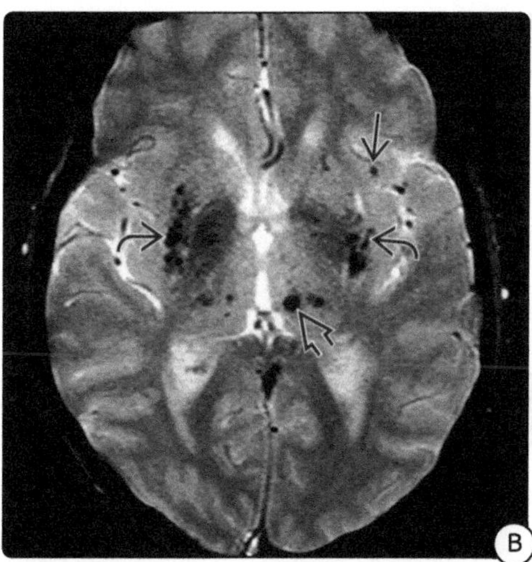

***(32-7B)** Numerous hypointensities in the basal ganglia ⮫ and thalami ⇨ and a single lesion in the left insular cortex ⇨ are present.*

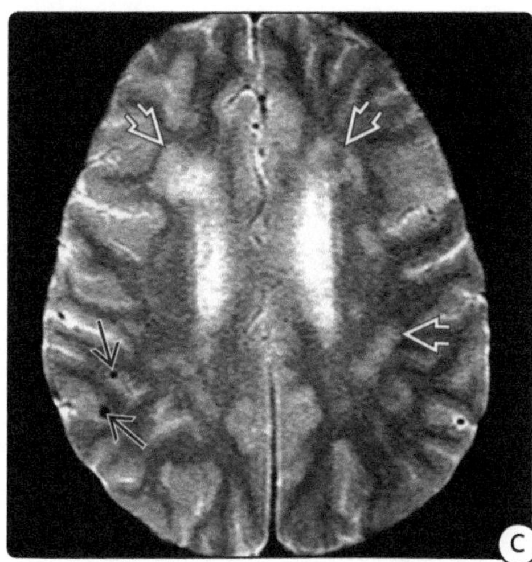

***(32-7C)** Scattered foci of gradient susceptibility in the cortex ⇨, extensive periventricular WM hyperintensities ➡ are present. Chronic HTN.*

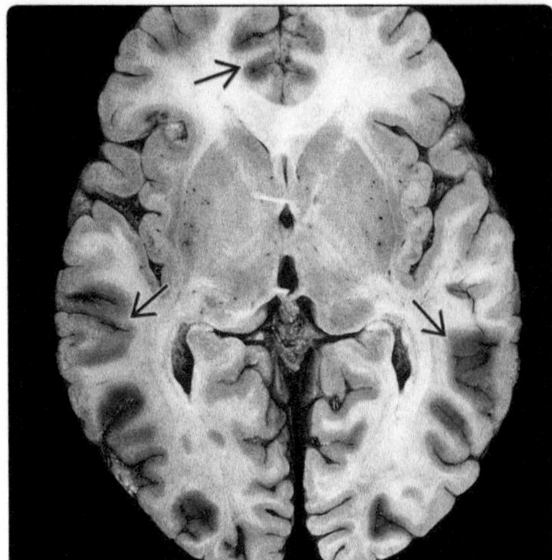

(32-8) Autopsy of severe hypoglycemia shows bilateral symmetric parietooccipital, frontal cortical necrosis ➡. (Courtesy R. Hewlett, MD.)

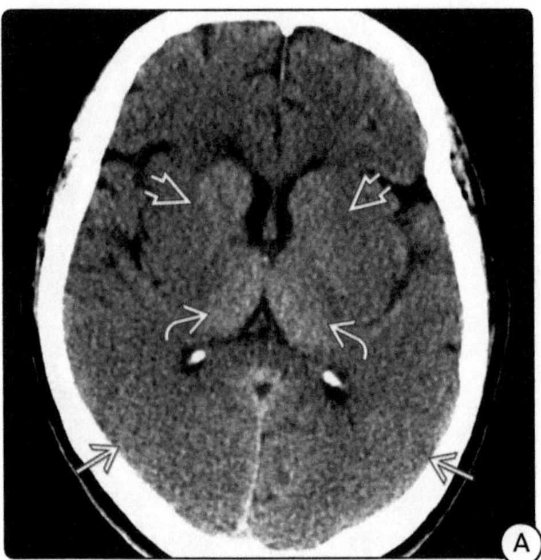

(32-9A) NECT shows typical changes of hypoglycemia with parietooccipital gyral swelling ➡, putamen hypodensity ➡, spared thalami ➡.

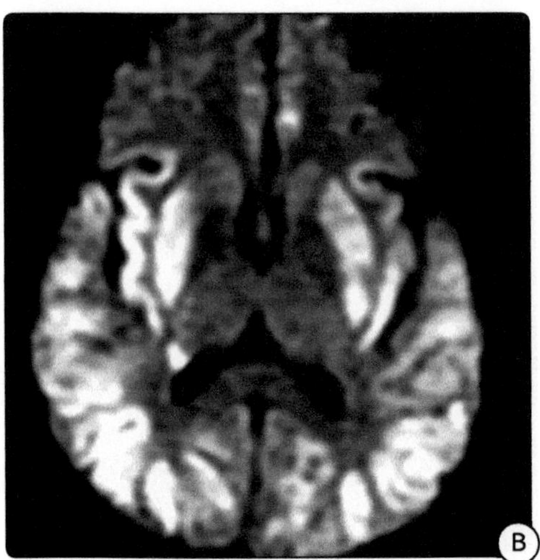

(32-9B) DWI MR in the same case of typical AHE shows restricted diffusion in parietooccipital cortex, putamina with thalamic and WM sparing.

rarely affect the brainstem or cerebellum. Hypertensive microhemorrhages are most common in the basal ganglia, pons, and cerebellum.

Cerebral autosomal dominant arteriopathy without subcortical infarcts and leukoencephalopathy (CADASIL) can also mimic CHtnE. CADASIL typically presents in younger patients and causes multiple subcortical lacunar infarcts. Lesions in the anterior temporal lobes and external capsules are classic imaging findings of CADASIL.

CHRONIC HYPERTENSIVE ENCEPHALOPATHY

Pathology
- Microvasculopathy
  - Arteriolosclerosis, lipohyalinosis
  - Myelin pallor, lacunar infarcts
  - Microbleeds (cerebellum, basal ganglia/thalami > cortex)

Clinical Issues
- Metabolic syndrome, headaches
- Can have "acute-on-chronic" HTN with encephalopathy

Imaging
- Diffuse patchy &/or confluent WM lesions
- Microbleeds on T2* (basal ganglia, cerebellum)

Differential Diagnosis
- Amyloid angiopathy (cortex > basal ganglia, cerebellum)
- CADASIL (younger patients, anterior temporal/external capsule WM lesions)

Glucose Disorders

The brain is a glucose glutton, consuming > 1/2 of the body's total glucose. Because the brain does not store excess energy as glycogen, CNS function is highly dependent on a steady, continuous supply of blood glucose (see next box).

Blood glucose levels are tightly regulated and are normally maintained within a narrow physiologic range. Disorders of glucose metabolism—both *hypo*glycemia and *hyper*glycemia—can injure the CNS.

The neurologic manifestations of deranged glucose metabolism range from mild, reversible focal deficits to status epilepticus, coma, and death. Because the clinical and imaging manifestations differ in neonates from those of older children and adults, hypoglycemia in these two age groups is discussed separately.

Pediatric/Adult Hypoglycemic Encephalopathy

Terminology

Hypoglycemia literally means low blood sugar and is caused by an imbalance between glucose supply and glucose utilization. Acute hypoglycemic brain injury is called hypoglycemic encephalopathy.

Etiology

Childhood hypoglycemic encephalopathy is most commonly associated with type 1 diabetes mellitus. In its most common adult setting—advanced type 2 diabetes—hypoglycemia typically results from the interplay between absolute or relative insulin excess and compromised glucose counterregulation; insulin in and of itself is not neurotoxic. Most cases of adult hypoglycemia occur as a side effect of diabetes treatment with insulin and sulfonylureas.

Pathology

Cortical necrosis is the most common gross finding in hypoglycemic encephalopathy. Although the entire cortical ribbon can be affected, the parietooccipital regions are usually the most severely involved **(32-8)**. Other especially vulnerable areas include the basal ganglia, hippocampi, and amygdalae. The thalami, WM, brainstem, and cerebellum are typically spared.

Clinical Issues

The typical hypoglycemic patient is an elderly diabetic on insulin replacement therapy with altered dietary glucose intake. Deliberate or accidental insulin overdose is more common in children and young or middle-aged adults.

Imaging

CT Findings. NECT scans typically show symmetrically hypodense parietal and occipital lobes. The putamina frequently appear hypodense, whereas the thalami are spared **(32-9A)**. In severe cases, diffuse cerebral edema with near-total sulcal effacement and blurred gray matter-white matter (GM-WM) interfaces can be seen.

MR Findings. T2/FLAIR hyperintensity in the parietooccipital cortex and basal ganglia is typical of acute hypoglycemic encephalopathy. The thalami, subcortical/deep WM, and cerebellum are generally spared. T2* scans generally show minimal or no "blooming" to suggest hemorrhage. Enhancement on T1 C+ is variable and, when present, usually mild.

DWI scans show restricted diffusion in the affected areas, predominately the posterior parietal and occipital cortex **(32-9B)**. Cytotoxic corpus callosum splenium lesions with restricted diffusion have also been reported in association with hypoglycemia.

Differential Diagnosis

The most important differential diagnosis of hypoglycemic encephalopathy is **hypoxic-ischemic encephalopathy** (HIE). HIE typically occurs following cardiac arrest or global hypoperfusion. In contrast to hypoglycemic encephalopathy, the thalami and cerebellum are often affected in HIE. **Acute cerebral ischemia-infarction** is wedge-shaped, involving both the cortex and underlying WM. **Acute hypertensive encephalopathy (PRES)** typically affects the parietooccipital cortex but spares most of the underlying WM and rarely restricts on DWI.

Neonatal/Infantile Hypoglycemia

Unlike older children and adults, neonates have lower absolute glucose demands and can utilize other substrates, such as lactate, to produce energy. Nevertheless, prolonged &/or severe hypoglycemia can result in devastating brain injury in newborn infants.

Neonatal/infantile hypoglycemic encephalopathy typically presents in the first 3 days of life, usually within the first 24 hours, and is most often caused by maternal diabetes with poor glycemic control. Uncontrolled maternal diabetes leads to chronic fetal hyperglycemia in utero. This results in *transient* neonatal hyperinsulinemia and hypoglycemia of varying severity. Congenital hyperinsulinism (HI) is the most common, most severe cause of *persistent* hypoglycemia in neonates and children.

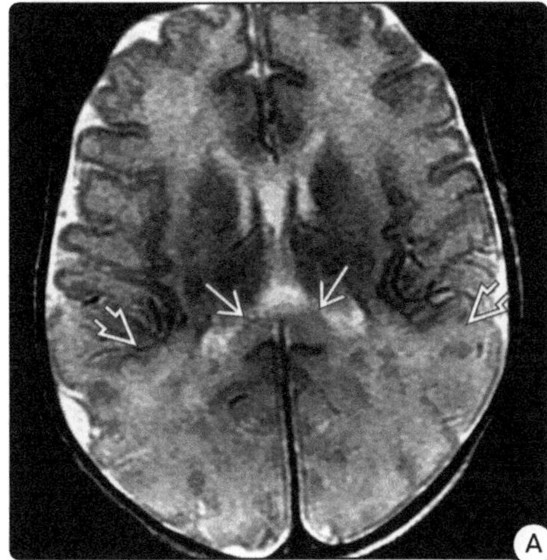

***(32-10A)** T2 MR in 5-day-old hypoglycemic infant shows edematous, hyperintense parietooccipital lobes ➡, corpus callosum splenium ➡.*

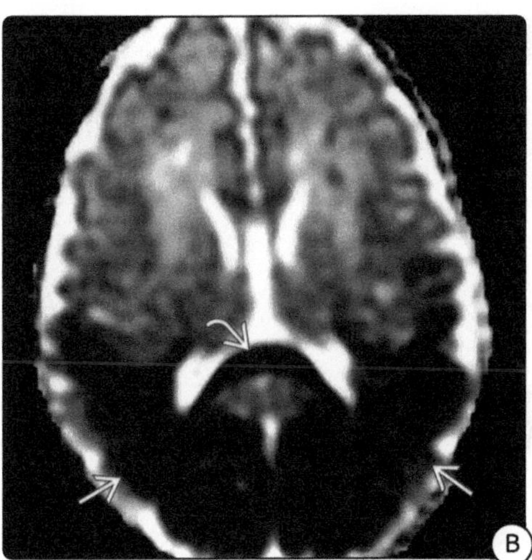

***(32-10B)** ADC shows profound restricted diffusion in the parietal and occipital lobes ➡ and corpus callosum splenium ➡.*

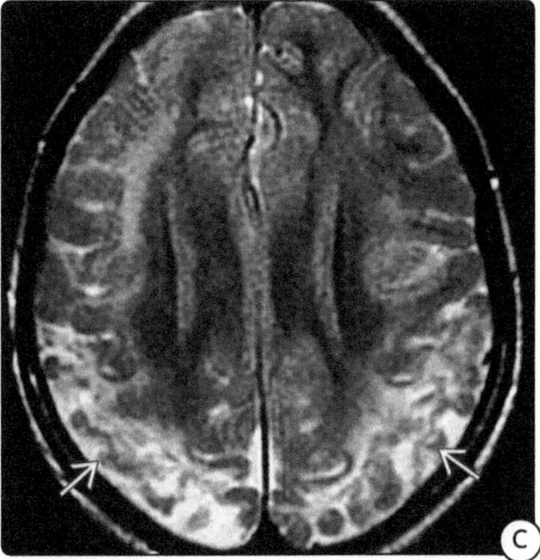

***(32-10C)** T2 MR at 1 year shows shrunken, hyperintense parietooccipital lobes with cortical loss and encephalomalacic-appearing WM ➡.*

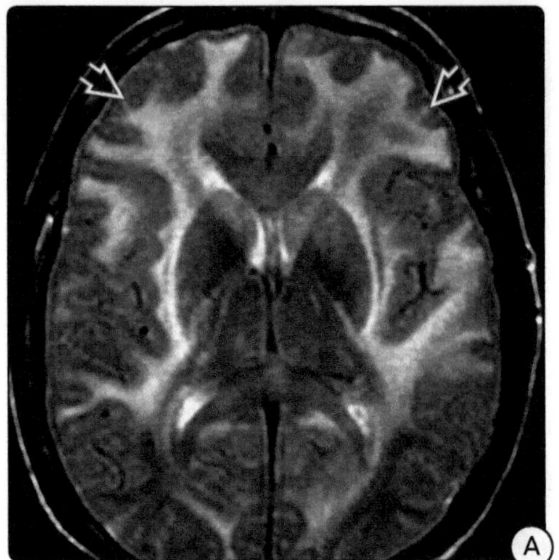
(32-11A) T2 MR of acute Hashimoto encephalopathy shows confluent, symmetric hyperintensity in the subcortical, deep WM ➡.

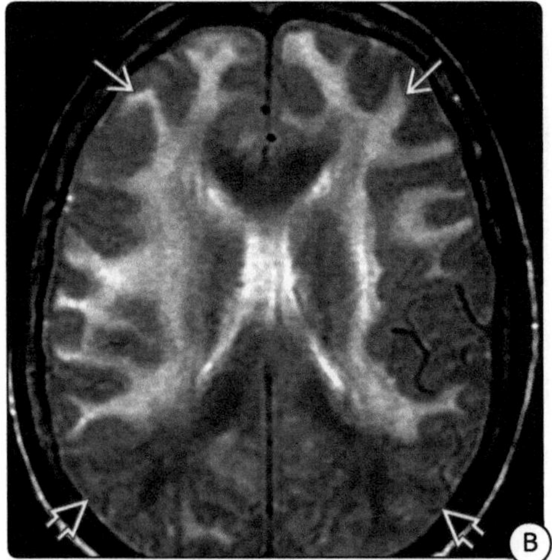
(32-11B) More cephalad T2 MR shows the frontoparietal dominance of WM edema ➡. Occipital lobes ➡ are largely spared.

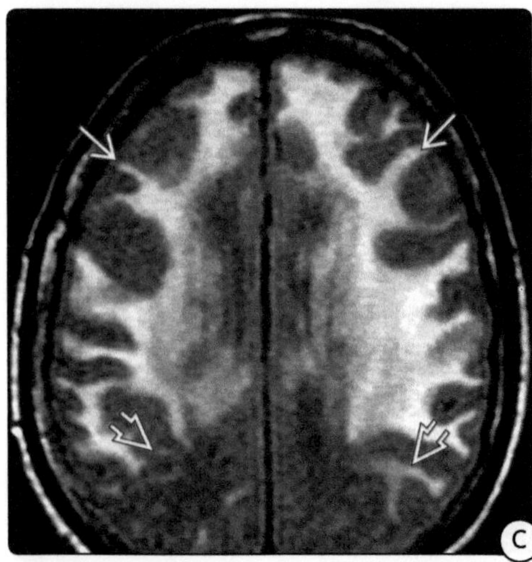
(32-11C) FLAIR MR through corona radiata shows frontal subcortical/deep WM edema ➡ with marked sparing of the occipital lobes ➡.

MR scans in the acute stages of neonatal hypoglycemic encephalopathy show T2/FLAIR hyperintensity and restricted diffusion in the parietooccipital cortex, subcortical WM, and corpus callosum splenium **(32-10)**.

As with older children and adults, the major differential diagnosis of neonatal hypoglycemic encephalopathy is **term hypoxic-ischemic injury** (HII). Hypoglycemic encephalopathy and HII often coexist, potentiating the extent of brain injury. Imaging findings in the two disorders may be indistinguishable.

Inherited mitochondrial disorders, such as **mitochondrial encephalopathy with lactic acidosis and stroke-like episodes** (MELAS), may present with cortical swelling that spares the underlying WM. MELAS is rarely bilaterally symmetric and demonstrates much more markedly elevated lactate on MRS.

HYPOGLYCEMIA

General Concepts
- Imbalance between glucose supply, utilization → hypoglycemia
- Can be mild, transient, asymptomatic
- Extent of brain injury depends on
  - Degree, duration of hypoglycemia
  - CBF, glucose utilization
  - Availability/utilization of alternative energy sources (e.g., lactate)
  - Exacerbating factors (e.g., hypoxia)
  - Recognition, prompt/appropriate treatment

Pediatric/Adult Hypoglycemia
- Etiology
  - Usually associated with diabetes
  - Absolute/relative insulin excess or glucose insufficiency
  - Energy production/O_2 utilization ↓, excitotoxic neurotransmitters ↑
- Pathology
  - Cortical necrosis
- Imaging
  - Hypodense/hyperintense parietooccipital cortex, basal ganglia
  - WM, thalami, cerebellum generally spared
  - Restricted diffusion common
  - May cause reversible corpus callosum splenium lesion

Neonatal/Infantile Hypoglycemia
- Etiology
  - Most common cause of transient hypoglycemia = maternal diabetes
  - Fetal hyperglycemia → neonatal hyperinsulinemia → hypoglycemia
  - Most common cause of severe, persistent hypoglycemia = congenital hyperinsulinemia (KATP mutation in 60%)
- Clinical issues
  - Usually presents in first 3 postnatal days
  - Glucose levels variable
- Imaging
  - Often similar to adult (posterior predominance)
  - Different: Subcortical WM, thalami often involved
- Differential diagnosis
  - Term hypoxic-ischemic encephalopathy
  - Mitochondrial encephalopathy (MELAS)

Hyperglycemia-Associated Disorders

Hyperglycemia-induced brain injury can be chronic or acute. With the worldwide rise in obesity and the soaring prevalence of diabetes mellitus type 2 (DM2), the effects of *chronic* hyperglycemia on the brain are increasingly recognized. Patients with DM2 have accelerated arteriolosclerosis and lipohyalinosis with silent infarcts, brain volume loss, and decreased cognitive functioning.

MR shows increased numbers of T2/FLAIR subcortical and periventricular hyperintensities, especially in the frontal WM, pons, and cerebellum. DTI demonstrates loss of microstructural integrity with decreased FA. Elevated myoinositol on MRS reflects gliosis, an indicator of brain injury.

Acute hyperglycemic brain injury can manifest as diabetic ketoacidosis (DKA). Imaging is nonspecific, with vasogenic cerebral edema the most common abnormality. Hyperglycemic hyperosmolar state with over-rapid correction may also develop osmotic demyelination with typical findings of central pontine myelinolysis.

Thyroid Disorders

Thyroid disorders are relatively common metabolic disturbances that are usually mild and rarely affect brain function. However, several imaging findings—some of them striking—have been associated with thyroid disease. Some can be mistaken for more serious disease (e.g., hypothyroid-induced pituitary hyperplasia mimicking pituitary adenoma), and a few (e.g., Hashimoto encephalopathy) can be life threatening.

Acquired Hypothyroid Disorders

Acquired hypothyroidism is much more common than the congenital variety. Acquired hypothyroidism has two important imaging manifestations: **Pituitary hyperplasia** and **Hashimoto thyroiditis/encephalopathy**.

Pituitary Hyperplasia

Physiologically enlarged pituitary glands are common in young menstruating female patients and pregnant/lactating female patients. *Non*physiologic increase in pituitary volume—pathologic pituitary enlargement—is much less common and typically occurs in response to end-organ failure.

Both physiologic and nonphysiologic pituitary hyperplasia are discussed in detail in Chapter 25. Most cases of hypothyroid-induced pituitary hyperplasia reverse with thyroid hormone replacement therapy (see Fig. 25-5). Caution: Any prepubescent male patient thought to harbor a "pituitary macroadenoma" on imaging studies should undergo comprehensive endocrine evaluation, as macroadenomas are exceptionally rare in this age group!

Hashimoto Encephalopathy

Hashimoto encephalopathy is a rare but treatable condition typically associated with Hashimoto thyroiditis. Hashimoto encephalitis is also called "steroid-responsive encephalopathy with autoimmune thyroiditis." It is a well-recognized neurologic complication of autoimmune thyroid disease and is the most common cause of acquired hypothyroidism.

Hashimoto encephalopathy occurs in both children and adults. Psychiatric symptoms ("myxedema madness") are common. Approximately 50% of patients demonstrate imaging abnormalities. The most typical MR findings are diffuse confluent or focal T2/FLAIR hyperintensities in the subcortical and deep periventricular WM with sparing of the occipital lobes **(32-11)**.

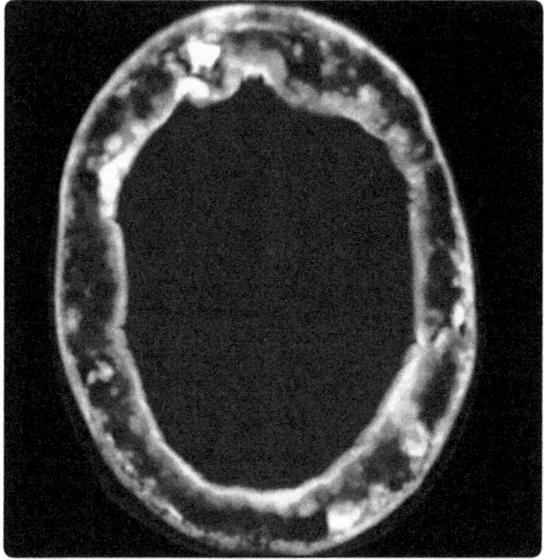

***(32-12)** NECT of the skull in a patient with HPTH shows the characteristic alternating salt and pepper foci of resorption and sclerosis.*

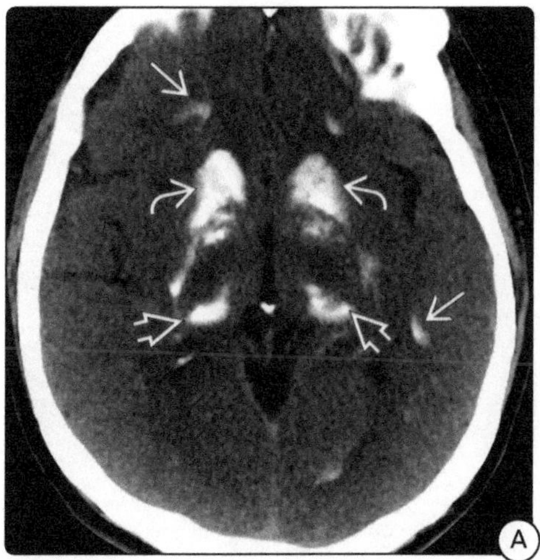

***(32-13A)** NECT in a 54-year-old man with hyperparathyroidism shows extensive symmetric Ca^{++} in basal ganglia ➡, thalami ➡, cortex ➡.*

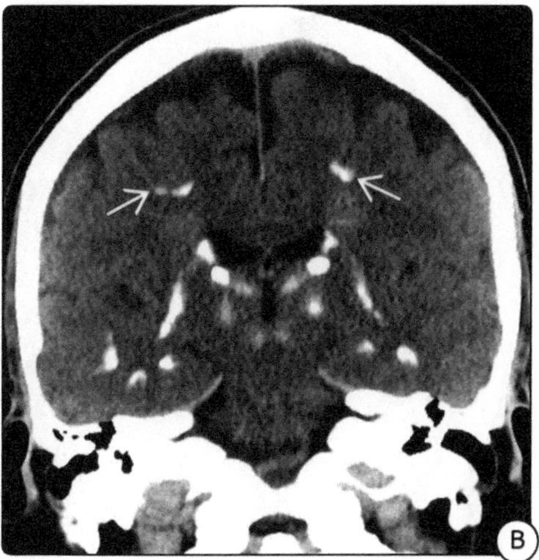

***(32-13B)** Coronal NECT in the same case shows how symmetric the basal Ca^{++} is. Note GM-WM interface calcifications ➡.*

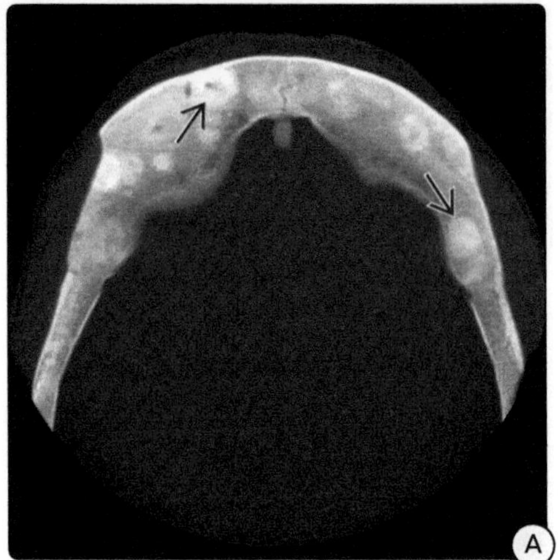

***(32-14A)** Axial bone CT in a patient with 2° HPTH shows leontiasis ossea with marked calvarial thickening, focal sclerotic "brown tumors" ➩.*

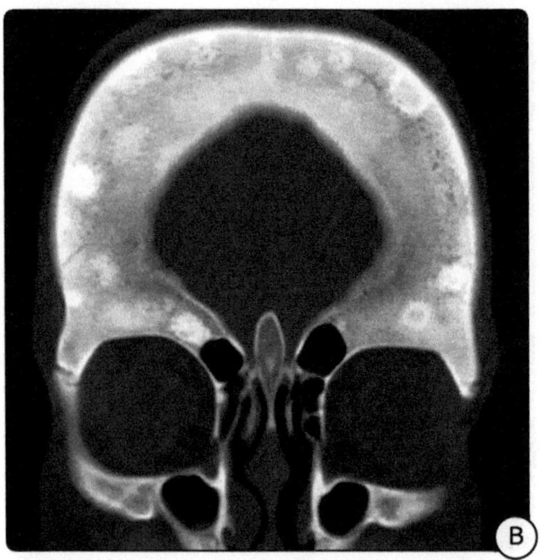

***(32-14B)** Coronal bone CT in the same patient demonstrates the striking calvarial thickening.*

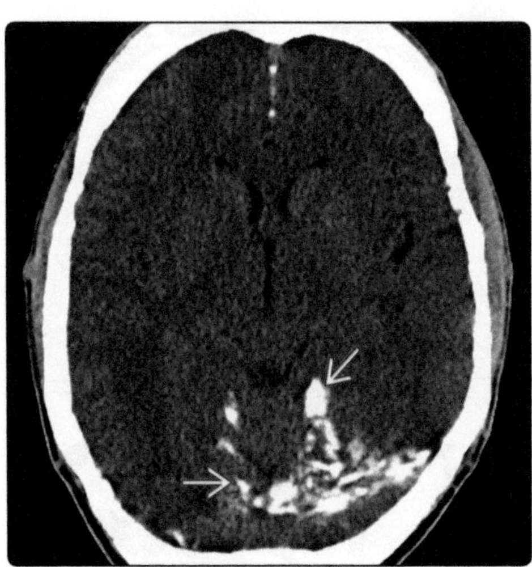

***(32-15)** NECT in a 31-year-old man with ESRD shows markedly thickened, plaque-like deposits along the tentorium ➡.*

Hyperthyroidism

The most common manifestation of hyperthyroidism in the head and neck is thyroid ophthalmopathy (Graves disease). Brain involvement in hyperthyroidism occurs but is very rare. A few cases of **acute idiopathic intracranial hypertension** ("pseudotumor cerebri") associated with hyperthyroidism have been reported.

Because of its effect on factor VIII activity, hyperthyroidism has also been reported as an independent risk factor for **dural venous sinus thrombosis**. Graves disease has been reported as a rare cause of **transient corpus callosum splenium hyperintensity** and an **MS-like multiphasic demyelinating autoimmune syndrome**.

Parathyroid and Related Disorders

Metabolic abnormalities related to parathyroid hormone dysfunction include primary and secondary hyperparathyroidism as well as hypoparathyroidism, pseudohypoparathyroidism, and pseudo-pseudohypoparathyroidism.

Hyperparathyroidism

The parathyroid glands control calcium metabolism by producing parathyroid hormone (PTH). Hyperparathyroidism (HPTH) is the classic disease of bone resorption, so imaging abnormalities may be seen in both the skull and brain.

HPTH can be an acquired (common) or inherited disorder (rare). HPTH can also be primary, secondary, or even tertiary. Because of the increasing number of patients on dialysis, the most common type is now secondary HPTH.

Primary Hyperparathyroidism

1° HPTH is most common in middle-aged to older adults and relatively rare in children. There is a striking female predominance. 1° HPTH is characterized by hypercalcemia and hypophosphatemia (serum calcium is elevated; serum phosphorus is normal or decreased). HPTH is usually asymptomatic. General signs of symptomatic HPTH have been characterized as "stones, bones, abdominal groans, and psychic moans."

Bone CT demonstrates diffuse patchy **salt and pepper lesions** in the skull. Foci of bone resorption are interspersed with variable patchy sclerosis. The most common findings in the brain are **basal ganglia calcifications** on NECT. Bilateral symmetric deposits in the globi pallidi, putamen, and caudate nuclei are typical. The thalami, subcortical WM, and dentate nuclei may also be affected.

MR shows symmetric T1 shortening and T2 hypointensity in the basal ganglia. Mild to moderate "blooming" on T2* (GRE, SWI) sequences is typical. **"Brown tumors"**—solitary or multiple nonneoplastic lesions in the skull—are common.

Secondary Hyperparathyroidism

The most common cause of 2° HPTH is chronic renal disease (CRD). The majority of dialysis patients eventually develop 2° HPTH. Other etiologies of 2° HPTH include dietary calcium deficiency, vitamin D disorders, disrupted phosphate metabolism, and hypomagnesemia.

Most patients with 2° HPTH are older than 40 years at the time of initial diagnosis. Serum calcium is normal or low, serum phosphorus is increased, and calcium-phosphate product is elevated. Vitamin D is low, almost always secondary to renal disease rather than dietary deficiency.

A common manifestation of CRD is renal osteodystrophy. Massive thickening of the calvarium and skull base narrows neural and vascular channels. Progressive cranial nerve involvement—most commonly compressive optic neuropathy—and carotid stenosis with ischemic symptoms are typical.

2° HPTH primarily affects the skull and dura; the brain parenchyma itself is usually normal. NECT scans show markedly thickened skull and facial bones, a condition sometimes referred to as **"uremic leontiasis ossea"** or "big head disease" **(32-14)**.

"Brown tumors" can be seen in both 1° HPTH and 2° HPTH. Fibrous replacement, hemorrhage, and necrosis lead to formation of brownish-appearing cysts. Solitary or multiple "brown tumors" are seen on bone CT as focal expansile lytic lesions with nonsclerotic margins. Signal intensity on MR is highly variable, reflecting the age and amount of hemorrhage as well as the presence of fibrous tissue and cyst formation.

The classic intracranial finding in 2° HPTH is unusually extensive, **plaque-like dural thickening (32-15)**. Longstanding CRD can also result in extensive **"pipestem" calcifications** in the internal and external carotid arteries.

Hypoparathyroid Disorders

Three types of hypoparathyroidism are recognized: Hypoparathyroidism (HP), pseudohypoparathyroidism (PHP), and pseudo-pseudohypoparathyroidism (PPHP). All three disorders share common features on brain imaging, although their clinical presentation and laboratory findings vary.

HP is characterized by brain calcifications. The basal ganglia and thalami are the most common sites **(32-16)** followed by the cerebrum and cerebellum.

PHP is characterized by *elevated* PTH levels and PTH-resistant hypocalcemia and hyperphosphatemia. Bilateral symmetric calcifications in the basal ganglia and thalami **(32-17)**, cerebellar hemispheres, subcortical WM, and occasionally the cerebral cortex are typical findings in both PHP and PPHP. **PPHP** typically shows no laboratory abnormalities, so calcium and phosphate levels are normal.

PARATHYROID DISORDERS

Hyperparathyroidism
- 1° hyperparathyroidism (parathyroid adenomas)
  - Salt and pepper skull, "brown tumors"
  - Basal ganglia Ca^{++}
- 2° (chronic renal failure)
  - Thick skull, face ("big head" disease) ± brown tumors
  - Plaque-like dural thickening, Ca^{++}

Hypoparathyroid Disorders
- 3 types (distinguished by clinical, laboratory findings)
  - Hypoparathyroidism
  - Pseudohypoparathyroidism
  - Pseudo-pseudohypoparathyroidism
- All have Ca^{++} in basal ganglia > cerebrum, cerebellum

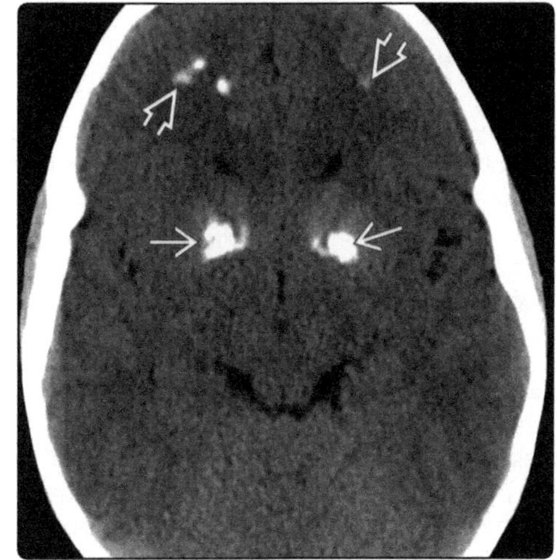

***(32-16)** NECT in 7y with hypoparathyroidism shows calcifications in the globi pallidi ➡ with smaller calcific foci at the GM-WM interfaces ➡.*

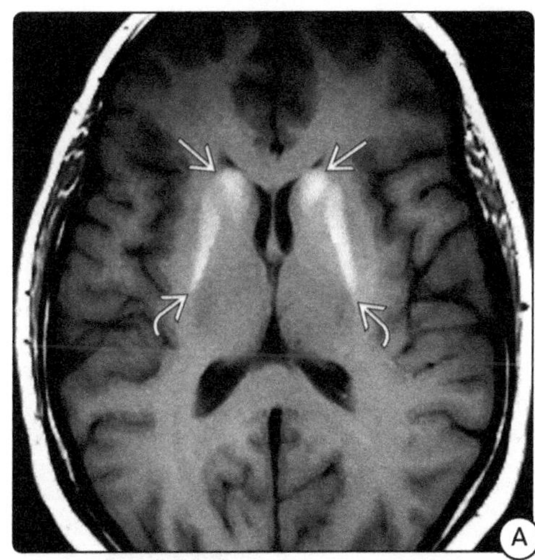

***(32-17A)** Axial T1 MR in 34y woman with PPHP on calcitriol shows symmetric T1 shortening in both caudate nuclei ➡ and putamina ➡.*

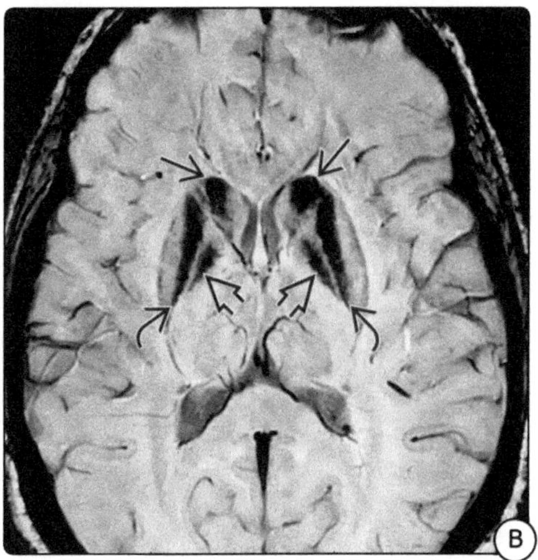

***(32-17B)** T2* SWI shows symmetric hypointensity in both caudate nuclei ➡, putamina ➡, and the globi pallidi ➡. (Courtesy P. Hildenbrand, MD.)*

Primary Familial Brain Calcification (Fahr Disease)

Primary familial brain calcification (PFBC), formerly termed Fahr disease, is an inherited disorder that results in striking brain calcifications. Calcium deposition begins in the third decade, but symptoms develop one or two decades later, usually between ages 30 and 60 years. Schizophrenic-like psychosis in young adults and extrapyramidal symptoms with subcortical dementia in patients over the age of 50 are typical.

NECT discloses extensive bilateral, relatively symmetric basal ganglia calcification. The lateral globus pallidus (GP) is the most severely affected with relative sparing of the medial GP. The putamen, caudate, thalami, dentate nuclei of the cerebellum, and both the cerebral and cerebellar WM (including the internal capsule) are commonly affected **(32-18)**.

MR signal intensity varies according to disease stage and the amount of calcification and heavy metal deposition. Calcification is typically hyperintense on T1WI **(32-19A)** **(32-19C)** but can be quite variable on T2WI. T2/FLAIR scans may appear normal or mildly abnormal. They may also show extensive foci of T2 prolongation in the cerebral WM that can be so striking as to mimic toxic/metabolic demyelination **(32-19D)**.

T2* (GRE, SWI) scans show profound susceptibility changes with "blooming" hypointensity secondary to iron deposition **(32-19B)**. Fahr disease does not enhance on T1 C+ sequences.

The major differential diagnosis of PFBC is normal **physiologic calcification of the basal ganglia**. Age-related ("senescent") calcification in the basal ganglia is common, typically localized in the *medial* GP. PFBC has much heavier, far more extensive calcification.

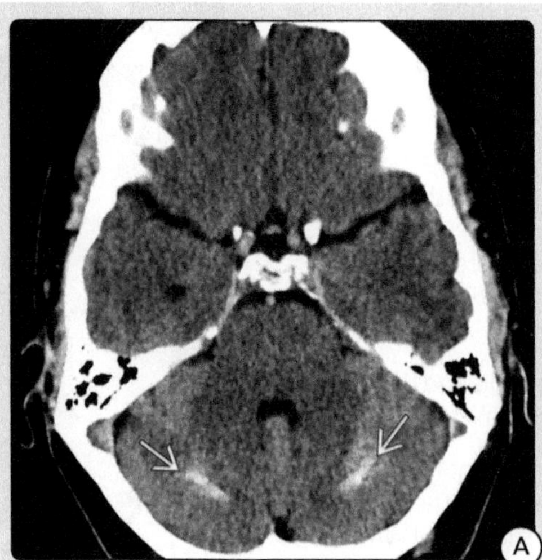

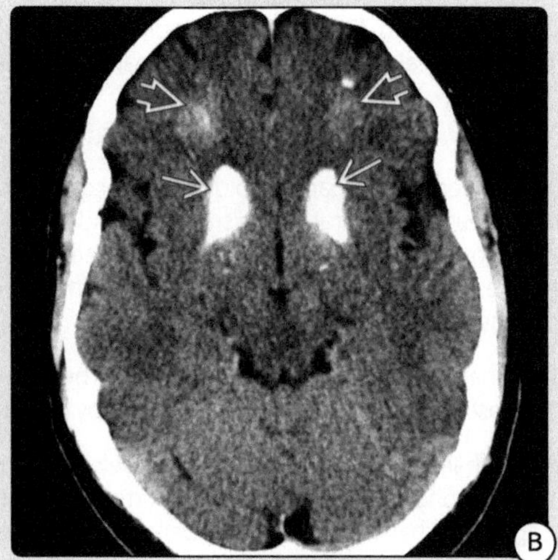

***(32-18A)** Series of axial NECT scans in a 51-year-old man with Fahr disease shows bilaterally symmetric calcifications in the cerebellar white matter ➡. **(32-18B)** NECT shows very dense calcifications in both caudate nuclei and globi pallidi ➡, as well as more faint calcification in the frontal white matter ➡.*

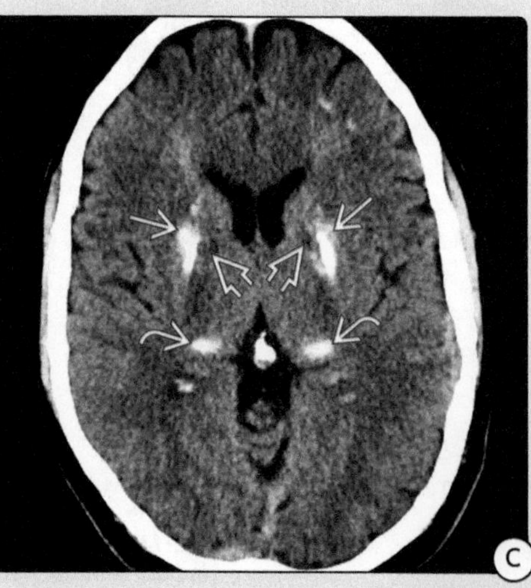

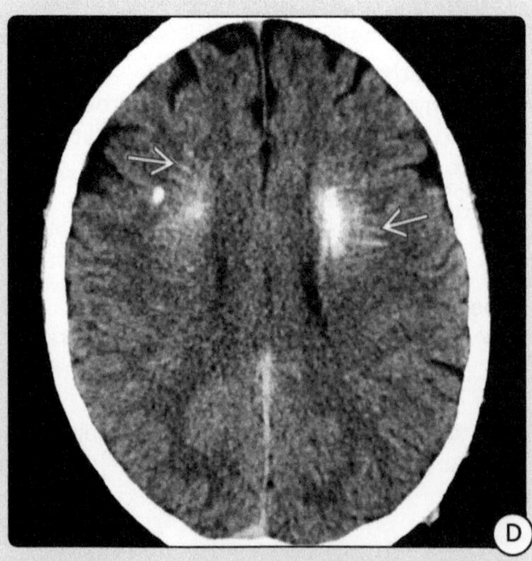

***(32-18C)** More cephalad NECT in the same patient shows calcification in the putamina and lateral globi pallidi ➡ with relative sparing of the most medial GP ➡. Calcification is present in the pulvinars of both thalami ➡. Punctate calcification is seen in the cerebral WM. **(32-18D)** NECT shows linear calcification extending perpendicularly from the caudate nuclei into the cerebral white matter ➡.*

PRIMARY FAMILIAL BRAIN CALCIFICATION

Pathoetiology, Clinical Features
- a.k.a. Fahr disease
- Caused by 4 gene mutations (*SLC20A2* most common)
- Usually presents between 30 and 60 years
  - Extrapyramidal symptoms, dementia

Imaging Findings
- NECT
  - Extensive bilateral basal ganglia Ca^{++}
  - Putamen, caudate, thalami, dentate nuclei
  - WM of hemispheres, cerebellum
- MR
  - T1 shortening in areas of calcification
  - ± T2/FLAIR WM hyperintensity, cysts
  - Extensive "blooming" on T2* (GRE/SWI)
  - DDx = physiologic Ca^{++}, PHP/PPHP

Seizures and Related Disorders

Seizures can be precipitated by many infective, metabolic, toxic, developmental, neoplastic, or degenerative conditions and can affect numerous different areas of the brain. We will look at the imaging manifestations of two classic disorders, the effects of (1) chronic repeated seizures (mesial temporal sclerosis) and (2) prolonged acute seizure activity (status epilepticus).

We then discuss a recently described abnormality that can be seen with seizures (as well as a variety of other disorders), cytotoxic lesion of the corpus callosum. The section concludes with a consideration of imaging findings in transient global amnesia, which specifically affects the hippocampus.

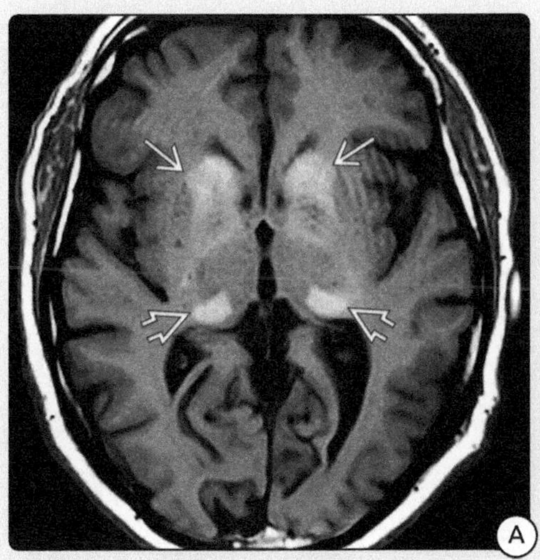

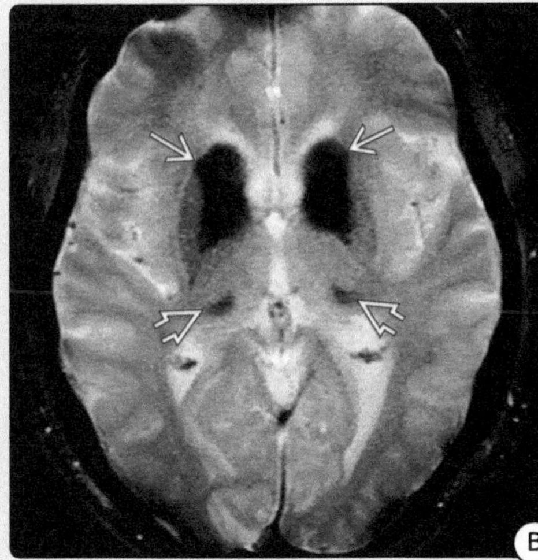

***(32-19A)** Axial T1 MR in a 67-year-old man with epilepsy and known Fahr disease shows symmetric T1 shortening in the basal ganglia ➡ and pulvinars ➡ of both thalami. **(32-19B)** T2* GRE in the same case shows dense susceptibility "blooming" in the basal ganglia ➡ and thalami ➡ corresponding to the areas of T1 shortening.*

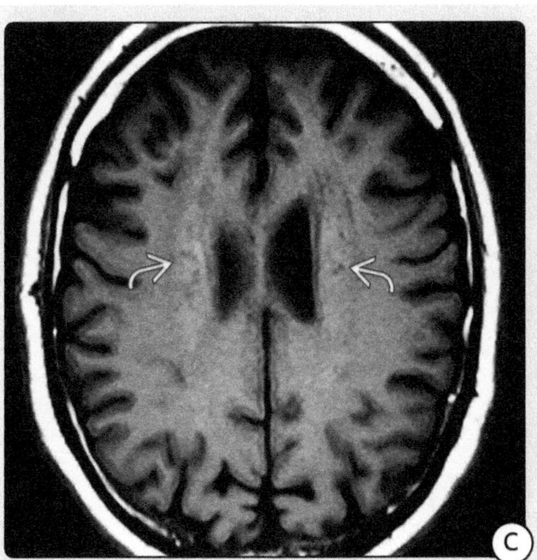

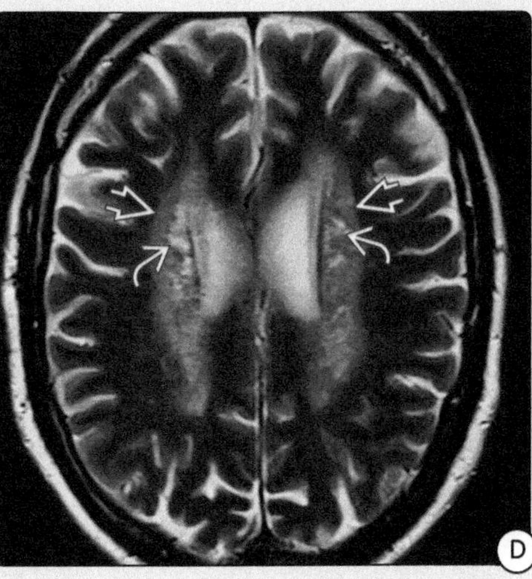

***(32-19C)** More cephalad T1 MR in the same case shows mixed foci of T1 shortening and hypointensity in the caudate nuclei and deep periventricular white matter ➡. **(32-19D)** T2 MR in the same case shows extensive confluent areas of T2 hyperintensity in the deep WM ➡ intermixed with areas of cystic degeneration ➡ and hypointense foci. This pattern of WM cysts with leukodystrophy is characteristic for PDGFB mutation.*

Mesial Temporal (Hippocampal) Sclerosis

Mesial temporal sclerosis (MTS), a.k.a. hippocampal sclerosis (HS) **(32-20)**, is the most common type of localization-related epilepsy and accounts for the majority of patients undergoing temporal lobectomy for seizure disorder.

Etiology and Pathology

A variety of events, such as trauma or infection, may precipitate intractable complex partial seizures **(32-21)**. The end result is MTS. MTS is characterized grossly by atrophy of the hippocampus and adjacent structures. The hippocampal body—particularly the CA1 and CA4 areas—is the most susceptible to hypoxic-ischemic damage, but all regions of the hippocampus can be affected. Approximately 15-20% of cases are bilateral but usually asymmetric.

Clinical Issues

Nearly 10% of all individuals experience a seizure in their lifetime. Two-thirds of these are nonrecurrent febrile/nonfebrile seizures. Peak prevalence is bimodal (< 1 year and > 55 years of age). One-third of patients develop repeated seizures ("epilepsy").

Imaging

MR Findings. Imaging markers of MTS are found in 60-70% of patients with temporal lobe epilepsy (TLE). True coronal IR or 3D SPGR sequences show a shrunken hippocampus with atrophy of the ipsilateral fornix and widening of the adjacent temporal horn &/or choroid fissure. Abnormal T2/FLAIR hyperintensity with obscuration of the internal hippocampal architecture is typical **(32-21)**. MTS typically does not enhance following contrast administration.

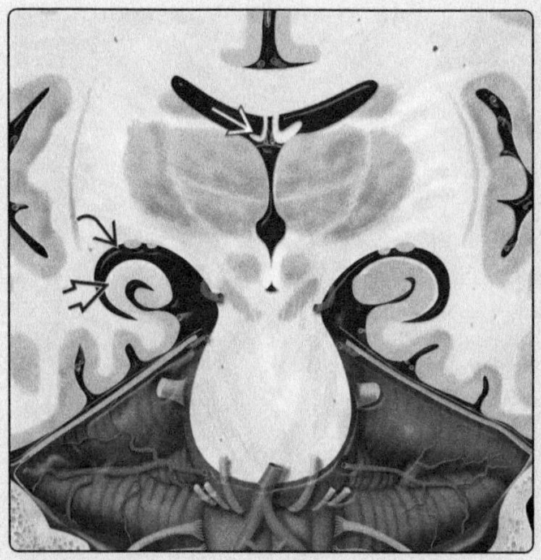

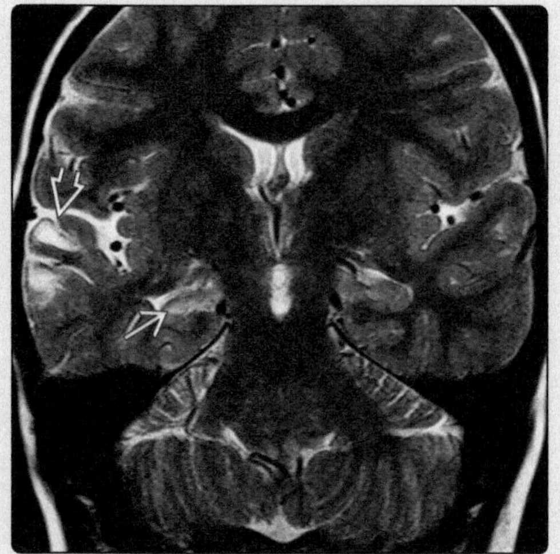

***(32-20)** Coronal graphic depicts typical mesial temporal sclerosis. R hippocampus ⇒ is atrophied, sclerotic with loss of normal internal architecture. R temporal horn ⇒ is enlarged, ipsilateral fornix ➡ is small. **(32-21)** Coronal T2 MR in 27y man with history of intractable epilepsy, remote closed head trauma shows temporal lobe encephalomalacia ➡. Shrunken, hyperintense R hippocampus ➡ is consistent with MTS.*

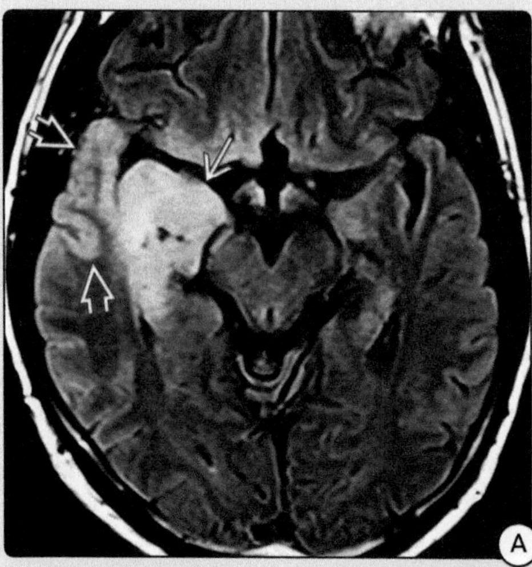

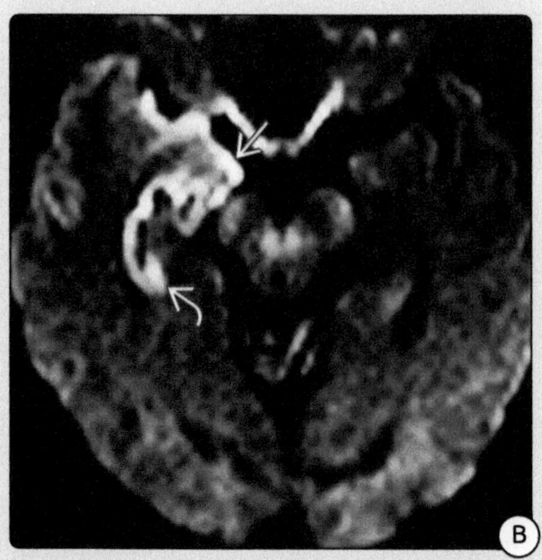

***(32-22A)** Axial FLAIR MR in a 58-year-old man with new onset of drug-refractory seizures shows mass-like hyperintensity in the right medial temporal lobe ➡. Note hyperintensity of the lateral temporal lobe cortex ➡. **(32-22B)** DWI MR shows restricted diffusion in the uncus ➡ and hippocampus ➡ of the right temporal lobe. EEG confirmed temporal lobe epilepsy. Biopsy and resection revealed diffusely infiltrating astrocytoma.*

Nuclear Medicine Findings. FDG PET is one of the most sensitive imaging procedures for diagnosing MTS. Temporal lobe hypometabolism is the typical finding. SPECT shows hyperperfusion in the epileptogenic zone during seizure activity; hypoperfusion in the interictal period is common.

Differential Diagnosis

The major differential diagnosis of MTS is status epilepticus. **Status epilepticus** can be subclinical and may cause transient gyral edema with T2/FLAIR hyperintensity &/or enhancement in the affected cortex as well as the hippocampus.

A **low-grade glioma** (WHO grade II astrocytoma, oligodendroglioma, or oligoastrocytoma) in the temporal lobe can cause drug-resistant TLE **(32-22A)**. Gliomas are usually T2/FLAIR hyperintense and cause mass effect, not volume loss. Cortically based neoplasms associated with TLE include **dysembryoplastic neuroepithelial tumor (DNET)**. DNET is typically a well-demarcated, "bubbly" mass that is often associated with adjacent cortical dysplasia. **Cortical dysplasia** is isointense with GM but frequently causes T2 hyperintensity in the underlying temporal lobe WM.

Cystic-appearing lesions in the temporal lobe that are hyperintense on T2WI include **prominent perivascular spaces, hippocampal sulcus remnants**, and **choroid fissure cysts**. These "leave me alone" lesions all behave like CSF and suppress on FLAIR.

Status Epilepticus

Etiology and Pathophysiology

Status epilepticus (SE) is a prolonged (> 30 minutes), continuously active seizure with EEG-demonstrated seizure activity. SE can be focal or generalized, clinical or subclinical (silent). Generalized convulsive SE is potentially life threatening if not controlled.

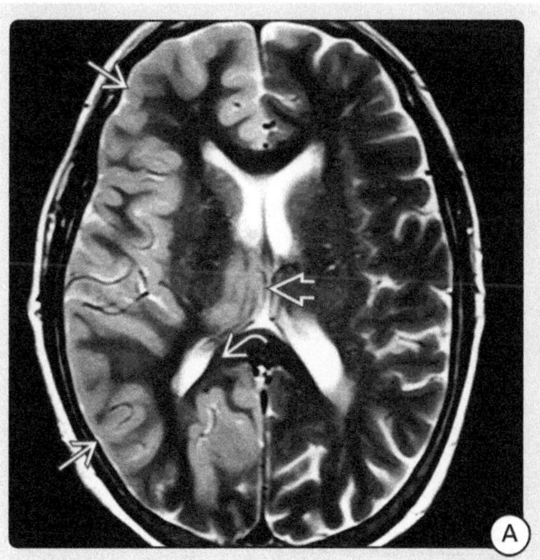

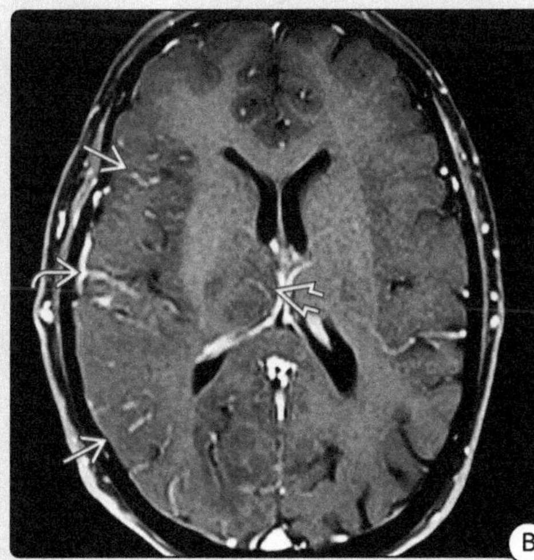

***(32-23A)** T2 MR in a 52-year-old woman in status epilepticus for 24 hours shows diffuse gyral ➡ and right thalamic ➡ swelling and hyperintensity. The WM in the parietal lobe and corpus callosum ➡ is subtly abnormal. **(32-23B)** T1 C+ FS MR shows corresponding cortical, thalamic ➡ hypointensity. Note engorgement of right cortical vessels ➡ and draining veins ➡ compared with the normal left side.*

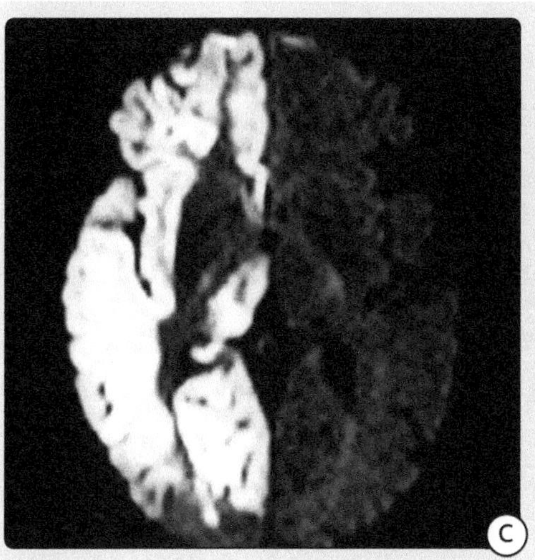

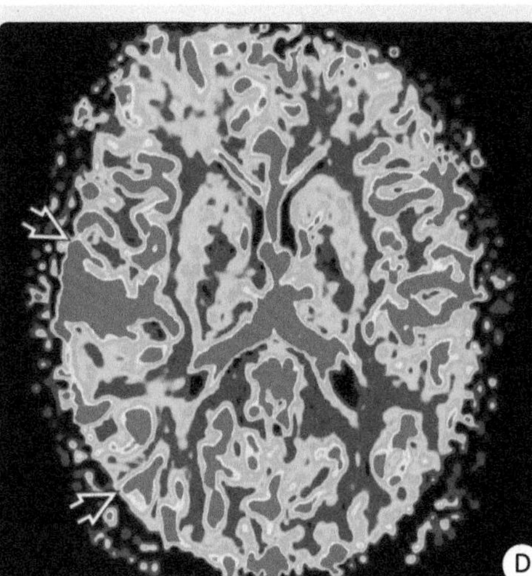

***(32-23C)** DWI MR shows markedly restricted diffusion in the right hemisphere cortex, subcortical WM, and thalamus. **(32-23D)** The rCBV map shows increased blood volume throughout the right hemisphere ➡ compared with the left.*

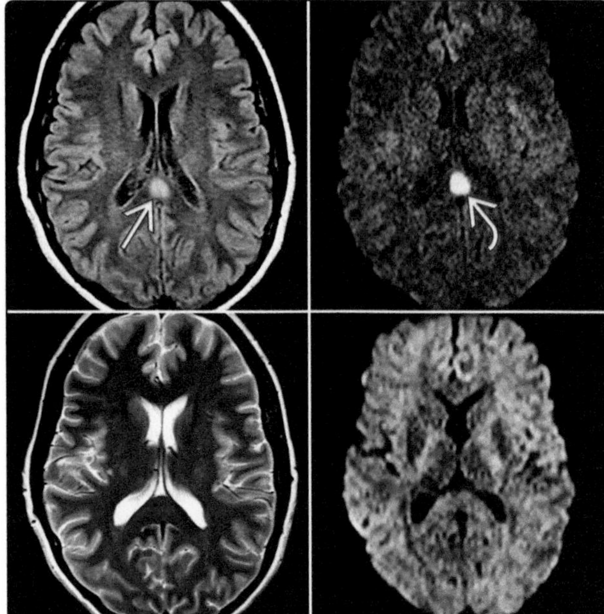

(32-24) A patient taken off antiseizure medications 3 weeks prior to imaging shows round FLAIR hyperintense lesion ➡ in CC splenium (top L) that restricts on DWI ➡ (top R). Repeat scan 2 weeks later shows that the lesions have resolved. This is CLCC.

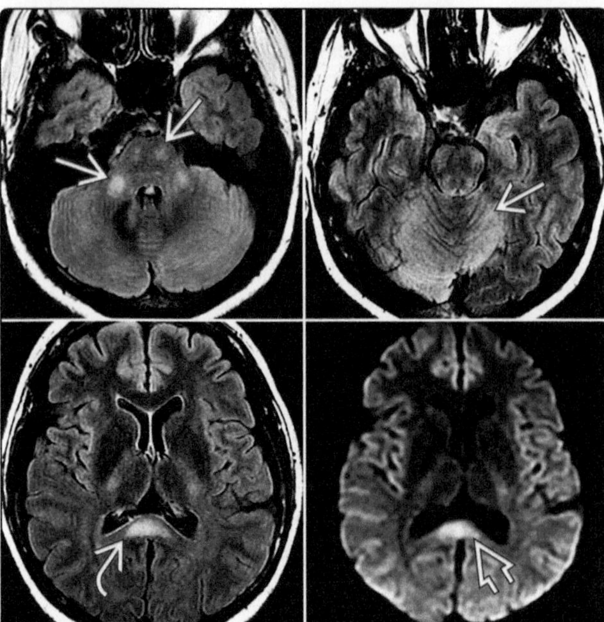

(32-25) Series of FLAIR MR scans in viral encephalitis shows lesions ➡ in pons, peduncles, and cerebellar hemisphere. Corpus callosum splenium lesion ➡ restricts on DWI ➡. This is virus-associated CLCC.

Prolonged ictal activity induces hypermetabolism with increased glucose utilization. Perfusion increases but is still insufficient to match glucose demand. The result is compromised cellular energy production, cytotoxic cell swelling, and vasogenic edema. With prolonged severe seizure activity, the blood-brain barrier may become permeable, permitting leakage of fluid and macromolecules into the extracellular spaces.

Imaging

CT Findings. Initial NECT scans may be normal or show gyral swelling with sulcal effacement, parenchymal hypodensity, and lack of GM-WM differentiation.

MR Findings. Periictal MR shows T2/FLAIR hyperintensity with gyral swelling **(32-23A)**. Subcortical and deep WM is relatively spared. Ipsilateral thalamic hyperintensity is common in SE.

Gyriform enhancement on T1 C+ varies from none to striking **(32-23B)**. DWI may show restricted diffusion with uni- or bilateral hippocampal, thalamic, and cortical lesions **(32-23C)**.

Follow-up scans in severe cases may show permanent abnormalities, including focal brain atrophy, cortical laminar necrosis, and mesial temporal sclerosis.

Differential Diagnosis

The major differential diagnosis of periictal brain swelling is **acute cerebral ischemia-infarction**. Acute cerebral ischemia occurs in a typical vascular territorial distribution, is wedge-shaped (involving both GM and WM), and is positive on DWI *before* T2/FLAIR hyperintensity develops. In ongoing SE, DWI and T2 signal changes typically occur simultaneously.

Cerebritis may cause a T2-/FLAIR-hyperintense mass that restricts on DWI. Cerebritis typically involves the subcortical WM as well as the cortex. Acute onset **of mitochondrial encephalopathy with lactic acidosis and stroke-like episodes** (MELAS) may affect the cortex in a nonvascular distribution.

Cytotoxic Lesions of the Corpus Callosum

Terminology and Etiology

Cytotoxic lesions of the corpus callosum (CLCCs) are acquired lesions that have been associated with a number of different entities. Because they are (1) often reversible and (2) most common in the corpus callosum splenium, they have also been called transient or reversible splenial lesions.

Most investigators believe CLCCs are a cytokinopathy with secondary excitotoxic glutaminergic-associated intracellular edema. The corpus callosum—especially the splenium—has a high density of excitatory amino acid, toxin, and drug receptors and is hence more vulnerable to the development of cytotoxic edema.

Associated Conditions

The most common causes of CLCCs are drug associated. CLCCs were initially reported as a reversible phenomenon associated with the use and subsequent withdrawal of antiepileptic drugs (e.g., carbamazepine). Other drugs, such as metronidazole, have been associated with CLCCs.

The second most common cause of CLCC is infection, usually a viral encephalitis that may also cause a mild febrile encephalopathy. Influenza virus, measles, human herpesvirus-6, West Nile virus, Epstein-Barr virus, varicella-zoster virus, mumps, and adenoviruses have all been reported with CLCCs.

Metabolic derangements, such as hypoglycemia and hypernatremia, acute alcohol poisoning, malnutrition, and vitamin B12 deficiency, are the third most common group of CLCC-associated disorders.

Miscellaneous reported associations include migraine headache, trauma, high-altitude cerebral edema, systemic lupus erythematosus, internal cerebral vein occlusion, Charcot-Marie-Tooth disease, and neoplasms.

Imaging

Typical CLCCs are round to ovoid homogeneous, nonhemorrhagic lesions centered in the corpus callosum splenium. They are mildly hypointense on T1WI, hyperintense on T2/FLAIR, do not enhance, and demonstrate restricted diffusion **(32-24)** **(32-25)**. A variant type of CLCC that involves the entire corpus callosum splenium and extending into the forceps major has been termed the "boomerang" sign. Rarely, CLCCs extend anteriorly from the splenium into the corpus callosum body.

Most CLCCs resolve spontaneously and disappear completely within a few days or weeks. Follow-up imaging studies are typically normal.

CYTOTOXIC LESIONS OF THE CORPUS CALLOSUM

Pathoetiology
- Cytokinopathy with glutamate-induced intracellular edema
- Associated with
  - Seizures
  - Drugs (antiepileptic, metronidazole, etc.)
  - Infections (often but not invariably viral)
  - Metabolic disorders (alcohol, Wernicke, osmotic)
  - Neoplasms, chemotherapy
  - Trauma

Clinical Features
- Usually asymptomatic, incidental
- Typically (but not invariably) resolves spontaneously

Imaging Findings
- Round, ovoid, or "boomerang-shaped" lesion
- Splenium > > > body, central > > eccentric
- T2/FLAIR hyperintense
- Restricts on DWI
- Does not enhance

Transient Global Amnesia

Terminology and Clinical Features

Transient global amnesia (TGA) is a unique neurologic disorder characterized by (1) sudden memory loss without other signs of cognitive or neurologic impairment and (2) complete clinical recovery within 24 hours. The underlying etiology of TGA is unknown.

Most TGA patients are between 50 and 70 years old; TGA is rare under the age of 40. Isolated anterograde amnesia with preserved alertness, attention, and personal identity are consistent features. EEGs are normal in 80-90% of cases with the remainder showing minor nonepileptiform activity. Symptoms resolve in 24 hours or less. Recurrences are relatively rare.

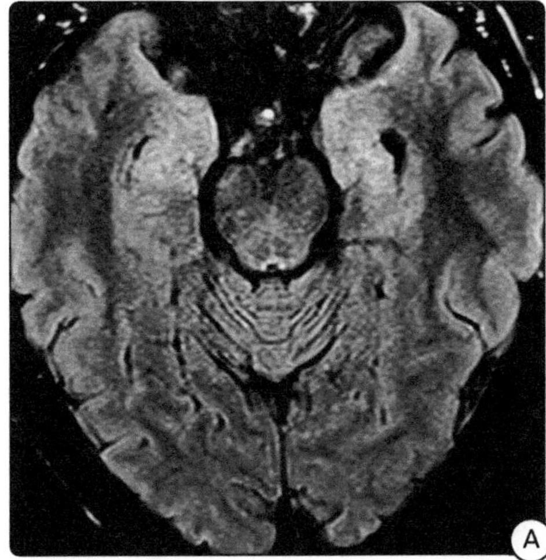

(32-26A) Axial FLAIR MR in a 70-year-old woman with sudden onset of confusion and amnesia is normal.

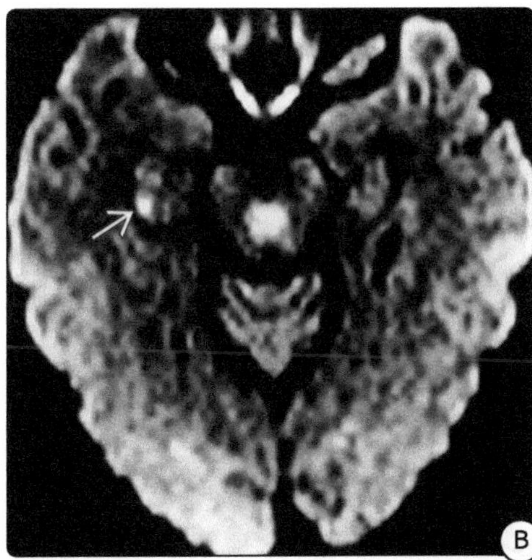

(32-26B) DWI MR shows small focus of restricted diffusion in the right hippocampus ➡. Symptoms resolved; follow-up scan was normal. This is TGA.

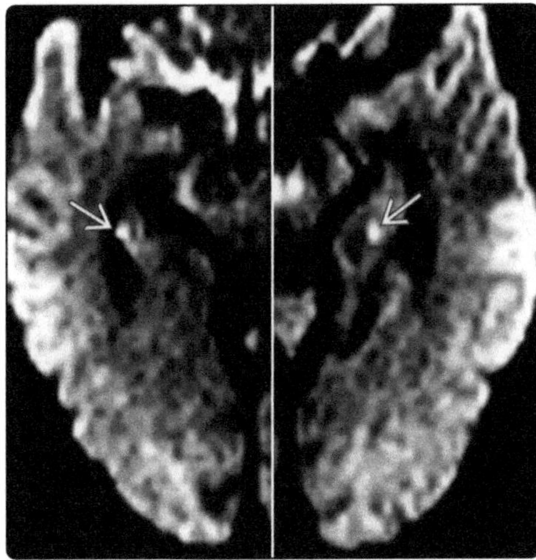

(32-27) DWI MR in 65-year-old man with sudden anterograde memory loss shows foci of restricted diffusion in both hippocampi ➡. This is TGA.

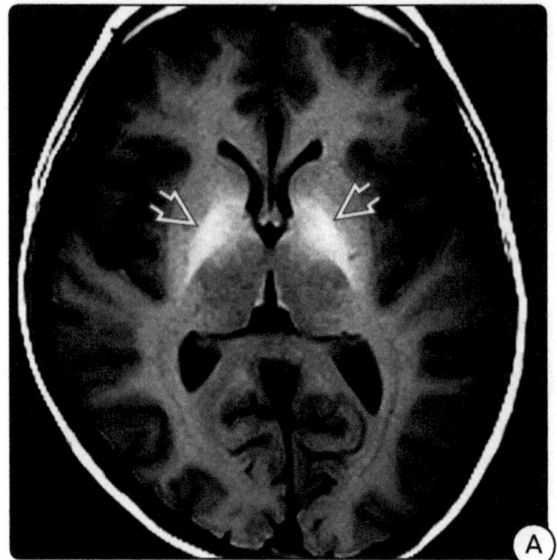

(32-28A) *T1 MR in chronic liver failure with acute onset of encephalopathy shows striking, symmetric T1 shortening in the globi pallidi ⇨.*

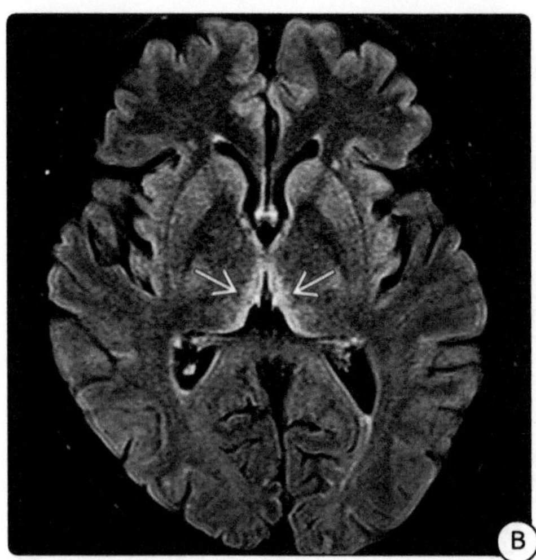

(32-28B) *Axial FLAIR MR in the same case shows symmetric hyperintensity ⇨ in the medial thalami around the 3rd ventricle.*

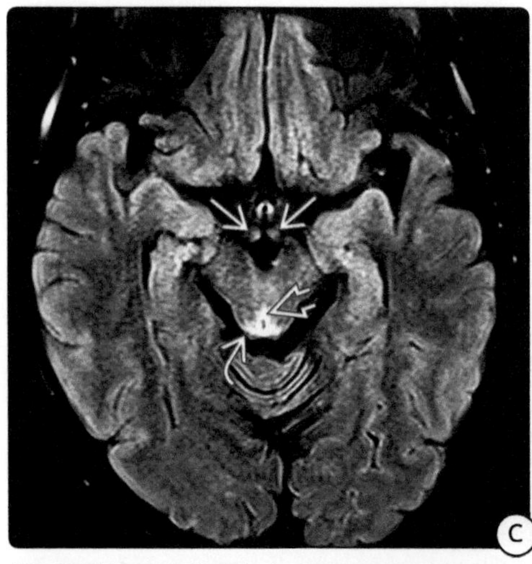

(32-28C) *Hyperintensity in periaqueductal gray ⇨, tectum ⇨, both mammillary bodies ⇨. Acute WE superimposed on chronic liver failure.*

Imaging

CT scans are invariably normal, and standard MR sequences (T2/FLAIR) typically show no abnormalities. DWI shows punctate or dot-like foci of restricted diffusion in the CA1 area of the hippocampus, along the lateral aspect of the hippocampus just medial to the temporal horn. Lesions can be single (55%) **(32-26)** or multiple (45%), unilateral (50-55%), or bilateral (45-50%) **(32-27)**. The body of the hippocampus is most commonly involved followed by the head.

DWI abnormalities in TGA increase significantly with time following symptom onset. Between 0-6 hours, 34% show foci of restricted diffusion. This increases to 62% in patients imaged between 6 and 12 hours and to 67% of patients between 12 and 24 hours. By day three, 75% of patients demonstrate abnormalities. Follow-up scans typically show complete resolution by day 10.

Differential Diagnosis

The two major differential diagnoses of TGA are stroke and seizure. Their exclusive location in the hippocampus mitigates against typical embolic infarcts. However, acute **isolated punctate hippocampal infarction** can be indistinguishable from TGA based on imaging studies alone.

Seizures can cause transient diffusion restriction but typically involve moderate to large areas of the cortex. The dot-like lesions in TGA are distinctly different from the cortical gyriform ribbons of restricted diffusion seen in **status epilepticus** and the posterior-predominant lesions seen in **hypoglycemic seizures**.

Miscellaneous Disorders

Hepatic Encephalopathy

Hepatic encephalopathy (HE) is an important cause of morbidity and mortality in patients with severe liver disease. HE is classified into three main groups: Minimal HE (a.k.a. latent or subclinical HE), chronic HE, and acute HE.

Although the precise mechanisms responsible for HE remain elusive, elevated blood and brain ammonia levels have been strongly implicated in the pathogenesis of HE.

Ammonia is metabolized primarily in the liver via the urea cycle. When the metabolic capacity of the liver is severely diminished, ammonia detoxification is compromised. Nitrogenous wastes accumulate and easily cross the blood-brain barrier. Ammonia and its principal metabolite, glutamine, interfere with brain mitochondrial metabolism and energy production. Increased osmolarity in the astrocytes causes swelling and loss of autoregulation and results in cerebral edema.

We first discuss chronic HE, then focus on the acute manifestations of liver failure and its most fulminant manifestation, hyperammonemic encephalopathy.

Chronic Hepatic Encephalopathy

Chronic HE is a potentially reversible clinical syndrome that occurs in the setting of chronic severe liver dysfunction. Both children and adults are affected. Most patients have a longstanding history of cirrhosis, often accompanied by portal hypertension and portosystemic shunting.

NECT scans are typically normal or show mild volume loss. In the vast majority of cases, MR scans show bilateral symmetric hyperintensity in the globi pallidi and substantia nigra on T1WI, probably secondary to manganese deposition **(32-28A)**. T1 hyperintensity has also been reported in the pituitary gland and hypothalamus but is less common. The T1 hyperintensity in the striatopallidal system may decrease or even disappear completely after liver transplantation.

Acute-on-Chronic Liver Failure

Acute-on-chronic liver failure (ACLF) is acute deterioration in liver function in an individual with preexisting chronic liver disease, commonly cirrhosis. Hepatic and extrahepatic organ failure—often renal dysfunction—is common in ACLF and is associated with substantial short-term mortality. Precipitating factors include bacterial and viral infections, alcoholic hepatitis, and surgery. In > 40% of cases, no precipitating event is identified.

Changes in consciousness as a result of acute HE are common and range from mild confusion to coma. Imaging reflects a combination of chronic liver disease and superimposed changes of acute liver dysfunction, such as hyperammonemia with cortical edema or Wernicke encephalopathy **(32-28)**.

Acute Hepatic Encephalopathy and Hyperammonemia

Terminology. Acute HE (AHE) is caused by hyperammonemia, which can be both hepatic *and* nonhepatic. Hyperammonemia, systemic inflammation (including sepsis, bacterial translocation, and insulin resistance), and oxidative stress are key factors mediating clinical deterioration.

Etiology. Although acute hepatic decompensation is the most common cause of hyperammonemia in adults, drug toxicity is also an important consideration. Valproate, asparaginase, acetaminophen, and chemotherapy have all been implicated in the development of hyperammonemic encephalopathy. Other important nonhepatic causes of hyperammonemia include hematologic disease, parenteral nutrition, bone marrow transplantation, urinary tract infection, and fulminant viral hepatitis.

Inherited urea cycle abnormalities or organic acidemias, such as citrullinemia and ornithine transcarbamylase deficiency, are other potential causes of acute hyperammonemic encephalopathy (see Chapter 31).

Imaging. Bilaterally symmetric T2/FLAIR hyperintensity in the insular cortex, cingulate gyri, and basal ganglia is typical, as is relative sparing of the perirolandic and occipital regions (see Fig. 31-34). The hemispheric WM is typically spared. AHE restricts strongly on DWI.

Differential Diagnosis. The major differential diagnoses of AHE/hyperammonemia are hypoxic-ischemic encephalopathy, hypoglycemia, status epilepticus, and Wernicke encephalopathy. **Hypoxic-ischemic encephalopathy** may be difficult to distinguish from AHE on imaging alone. Symmetric involvement of the insular cortex and cingulate gyri should suggest AHE.

Hypoglycemia is a common comorbidity in patients with chronic HE. Acute hypoglycemia typically affects the parietooccipital GM, whereas early AHE may spare the posterior cortex. Serum glucose is low, and ammonia is normal. **Status epilepticus** is usually unilateral, and, although the thalamus is often involved, the basal ganglia are generally spared. **Wernicke encephalopathy** affects the medial thalami, mammillary bodies, tectal plate, and periaqueductal GM. The cerebral cortex and basal ganglia are less commonly involved.

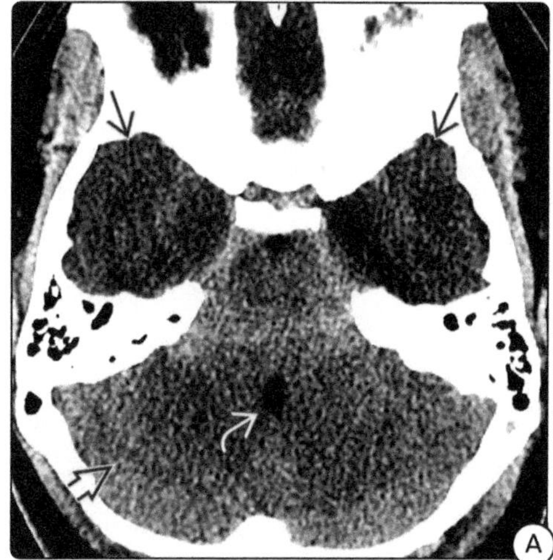

***(32-29A)** NECT of heatstroke 6 days after admission shows swollen temporal lobes ➡, cerebellum ➡, compressed 4th ventricle ➡.*

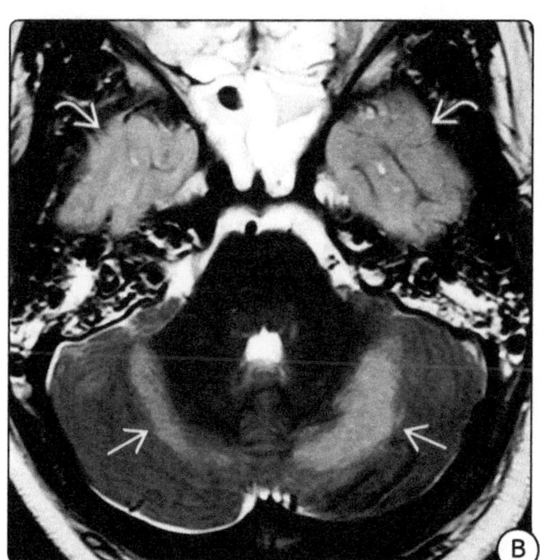

***(32-29B)** T2 MR shows diffuse swelling and hyperintensity of both temporal lobes ➡. The cerebellar white matter is also hyperintense ➡.*

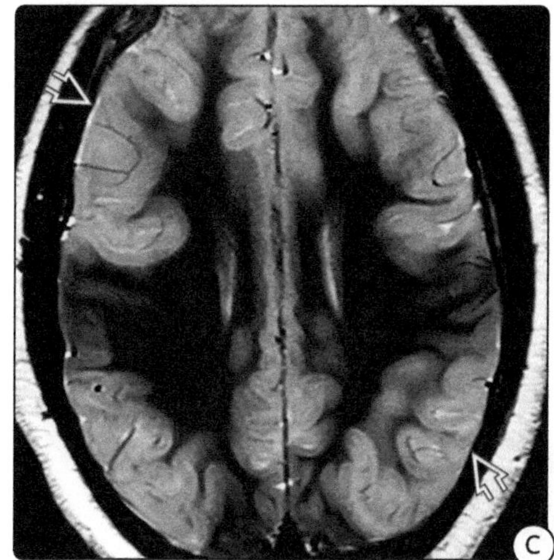

***(32-29C)** More cephalad T2 MR shows diffuse cortical hyperintensity ➡. This is heat stroke. (Courtesy P. Hudgins, MD.)*

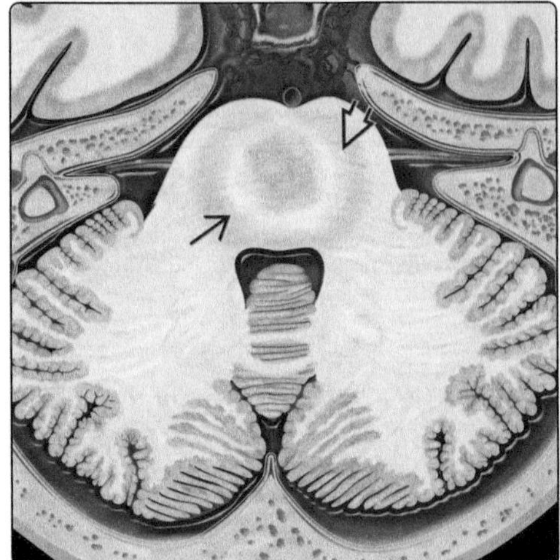
(32-30) Graphic shows acute osmotic central pontine demyelination . Note sparing of peripheral WM, traversing corticospinal tracts .

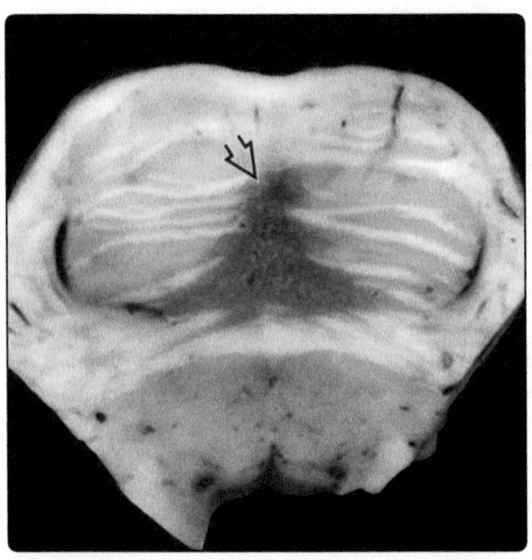
(32-31) Autopsied remote CPM shows triangular shape of brown discolored demyelination in the central pons. (From Agamanolis DP, op cit.)

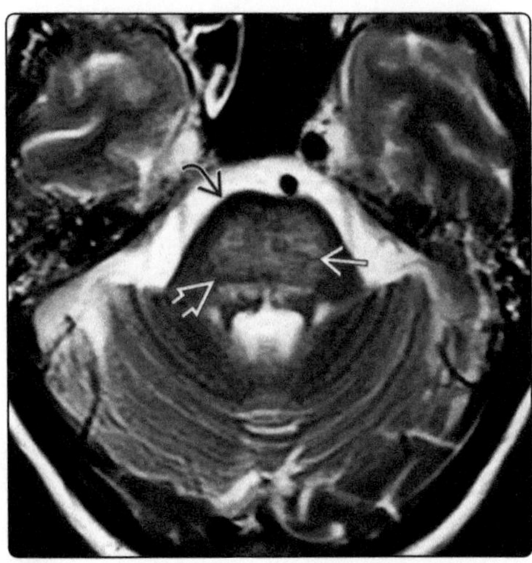
(32-32) T2 MR shows CPM . The peripheral pons is spared as are the corticospinal tracts and transverse pontine fibers .

Hyperthermic Encephalopathy

Acute heat-related illness is a spectrum of disorders that ranges from minor heat cramps and heat exhaustion to life-threatening heat stroke. It can cause delirium, seizures, and coma.

Heat stroke is defined clinically as a core body temperature exceeding 40°C. Risk factors include high ambient temperature and humidity, dehydration, alcohol abuse, and some medications (antihypertensive or psychiatric). Both ends of the age spectrum—infants and the very old—are especially susceptible. Morbidity and mortality in patients suffering from heat stroke range between 10% and 50%.

Purkinje cells in the cerebellum are especially susceptible to thermic injury. MR may demonstrate T2/FLAIR hyperintensity in the cerebellum, basal ganglia/thalami, hippocampus, and cerebral cortex **(32-29)**. Restricted diffusion in the affected areas is common.

Osmotic Encephalopathy

The most common hypoosmolar state is hyponatremia, and the most common osmotic encephalopathy is **osmotic demyelination syndrome** (ODS).

Terminology and Etiology

ODS was formerly called **central pontine myelinolysis** (when it affected only the pons) or, if it involved both the pons and **extrapontine myelinolysis**, osmotic myelinolysis. ODS is now the preferred term.

ODS occurs with osmotic stress, classically occurring when wide fluxes in serum sodium levels are induced by too-rapid correction of hyponatremia. ODS occurs with other disorders, such as organ transplantation (particularly liver), hemodialysis, and correction of hypoglycemia.

Pathology

ODS is traditionally considered primarily a pontine lesion **(32-30) (32-31)**. However, multifocal involvement is common and typical. Only 50% of ODS cases have isolated pontine lesions. In 30% of cases, myelinolytic foci occur both outside and inside the pons. The basal ganglia and hemispheric WM are common sites. WM demyelination is exclusively extrapontine in 20-25% of cases.

Other parts of the CNS that can be involved in ODS include the cerebellum (especially the middle cerebellar peduncles), basal ganglia, thalami, lateral geniculate body, and hemispheric WM. Some ODS cases involve the cortex.

Grossly, the central pons is abnormally soft and exhibits a rhomboid or trident-shaped area of grayish tan discoloration. The peripheral pons is spared. Laminar cortical necrosis can occur in ODS, either primarily or in association with hypoxia or anoxia. In such cases, the affected cortex appears soft and pale.

Clinical Issues

ODS is rare. It can occur at any age but is most common in middle-aged patients (peak = 30-60 years). Pediatric patients with ODS typically have diabetes or anorexia. The most common presenting symptoms of ODS are altered mental status and seizures. ODS outcome varies significantly, ranging from complete recovery to coma, "locked in" syndrome and death.

ODS may also occur (1) in normonatremic patients and (2) independent of changes in serum sodium!

Imaging

Imaging findings in ODS typically lag one or two weeks behind clinical symptoms.

CT Findings. NECT scans can be normal or show hypodensity in the affected areas, particularly the central pons **(32-33A)**.

MR Findings. Standard MR sequences may be normal in the first several days. Eventually, ODS becomes hypointense on T1WI **(32-33B)** and hyperintense on T2/FLAIR **(32-33C)**. The lesions are typically well demarcated and symmetric. Pontine ODS is often round or sometimes trident-shaped **(32-31)**. The peripheral pons, corticospinal tracts, and transverse pontine fibers are spared **(32-32)**. Involvement of the basal ganglia and hemispheric WM or cortex is seen in at least 1/2 of all cases ("extrapontine myelinolysis") **(32-35)**.

DWI is the most sensitive sequence for acute ODS and can demonstrate restricted diffusion when other sequences are normal **(32-34D)** **(32-35)**. DTI shows disruption of central pontine WM with sparing of peripheral, transverse tracts.

In ~ 20% of acute ODS cases, enhancement in midline and rim of affected region may form a distinct trident-shaped lesion. Late acute or subacute ODS lesions may demonstrate moderate confluent enhancement on T1 C+ **(32-34)**. Enhancement typically resolves within a few weeks after onset.

Differential Diagnosis

The major differential diagnosis of "central" ODS is pontine ischemia-infarction. **Basilar perforating artery infarcts** involve the surface of the pons and are usually asymmetric. **Demyelinating disease** can involve the pons but is rarely symmetric.

The major differential diagnosis of extrapontine ODS with basal ganglia &/or cortical involvement is metabolic disease. **Hypertensive encephalopathy** (PRES) can involve the pons but does not spare the peripheral WM tracts. The basal ganglia are affected in **Wilson disease** and **mitochondrial disorders**, but the pons is less commonly involved.

OSMOTIC DEMYELINATION SYNDROMES

Terminology, Etiology
- ODS (formerly pontine, extrapontine myelinolysis)
- Serum hypotonicity → cells lose osmoles, shrink
- Oligodendrocytes especially vulnerable to osmotic stress
- Note: Can occur without serum sodium disturbances!

Location
- 50% pons (spares periphery, transverse pontine tracts)
- 30% pons + extrapontine (basal ganglia, thalami, WM)
- 20-25% exclusively extrapontine
- ± cortical laminar necrosis

Imaging
- Hypointense on T1, hyperintense on T2
    - "Trident" sign on T2WI, T1 C+ in acute ODS
- May restrict on DWI

Selected References: The complete reference list is available on the Expert Consult™ eBook version included with purchase.

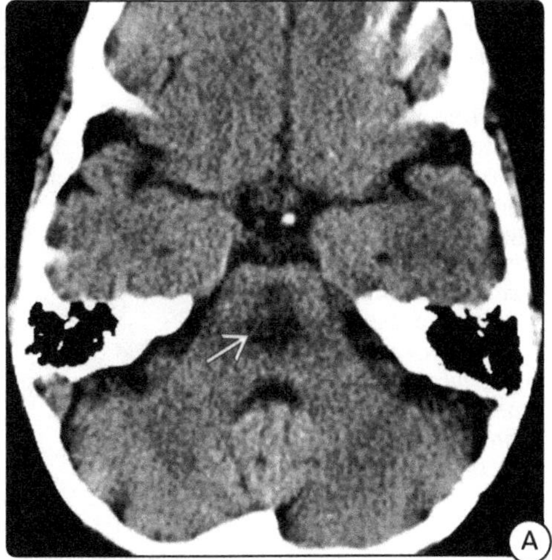

***(32-33A)** NECT in a 37-year-old woman with osmotic demyelination syndrome shows a triangular central pontine hypodensity ➡.*

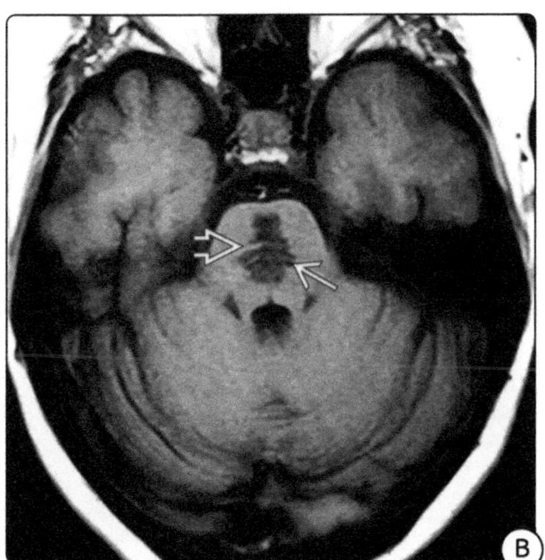

***(32-33B)** T1 MR shows that the lesion is hypointense ➡. Transverse pontine fibers are spared, seen here as lines of preserved brain ➡.*

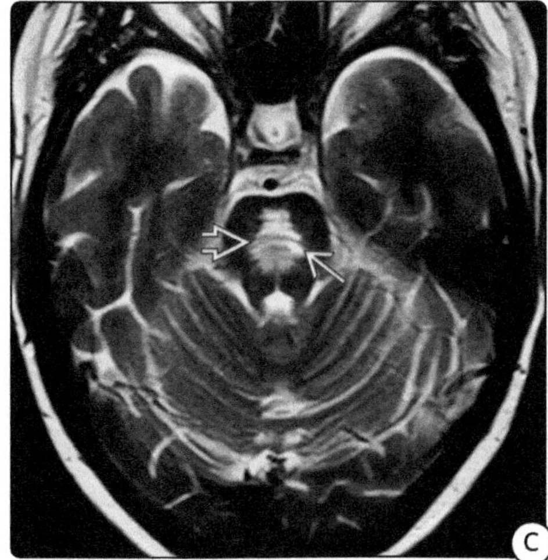

***(32-33C)** T2 MR through the upper pons shows the lesion ➡ with "stripes" of preserved myelinated transverse pontine tracts ➡.*

(32-34A) Sagittal T1 MR shows a 44-year-old alcoholic man with vomiting, seizures, and acutely altered mental status. The central pons is slightly swollen and hypointense, whereas the peripheral pons is spared. (32-34B) T2 MR in the same patient shows symmetric central hyperintensity with sparing of the peripheral pons and corticospinal tracts.

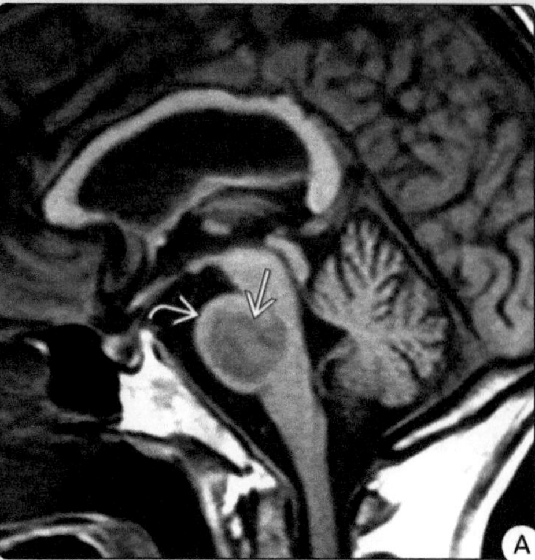

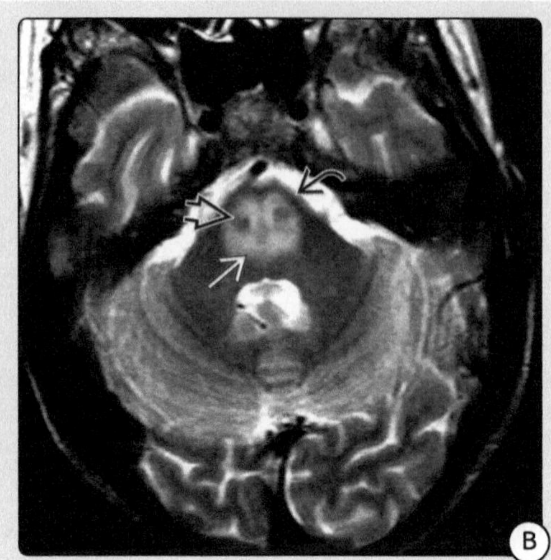

(32-34C) Axial T1 C+ MR in the same patient shows patchy but symmetric enhancement in the affected WM with sparing of the corticospinal tracts. (32-34D) DWI MR in the same patient shows acutely restricted diffusion. ODS with acute demyelination can both enhance and restrict.

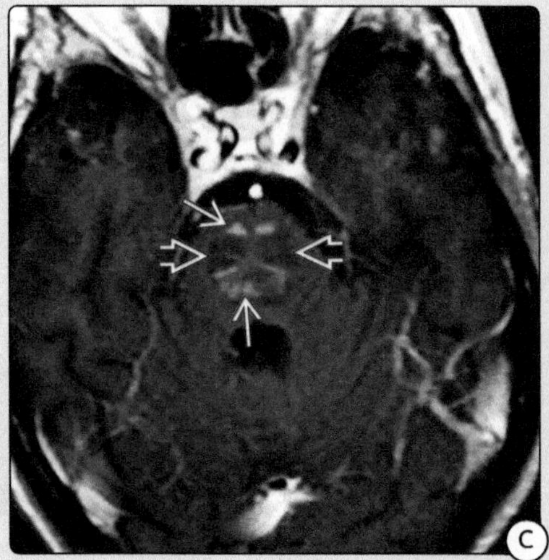

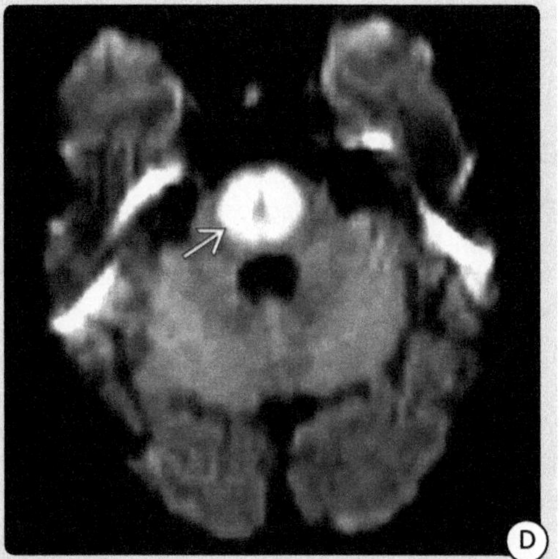

(32-35A) A variant case of ODS is illustrated by this axial FLAIR MR in a 56-year-old man with confusion after rapid correction of hyponatremia. Note hyperintensity in the basal ganglia and both thalami. (32-35B) DWI MR shows that the cortex is also diffusely but somewhat asymmetrically affected. Cortical laminar necrosis can sometimes be seen in ODS.

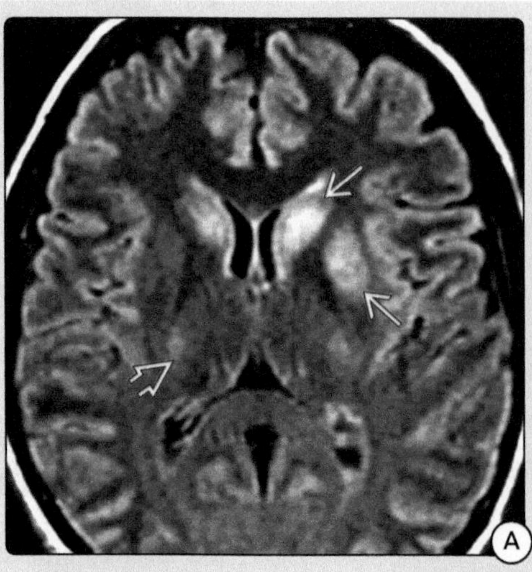

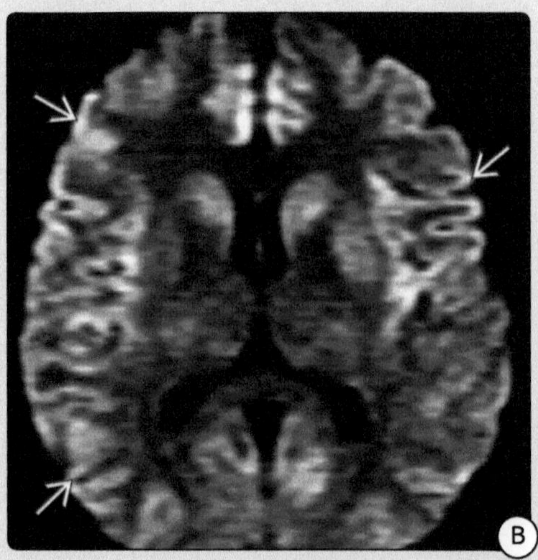

Dementias and Brain Degenerations

One in three adults over 85 years old suffers from Alzheimer disease (AD) or other forms of dementia. New treatments to slow progression of this devastating disease are being developed; most rely on early identification of at-risk individuals before clinical symptoms emerge.

Innovative technologies, such as tau imaging and MR connectivity analyses, represent new, exciting frontiers in the early identification of dementing disorders. While some illustrative case examples are included here, the overall purpose of this chapter is to discuss normal and abnormal brain aging changes on imaging modalities that are generally available to practicing neuroradiologists.

After our discussion of the normal aging brain, we turn our attention to dementias and brain degenerative disorders. **Dementia** is a loss of brain function that affects memory, thinking, language, judgment, and behavior. Dementia has many causes but most often occurs secondary to degenerative processes in the brain.

Neurodegeneration occurs when neurons in specific parts of the brain, spinal cord, or peripheral nerves die. Although dementia always involves brain degeneration, not all neurodegenerative disorders are dementing illnesses. Some neurodegenerative disorders (e.g., Parkinson disease) can have associated dementia, but most do not.

The Normal Aging Brain

Introduction to the Normal Aging Brain

Age-related changes take place in virtually all parts of the brain and occur at all ages. Understanding the biology and imaging of normal aging is a prerequisite to understanding the pathobiology of degenerative brain diseases.

Terminology

The term **"normal aging brain"** as used in this chapter refers to the spectrum of normal age-related neuroimaging findings as delineated by longitudinal population-based studies, such as the Rotterdam Scan Study (RSS).

Genetics

Genetic factors definitely affect brain aging and contribute to age-related cognitive decline. Apolipoprotein E (specifically *APOE*-ε4) and other risk-

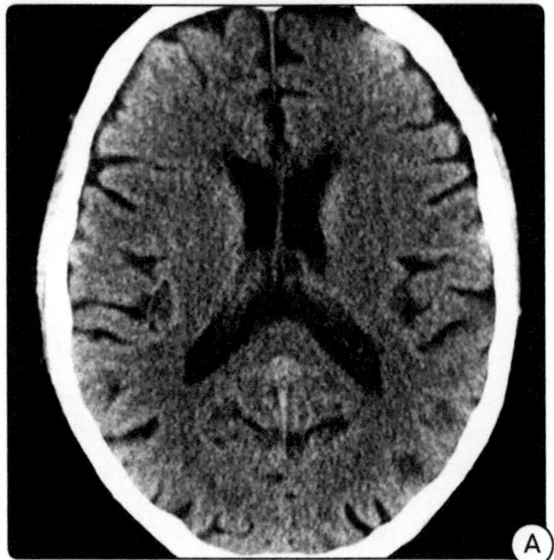

(33-1A) NECT in a 71-year-old cognitively intact man shows mildly enlarged ventricles and sulci with normal-appearing white matter.

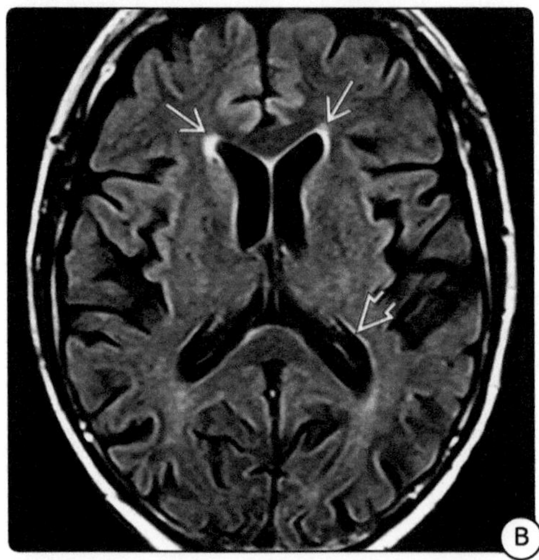

(33-1B) FLAIR MR in the same patient shows frontal periventricular "caps" ➡ and a thin hyperintense rim around the lateral ventricles ➡.

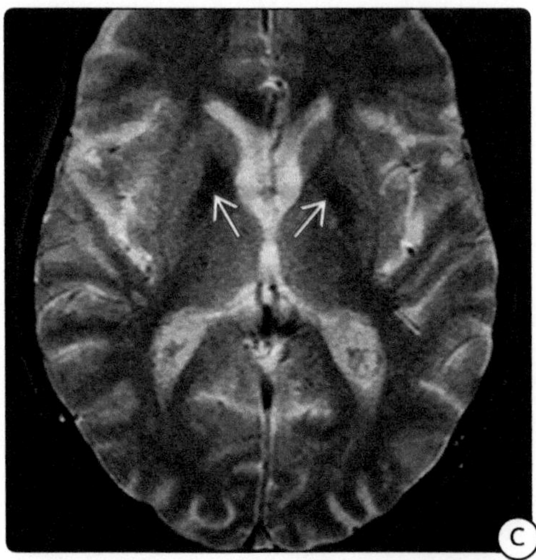

(33-1C) T2* GRE shows hypointensity in GPs ➡ but not in putamina or thalami. No microbleeds are present. Normal "successfully" aging brain.

associated single-nucleotide polymorphisms are genetic variants that are robustly associated with brain pathology on MR. Epigenetic dysregulation has also been identified as a pivotal player in aging as well as age-related cognitive decline and degenerative disorders.

Pathology

Gross Pathology. Overall brain volume decreases with advancing age and is indicated by a relative increase in the size of the CSF spaces. Widened sulci with proportionate enlargement of the ventricles are common. Although minor thinning of the cortical mantle occurs with aging, the predominant neuroanatomic changes occur in the subcortical white matter (WM).

Microscopic Features. The subcortical WM demonstrates decreased numbers of myelinated fibers, increased extracellular space, and gliosis. Perivascular (Virchow-Robin) spaces in the subcortical and basal ganglia enlarge.

Three histologic markers are associated with dementias: **Senile plaques (SPs), neurofibrillary tangles (NFTs)**, and **Lewy bodies**. **SPs** are extracellular amyloid deposits that accumulate in cerebral gray matter. Nearly 1/2 of cognitively intact older individuals demonstrate moderate or frequent SP density.

NFTs are caused by tau aggregations within neurons. **Lewy bodies** are intraneuronal clumps of α-synuclein and ubiquitin proteins. They are found in 5-10% of cognitively intact individuals.

Clinical Issues

Although the incidence of dementias increases dramatically with aging, nearly 2/3 of patients over 85 years of age remain neurologically intact and cognitively normal.

Imaging the Normal Aging Brain

Imaging plays an increasingly central role in evaluating older patients for "altered mental status" and early signs of dementia.

CT Findings

Screening NECT scans are often obtained in older patients for nonspecific indications, such as "altered mental status." The normal aging brain demonstrates mildly enlarged ventricles and widened sulci on NECT scans **(33-1A)**. A few scattered patchy WM hypodensities are common, but confluent subcortical hypointensities, especially around the atria of the lateral ventricles, are a marker of arteriolosclerosis ("microvascular disease").

MR Findings

T1WI. T1-weighted images show mild but symmetric ventricular enlargement and proportionate prominence of the subarachnoid spaces.

T2/FLAIR. White matter hyperintensities (WMHs) and lacunar infarcts on T2/FLAIR scans are highly prevalent in the elderly. They are associated with cardiovascular risk factors, such as diabetes and hyperlipidemia. "Successfully" aging brains may demonstrate a few scattered nonconfluent WMHs (a reasonable number is one WMH per decade, but the prevalence rises more steeply after age 50).

Perivascular spaces increase in prevalence and size with aging and are seen on T2WI as well-delineated round, ovoid, or linear CSF-like collections in the basal ganglia, subcortical WM, midbrain, etc. (see Chapter 28) **(33-1)**. PVSs suppress completely on FLAIR. Between 25% and 30% may display a thin, smooth, hyperintense rim. Lacunar infarcts typically demonstrate an irregular hyperintense rim around the lesions.

FLAIR scans in normal older patients demonstrate a smooth, thin, periventricular hyperintense rim around the lateral ventricles that probably represents increased extracellular interstitial fluid in the subependymal WM **(33-1B)**. A "cap" of hyperintensity around the frontal horns is common and normal.

T2* (GRE, SWI). Ferric iron deposition in the basal ganglia increases with age and is best demonstrated on T2* sequences. Hypointensity on T2* scans is normal in the medial globus pallidus **(33-1C)**. Putaminal hypointensity is typically less prominent until the eighth decade. The caudate nucleus shows a scarce iron load at any age. The thalamus does not normally exhibit any hypointensity on T2* sequences.

Microbleeds on T2* scans are common in the aging brain. GRE and SWI sequences demonstrate cerebral microbleeds in 20% of patients over age 60 years and 1/3 of patients aged 80 years and older. Although common and therefore *statistically* "normal," microbleeds are not characteristic of *successful* brain aging. Basal ganglia and cerebellar microbleeds are usually indicative of chronic hypertensive encephalopathy. Lobar and cortical microbleeds are typical of amyloid angiopathy and are associated with worse cognitive performance.

Differential Diagnosis

The correlation between cognitive performance and brain imaging is complex and difficult to determine. Therefore, the major differential diagnosis of a normal aging brain is **mild cognitive impairment** and early "preclinical" **AD**. WMHs are markers of microvascular disease, so there is considerable overlap between normal brains and those with **subcortical arteriosclerotic encephalopathy**.

Dementias

The three most common dementias are **Alzheimer disease (AD), dementia with Lewy bodies**, and **vascular dementia (VaD)**. Together, they account for the vast majority of all dementia cases. Less frequent causes include **frontotemporal lobar degeneration** (formerly known as Pick disease) and **corticobasal degeneration**. It can be difficult to distinguish between the various dementia syndromes because clinical features frequently overlap and so-called mixed dementias are common.

Alzheimer Disease

Alzheimer disease (AD) remains the only leading cause of death for which no disease-modifying treatment currently exists and age is by far the greatest risk factor. At least 1/3 of older individuals in the USA will die with dementia, largely due to AD.

Terminology

AD is a progressive neurodegenerative condition that leads to cognitive decline, impaired ability to perform the activities of daily living, and a range of behavioral and psychologic conditions.

There is increasing evidence that AD represents a continuum of severity. The pathogenic process is prolonged and may extend over several decades. A prodromal **preclinical/asymptomatic disease** (i.e., pathology is present, but cognition remains intact) may exist for years before evidence of **mild cognitive impairment** (MCI) develops.

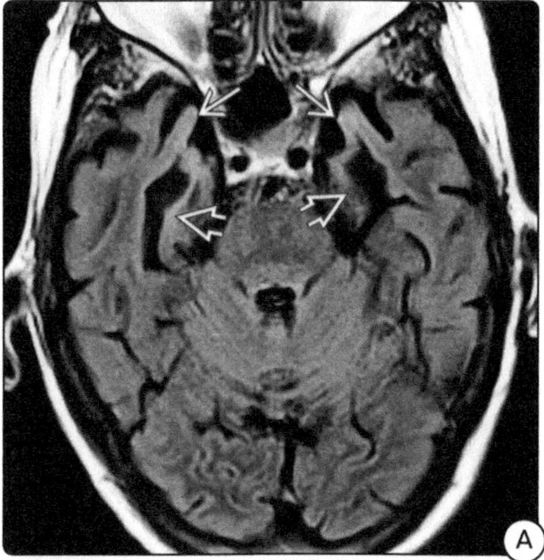

***(33-2A)** FLAIR in 67yF with clinically definite AD shows markedly severely shrunken, hyperintense hippocampi ➡ and medial temporal lobes ➡.*

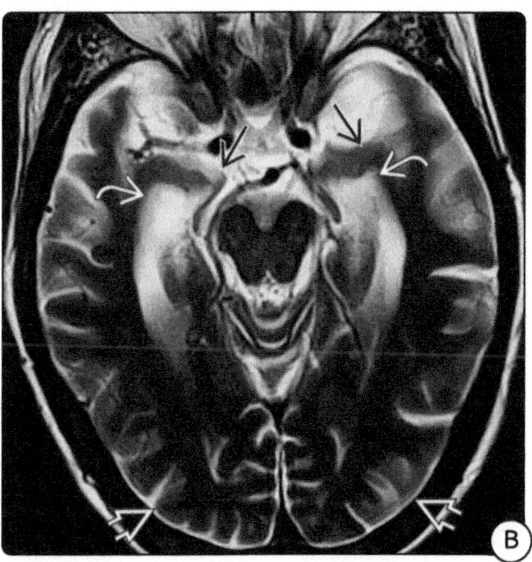

***(33-2B)** T2 MR shows enlarged temporal horns ➡, volume loss in the temporal lobes ➡, and normal-appearing occipital lobes ➡.*

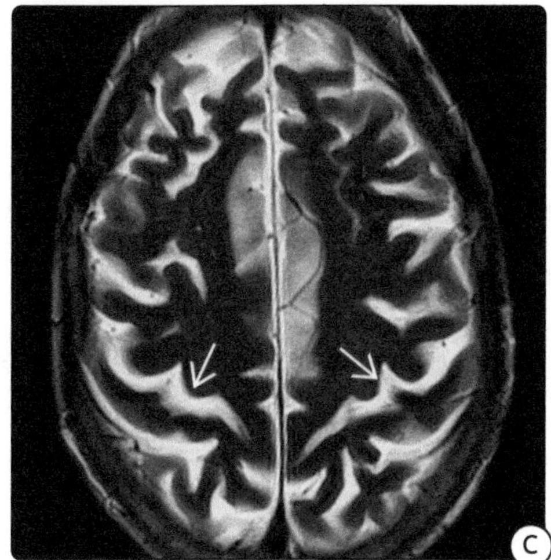

***(33-2C)** Scan through the upper cerebral hemispheres shows symmetric parietal lobe atrophy with enlarged central sulci ➡.*

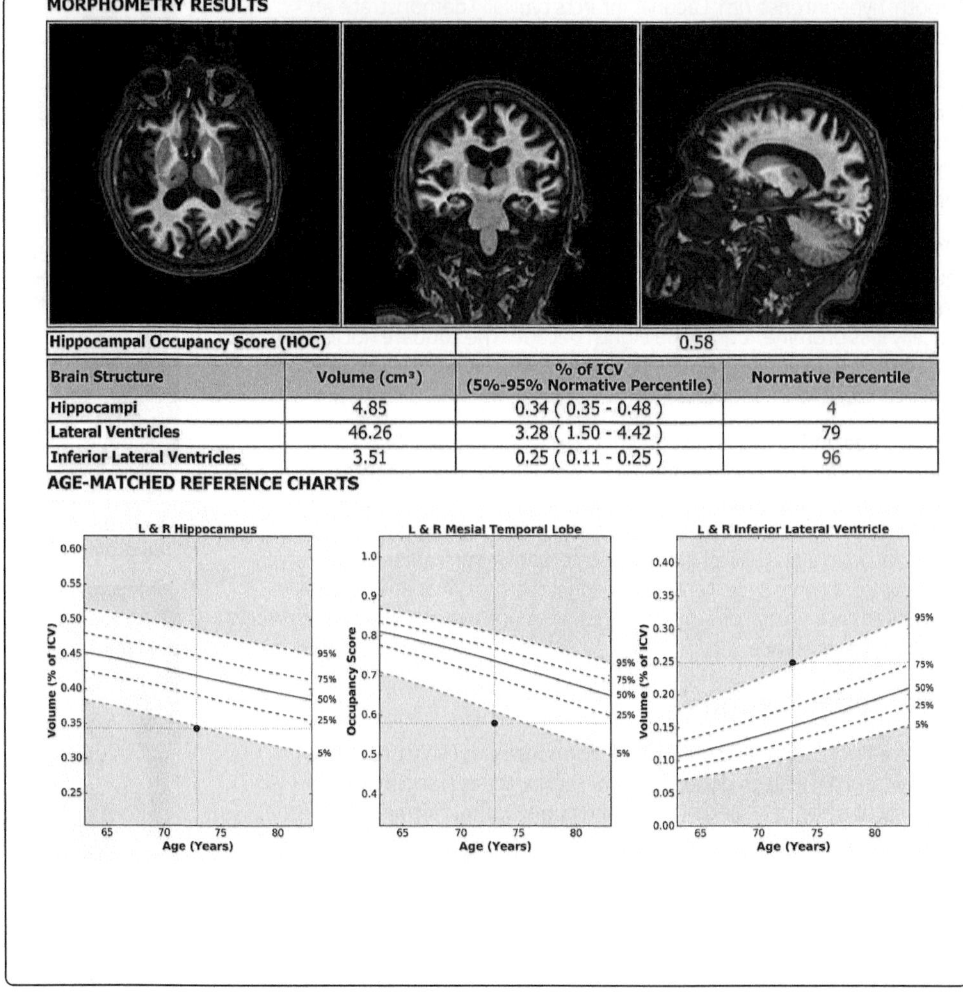
MORPHOMETRY RESULTS

Hippocampal Occupancy Score (HOC)		0.58	
Brain Structure	**Volume (cm³)**	**% of ICV (5%-95% Normative Percentile)**	**Normative Percentile**
Hippocampi	4.85	0.34 (0.35 - 0.48)	4
Lateral Ventricles	46.26	3.28 (1.50 - 4.42)	79
Inferior Lateral Ventricles	3.51	0.25 (0.11 - 0.25)	96

AGE-MATCHED REFERENCE CHARTS

***(33-3)** NeuroQuant morphometry obtained using thin-section MP-RAGE and age-matched controls shows a hippocampal occupancy score (HOC) of 0.58. The hippocampal volumes are at the 4th percentile, and the inferior lateral ventricle volumes are at the 96th percentile for age. The mesial temporal lobes are > 2 standard deviations below normal.*

Etiology

General Concepts. AD is characterized by an "amyloid cascade." Reduced clearance of amyloid-β (Aβ) results in its aggregation in neurons. The **Aβ**42 residue is both insoluble and highly neurotoxic. Aβ42 clumps form **senile plaques** in the cortical gray matter. Aβ42 deposits also thicken the walls of cortical and leptomeningeal arterioles, causing **amyloid angiopathy**.

Another key feature of AD is **tauopathy**. Abnormal phosphorylation of a microtubule-associated protein known as "tau" eventually leads to the development of **neurofibrillary tangles** and **neuronal death**.

Genetics. Approximately 10% of AD cases have a strong family history of the disorder. The ε4 allele is the ancestral form of apolipoprotein E (*APOE*) and is associated with both higher absorption of cholesterol at the intestinal level and higher plasma cholesterol levels in carriers. Both the ε4 and *MTHFR* polymorphisms are known risk factors for late-onset AD (the most common type) and cerebrovascular disease (including VaD; see later discussion).

Pathology

Gross Pathology. Brains affected by AD show generalized (whole-brain) atrophy with shrunken gyri, widened sulci, and ventricular expansion (especially the temporal horns). Changes are most marked in the medial temporal and parietal lobes **(33-5)**. The frontal lobes are commonly involved, whereas the occipital lobes and motor cortex are relatively spared.

Microscopic Features. The three characteristic histologic hallmarks of AD are senile plaques, neurofibrillary tangles, and exaggerated neuronal loss. All are characteristic of—but none is specific for—AD.

AD also often coexists with other pathologies, such as vascular disease or Lewy bodies. Variable amounts of amyloid deposition in arterioles of the cortex and leptomeninges (amyloid angiopathy) are present in over 90% of AD cases.

Staging, Grading, and Classification. One of the most widely used systems—the Braak and Braak system—is based on the topographic distribution of neurofibrillary tangles and neuropil threads with grades from 1 to 6.

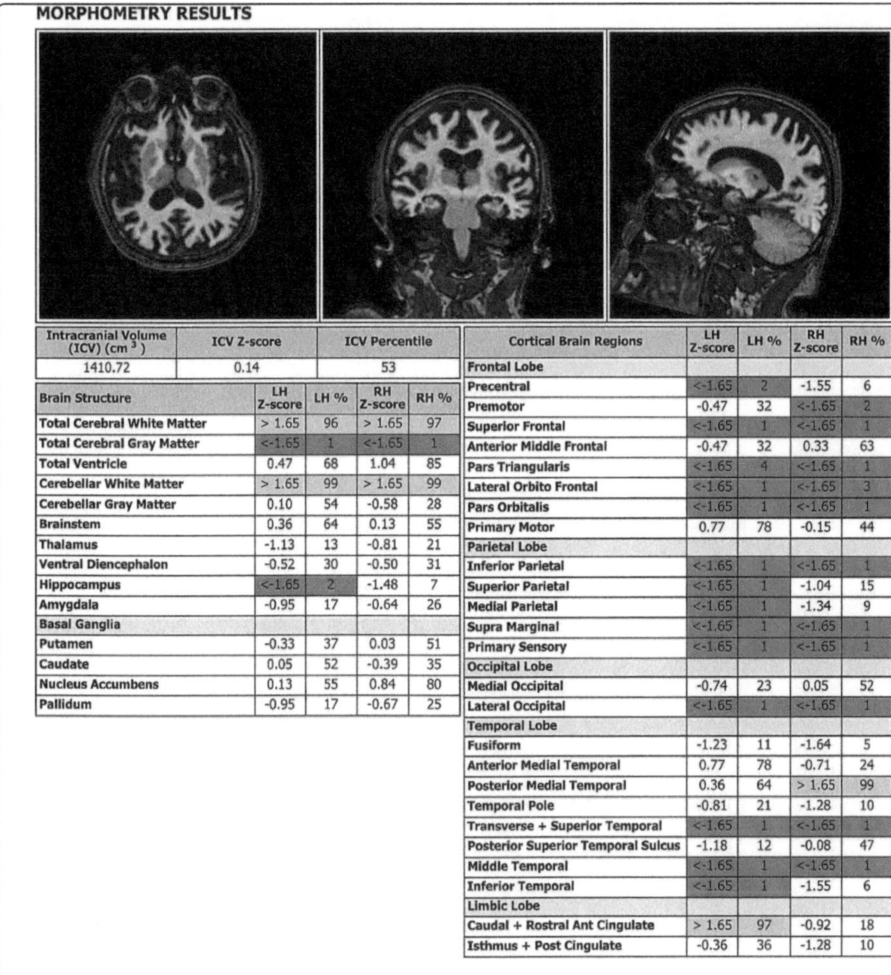
MORPHOMETRY RESULTS

Intracranial Volume (ICV) (cm ^{3})	ICV Z-score	ICV Percentile
1410.72	0.14	53

Brain Structure	LH Z-score	LH %	RH Z-score	RH %
Total Cerebral White Matter	> 1.65	96	> 1.65	97
Total Cerebral Gray Matter	<-1.65	1	<-1.65	1
Total Ventricle	0.47	68	1.04	85
Cerebellar White Matter	> 1.65	99	> 1.65	99
Cerebellar Gray Matter	0.10	54	-0.58	28
Brainstem	0.36	64	0.13	55
Thalamus	-1.13	13	-0.81	21
Ventral Diencephalon	-0.52	30	-0.50	31
Hippocampus	<-1.65	2	-1.48	7
Amygdala	-0.95	17	-0.64	26
Basal Ganglia				
Putamen	-0.33	37	0.03	51
Caudate	0.05	52	-0.39	35
Nucleus Accumbens	0.13	55	0.84	80
Pallidum	-0.95	17	-0.67	25

Cortical Brain Regions	LH Z-score	LH %	RH Z-score	RH %
Frontal Lobe				
Precentral	<-1.65	2	-1.55	6
Premotor	-0.47	32	<-1.65	2
Superior Frontal	<-1.65	1	<-1.65	1
Anterior Middle Frontal	-0.47	32	0.33	63
Pars Triangularis	<-1.65	4	<-1.65	1
Lateral Orbito Frontal	<-1.65	1	<-1.65	3
Pars Orbitalis	<-1.65	1	<-1.65	1
Primary Motor	0.77	78	-0.15	44
Parietal Lobe				
Inferior Parietal	<-1.65	1	<-1.65	1
Superior Parietal	<-1.65	1	-1.04	15
Medial Parietal	<-1.65	1	-1.34	9
Supra Marginal	<-1.65	1	<-1.65	1
Primary Sensory	<-1.65	1	<-1.65	1
Occipital Lobe				
Medial Occipital	-0.74	23	0.05	52
Lateral Occipital	<-1.65	1	<-1.65	1
Temporal Lobe				
Fusiform	-1.23	11	-1.64	5
Anterior Medial Temporal	0.77	78	-0.71	24
Posterior Medial Temporal	0.36	64	> 1.65	99
Temporal Pole	-0.81	21	-1.28	10
Transverse + Superior Temporal	<-1.65	1	<-1.65	1
Posterior Superior Temporal Sulcus	-1.18	12	-0.08	47
Middle Temporal	<-1.65	1	<-1.65	1
Inferior Temporal	<-1.65	1	-1.55	6
Limbic Lobe				
Caudal + Rostral Ant Cingulate	> 1.65	97	-0.92	18
Isthmus + Post Cingulate	-0.36	36	-1.28	10

(33-4) NeuroQuant morphometry results are of the same case illustrated on the previous page. Detailed analyses of total cerebral gray matter, hippocampi, and several cortical brain regions (frontal, parietal, temporal) are grossly abnormal, highlighted in red.

Clinical Issues

Epidemiology and Demographics. AD accounts for ~ 50-60% of all dementias. Age is the biggest risk factor for developing AD. The prevalence of AD is 1-2% at age 65 and increases by 15-25% each decade. In the "oldest-old" patients (> 90 years), mixed pathologies—typically AD plus VaD—predominate.

Diagnosis. AD represents a disease spectrum that ranges from cognitively normal individuals with elevated Aβ through those who exhibit the very first, minimal signs of cognitive impairment (MCI) to frank AD.

Historically, the *definitive* diagnosis of AD was made only by biopsy or autopsy. The *clinical* diagnosis of AD defines three levels of certainty: Possible, probable, and definite AD. The diagnosis of definite AD currently requires the clinical diagnosis of probable AD *plus* neuropathologic confirmation.

The Alzheimer Disease Neuroimaging Initiative (ADNI) standardized datasets are currently the most commonly used references for the computer-aided diagnosis of dementia.

Natural History. AD is a chronic disease. Progression is gradual, and patients live an average of 8-10 years after diagnosis. Between 5% and 10% of patients with MCI progress to probable AD each year.

Imaging

General Features. One of the most important goals of routine CT and MR is to identify specific abnormalities that could support the clinical diagnosis of AD. The other major role is to exclude alternative etiologies that can mimic AD clinically, i.e., "causes of reversible dementia" (see next page).

The introduction of radiotracers for the noninvasive in vivo quantification of Aβ burden in the brain has revolutionized the approach to the imaging evaluation of AD.

CT Findings. NECT is used to exclude potentially reversible or treatable causes of dementia, such as subdural hematoma, but are otherwise uninformative, especially in the early stages of AD. Medial temporal lobe atrophy is generally the earliest identifiable finding on CT.

MR Findings. The current role of conventional MR in the evaluation of patients with dementing disorders is to (1) exclude other causes of dementia, (2) identify region-specific patterns of brain volume loss (e.g., "lobar-predominant" atrophy), and (3) identify imaging markers of comorbid vascular disease, such as amyloid angiopathy.

The most common morphologic changes on standard MR are thinned gyri, widened sulci, and enlarged lateral ventricles.

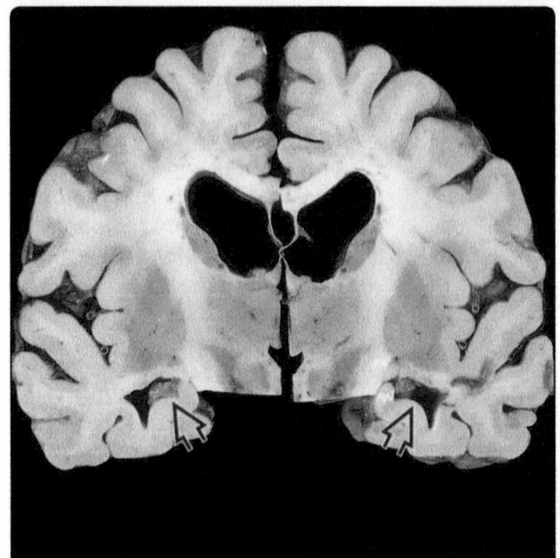

***(33-5)** Autopsy in proven early AD shows enlarged lateral ventricles. Hippocampi ⇨ appear mildly atrophic. (R. Hewlett, MD.)*

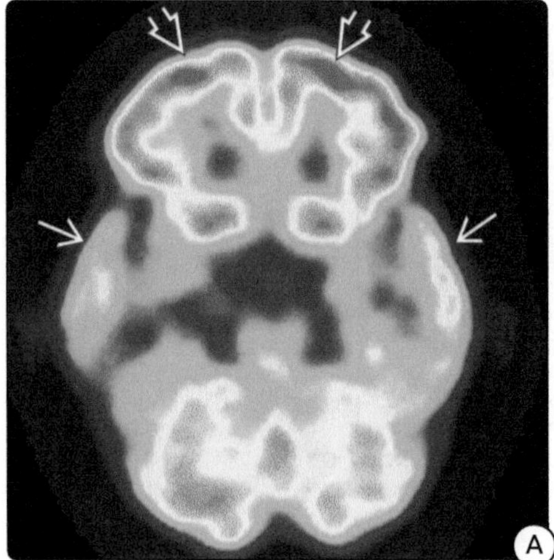

***(33-6A)** 18F FDG PET in AD shows markedly reduced metabolism in both temporal lobes ➡ with comparatively normal frontal lobes ⇨.*

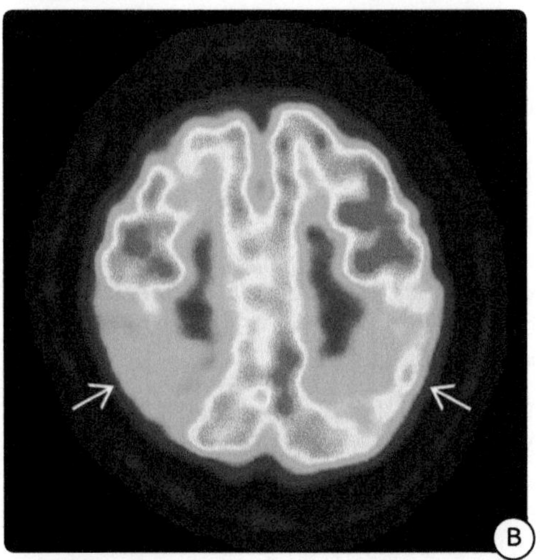

***(33-6B)** Parietal hypometabolism ➡ on cephalad PET shows temporal/parietal hypometabolism; preserved frontal activity is common.*

The medial temporal lobe—particularly the hippocampus and entorhinal cortex—are often disproportionately affected **(33-2)** as are the posterior cingulate gyri.

T1-weighted MP-RAGE data can be used to quantify regional brain atrophy using open-source (i.e., FreeSurfer), proprietary, or commercial (i.e., NeuroQuant) automated volumetric analyses **(33-3)**. 7T MR can identify abnormalities in the hippocampal subfields. The most consistent finding is reduction in CA1 volume (specifically CA1-SRLM) **(33-4)**.

T2* (GRE, SWI) sequences are much more sensitive than standard FSE in detecting cortical microhemorrhages that may suggest comorbid amyloid angiopathy.

Functional Neuroimaging. fMRI shows decrease in intensity &/or extent of activation in the frontal and temporal regions in cognitive tasks. pMR may demonstrate subtly reduced rCBV in the temporal and parietal lobes in MCI patients.

Nuclear Medicine. 18F FDG PET demonstrates areas of regional hypometabolism **(33-6)** and helps distinguish AD from other lobar-predominant dementias (e.g., frontotemporal lobar degeneration).

PET using amyloid-binding radiotracers, such as 11[C] PiB (Pittsburgh compound B), has emerged as one of the best techniques for early AD diagnosis. Aβ deposition occurs well before symptom onset and likely represents preclinical AD in asymptomatic individuals and prodromal AD in patients with MCI.

Differential Diagnosis

The most difficult distinction is differentiating **normal age-related degenerative processes** and early "preclinical" AD.

"Mixed dementias" are common, especially in patients over the age of 90 years old. **VaD** is the most common dementia associated with AD. Lacunar and cortical infarcts are typical findings in VaD. **Cerebral amyloid angiopathy** often coexists with AD. **Lewy bodies** are sometimes found in AD patients ("Lewy body variant of AD").

Frontotemporal lobar degeneration shows frontal &/or anterior temporal atrophy and hypometabolism; the parietal lobes are generally spared. **Dementia with Lewy bodies** typically demonstrates generalized, nonfocal hypometabolism. Patients with **corticobasal degeneration** have prominent extrapyramidal symptoms.

Causes of reversible dementia that can be identified on imaging studies include mass lesions, such as chronic subdural hematoma or neoplasm, vitamin deficiencies (thiamine, B12), endocrinopathy (e.g., hypothyroidism), and normal pressure hydrocephalus.

ALZHEIMER DISEASE

Pathoetiology
- Neurotoxic "amyloid cascade"
  - Aβ42 accumulation → senile plaques, amyloid angiopathy
- Tauopathy → neurofibrillary tangles, neuronal death

Clinical Issues
- Most common dementia (50-60% of all cases)
- Prevalence increases 15-25% per decade after 65 years
- Pathology begins *at least* 1 decade before clinical symptoms emerge
  - "Clinically normal" on preclinical Alzheimer cognitive composite
  - Aβ in clinically normal predicts significant longitudinal decline

Imaging
- Frontoparietal dominant lobar atrophy
  - Hippocampus, entorhinal cortex
  - FDG PET shows hypometabolism
  - Amyloid-binding markers, such as 11[C] PiB
- Amyloid angiopathy
  - Present in > 95% of cases
  - T2* cortical "blooming black dots"
  - With or without cortical siderosis

Differential Diagnosis
- Exclude reversible dementias!
  - Subdural hematoma
  - Normal pressure hydrocephalus
- DDx
  - Normal aging
  - Vascular dementia
  - Frontotemporal lobar degeneration
  - AD often mixed with other dementias (especially vascular)

Vascular Dementia

Cerebrovascular disease is a common cause of cognitive decline. The burden of "silent" microvascular disease and its long-term deleterious effect on cognition is becoming increasingly well recognized, as is its link with AD as a significant comorbidity.

Terminology

Vascular dementia (VaD) is sometimes also called multiinfarct dementia, vascular cognitive disorder, vascular cognitive impairment, subcortical ischemic VaD, and poststroke dementia.

Etiology

Inherited Vascular Dementias. Monogenic disorders are estimated to cause ~ 5% of all strokes and 10% of VaDs. The most common inherited disorders that can cause VaD are CADASIL and Fabry disease.

Sporadic Vascular Dementias. Most cases of VaD are sporadic and caused by the cumulative burden of cerebrovascular lesions. Risk factors for VaD include hypertension, dyslipidemia, and smoking. Mutations in the *MTHFR* gene correlate with elevated levels of plasma homocysteine and are associated with both AD and vasculogenic cognitive impairment.

Pathology

Gross Pathology. The most common readily identifiable gross finding in VaD is multiple infarcts with focal atrophy **(33-7)**. Multiple subcortical lacunar

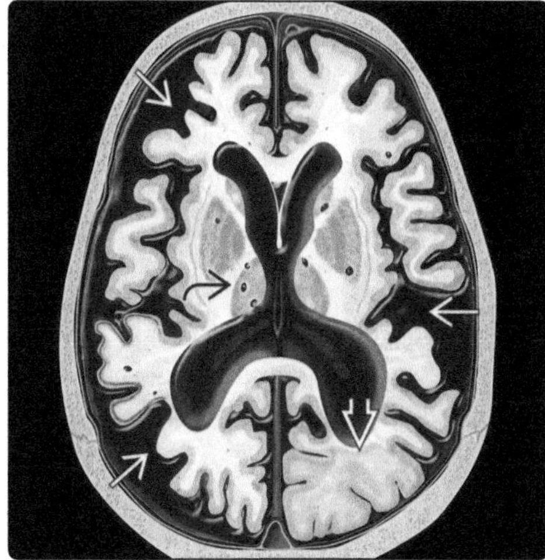

***(33-7)** Graphic of VaD shows multiple chronic infarcts ➡, acute left occipital lobe infarct ⇨, and small basal ganglia lacunar infarcts ↪.*

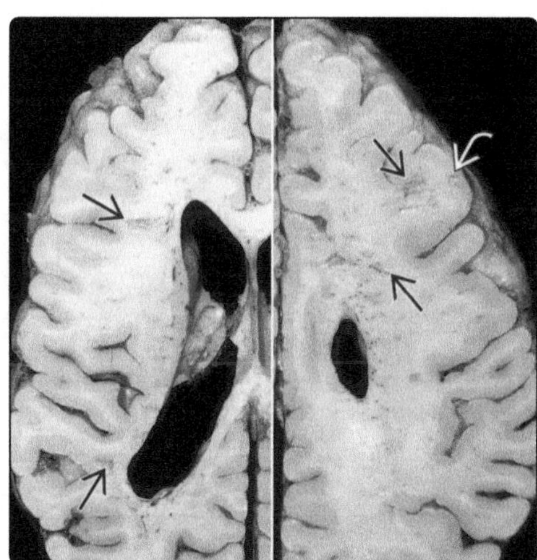

***(33-8)** VaD shows multiple WM ➡, cortical ↪ lacunae at the level of the lateral ventricle (L), corona radiata (R). (Courtesy R. Hewlett, MD.)*

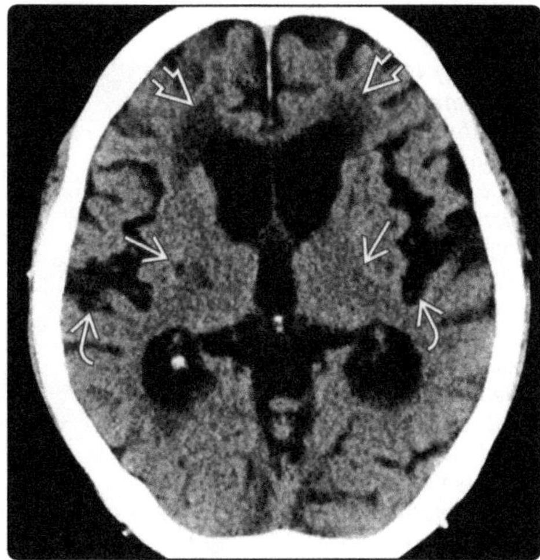

***(33-9)** NECT in 72-year-old man with VaD shows enlarged ventricles, sulci ↪, white matter rarefaction ⇨, and old lacunar infarcts ➡.*

infarcts **(33-8)** &/or widespread WM ischemia are more common than cortical branch occlusions or large territorial infarcts **(33-32)**.

Microscopic Features. Arteriolosclerosis and **amyloid angiopathy** are the major underlying pathologies in VaD. So-called **microinfarcts**—minute foci of neuronal loss, gliosis, pallor, or frank cystic degeneration—are seen at autopsy in nearly 2/3 of patients with VaD and > 1/2 of all cases with other dementing disorders (e.g., AD, dementia with Lewy bodies). Lesions are found in all brain regions and are especially common in the cortex, subcortical WM, and basal ganglia.

Clinical Issues

Epidemiology and Demographics. VaD is the second most common cause of dementia (after AD) and accounts for ~ 10% of all dementia cases in developed countries. VaD is a common component of "mixed" dementias and is especially prevalent in patients with AD.

The incidence of VaD increases with age. Risk factors include hypertension, diabetes, dyslipidemia, and smoking. There is a moderate male predominance.

Natural History. Progressive, episodic, stepwise neurologic deterioration interspersed with intervals of relative clinical stabilization is the typical pattern of VaD.

Imaging

General Features. The general imaging features of VaD are those of multifocal infarcts and WM ischemia.

CT Findings. NECT scans often show generalized volume loss with multiple cortical, subcortical, and basal ganglia infarcts. Patchy or confluent hypodensities in the subcortical and deep

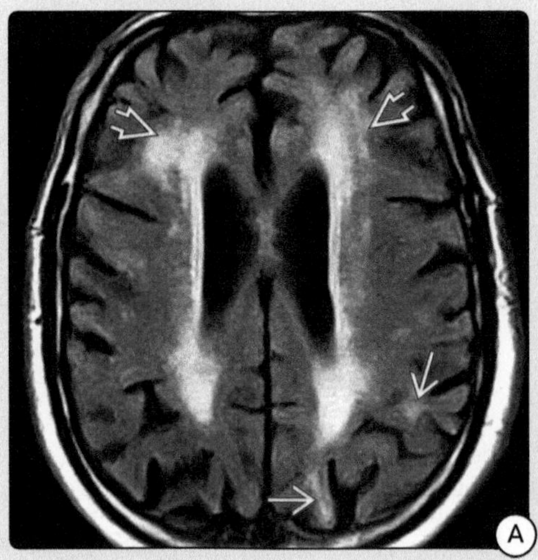

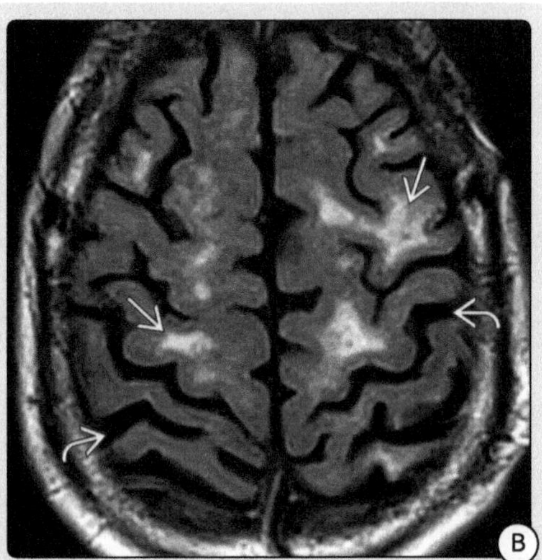

(33-10A) FLAIR MR in a 76-year-old normotensive demented man shows multifocal confluent hyperintensities in the subcortical ➡, deep periventricular WM ➡. (33-10B) More cephalad FLAIR MR in the same patient shows significant lesion burden in the subcortical WM ➡. Note enlarged parietal sulci ➡.

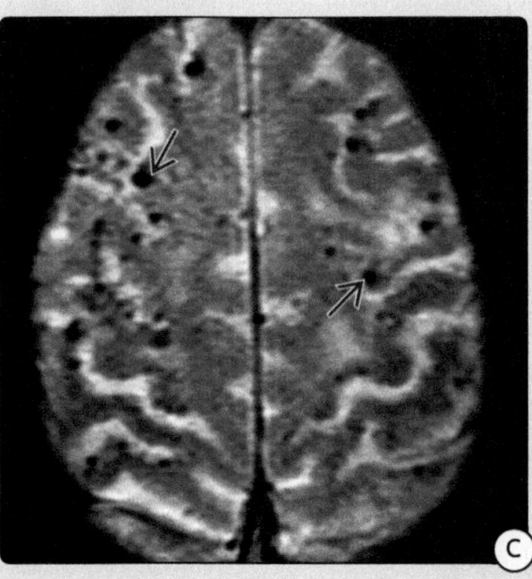

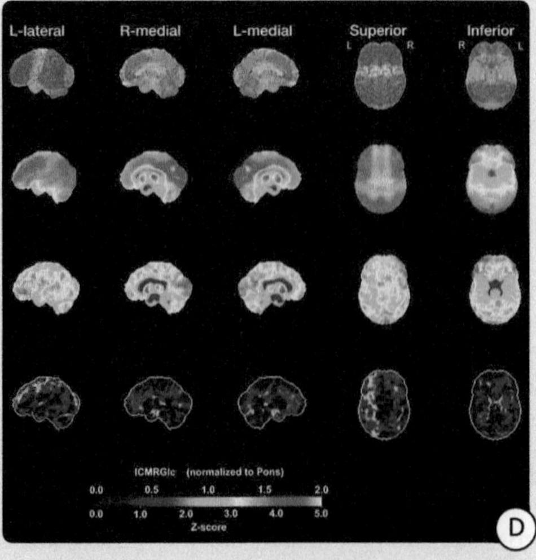

(33-10C) T2 GRE MR in the same patient shows multifocal cortical "blooming" hypointensities ➡ characteristic of cerebral amyloid angiopathy. (33-10D) PET scan in the same patient shows multifocal areas of decreased glucose metabolism (3rd row) compared with age-matched normal controls (2nd row). Z-score map (bottom row) shows the diffuse nature of the lesions seen in VaD. (Courtesy N. Foster, MD.)*

periventricular WM, especially around the atria of the lateral ventricles, are typical.

MR Findings. T1WI often shows greater than expected generalized volume loss. Multiple hypointensities in the basal ganglia and deep WM are typical. Focal cortical and large territorial infarcts with encephalomalacia can be identified in many cases.

T2/FLAIR scans show multifocal diffuse and confluent hyperintensities in the basal ganglia and cerebral WM. The cortex and subcortical WM are commonly affected **(33-10)**. T2* sequences may demonstrate multiple "blooming" hypointensities in the cortex and along the pial surface of the hemispheres **(33-10)**.

Nuclear Medicine. FDG PET shows multiple diffusely distributed areas of hypometabolism, generally without specific lobar predominance **(33-10D)**.

Differential Diagnosis

The major differential diagnosis of VaD is **Alzheimer disease**. The two disorders overlap and often coexist. AD typically shows striking and selective volume loss in the temporal lobes, especially the hippocampi. The basal ganglia are typically spared in AD, whereas they are often affected in VaD.

CADASIL is the most common *inherited* cause of VaD. Onset is typically earlier than in *sporadic* VaD. Anterior temporal and external capsule lesions are highly suggestive of CADASIL.

Frontotemporal lobar degeneration (FTLD) is characterized by early onset of behavior changes, whereas visuospatial skills remain relatively unaffected. Frontotemporal atrophy with knife-like gyri is typical. **Dementia with Lewy bodies** (DLB) may be difficult to distinguish from VaD without biopsy. **Cerebral amyloid angiopathy** commonly coexists with both AD and VaD and may be indistinguishable without biopsy.

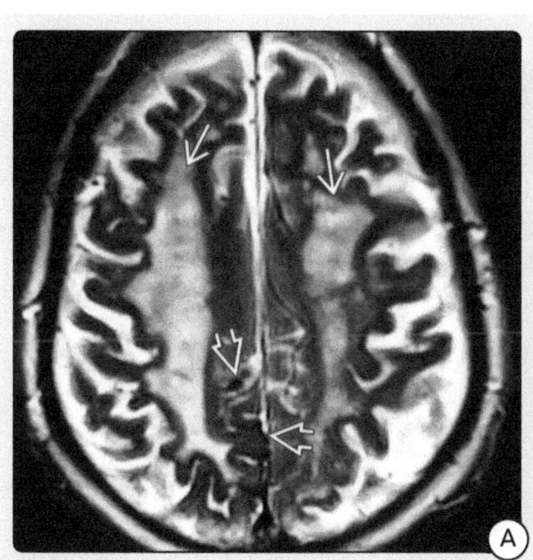

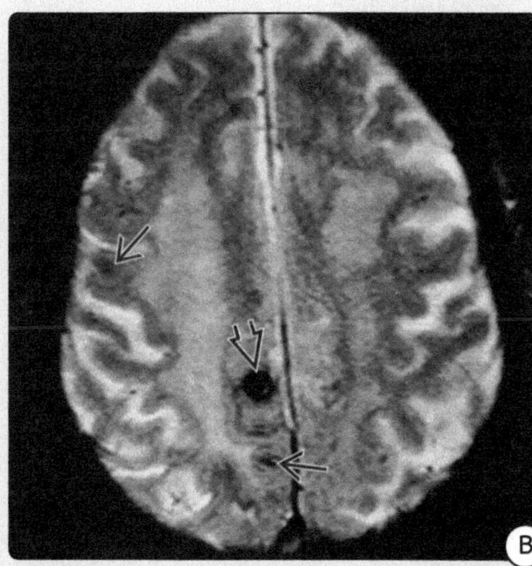

***(33-11A)** Axial T2 MR in a 76-year-old woman with a history of multiple strokes and clinical diagnosis of VaD shows generalized volume loss with confluent subcortical WM hyperintensity ➡. Insensitivity of FSE scans to hemorrhage is demonstrated by this case; only faint hypointensities ➡ can be identified. **(33-11B)** T2* GRE shows a round, focal "blooming" lesion ➡ with several faint linear hypointensities ➡.*

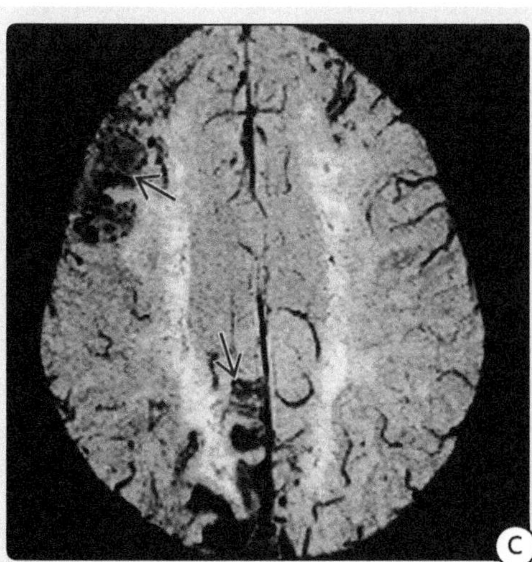

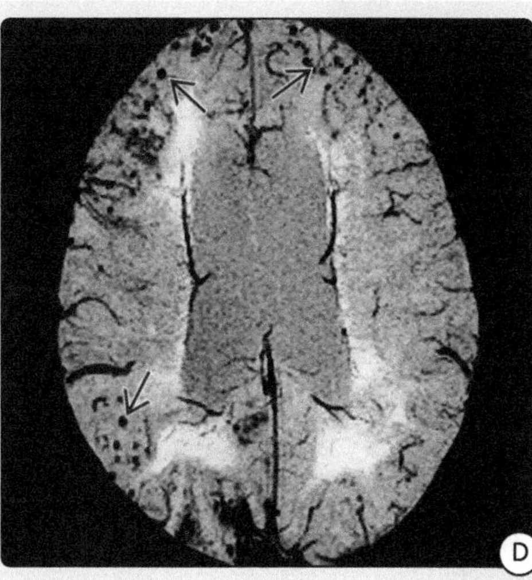

***(33-11C)** T2* SWI sequence in the same patient shows much more extensive confluent cortical and pial hypointensities ➡. **(33-11D)** Lower T2* SWI scan shows multiple tiny cortical "black dots" ➡ characteristic of amyloid angiopathy, the underlying cause of this patient's vascular dementia. T2* sequences should be an integral part of all MR protocols in patients with dementia.*

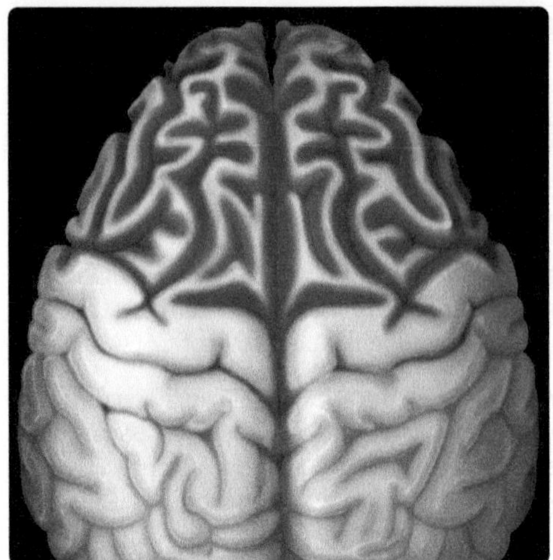
(33-12) Graphic shows frontal atrophy in late-stage FTLD with "knife-like" gyri. Parietooccipital lobes are spared.

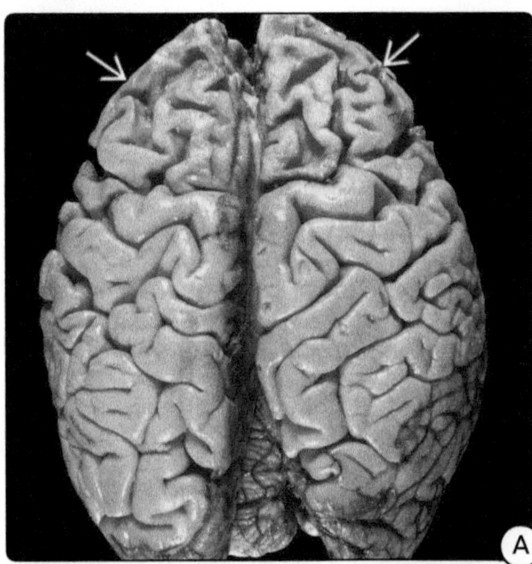
(33-13A) Autopsy of FTLD shows striking atrophy of the frontal gyri ➡ and normal-appearing parietal and occipital lobes.

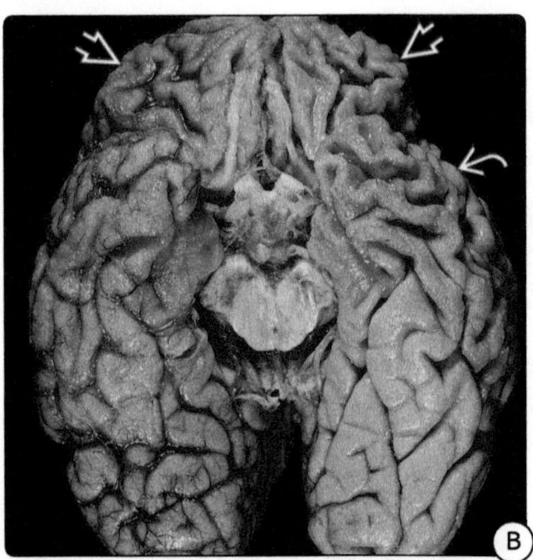
(33-13B) Submentovertex view in the same case shows striking frontal ➡ and temporal lobe atrophy ➡. (Courtesy R. Hewlett, MD.)

VASCULAR DEMENTIA: IMAGING AND DIFFERENTIAL DIAGNOSIS

Imaging

- General features
  - Multifocal infarcts (lacunae, cortical > large territorial)
  - WM ischemia (patchy &/or confluent T2/FLAIR hyperintensities)
  - T2* "blooming black dots" (amyloid or HTN)

Differential Diagnosis

- Alzheimer disease
- CADASIL (most common *inherited* VaD)
- FTLD
- Lewy body disease
- Cerebral amyloid angiopathy 7

Frontotemporal Lobar Degeneration

Terminology

Frontotemporal lobar degeneration (FTLD) is a clinically, pathologically, and genetically heterogeneous group of disorders—sometimes called frontotemporal dementias (FTDs)—that principally affect the frontal and temporal lobes. The FTLD spectrum also includes Parkinson disease with dementia and ALS.

Etiology

Genetics. Mutations in three major genes, *MAPT*, *GRN*, and *C9orf72*, account for most cases of FTLD. Tau protein is the product of *MAPT*, and abnormal tau accumulation in neurons &/or glia is known as Pick bodies.

Pathology

Gross Pathology. FTLDs are characterized by severe frontotemporal atrophy with neuronal loss, gliosis, and spongiosis of the superficial cortical layers **(33-12)**. The affected gyri are thinned and narrowed, causing the typical appearance of "knife-like" gyri **(33-13)**. The posterior brain regions, especially the occipital poles, are relatively spared until very late in the disease process **(33-13)**.

Microscopic Features. The three principal FTLD histologies are characterized by neuronal accumulations of aggregated proteins. They are (1) tau, (2) TDP-43, and (3) FUS proteins. Intraneuronal tau occurs as either Pick bodies or neurofibrillary tangle-like structures.

Clinical Issues

Epidemiology and Demographics. FTLD is the second most common cause of "presenile dementia," accounting for 20% of all cases in patients under the age of 65 years. FTLD is the third most common overall cause of dementia (after AD and VaD), constituting 10-25% of all dementia cases. Average age at disease onset is typically around 60 years, younger than seen in AD and other neurodegenerative disorders.

Presentation. Three different *clinical* subtypes of FTLD are recognized. The most common is **behavioral-variant frontotemporal dementia** (bvFTD), which accounts for > 1/2 of all cases. The second, less common syndrome is **semantic dementia** (SD). The third clinical syndrome is termed **progressive nonfluent aphasia** (PNFA).

Imaging

General Features. Neuroimaging features of the FTDs should be assessed according to whether they produce focal temporal or extratemporal (e.g., frontal) atrophy, whether the pattern is relatively symmetric or strongly asymmetric, and which side (left vs. right) is most severely affected.

CT Findings. Abnormalities on CT represent late-stage FTLD. Severe symmetric atrophy of the frontal lobes with lesser volume loss in the temporal lobes is the most common finding.

MR Findings. Whereas standard T1 scans may show generalized frontotemporal volume loss, voxel-based morphometry can discriminate between various *pathologic* subtypes. For example, FTLD-tau is associated with strongly asymmetric atrophy involving the temporal &/or extratemporal (i.e., frontal) regions.

Clinical FTLD subtypes also correlate with frontal-vs.-temporal and left-vs.-right atrophy predominance. The SD subtype shows bilateral temporal volume loss but little or no frontal atrophy **(33-14)**. bvFTD and PNFA both demonstrate bilateral frontal and temporal volume loss, but the right hemisphere is most affected in bvFTD, whereas left-sided volume loss dominates in PNFA.

Nuclear Medicine Findings. FDG PET scans show hypoperfusion and hypometabolism in the frontal and temporal lobes.

Differential Diagnosis. The major differential diagnoses of FTLD are AD (parietal lobe, hippocampi more than frontal) and VaD (WM, basal ganglia lacunae).

FRONTOTEMPORAL LOBAR DEGENERATION

Pathology
- 3 major types
  - FT:D-tau (45%)
  - FTLD-TDP (50%)
  - FTLD-FUS (5%)

Clinical Issues
- 2nd most common cause of "presenile" dementia
- Accounts for 20% of all cases < 65 years of age
- 3 major subtypes
  - Behavioral variant (bvFTD)
  - Semantic dementia (SD)
  - Progressive nonfluent aphasia (PNFA)

Imaging
- Classify atrophy (volumetric MR best)
  - Temporal vs. extratemporal (frontal) predominance
  - Symmetric or asymmetric
- 18F FDG PET
  - Frontotemporal hypometabolism

Differential Diagnosis
- Alzheimer disease (parietal, temporal > frontotemporal)
- Vascular dementia
  - Multifocal infarcts
  - WM ischemic changes

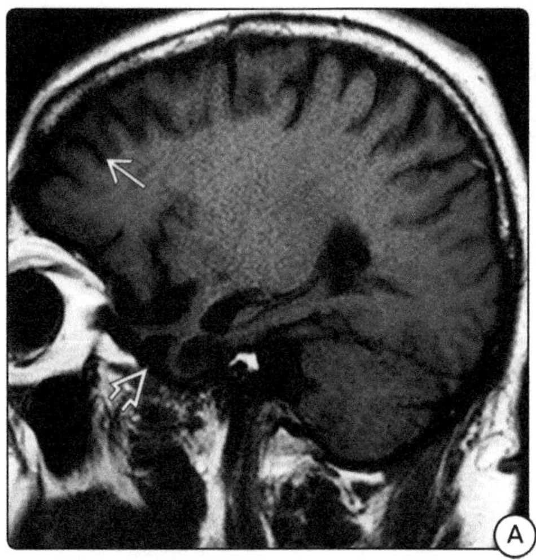

***(33-14A)** Sagittal T1 MR in 63y demented man shows striking temporal lobe volume loss with relatively well-preserved frontal gyri.*

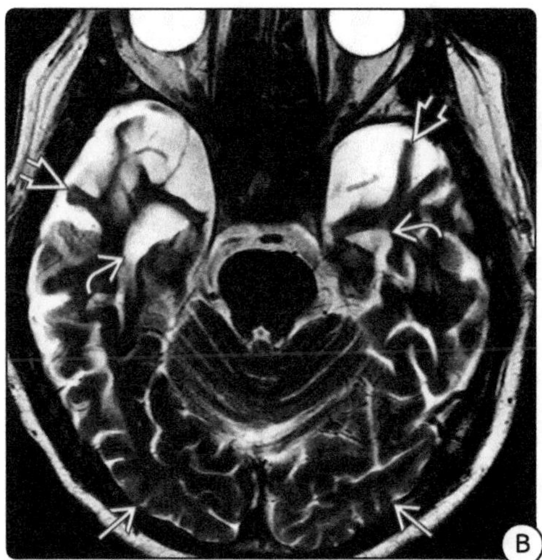

***(33-14B)** T2 MR shows symmetric temporal lobe atrophy, knife-like gyri, large temporal horns, normal occipital lobes. SD FTLD subtype.*

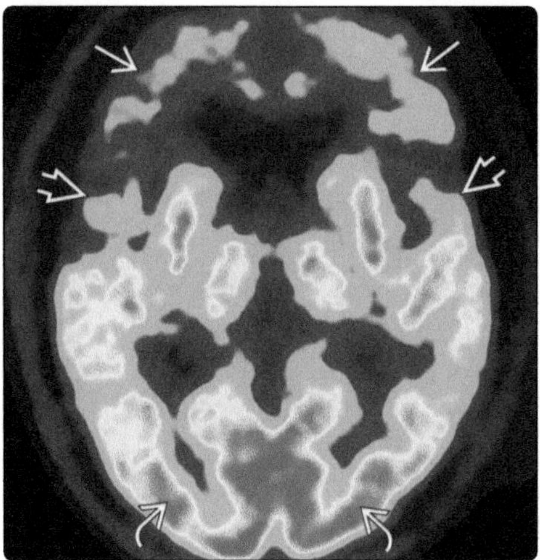

***(33-15)** FDG PET in FTLD shows severe frontal, moderate temporal lobe hypometabolism. Both occipital lobes appear normal.*

(33-16) sCJD shows caudate, anterior basal ganglia atrophy, cortical thinning especially in the occipital lobes. (Courtesy R. Hewlett, MD.)

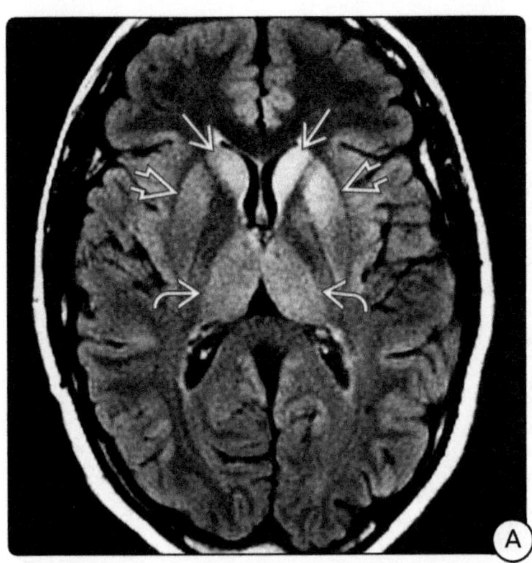

(33-17A) Axial FLAIR MR shows classic findings of sCJD with hyperintense caudate nuclei, anterior putamina, and thalami.

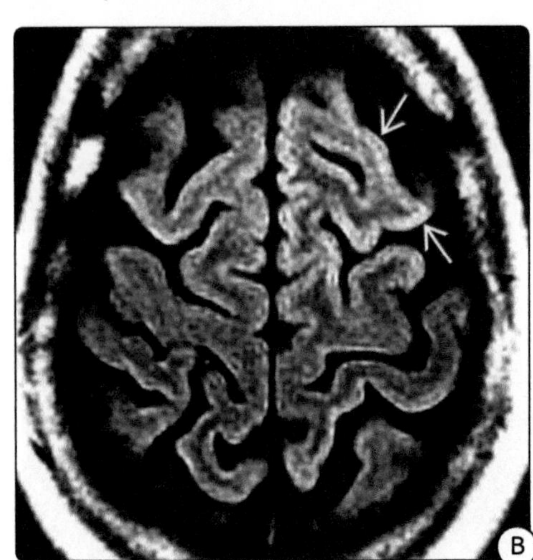

(33-17B) More cephalad FLAIR MR shows subtle hyperintensity in the left frontal cortex. This is autopsy-proven sCJD.

Miscellaneous Dementias

Creutzfeldt-Jakob Disease

Transmissible spongiform encephalopathies (TSEs), a.k.a. **prion diseases**, are a group of neurodegenerative disorders that includes **Creutzfeldt-Jakob disease** (CJD). Animal TSEs include bovine spongiform encephalopathy ("mad cow" disease).

CJD is the most common human TSE and has a worldwide distribution. CJD is unique, as it is both an infectious and neurogenetic dementing disorder. CJD is the archetypal human TSE.

Etiology. CJD is a rapidly progressive neurodegenerative disorder caused by an abnormal, misfolded prion protein, PrP(Sc). The abnormal form propagates itself by recruiting its normal isoform and imposing its conformation on the homologous host cell protein. *The conformational conversion of PrP(C) to PrP(Sc) is the fundamental event underlying all prion diseases.*

Four types of CJD are recognized: **Sporadic** (sCJD), **familial** or **genetic** (gCJD), **iatrogenic** (iCJD), and **variant** (vCJD). sCJD is the most common type. gCJD is caused by diverse mutations in the *PRNP* gene. iCJD is caused by prion-contaminated materials (e.g., surgical instruments, dura mater grafts). vCJD typically results from the transmission of bovine spongiform encephalopathy from cattle to humans.

Pathology. Gross pathology shows ventricular enlargement, caudate atrophy, and variable cortex volume loss **(33-16)** with relative sparing of the WM. The classic triad of histopathologic findings is marked neuronal loss, spongiform change, and striking astrogliosis. PrP(Sc) immunoreactivity is the gold standard for the neuropathologic diagnosis of human prion diseases.

HUMAN PRION DISEASES

Sporadic (Idiopathic) Prion Diseases (85%)
- sCJD
- Sporadic fatal insomnia, variably protease-sensitive prionopathy

Acquired (Infectious) Prion Diseases (2-5%)
- iCJD (due to medical interventions)
- Kuru
- vCJD

Familial (Inherited/Genetic) Prion Diseases (5-15%)
- iCJD
- Gerstmann-Sträussler-Scheinker syndrome
- Fatal familial insomnia

Epidemiology and Demographics. CJD now accounts for > 90% of all human prion diseases. Approximately 85% of CJD cases are sporadic (sCJD). Peak age of onset is 55-75 years. gCJD causes most of the remaining cases (5-15%). vCJD and iCJD are now rare.

Clinical Issues. CJD is a progressive, fatal illness. Over 90% of patients progress from normal function to death in under a year. Median survival is ~ 4 months, although vCJD progresses more slowly.

Several clinicopathologic subtypes of sCJD have been identified. In the most common subtype, rapidly worsening dementia is followed by myoclonic jerks and akinetic mutism. In 2/3 of sCJD cases, EEG shows a characteristic pattern of periodic bi- or triphasic complexes. The **Heidenhain variant** occurs as pure visual impairment leading to cortical blindness.

Imaging. CJD primarily involves the gray matter structures of the brain. MR with DWI is the imaging procedure of choice. T1 scans are often normal but may show faint hyperintensities in the posterior thalami **(33-19)**. FLAIR hyperintensity or restricted diffusion in the caudate nucleus and putamen or in at least two cortical regions (temporal-parietal-occipital "cortical ribboning") are considered highly sensitive and specific (96% and 93%, respectively) for the diagnosis of sCJD **(33-17)**. Occipital lobe involvement predominates in the Heidenhain variant.

T2/FLAIR hyperintensity in the posterior thalamus ("pulvinar" sign) or posteromedial thalamus ("hockey stick" sign) is seen in 90% of vCJD cases but can also occur in sCJD **(33-18)**. CJD does not enhance on T1 C+.

Differential Diagnosis. CJD must be distinguished from other causes of rapidly progressive dementia, such as **viral encephalitis, paraneoplastic limbic encephalitis**, and **autoimmune-mediated inflammatory disorders**, such as LGI1, NMDAR, or GABA encephalopathies. These CJD "mimics" can usually be excluded with appropriate serologic examination.

Other dementias, such as **Alzheimer disease** and **frontotemporal lobar degeneration**, are more insidiously progressive. The basal ganglia involvement in CJD is a helpful differentiating feature. Unlike most dementing diseases, CJD also shows striking diffusion restriction.

CREUTZFELDT-JAKOB DISEASE

Pathology and Etiology

- Most common human transmissible spongiform encephalopathy
- CJD is prion disease
  - Proteinaceous particles without DNA, RNA ("prions")
  - Misfolded isoform PrP(Sc) of normal host PrP(C)
  - Propagated by conformational conversion of PrP(C) to PrP(Sc)
- 4 CJD types recognized
  - Sporadic (sCJD) (85%)
  - Genetic/familial (gCJD) (5-15%)
  - Iatrogenic (iCJD) (2-5%)
  - Variant (vCJD, "mad cow" disease) (< 1%)

Clinical Issues

- Peak age = 55-75 years
- Rapidly progressive dementia, death in sCJD within 4 months

Imaging

- T2/FLAIR hyperintensity
  - Basal ganglia, thalami, cortex
  - "Pulvinar" sign: Posterior thalami
  - "Hockey stick" sign: Posteromedial thalami
  - Occipital cortex in Heidenhain variant
- Restricted diffusion

Degenerative Disorders

In this section, we consider a range of brain degenerations. Although some [such as Parkinson disease (PD)] can be associated with dementia, most are not. Because PD occurs more often as a movement disorder than a dementing illness, it is discussed with other degenerative diseases.

The use of deep brain stimulators (DBSs) in treating patients with disabling akinetic-rigid PD is increasingly common, so a brief review of the dopaminergic striatonigral system and its relevant anatomy will be helpful before we discuss PD.

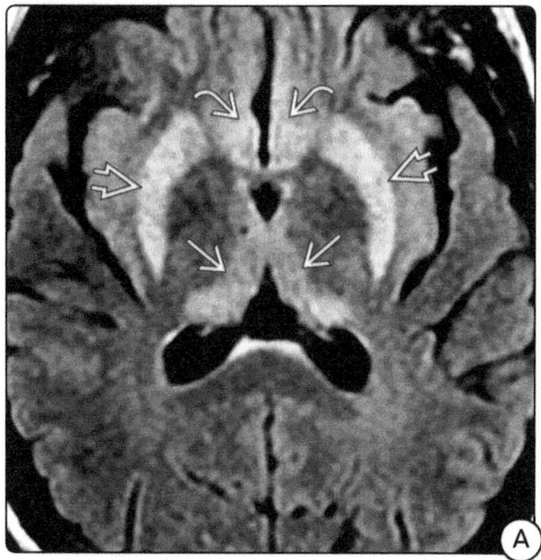

(33-18A) FLAIR in sCJD shows the classic "hockey stick" sign in thalami ➡. Anterior caudate nuclei ➡ and both putamina ➡ are also involved.

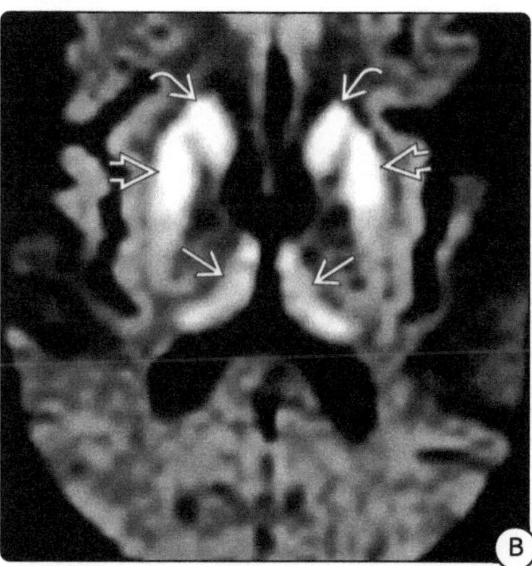

(33-18B) DWI MR shows corresponding strong diffusion restriction in the posteromedial thalami ➡, caudate nuclei ➡, and putamina ➡.

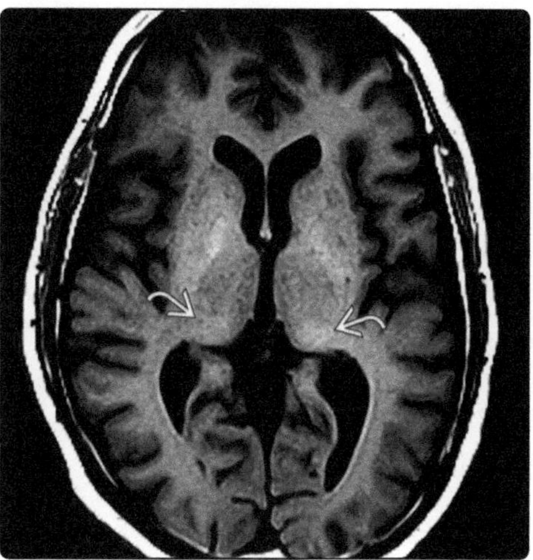

(33-19) Axial T1 MR in a 64-year-old man with biopsy-proven sCJD shows faint hyperintensities ➡ in the pulvinars of both thalami.

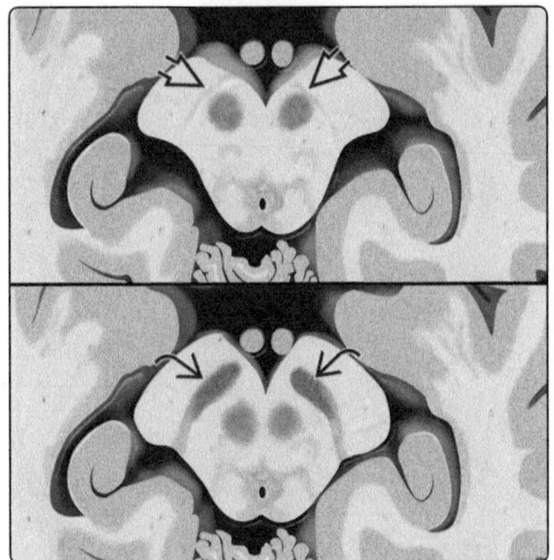

(33-20) PD midbrain atrophy, SN narrowed, depigmented ; pars compacta between red nuclei, SN ↓ (top). Normal STN on bottom.

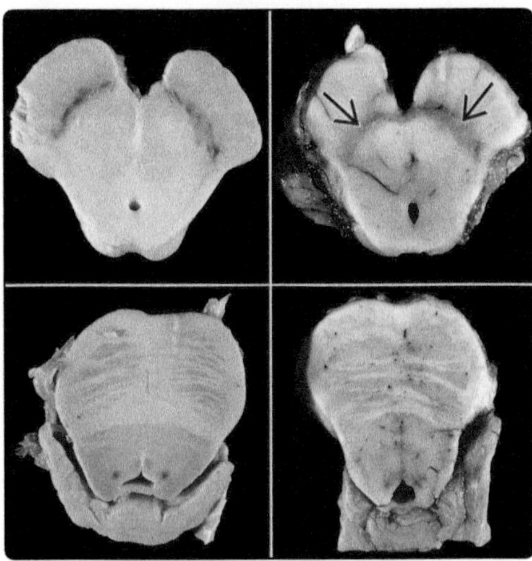

(33-21) Normal midbrain (L) PD (R). Midbrain volume loss in PD, abnormal pallor of the substantia nigra . (Courtesy R. Hewlett, MD.)

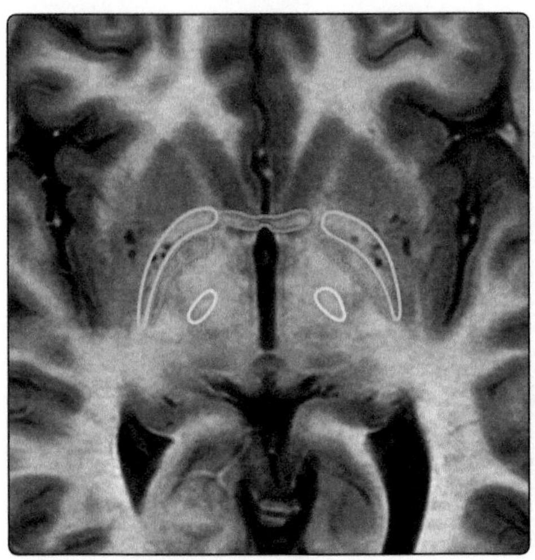

(33-22) Normal 3T T1 MR shows approximate locations of globus pallidus externa (green), interna (red), and subthalamic nuclei (orange).

Parkinson Disease

Terminology

Parkinson disease (PD) is a neurodegenerative disorder. The constellation of resting tremor, bradykinesia, and rigidity is often termed **parkinsonism**. When PD is accompanied by dementia, it is referred to as **Parkinson disease dementia** (PDD). PDD is a synucleinopathy like Lewy body dementia.

Etiology

Aging is the most significant known risk factor for PD. Degeneration of dopaminergic neurons in the SNPc reduces dopaminergic input to the striatum. By the time clinical symptoms develop, over 60% of dopaminergic neurons are lost and 80% of striatal dopamine is already depleted.

Between 10-20% of cases of PD are familial, but most are sporadic. The vast majority of cases are genetically complex but only 5-10% of patients have a monogenic form of PD.

Pathology

Gross Pathology. The midbrain may appear mildly atrophic with a splayed or "butterfly" configuration of the cerebral peduncles **(33-21)**. Depigmentation of the substantia nigra is a common pathologic feature of PD **(33-21)**.

Microscopic Features. The two histopathologic hallmarks of PD are (1) severe depletion of dopaminergic neurons in the pars compacta of the substantia nigra and (2) the presence of Lewy bodies (LBs) in the surviving neurons.

Clinical Issues

Epidemiology and Demographics. PD is both the most common movement disorder and the most common of the Lewy body diseases. Peak age at onset is 60 years. PD typically follows a slowly progressive course with an overall mean duration of 13 years.

Presentation. PD diagnosis depends on a constellation of symptoms. The three cardinal clinical features of PD are (1) resting tremor, (2) rigidity, and (3) bradykinesia (slowness in executing movements). Other classic symptoms are "pill-rolling" tremor, "cogwheel" or "lead pipe" rigidity. Dementia eventually develops in 40% of PD patients.

Treatment Options. A number of medications are available to control PD symptoms. Levodopa was introduced > 40 years ago and remains the most efficacious treatment.

Deep brain stimulation (DBS) has become the preferred technique for treating a gamut of advanced PD-related symptoms. As the subthalamic nucleus is often difficult to identify on standard MR, many neurosurgeons identify the red nucleus and position the DBSs slightly anterolateral to it.

High-frequency ultrasound (HIFU) is a new ablative therapy for PD and essential tremor.

Imaging

CT Findings. CT is used primarily following DBS placement to evaluate electrode position and to check for surgical complications. The subthalamic nucleus (STN) is the usual target and electrode tips are located ~ 9 mm from the midline, just inside the upper margin of the cerebral peduncles **(33-22)**. Complications are rare and include hemorrhage and ischemia. Transient inflammation may develop, appearing within a few weeks as hypodensity around the electrodes. Changes gradually resolve.

MR Findings. Mild midbrain volume loss with a "butterfly" configuration can be seen at 1.5T in some *late*-stage cases of PD. Findings that may support the diagnosis of PD include thinning of the pars compacta (with "touching" RNs and "smudging" of the SNs) **(33-23)** and loss of normal SN hyperintensity on T1WI.

Nuclear Medicine. The most sensitive imaging techniques for an *early* diagnosis of parkinsonian syndromes are SPECT and PET. DaT-SPECT is used to assess integrity of presynaptic dopaminergic nerve cells in patients with movement disorders **(33-24)**. Decreased uptake of I-123 FP-CIT is considered highly suggestive of PD **(33-25)** but is also seen in other parkinsonian degenerations.

Differential Diagnosis

DaT-SPECT imaging enables differentiation of neurodegenerative causes of parkinsonism from other movement or tremor disorders in which the study is typically normal. When dementia is present, the major differential diagnosis of PDD is **dementia with Lewy bodies**.

PARKINSON DISEASE

Etiology and Pathology

- Degeneration of dopaminergic neurons in SNPc
  - Reduced dopaminergic input to striatum
  - 60% of SNPc neurons lost
  - 80% striatal dopamine depleted before clinical PD develops
- Substantia nigra (SN) becomes depigmented
- Pars compacta thins
- Synucleinopathy with Lewy bodies develops
  - PD is most common Lewy body disease

Clinical Issues

- Peak age = 60 years
- 3 cardinal features
  - Resting tremor
  - Rigidity
  - Bradykinesia

Treatment Options

- Medical
  - Levodopa (L-dopa), other drugs
- Surgical
  - Deep brain stimulation (DBS)
  - Electrodes implanted into subthalamic nuclei
  - Should be ≈ 9 mm from midline
  - Just inside upper margin of cerebral peduncles
  - Complications = ischemia, hemorrhage, transient inflammation around electrodes

Imaging

- Difficult to diagnose on standard MR
  - ± midbrain atrophy
  - ± thinned, irregular SN
  - ± "touching" SN, red nuclei
- Dopamine transporter (DaT) imaging
  - PET or SPECT can show decreased uptake

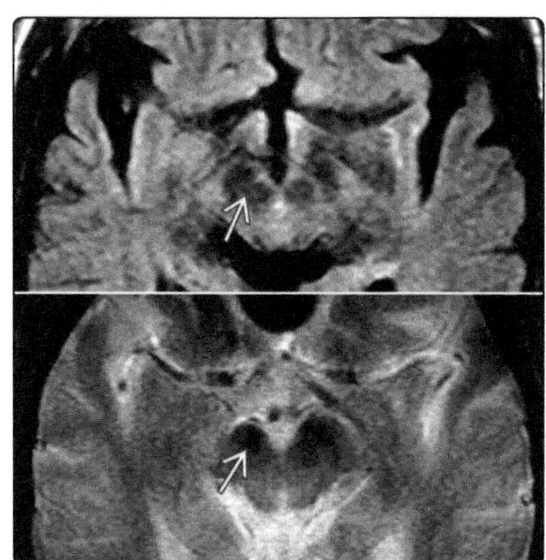

***(33-23)** FLAIR (top), T2* GRE (bottom) in PD shows mild midbrain atrophy with narrowed SNPc ➡ between substantia nigra, red nucleus.*

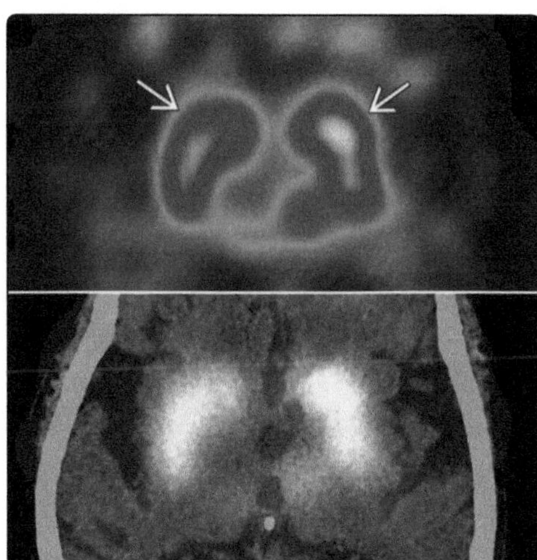

***(33-24)** Normal DaT scan (top) with double "comma-shaped" configuration ➡. (Bottom) Fused PET/CT is negative for Parkinson disease.*

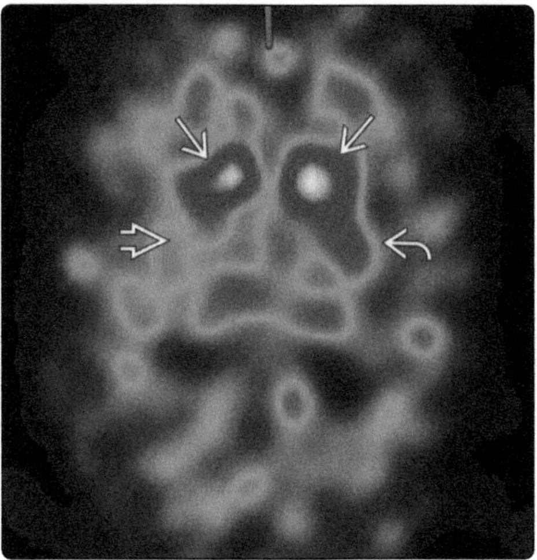

***(33-25)** DaT scan in PD shows normal caudate heads ➡, absent uptake in R putamen ➡, and markedly reduced uptake in the left putamen ➡.*

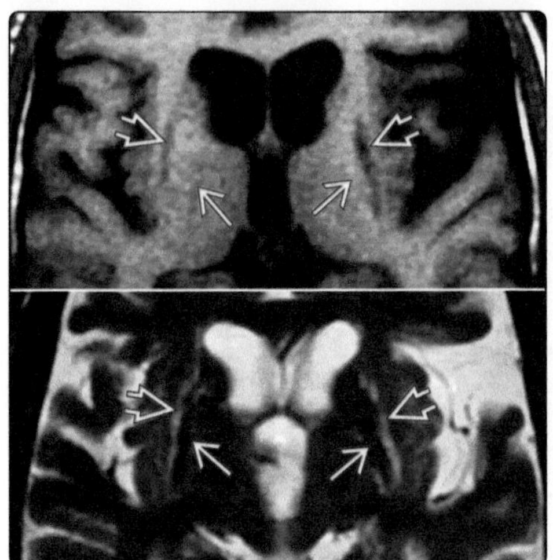

(33-26) MSA-P shows large ventricles/sulci and thinned, atrophic putamina ➡ with an irregular lateral rim of hypo- and hyperintensity ⇨.

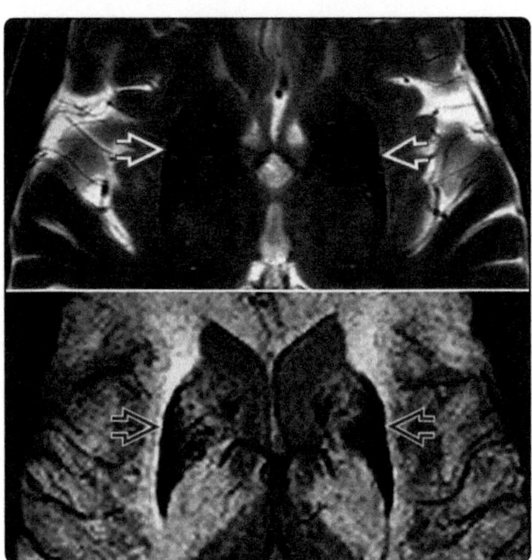

(33-27) MSA-P shows putaminal hypointensity on T2 MR ➡, SWI with shrunken, hypointense putamina and irregular lateral margins ⇨.

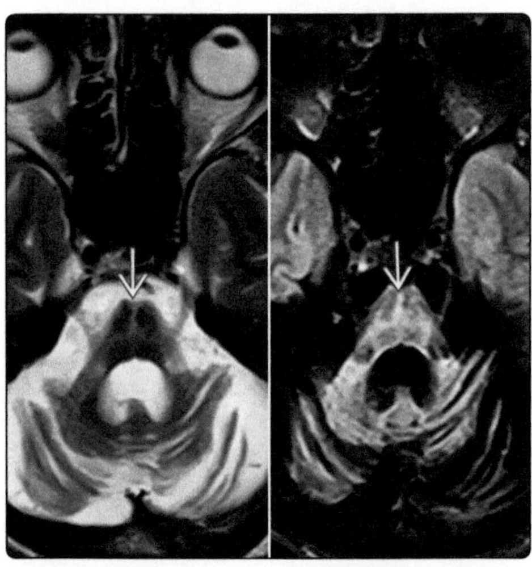

(33-28) (L) T2 and (R) FLAIR MR in MSA-C show severe pontine, cerebellar atrophy with a distinct hyperintense "hot cross bun" sign ➡.

Multiple System Atrophy

Terminology

Multiple system atrophy (MSA) is an adult-onset sporadic neurodegenerative disorder that is one of the more common **Parkinson-plus** syndromes. There are three MSA subtypes. When extrapyramidal (i.e., parkinsonian) symptoms predominate, the disease is designated **MSA-P**. If cerebellar symptoms such as ataxia predominate, the disorder is designated **MSA-C**. MSA with signs of autonomic failure (**MSA-A**) is the rarest subtype.

Pathology

Gross pathology shows two distinct atrophy patterns. MSA-P shows depigmentation and pallor of the substantia nigra. The putamen may be atrophic and show a grayish discoloration secondary to lipofuscin pigment accumulation. In MSA-C, marked volume loss in the cerebellum, pons, middle cerebellar peduncles (MCPs), and medulla gives the pons a "beaked" appearance. MSA-A may demonstrate a combination of these patterns. Like PD and DLB, MSA is a synucleinopathy.

Clinical Issues

Mean age of onset is 58 years; mean disease duration is 5.8 years.

Parkinson-like features are present in 85-90% of all MSA patients, regardless of subtype. Nearly 2/3 of MSA cases are classified as parkinsonian type (MSA-P) and 32% as MSA-C. Less than 5% of MSA patients have MSA-A.

Imaging

CT Findings. NECT scans in MSA-C show cerebellar atrophy with the hemispheres more severely affected than the vermis. A small flattened pons and an enlarged fourth ventricle are common associated findings. Cortical atrophy—especially involving the frontal and parietal lobes—may be present. Findings in MSA-P are less obvious; NECT may demonstrate shrunken putamina with flattened lateral margins.

MR Findings

MSA-P. In patients with MSA-P, the putamina appear small and hypointense on T2WI and often have a somewhat irregular high signal intensity rim along their lateral borders on 1.5T scans (**"hyperintense putaminal rim"** sign) **(33-26)**. This finding is nonspecific, as it can be seen in some cases of CBD as well as in > 1/3 of normal patients.

T2* (GRE, SWI) scans show significantly higher iron deposition in the putamen compared with both age-matched controls and patients with PD **(33-27)**. DTI shows decreased FA in the pons and middle cerebellar peduncle.

MSA-C. T1 scans in MSA-C show a shrunken pons and medulla, symmetric cerebellar atrophy, small concave-appearing MCPs, and an enlarged fourth ventricle.

T2/FLAIR scans demonstrate a cruciform hyperintensity in the pons termed the **"hot cross bun"** sign **(33-28)**. The "hot cross bun" sign results from selective loss of myelinated transverse pontocerebellar fibers and neurons in the pontine raphe.

Nuclear Medicine. DaT scans are usually normal in MSA.

Differential Diagnosis

The major differential diagnosis of MSA is **Parkinson disease**. Clinical findings often overlap. Imaging shows that the width of the middle cerebellar peduncles is diminished in MSA-C but not PD. Putaminal iron deposition appears earlier and is more prominent in MSA-P compared with PD. DTI also shows decreased FA in the middle cerebral peduncles in MSA-P.

Progressive Supranuclear Palsy

Terminology

Progressive supranuclear palsy (PSP) is a neurodegenerative disease characterized by supranuclear gaze palsy, postural instability, and mild dementia.

Etiology and Pathology

PSP is a **tauopathy**. PSP shares many clinical, pathologic, and genetic features with other tau-related diseases, such as tau-positive frontotemporal lobar degeneration (FTLD).

The major gross pathologic findings are substantia nigra depigmentation and midbrain atrophy. Variable atrophy of the pallidum, thalamus, and subthalamic nucleus together with mild symmetric frontal volume loss may also be present **(33-29)** **(33-30)**.

Clinical Issues

PSP is the second most common form of parkinsonism (after idiopathic PD) and is the most common of the so-called Parkinson-plus syndromes.

PSP symptom onset is insidious, typically beginning in the sixth or seventh decade. Peak onset is 63 years, and no cases have been reported in patients under the age of 40 years.

Imaging

CT Findings. NECT scans show variable midbrain volume loss with prominent interpeduncular and ambient cisterns. Mild to moderate ventricular enlargement is common.

MR Findings. Sagittal T1- and T2-weighted images show midbrain atrophy with a concave upper surface (the **"penguin"** or **"hummingbird" sign**) **(33-31)**. Axial scans show a widened interpeduncular angle and abnormal concavity of the midbrain tegmentum.

The quadrigeminal plate is often thinned, especially the superior colliculi. Cerebellar atrophy is common, and the *superior* cerebellar peduncles also frequently appear atrophic.

Differential Diagnosis

The major differential diagnosis includes **other tauopathies**, such as some FTLD subtypes. All share common molecular mechanisms and are therefore probably part of the same disease spectrum. **AD**, **PD**, and **MSA-P** usually do not exhibit severe atrophy of the superior colliculi that is seen with PSP.

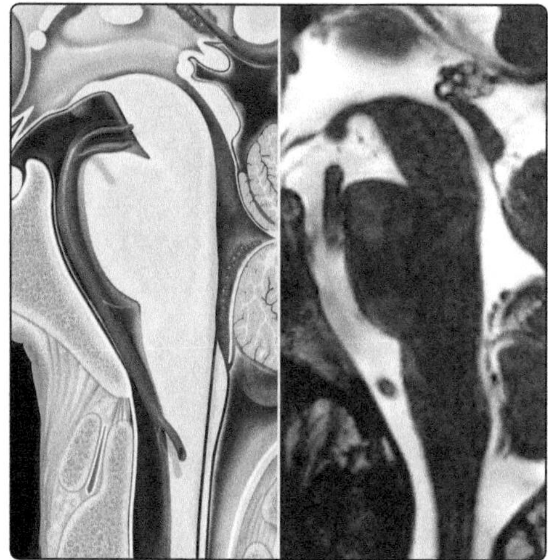

***(33-29)** Sagittal graphic (L) and high-resolution T2 MR (R) together show normal midbrain and pons.*

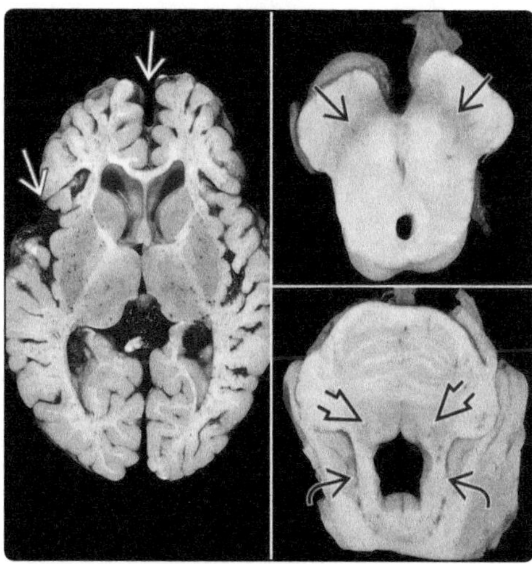

***(33-30)** PSP with frontotemporal atrophy ➡, depigmented SN ➡, locus ceruleus ➡, small superior cerebellar peduncles ➡. (R. Hewlett.)*

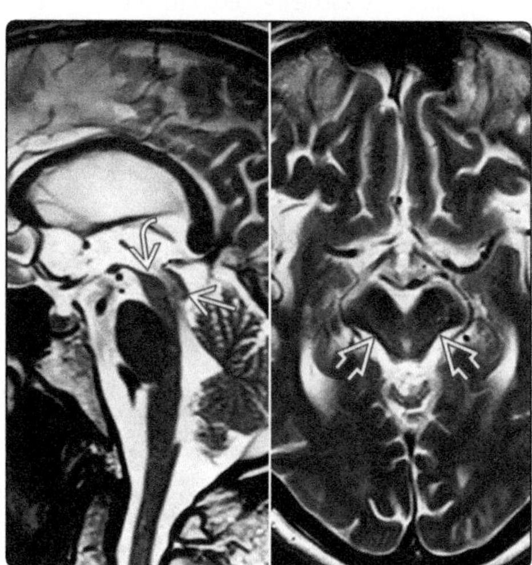

***(33-31)** PSP shows small midbrain with upper concavity and "penguin" or "hummingbird" sign ➡, tectal atrophy ➡, and concave midbrain ➡.*

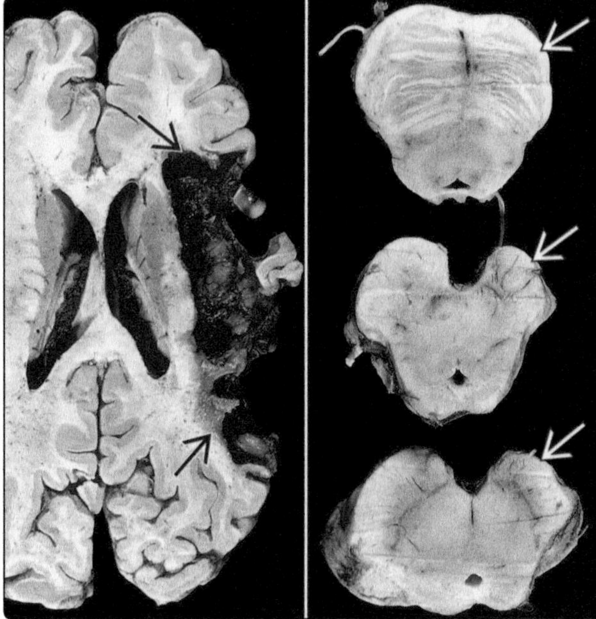

(33-32) Autopsy specimen from a patient with chronic WaD following large left MCA infarct ⇒ shows volume loss in the left cerebral peduncle and upper pons ➡. (Courtesy R. Hewlett, MD.)

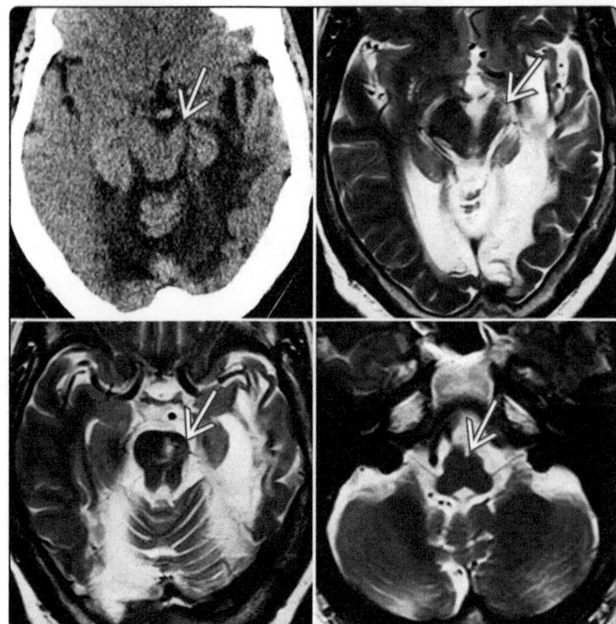

(33-33) NECT (upper left) and a series of T2 scans demonstrate changes of chronic WaD following major territorial infarction. Note atrophy of the left cerebral peduncle, upper pons, and midbrain ➡.

Wallerian Degeneration

Terminology

Wallerian degeneration (WaD) is an intrinsic anterograde degeneration of distal axons and their myelin sheaths caused by detachment from—or injury to—their proximal axons or cell bodies.

Etiology

In the brain, WaD most often occurs after trauma, infarction, demyelinating disease, or surgical resection. Descending WM tracts ipsilateral to the injured neurons degenerate—but not immediately. Axons may stay morphologically stable for the first 24-72 hours. The distal part of the axon then undergoes progressive fragmentation that proceeds directionally along the axon stump.

Pathology

Virtually any WM tract or nerve in the brain, spinal cord, or peripheral nervous system can exhibit changes of WaD. The descending corticospinal tract (CST) is the most common site of visible brain involvement. In chronic WaD, midbrain and pons volume loss ipsilateral to a destructive lesion (e.g., a large territorial infarct) are grossly visible **(33-32)**.

Imaging

CT Findings. Chronic changes of WaD include foci of frank encephalomalacia with volume loss of the ipsilateral peduncle, rostral pons, and medullary pyramid **(33-33)**.

MR Findings. The development of visible WaD following stroke, trauma, or surgery is unpredictable. Fewer than 1/2 of all patients with motor deficits following acute cerebral infarction demonstrate T2/FLAIR hyperintensities or diffusion restriction in the CST that might herald WaD. Transient restricted diffusion in the CST may develop in acute ischemic stroke within 48-72 hours.

When it does develop, T2/FLAIR hyperintensity along the CST ipsilateral to the damaged cortex may occur as early as three days after major stroke onset ("pre-wallerian degeneration") but more typically becomes visible between three and four weeks later **(33-33)**. The hyperintensity may be transient or permanent.

Other WM tracts can undergo WaD with an insult to their neuronal cell bodies. These include the corticopontocerebellar tract, dentate-rubro-olivary pathway (Guillain-Mollaret triangle), posterior column of the spinal cord, limbic circuit, and optic pathway.

Differential Diagnosis

The major differential diagnosis of WaD is primary neurodegenerative disease. The T2/FLAIR hyperintensity sometimes seen in **amyotrophic lateral sclerosis** is bilateral and extends from the subcortical WM adjacent to the motor cortex into the brainstem. High-grade infiltrating primary brain tumors (typically **anaplastic astrocytoma** or **glioblastoma multiforme**) infiltrate along compact WM tracts but cause expansion, not atrophy.

Hypertrophic Olivary Degeneration

Anatomy of the Medulla and Guillain-Mollaret Triangle

The **Guillain-Mollaret triangle** consists of the **ipsilateral inferior olivary nucleus** (ION), **contralateral dentate nucleus** (DN), and **ipsilateral red nucleus** (RN) together with their three connecting neural pathways, i.e., the **olivocerebellar tract, dentatorubral tract,** and **central tegmental tract**.

Olivocerebellar fibers from the ipsilateral ION cross the midline through the inferior cerebellar peduncle, connecting it with the contralateral DN and cerebellar cortex. Dentatorubral fibers then enter the superior cerebellar peduncle (brachium conjunctivum) and decussate in the midbrain to connect to the opposite RN. The ipsilateral central tegmental tract then descends from the RN to the ipsilateral ION, completing the Guillain-Mollaret triangle **(33-34)**.

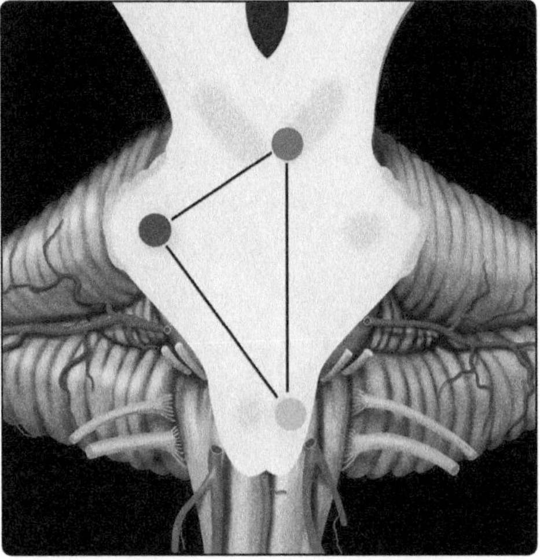

***(33-34)** Guillain-Mollaret triangle = ipsilateral olivary nucleus (green), contralateral dentate nucleus (blue), ipsilateral red nucleus (red).*

Terminology

Hypertrophic olivary degeneration (HOD) is a transsynaptic degeneration caused by injury to the dentato-rubro-olivary pathway. Interruption of the dentato-rubro-olivary pathway at any point can cause HOD, which can be uni- (75%) or bilateral (25%).

Etiology

Unlike other degenerations, in hypertrophic olivary degeneration, the degenerating structure (the olive) becomes hypertrophic rather than atrophic. Cerebellar symptoms and olivary hypertrophy typically develop many months after the inciting event.

The primary causative lesion in developing HOD is often **hemorrhage**, either from hypertension, surgery, vascular malformation, or trauma. **Pontomesencephalic stroke** also occasionally causes HOD. **Postoperative pediatric cerebellar mutism** (POPCMS) is a well-recognized complication that affects children undergoing posterior fossa brain tumor resection. Interruption of the dentato-thalamo-cortical pathway is recognized as its anatomic substrate. The proximal structures of the DTC pathway also form a segment of the Guillain-Mollaret triangle, so bilateral HOD is common in patients with POPCMS.

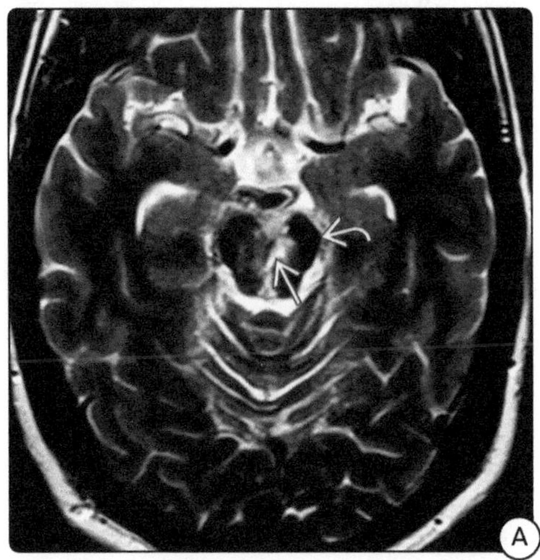

***(33-35A)** T2 MR in 24-year-old man shows palatal myoclonus from remote midbrain infarct ➡. Note volume loss in the left side of midbrain ➡.*

Pathology

Location. Three distinct patterns develop, all related to the location of the inciting lesion. In **ipsilateral HOD**, the primary lesion is limited to the central tegmental tract of the brainstem. In **contralateral HOD**, the primary lesion is located within the cerebellum (either the DN or the superior cerebellar peduncle). In **bilateral HOD**, the lesion involves both the central tegmental tract and the superior cerebellar peduncle.

Gross Pathology. Olivary hypertrophy is seen grossly as asymmetric enlargement of the anterior medulla. In chronic HOD, the ipsilateral ION and contralateral cerebellar cortex may be shrunken and atrophic.

Microscopic Features. Interruption of the Guillain-Mollaret triangle functionally deafferents the olive. The result is vacuolar cytoplasmic degeneration, neuronal enlargement, and proliferation of gemistocytic astrocytes. The enlarged neurons and proliferating astrocytes cause the initial hypertrophy. Over time, the affected olive atrophies.

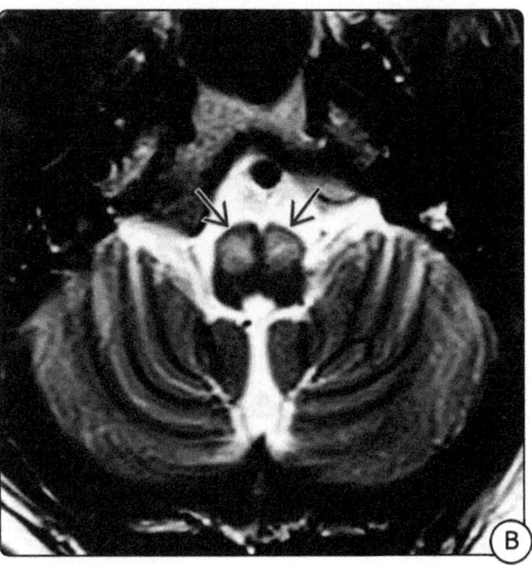

***(33-35B)** T2 MR shows expansion, hyperintensity of both olives ➡. This is acute hypertrophic olivary degeneration.*

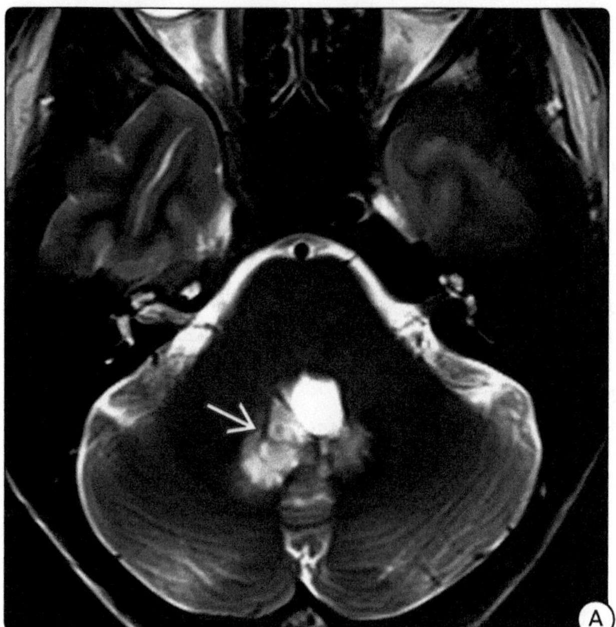

***(33-36A)** Axial T2 MR in a patient who developed palatal myoclonus 6 months after medulloblastoma resection shows surgical changes in the right dentate nucleus ➡.*

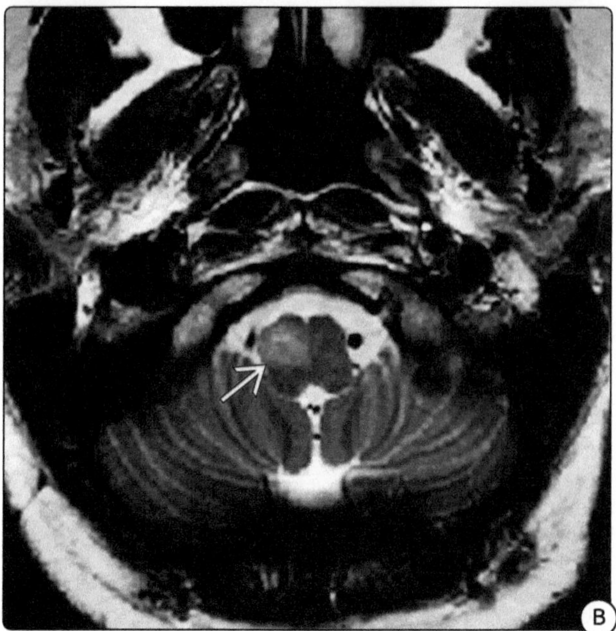

***(33-36B)** Axial T2 MR through the medulla in the same patient shows unilateral hypertrophic olivary degeneration ➡.*

HYPERTROPHIC OLIVARY DEGENERATION

Etiology
- Interruption of Guillain-Mollaret triangle

Pathology
- Inferior olives hypertrophy
  - Can be uni- or bilateral
  - Ipsi- or contralateral to primary lesion

Imaging
- Maximum hypertrophy at 5-15 months
  - Usually resolves in 1-3 years
  - Then ION atrophies
- ION T2/FLAIR hyperintensity
- Does not enhance

Differential Diagnosis
- Multiple sclerosis, neoplasm
- Perforating artery infarct
- Metronidazole neurotoxicity

Clinical Issues

HOD is rare. It has been reported in patients of all ages, from young children to the elderly. The classic clinical presentation of HOD is palatal myoclonus, typically developing 4-12 months following the brain insult.

Imaging

The development of HOD is a delayed process. Although changes can sometimes be detected within three or four weeks after the initial insult, maximum hypertrophy occurs between 5 and 15 months. The hypertrophy typically resolves in 1-3 years, and the ION eventually becomes atrophic.

T1 scans are usually normal or show mild enlargement of the ION. T2/FLAIR hyperintensity without enlargement of the ION occurs in 4-6 months but may be detectable as early as three weeks after the initial insult.

Between 6 months and several years later, the ION appears both hyperintense and hypertrophied **(33-35B)** **(33-36)**. HOD does not enhance on T1 C+. The hypertrophy typically resolves and atrophy ensues, but the hyperintensity may persist indefinitely.

Differential Diagnosis

Other lesions with T2/FLAIR hyperintensity in the anterior medulla include **demyelinating disease, neoplasm**, and **perforating artery infarction. Metronidazole neurotoxicity** exhibits bilateral, symmetric T2-/FLAIR-hyperintense lesions in the corpus callosum splenium and RN as well as the caudate, lentiform, olivary, and dentate nuclei.

Selected References: The complete reference list is available on the Expert Consult™ eBook version included with purchase.

Hydrocephalus and CSF Disorders

The brain CSF spaces include the ventricular system—a series of interconnected, CSF-filled cavities—and the subarachnoid space. This chapter begins with a brief discussion of the normal ventricles and CSF spaces.

We describe normal variants, which should not be mistaken for disease, then turn our attention to hydrocephalus and the manifestations of elevated CSF pressure, including idiopathic intracranial hypertension ("pseudotumor cerebri"). We close the chapter with a discussion of CSF leaks and intracranial hypotension.

Normal Anatomy of the Ventricles and Cisterns

Ventricular System

The ventricular system is composed of four interconnected ependyma-lined cavities that lie deep within the brain **(34-3)**. The paired lateral ventricles communicate with the third ventricle via the Y-shaped foramen of Monro. The third ventricle communicates with the fourth ventricle via the cerebral aqueduct (of Sylvius). In turn, the fourth ventricle communicates with the subarachnoid space (SAS).

Choroid Plexus, CSF, and Brain Interstitial Fluid

The CSF space is a dynamic pressure system with a hydrostatic balance between CSF production and absorption. The choroid plexus (CP) has two major functions: CSF production and maintenance of the blood-CSF barrier. In adult humans, the CP epithelium forms CSF at the rate of ~ 0.4 mL per minute or ~ 500-600 mL every 24 hours. CSF is turned over about four times a day, allowing for the removal of waste products.

Brain interstitial fluid (ISF) in the extracellular spaces is also a significant extrachoroidal source of CSF.

The CP maintains the blood-CSF barrier via tight junctions between epithelial cells. The exchange of substances between the brain ISF and the CSF across the blood-CSF barrier is highly regulated. Specialized subpopulations of CP epithelial cells are responsible for the transfer of plasma proteins from blood to the CSF.

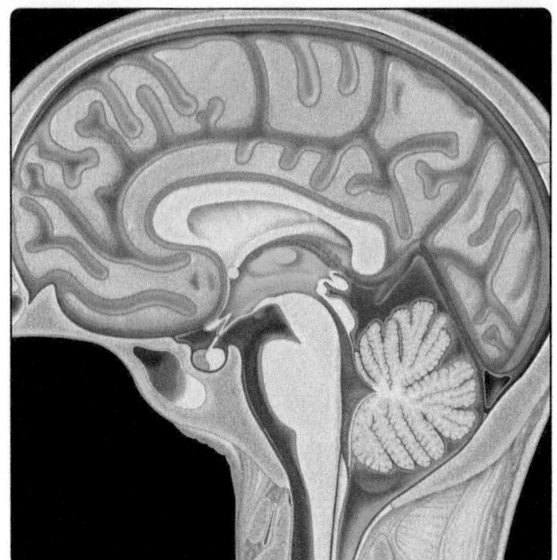

(34-1) Sagittal graphic depicts subarachnoid spaces with CSF (blue) between arachnoid (purple) and pia (orange).

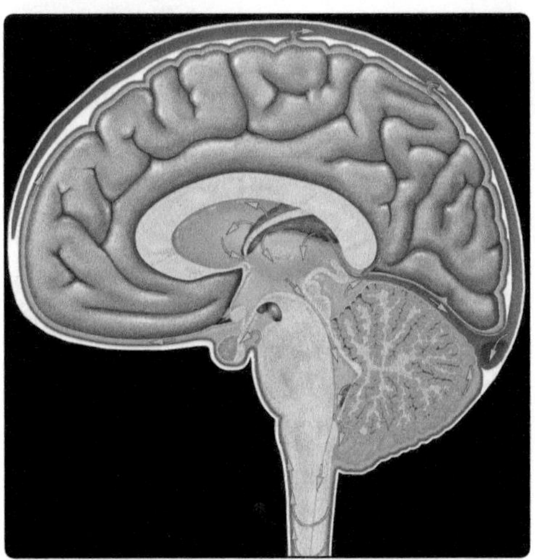

(34-2) Classic model of CSF produced by choroid plexus, flowing in a unidirectional manner and absorbed by arachnoid granulations.

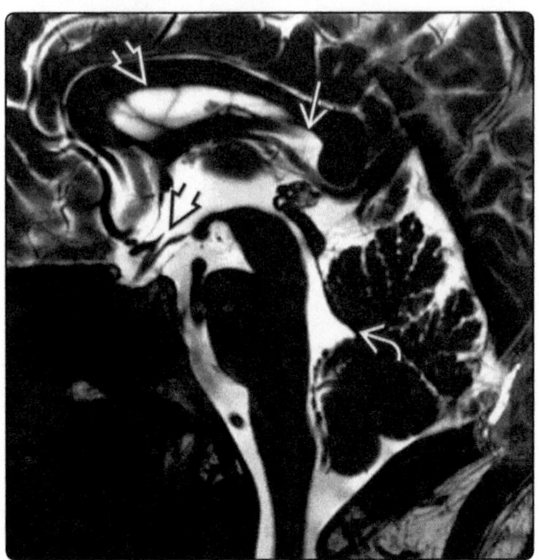

(34-3) T2 MR shows lateral ventricle ➡, velum interpositum ➡, anterior 3rd ventricle recesses ➡, fastigium of the 4th ventricle ➡.

CSF Circulation and Homeostasis

Traditional Model of CSF Homeostasis. The longstanding, classic model of CSF homeostasis was based on the *circulation theory* in which the majority of CSF is produced by the CP, then circulates from the ventricles into the SASs **(34-1)**. In this model, CSF flow in the ventricular cavities is unidirectional and rostrocaudal. CSF exits the fourth ventricle into the SASs through the medial foramen (of Magendie) and the two lateral foramina (of Luschka), which form the only natural communications between the ventricles and the SAS **(34-2)**.

Updated Model of CSF and ISF Homeostasis. New evidence suggests that the traditional model of CSF production, circulation, and function is too simplistic and much more complex than previously thought. It is now recognized that CSF plays an essential role in the maintenance of brain ISF homeostasis and that the two are intimately interrelated in maintaining normal brain function. The main sources of ISF are the blood and CSF.

In the updated CSF-ISF model, the brain perivascular spaces (PVSs) (Virchow-Robin) and paravascular spaces play a critical role in CSF homeostasis. The PVSs form a key component of the brain's "protolymphatic" or *"glymphatic" system*. The PVSs are lined with leptomeningeal (pial) cells that coat the PVSs as well as arteries and veins in the SAS, thus separating CSF in the SAS from the brain parenchyma and PVSs.

ISF diffuses through the brain's extracellular spaces and then drains via bulk flow along the basement membranes of cerebral capillaries. ISF circulation likely occurs through the water-selective aquaporin (AQP) channels of the glymphatic system, key factors in regulating ECS water homeostasis. AQP4 is highly expressed in astrocytic end-feet and also appears to be crucial for fluid exchange between the CSF and ISF.

Finally, in this model of CSF and ISF homeostasis, drainage of extracellular fluids in the CNS and integrity of the brain glymphatic system is important for not only volume regulation but also clearance of waste products, such as amyloid-β (Aβ) from the brain parenchyma.

Subarachnoid Spaces/Cisterns

The **subarachnoid spaces** (SASs) lie between the pia and arachnoid **(34-1)**. The **sulci** are small, thin SASs that are interposed between the gyral folds. Focal expansions of the SASs form the brain CSF cisterns. Numerous pial-covered septa cross the SASs from the brain to the arachnoid, which is loosely attached to the inner layer of the dura. All SASs normally communicate freely with each other and the ventricular system.

Normal Variants

Age-Related Changes

Increase in lateral ventricular volume is a constant, linear function of age throughout life.

Asymmetric Lateral Ventricles

Asymmetric lateral ventricles can be identified on imaging studies in ~ 5-10% of normal patients. The asymmetry is typically mild to moderate. Bowing, deviation, or displacement of the septi pellucidi across the midline is common; by itself, it neither indicates pathology nor implicates an etiology for nonspecific headache.

Cavum Septi Pellucidi and Vergae

A **cavum septi pellucidi** (CSP) is a fluid-filled cavity that lies between the frontal horns of the lateral ventricles **(34-4)**. A **cavum vergae** (CV) is an elongated finger-like posterior extension from the CSP that lies between the fornices **(34-5)**.

A CSP may occur in isolation, but a CV occurs only in combination with a CSP. When the two occur together, the correct Latin terminology is "cavum septi pellucidi et vergae." In common usage, the combination is often referred to simply as a CSP.

The appearance of CSPs and CVs on CT and MR varies from an almost inapparent, slit-like cavity to a prominent collection measuring several millimeters in diameter. A CSP is isodense with CSF on NECT and follows CSF signal intensity exactly on MR. It suppresses completely on FLAIR.

Cavum Velum Interpositum

The velum interpositum (VI) is a thin translucent membrane formed by two infolded layers of pia-arachnoid. The VI extends laterally over the thalami to become continuous with the choroid plexus of the lateral ventricles. Together with the fornices, the VI forms the roof of the third ventricle.

The VI is often CSF filled and open posteriorly, communicating directly with the quadrigeminal cistern. In such cases, it is called a cavum velum interpositum (CVI) **(34-6)**. A CVI is considered a normal anatomic variant.

On imaging studies, a CVI appears as a triangular CSF space that curves over the thalami between the lateral ventricles. Its apex points toward the foramen of Monro **(34-7)**. A CVI is isodense with CSF on NECT and isointense on all MR sequences. It suppresses completely on FLAIR, does not enhance, and does not restrict on DWI.

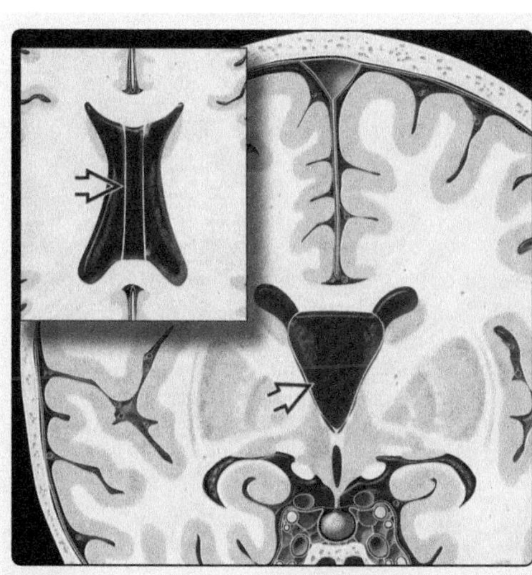

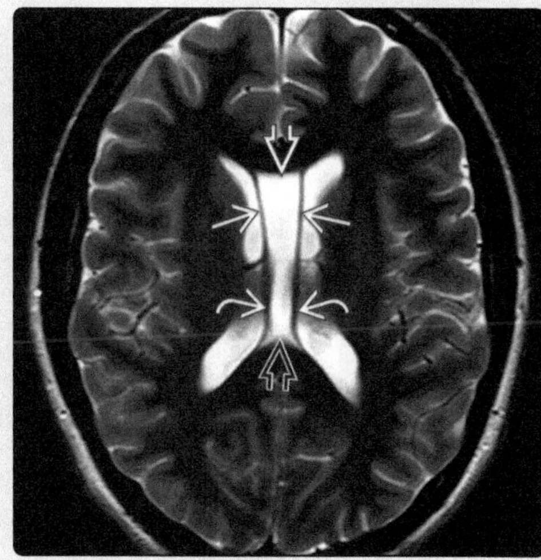

***(34-4)** Coronal graphic with axial inset shows classic cavum septi pellucidi (CSP) with cavum vergae (CV). The CSP appears triangular on the coronal image but finger-like on the axial view. (34-5) Axial T2 MR shows a CSP with CV. The leaves of the septum pellucidum and bodies of the fornices are splayed apart by a contiguous CSF-containing cavity that lies between them. The CSP and CV are continuous in this normal variant.*

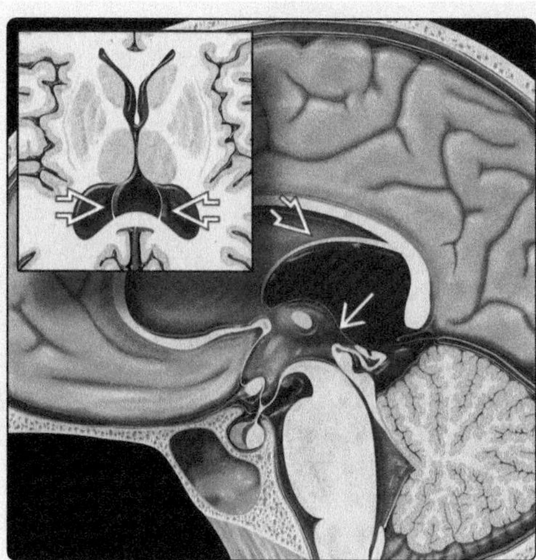

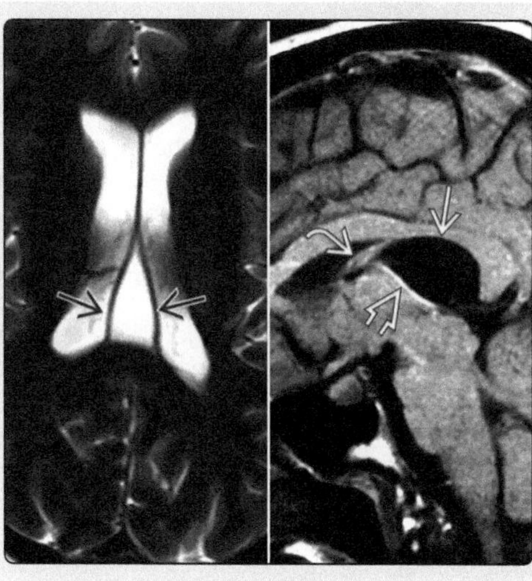

***(34-6)** Sagittal graphic with axial inset shows a cavum vellum interpositum (CVI). Note the elevation and splaying of the fornices. Also noted is the inferior displacement of the internal cerebral veins and 3rd ventricle. (34-7) On axial T2 MR (L), a CVI is triangular and separates the fornices. On the sagittal image (R), CVI flattens the internal cerebral vein inferiorly but elevates and displaces the fornix superiorly.*

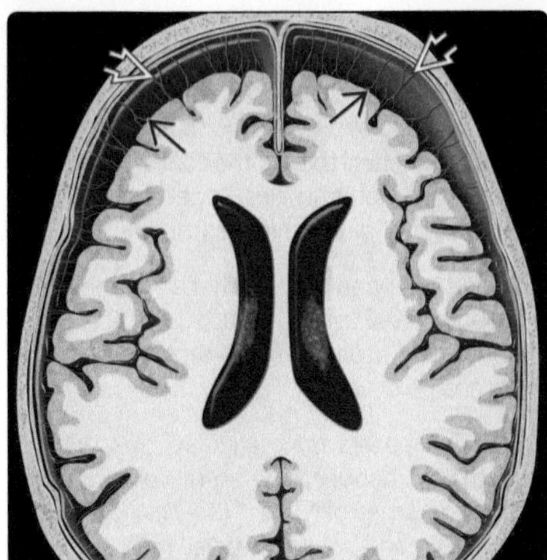

***(34-8)** Graphic depicts benign enlarged frontal SASs ⇨. Posterior SASs are normal. Note cortical veins crossing the prominent SASs ➡.*

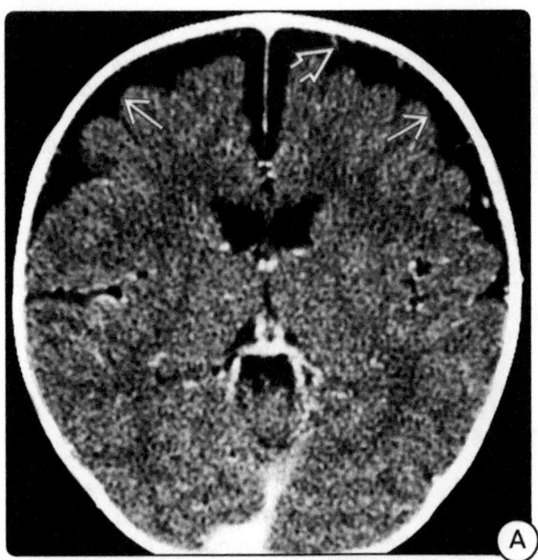

***(34-9A)** CECT in a 7-month-old infant shows prominent bifrontal, interhemispheric subarachnoid spaces ➡ and bridging veins ➡.*

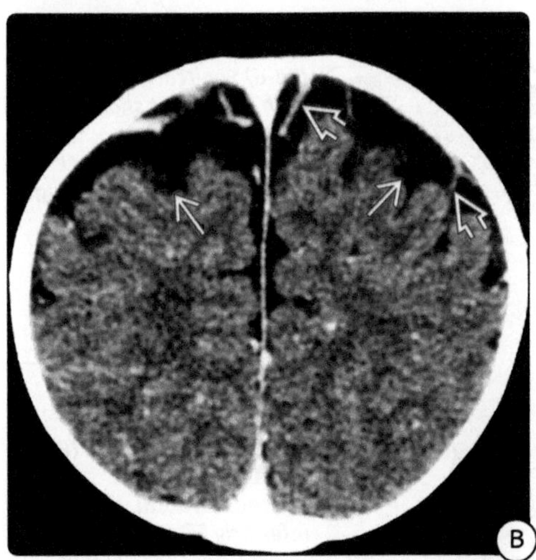

***(34-9B)** More cephalad CECT in the same patient shows fluid collections ➡, bridging veins ➡. These are benign enlarged SASs of infancy.*

Enlarged Subarachnoid Spaces

Enlarged subarachnoid spaces (SASs) occur in three conditions: Extraventricular obstructive ("communicating") hydrocephalus, brain atrophy, and benign enlargement of the SASs **(34-8)**. Communicating hydrocephalus (both the intra- and extraventricular types) is discussed below. Brain volume loss is a manifestation of both normal aging and brain degeneration. In this section, we discuss benign physiologic enlargement of the SAS.

Terminology

Idiopathic enlargement of the SASs with normal to slightly increased ventricular size is common in infants. Large CSF spaces in developmentally and neurologically normal children with or without macrocephaly is termed **benign enlargement of the SASs (BESS)**.

Etiology and Pathology

The etiology of benign enlarged SASs in infants is unknown but probably related to immature CSF drainage pathways. Approximately 80% of infants with benign enlarged SASs have a family history of macrocephaly.

Grossly, the SASs appear deep and unusually prominent but otherwise normal. There are no subdural membranes present that would suggest chronic subdural hematomas or effusions.

Clinical Issues

Benign enlarged SASs typically present between 3 and 8 months. There is a 4:1 M:F predominance. There are no findings indicative of elevated intracranial pressure (ICP) or nonaccidental trauma.

Benign enlargement of the SASs is reported on 2-65% of imaging studies for macrocrania in children under 1 year of age. BESS is a self-limited phenomenon that typically resolves by 12-24 months without intervention. The associated macrocephaly may resolve by 2 years, but it often levels off, remaining at the 98th percentile.

Imaging

Bifrontal and anterior interhemispheric SASs are > 5 mm in diameter **(34-9A)**. The suprasellar/chiasmatic cistern and sylvian fissures are also prominent. The lateral and third ventricles can be mildly enlarged. CECT scans demonstrate bridging veins traversing the SAS **(34-9B)**. There is *no* evidence of thickened enhancing membranes to suggest subdural hematoma or hygroma.

Fluid in the enlarged frontal SASs exactly parallels CSF on all MR sequences because it *is* CSF. The fluid suppresses completely on FLAIR. Bridging veins can be seen crossing the prominent SASs on T1 C+.

Differential Diagnosis

The major differential diagnoses of benign enlarged SASs are atrophy, extraventricular obstructive hydrocephalus, and nonaccidental trauma. Occasionally, infants with benign enlarged SASs have minor superimposed hemorrhagic subdural collections similar to those sometimes observed with arachnoid cysts. In such infants, **abusive head trauma** must be a consideration until careful screening discloses no substantiating evidence of inflicted injury.

Hydrocephalus

The term "hydrocephalus" literally means "water head." The term "ventriculomegaly" means enlargement of the ventricular system. Remember: The terms **"hydrocephalus" and "ventriculomegaly" are descriptive findings, not a diagnosis!** The role of imaging is to **find the etiology of the ventricular enlargement**.

Hydrocephalus has traditionally been regarded as an abnormality in the formation, flow, or resorption of CSF. If normal CSF flow is impeded by a blockage within the ventricular system, CSF production continues and the ventricles enlarge. In the classic model, hydrocephalus can also result from an imbalance between CSF production and absorption. When CSF absorption through the arachnoid granulations is compromised, the ventricles enlarge and hydrocephalus results. Absorption can be blocked at any level within the subarachnoid cisterns, e.g., within the cisterna magna, at the basilar cisterns, or along the cerebral convexities.

In the newest attempt to understand the development of hydrocephalus, aquaporin (AQP)-mediated brain water homeostasis &/or clearance of both CSF and ISF into the PVSs and blood are compromised. The molecular mechanisms that drive AQP4 modifications in hydrocephalus that fail to facilitate removal of excess water are still relatively unknown.

Terminology

We follow the common approach of subclassifying hydrocephalus by the *presumed* site of CSF obstruction, i.e., inside [**intraventricular obstructive hydrocephalus** (IVOH)] or outside the ventricles [**extraventricular obstructive hydrocephalus** (EVOH)]. The outdated term "ex vacuo hydrocephalus," referring to ventricular and cisternal enlargement caused by parenchymal volume loss, is no longer used.

Etiology

When abnormally large cerebral ventricles are identified on imaging studies, the diagnostic imperative is to find the cause of the hydrocephalus.

In the pediatric age group, a majority of cases are caused by congenital defects of the CSF pathway. Adult-onset hydrocephalus is usually secondary to different pathologies that encompass a heterogeneous group of disorders, such as intracranial hemorrhage and neoplasms.

Intraventricular Obstructive Hydrocephalus

Terminology

IVOH is used to designate physical obstruction at or proximal to the fourth ventricular outlet foramina. The term "noncommunicating hydrocephalus" is no longer used.

Etiology

General Concepts. IVOH can be **congenital** or **acquired**, **acute** (aIVOH) or **chronic** (cIVOH). Congenital IVOH occurs with disorders such as aqueductal stenosis.

When the ventricles become obstructed, CSF outflow is impeded. As CSF production continues, the ventricles expand. As the ventricles expand, increased pressure is exerted on the adjacent brain parenchyma. Increased intraparenchymal pressure compromises cerebral blood flow, reducing brain perfusion. The increased pressure also compresses the subependymal veins,

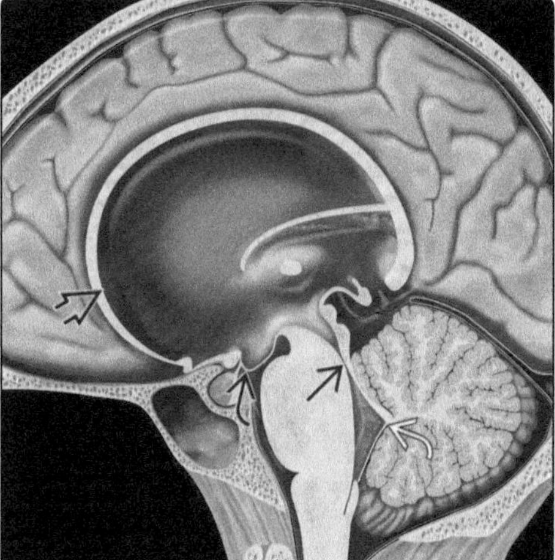

***(34-10)** Note aqueductal stenosis ⇒, IVOH with enlarged lateral ⇒, 3rd ⇒ ventricles, stretched corpus callosum, normal 4th ventricle ⇒.*

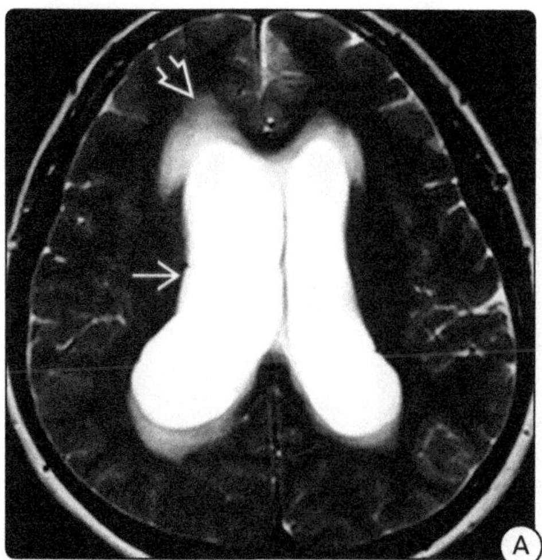

***(34-11A)** Axial T2 MR in patient with severe headaches shows large lateral ventricles ⇒ with extensive periventricular fluid accumulation ⇒.*

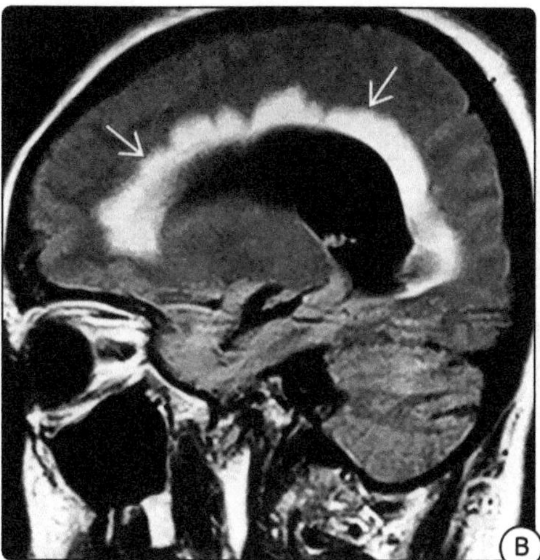

***(34-11B)** Sagittal FLAIR MR shows hyperintense "fingers" ⇒ extending along the entire margin of the lateral ventricle, acute IVOH.*

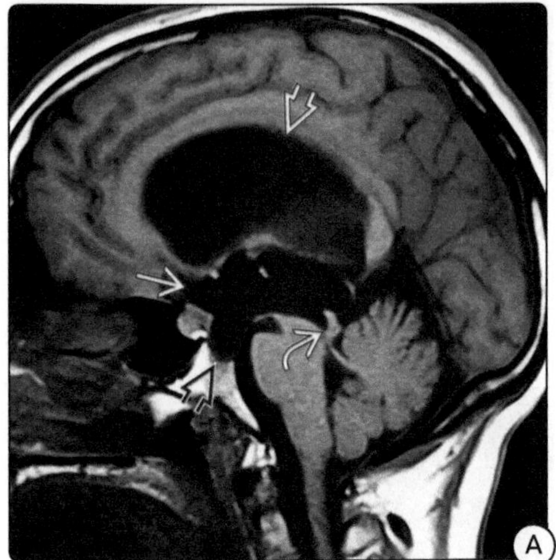

(34-12A) T1WI in a 22y woman with longstanding aqueductal stenosis ➡ shows enlarged lateral ➡, 3rd ➡ ventricles with remodeled clivus ⇨.

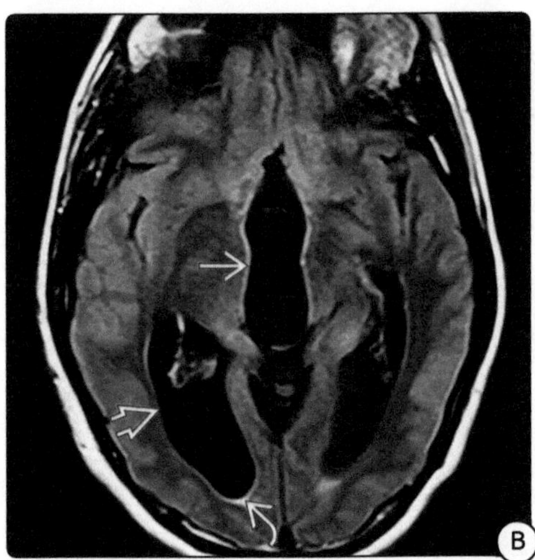

(34-12B) Axial FLAIR MR shows enlarged 3rd ➡, lateral ➡ ventricles with minimal hyperintense rim ➡.

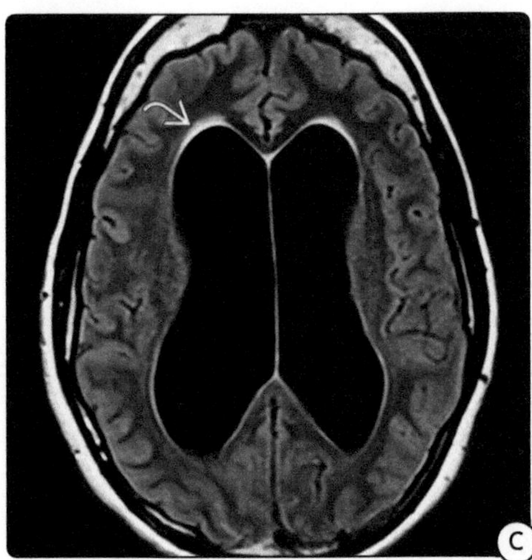

(34-12C) More cephalad FLAIR MR shows marked, symmetrically enlarged ventricles, thin fluid rim ➡. This is chronic compensated IVOH.

which reduces absorption of brain interstitial fluid via the deep medullary veins and perivascular spaces. The result is **periventricular interstitial edema**. Whether the edema results from CSF extruding across the ventricular ependyma (**"transependymal CSF flow"**) or accumulation of brain extracellular fluid is unknown.

In chronic "compensated" IVOH, the ventricles expand slowly enough that CSF homeostasis is relatively maintained. Periventricular interstitial edema is minimal or absent.

Pathology

Grossly, the ventricles proximal to the obstruction appear ballooned **(34-10)**. The ependyma is thinned and may be focally disrupted or even absent. The corpus callosum (CC) is thinned and compressed superiorly against the falx cerebri. The ependymal lining is discontinuous or inapparent, the periventricular extracellular space is increased, and the surrounding white matter (WM) is rarefied and stains pale.

Clinical Issues

The presentation of IVOH varies with acuity and severity. Headache is the most common overall symptom, and papilledema is the most common sign. Nausea, vomiting, and CNVI palsy are also common with aIVOH.

Most cases are typically progressive unless treated. Untreated severe aIVOH can result in brain herniation with coma and even death. Some patients with slowly developing compensated IVOH may not present until late in adult life (e.g., the recently recognized syndrome of late-onset aqueductal stenosis).

CSF diversion (shunt, ventriculostomy, endoscopic fenestration of the third ventricle floor) is common, often performed as a first step before definitive treatment of the obstruction (e.g., removal of a colloid cyst or resection of an intraventricular neoplasm).

Imaging

CT Findings. Imaging findings vary with acuity and severity. NECT scans in aIVOH demonstrate enlarged lateral and third ventricles, whereas the size of the fourth ventricle varies. The temporal horns are prominent, the frontal horns are "rounded," and the margins of the ventricles appear indistinct or "blurred." Periventricular fluid—whether from compromised drainage of interstitial fluid or transependymal CSF migration—causes a "halo" of low density in the adjacent WM. The sulci and basal cisterns appear compressed or indistinct.

MR Findings. Axial T1WI shows that both lateral ventricles are symmetrically enlarged. On sagittal views, the CC appears thinned and stretched superiorly **(34-18A)**, whereas the fornices and internal cerebral veins are displaced inferiorly.

In aIVOH, T2 scans may demonstrate "fingers" of CSF-like hyperintensity extending outward from the lateral ventricles into the surrounding WM **(34-11A)**. Fluid in the periventricular "halo" does not suppress on FLAIR **(34-11B)**. In longstanding chronic "compensated" hydrocephalus, the ventricles appear enlarged and the WM attenuated but without a thick periventricular "halo" **(34-12)**.

Complications of Hydrocephalus. In severe cases of IVOH, the CC becomes compressed against the free inferior margin of the falx **(34-13)** **(34-14)**. This can cause pressure necrosis and loss of callosal axons, the so-called **corpus callosum impingement syndrome** (CCIS) **(34-18C)**. In acute CCIS, the CC may initially appear swollen and hyperintense on T2WI and FLAIR. Subacute and chronic changes are seen as encephalomalacic foci in a shrunken, atrophic-appearing CC. In 15% of treated IVOH cases, the CC shows T2/FLAIR hyperintensity after decompression. In rare cases, the hyperintensity extends beyond the CC itself into the periventricular WM **(34-15)**.

Massive ventricular enlargement may weaken the medial wall of the lateral ventricle enough that a pulsion-type diverticulum of CSF extrudes through the inferomedial wall of the atrium. Such **medial atrial diverticula** may cause significant mass effect on the posterior third ventricle, tectal plate, and aqueduct. Large atrial diverticula can herniate inferiorly through the tentorial incisura into the posterior fossa, compressing the vermis and fourth ventricle.

Differential Diagnosis

The major differential diagnosis of IVOH is **extraventricular obstructive hydrocephalus**. **Parenchymal volume loss** causes secondary dilatation of the ventricles (ventriculomegaly) with proportional enlargement of the surface sulci and cisterns.

A helpful feature to distinguish obstructive hydrocephalus from atrophy is the appearance of the temporal horns. In obstructive hydrocephalus, they appear rounded and moderately to strikingly enlarged. Even with relatively severe volume loss, the temporal horns retain their normal kidney bean shape and are only minimally to moderately enlarged.

Normal pressure hydrocephalus is typically a disorder of older adults and is typified clinically by progressive dementia, gait disturbance, and incontinence. The ventricles often appear disproportionately enlarged relative to the sulci and cisterns.

INTRAVENTRICULAR OBSTRUCTIVE HYDROCEPHALUS

Terminology, Etiology
- Proximal to 4th ventricle outlet foramina
- Can be congenital or acquired, acute or chronic
  - Postinflammation/posthemorrhage
  - Obstructing intraventricular mass

Acute Obstructive Hydrocephalus
- Ventricles proximal to obstruction are ballooned
- "Blurred" margins of ventricles
- Periventricular fluid accumulation (CSF, ISF, or both)
  - "Halo" ± "fingers" of fluid around ventricles
  - T2 hyperintense; does not suppress on FLAIR

Chronic Compensated Obstructive Hydrocephalus
- Large ventricles, no periventricular "halo"
- ± callosal impingement, atrial diverticula

Extraventricular Obstructive Hydrocephalus

Terminology

In extraventricular obstructive hydrocephalus (EVOH), the obstruction is located *outside* the ventricular system.

Etiology

The obstruction causing EVOH can be located at any level from the fourth ventricular outlet foramina to the arachnoid granulations. Subarachnoid hemorrhage—whether traumatic or aneurysmal—is the most frequent cause. Other common etiologies include purulent meningitis, granulomatous meningitis, and disseminated CSF metastases.

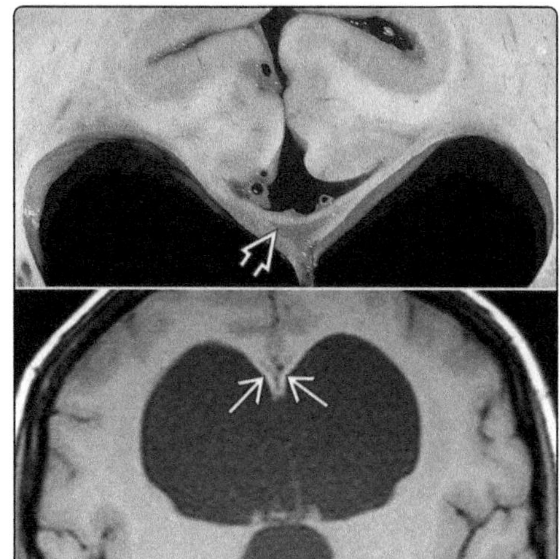

***(34-13)** (Top) IVOH, thinned encephalomalacic CC ➡ is caused by falx impingement. (Bottom) T1 MR shows CC impingement ➡.*

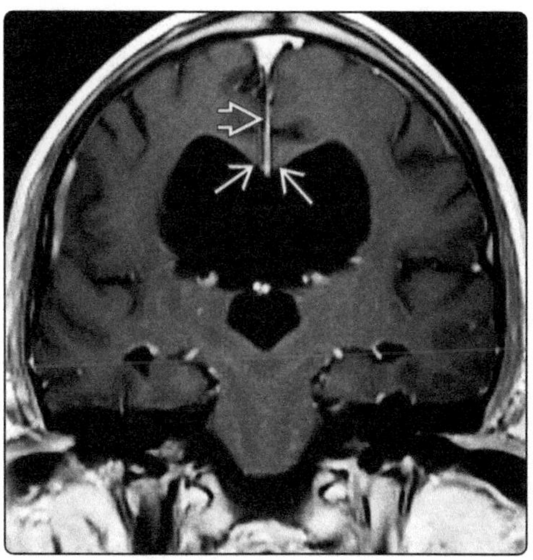

***(34-14)** Coronal T1 C+ MR of longstanding IVOH shows the lateral ventricles ➡, corpus callosum are forced upward against the falx cerebri ➡.*

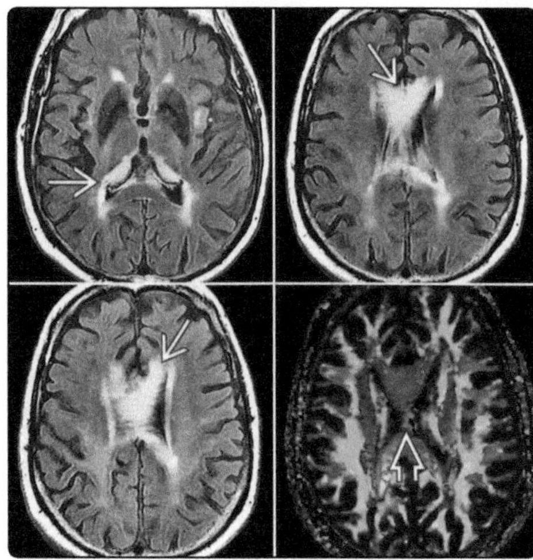

***(34-15)** CCIS with decompression, postshunt FLAIR shows hyperintensity in CC, periventricular WM ➡, disrupted fibers on DTI ➡.*

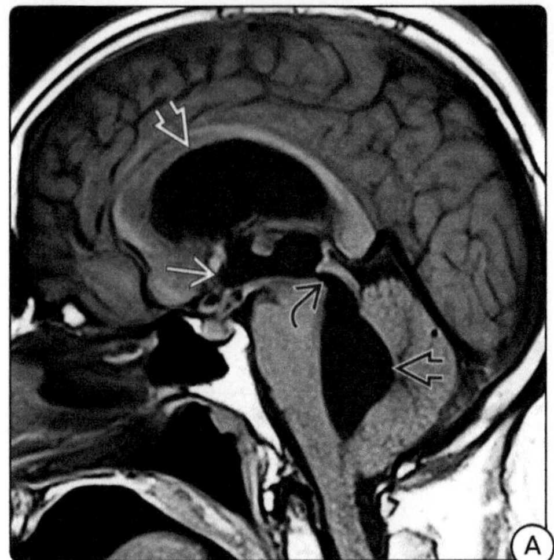

***(34-16A)** T1WI in patient with headaches, remote history of meningitis shows enlarged 4th ➲, 3rd ➔, lateral ➔ ventricles and aqueduct ↗.*

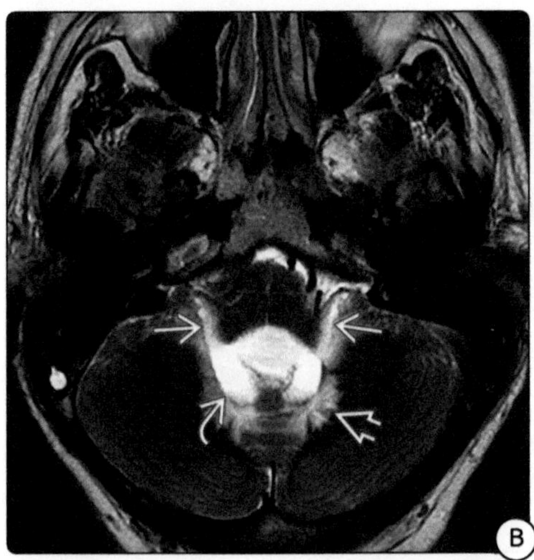

***(34-16B)** T2 MR shows marked enlargement of 4th ventricle ➔, including lateral recesses ➔, CSF migration into the adjacent cerebellum ➔.*

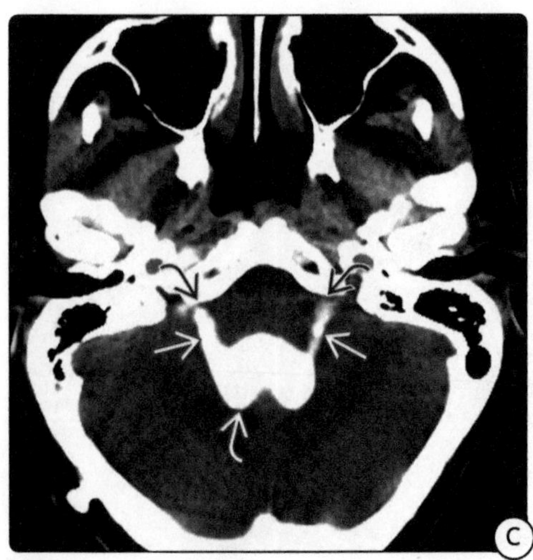

***(34-16C)** Contrast injected via ventriculostomy fills 4th ventricle ➔, lateral recesses ➔ but is obstructed at the outlet foramina ↗. EVOH.*

EXTRAVENTRICULAR OBSTRUCTIVE HYDROCEPHALUS

Terminology
- Formerly called "communicating" hydrocephalus
- Obstruction outside ventricular system
  - Any site from 4th ventricle foramina to arachnoid granulations

Etiology
- Most common
  - Subarachnoid hemorrhage (aneurysm > trauma)
- Less common
  - Meningitis (bacterial, granulomatous)
  - Metastases

Imaging
- > 50% show no discernible etiology
- Use CISS to look for obstructing membranes

Imaging

The classic appearance of EVOH on NECT scans is that of symmetric, proportionally enlarged lateral, third, and fourth ventricles. CECT scans may demonstrate enhancement in cases of EVOH secondary to infection or neoplasm.

The same imaging sequences used in IVOH apply to the evaluation of EVOH **(34-16)**. If the hydrocephalus is caused by acute subarachnoid hemorrhage or meningitis, the CSF appears "dirty" on T1WI and hyperintense on FLAIR. T1 C+ scans may demonstrate sulcal-cisternal enhancement.

In contrast to IVOH, > 1/2 of EVOH cases have no discernible cause for the obstruction on standard MR sequences. In such cases, it is especially important to identify subtle thin membranes that may be causing the extraventricular obstruction.

Overproduction Hydrocephalus

Overproduction hydrocephalus is uncommon and results from excessive CSF formation. **Choroid plexus papillomas** (CPPs) are the most common cause of overproduction hydrocephalus (see Fig. 18-17). **Diffuse villous hyperplasia of the choroid plexus** (DVHCP) is a rare cause of overproduction hydrocephalus. Imaging studies in DVHCP show severe hydrocephalus with massive enlargement of the entire choroid plexus.

Normal Pressure Hydrocephalus

There are no currently accepted evidence-based guidelines for either the diagnosis or treatment of normal pressure hydrocephalus (NPH). In this section, we briefly review the syndrome and summarize the spectrum of imaging findings that—in conjunction with clinical history and neurologic examination—may suggest the diagnosis.

Terminology

NPH is characterized by ventriculomegaly with normal CSF pressure but altered CSF hydrodynamics. **Primary** or **idiopathic NPH** (iNPH) is distinguished from **secondary NPH** (sNPH) in which there is a known antecedent, such as subarachnoid hemorrhage, traumatic brain injury, or meningitis.

Etiology

The pathogenesis of NPH is poorly understood and remains controversial. Recent studies of NPH suggest altered CSF dynamics (production, kinetics, reabsorption), and ISF stasis disrupts the balance between hydrostatic and osmotic pressures, reversing ISF flow and causing ventricular enlargement.

Pathology

The ventricles appear grossly enlarged. The periventricular WM often appears abnormal with or without frank lacunar infarction. Neurofibrillary tangles and other microscopic changes typically found in Alzheimer disease are seen in 20% of cases.

Clinical Issues

NPH accounts for ~ 5-6% of all dementias. The nature and severity of symptoms as well as the disease course vary. Impaired gait and balance are the typical initial symptoms. The classic triad of dementia, gait disturbance, and urinary incontinence is present in a minority of patients and typically represents advanced disease.

Some patients initially respond dramatically to ventricular shunting ("shunt-responsive" NPH). The favorable response to shunting varies from ~ 35-40% in patients with clinically "possible" NPH to 65% in patients diagnosed with "probable" NPH.

Imaging

General Features. Imaging studies in suspected NPH are necessary but insufficient to establish the definitive diagnosis of NPH. The goal of identifying patients who are likely to improve following ventriculoperitoneal shunting likewise remains elusive.

The most common general imaging feature of NPH is ventriculomegaly that appears out of proportion to sulcal enlargement ("ventriculosulcal disproportion").

CT Findings. NECT scans show enlarged lateral ventricles with rounded frontal horns. The third ventricle is moderately enlarged, whereas the fourth ventricle appears relatively normal. Compared with the degree of ventriculomegaly, generalized sulcal enlargement is mild. Periventricular hypodensity is common and often represents a combination of increased interstitial fluid and WM rarefaction secondary to microvascular disease.

MR Findings. T1 scans show large lateral ventricles. The convexity and medial subarachnoid spaces may appear decreased or "tight," whereas the basal cisterns and sylvian fissures are often enlarged. The corpus callosum is usually thinned. Most patients have a mild to moderate periventricular "halo" on T2/FLAIR **(34-18)**.

A prominent, exaggerated "hyperdynamic" aqueductal "flow void" may be present. Recent studies show some NPH patients have hyperdynamic CSF flow with increased velocity and volume in *both* systole and diastole. Net flow direction is caudocranial, the reverse of normal.

Nuclear Medicine. Prominent ventricular activity at 24 hours on In-111 DTPA cisternography is considered a relatively good indicator of NPH. 18F FDG PET shows decreased regional cerebral metabolism.

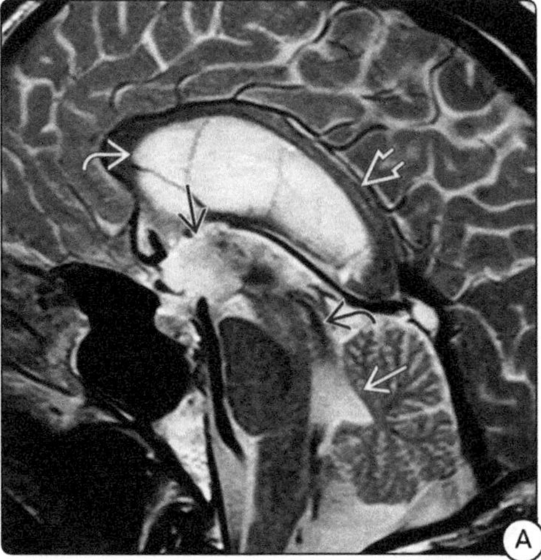

***(34-17A)** T2 MR shows large lateral ➡, 3rd ➡, 4th ➡ ventricles, exaggerated aqueductal "flow void" ➡, thin hyperintense corpus callosum ➡.*

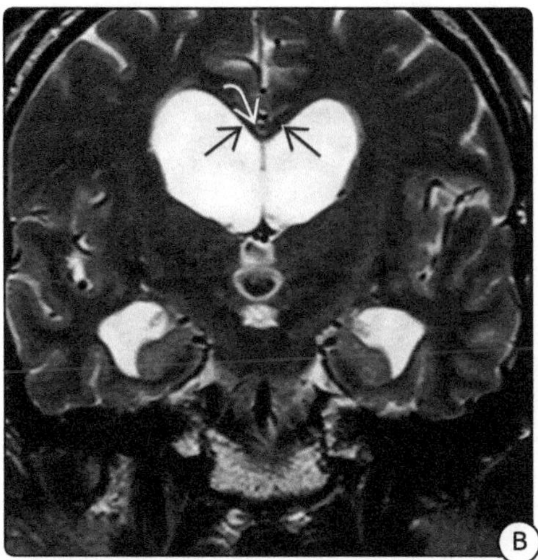

***(34-17B)** Coronal T2 MR shows enlarged lateral ventricles ➡ push encephalomalacic corpus callosum against falx ➡ (see Fig. 34-13).*

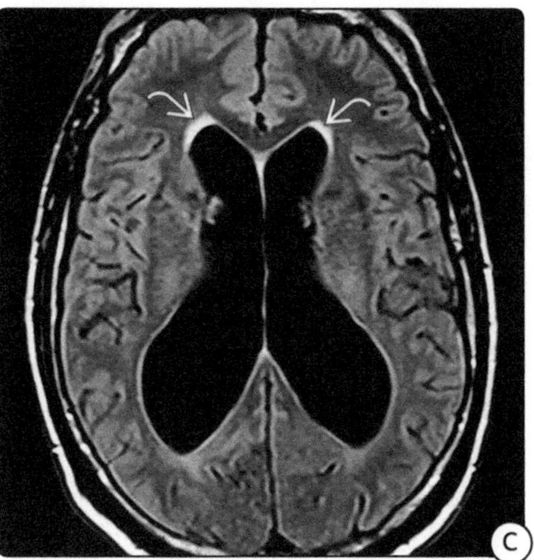

***(34-17C)** FLAIR shows thin rim of periventricular fluid accumulation ➡. Aqueductal stroke volume was 72 µL. This is shunt-responsive NPH.*

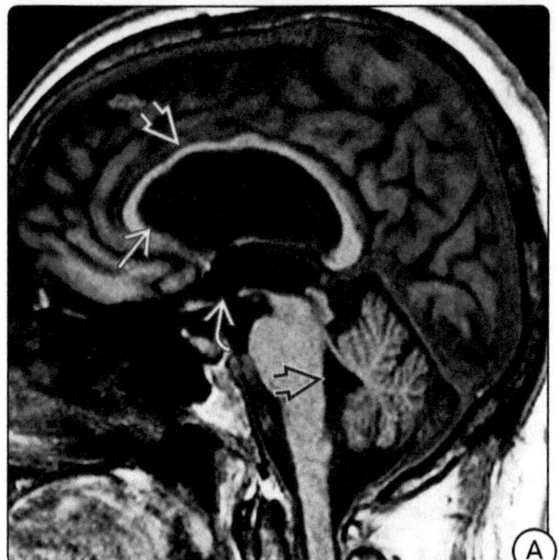

***(34-18A)** MP-RAGE in 72y man with NPH shows large lateral ➡, 3rd ➡, 4th ➡ ventricles. Corpus callosum ➡ is stretched and thinned.*

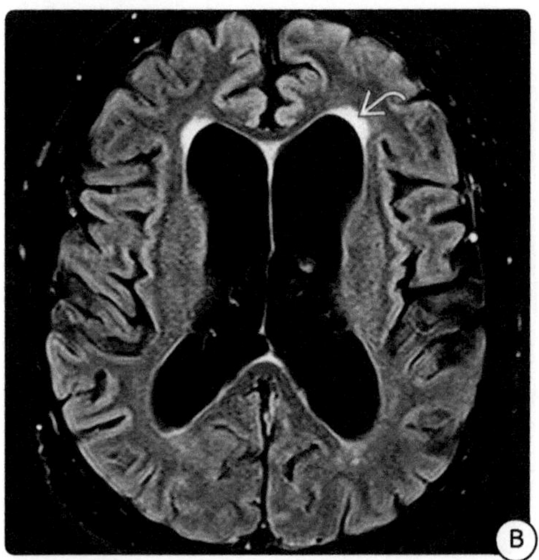

***(34-18B)** FLAIR MR shows enlarged lateral ventricles, normal sulci. Prominent hyperintense rim ➡ surrounds the ventricles.*

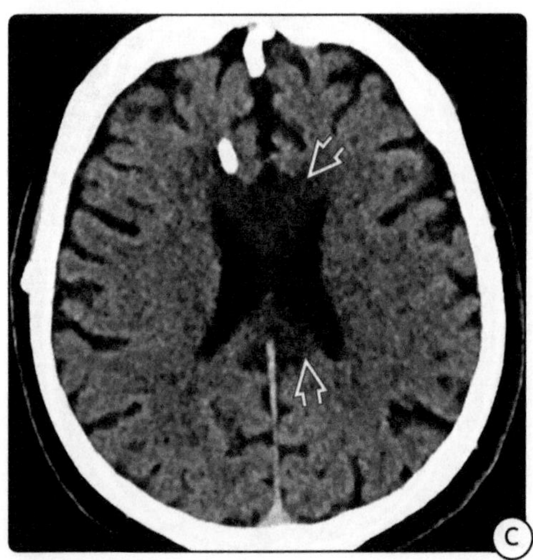

***(34-18C)** Follow-up NECT after shunting shows the hypodense corpus callosum ➡. This is NPH with callosal impingement syndrome.*

Differential Diagnosis

A major difficulty in diagnosing NPH is distinguishing it from other neurodegenerative disorders, such as **Alzheimer disease**, **vascular dementia**, and **age-related atrophy**. Recent studies suggest CSF biomarkers, such as AQP4, T-tau, and Aβ40, may be helpful in separating NPH from cognitive and movement disorder mimics.

Arrested Hydrocephalus

Arrested hydrocephalus (AH) has also been called compensated hydrocephalus, ventriculomegaly of adulthood, and late-onset idiopathic aqueductal stenosis. Patients rarely present with symptoms or stigmata of elevated ICP, and the diagnosis of hydrocephalus is often incidental and unexpected. Moderate to severe triventricular enlargement without evidence for periventricular fluid accumulation is present on imaging studies and may remain stable for years.

Idiopathic Intracranial Hypertension

Terminology

Idiopathic intracranial hypertension (IIH) is preferred to the term **pseudotumor cerebri**. IIH is characterized by unexplained elevation of ICP not related to an intracranial mass lesion, a meningeal process, or cerebral venous thrombosis. Patients with a known cause of elevated ICP (e.g., dural venous sinus stenosis) are nonetheless still classified as having IIH.

Etiology and Pathology

The precise etiology of IIH is unknown. An obese phenotype with elevated body mass index is common. Disturbed CSF-ISF drainage through the "glymphatic pathway" has been invoked by some investigators.

It is unclear whether the dural venous sinus stenosis found in the vast majority of IIH patients is a cause (from venous outflow obstruction) or an effect (from extrinsic compression) of elevated ICP, or both.

Clinical Issues

Classically, IIH presents in overweight women who are 20-45 years of age, although recent studies have confirmed a rising incidence in obese children, especially girls.

Headache is the most constant symptom (90-95%) followed by tinnitus and visual disturbances. Papilledema is the most common sign on neurologic examination **(34-19)**. Cranial nerve deficits, usually limited to CNVI, are common.

The definitive diagnosis of IIH is established by lumbar puncture, which demonstrates elevated ICP (> 200 mm H_2O in adults or 280 mm H_2O in children) with normal CSF composition.

Visual loss is the major morbidity in IIH. In fulminant IIH, visual loss can progress rapidly and become irreversible **(34-19)**. Serial CSF removal (10-20 mL at initial LP) often temporarily ameliorates IIH-associated headache. Venous sinus stenting in patients who have transverse sinus stenosis has been successful in improving symptoms and reducing papilledema in some cases.

Imaging

Neuroimaging is used to (1) exclude identifiable causes of increased ICP (e.g., neoplasm or obstructive hydrocephalus) and (2) detect findings associated with IIH.

The most significant imaging findings of IIH include **flattening of the posterior globes, distension of the perioptic subarachnoid space with or without a tortuous optic nerve, intraocular optic nerve protrusion, partial empty sella**, and **transverse venous sinus stenosis** on CTV/MRV or DSA **(34-20) (34-21)**. The presence of one or a combination of these signs—especially transverse sinus stenosis—significantly increases the odds of IIH, but their absence does not rule out IIH.

The prevalence of other reported findings, such as slit-like or "pinched" ventricles (10%), "tight" subarachnoid spaces (small sulci and cisterns), and inferiorly displaced tonsils, may be present. Cerebellar tonsillar ectopia may be present and sometimes even "peg-like" in configuration, mimicking Chiari 1 malformation or intracranial *hypo*tension.

Meningoceles or cephaloceles protruding through osseous-dural defects in the skull base are common, especially in extremely obese patients. CSF leaks are common, and CT or gadolinium MR cisternography may identify which of several bony defects is leaking.

Differential Diagnosis

The most important differential diagnosis in patients with suspected IIH is **secondary intracranial hypertension** (i.e., increased ICP with an identifiable cause). Ventriculomegaly is more common in secondary intracranial hypertension, whereas the ventricles are usually normal to small in IIH.

Dural sinus thrombosis is another important consideration. T2* (GRE, SWI) shows "blooming" thrombus in the affected sinuses. MRV and CTV demonstrate a cigar-shaped, long-segment clot.

IDIOPATHIC INTRACRANIAL HYPERTENSION

Terminology and Etiology

- a.k.a. benign intracranial hypertension
- Often no cause identified (idiopathic)

Clinical Issues

- F > M; obesity = definite risk
- Peak: 20-45 years
- Headache, tinnitus, vision loss, LP > 200 mm H_2O

Imaging

- Dilated optic nerve sheaths
- Intraoptic disc protrusion
- Flat posterior globe
- Partial empty sella
- "Tight" brain, ± tonsillar herniation
- ± dural sinus thrombosis, stenosis

CSF Shunts and Complications

Imaging is a key component in evaluating patients with CSF diversions. Shunt failure can result in either enlarging or collapsing ventricles. The most common imaging manifestation of shunt failure is enlarging ventricles. CT is generally the preferred technique to assess patients with intracranial shunt catheters. Alternative modalities include transfontanelle ultrasound and new

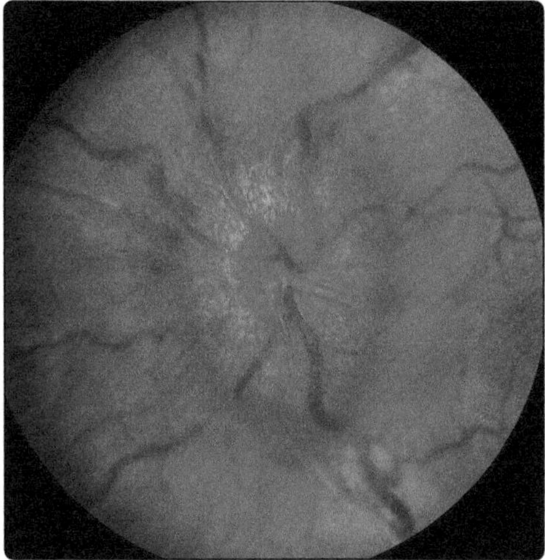

(34-19) Funduscopic image shows findings of severe papilledema with elevated, blurred optic disc. (From K. Digre, MD, Imaging in Neurology.)

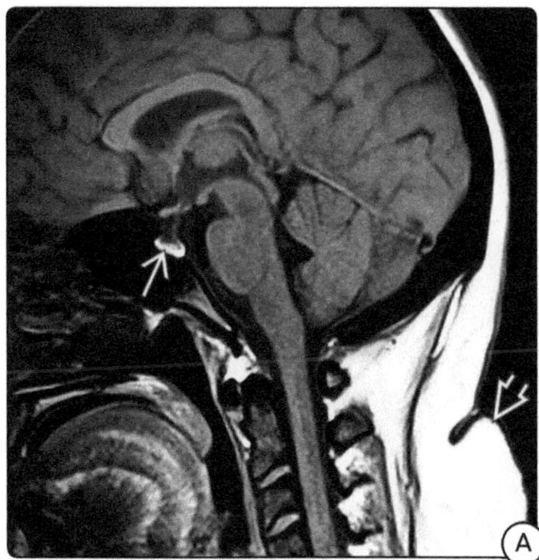

(34-20A) Sagittal T1 MR in a 33y obese woman shows excessive subcutaneous fat ➡ and a partial empty sella ➡.

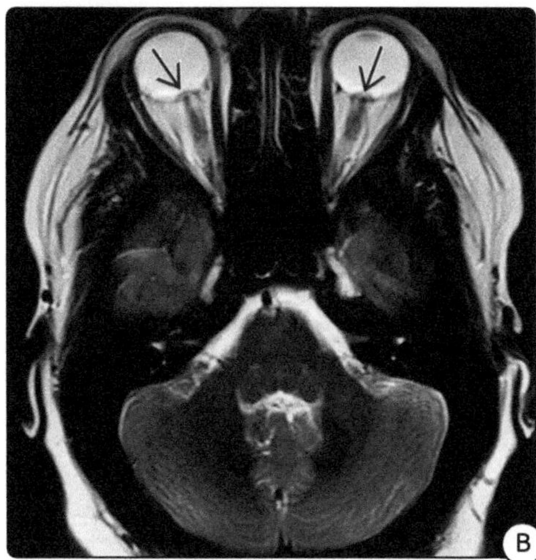

(34-20B) T2 MR shows flattening of the globes, intraocular protrusion of optic nerve heads ➡. At LP, the OP was 440 mm H_2O. This was IIH.

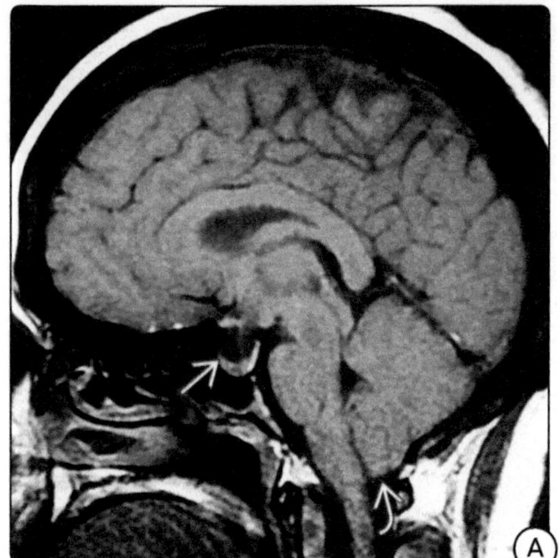

(34-21A) *T1 MR in 30y woman with severe headaches shows partial empty sella ➡ and mild tonsillar descent ➡.*

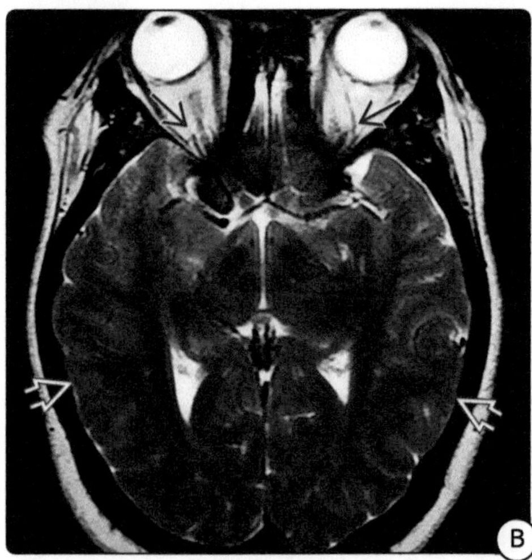

(34-21B) *T2 MR shows subtle dilatation of optic nerve sheaths ➡ and relative lack of CSF-filled sulci over brain surfaces ➡.*

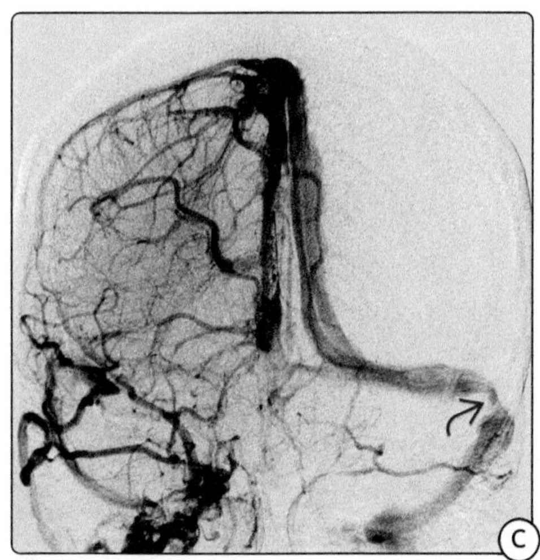

(34-21C) *AP DSA shows left transverse sinus stenosis ➡ with 10 mm Hg gradient. Stenting resolved the patient's headaches.*

rapid MR techniques, such as fast steady-state gradient-recalled-echo (SS-GRE) sequences.

Some shunted hydrocephalus patients exhibit clinical signs of shunt failure without evidence of ventricular enlargement, a condition called **slit ventricle syndrome** (SVS). Comparison to prior imaging studies is essential. NECT scans show that one or both lateral ventricles are small or slit-like.

CSF Leaks and Sequelae

CSF Leaks

CSF leaks can occur in patients of all ages. Trauma, prior skull base operation, and sinonasal surgery are common antecedents. Spontaneous CSF leaks usually develop in middle-aged obese women with idiopathic intracranial hypertension and are most commonly associated with arachnoid granulations in the lateral sphenoid sinus.

Bone CT with multiplanar reformations is the procedure of choice and may obviate the need for invasive CT cisternography. A bone defect, with or without an air-fluid level in the adjacent sinus, is the typical finding. Defects under 3 or 4 mm may be difficult to detect, especially in areas where the bone is normally very thin.

MR is generally used only if CT is negative or the presence of brain parenchyma within a cephalocele is suspected. T2 scans disclose an osseous defect with fluid in the adjacent sinus cavity.

Intracranial Hypotension

Terminology

Intracranial hypotension is also known as **CSF hypovolemia syndrome**.

Etiology and Pathology

Intracranial hypotension can be spontaneous (SIH) or acquired. Common antecedent causes include lumbar puncture, spinal surgery, and trauma.

Spinal meningeal diverticula can rupture suddenly and may be responsible for many cases of "spontaneous" intracranial hypotension. In contrast to idiopathic intracranial hypertension, skull base CSF leaks rarely cause SIH.

CSF hypovolemia and hypotension (lumbar OP < 60 mm H_2O) result in venous and dural interstitial engorgement with brain descent ("sagging") **(34-22)**. Patients with Marfan and Ehlers-Danlos syndromes have abnormal connective tissue and an increased risk of CSF rupture through the congenitally weakened dura.

Clinical Issues

Symptoms range widely, from mild headache to coma. The classic presentation is severe orthostatic headache that is relieved by lying down. Most cases of SIH resolve spontaneously. Severe cases may present with progressive encephalopathy and, in rare cases, severe unrelieved brain descent can result in coma or even death.

Treatment is aimed at restoring CSF volume. Fluid replacement and bed rest can be sufficient in many cases. In others, epidural blood patch or surgical repair may be required.

Epidural blood patch is often performed on the basis of clinical and brain imaging findings alone. If low- and high-volume patches are unsuccessful, further studies may be necessary to localize precisely the level of the CSF leak.

Imaging

Imaging is key to the diagnosis, sometimes providing the first insight into the cause of often puzzling symptoms.

Although CT is often obtained as an initial screening study in patients with severe or intractable headache, MR of the brain and spine is the procedure of choice to evaluate possible SIH.

Between 90-95% of SIH patients have one or more key findings on standard MR scans. A spectrum of findings occurs with SIH; only rarely are *all* imaging signs present in the same patient!

CT Findings. CT scans in SIH are often normal. The most obvious findings are subdural fluid collections. Subtle CT clues to the presence of SIH include effacement of the basal cisterns (especially the suprasellar subarachnoid space), medial herniation of the temporal lobes into the tentorial incisura, small ventricles with medial deviation of the atria of the lateral ventricles, and a "fat" pons.

MR Findings

T1WI. Sagittal T1 scans show brain descent in ~ 1/2 of all cases **(34-23)**. Midbrain "sagging" with the midbrain displaced below the level of the dorsum sellae, decreased angle between the peduncles and pons below 50°, shortened pontomammillary distance below 5.5 mm, and flattening of the pons against the clivus are typical findings **(34-24)**. Caudal displacement of the tonsils is common but not invariably present.

The optic chiasm and hypothalamus are often draped over the sella, effacing the suprasellar cistern. The pituitary gland appears enlarged in at least 50% of all cases **(34-22) (34-23)**.

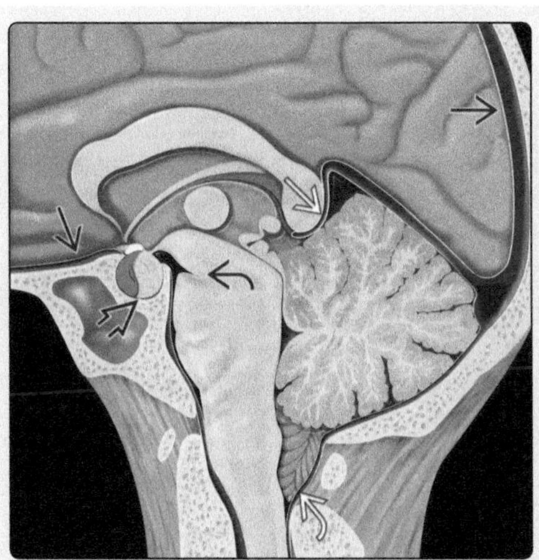

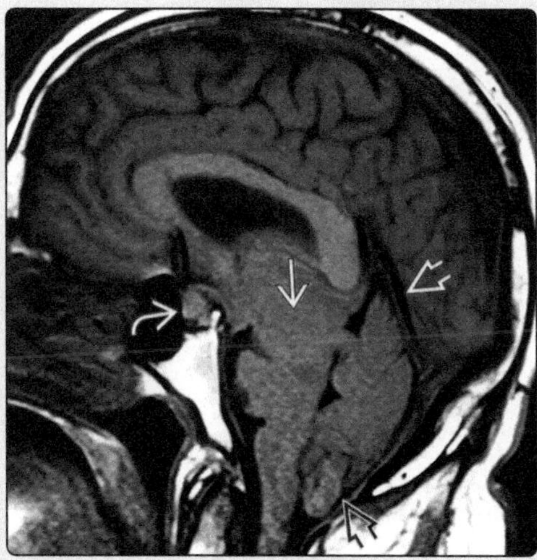

***(34-22)** Intracranial hypotension (ICH) is shown with distended dural sinuses ⇒, enlarged pituitary ⇒, and herniated tonsils ⇒. Central brain descent causes midbrain "slumping," inferiorly displaced pons, "closed" pons-midbrain angle ⇒, splenium depressing ICV/V of G junction ⇒. **(34-23)** Sagittal T1 MR in patient with severe ICH shows severe midbrain, pons sagging ⇒, fat pituitary ⇒, low-lying tonsils ⇒, and prominent venous sinuses ⇒.*

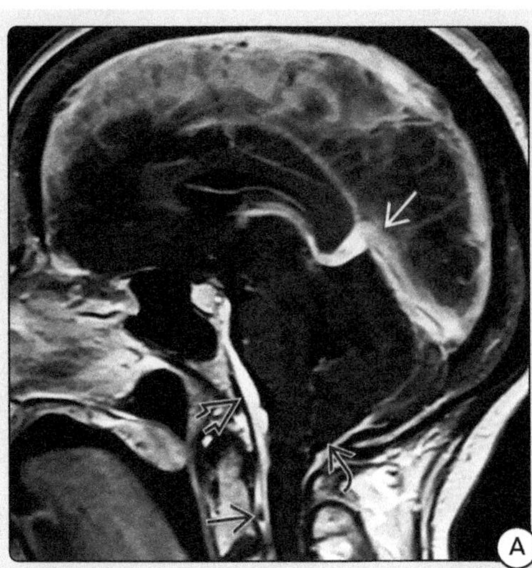

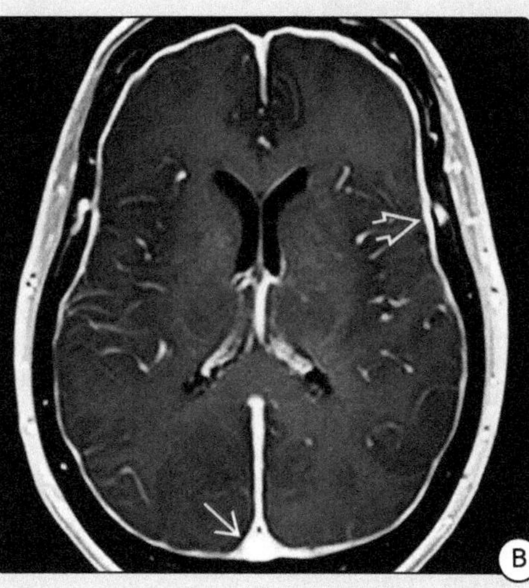

***(34-24A)** Sagittal T1 C+ MR in a 58y woman with postural headaches shows extensive dura-arachnoid thickening, enhancement ⇒ that extends into the upper cervical spine ⇒. Midbrain slumping and tonsillar herniation ⇒ are minimal. Venous sinuses are engorged ⇒. **(34-24B)** Axial T1 C+ MR shows venous engorgement ⇒, diffuse dura-arachnoid thickening, and enhancement ⇒. ICH is secondary to spinal CSF leak (not shown).*

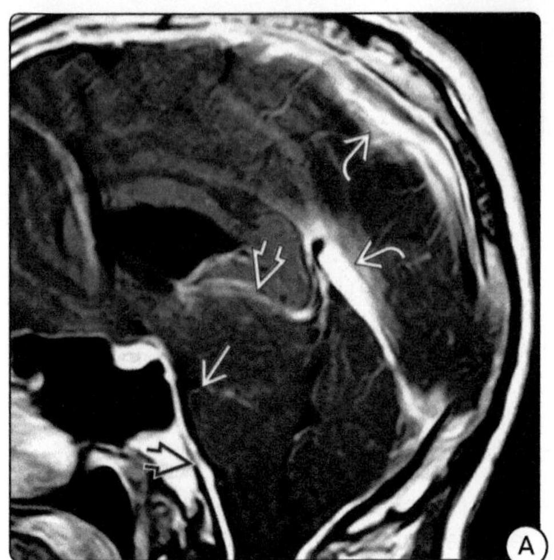

(34-25A) ***Note intracranial hypotension, midbrain "slumping," compressed pons ➡, flattened ICVs ➡, dural distension ➡, enhancement ➡.***

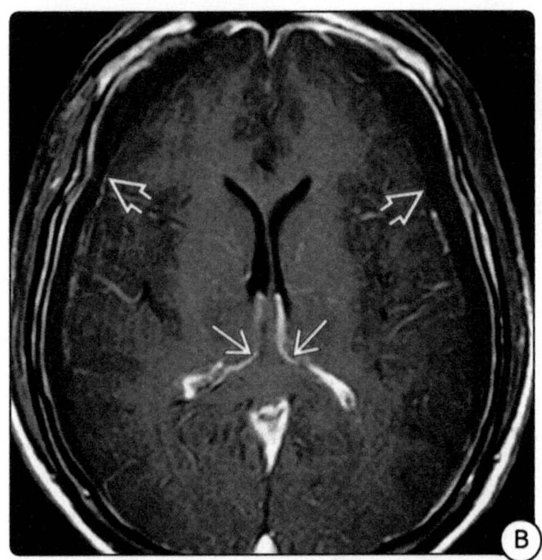

(34-25B) ***T1 C+ FS MR demonstrates medially displaced ICVs and ventricles ➡ and bilateral SDHs ➡.***

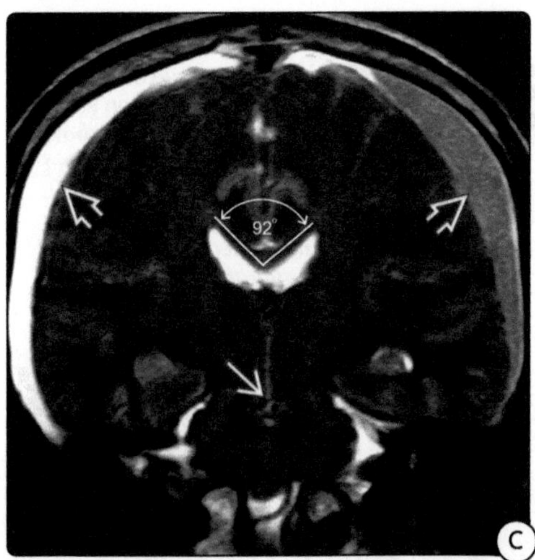

(34-25C) ***Coronal T2 MR shows 3rd ventricle ➡ displaced through tentorial incisura, SDHs of different ages ➡, and "closed" ventricular angle.***

Axial scans show that the basal cisterns are effaced. The pons often appears elongated and "fat." Midbrain anatomy is distorted with decreased width and increased anteroposterior diameter. The temporal lobes are displaced medially over the tentorium into the incisura. The lateral ventricles are usually small and distorted, as they are pulled medially and inferiorly by the brain "sagging" **(34-25)**.

In cases with severe brain descent, coronal scans may show that the angle between the roof of the lateral ventricles progressively decreases (< 120°) as brain sagging increases **(34-25C)**. The dural sinuses often appear distended with outwardly convex margins and exaggerated "flow voids." 15-50% of cases have subdural fluid collections (hygromas > hematomas) **(34-25)**.

T2/FLAIR. The slit-like third ventricle is displaced downward and, on axial scans, appears almost superimposed on the midbrain and hypothalamus.

T1 C+. One of the most consistent findings in SIH, seen in 80-85% of cases, is diffuse dural thickening with intense enhancement. Linear dural thickening may extend into the internal auditory canals, down the clivus, and through the foramen magnum into the upper cervical canal **(34-24)**.

T2* (GRE, SWI). Tearing of bridging veins caused by brain sagging can result in subarachnoid hemorrhage and superficial siderosis.

Differential Diagnosis

The major DDx of intracranial hypotension is **Chiari 1 malformation**. In Chiari 1, the only intracranial abnormality is displaced tonsils. Other findings of SIH are absent. *Mistaking SIH for Chiari 1 on imaging studies can lead to decompressive surgery, worsening CSF hypovolemia, and clinical deterioration!*

INTRACRANIAL HYPOTENSION

Etiology and Pathology
- CSF hypovolemia leads to brain "sags," dural/venous sinuses increase
- Can be spontaneous (idiopathic) or acquired

Clinical Issues
- Most common symptom = headache
  - ± orthostatic
- Severe intracranial hypotension can cause coma, even death

MR Findings
- Common
  - Midbrain "sags" down
  - Angle between midbrain, pons decreases (< 50°)
  - Pontomammillary distance: < 5.5 mm
  - Optic chiasm/hypothalamus draped over prominent pituitary
  - Diffusely thickened enhancing dura (reduced with time)
  - "Fat" pituitary
- Less common
  - Pons, midbrain may appear "fat"
  - ± tonsils displaced downward
  - Effaced cisterns/sulci
  - Small lateral ventricles ± atria "tugged" inferomedially
  - ± subdural collections (hygromas > frank hematomas)
  - Enlarged dural sinuses with outwardly bulging (convex) margins
- Rare but important
  - Ventricular angle on coronal imaging decreases
  - Torn bridging cortical veins
  - Subarachnoid hemorrhage, superficial siderosis

Selected References: The complete reference list is available on the Expert Consult™ eBook version included with purchase.

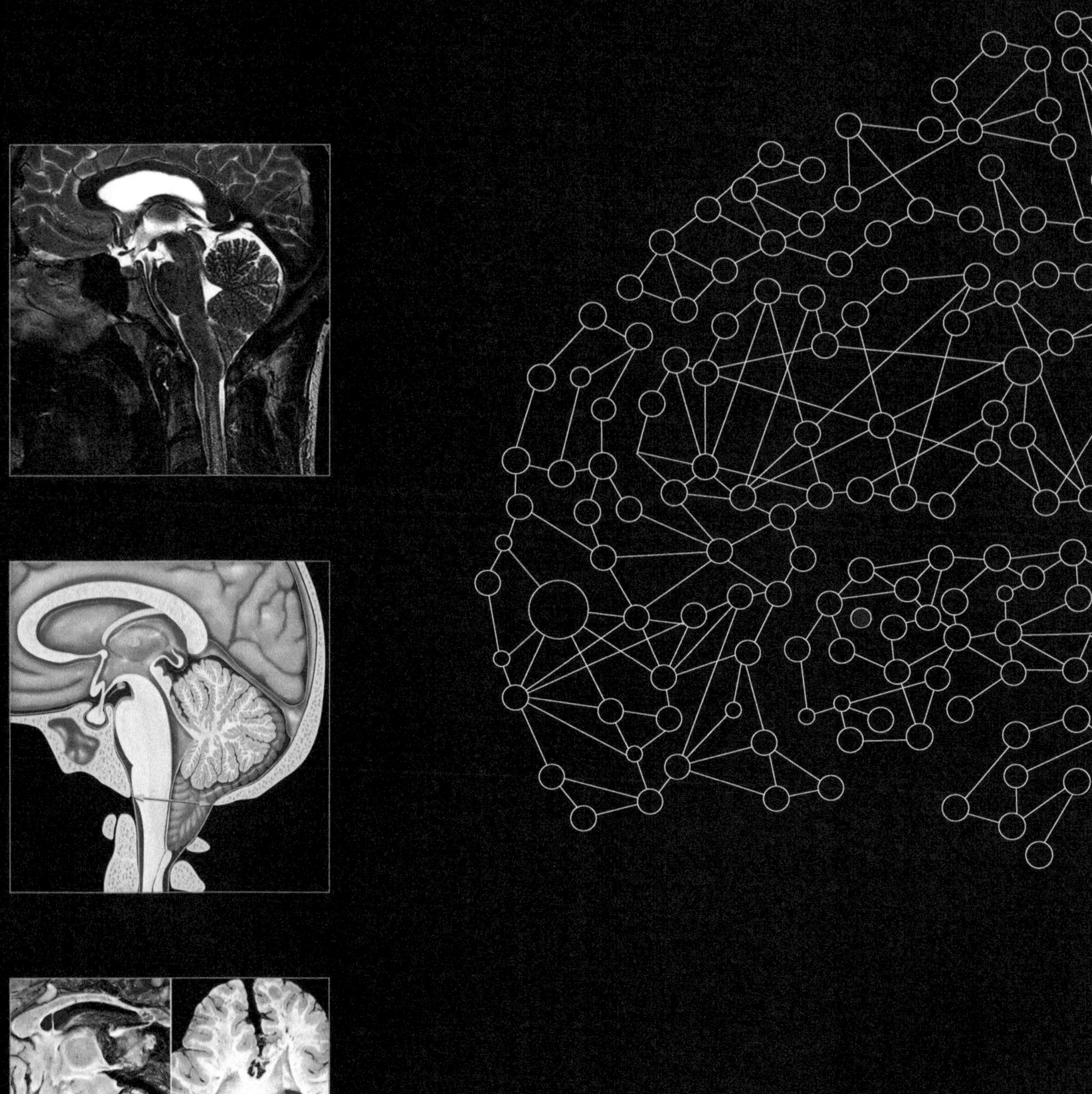

Section 6

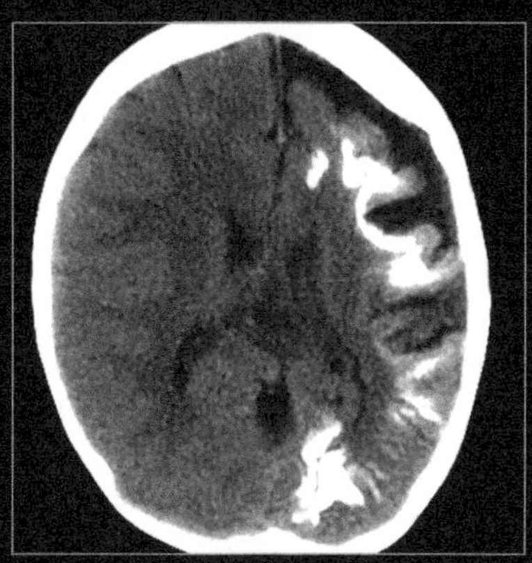

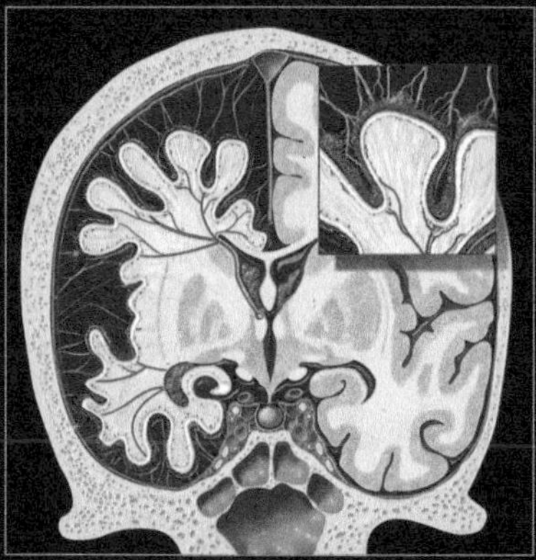

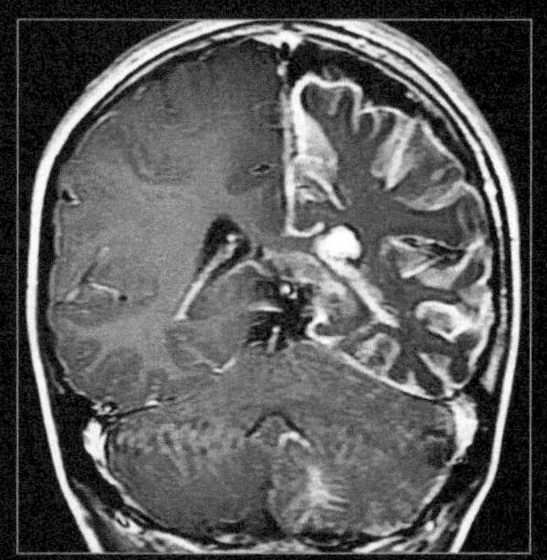

Section 6

Congenital Malformations of the Skull and Brain

Embryology and Approach to Congenital Malformations

A basic knowledge of normal brain development and maturation provides the essential foundation for understanding congenital malformations, the subject of the final part of this book.

Here, we briefly consider normal development of the cerebral hemispheres and cerebellum. We first focus on the basics of neurulation and neural tube closure, then turn our attention to how the neural tube flexes, bends, and evolves into the forebrain, midbrain, and hindbrain. Developmental errors and the resulting malformations that may occur at each stage are briefly summarized.

Cerebral hemisphere growth and elaboration into lobes, development of sulci and gyri, patterns of gray matter migration, and layering of the neocortex are all succinctly delineated.

Cerebral Hemisphere Formation

The major embryologic events in brain development begin with neurulation, neuronal proliferation, and neuronal migration. The processes of operculization, gyral and sulcal development, and the earliest steps in myelination all take place later, between gestational weeks 11 and birth.

Neurulation

Neural Tube and Brain Vesicles

The **neural plate** develops at the cranial end of the embryo as a thickening of ectoderm on either side of the midline. The neural plate then indents and thickens laterally, forming the **neural folds**. The neural folds bend upward, meet in the midline, and then fuse to form the **neural tube**. The primitive **notochord** lies ventral to the neural tube. **Neural crest** cells are extruded and migrate laterally. The neural tube forms the brain and spinal cord, whereas the neural crest gives rise to peripheral nerves, roots, and ganglia of the autonomic nervous system **(35-1)**.

The neural tube closes, beginning in the middle and proceeding bidirectionally in a zipper-like fashion along the length of the embryo **(35-2)**.

As the neural tube closes, the neuroectoderm (which will form the CNS) separates from the cutaneous ectoderm in a process known as disjunction. Upon completion of disjunction, the cutaneous ectoderm fuses in the midline, dorsal to the closed neural tube. The brain grows rapidly and begins to bend, forming several flexures. The embryonic brain eventually has five definitive vesicles **(35-3)**.

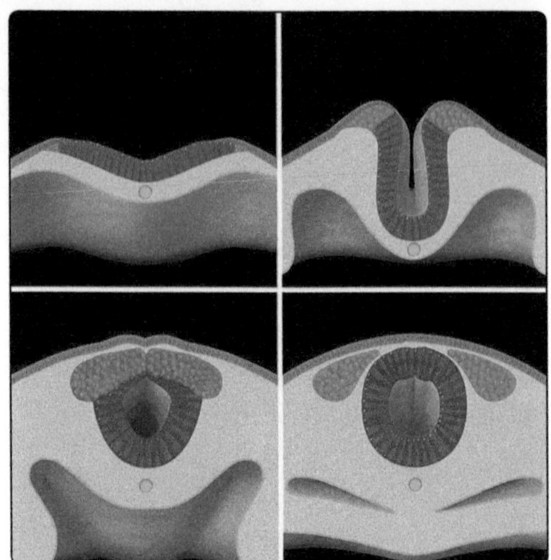

(35-1) *Neural plate (red) forms, folds, & fuses in midline. Neural, cutaneous ectoderm separate. Notochord (green), neural crest (blue) are shown.*

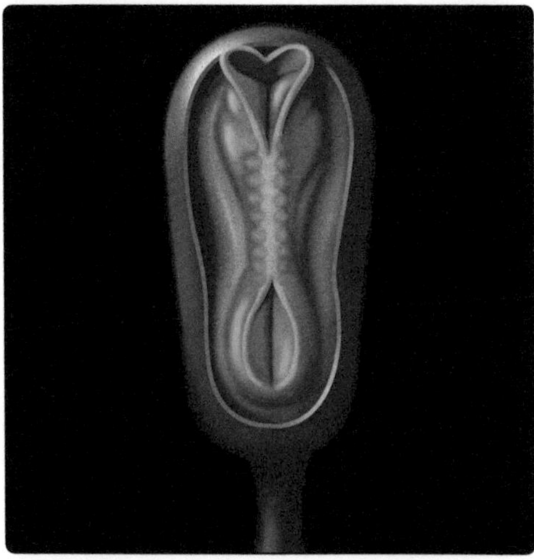

(35-2) *The neural tube closes in a bidirectional zipper-like manner, starting in the middle and proceeding toward both ends.*

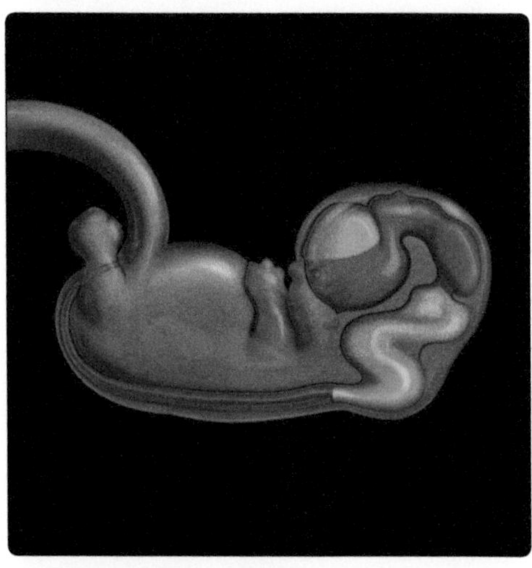

(35-3) *Brain flexures with telencephalon (green), diencephalon (red), mesencephalon (purple), metencephalon (yellow).*

Neurulation Errors

Errors in neurulation result in a spectrum of congenital anomalies. The most severe is **anencephaly** (essentially complete absence of the cerebral hemispheres). Various types of **cephaloceles** also result from abnormalities of neurulation.

Incomplete closure of the posterior neuropore results in **spina bifida**. If the neuroectoderm fails to separate completely from the cutaneous ectoderm, **myelomeningocele** results. Abnormal neurulation of the hindbrain leads to a **Chiari 2 malformation**.

Neuronal Proliferation

Embryonic Stem Cells

*Pluri*potent embryonic stem cells are derived from the inner cell mass of the 4- to 5-day blastocyst. These cells are able to proliferate and differentiate into all three germ layers (ectoderm, mesoderm, endoderm). MicroRNAs seem to play an important role as genetic regulators of stem cell development, differentiation, growth, and neurogenesis.

Histogenesis of Neurons and Glia

As the cerebral vesicles develop and expand, layers of stem cells arise around the primitive ventricular ependyma, forming the germinal matrix. These neural stem cells (NSCs) are *multi*potent cells that generate the main CNS phenotypes, i.e., neurons, astrocytes, and oligodendrocytes. NSCs are found primarily in the germinal zones.

*Pluri*potent NSCs in the germinal matrix give rise to "primitive" or "young" **neurons** that migrate outward to form the cortical mantle zone (precursor of the definitive cortex). Axons from the migrating neurons form an intermediate zone between the germinal matrix and cortical mantle that will eventually become the cerebral white matter.

Some NSCs become specialized **radial glial cells** (RGCs) that will eventually span the entire hemisphere from the ventricular ependyma to the pia. RGCs can give rise to both neurons and glia. Elongated cell bodies of the RGCs serve as a "rope ladder" that guides migrating neurons from the germinal matrix to the cortex.

Errors in Histogenesis

Errors in histogenesis and differentiation result in a number of embryonal neoplasms, including medulloblastoma and primitive neuroectodermal tumors. Problems with NSC proliferation and differentiation also contribute to malformations of cortical development.

Neuronal Migration

Understanding how neurons are formed, migrate, organize, and then connect is essential to recognizing and understanding malformations of cortical development (MCDs).

Genesis of Cortical Neurons

Once the "young" neurons have been generated in the germinal matrix, they must leave their "home" to reach their final destination (the cortex). The definitive cerebral cortex develops through a highly ordered process of neuronal proliferation, migration, and differentiation.

Neuronal Migration

Migration of newly proliferated neurons occurs along scaffolding provided by the RGCs. Neurons travel from the germinal zone to the cortical mantle in a generally "inside-out" sequence. Cells initially form the deepest layer of the cortex with each successive migration ascending farther outward and progressively forming more superficial layers. Each migrating group passes through layers already laid down by the earlier-arriving cells.

Peak neuronal migration occurs between 11-15 fetal weeks, although migration continues up to 35 weeks.

Errors in Neuronal Migration and Cortical Organization

The primary result of errors at these stages are **malformations of cortical development**. Problems with NSC proliferation or differentiation, migration, and cortical organization can all result in developmental anomalies of the neocortex. Examples include **microcephaly, megalencephaly, heterotopias, cortical dysplasias**, and **lissencephaly**.

Operculization, Sulcation, and Gyration

Lobulation and Operculization

The hemispheres are initially almost featureless; the cortex is thin and smooth. As the hemispheres elongate and rotate, they assume a "C" shape with the caudal ends turning ventrally to form the temporal lobes.

Sulcation and Gyration

Sulcation and gyration occurs relatively late in embryonic development. Shallow triangular surface indentations along the sides of the hemisphere—the beginnings of the lateral cerebral (sylvian) fissures—first appear between the fourth and fifth fetal months **(35-4)**.

After the sylvian fissures form **(35-6)**, multiple secondary and tertiary gyri develop **(35-5)**. Gyral development occurs most rapidly around the sensorimotor and visual pathways.

Anomalies in Sulcation and Gyration

Developmental errors in operculization, sulcation, and gyration are relatively uncommon. **Microcephaly** with simplified gyral pattern and **microlissencephaly** are representative anomalies that have too few gyri and abnormally shallow sulci.

Myelination

Myelination occurs in an orderly, predictable manner and can be detected as early as 20 fetal weeks. In general, myelination proceeds from **inferior to superior**, from **back to front**, and from **central to peripheral**.

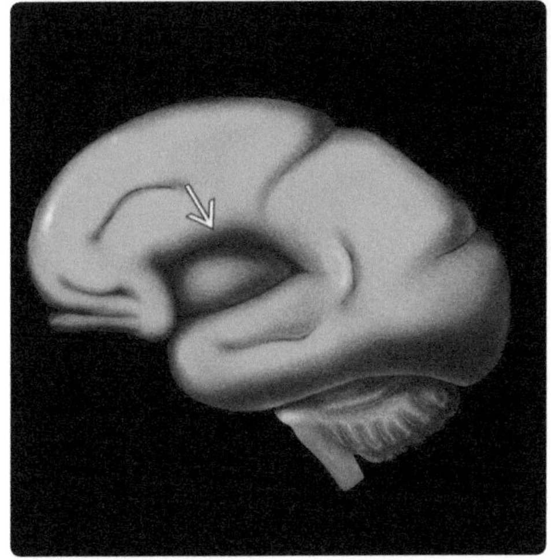

***(35-4)** 22-week fetal brain is mostly agyric with shallow lateral cerebral (sylvian) fissures ➡.*

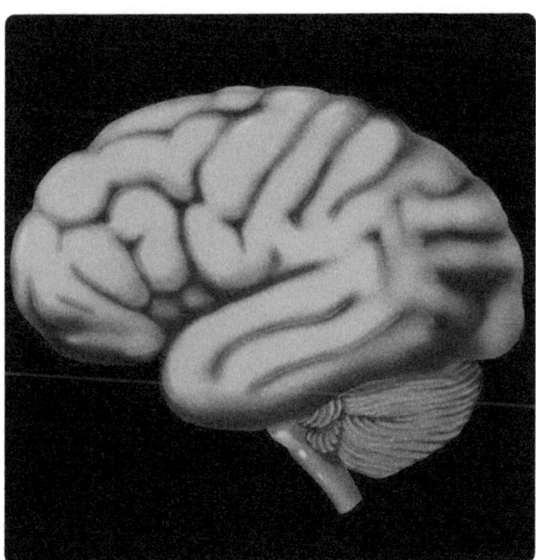

***(35-5)** Multiple secondary and tertiary gyri then develop, and the number and complexity of the cerebellar folia increase.*

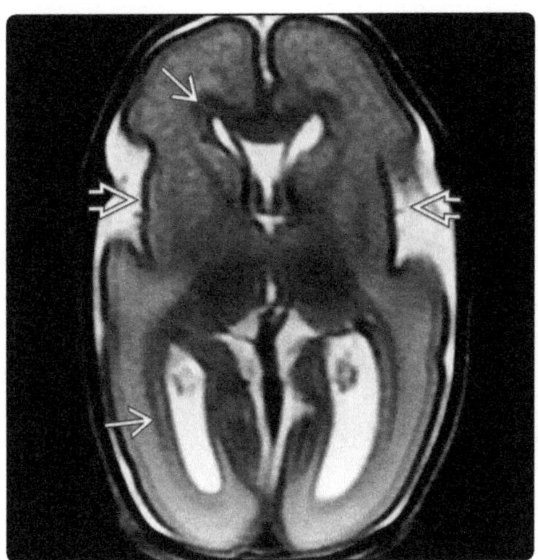

***(35-6)** T2 MR in 26-week-old preemie: Sylvian fissures ➡ are just beginning to form. Germinal matrix ➡ surrounds lateral ventricles.*

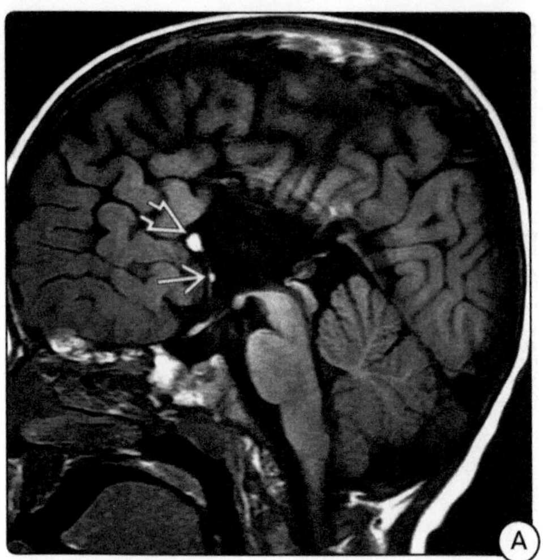

(35-7A) Sagittal midline T1 MR shows classic callosal agenesis. The anterior commissure ➡ is present, as is a tiny remnant of the genu ➡.

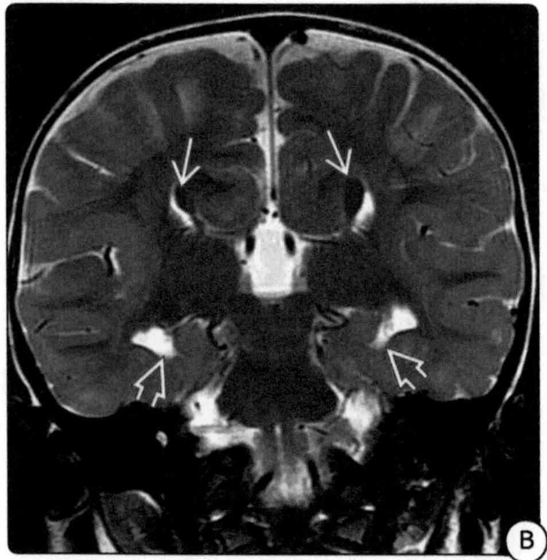

(35-7B) Coronal T2 MR shows Probst bundles ➡ indenting the lateral ventricles. Note vertically oriented hippocampi ➡.

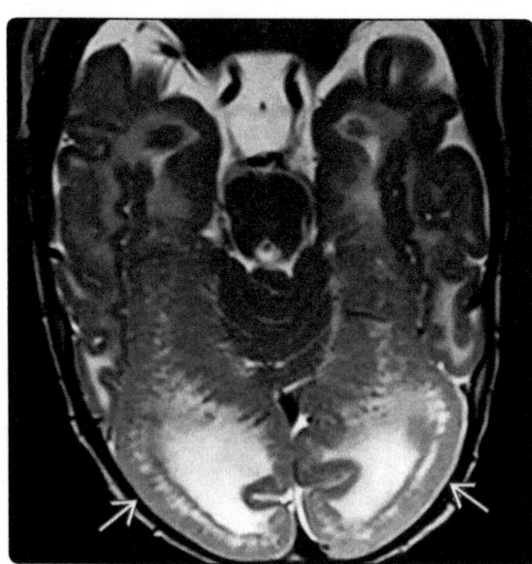

(35-8) Axial T2 MR shows "cobblestone" lissencephaly in both occipital poles ➡. (Courtesy M. Warmuth-Metz, MD.)

Imaging Approach to Brain Malformations

Technical Considerations

CT

Clinicians sometimes order NECT scans as an initial screening procedure in a patient with seizures or suspected brain malformation. Although parenchymal calcifications, ventricular size/configuration, and major abnormalities can be identified, subtle abnormalities, such as cortical dysplasia, are difficult to detect and easy to overlook.

Bone CT is helpful in depicting midline facial defects, synostoses, and anomalies of endochondral bone.

MR

MR is the procedure of choice. The two most important factors are gray matter-white matter differentiation and high spatial resolution. Many pediatric neuroradiologists recommend a sagittal T1 or T1 FLAIR sequence, volumetric T1 sequences (e.g., MP-RAGE), and sagittal and coronal heavily T2-weighted sequences with very long TR/TEs. 3D imaging acquisitions allow isotropic orthogonal reformations.

A T2* sequence (GRE, SWI) can be a helpful addition if abnormal mineralization or vascular anomaly is suspected. DTI tractography is valuable when commissural anomalies are identified on initial sequences.

Contrast-enhanced T1 and FLAIR sequences are generally optional, as they add little useful information in most congenital malformations. However, they can be very helpful in delineating associated vascular anomalies. DWI and MRS are useful in evaluating mass lesions and inborn errors of metabolism.

Image Analysis

The following approach to analyzing imaging studies is modified and adapted from A. James Barkovich's guidelines on imaging evaluation of the pediatric brain (see reference cited in Chapter 36).

Sagittal Images

Begin with the midline section and examine the craniofacial proportion. At birth, the ratio of calvarium to face should be 5:1 or 6:1. At 2 years, it should be 2.5:1. In adults and children over the age of 10 years, it should be ~ 1.5:1. Assess myelination of midline structures, such as the corpus callosum and brainstem.

The most common of all brain malformations are anomalies of the cerebral commissures (especially the corpus callosum), which can be readily identified on sagittal T1 scans **(35-7A)**. Commissural anomalies are also the most common malformation associated with other anomalies and syndromes, so, if you see one, keep looking! Look for abnormalities of the pituitary gland and hypothalamus. Evaluate the size and shape of the third ventricle, especially its anterior recesses.

Look for other lesions, such as lipomas and cysts. These are often midline or paramidline and can be readily identified. The midline sagittal scan also permits a very nice evaluation of the posterior fossa structures. Does the fourth ventricle appear normal? Can you find its dorsally pointing fastigium?

Evaluate the position of the tonsils and the craniovertebral junction for anomalies.

If the lateral and third ventricles are large and the fourth ventricle appears normal, look for a funnel-shaped aqueduct indicating aqueductal stenosis. If you see aqueductal stenosis, look at the quadrigeminal plate carefully to see whether the cause might be a low-grade tectal glioma.

Sagittal images are also especially useful in evaluating the cerebral cortex. Is the cortex too thick? Too thin? Irregular? "Lumpy-bumpy"? Anomalies of cortical development, such as pachygyria and cortical dysplasia associated with brain clefting ("schizencephaly"), are often most easily identified on sagittal images. Finally, note the position and size of the vein of Galen, straight sinus, and torcular Herophili.

Coronal Images

Cortical dysplasias are often bilateral and most frequently cluster around the sylvian fissure. Coronal scans make side-to-side comparison relatively easy. Follow the interhemispheric fissure (IHF) all the way from front to back. If the hemispheres are in contiguity across the midline, holoprosencephaly is present. If the IHF appears irregular and the gyri "interdigitate" across the midline, the patient almost certainly has a Chiari 2 malformation.

Evaluate the size, shape, and position of the ventricles. If the third ventricle appears "high riding" and the frontal horns of the lateral ventricles look like a "Viking helmet," corpus callosum dysgenesis is present **(35-7B)**.

If the frontal horns appear squared-off or box-like, look carefully for an absent cavum septi pellucidi. Absent cavum septi pellucidi is seen in septo-optic dysplasia (SOD) and often occurs with callosal dysplasia or schizencephaly. If absent septi pellucidi is noted, look for fusion of the anterior columns of the fornix.

Carefully evaluate the temporal horns and hippocampi to make sure that they are normally folded and oriented horizontally (not vertically, as often occurs with holoprosencephaly, lissencephaly, callosal anomalies, and malformations of cortical development).

Axial Images

The combination of a true T1WI together with a long TR/TE T2WI is necessary in evaluating all cases of delayed development to assess myelin maturation. The thickness and configuration of the cortical mantle are well seen **(35-8)**. The size, shape, and configuration of the ventricles is easily evaluated on these sequences.

After 6-8 months of age, FLAIR sequences are especially useful in evaluating abnormalities such as focal or Taylor cortical dysplasia and the flame-shaped subcortical white matter hyperintensities seen in tuberous sclerosis complex **(35-9)**.

Don't forget the posterior fossa! The fourth ventricle in the axial plane is normally shaped like a kidney bean on its side. If the vermis is absent and the cerebellar hemispheres appear continuous from side to side, rhombencephalosynapsis is present **(35-10)**. If the fourth ventricle and superior cerebellar peduncles resemble a molar tooth, then a molar tooth malformation is present **(35-11)**.

Selected References: The complete reference list is available on the Expert Consult™ eBook version included with purchase.

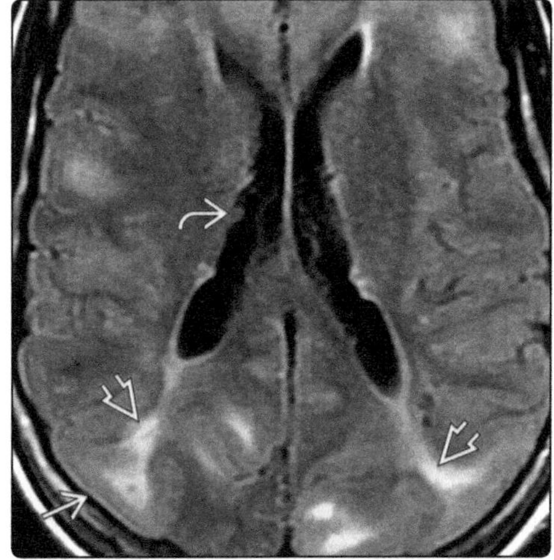

***(35-9)** FLAIR MR shows subependymal nodules ➡ and cortical tubers ➡ with subcortical hyperintensities ➡ of tuberous sclerosis.*

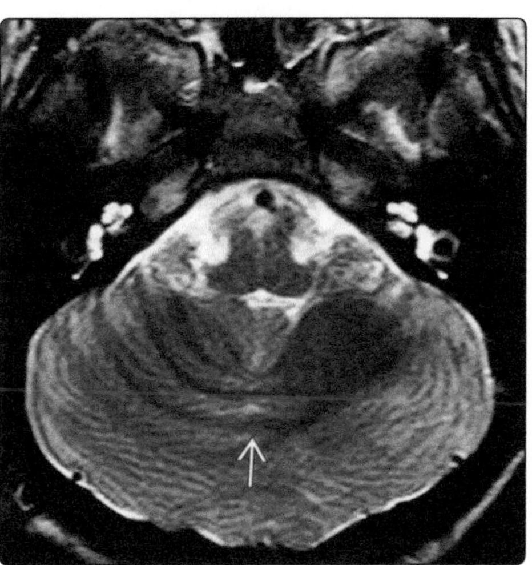

***(35-10)** T2WI of rhombencephalosynapsis shows continuity of cerebellar hemispheres across the midline ➡. (Courtesy M. Warmuth-Metz, MD.)*

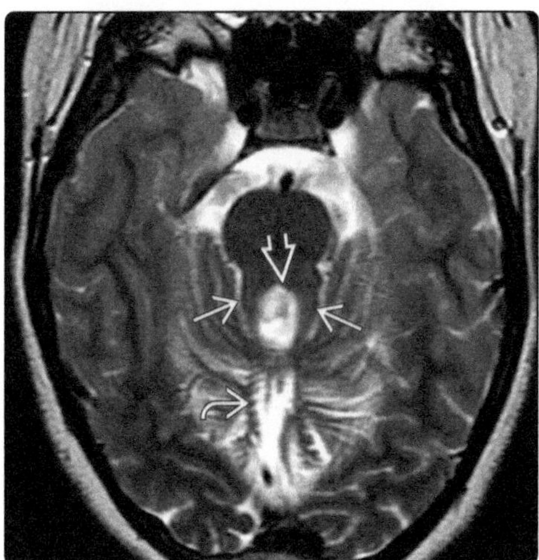

***(35-11)** T2WI shows "molar tooth" anomaly, elongated upper 4th ventricle ➡, thick superior cerebellar peduncles ➡, and "split" vermis ➡.*

Posterior Fossa Malformations

Neural structures in the midbrain and posterior fossa are derived from three sources: (1) The embryonic mesencephalon gives rise to midbrain structures. (2) The embryonic hindbrain (rhombencephalon) gives rise to the posterior fossa structures. (3) Mesodermal elements give rise to the meninges and bone that surround and protect these neural structures. Developmental errors can give rise to a spectrum of midbrain and hindbrain malformations.

Chiari Malformations

Introduction to Chiari Malformations

Chiari 1 and 2 are pathogenetically distinct disorders. **Chiari 1** is inferior dislocation of the cerebellar tonsils **(36-1)**. **Chiari 2** is herniation of the medulla and vermis and is always associated with myelodysplasia (spinal cord anomalies) **(36-6)**. **Chiari 3** is characterized by herniation of posterior fossa contents through a low occipitocervical bony defect.

Chiari 1

Terminology

Chiari 1 malformation (CM1) is defined as caudal cerebellar tonsillar ectopia. The precise distance of the tonsils below the foramen magnum (FM) required to diagnose CM1 is not agreed upon. Some investigators consider tonsillar ectopia measuring ≥ 5 mm as sufficient to establish the diagnosis of CM1. However, most insist additional abnormalities, such as tonsillar deformity, obliterated retrotonsillar CSF spaces, or altered CSF flow dynamics should also be present.

Overview

Abnormalities of the cervical spinal cord are common in CM1. A complex CSF-filled cavity with multiple septations of spongy glial tissue is typical. *Glia*-lined cord cavitations are generally referred to as **syringomyelia**. The term **hydromyelia** refers to an *ependyma*-lined expansion of the central canal. In CM1, extensive areas of ependymal denuding and astrocytic scarring make it difficult to distinguish between hydro- and syringomyelia even on histologic examination. Therefore, these nonneoplastic, septated, paracentral, fluid-containing cavitations are often referred to as **hydrosyringomyelia** or simply syrinx.

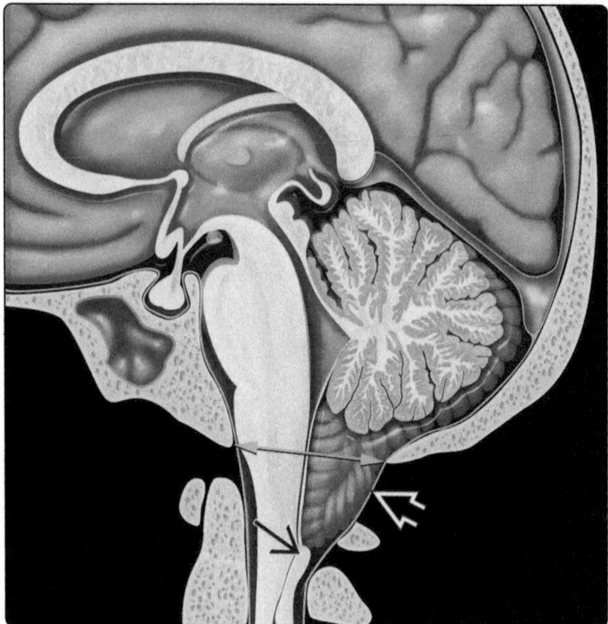

(36-1) Chiari 1 malformation (CM1) shows the basion-opisthion line in green. Note the low-lying, pointed tonsil with vertically oriented folia ➡. The nucleus gracilis ⇨ is inferiorly displaced.

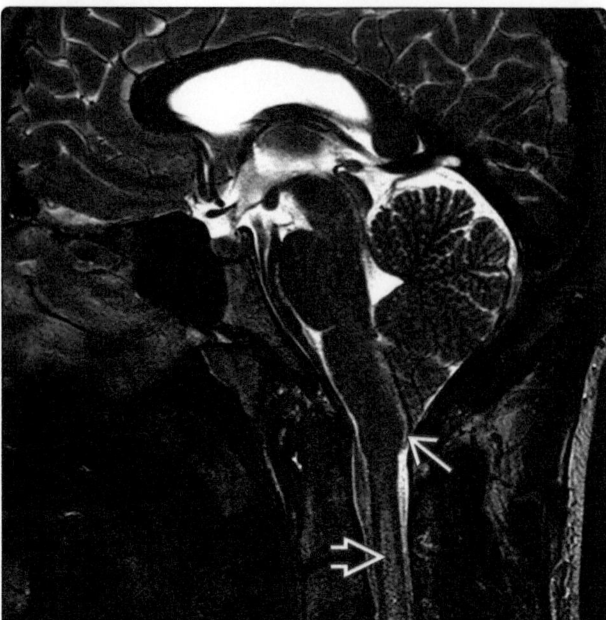

(36-2) Sagittal T2 MR in a 23-year-old man with classic CM1 shows a low-lying, pointed tonsil ➡ and normal-sized posterior fossa. Cord T2 hyperintensity ➡ represents the "presyrinx" state.

Etiology

Abnormal Posterior Fossa. Many—but by no means all—patients with CM1 demonstrate abnormal geometry of the bony posterior fossa (*"normal-sized hindbrain housed in a too-small bony envelope"*). Various combinations of congenitally reduced clival length, shortened basiocciput, and craniovertebral junction (CVJ) fusion anomalies may all result in diminished posterior cranial fossa depth &/or an abnormally small posterior fossa volume.

Altered CSF Dynamics. Syringomyelia is present in 40-80% of individuals with symptomatic CM1. Systolic piston-like descent of impacted tonsils may create abnormal intraspinal CSF pressure waves, which, in turn, could result in the development of hydrosyringomyelia in the upper cervical cord.

Pathology

Grossly, the herniated tonsils in CM1 are inferiorly displaced and grooved by impaction against the opisthion **(36-3)**. They often appear firm and sclerotic. Arachnoid thickening and adhesions around the CVJ are common.

Clinical Issues

Epidemiology and Demographics. CM1 is the most common of the Chiari malformations and can be identified in patients of all ages. CM1 can be identified in 3.6% of children undergoing routine brain or cervical spine MR.

Presentation. 1/3 to 1/2 of all patients with CM1 on imaging are asymptomatic at the time of diagnosis.

Presentation of symptomatic CM1 differs with age. Children who are 2 years and younger most commonly present with oropharyngeal dysfunction (nearly 80%). Those between 3 and 5 years present with headache (57%) or scoliosis (38%). Children with holocord syringohydromyelia demonstrate altered pain, temperature, and vibratory sensation.

Natural History. Many patients remain asymptomatic. Some investigators believe that the degree of tonsillar ectopia in CM1 gradually increases with time and is associated with a greater likelihood of becoming symptomatic.

Treatment Options. Asymptomatic tonsillar ectopia in the absence of an associated syrinx or scoliosis is usually not treated. Surgical treatment of symptomatic CM1 attempts to restore normal CSF fluid dynamics at the FM.

Imaging

General Features. The basion-opisthion line (BOL) is a line drawn from the tip of the clivus to the posterior rim of the FM **(36-1)**. Measuring the distance from this line to the inferior margin of the cerebellar tonsils on sagittal MR defines tonsillar position.

Midline tonsillar descent 5 mm or more below the BOL—often considered diagnostic of CM1—is by itself a poor criterion for definitive diagnosis. Tonsils 6 mm below the FM are common during the first decade of life. Almost 15% of normal patients have tonsils that lie 1-4 mm below the FM, and 0.5-1.0% have tonsils that project 5 mm into the upper cervical canal.

Great caution should be exercised in establishing a diagnosis of CM1, especially on the basis of borderline tonsillar ectopia alone. Unless (1) the tonsils appear compressed and pointed

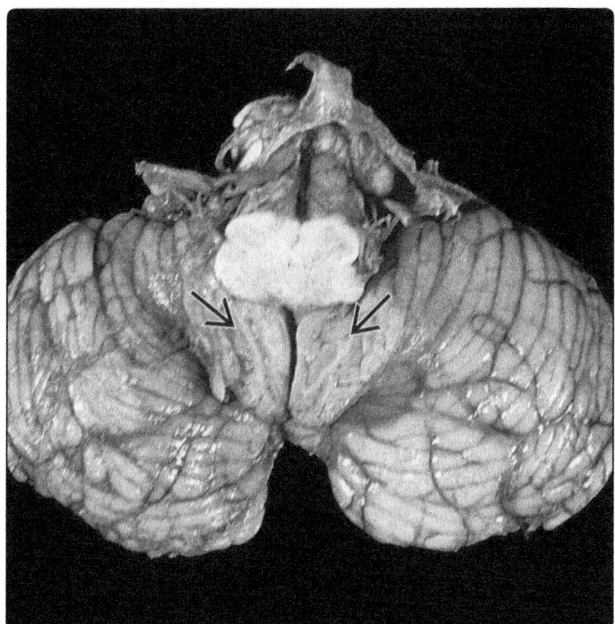

***(36-3)** Semiaxial view of an autopsy case shows CM1. Note inferiorly displaced tonsils with vertically oriented folia ➡. (Courtesy E. T. Hedley-Whyte, MD.)*

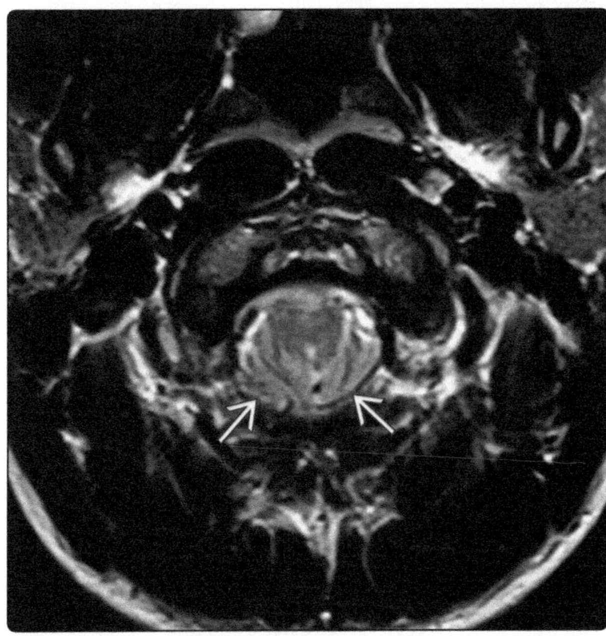

***(36-4)** Axial T2 MR in the same patient shows "crowded" foramen magnum with obliterated retrotonsillar CSF spaces ➡.*

(peg-like) instead of gently rounded **(36-2)**, (2) the tonsillar folia are angled obliquely or inferiorly (instead of horizontally), and (3) the retrocerebellar CSF spaces at the FM/C1 level are effaced **(36-4)**, the diagnosis may not be warranted. Low-lying tonsils that retain their rounded shapes and are surrounded by normal-appearing CSF spaces are usually asymptomatic and of no diagnostic significance.

CT Findings. NECT scans may reveal a "crowded" FM and effaced retrotonsillar CSF space. Bone CT often demonstrates a combination of undersized, shallow posterior cranial fossa, short clivus, and CVJ assimilation anomalies.

MR Findings. Sagittal T1 and T2 scans show "pointed" tonsils with more vertically oriented folia, obliterated retrocerebellar and premedullary subarachnoid spaces, and a "crowded" FM. The fourth ventricle usually appears normal. In some cases, the inferior fourth ventricle is mildly elongated, and the nucleus gracilis—which demarcates the end of the obex and beginning of the central canal—can appear slightly low lying **(36-5)**.

The proximal cervical spinal cord should be carefully examined for the presence of hydrosyringomyelia. T2/FLAIR parenchymal hyperintensity without frank cyst formation may indicate a "presyrinx" state.

Sagittal phase-contrast CSF flow studies show diminished or absent alternating bright (systolic) and dark (diastolic) signals behind the cervicomedullary junction. Any change in signal intensity of the cerebellar tonsils in cine mode suggests tonsillar pulsations **(36-5D)**.

Differential Diagnosis

Congenital tonsillar descent (CM1) must be distinguished from **normal variants** (mild uncomplicated tonsillar ectopia). The most important pathologic differential diagnosis is *acquired* tonsillar herniation caused by increased intracranial pressure **or** intracranial hypotension.

Increased intracranial pressure due to supratentorial mass effect with transmission of the pressure cone through the tentorial incisura can be easily distinguished from CM1. Signs of descending transtentorial herniation are present along with downward midbrain displacement. Tonsillar herniation in such cases is a secondary effect and should *not* be termed "acquired Chiari 1."

Intracranial hypotension shows a constellation of other findings besides inferiorly displaced tonsils. "Slumping" midbrain, enlarged pituitary gland, draping of the optic chiasm and hypothalamus over the dorsum sellae, subdural hematoma, engorged venous sinuses, and dura-arachnoid thickening and enhancement are typical abnormalities. *Mistaking intracranial hypotension for CM1 can have disastrous consequences, as surgical decompression may exacerbate brainstem "slumping."*

Approximately 20% of patients with **idiopathic intracranial hypertension** exhibit cerebellar tonsillar ectopia ≥ 5 mm. 50% have a peg-like tonsil configuration, and many have a low-lying obex. Looking for other signs of idiopathic intracranial hypertension (e.g., optic nerve head protrusion into the globe) is essential to avoid misdiagnosis as CM1.

CHIARI 1 IMAGING

General Features
- Caudal tonsillar ectopia [≥ 5 mm below foramen magnum (FM)]
- Pointed, peg-like tonsils with angled folia
- "Crowded" FM with effaced CSF spaces
- Diminished/absent CSF flow at posterior FM
- Syrinx prevalence
  - 10-20% asymptomatic
  - 40-80% symptomatic patients

Differential Diagnosis
- Normal "low-lying" tonsils (rounded, no disturbed CSF flow)
- Acquired herniation (elevated intracranial pressure, intracranial hypotension)

Chiari 2

Terminology and Definition

Chiari 2 malformation (CM2) is a complex hindbrain malformation that is almost always associated with myelodysplasia (myelomeningocele).

Etiology

General Concepts. CM2 is a disorder of neural tube closure but also involves paraxial mesodermal abnormalities of the skull and spine. A number of steps are required for proper neural tube closure and formation of the focal expansions that subsequently form the cerebral vesicles and ventricles. Skeletal elements of both the skull and vertebral column become "modeled" around the neural tube.

Only if the posterior neuropore closes will the developing ventricles expand sufficiently for a normal-sized posterior

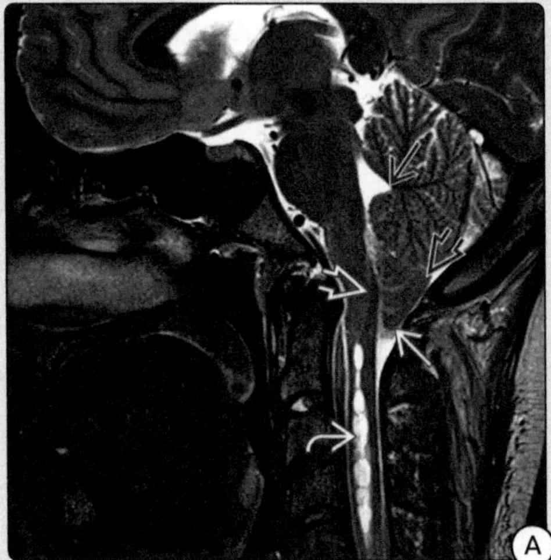

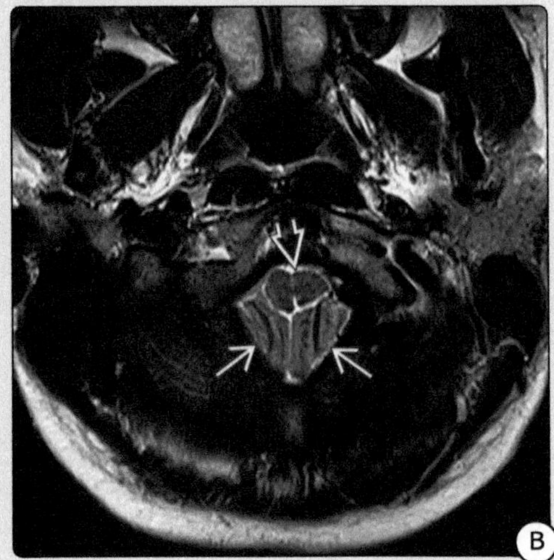

***(36-5A)** Sagittal T2 MR of CM1 shows "pointed" tonsil ➡, obliquely oriented tonsillar folia ➡. Multiple septations in a syrinx cavity are clearly seen ➡. The fastigium ➡ is normal, but the inferior 4th ventricle is somewhat elongated, and the nucleus gracilis ➡ is slightly low lying. **(36-5B)** T2WI in the same patient shows tonsils ➡ and a compressed and slightly deformed medulla ➡, giving the appearance of the "crowded" foramen magnum typical of CM1.*

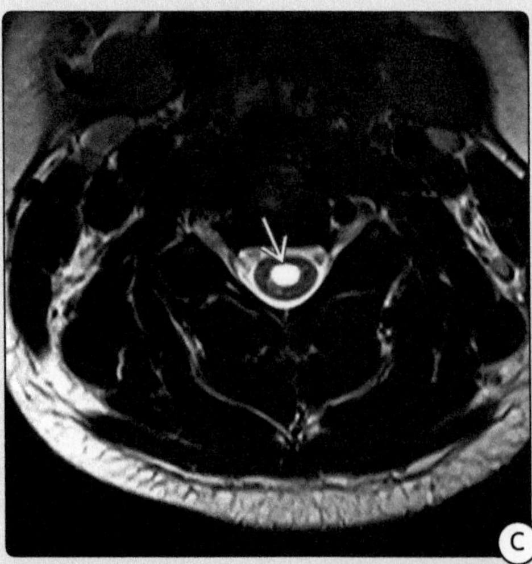

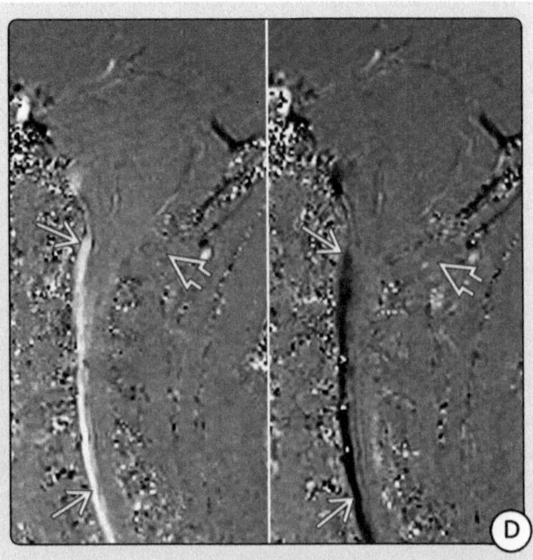

***(36-5C)** Axial T2 MR shows a well-demarcated CSF cavity ➡, typical of hydrosyringomelia. **(36-5D)** Sagittal phase-contrast CSF flow study in systole (L) and diastole (R) shows normal CSF flow ➡ in front of the cervicomedullary junction and no posterior flow in the foramen magnum ➡. Tonsillar "crowding" and adhesions prevent normal CSF circulation.*

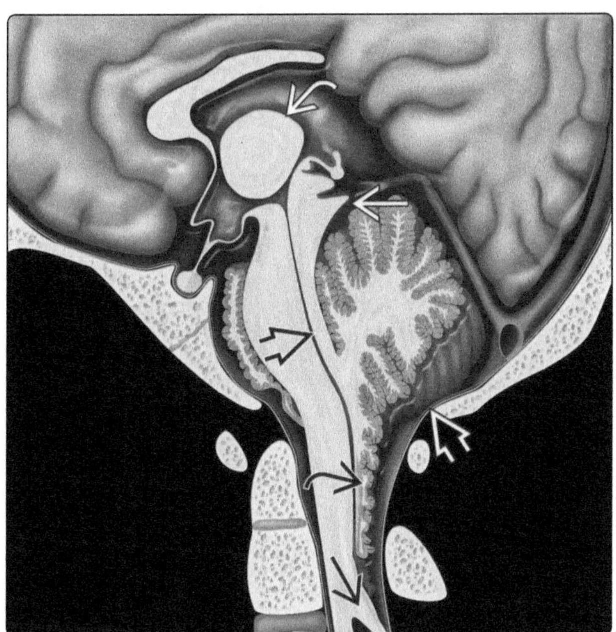

(36-6) ***Graphic shows CM2 with small posterior fossa ➡, large massa intermedia ➡, "beaked" tectum ➡, callosal dysgenesis, elongated 4th ventricle ➡ with "cascade" of inferiorly displaced nodulus ➡ and choroid plexus, and medullary spur ➡.***

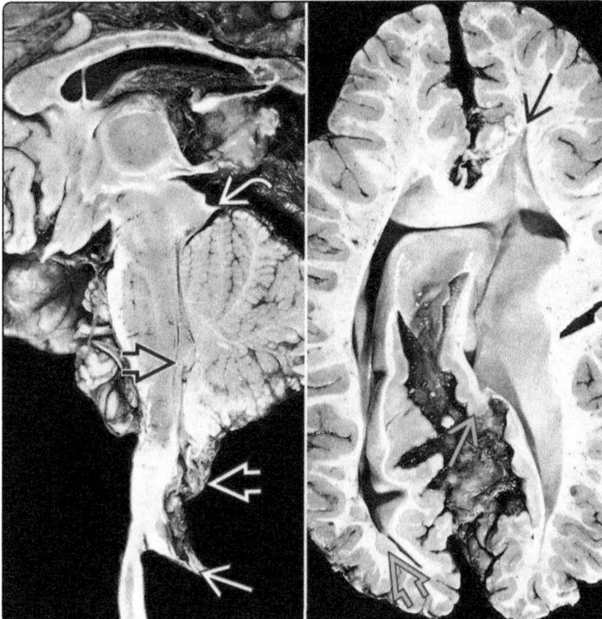

(36-7) ***(L) CM2 shows medullary spur ➡, nodulus ➡ behind medulla, elongated 4th ventricle ➡, "beaked" tectum ➡. (T. P. Naidich, MD.) (R) CM2 has stenogyria ➡, heterotopic GM ➡, "pointed" lateral ventricles ➡. (E. T. Hedley-Whyte, MD.)***

fossa to form around the hindbrain. If this does not happen, the cerebellum develops in a small posterior fossa with abnormally low tentorial attachments. The growing cerebellum is squeezed cephalad through the tentorial incisura and stretched inferiorly through the foramen magnum (FM).

Genetics. Nearly 1/2 of all neural tube closure anomalies have mutations on the methylene-tetra-hydrofolate reductase gene (*MTHFR*). Maternal folate deficiency and teratogens, such as anticonvulsants, have been linked to increased risk of CM2.

Pathology

Grossly, a broad spectrum of findings can be present in CM2. Myelomeningocele and a small posterior fossa with concave clivus and petrous pyramids are virtually always present **(36-6)**. The cerebellar vermis (typically the nodulus) is displaced inferiorly along the dorsal aspect of the cervical spinal cord. The fourth ventricle, pons, and medulla are elongated and partially dislocated into the cervical spinal canal. The lower medulla may be kinked.

Unlike CM1, supratentorial abnormalities are the rule in CM2, not the exception. Hydrocephalus is present in the majority of cases, and aqueductal stenosis is common. Corpus callosum dysgenesis and gray matter anomalies, such as polymicrogyria and heterotopias, are frequent **(36-7)**.

Clinical Issues

Epidemiology and Demographics. The overall prevalence of CM2 is 0.44 in 1,000 live births but has been decreasing with prophylactic maternal folate therapy. A dose of 4 mg per day reduces the risk of CM2 by at least 70%.

Presentation. CM2 is identified in utero with ultrasound or fetal screening for elevated α-fetoprotein. At birth, coexistent myelomeningocele and hydrocephalus are dominant clinical features in over 90% of cases. Lower cranial nerve deficits, apneic spells, and bulbar signs may be present. Lower extremity paralysis, sphincter dysfunction, and spasticity often develop later.

Treatment Options. Fetal repair of myelomeningocele is increasingly common and may reduce subsequent symptoms. Surgical repair within 72 hours following delivery reduces mortality and morbidity from the open dysraphism.

Imaging

CM2 affects many regions of the skull, brain, and spine, so a variety of imaging abnormalities may be seen.

Skull and Dura. The calvarial vault forms from membranous bone. With failure of neural tube closure and absence of fetal brain distension, normal induction of the calvarial membranous plates does not occur. Disorganized collections of collagen fibers and deficient radial growth of the developing calvarium ensue, resulting in **lacunar skull** (i.e., Lückenschädel) **(36-8)**. The skull defects ("craniofenestra") are caused by the mesenchymal abnormality and are *not* a consequence of increased intracranial pressure.

Focal calvarial thinning and a "scooped-out" appearance are typical imaging findings of lacunar skull. The calvarium appears thinned with numerous circular or oval lucent defects and shallow depressions. The craniofenestra diminish with age and typically resolve by 6 months, although some scalloping of the inner table often persists into adulthood.

A **small, shallow, bony posterior fossa** with low-lying transverse sinuses is almost always present in CM2. A **large, "gaping" FM** is common. **Concave petrous temporal bones** and a **short concave clivus** are often present **(36-9)**.

Dural abnormalities are common. A widened, open, **heart-shaped tentorial incisura** and **thinned, hypoplastic**, or **fenestrated falx** are frequent findings. The fenestrated falx allows gyri to cross the midline. Interdigitating gyri and the deficient falx result in the appearance of an **irregular interhemispheric fissure** on imaging studies **(36-9C) (36-10C)**.

Midbrain, Hindbrain, and Cerebellum. Hindbrain and cerebellum anomalies are a constant in CM2. The medulla and cerebellar vermis (*not* the tonsils!) are displaced downward into the upper cervical canal for a variable distance. The **inferiorly displaced cerebellar tissue** is typically the **nodulus** with variable contributions from the uvula and pyramid. A **cervicomedullary "kink"** with a **"medullary spur"** is common in the upper cervical canal but may lie as low as T1-4 in severe cases.

On sagittal T1 and T2 scans, the inferiorly displaced vermis, medulla, and choroid plexus form a **"cascade" of tissue** that protrudes downward through the gaping FM to lie behind the spinal cord. The superiorly herniated cerebellum may compress and deform the quadrigeminal plate, giving the appearance of a **"beaked" tectum (36-10A) (36-10B)**.

In addition to the cephalocaudal displacement of posterior fossa contents, the cerebellar hemispheres often curve anteromedially around the brainstem. In severe cases, the pons and medulla appear nearly engulfed by the "creeping" cerebellum on axial imaging studies.

***(36-8)** Autopsy case of lacunar (Lückenschädel) skull in CM2 shows multiple "scooped" out foci of thinned, almost translucent bone. (Courtesy R. Hewlett, MD.) **(36-9A)** NECT of CM2 shows small posterior fossa with concave petrous ridges, scalloped inner table, no visible 4th ventricle, and "creeping" cerebellar hemispheres almost enveloping an elongated, inferiorly stretched medulla.*

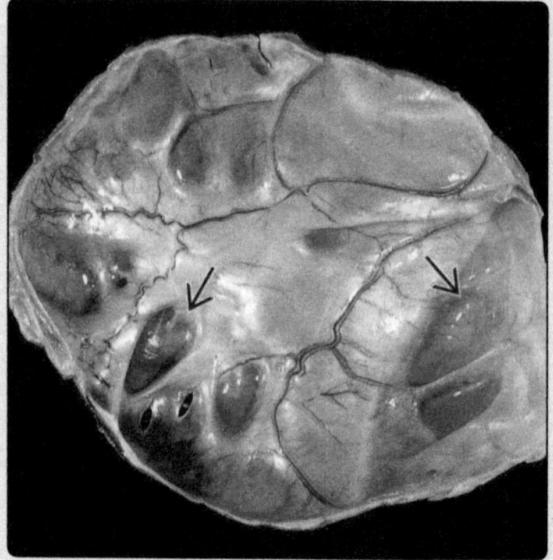

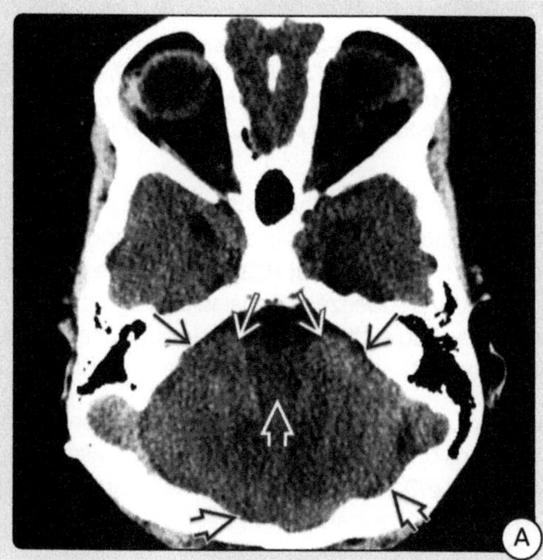

***(36-9B)** NECT in the same patient shows widely gaping, heart-shaped incisura with "towering" cerebellum protruding superiorly and mild "beaking" of the tectum. **(36-9C)** More cephalad scan in the same patient shows the typical "serrated" appearance of the interhemispheric fissure due to the interdigitating gyri typically seen in CM2.*

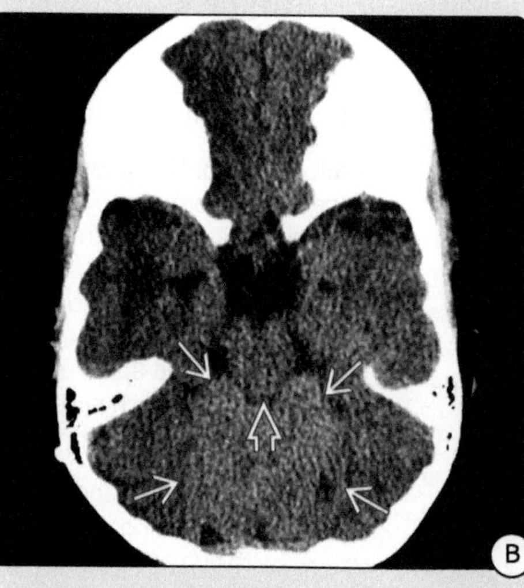

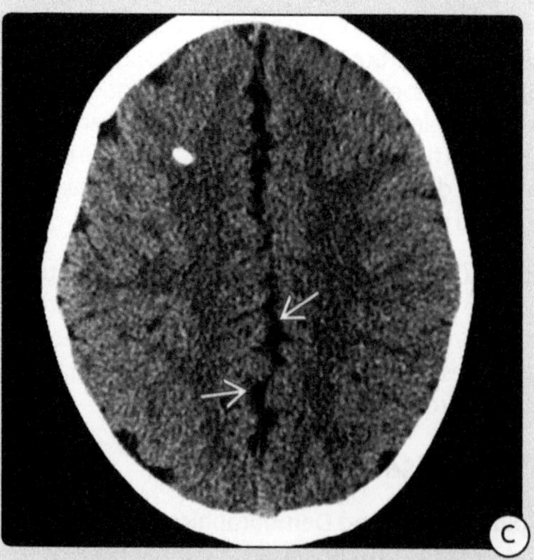

The cerebellar hemispheres and vermis are pushed upward through the incisura, giving the appearance of a **"towering" cerebellum** on coronal T1 and T2 scans **(36-10D)**.

Ventricles. Abnormalities of the ventricles are present in over 90% of CM2 patients. The fourth ventricle is caudally displaced, typically lacks a fastigium (dorsal point), and appears thin and elongated (**"soda straw" fourth ventricle**). The third ventricle is often large and has a very **prominent massa intermedia (36-10A)**.

The lateral ventricles vary in size and configuration. Hydrocephalus is almost always present at birth. The atria and occipital horns are often disproportionately enlarged (**"colpocephaly"**), suggesting the presence of callosal and forceps major dysgenesis.

Following shunting, the lateral ventricles frequently retain a **serrated** or **scalloped appearance**. A large CSF space between the occipital lobes often persists.

Cerebral Hemispheres. Malformations of cortical development, such as **polymicrogyria**, contracted narrow gyri (**"stenogyria"**) **(36-10B)**, and **heterotopic gray matter**, are frequent associated findings.

Callosal dysgenesis is found in nearly 2/3 of all cases, and **abnormalities of the fornices** are also common.

Spine and Spinal Cord. Open spinal dysraphism with **myelomeningocele** is present in almost all cases of CM2. **Hydrosyringomyelia** is seen in 50%.

Differential Diagnosis

The major differential diagnosis of CM2 is other Chiari malformations.

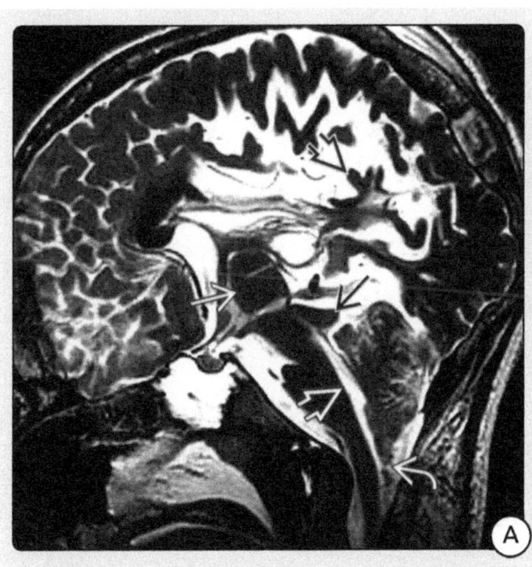

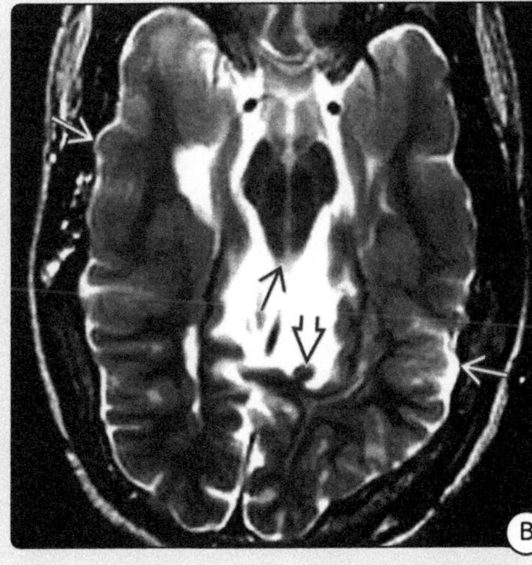

***(36-10A)** Sagittal MR in a 13y patient demonstrates many features of CM2, including small posterior fossa, elongated "soda straw" 4th ventricle ➡, "cascade" of vermis/choroid plexus behind the medulla ➡, "beaked" tectum ➡, large massa intermedia ➡, and multiple gyral malformations ("stenogyria") ➡. **(36-10B)** Axial T2 MR shows "beaked" tectum ➡, stenogyria ➡, and scalloped calvarium ➡.*

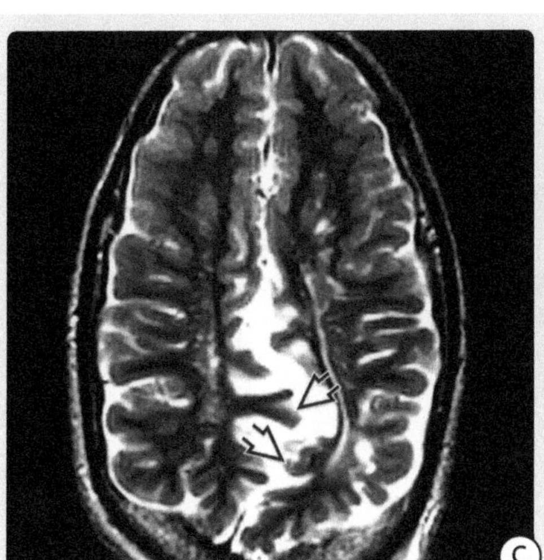

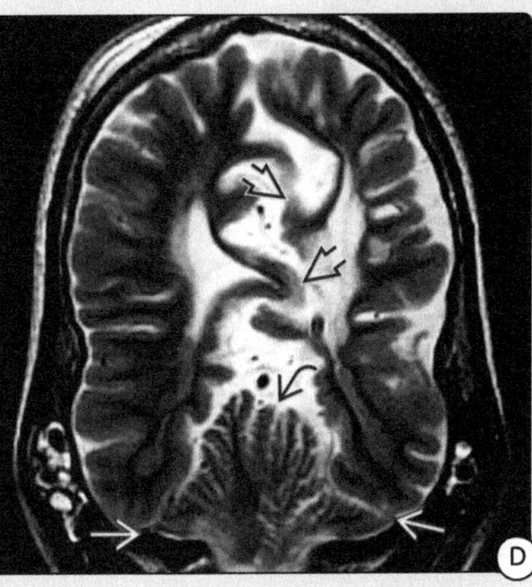

***(36-10C)** Axial T2 MR shows fenestrated falx with shortened interdigitating gyri ➡, irregular "serrated" appearance to interhemispheric fissure. **(36-10D)** Coronal T2 MR shows low-lying transverse sinuses ➡ with a very small posterior fossa, "towering" cerebellum ➡ that protrudes upward through the tentorial incisura, and interdigitating gyri ➡, giving a "serrated" appearance to the interhemispheric fissure.*

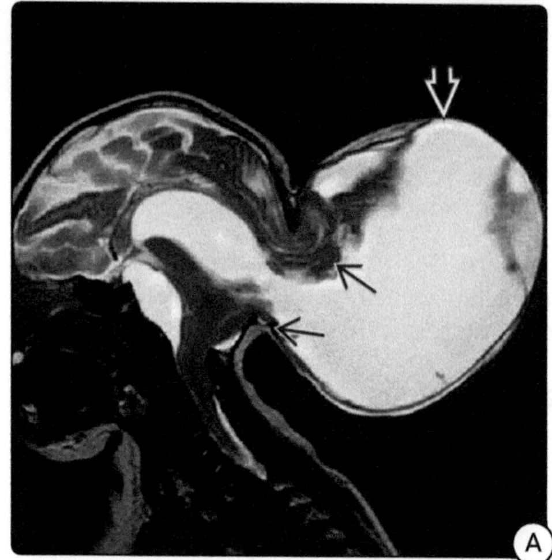

(36-11A) Sagittal T2 shows CM3 with cephalocele ➡ that contains herniated dysplastic brain ➡ and CSF in continuity with a lateral ventricle.

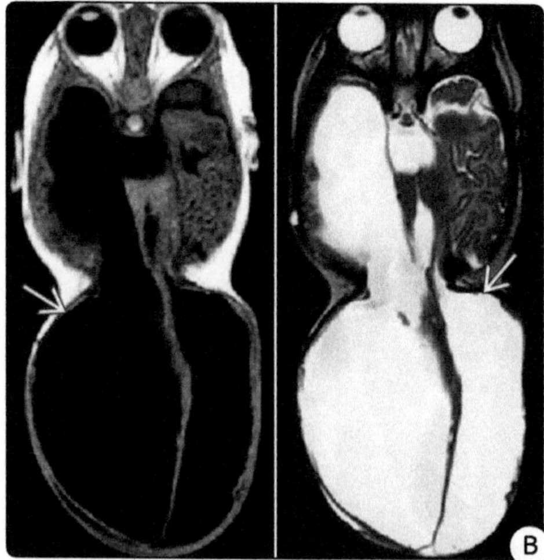

(36-11B) Axial T1 (L), T2 (R) MRs in the same patient show extension of the lateral ventricles ➡ into the cephalocele.

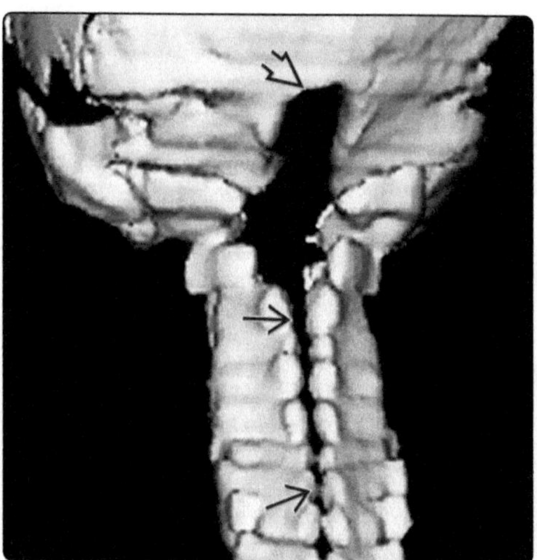

(36-12) CM3 is shown with extensive cranium bifidum extending from the occipital bone ➡ through the entire cervical spine ➡.

In **Chiari 1**, it is the tonsils (not the vermis) that are herniated inferiorly. Myelomeningocele is absent, and, other than being somewhat small, the posterior fossa and its contents appear relatively normal.

If findings of CM2 plus a low occipital or high cervical cephalocele are present, the diagnosis is **Chiari 3**.

CHIARI 2 MALFORMATION

Pathoetiology

- Complex hindbrain malformation with myelomeningocele
  - Posterior neuropore closure disorder
  - Developing vesicles fail to expand
  - Paraxial mesodermal abnormalities (skull, spine)
- Result = "too small" bony posterior fossa

Clinical Issues

- Prevalence reduced with maternal folate
- Myelomeningocele, hydrocephalus dominate clinical picture at birth

Imaging Findings

- Myelomeningocele (almost always)
- Lacunar skull
- Small posterior fossa
- Abnormal dura (gaping FM, heart-shaped incisura, fenestrated falx)
- Inferiorly displaced medulla, vermis lead to "cascade" of tissue
- Cervicomedullary "kink," medullary "spur"
- "Towering" and "creeping" cerebellum
- "Soda straw" 4th ventricle
- Prominent massa intermedia
- Hydrocephalus, shunted ventricles appear scalloped
- Callosal dysgenesis
- Stenogyria, gray matter heterotopias

Chiari 3

Chiari 3 malformation (CM3) is the rarest of the Chiari malformations. CM3 consists of a small posterior fossa with a caudally displaced brainstem and variable herniation of meninges/posterior fossa contents through a low occipital or upper cervical bony defect.

The cephalocele contains meninges together with variable amounts of brain tissue, vessels, and CSF spaces. The brain is often featureless, dysplastic-appearing, and disorganized with extensive gliosis and gray matter heterotopias.

NECT scans show bony features similar to those seen in CM2, i.e., a small posterior cranial fossa, short scalloped clivus, lacunar skull, a defect in the ventral chondral portion of the supraoccipital bone, and low cranium bifidum that may extend inferiorly to involve much of the cervical spine **(36-12)**.

MR best delineates sac contents, which often include dysplastic-appearing cerebellum &/or brainstem, as well as distorted CSF spaces and vessels. A deformed fourth and sometimes third ventricle can be partially found within the mass of herniated brain and meninges. Veins, dural sinuses, and even the basilar artery are sometimes "pulled" into the defect **(36-11)**.

Hindbrain Malformations

Cystic Posterior Fossa Anomalies and the Dandy-Walker Continuum

Terminology

The Dandy-Walker continuum (DWC) is a spectrum of anomalies that includes **Dandy-Walker malformation (DWM), vermian hypoplasia**, and **mega cisterna magna (MCM)**.

DWM affects both the cerebellum and overlying meninges. It consists of an enlarged posterior fossa (PF) with a high-inserting venous sinus confluence, large PF pia-ependyma-lined cyst extending dorsally from the fourth ventricle, and varying degrees of vermian and cerebellar hemispheric hypoplasia **(36-13)**.

In **vermian hypoplasia** (old term = Dandy-Walker variant), the vermis is rotated superiorly and the inferior vermis is hypoplastic with a "keyhole" opening into the cisterna magna via a gaping foramen of Magendie. The overall size of the PF is normal.

MCM is the mildest end of the DWC spectrum with an enlarged retrocerebellar CSF collection (> 10 mm). There is no mass effect on the cerebellar hemispheres or vermis. The vermis is well formed and normal. Cerebellar veins and elements of the falx cerebelli can be seen crossing through the MCM, and the adjacent bone can appear scalloped by pulsatile CSF in the MCM.

Etiology

Etiology and Genetics. Three main DWM causative genes have been identified: *FOXC1* and the linked *ZIC1* and *ZIC4* genes.

DWM is accompanied by > 18 types of chromosomal abnormality and co-occurs with > 40 genetic syndromes. In addition, DWM can arise as a result of maternal diabetes or fetal infection (e.g., cytomegalovirus or Zika virus).

Known clinical associations with DWM include PHACES, neurocutaneous melanosis, midline anomalies, and trisomy 18.

Pathology

Gross Pathology. Major findings in DWM are (1) an enlarged PF with (2) upward displacement of the tentorium and accompanying venous sinuses and (3) cystic dilatation of the fourth ventricle. Vermian abnormalities range from complete absence to varying degrees of hypoplasia. The PF cyst in DWM is typically lined by an outer layer of pia-arachnoid and an inner layer of ependyma.

DWM is frequently associated with other CNS anomalies. Almost 2/3 of patients have gyral abnormalities (e.g., pachy- or polymicrogyria and heterotopic GM). Callosal dysgenesis is common.

Clinical Issues

DWM is the most common congenital cerebellar malformation. The most common presentation of DWM is increased intracranial pressure secondary to hydrocephalus.

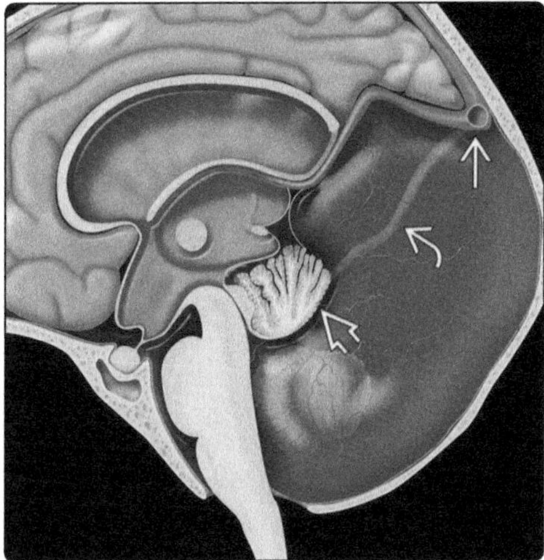

***(36-13)** Elevated torcular ➡, steeply angled TS ➡, superiorly rotated hypoplastic cerebellar vermis ➡, and hydrocephalus reveal DWM.*

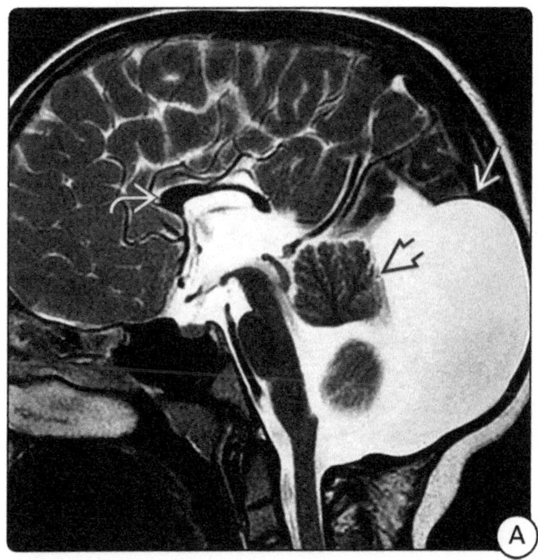

***(36-14A)** DWM shows large PF cyst elevating torcular ➡, superiorly rotated vermian remnant ➡, small pons, dysgenetic corpus callosum ➡.*

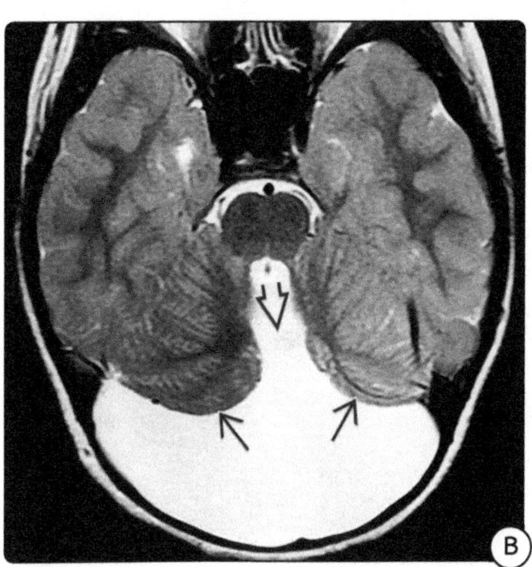

***(36-14B)** Axial T2 MR in DWM shows 4th ventricle open dorsally ➡ to the large PF cyst. Cerebellar hemispheres are small, "winged" anteriorly ➡.*

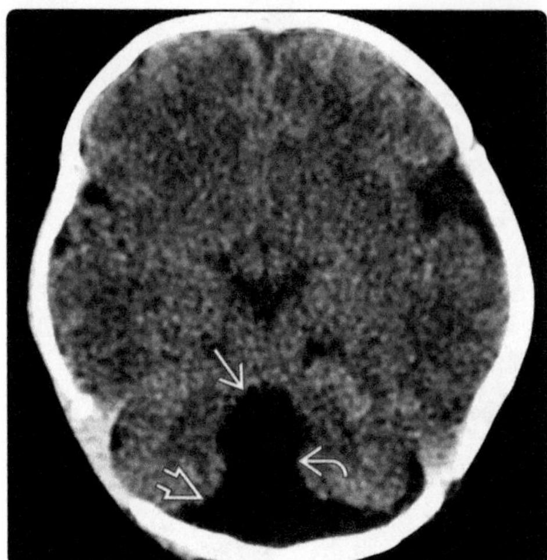

(36-15) NECT shows "keyhole" of vermian hypoplasia + large 4th v ➡ opening into cisterna magna ➡ via gaping foramen of Magendie ➡.

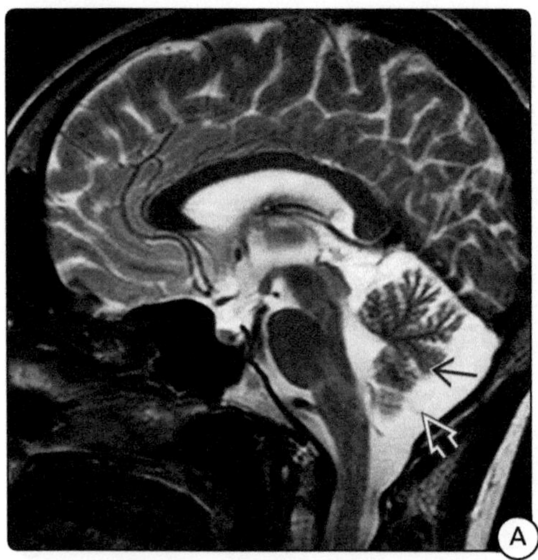

(36-16A) Sagittal T2 MR shows a very prominent cisterna magna ➡, somewhat hypoplastic-appearing inferior vermis ➡. This is DWC-VH.

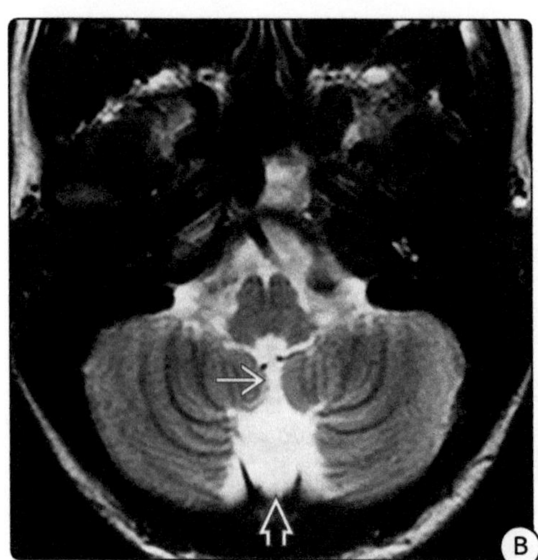

(36-16B) T2 MR shows large cisterna magna ➡, vermian hypoplasia, wide foramen of Magendie ➡. Mild DWC with mega cisterna magna (MCM).

Imaging

The spectrum of imaging abnormalities in DWM is broad, affecting—to varying degrees—the skull and dura, ventricles and CSF spaces, and brain.

Skull and Dura, Venous Sinuses. In contrast to CM2 in which the PF is abnormally small, the PF in DWM is strikingly enlarged. The straight sinus, sinus confluence, and tentorial apex are elevated above the lambdoid suture ("lambdoid-torcular inversion"). The transverse sinuses descend at a steep angle from the torcular Herophili toward the sigmoid sinuses **(36-13)**.

The occipital bone may appear scalloped, focally thinned, and remodeled (may be present in all forms of DWM). Retrocerebellar CSF cysts (formerly termed "mega cisterna magna") **(36-17)** often demonstrate partially infolded dura-arachnoid (falx cerebelli) on axial T2 scans. The falx cerebelli is usually absent in DWM.

Ventricles and Cisterns. The floor of the fourth ventricle is present and appears normal in DWM. The fastigium and choroid plexus are absent. The fourth ventricle opens dorsally to a variably sized CSF-containing cyst that balloons posteriorly behind and between the cerebellar hemisphere remnants.

Generalized obstructive hydrocephalus is present in over 80% of neonates with DWM at birth. If callosal dysgenesis is present, the lateral ventricles are widely separated and may have unusually prominent occipital horns (colpocephaly).

In DWC (previously called Dandy-Walker "variant"), the fourth ventricle has a "keyhole" configuration on axial imaging caused by a widely patent vallecula that communicates with a prominent cisterna magna **(36-15)**.

Brainstem, Cerebellum, and Vermis. The brainstem appears normal in mild forms of DWM but often appears somewhat small in moderate to more severe DWM.

Varying degrees of vermian hypoplasia are seen in DWM **(36-16)**. The inferior lobules are often hypoplastic in mild DWC. In classic DWM, the vermian remnant is rotated and elevated above the large PF cyst **(36-14A)**.

The cerebellar hemispheres are hypoplastic in DWM. In severe cases of DWM, the cerebellar remnants appear "winged" outward and displaced anterolaterally **(36-14B)**.

Associated Abnormalities. Other CNS abnormalities are present in 70% of DWM. The most common finding is callosal agenesis or dysgenesis. A dorsal interhemispheric cyst may be present. Gray matter abnormalities (e.g., heterotopias, clefts, and pachy- and polymicrogyria) are common associated abnormalities.

Differential Diagnosis

Because Dandy-Walker really is a spectrum, there are many "in between" cases. From a clinical perspective, it is most important for the radiologist to specifically describe vermian, cerebellar, and any coexisting supratentorial anomalies (see previous shaded box).

A **retrocerebellar arachnoid cyst** is not part of DWC. It is a midline arachnoid-lined cyst located behind the vermis and fourth ventricle that does not communicate with the latter. Although there may be mass effect on the cerebellum, there is no associated hydrocephalus and no communication with the fourth ventricle. The cerebellum otherwise appears normal. Veins and a falx cerebelli do not traverse the CSF collection.

In the absence of other findings, a prominent retrocerebellar CSF collection > 10 mm with crossing vessels and a traversing falx cerebelli is most often a **mega cisterna magna** (MCM), a normal variant that is of no clinical significance **(36-16)**.

DANDY-WALKER CONTINUUM (DWC): DIFFERENTIAL DIAGNOSIS

Dandy-Walker Malformation (DWM)
- Large posterior fossa (PF)
  - Torcular-lambdoid inversion
- Cyst extending posteriorly from 4th ventricle
- Vermian agenesis or hypogenesis
- Cerebellar hemispheres often hypoplastic
  - May appear "winged" outward, displaced anterolaterally

Vermian Hypoplasia (VH)
- Old term = Dandy-Walker variant
- Reduced vermian tissue below fastigium-declive line
- Superior rotation of vermis
  - Increased tegmento-vermian angle (18-45°)
- PF normal size

Mega Cisterna Magna (MCM)
- Enlarged retrocerebellar CSF (> 10 mm)
- No mass effect on vermis or cerebellum
- Normal vermis
- Fluid crossed by veins, falx cerebelli
- May scallop, remodel occiput**
  - **All categories in DWC may "scallop" inner occipital bone

Arachnoid Cyst
- Not truly in Dandy-Walker continuum
  - Cerebellopontine angle > retrovermian
- No communication with 4th ventricle
- No crossing veins or falx cerebelli
- Causes mass effect

Miscellaneous Malformations

Several less common PF malformations are largely defined by imaging features. These include rhombencephalosynapsis, Joubert syndrome, and cerebellar hypoplasias/dysplasias.

Rhombencephalosynapsis

Rhombencephalosynapsis is a midline brain malformation characterized by (1) a "missing" cerebellar vermis and (2) apparent fusion of the cerebellar hemispheres. Dorsal midline continuity of the cerebellar hemispheres is characteristic. The tonsils, dentate nuclei, and superior cerebellar peduncles are usually fused.

Sagittal MR scans show an upwardly rounded fastigial recess of the fourth ventricle and lack of the normal midline foliar pattern of the vermis. Coronal and axial images show transverse folia and continuity of the cerebellar white matter across the midline **(36-18)**. Images through the rostral fourth ventricle may demonstrate a diamond or pointed shape.

Aqueductal stenosis and hydrocephalus are common. Absent cavum septi pellucidi is seen in 1/2 of all cases. The thalami, fornices, and tectum may be partially or completely fused. Other forebrain anomalies include absent olfactory bulbs and corpus callosum dysgenesis.

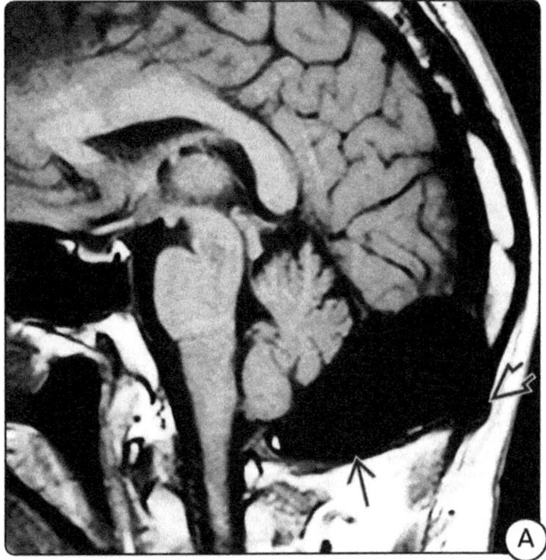

***(36-17A)** Sagittal T1 MR shows mild DWC (MCM). Note thinned ⇒, scalloped ⇒ occipital bone. Pons, vermis, 4th ventricle are normal.*

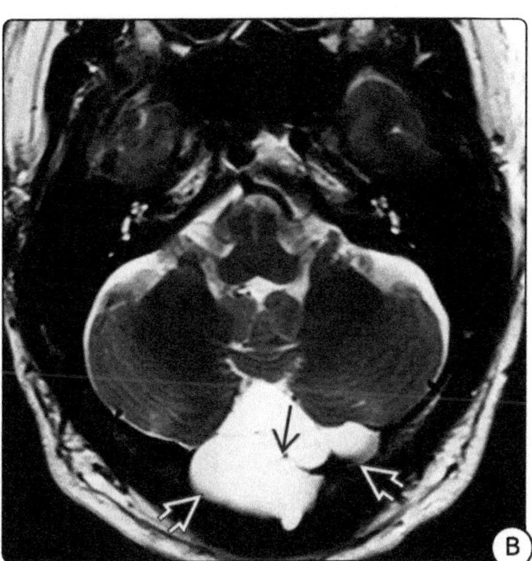

***(36-17B)** Axial T2 MR in the same patient shows bone "scalloping" ⇒ and partially infolded dura-arachnoid of falx cerebelli ⇒.*

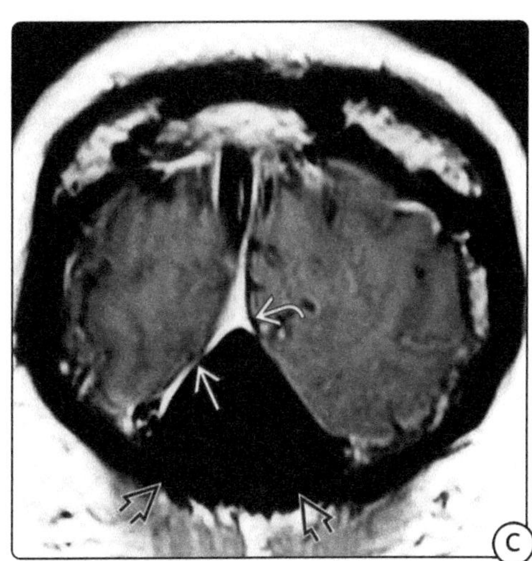

***(36-17C)** Coronal T1 C+ MR shows that MCM ⇒ can elevate the posterior tentorium ⇒ and torcular Herophili ⇒.*

Joubert Syndrome and Related Disorders

Joubert syndrome (JS) and related disorders (JSRD) are a group of syndromes in which the hallmark is the "molar tooth" sign, a complex mid- and hindbrain malformation that resembles a molar tooth on axial MR scans. Multiple syndromes exhibit "molar tooth" posterior fossa malformations, so genetic analysis may be required to distinguish among different JSRD subtypes.

Midline sagittal MR scans show a small dysmorphic vermis. The fourth ventricle appears deformed with a thin upwardly convex roof and an elongated, rounded fastigium **(36-20A)**.

Axial scans demonstrate the classic "molar tooth" appearance with foreshortened midbrain, narrow isthmus, deep interpeduncular fossa, and thickened superior cerebellar peduncles surrounding an oblong or diamond-shaped fourth ventricle **(36-20B)**. The superior vermis is clefted, and the cisterna magna may appear enlarged.

The major imaging differential diagnosis of JSRD is **vermian and pontocerebellar hypoplasia** in which the vermis is small but not clefted. In **rhombencephalosynapsis**, the cerebellar hemispheres and dentate nuclei are fused across the midline, not split.

Cerebellar Hypoplasia and Unclassified Dysplasias

Unclassified cerebellar dysplasias are not associated with other known malformations or syndromes, such as JS or DWC. In severe cases of cerebellar hypoplasia, the cerebellar hemispheres and vermis are almost completely absent, and the pons is hypoplastic.

Selected References: The complete reference list is available on the Expert Consult™ eBook version included with purchase.

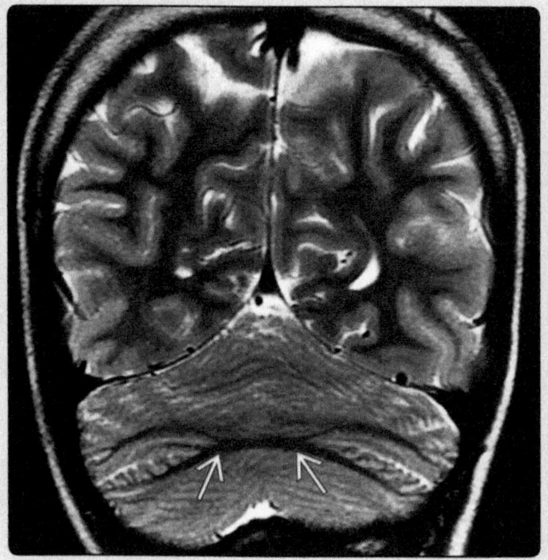

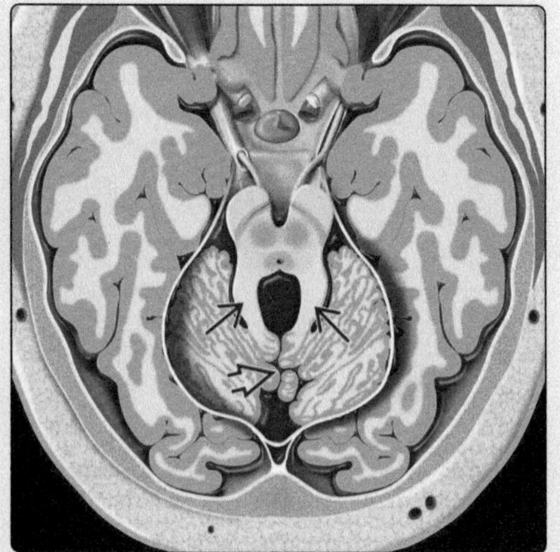

***(36-18)** Coronal T2 MR shows classic rhombencephalosynapsis. Note absent vermis, transversely oriented folia, and continuity of cerebellar white matter across the midline ➡. **(36-19)** Axial graphic shows Joubert malformation. Thickened superior cerebellar peduncles ➡ around an elongated 4th ventricle form the classic "molar tooth" sign. Note cleft cerebellar vermis ➡.*

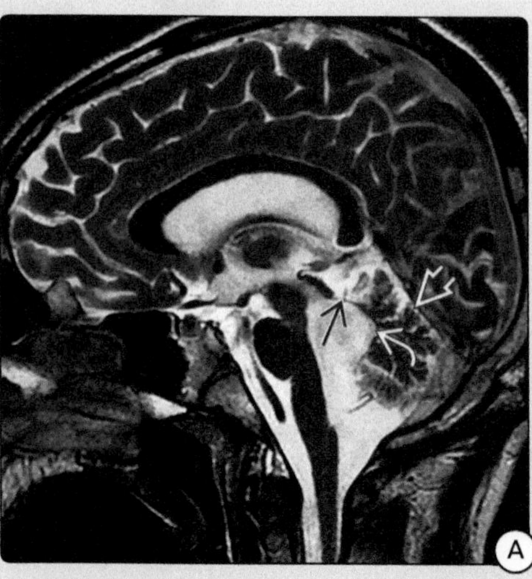

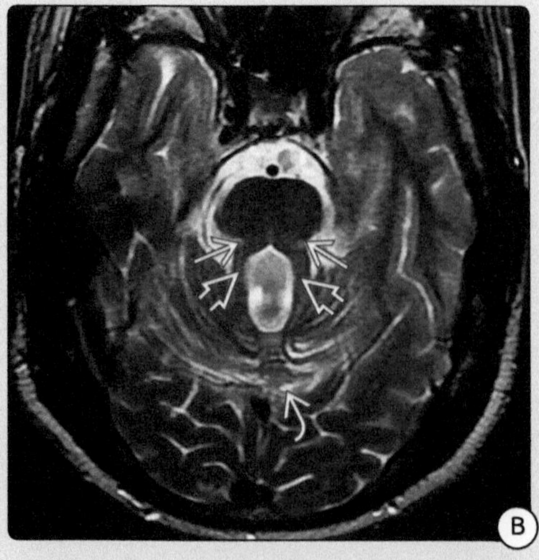

***(36-20A)** Sagittal T2 MR in a patient with classic Joubert shows small misshapen vermis ➡, upwardly convex superior 4th ventricle ➡, rounded enlarged fastigial point ➡. **(36-20B)** Axial MR in the same patient shows "molar tooth" sign, foreshortened midbrain with narrow isthmus ➡, thick superior cerebellar peduncles ➡ surrounding an elongated 4th ventricle, and disorganized cleft vermis ➡.*

Commissural and Cortical Maldevelopment

Corpus callosum dysgenesis and malformations of cortical development (MCDs) are two of the most important congenital brain anomalies. Anomalies of the cerebral commissures are the most common of all congenital brain malformations, and corpus callosum dysgenesis is the single most common malformation that accompanies other developmental brain anomalies.

Cortical malformations arise when migrating precursor cells fail to reach their target destinations. MCDs are intrinsically epileptogenic and may be responsible for 25-40% of all medically refractory childhood epilepsies.

Commissural Anomalies

Callosal Dysgenesis Spectrum

Terminology

The corpus callosum (CC) can be completely absent (agenesis) **(37-1)** or partially formed (hypogenesis). **Complete CC agenesis** is almost always accompanied by the absence of the hippocampal commissure (HC). The anterior commissure (AC), which forms three weeks earlier than the CC, is usually present and normal. If the CC is hypogenetic, the posterior segments and the inferior genu and rostrum are usually absent.

Pathology

In *complete* CC agenesis, all five segments are missing. The **cingulate gyrus** is absent on sagittal sections, whereas the hemispheres demonstrate a radiating **"spoke-wheel" gyral pattern** extending perpendicularly to the roof of the third ventricle **(37-3)**.

On coronal sections, the **"high-riding" third ventricle** looks as if it opens directly into the interhemispheric fissure. It is actually covered by a thin membranous roof that bulges into the interhemispheric fissure, displacing the fornices laterally. The lateral ventricles have upturned, pointed corners **(37-1)**.

A prominent longitudinal white matter (WM) tract called the **Probst bundle** is situated just inside the apex of each ventricle **(37-1)**. These bundles consist of the misdirected commissural fibers, which should have crossed the midline but instead course from front to back, indenting the medial walls of the lateral ventricles.

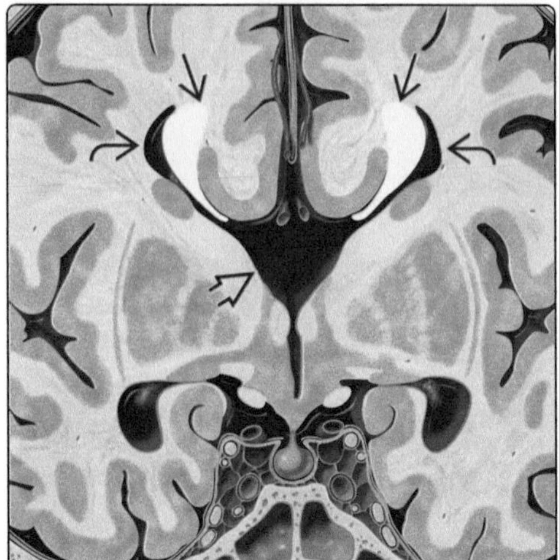

***(37-1)** Agenesis of CC (ACC) shows "Viking helmet," "high-riding" 3rd ventricle ⇨, pointed lateral ventricles ⇨, and Probst bundles ⇨.*

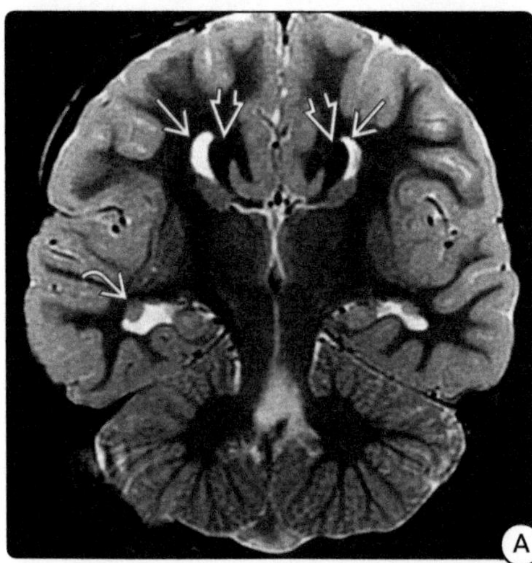

***(37-2A)** Coronal T2 MR shows "Viking helmet" of ACC with curving, upturned lateral ventricles ➡, Probst bundles ➡, and heterotopic GM ➡.*

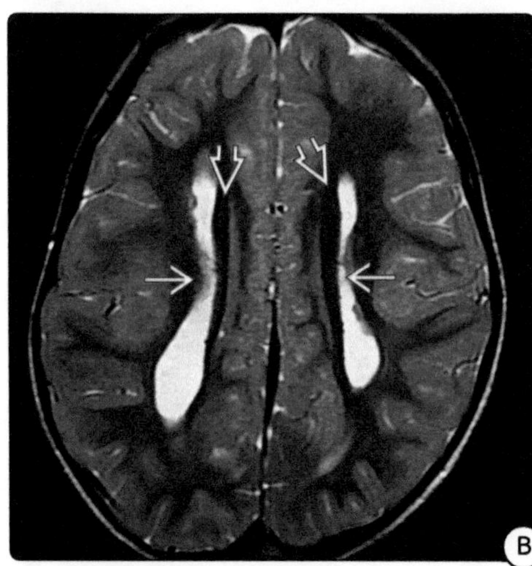

***(37-2B)** Axial MR shows parallel, "nonconverging" lateral ventricles ➡ and Probst bundles ➡.*

Axial sections show that the lateral ventricles are parallel and nonconverging. The occipital horns are often disproportionately dilated, a condition termed "colpocephaly."

The gross pathology of CC *hypogenesis* varies according to which segments are missing. The splenium is usually small or absent.

Clinical Issues

CC dysgenesis is the most common of all CNS malformations and are present in 3-5% of individuals with neurodevelopmental disorders.

Minor CC dysgenesis/hypogenesis is often discovered incidentally on imaging studies or at autopsy. Major commissural malformations are associated with seizures, developmental delay, and symptoms secondary to disruptions of the hypothalamic-pituitary axis.

CALLOSAL DYSGENESIS: PATHOETIOLOGY AND CLINICAL ISSUES

Terminology

- Complete absence of corpus callosum (CC) = agenesis
  - Hippocampal commissure (HC) absent
  - Anterior commissure (AC) often present
  - All 3 absent = tricommissural agenesis
- Hypogenetic, dysgenetic CC
  - Rostrum, splenium often absent in partial agenesis
  - Partial posterior agenesis = HC, splenium, ± posterior body

Clinical Issues

- Most common CNS malformation
- Found in 3-5% of neurodevelopmental disorders

Imaging

MR Findings. Sagittal T1 and T2 scans best demonstrate complete CC absence or partial dysgenesis.

Complete Corpus Callosum Agenesis. With complete agenesis, the third ventricle appears continuous with the interhemispheric fissure and is surrounded dorsally by fingers of radiating gyri that "point" toward the third ventricle on sagittal images **(37-4)**. Associated findings include a variable midline interhemispheric cyst and azygous anterior cerebral artery.

Axial scans demonstrate the parallel lateral ventricles especially well. The prominent myelinated tracts of the Probst bundles can appear quite prominent **(37-2B)**.

Coronal scans show a "Viking helmet" or "moose head" appearance caused by the curved, upwardly pointed lateral ventricles and "high-riding" third ventricle that expands into the interhemispheric fissure. The Probst bundles are seen as densely myelinated tracts lying just inside the lateral ventricle bodies. The hippocampi appear abnormally rounded and vertically oriented. Moderately enlarged temporal horns are common. Look for malformations, such as heterotopic gray matter (GM) **(37-2A)**.

DTI is especially helpful in depicting CC agenesis. The normal red (right-to-left encoded) color of the CC is absent. Instead, prominent front-to-back (green) tracts of the Probst bundles are seen.

Corpus Callosum Hypogenesis. In partial agenesis, the rostrum and splenium are usually absent **(37-5)**, and the remaining genu and body often have a "blocky," thickened appearance. The hippocampal commissure is typically absent, but the AC is generally preserved and often appears quite normal or even larger than usual.

CALLOSAL DYSGENESIS: IMAGING

Sagittal
- Partial or complete CC agenesis
- 3rd ventricle appears "open" to interhemispheric fissure
- Cingulate gyrus absent → gyri "radiate" outward from 3rd ventricle

Axial
- Lateral ventricles parallel, nonconverging, widely separated
- Probst bundles = WM along medial margins of lateral ventricles

Coronal
- "Viking helmet" or "moose head" appearance
- "High-riding" 3rd ventricle
- Pointed, upcurving lateral ventricles
- Probst bundles

Associated Anomalies and Syndromes

Although CC dysgenesis can occur as an isolated phenomenon, CC anomalies are the single most common malformation associated with *other* CNS anomalies and syndromes. **Chiari 2 malformation, Dandy-Walker spectrum**, syndromic **craniosynostoses, hypothalamic-pituitary** anomalies and **malformations of cortical development (37-2)** all have an increased prevalence of CC anomalies.

Anomalies of the cerebral commissures have been described in nearly 200 different syndromes! Striking examples include **Aicardi syndrome** where callosal agenesis is the most common anatomic abnormality.

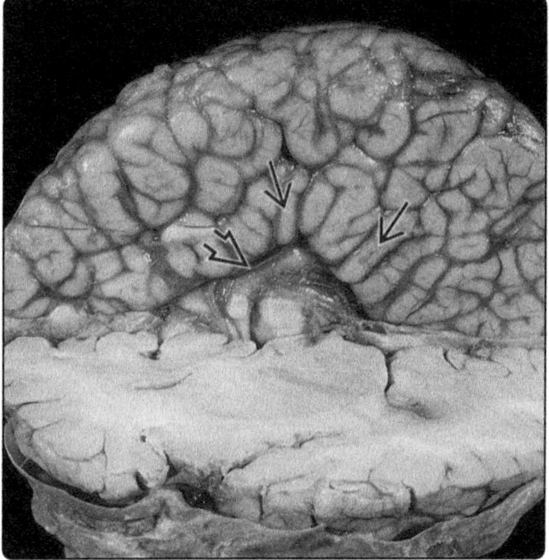

***(37-3)** ACC in Aicardi syndrome shows "radiating" gyri ➙ converging on "high-riding" 3rd ventricle ➙. (Courtesy R. Hewlett, MD.)*

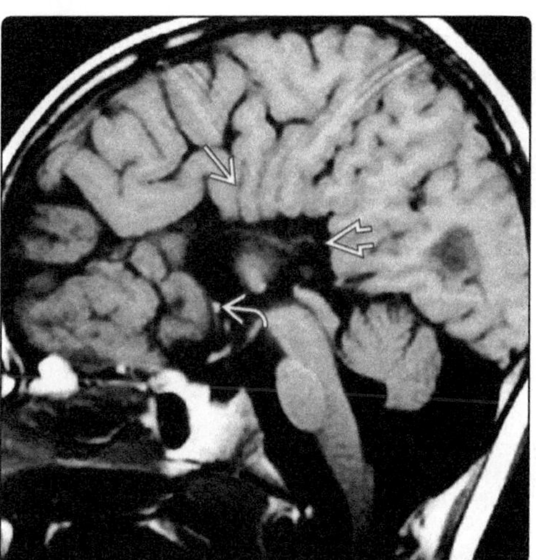

***(37-4)** "Spoke-wheel" gyri ➙ converge on 3rd ventricle ➙. Anterior commissure is normal ➙. Hippocampal commissure is absent. This is ACC.*

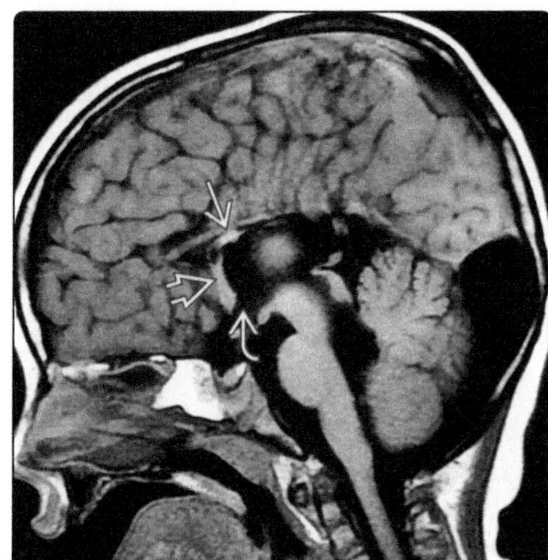

***(37-5)** Genu ➙, remnant of body ➙ are present. Rostrum ➙, splenium are absent. This is CC hypogenesis.*

Malformations of Cortical Development

Focal Cortical Dysplasias

Focal cortical dysplasias (FCDs) are a common cause of medically refractory epilepsy in both children and adults. Surgical resection is an increasingly important treatment option, so recognition and accurate delineation of FCD on imaging studies are key to successful patient management.

Terminology and International League Against Epilepsy (ILAE) Classification

FCDs—sometimes called **Taylor cortical dysplasia**—are localized regions of nonneoplastic malformed GM.

FCD type I is an isolated malformation with abnormal cortical layering that demonstrates either vertical (radial) persistence of developmental microcolumns (FCD type Ia) or loss of the horizontal hexalaminar structure (FCD type Ib) in one or multiple lobes. FCD type Ic is characterized by both patterns of abnormal cortical layering.

FCD type II is an isolated lesion characterized by altered cortical layering and dysmorphic neurons either without (type IIa) or with **balloon** (type IIb) **cells**. Type II is the most common type of FCD.

The third type of FCD, **FCD type III**, is a postmigrational disorder associated with principal pathologies, such as ischemia, infection, trauma, etc. In such cases, cytoarchitectural abnormalities occur together with hippocampal sclerosis (FCD type IIIa), epilepsy-associated tumors (FCD type IIIb), vascular

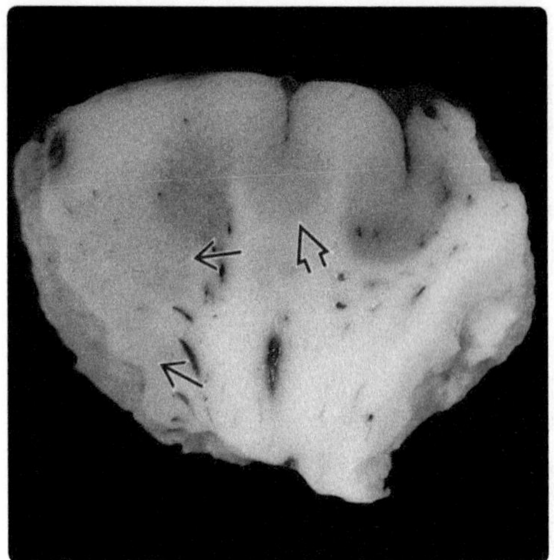

(37-6) Classic "funnel-shaped" area of thickened cortex, blurred gray-white interface ⇨ in FCD. Contrast with normal sulcus and gyrus ⇨.

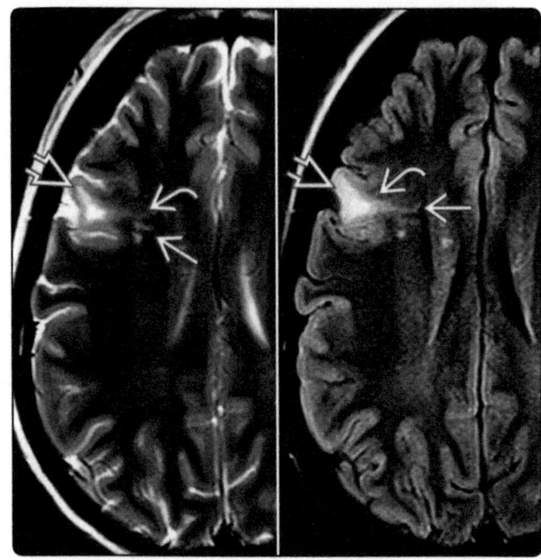

(37-7) FCDIIb with funnel shape ⇨, indistinct GM-WM ⇨, curvilinear hyperintense foci ⇨ extending toward the lateral ventricle is shown.

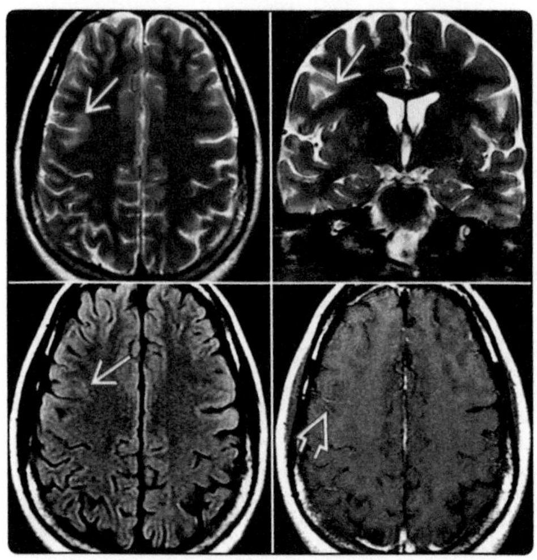

(37-8) Note FCD ⇨. Signal intensity is similar to GM. T1 C+ shows enhancement of "primitive" cortical veins ⇨. (Courtesy P. Hildenbrand, MD.)

malformations (FCD type IIIc), or—in the case of FCD type IIId—other epileptogenic lesions acquired in early life.

Etiology

The most convincing data implicate mammalian target of rapamycin (mTOR) cascade abnormalities as the cause of FCD. FCD type IIb specimens typically have sequence alterations in the *TSC1* (hamartin) gene and resemble the cortical tubers in tuberous sclerosis complex (TSC). Extensive cortical malformations can also be caused by prenatal infections

Pathology

Mildly thickened, slightly firm cortex with poor demarcation from the underlying WM is characteristic **(37-6)**. The histopathologic hallmarks of FCD are disorganized cytoarchitecture and neurons with abnormal shape, size, and orientation. Prominent balloon cells are typical of type IIb. These balloon cells are histologically identical to giant cells in the tubers from TSC patients.

Clinical Issues

FCDs are the single most common cause of severe early-onset drug-resistant epilepsy in children and young adults. FCD type II is found in 15-20% of patients undergoing surgery for medically resistant chronic epilepsy.

Imaging

MR of FCD type IIb shows a localized area of increased cortical thickness and a funnel-shaped area of blurred gray-white interface at the bottom of a sulcus, the **"transmantle MR" sign** **(37-7)**. Signal intensity varies with age. In older patients, FCD appears as a wedge-shaped area of T2/FLAIR hyperintensity extending from the bottom of a sulcus into the subcortical and deep WM **(37-8)**.

A subcortical linear or curvilinear focus of T2/FLAIR hyperintensity sometimes extends toward the superolateral margin of the lateral ventricle **(37-7)**. FCD type IIb does not enhance on T1 C+.

Differential Diagnosis

The major differential diagnosis of FCD (especially type IIb) includes epilepsy-associated **neoplasm** (e.g., dysembryoplastic neuroepithelial tumor, ganglioglioma, diffuse astrocytoma) and tuberous sclerosis. Cortical lesions in **tuberous sclerosis complex** can look very similar to FCD type IIb. TSC usually demonstrates other imaging stigmata, such as subependymal nodules.

FOCAL CORTICAL DYSPLASIA

ILAE Classification

- Most common type is FCD II
  - FCD IIa = without balloon cells
  - FCD IIb = with balloon cells (most common)

Pathology and Clinical Issues

- Mass-like with thickened cortex, indistinct GM-WM junction
- Most common cause of refractory epilepsy

Imaging

- Focal/wedge-shaped mass, blurred GM-WM interface
- Subcortical T2/FLAIR hyperintensity

Abnormalities of Neuronal Migration

The most common abnormalities of neuronal migration are GM heterotopias and lissencephaly spectrum disorders.

Heterotopias

Arrest of normal neuronal migration along the radial glial cells can result in grossly visible masses of "heterotopic" GM. These collections come in many shapes and sizes and can be found virtually anywhere between the ventricles and the pia. They can be solitary or multifocal and exist either as an isolated phenomenon or in association with other malformations.

Periventricular Nodular Heterotopia

Periventricular nodular heterotopia (PVNH) is the most common form of cortical malformation in adults. Here, one or more subependymal nodules of GM line the lateral walls of the ventricles **(37-9)**. PVNH can be unilateral or bilateral, focal or diffuse. Collections of round or ovoid nodules indent the lateral walls of the ventricles, giving them a distinctive "lumpy-bumpy" appearance.

PVNH follows GM in density/signal intensity and does not enhance following contrast administration **(37-10)**. The overlying cortex often appears thinned, but sulcation and gyration are typically normal.

The major differential diagnosis of PVNH is the subependymal nodules of **tuberous sclerosis**.

Subcortical Heterotopias

Subcortical heterotopias are malformations in which large, focal, mass-like collections of neurons are found in the deep cerebral WM anywhere from the ependyma to the cortex **(37-11)**. The involved portion of the affected hemisphere is abnormally small, and the overlying cortex appears thin and sometimes dysplastic **(37-12)**.

In other forms of heterotopia, focal masses of ectopic GM occur in linear or swirling curved columns of neurons that extend through normal-appearing WM from the ependyma to the pia. The overlying cortex is thin, and the underlying ventricle often appears distorted **(37-13)**. The masses follow GM on all sequences, do not demonstrate edema, and do not enhance.

Occasionally, ribbon-like bands of heterotopic GM (**subcortical band heterotopia**) form partway between the lateral ventricles and cortex **(37-14)**. Although these have been described with megalencephaly and polymicrogyria, most are probably part of the "double cortex" form of lissencephaly.

Lissencephaly Spectrum

Malformations due to widespread abnormal transmantle migration include **agyria, pachygyria**, and **band heterotopia**. All are part of the **lissencephaly spectrum**.

Terminology

The term lissencephaly (LIS) literally means "smooth brain." The spectrum of LISs ranges from severe (agyria) to milder forms, including abnormally broad

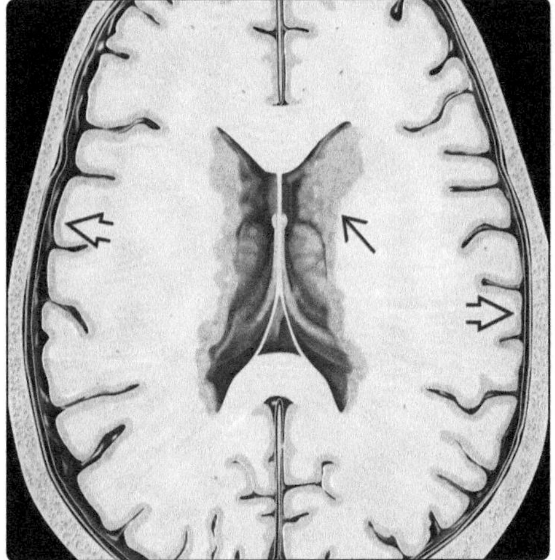

***(37-9)** Extensive subependymal heterotopia ➡ lines the lateral ventricles. The gray matter cortical ribbon is thin ➡ & sulci are shallow.*

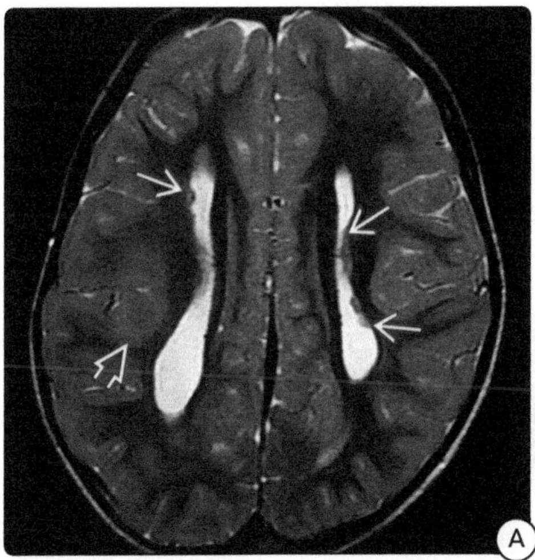

***(37-10A)** Axial T2 MR shows multiple foci of subependymal heterotopic GM ➡ and cortical dysplasia ➡. CC is absent.*

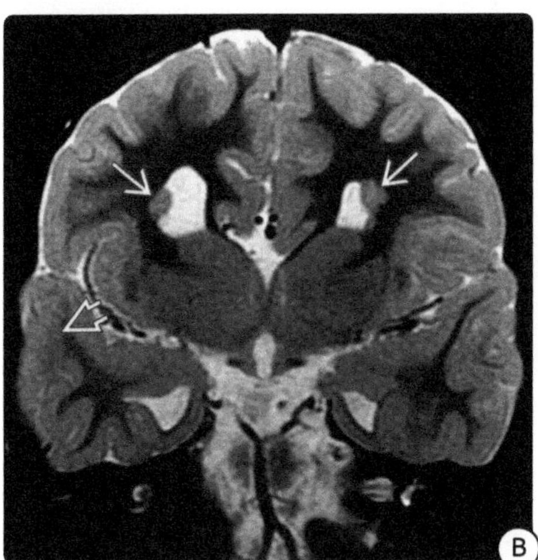

***(37-10B)** Coronal T2 MR demonstrates subependymal heterotopias ➡ and pachy- and polymicrogyria ➡.*

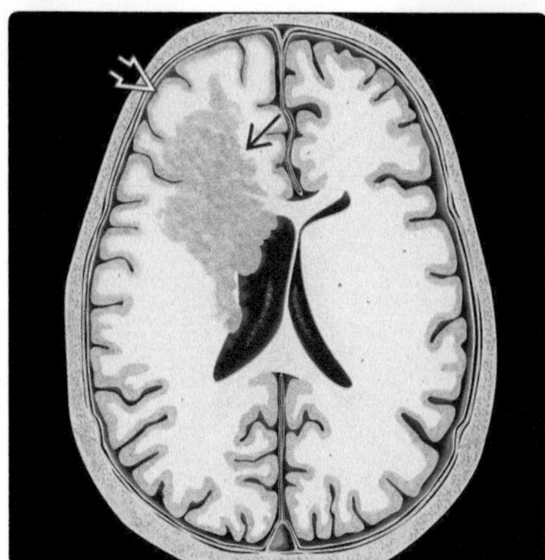

(37-11) Graphic depicts subcortical heterotopia. The large, focal, mass-like collection of gray matter ➡, thin overlying cortex ➡ are typical.

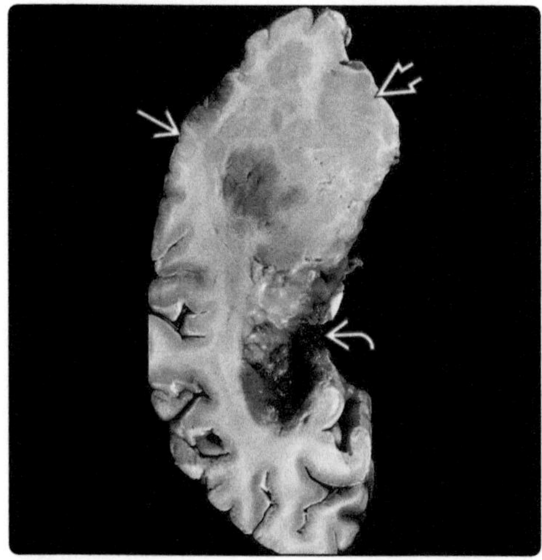

(37-12) Autopsy shows dysplastic lateral ventricle ➡, mass-like GM heterotopias ➡ under thin, polymicrogyric cortex ➡. (AFIP Archives.)

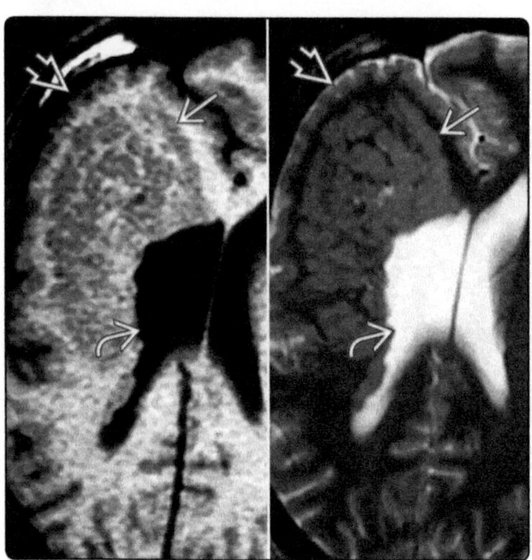

(37-13) T1 (L), T2 (R) show mass of heterotopic GM ➡, thin overlying cortex ➡, deformed underlying ventricle ➡ mimicking neoplasm.

folds (pachygyria) or a heterotopic layer of GM embedded in the WM below the cortex (subcortical band heterotopia).

In classic LIS (cLIS), the brain surface lacks normal sulcation and gyration. **cLIS** is also called **type 1 lissencephaly** or **four-layer lissencephaly** to differentiate it from cobblestone cortical malformation. Agyria is defined as a thick cortex with absence of surface gyri (**"complete" lissencephaly**).

True agyria with complete loss of all gyri is relatively uncommon. Most cases of cLIS show parietooccipital agyria with some areas of broad, flat gyri ("pachygyria") and shallow sulci along the inferior frontal and temporal lobes (**"incomplete" LIS**). **Subcortical band heterotopia** is also called **"double cortex" syndrome** and is the mildest form of cLIS.

Etiology

cLIS is caused by mutation in genes that regulate the outward migration of neuroblasts from the subependymal ventricular zone. Guided by radial glial fibers, postmitotic neuroblasts normally migrate outward to populate the cortical plate.

Pathology

In cLIS, the external surface of the brain shows a marked lack of gyri and sulci. In the most severe forms, the cerebral hemispheres are smooth with poor operculization and underdeveloped sylvian fissures. In cLIS, the normal six-layer cortex is replaced by a thick four-layer cortex. Coronal sections demonstrate a markedly thickened cerebral cortex with broad gyri and reduced volume of the underlying WM .

Clinical Issues

Patients with cLIS typically exhibit moderate to severe developmental delay, impaired neuromotor functions, variable mental retardation, and seizures. Patients with band heterotopia are almost always female.

Imaging

General Features. Imaging in patients with complete cLIS (agyria) shows a smooth, featureless brain surface with shallow sylvian fissures and large ventricles **(37-15)**. The cortex is thickened, and the WM is diminished in volume. The normal finger-like interdigitations between the cortical GM and subcortical WM are absent. In some cases, the cerebellum appears hypoplastic.

CT Findings. Axial NECT scans in cLIS show an "hourglass" or "figure-eight" appearance caused by the flat brain surface and shallow, wide sylvian fissures. A thick band of relatively well-delineated dense cortex surrounds a thinner, smooth band of WM.

CECT scans show prominent "primitive-appearing" veins running in the shallow sylvian fissures and coursing over the thickened cortices.

MR Findings

Classic Lissencephaly. In **cLIS**, T1 scans show a smooth cortical surface, a thick band of deep GM that is sharply demarcated from the underlying WM, and large ventricles **(37-15)**. T2 sequences are best to distinguish the separate cortical layers. A thin outer cellular layer that is isointense with GM covers a hyperintense "cell-sparse" layer. The WM layer is smooth and reduced in volume. A deeper, thick layer of arrested migrating neurons is common and may mimic band heterotopia. Callosal hypogenesis is common in cLIS.

Variant Lissencephaly. In **vLIS**, sulcation is reduced, and the cortex appears thick (although not as thick as in cLIS).

Band Heterotopia or "Double Cortex" Syndrome. In **band heterotopia**, a band of smooth GM is separated from a relatively thicker, more gyriform cortex by a layer of normal-appearing WM.

MR scans show a more normal gyral pattern with relatively thicker cortex. The distinguishing feature of band heterotopia is its "double cortex," a homogeneous layer of GM separated from the ventricles and cerebral cortex by layers of normal-appearing WM **(37-16)**.

Differential Diagnosis

Extremely premature brain is smooth at 24-26 gestational weeks and normally has a "lissencephalic" appearance. Full sulcation and gyration do not develop completely until ~ 40 weeks. **Pachygyria** is more localized, often multifocal, and usually asymmetric. In contrast to cLIS, the GM-WM junction along the thickened cortex is indistinct. **Cytomegalovirus**-associated LIS demonstrates periventricular calcifications.

LISSENCEPHALY SPECTRUM

Classic Lissencephaly (cLIS)
- Pathology: Thick, 4-layer cortex
  - Thin subpial layer
  - Thin outer cortex
  - "Cell-sparse" zone
  - Broad inner band of disorganized neurons
- Clinical issues
  - cLIS + severe facial anomalies = Miller-Dieker
- Imaging
  - Smooth, "hourglass" brain
  - Flat surface, shallow "open" sylvian fissures

Band Heterotopia ("Double Cortex")
- Clinical issues
  - Almost always in female patients
- Imaging: Looks like "double cortex"
  - Thin, gyriform cortex
  - Normal-appearing WM under cortex
  - Smooth inner band of GM
  - Normal-appearing periventricular WM

Differential Diagnosis
- Extremely premature brain
  - cLIS looks like 20- to 24-week fetal brain
- Microcephaly with simplified gyral pattern
  - Brain size ≥ 3 standard deviations below normal
- Cobblestone lissencephalies (type 2 LIS)
  - Associated with congenital muscular dystrophies
  - "Pebbly" (cobblestone) surface, not smooth
- Pachygyria
  - More localized, often multifocal
  - GM-WM interface indistinct
- Congenital cytomegalovirus
  - Often microcephalic
  - Smooth brain, periventricular Ca^{++}

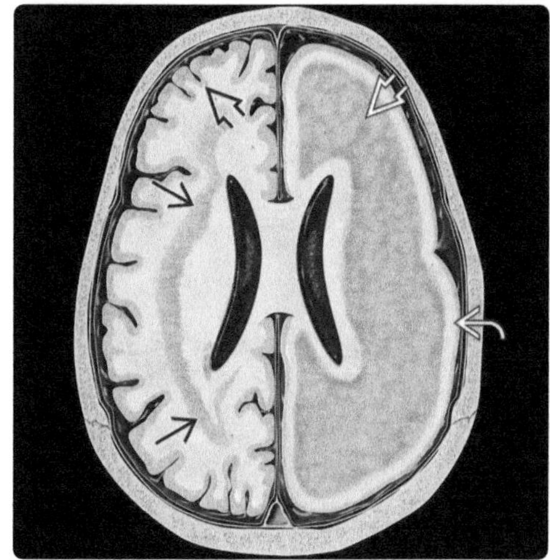

(37-14) *cLIS on L shows thick subcortical GM band ➡, thin cortex ➡. R = band heterotopia ("double cortex") ➡ with thin outer cortex ➡.*

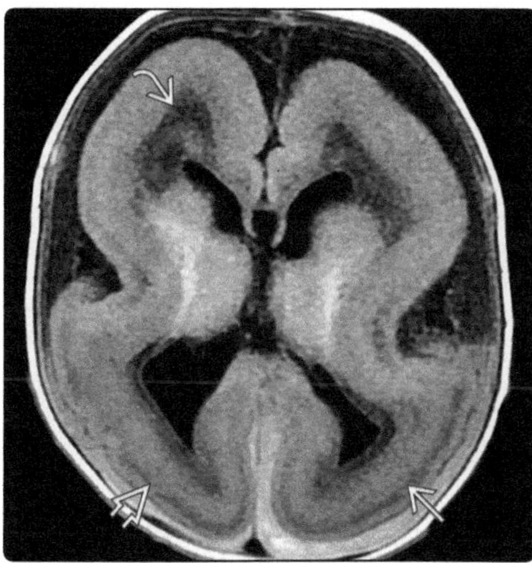

(37-15) *T1 MR of cLIS shows flat gyri, thick inner layers of GM ➡ separated by hypointense cell sparse layer ➡, reduced WM volume ➡.*

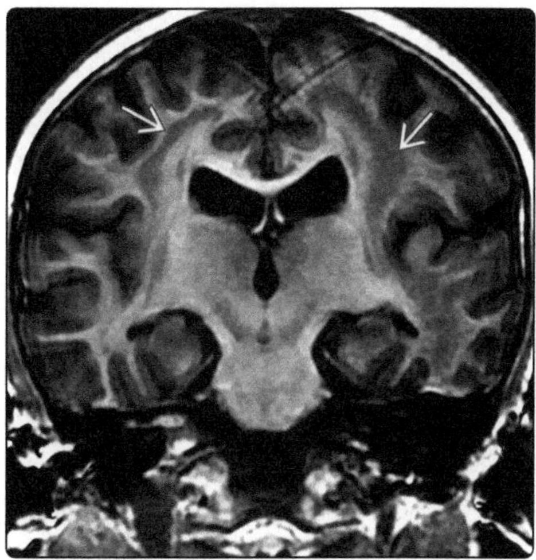

(37-16) *Coronal SPGR nicely demonstrates bilateral homogeneous-appearing bands of subcortical heterotopic gray matter ➡.*

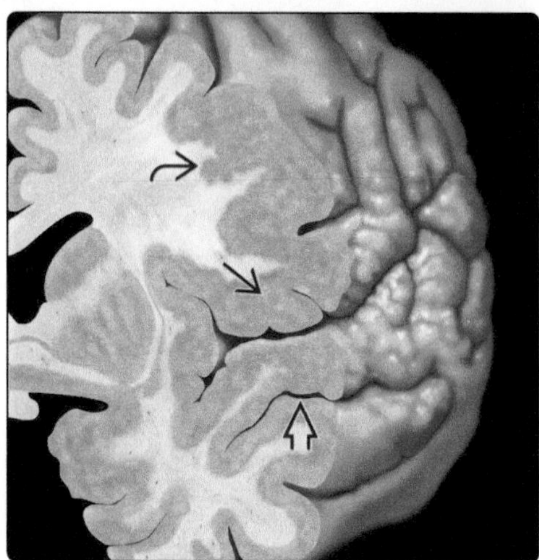

(37-17) Thick "pebbly" polymicrogyria in frontal ➡, temporal ➡ lobes. Note abnormal sulcation, irregular cortical-white matter interface ➡.

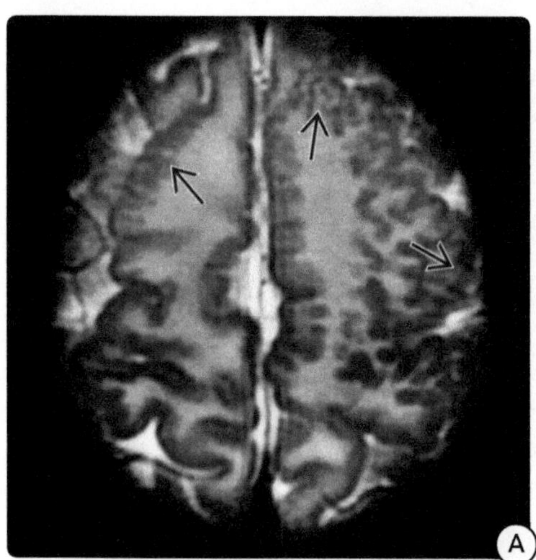

(37-18A) T2 MR in a 2-w/o infant shows multiple foci of polymicrogyria ➡. The left hemisphere is much more severely affected than the right.

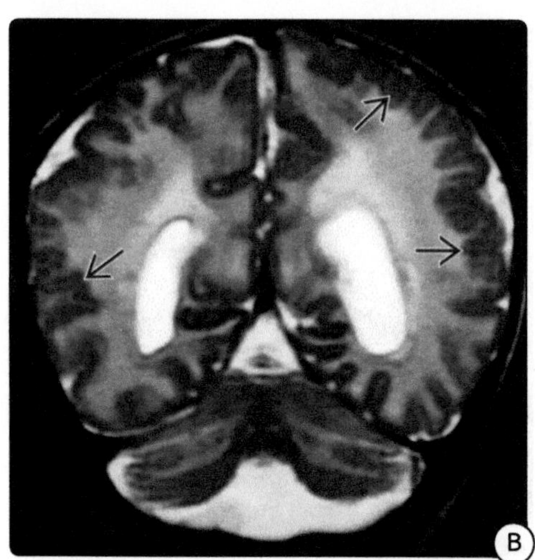

(37-18B) Coronal T2 MR shows polymicrogyria ➡. The appearance of multiple tiny nodules of gray matter piled on top of gyri is characteristic.

Malformations Secondary to Abnormal Postmigrational Development

The third major group of cortical malformations is secondary to abnormal postmigrational development and typically reflects infectious or ischemic insults. This group was formerly designated "abnormalities of cortical organization." It is currently divided into several subtypes of polymicrogyria (PMG) according to whether clefts (schizencephaly) are present and whether they occur as part of a recognized multiple malformation syndrome or an inherited metabolic disorder.

Polymicrogyria

The signature feature of PMG is an irregular cortex with numerous small convolutions and shallow or obliterated sulci. The appearance is that of tiny miniature gyri piled on top of other disorganized gyri **(37-17)**.

Etiology

Mutations in the tubulin genes are common. The phenotypic spectrum of *TUBA1A* mutations includes bilateral perisylvian PMG with dysmorphic basal ganglia, cerebellar vermis dysplasia, and pontine hypoplasia.

Encephaloclastic insults such as infection (e.g., TORCH, Zika virus infection), intrauterine vascular accident (e.g., middle cerebral artery occlusion), trauma, and metabolic disorders have also been implicated in the development of PMG.

Pathology

PMG can involve a single gyrus or most of an entire cerebral hemisphere. It can be uni- or bilateral, symmetric or asymmetric, and focal or diffuse.

Bilateral perisylvian PMG is the most common location (61% of cases). Generalized (13%), frontal (5%), and parasagittal parietooccipital (3%) sites are less common. Associated periventricular GM heterotopias are found in 11% of cases, and other anomalies, such as schizencephaly, are common.

Clinical Issues

PMG can present at any age. PMG is the most common imaging abnormality seen in infants with congenital cytomegalovirus infection. Symptoms depend on the location and extent of PMG, ranging from global developmental delay to focal neurologic deficit(s) and seizures.

Imaging

Multiplanar MR with high-resolution thin sections is required for complete delineation and detection of subtle lesions. Thickened or overfolded cortex with nodular surfaces and irregular "stippled" GM-WM interfaces are the most characteristic findings **(37-18)**. The basal ganglia often appear dysmorphic.

Differential Diagnosis

The major differential diagnosis of PMG is **type 2 lissencephaly** (cobblestone malformation). The absence of congenital muscular dystrophy and "Z-shaped" brainstem is a helpful clinical distinction.

Sometimes, **pachygyria** can be confused with PMG. The cortex in PMG is thin, nodular, and excessively folded. In **focal cortical dysplasia**, the GM is thickened, and the GM-WM interface is blurred.

In **schizencephaly**, the dysplastic cortex lining the cleft may appear "pebbled," but the cleft distinguishes it from PMG.

Schizencephaly

Schizencephaly (literally meaning "split brain") is a GM-lined cleft that extends from the ventricular ependyma to the pial surface of the cortex. The cleft spans the full thickness of the affected hemisphere **(37-19)**. Destructive vascular lesions (e.g., middle cerebral artery occlusion) and infections (e.g., TORCH) occurring before 28 fetal weeks are considered likely etiologies.

A schizencephalic brain exhibits a deep cleft that extends from its surface to the ventricle. The cleft is surrounded and lined by disorganized, dysmorphic-appearing GM. The "lips" of the cleft can be fused or closely apposed ("closed lip" schizencephaly) or appear widely separated ("open lip" schizencephaly). Clefts may be associated with a range of other macroscopic abnormalities involving the septi pellucidi, corpus callosum, optic chiasm, and hippocampus.

The key imaging features of schizencephaly are (1) a CSF-filled defect extending from the ventricle wall to the pial surface and (2) dysplastic GM lining the cleft.

Imaging studies typically show a focal V-shaped outpouching or "dimple" of CSF extending outward from the lateral ventricle **(37-20)**. The clefts can be uni- (60%) or bilateral (40%) with prominent ("open lip") or barely visible ("closed lip") **(37-20)**.

MR is more sensitive than CT, especially in delineating associated abnormalities, such as cortical dysplasia (polymicrogyria, pachygyria) and heterotopic GM. The cleft follows CSF signal intensity on all sequences **(37-21)**.

The differential diagnosis of CSF-filled brain defects includes both developmental and destructive lesions. The major differential diagnosis of schizencephaly is **porencephaly**. In porencephaly, the cleft is lined by gliotic WM, not dysplastic GM.

Transmantle **heterotopia** or deeply infolded **polymicrogyria** may be difficult to distinguish from schizencephaly with closed, nearly fused "lips." High-resolution T2WI or thin-section T1-weighted sequences with 3D reformatting and shaded surface displays are helpful in differentiating these entities. An **arachnoid cyst** displaces the adjacent cortex, which is otherwise normal in appearance.

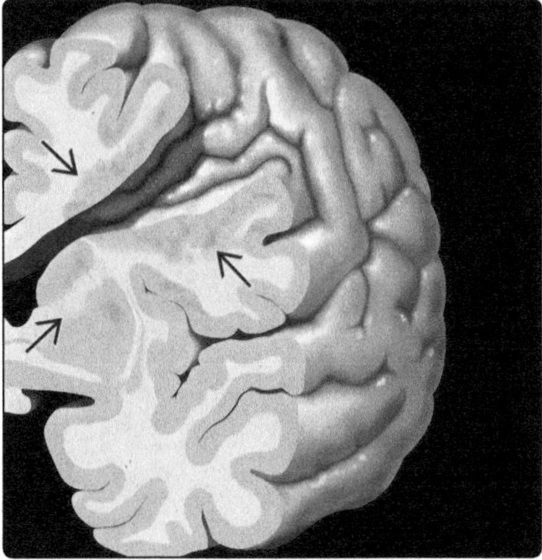

***(37-19)** "Open lip" schizencephaly is shown with irregular GM-WM interface of the cortex lining the cleft ➡, indicating its dysplastic nature.*

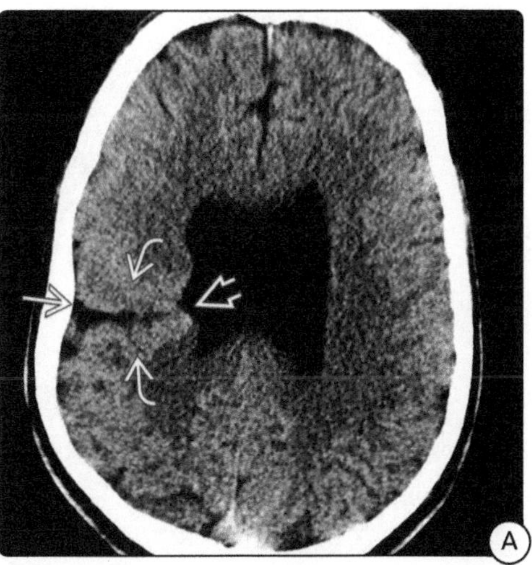

***(37-20A)** Unilateral schizencephaly is shown with outpouching of CSF from the lateral ventricle ➡. Cleft of CSF ➡ is lined with dysplastic GM ➡.*

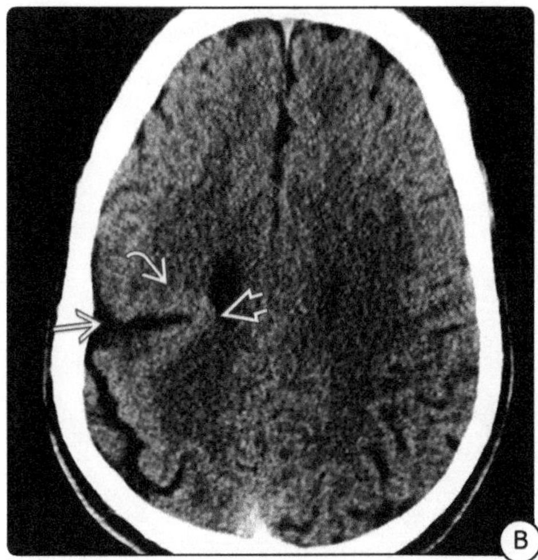

***(37-20B)** More cephalad scan shows cleft ➡ and dysplastic GM ➡ extending to ventricular ependyma ➡.*

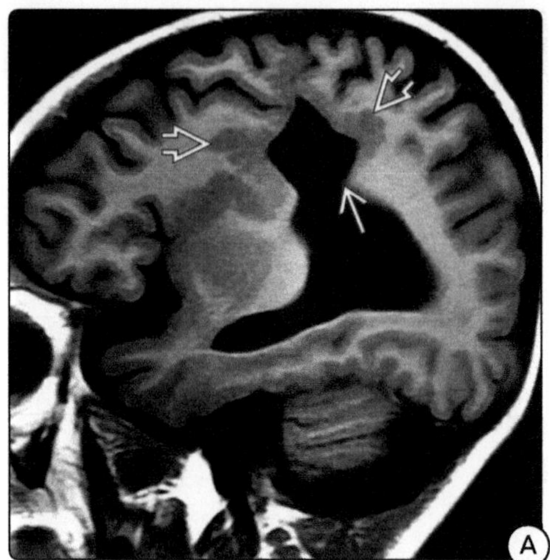

***(37-21A)** T1 MR shows CSF-filled cleft ➡ extending superiorly from lateral ventricle. Cleft is lined with dysplastic-appearing gray matter ⇨.*

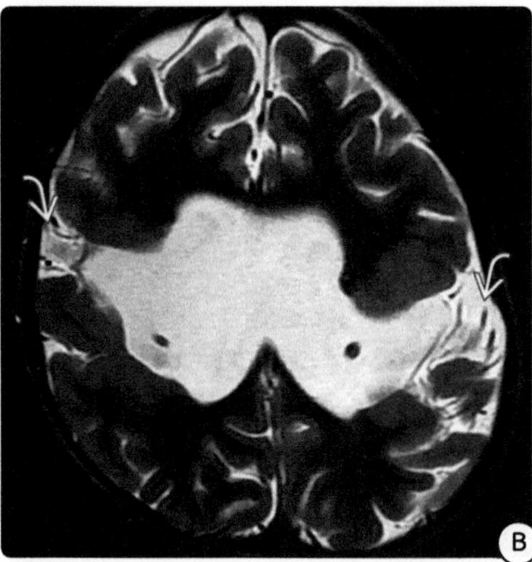

***(37-21B)** T2 MR shows open clefts with prominent "flow voids" ➡ from primitive cortical veins that commonly accompany schizencephaly.*

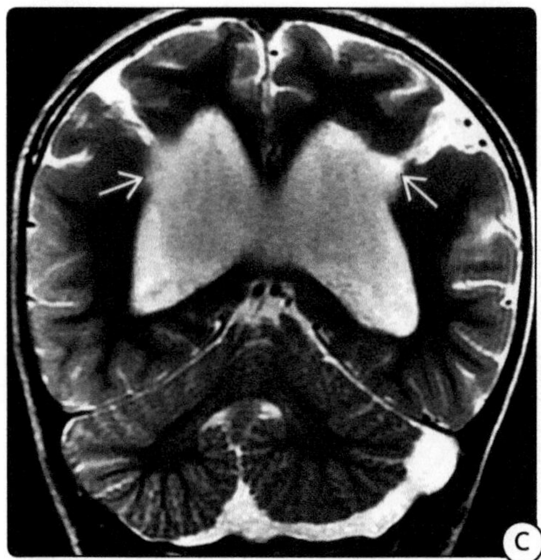

***(37-21C)** Coronal T2 MR shows the pointed "nipples" ➡ of CSF that extend outward from the ventricles into the schizencephalic clefts.*

POSTMIGRATION DISORDERS

Polymicrogyria
- Etiology
  - Inherited (tubulin gene mutations): Encephaloclastic
  - Acquired (infection, intrauterine vascular accident)
- Pathology
  - Irregular "pebbly" cortex
  - Can be uni- or bilateral
  - Symmetric or asymmetric
  - Focal or diffuse
  - Miniature gyri "piled on top of gyri"
- Imaging
  - Bilateral perisylvian most common location
  - Thickened cortex, nodular surfaces
  - Irregular GM-WM interfaces
- Differential diagnosis
  - Type 2 lissencephaly (no congenital muscular dystrophy, Z-shaped brainstem)

Schizencephaly
- Etiology
  - Encephaloclastic (TORCH, vascular accident)
- Pathology
  - Full-thickness CSF-containing cleft from ventricle to pia
  - CSF cleft can be closed, open
  - Uni- or bilateral
- Imaging
  - Look for "nipple" outpouching of CSF from ventricle
  - Cleft lined by dysmorphic GM
  - Follows cortex on all sequences
- Differential diagnosis
  - Transmantle heterotopic (no CSF cleft)

Selected References: The complete reference list is available on the Expert Consult™ eBook version included with purchase.

Holoprosencephalies, Related Disorders, and Mimics

Holoprosencephalies and variants such as syntelencephaly are classified as anomalies of ventral prosencephalon development. Other anomalies of the ventral prosencephalon include septo-optic dysplasia (with or without anomalies of the hypothalamic-pituitary axis) and arrhinencephaly, both of which are discussed in this chapter.

We conclude the chapter with a brief discussion of hydranencephaly, an in utero acquired destruction of the cerebral hemispheres that can sometimes be confused with alobar holoprosencephaly or severe "open lip" schizencephaly.

Holoprosencephaly

Holoprosencephaly (HPE) spans a continuum from alobar to lobar forms. Although each is delineated separately, keep in mind that the HPEs are really a spectrum with no clear boundaries that reliably distinguish one type from another.

Overview and Etiology

The fetal forebrain starts as a featureless, mostly fluid-filled sac. Outpouchings from the neural tube initially form a single central fluid-filled cavity ("monoventricle"). The fetal forebrain and monoventricle subsequently divide into the two cerebral hemispheres, also forming the definitive ventricles. Failure of this process leads to HPE. "Holoprosencephaly" literally means a single ("holo") ventricle involving the embryonic forebrain (prosencephalon).

HPE is divided into three subtypes based on severity, although HPE is a continuum that ranges from the most severe type (**alobar** HPE) to milder **lobar** forms. In the most severe forms, a central monoventricle is present and structures such as the basal ganglia are fused in the midline.

An intermediate type, **semilobar** HPE, is more severe than alobar HPE but not nearly as well differentiated as the lobar variety. The distinction between these three forms is based primarily on the presence or absence of a midline fissure separating the hemispheres.

Clinical Issues

HPE is the most common human forebrain malformation. Craniofacial malformations, such as cyclopia or single proboscis, hypotelorism, nasal anomalies, and facial clefts, occur in ~ 75-80% of cases. The statement "the face predicts the brain" means that the most severe facial defects generally are found with the most severe intracranial anomalies.

Nearly 3/4 of HPE patients have endocrinopathies. Pituitary insufficiency and congenital anosmia with absent CNI ("arrhinencephaly") are other common clinical features of HPE.

General Imaging Features

Imaging findings range from a pancake-like holosphere with central monoventricle (alobar HPE) to well-differentiated, almost completely separated hemispheres with minimal abnormalities (lobar HPE). The septum pellucidum is absent in all cases of HPE.

Alobar Holoprosencephaly

Terminology and Pathology

Alobar HPE (aHPE) is the most severe form of HPE. No midline fissure divides the brain into two separate cerebral hemispheres and no identifiable lobes are seen. The basal ganglia are fused. The falx and sagittal sinus are absent, as are the olfactory bulbs and tracts.

The brain configuration varies from flat ("pancake") to cup- or ball-shaped. The sylvian fissures are unformed, and the brain surface often appears completely agyric or minimally sulcated with shallow sulci and flat, disordered gyri **(38-1)**.

Cut sections demonstrate a single crescent-shaped monoventricle that opens dorsally into a large CSF-filled dorsal cyst.

***(38-1)** Autopsy of alobar holoprosencephaly (HPE) shows large dorsal cyst ⇨, fused thalami ➡, and rudimentary hemispheres ➡ with minimal sulcation and gyration. **(38-2)** NECT scan shows alobar HPE. Small rim of cortex ➡ surrounds "horseshoe" central monoventricle ➡. Thalami are fused ➡.*

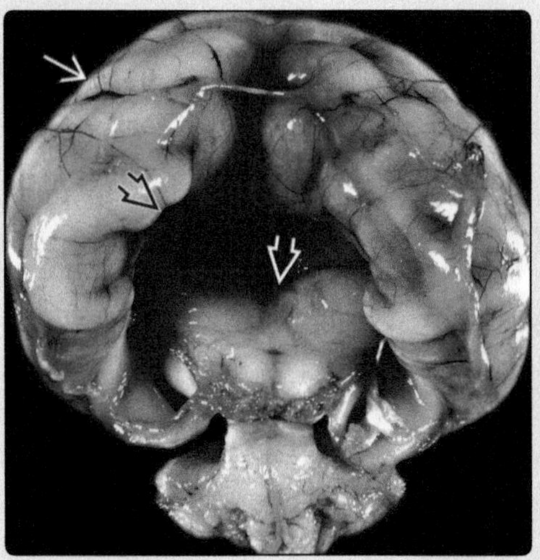

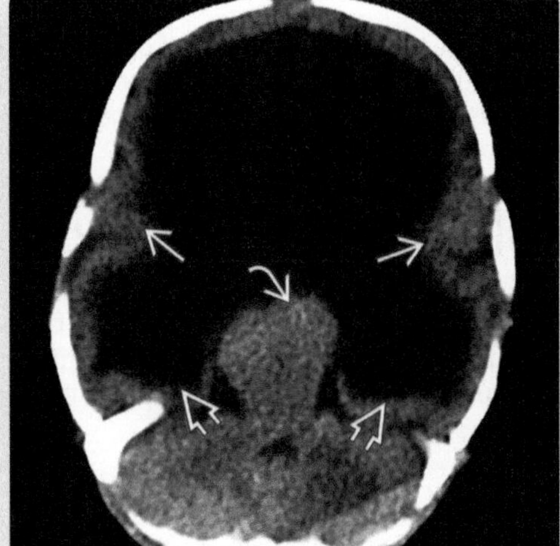

***(38-3)** Coronal autopsy of severe sHPE shows H-shaped central ventricle with primitive-appearing temporal horns ⇨, fused BG ➡, and rudimentary interhemispheric fissure ➡. (Courtesy R. Hewlett, MD.) **(38-4)** Axial T2 MR shows severe sHPE with rudimentary posterior interhemispheric fissure ➡, primitive ventricular horns ➡, and anterior midline fusion. Diffuse frontal migration arrest with subcortical heterotopic GM ➡ is also present.*

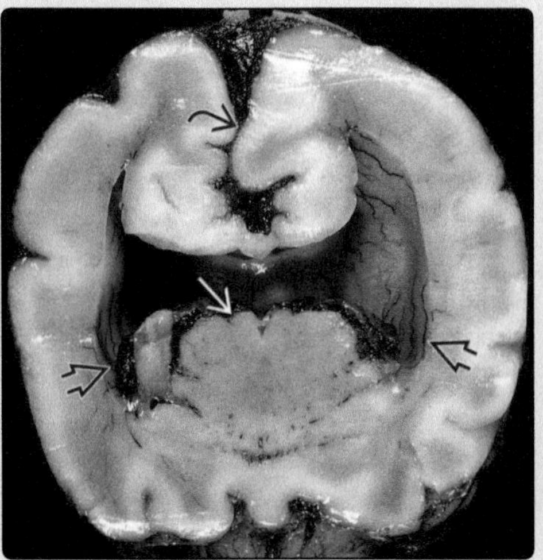

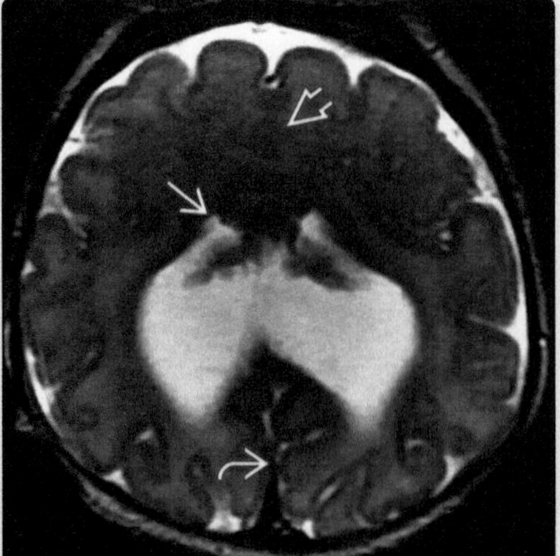

Clinical Issues

aHPE has a high intrauterine lethality and stillbirth rate. Prognosis in surviving infants is poor. At least 1/2 of all patients with aHPE die in < 5 months, and 80% die before 1 year of age.

Imaging

The cardinal feature of aHPE is a CSF-filled, horseshoe-shaped cavity **(38-2)** ("central monoventricle") that is often continuous posteriorly with a large dorsal cyst. Severe facial anomalies, such as cyclopia and proboscis, are common.

The septi pellucidi and third ventricle are absent, as are the falx cerebri and interhemispheric fissure. The brain is completely fused across the midline without evidence of an anterior interhemispheric fissure. The brain appears thin and almost agyric, although a few shallow sulci may be present. The basal ganglia are small and fused across the midline. There are no discernible commissures. Associated vascular anomalies, such as azygous anterior cerebral artery, are common.

Differential Diagnosis

The major differential diagnosis of aHPE is **hydranencephaly**. In hydranencephaly, the face is normal. A falx is present, but most of the cerebral tissue has been destroyed, usually by an intrauterine vascular accident or infection.

Semilobar Holoprosencephaly

Terminology and Pathology

Semilobar HPE (sHPE) is intermediate in severity between alobar HPE and lobar HPE. A gradation of findings is present. The most severe sHPE shows a rudimentary interhemispheric fissure and incomplete falx **(38-3)**. The temporal horns of the

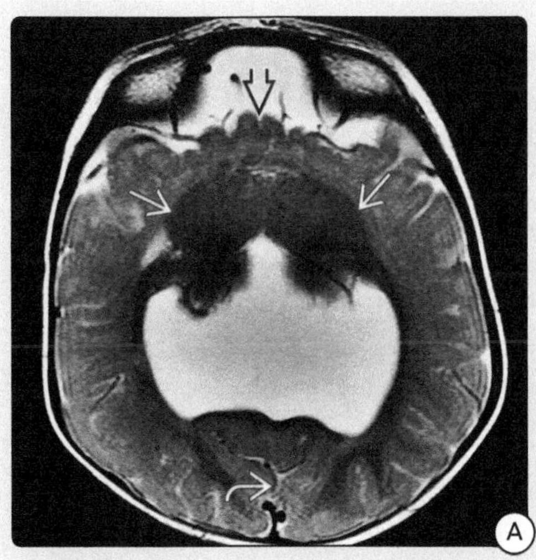

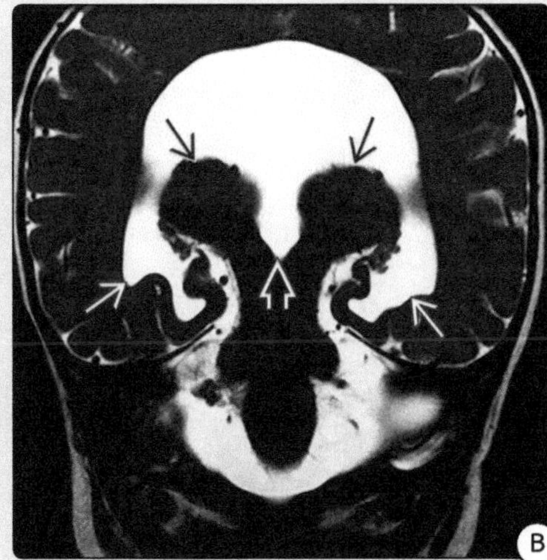

***(38-5A)** T2 MR in sHPE shows fused basal ganglia ➡, rudimentary posterior interhemispheric fissure ➡, and absence of anterior interhemispheric fissure with the brain fused across the midline ➡. **(38-5B)** Coronal T2 MR shows the monoventricle with rudimentary temporal horns ➡. A partially formed 3rd ventricle ➡ separates the thalami ➡. The interhemispheric fissure is absent.*

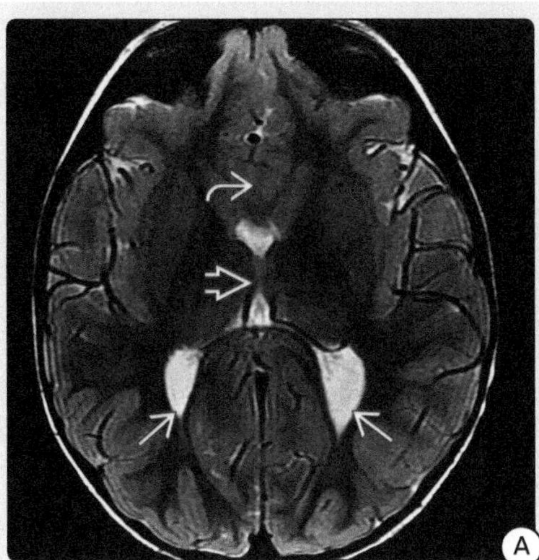

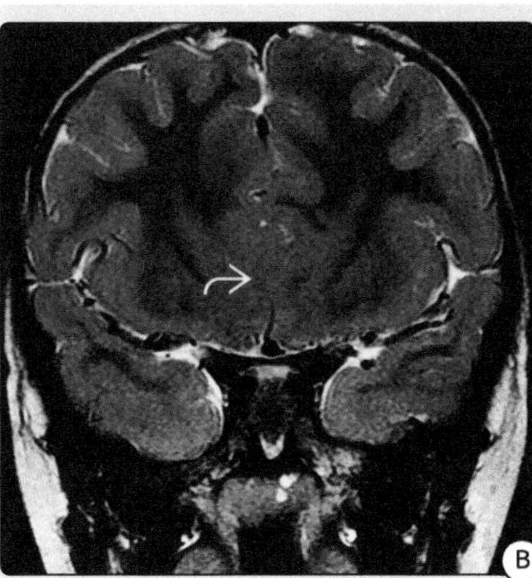

***(38-6A)** Axial T2 MR of lobar HPE shows well-developed occipital horns ➡, 3rd ventricle ➡, and minimal anterior midline fusion ➡. **(38-6B)** Coronal T2 MR shows that the anteroinferior frontal cortex is fused across the midline ➡.*

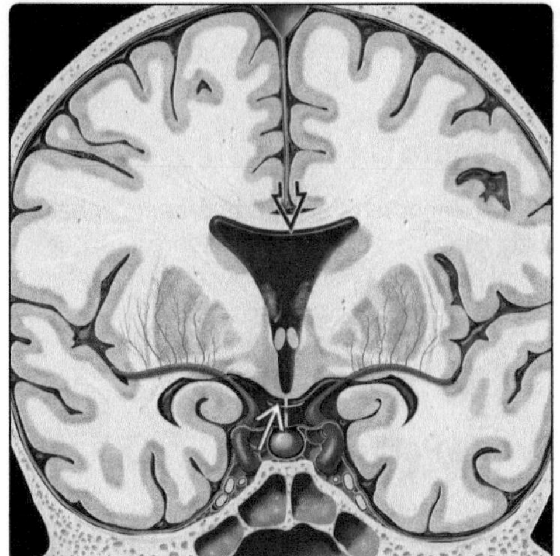

(38-7) Coronal graphic shows SOD with absent cavum septi pellucidi with flat-roofed anterior horns ⇒ and small optic chiasm ➡.

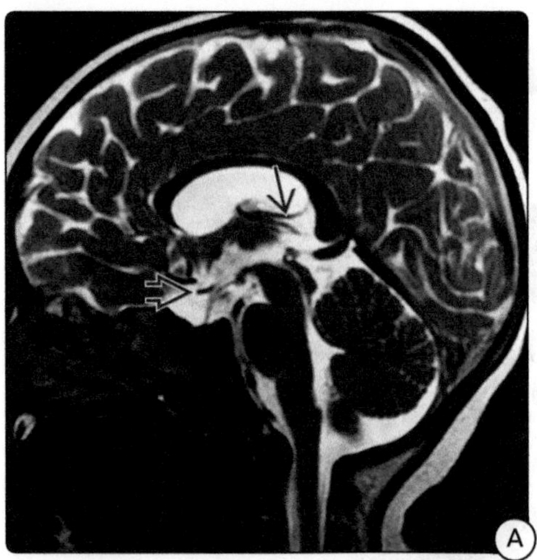

(38-8A) Sagittal T2 MR of SOD shows an empty-appearing lateral ventricle with low-lying fornix ➡. The optic chiasm ⇒ appears small.

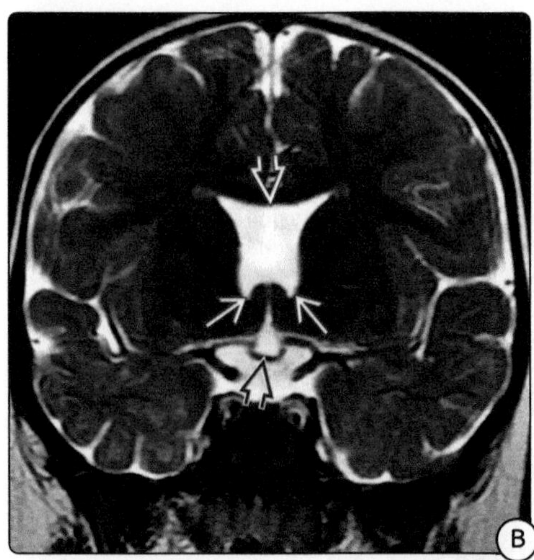

(38-8B) Coronal T2 MR shows hypoplastic optic chiasm ⇒, absent septi pellucidi ➡, and box-like or "squared-off" appearance of frontal horns ➡.

lateral ventricle may be partially formed, but the septi pellucidi are absent. A dorsal cyst is often present.

Imaging

With progressively better-differentiated sHPE, more of the interhemispheric fissure appears formed **(38-4)**. The deep nuclei exhibit various degrees of separation. If a rudimentary third ventricle is present, the thalami may be partially separated. The basal ganglia and hypothalami are still largely fused **(38-5)**. The caudate heads are continuous across the midline.

A corpus callosum splenium is present, but the body and genu are absent. Associated abnormalities include a dorsal cyst (present in 1/3 of cases) and vascular anomalies, such as azygous anterior cerebral artery and rudimentary deep veins.

Differential Diagnosis

The major differential diagnoses of sHPE are **alobar HPE and lobar HPE**, depending on the severity of the sHPE.

Lobar Holoprosencephaly

Terminology and Pathology

Lobar HPE is the best differentiated of the HPEs. The interhemispheric fissure and falx are clearly developed. The third ventricle and lateral ventricular horns are generally well formed, although the septi pellucidi are absent and the frontal horns almost always appear dysmorphic. The hippocampi are present but often more vertically oriented than normal.

Clinical Issues

Patients with lobar HPE are less severely affected compared with individuals with sHPE. Mild developmental delay, hypothalamic-pituitary dysfunction, and visual disturbances are the most common symptoms.

Imaging

In lobar HPE, the cerebral hemispheres—including the thalami and most of the basal ganglia—are mostly separated. At least some of the most rostral and ventral portions of the frontal lobes are continuous across the midline **(38-6)**. The anterior columns of the fornix are fused. The thalami and basal ganglia are separated, although the caudate heads may remain fused.

The frontal horns of the lateral ventricles are present but dysplastic-appearing. The temporal and occipital horns are better defined, and the third ventricle generally appears normal. There are no septi pellucidi.

The corpus callosum is present and can be normal, incomplete, or hypoplastic. The splenium and most of the body can usually be identified, although the genu and rostrum are often absent. In contrast to isolated or syndromic corpus callosum dysgenesis, there are no Probst bundles in any of the HPEs.

The walls of the hypothalamus remain unseparated, and the optic chiasm is often smaller than normal. The olfactory bulbs are present in well-differentiated lobar HPE. The pituitary gland can be flattened, hypoplastic, or ectopic. Associated vascular anomalies include an azygous anterior cerebral artery.

Differential Diagnosis

The major differential diagnosis of lobar HPE is **septo-optic dysplasia** (SOD). Some authors consider SOD the best differentiated of the HPE spectrum. In contrast to lobar HPE, the frontal horns are well formed in SOD. **Arrhinencephaly** may resemble lobar HPE, but the olfactory bulbs are usually present in lobar HPE.

In the rare **middle interhemispheric variant of HPE** (syntelencephaly), the corpus callosum genu and splenium are formed; however, the *body* is missing, and the posterior frontal lobes are continuous across the midline.

Related Midline Disorders

Septo-Optic Dysplasia

Terminology and Pathology

Some authors consider septo-optic dysplasia (SOD) simply a very well-differentiated form of lobar holoprosencephaly (HPE). Two cardinal pathologic features define SOD: (1) Absence of the septum pellucidum and (2) optic nerve hypoplasia **(38-7)**. There is no ventral midline fusion.

Clinical Issues

The most common clinical feature of SOD is visual impairment. Nearly 2/3 of SOD patients also develop endocrine abnormalities from hypothalamic-pituitary insufficiency (e.g., hypoglycemic seizures).

Imaging

Thin-section coronal T1- and T2-weighted images show absent or hypoplastic septi pellucidi. The frontal horns appear "squared-off" or box-like with distinct inferior pointing **(38-8B)**. The optic chiasm and one or both optic nerves appear small in most cases **(38-8)**. Sagittal images show that the septi pellucidi are absent and the fornices are low lying, giving the lateral ventricles an "empty" appearance **(38-8A)**. The optic nerves and chiasm are hypoplastic.

Isolated absence of the septi pellucidi is relatively rare, so look carefully for other anomalies like malformations of cortical development (e.g., heterotopias, schizencephaly, and polymicrogyria). Others exhibit a small pituitary gland with thin or absent stalk and an ectopic neurohypophysis. Olfactory tract/bulb hypoplasia and incomplete hippocampal rotation are common.

SEPTO-OPTIC DYSPLASIA: IMAGING

Imaging Findings
- Absent septum pellucidum
  - "Squared-off" frontal horns, pointed inferiorly on coronal T2WI
- Hypoplastic optic nerves, chiasm
- Look for
  - Malformations of cortical development
  - Thin stalk, small gland, ectopic posterior pituitary

Differential Diagnosis

The major differential diagnosis of SOD is well-differentiated **lobar HPE**. The cerebral hemispheres and basal ganglia are completely separated in SOD.

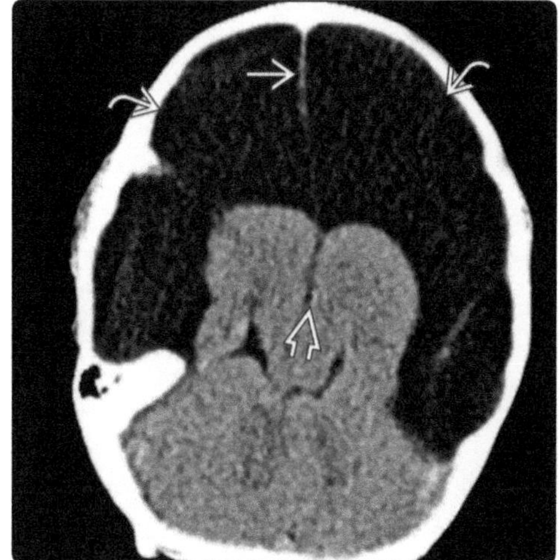

(38-9) *NECT of hydranencephaly shows basal ganglia/thalami are separated ➡, falx is present ➡. No brain is visible over CSF-filled cavities ➡.*

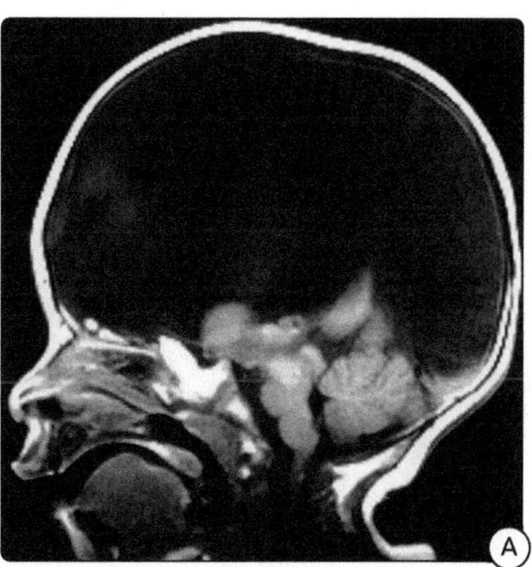

(38-10A) *T1 MR shows hydranencephaly with macrocephaly; CSF fills the supratentorial spaces. Brainstem and cerebellum are normal.*

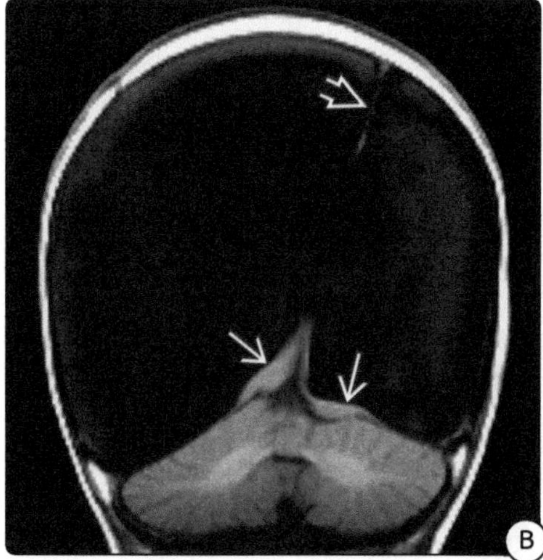

(38-10B) *Coronal T1 MR shows CSF-filled cranial vault & only tiny remnants of brain ➡. A falx is present ➡. (Courtesy A. Illner, MD.)*

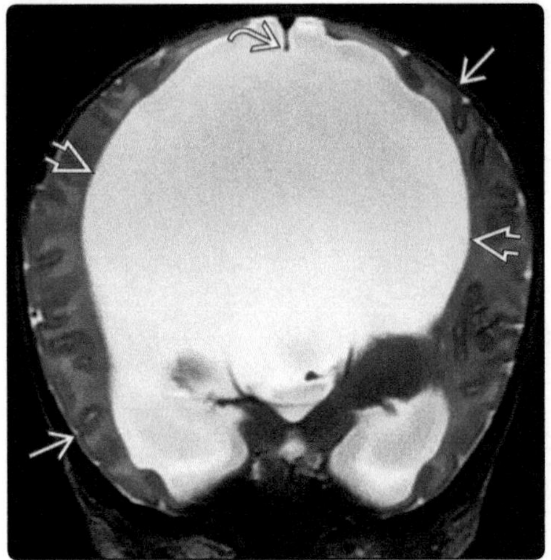

(38-11) Coronal T2 MR shows maximal obstructive hydrocephalus ➡, rim of compressed but normal brain ➡. Falx ➡ is present.

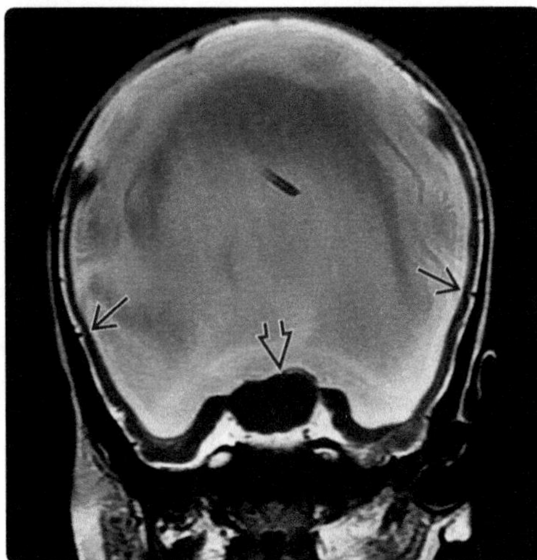

(38-12) T2 MR shows aHPE, horseshoe-shaped monoventricle, fused basal ganglia ➡, absent falx, thin dysplastic-appearing brain ➡.

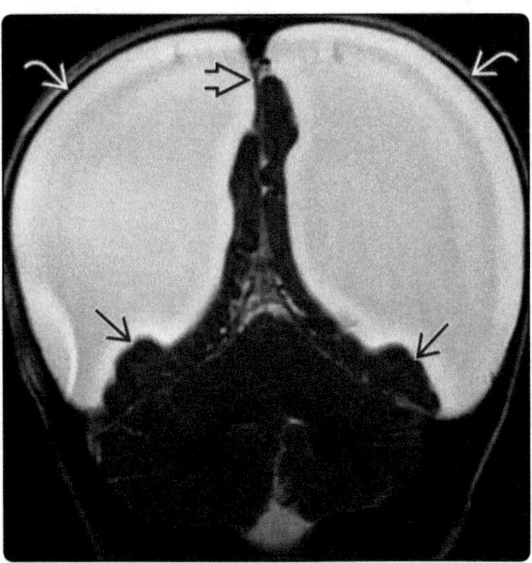

(38-13) Huge "open" lip schizencephaly with dysplastic brain lining clefts ➡, no cortex external to clefts ➡. Falx ➡ is present.

Holoprosencephaly Mimics

Hydranencephaly

Although some authors consider hydranencephaly a congenital malformation, it is actually the consequence of severe brain destruction in utero. It is important to recognize and distinguish hydranencephaly from other disorders, such as alobar holoprosencephaly or maximal hydrocephalus.

In hydranencephaly, the cerebral hemispheres are completely or almost completely missing. Instead, a membranous sac filled with CSF, glial tissue, and ependyma is present.

NECT scans show that CSF almost completely fills the supratentorial space. The falx cerebri is generally intact and appears to "float" in the water-filled cranial vault **(38-9)**. The basal ganglia are present and separated. Small remnants of the medial frontal and parietooccipital cortex can be present.

MR demonstrates a largely absent cerebral mantle **(38-10A)**. The falx is easily identified **(38-10B)**. The fluid-filled spaces follow CSF on all sequences, although some signal heterogeneity is often present secondary to CSF pulsations.

The most important differential diagnosis of hydranencephaly **(38-10)** is severe, "maximal" **obstructive hydrocephalus** (OH). In severe OH (e.g., secondary to aqueductal stenosis), a thin cortex can be seen compressed against the dura and inner table of the calvarium **(38-11)**.

In **alobar holoprosencephaly**, the falx and interhemispheric fissure are absent. The basal ganglia are fused **(38-12)**. Severe **bilateral "open lip" schizencephaly** has large transmantle CSF clefts that are lined with dysplastic-appearing cortex **(38-13)**. There is no cortex external to the huge open clefts. The falx and tentorium are normal.

DIFFERENTIAL DIAGNOSIS OF "WATER-BAG" BRAIN

"Maximal" Obstructive Hydrocephalus
- Large head
- Thinned but normal cortex
- Massively enlarged ventricles
  - Normal horns
- Falx present
- Basal ganglia separated

Alobar Holoprosencephaly
- Small head
- Smooth or minimally sulcated brain
- "Horseshoe" monoventricle
- Absent falx, interhemispheric fissure
- Basal ganglia fused

"Open Lip" Schizencephaly
- Remnant "nubbins" of brain
- No cortex external to huge "open" clefts
- Dysplastic cortex lines sides of open cleft
- Falx, interhemispheric fissure present
- Basal ganglia separated

Selected References: The complete reference list is available on the Expert Consult™ eBook version included with purchase.

Familial Cancer Predisposition Syndromes

***The term cancer predisposition syndrome** is used to describe familial cancers in which a clear mode of inheritance can be established. The 2016 WHO classifies these as **familial tumor syndromes**.*

The term **neurocutaneous syndromes** denotes a group of CNS disorders that are characterized by brain malformations or neoplasms and skin/eye lesions.

Most—but not all—neurocutaneous syndromes are inherited. Most—but not all—are associated with a distinct predilection to develop CNS neoplasms; these have also been called **inherited cancer syndromes**. Most—but again, not all—of these also have characteristic cutaneous lesions. Many—but not all—also have prominent visceral and connective tissue abnormalities.

In this chapter, we consider familial tumor syndromes that involve the nervous system, beginning with the neurofibromatoses. Major attention is also directed to tuberous sclerosis, von Hippel-Lindau disease, and Li-Fraumeni syndrome.

Neurofibromatosis

Although they are the most common CNS tumor predisposition syndromes, neurofibromatoses are multisystem disorders with both neoplastic and nonneoplastic manifestations. Two types of neurofibromatosis are widely recognized: Neurofibromatosis type 1 (NF1) and neurofibromatosis type 2 (NF2).

Neurofibromatosis Type 1

Etiology

Genetics. Neurofibromatosis type 1 (NF1) is an autosomal dominant disorder with variable expression, a high rate of new mutations, and virtually 100% penetrance by age 20.

NF1 is caused by mutation of the *NF1* gene on chromosome 17q11.2. Mutations inactivate the gene that encodes the tumor suppressor protein, **neurofibromin**. Neurofibromin also acts as a regulator of neural stem cell proliferation and differentiation; it is required for normal glial and neuronal development.

Approximately 1/2 of all NF1 cases are familial. Nearly 50% are sporadic ("de novo") and represent new mutations. NF1 patients already harboring a heterozygous germline *NF1* mutation develop neurofibromas upon somatic mutation of the second (wild-type) *NF1* allele.

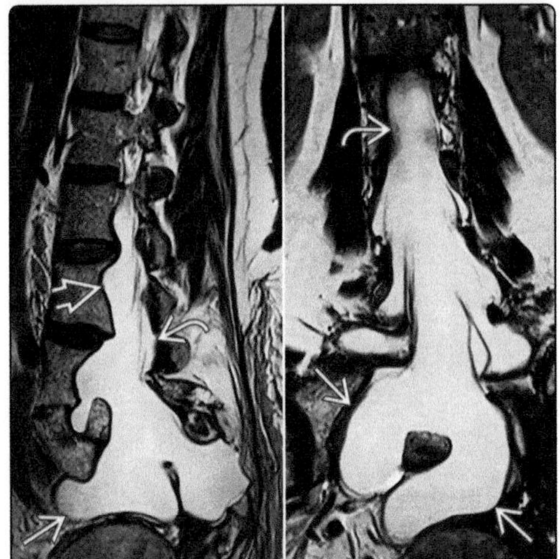

***(39-1)** Sagittal (L), coronal (R) T2 MRs show NF1 dural ectasia ➡ causing posterior vertebral scalloping ➡ and extensive meningoceles ➡.*

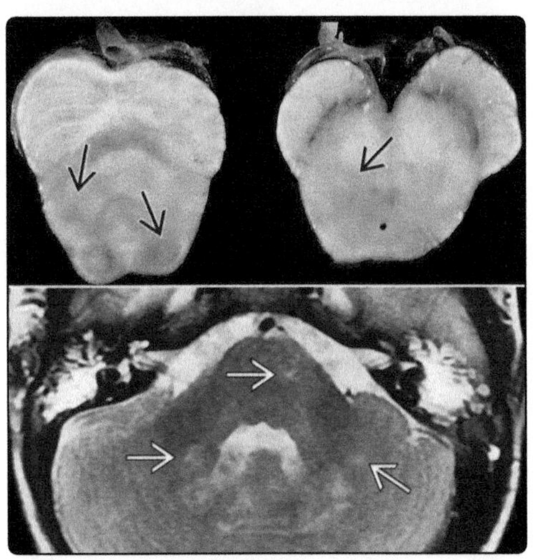

***(39-2)** (Top) Autopsied NF1 shows foci of discolored WM ➡ (AFIP). (Bottom) T2 MR shows hyperintense lesions ➡ in pons, cerebellum.*

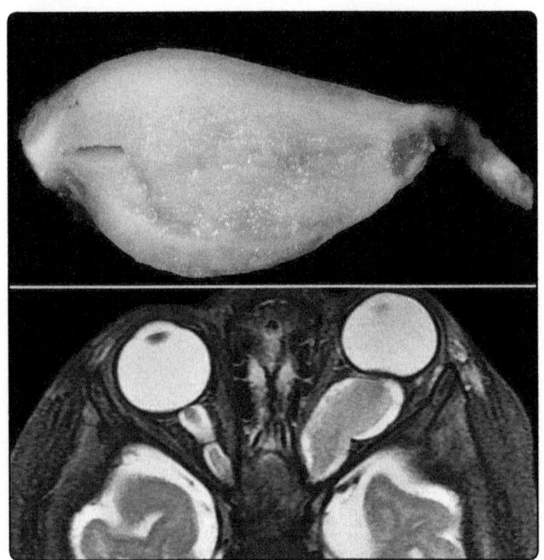

***(39-3)** Optic nerve glioma in NF1 (top), axial T2 MR (bottom) show fusiform enlargement of optic nerve. Nerve sheaths are partly patulous.*

Pathology

CNS lesions are found in 15-20% of patients. A variety of nonneoplastic lesions as well as benign and malignant tumors are associated with NF1. An increased risk of non-CNS malignancies also occurs in NF1 patients.

Nonneoplastic CNS Lesions. Multiple waxing and waning **dysplastic white matter (WM) lesions** on T2/FLAIR are commonly identified in patients with NF1. Histopathologically, these lesions represent zones of myelin vacuolization and dysgenesis, not hamartomas **(39-2)**. These lesions follow a benign course, initially waxing and then regressing by 20 years.

Dural ectasia may cause dilatation of the optic nerve sheaths, Meckel cave, or internal auditory canals. Arteriopathy occurs in at least 6% of cases. The most common manifestation is progressive intimal fibrosis of the supraclinoid internal carotid arteries, resulting in **moyamoya**.

CNS Neoplasms. CNS tumors occur in ~ 20% of individuals with NF1. Benign NF1-related neoplasms include neurofibromas. Malignant tumors include malignant peripheral nerve sheath tumors and gliomas.

Neurofibromas. A spectrum of NF1-associated neurofibromas occurs. **Dermal neurofibromas** arise within a peripheral nerve and appear as soft, well-circumscribed pedunculated or sessile lesions. Most patients develop more tumors as they age, and some have literally thousands of dermal neurofibromas. More than 95% of adults with NF1 have at least one lesion.

Plexiform neurofibromas (PNFs) are distinct from dermal neurofibromas and are virtually pathognomonic of NF1. PNFs develop in 30-50% of individuals with NF1.

PNFs are generally large bulky tumors usually associated with major nerve trunks and plexuses. PNFs are rope-like, diffusely infiltrating, noncircumscribed transspatial lesions that resemble a bag of worms **(39-5)**. The scalp and orbit are common sites for PNFs. Spinal neurofibromas and PNFs are found in ~ 40% of patients with NF1.

Malignant Peripheral Nerve Sheath Tumors. Although most PNFs remain benign, 10-15% become malignant. Individuals with NF1 have an 8-13% cumulative lifetime risk of developing a **malignant peripheral nerve sheath tumor** (MPNST) from a PNF. MPNST is an aggressive, deadly tumor with a high rate of metastases and poor overall prognosis.

Gliomas. The overwhelming majority of CNS neoplasms in NF1 are grade I **pilocytic astrocytomas** (PAs). Approximately 80% of NF1 PAs arise in the optic pathway, 15% occur in the brainstem, and 5% occur in other regions.

Optic pathway gliomas (OPGs) occur in 15-20% of patients with NF1 and can be uni- or bilateral **(39-4)**. Any part of the optic pathway can be involved. Some OPGs affect just the optic nerve, whereas others involve the optic chiasm and optic tracts.

NF1-associated gliomas of the medulla, tectum, and pons are typically indolent neoplasms. Approximately 20% are malignant (WHO grades II-IV). These include **diffusely infiltrating ("low-grade") fibrillary astrocytoma, anaplastic astrocytoma**, and **glioblastoma**.

Non-CNS Neoplasms. NF1 is associated with an increased risk of leukemia (especially juvenile myelomonocytic leukemia and myelodysplastic syndromes), gastrointestinal stromal tumors (6%), and adrenal or extraadrenal pheochromocytoma (0.1-5.0%).

NF1-ASSOCIATED NEOPLASMS

Common
- Dermal neurofibromas (95% of adults)
- Plexiform neurofibromas (PNFs) (30-50%)
- Spinal neurofibromas

Less Common
- Pilocytic astrocytoma (80% of gliomas)
  - 80% in optic pathway (15-20% of NF1 patients)
  - 15% in brainstem
  - 5% in other locations (cerebellum, cerebral hemispheres)
- Other astrocytomas (20%)
  - Diffusely infiltrating fibrillary astrocytoma (WHO grade II)
  - Anaplastic astrocytoma (WHO grade III)
  - Glioblastoma (WHO grade IV)

Rare but Important
- Malignant peripheral nerve sheath tumor
  - Develops in 8-13% of PNFs
- Juvenile chronic myeloid leukemia
- Gastrointestinal stromal tumor
- Pheochromocytoma

Clinical Issues

Presentation. NF1 is one of the most common CNS single-gene disorders, affecting 1:3,000 live births.

Characteristic features include cutaneous neurofibromas (present in almost all adults with NF1), hyperpigmentary skin abnormalities with café au lait macules (95%), inguinal/axillary freckling (65-85%), and iris hamartomas or Lisch nodules. Funduscopic examination using near-infrared reflectance demonstrates bright patchy choroidal nodules in 70% of pediatric patients and 80% of adults.

Other less common NF1-associated features include distinctive skeletal abnormalities, such as sphenoid dysplasia (3-11%), long bone deformities (1-4%), pseudarthroses, and progressive kyphoscoliosis. Cardiovascular anomalies occur in ~ 25% of individuals with NF1. Conotruncal cardiac defects, pulmonary valvular stenosis, and arterial hyperplasia are typical anomalies.

Clinical Diagnosis. Molecular diagnostic testing distinguishes NF1 from other disorders that share similar phenotypic features. With the exception of PNF, most clinical stigmata of NF1 also occur in other disorders (e.g., multiple café au lait macules in McCune-Albright syndrome). Consensus criteria for the clinical diagnosis of NF1 are summarized in the next box.

Natural History. Prognosis in NF1 is variable and relates to its specific manifestations. Increased mortality is related to MPNST, glioma, and cardiovascular disease.

The foci of myelin vacuolization increase in number and size over the first decade, then regress, and eventually disappear. They are rarely identified in adults.

Imaging

Nonneoplastic CNS Lesions. Bone dysplasias occur in the skull, spine, and long bones (e.g., pseudarthroses). NECT scans may demonstrate a hypoplastic sphenoid wing and enlarged middle cranial fossa, with or without an associated arachnoid cyst. Protrusion of the anterior temporal

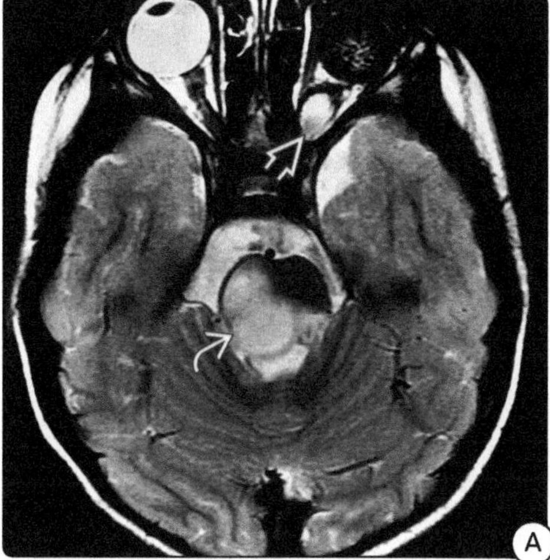

***(39-4A)** T2 MR in NF1 shows enlarged hyperintense left optic nerve ➡, hyperintense mass ➡ in the pons.*

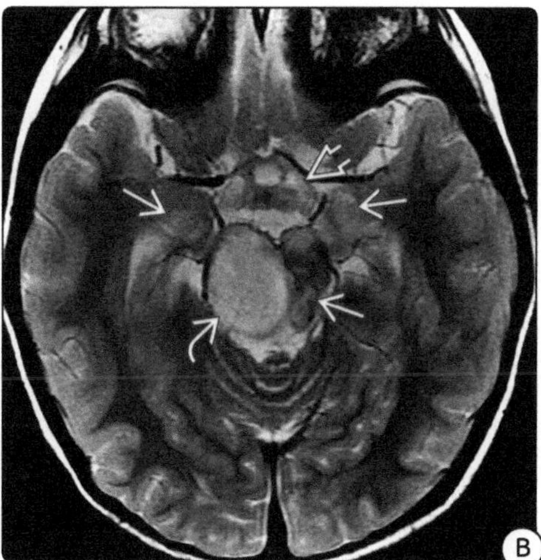

***(39-4B)** Note enlarged optic chiasm ➡, midbrain mass ➡, FASIs are in both medial temporal lobes and the left midbrain ➡.*

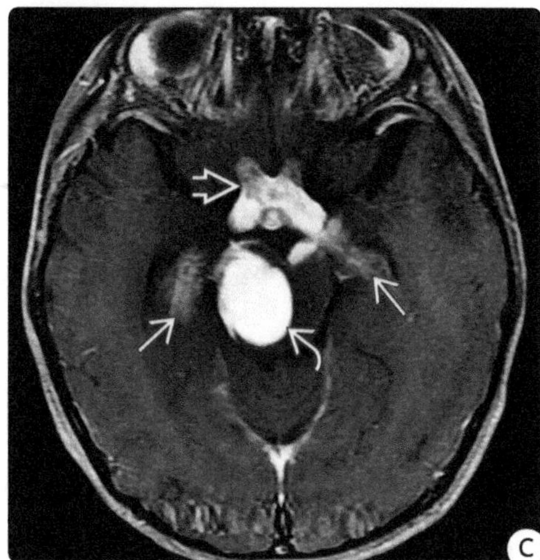

***(39-4C)** T1 C+ FS MR shows intense enhancement in the enlarged optic chiasm ➡, medial temporal lobes ➡, and midbrain ➡. OPG.*

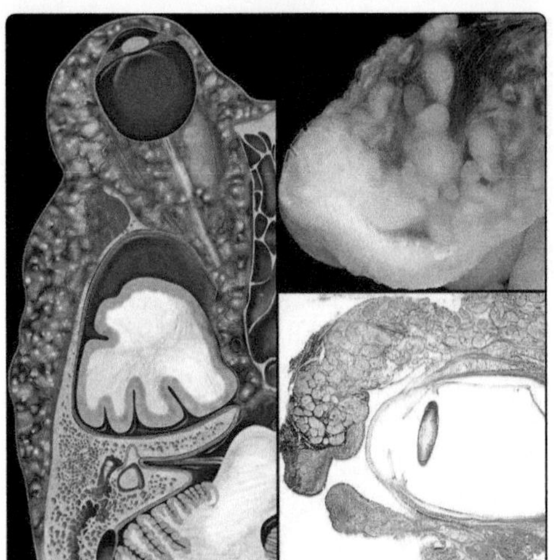

(39-5) *Graphic (L), surgical specimens (AFIP Archives) (R) show typical plexiform neurofibroma of orbit, eyelid, and scalp.*

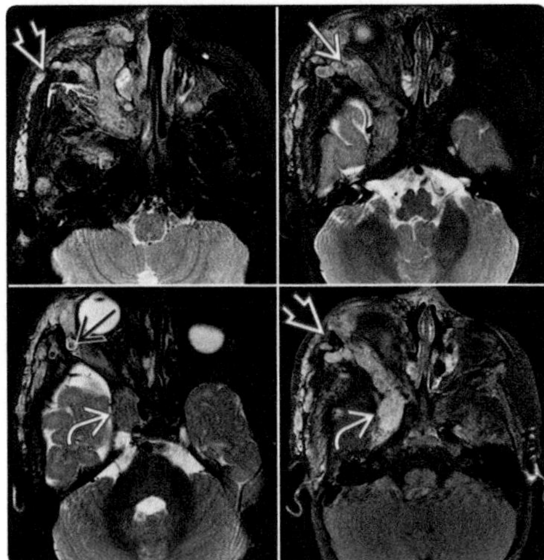

(39-6) *Plexiform neurofibroma infiltrates orbit ➡, masticator space ➡, cavernous sinus ➡. This is a typical target appearance ➡.*

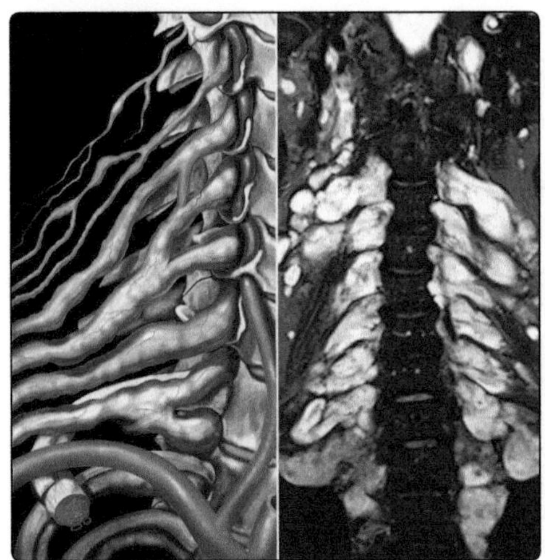

(39-7) *Plexiform neurofibroma involving cervical nerve roots is depicted in the graphic (L) and on a coronal STIR scan (R).*

lobe may result in ipsilateral proptosis. The globe is frequently enlarged ("buphthalmos"), and a plexiform neurofibroma is often present **(39-5)**.

Dural dysplasia with patulous spinal dura as well as enlarged optic nerve sheaths, internal auditory canals, and Meckel caves can occur.

Dysplastic WM lesions (often termed "FASIs" for **f**oci of **a**bnormal **s**ignal **i**ntensity) are seen as multifocal hyperintensities on T2/FLAIR imaging. These foci represent zones of myelin vacuolization and are seen in 70% of children with NF1. They generally increase in size and number until ~ 10 years of age but then wane and disappear **(39-4)**.

The most common sites are the globi pallidi (GP), centrum semiovale, cerebellar WM, dentate nuclei, thalamus, and brainstem **(39-2)**. Most are smaller than 2 cm in diameter. Most FASIs are iso- or minimally hypointense on T1WI, although GP lesions are often mildly hyperintense. FASIs do not enhance following contrast administration.

Relentless endothelial hyperplasia can cause progressive stenosis of the intracranial internal carotid arteries, resulting in a **moyamoya** pattern. Careful scrutiny of the intracranial vasculature demonstrates attenuation of the middle cerebral artery "flow voids."

CNS Neoplasms

Neurofibromas. Patients with **cutaneous neurofibromas** often demonstrate solitary or multifocal discrete round or ovoid scalp lesions that are hypointense to brain on T1WI and hyperintense on T2WI. A target sign with a hyperintense rim and relatively hypointense center is common. Strong but heterogeneous enhancement following contrast administration is typical.

PNFs are most common in the orbit, where they are seen as poorly marginated serpentine masses that infiltrate the orbit, extraocular muscles, and eyelids **(39-6)**. They often extend inferiorly into the pterygopalatine fossa and buccal spaces as well as superiorly into the adjacent scalp and masticator spaces. PNFs enhance strongly and resemble a "bag of worms."

Malignant Peripheral Nerve Sheath Tumors. **MPNSTs** arising within a PNF can be difficult to detect and to differentiate from the parent tumor. MPNSTs tend to be more heterogeneous in signal intensity, often exhibiting intratumoral cysts, perilesional edema, and peripheral enhancement.

Gliomas. The most common NF1-associated glioma is **pilocytic astrocytoma**. Optic pathway glioma (OPG) is the most frequent type and occurs as a diffuse, fusiform, or bulbous enlargement of one or both optic nerves **(39-3)**. Tumor may extend posteriorly into the optic chiasm, superiorly into the hypothalamus, and involve the optic tracts and lateral geniculate bodies. Extensive lesions can reach the cerebral peduncles and brainstem **(39-4)**.

Most OPGs are isointense with brain on T1WI and iso- to moderately hyperintense on T2WI. Enhancement on T1 C+ FS scans varies from none to striking.

NF1-associated **low-grade fibrillary astrocytomas** can be difficult to distinguish from FASIs. They are usually moderately hypointense on T1WI and hyperintense on T2WI and show progression on follow-up imaging.

Anaplastic astrocytoma and **glioblastoma multiforme** are more aggressive, more heterogeneous tumors that demonstrate relentless progression. A progressively enlarging mass that enhances following contrast administration in a child with NF1 should raise suspicion of malignant neoplasm.

NF1: IMAGING

Scalp/Skull, Meninges, and Orbit
- Dermal neurofibromas
  - Solitary/multifocal scalp nodules
  - Increases with age
  - Localized, well circumscribed
- Plexiform neurofibroma
  - Pathognomonic of NF1 (30-50% of cases)
  - Large, bulky infiltrative transspatial lesions
  - Scalp, face/neck, spine
  - Orbit lesions may extend into cavernous sinus
- Sphenoid wing dysplasia
  - Hypoplasia → enlarged orbital fissure
  - Enlarged middle fossa ± arachnoid cyst
  - Temporal lobe may protrude into orbit
- Dural ectasia
  - Tortuous optic nerve sheath
  - Patulous Meckel caves
  - Enlarged IACs

Brain
- Hyperintense T2/FLAIR WM foci
  - Wax in 1st decade, then wane
  - Rare in adults
- Astrocytomas
  - Most common: Pilocytic
  - Optic pathway, hypothalamus > brainstem
  - Malignant astrocytoma (anaplastic astrocytoma, glioblastoma multiforme) less common

Arteries
- Progressive ICA stenosis → moyamoya
- Fusiform ectasias, arteriovenous fistulas
  - Vertebral > carotid

Differential Diagnosis

In combination with appropriate clinical findings, the presence of FASIs on MR with or without OPG is diagnostic of NF1. Unusually large FASIs can cause mass effect and mimic **neoplasm** (i.e., pilocytic astrocytoma, diffuse astrocytoma). While FASIs and astrocytomas are both part of the NF1 spectrum, FASIs typically do not enhance.

Neurofibromatosis Type 2

Neurofibromatosis type 2 (NF2) is a distinct syndrome with totally different mutations, clinical features, and imaging findings. Neurofibromas characterize NF1 and are composed of Schwann cells plus fibroblasts. Schwannomas—especially bilateral vestibular schwannomas—are the major feature of NF2. Schwannomas contain only Schwann cells.

The associated neoplasms are also different from those in NF1. Astrocytomas are found in NF1, whereas ependymomas and meningiomas are the predominant tumors in NF2.

Etiology

General Concepts. Like NF1, NF2 is an autosomal dominant disorder. About 1/2 of all cases occur in individuals with no family history of NF2 and are caused by newly acquired germline mutations.

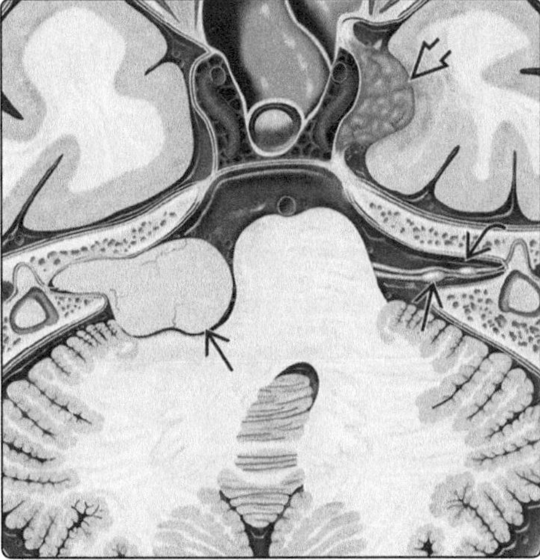

***(39-8)** Graphic depicts classic NF2 with bilateral vestibular schwannomas ⇒, facial schwannoma ⇒, and cavernous sinus meningioma ⇒.*

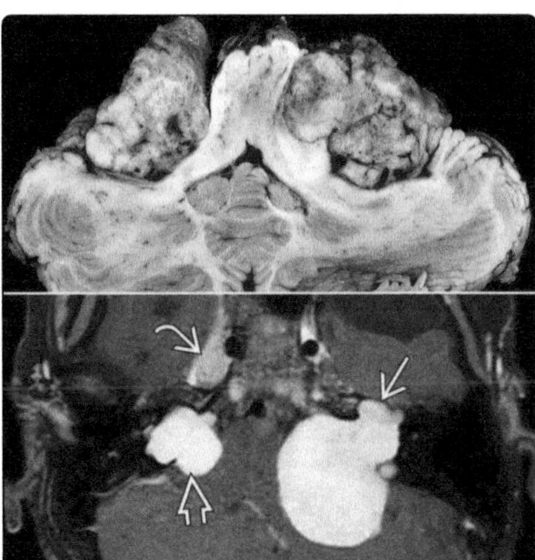

***(39-9)** (Top) Bilateral VSs in NF2. (A. Ersen, MD.) (Bottom) T1 C+ shows bilateral vestibular ⇒, facial ⇒, and right CNV ⇒ schwannomas.*

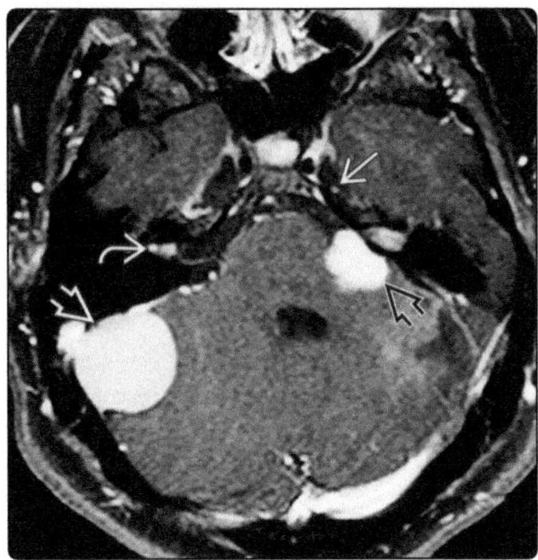

***(39-10)** T1 C+ FS MR shows large left ⇒, small right VSs ⇒, tiny CNV schwannoma in Meckel cave ⇒, right CPA meningioma ⇒. NF2.*

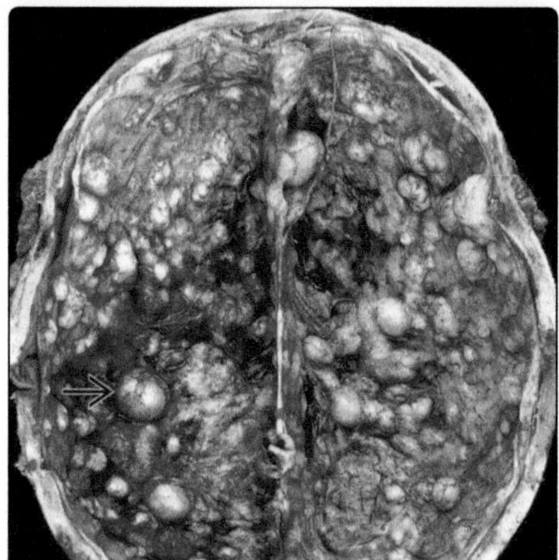

(39-11) Autopsy specimen demonstrates innumerable small meningiomas ➩, a common finding in NF2. (From DP: Neuropathology, 2e.)

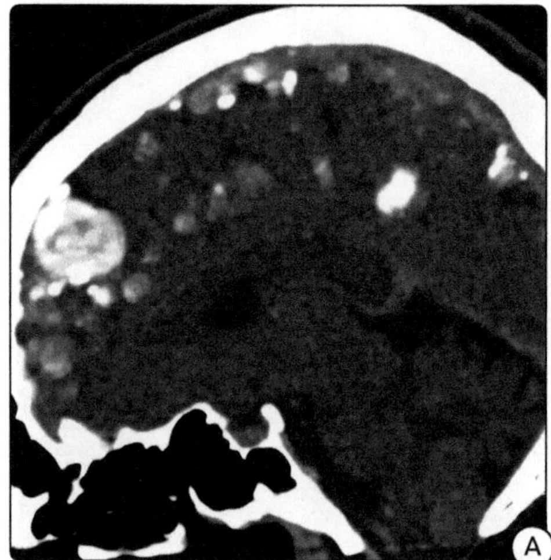

(39-12A) NECT shows hyperdense calcified masses that abut the dura and falx characteristic of NF2-associated meningiomatosis.

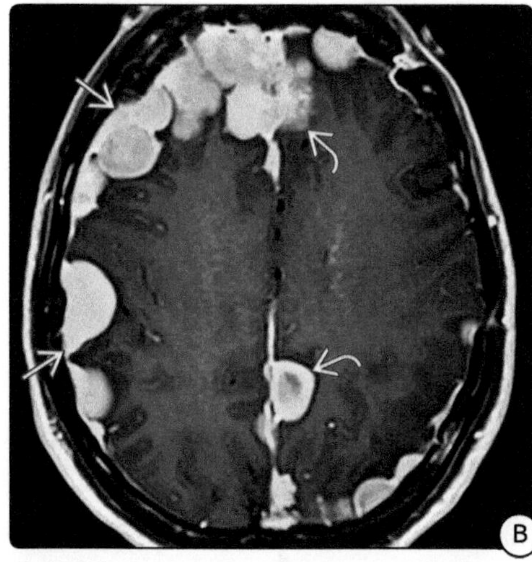

(39-12B) T1 C+ FS MR in the same case shows multiple meningiomas along the convexity ➡, falx ➢.

Genetics. NF2 is caused by mutations of the *NF2* gene on chromosome 22q12.2. The *NF2* gene encodes the protein merlin, which functions as a tumor suppressor gene. Inactivating *NF2* mutations cause predominantly benign neoplasms (schwannomas and meningiomas).
Biallelic *NF2* inactivation is also detected in the majority of sporadic meningiomas and nearly all schwannomas.

Pathology

Location. The most common NF2-related schwannomas are vestibular schwannomas (VSs) **(39-8)**. Approximately 50% of patients also have nonvestibular schwannomas (NVSs). The most common locations for NVSs are the trigeminal and oculomotor nerves. Trochlear and lower cranial nerve schwannomas occur but are rare.

Meningiomas occur in ~ 1/2 of all patients with NF2 and can be found anywhere in the skull and spine. The most frequent sites are along the falx and cerebral convexities.

Intracranial ependymomas are rare in NF2. Most are found in the spinal cord, especially within the cervical cord or at the cervicomedullary junction.

Size and Number. NF2-related schwannomas, meningiomas, and ependymomas are often multiple. The presence of bilateral VSs is pathognomonic of NF2 **(39-9)**.

Size varies from tiny to several centimeters. Innumerable tiny schwannomas ("tumorlets") throughout the cauda equina are seen in the majority of patients. Intramedullary ependymomas are often small; multiple tumors are present in nearly 60% of patients.

Gross Pathology. NF2 is characterized by multiple schwannomas, meningiomas, and ependymomas. Virtually all patients have bilateral VSs, the hallmark of NF2 **(39-9)**. Most schwannomas are well-delineated round or ovoid encapsulated masses that are attached to—but do not infiltrate—their parent nerves.

Multiple meningiomas are the second pathologic hallmark of NF2 **(39-11)**. They are found in ~ 50% of patients and may be the presenting feature (especially in children). Meningiomas appear as unencapsulated but sharply demarcated masses.

Microscopic Features. Schwannomas are composed of neoplastic Schwann cells. Areas of alternating high and low cellularity (Antoni A pattern) are admixed with foci that exhibit microcysts and myxoid changes (Antoni B pattern).

Staging, Grading, and Classification. NF2-associated schwannomas are WHO grade I tumors. Most NF2-associated meningiomas are also WHO grade I neoplasms. NF2-associated ependymomas—especially those in the spinal cord—are generally indolent and carry a favorable prognosis.

Clinical Issues

Presentation. NF2 is much less common than NF1. However, individuals with NF2 generally do not become symptomatic until the second to fourth decades; less than 20% of patients with NF2 present under the age of 15. Progressive sensorineural hearing loss, tinnitus, and difficulties with balance are typical. Other common symptoms include facial pain &/or paralysis, vertigo, and seizures.

Many NF2-related meningiomas are asymptomatic and discovered incidentally on imaging. Spinal cord ependymomas are asymptomatic in 75% of patients.

Clinical Diagnosis. The definitive diagnosis of NF2 is established genetically. Consensus criteria have been developed for the clinical diagnosis and are summarized in the box below.

NF2: DIAGNOSTIC CLINICAL FEATURES

Definite NF2

- Bilateral vestibular schwannomas (VSs)
- 1st-degree relative with NF2 *and* unilateral VS diagnosed before 30 years of age
- *Or* 1st-degree relative with NF2 *and* 2 of the following
  - Meningioma
  - Glioma
  - Schwannoma
  - Juvenile posterior subcapsular lenticular opacities or cataracts

Probable NF2

- Unilateral VS diagnosed < 30 years of age *and* 1 of the following
  - Meningioma
  - Glioma
  - Schwannoma
  - Juvenile posterior subcapsular lenticular opacities or cataracts
- ≥ 2 meningiomas *and* 1 of the following
  - 1 VS diagnosed < 30 years of age
  - 1 meningioma, glioma, schwannoma, or lens opacity

Natural History. NF2-associated intracranial neoplasms often demonstrate a "saltatory" growth pattern characterized by alternating periods of growth and quiescence. As new tumors can develop and radiographic progression and symptom development are unpredictable, continued surveillance is necessary. Current recommended MR surveillance includes imaging at 1, 5, and 10 years after surgery.

Imaging

General Features. The cardinal imaging feature of NF2 is bilateral vestibular schwannomas.

CT Findings. NECT scans typically demonstrate a mass in one or both cerebellopontine angle (CPA) cisterns. Both schwannomas and meningiomas are typically iso- to slightly hyperdense on NECT **(39-12A)** and exhibit strong enhancement following contrast administration.

Nonneoplastic choroid plexus calcifications in atypical locations (e.g., temporal horn) are a rare manifestation of NF2 but can be striking. Bone CT typically shows that one or both internal auditory canals are widened.

MR Findings. MR findings of NF2-related schwannomas and meningiomas are similar to those of their sporadic counterparts. If NF2 is suspected on the basis of brain imaging, the entire spine and spinal cord should be screened. High-resolution T2WI and contrast-enhanced sequences disclose asymptomatic tiny schwannomas **(39-13)** **(39-16)** and intramedullary ependymomas **(39-14)** in at least 1/2 of all individuals with NF2 **(39-15)**.

Differential Diagnosis

The major differential diagnosis of NF2 is **schwannomatosis**. Schwannomatosis is characterized by multiple nonvestibular schwannomas while meningiomas are less common in schwannomatosis. **Multiple meningiomatosis** is characterized by multifocal meningiomas without schwannomas.

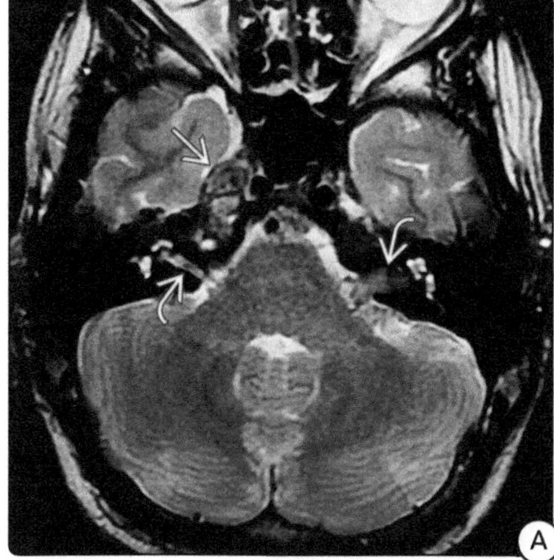

***(39-13A)** T2 MR in a 14-year-old boy with NF2 reveals lesions in the right cavernous sinus and both internal auditory canals (IACs).*

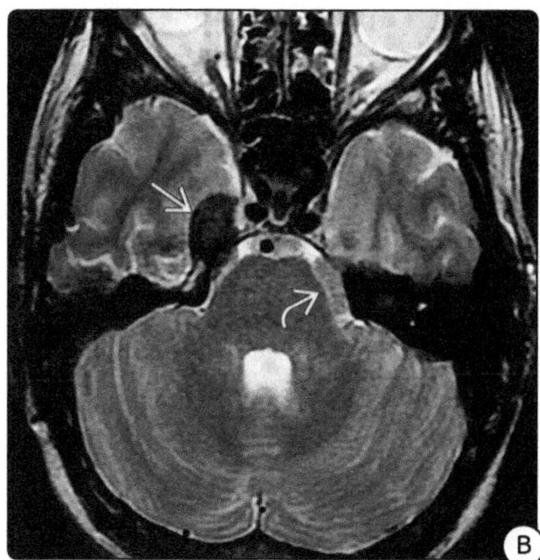

***(39-13B)** More cephalad T2WI in in the same case shows a hypodense mass in the right cavernous sinus and lesions in the left CPA cistern.*

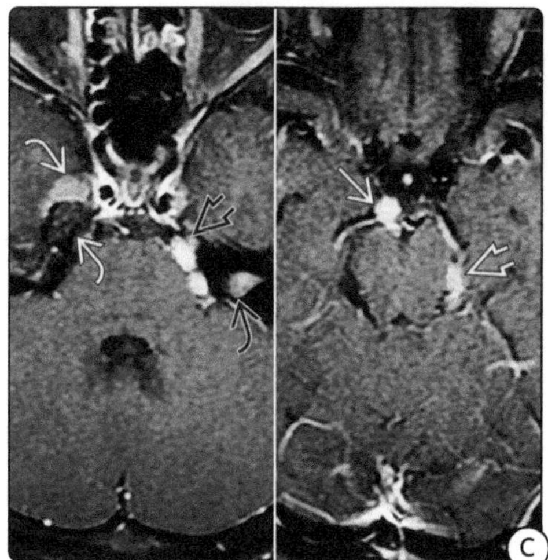

***(39-13C)** T1 C+ FS MRs show right cavernous sinus meningioma, CNIII, and left CNs IV, V, and VIII schwannomas.*

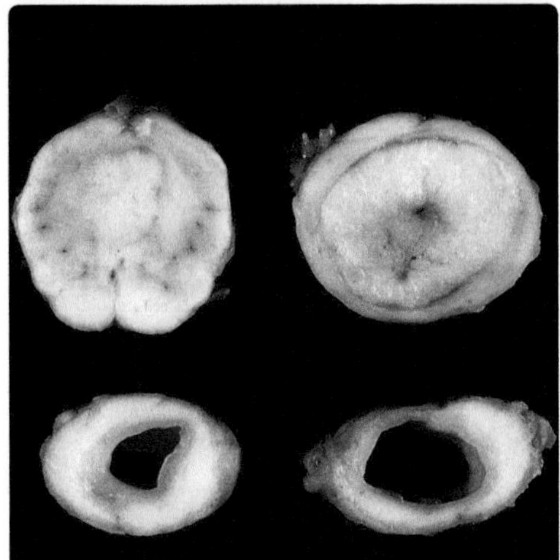

(39-14) Axial gross pathology in NF2 shows intramedullary ependymoma with cyst expanding cervical cord. (Courtesy R. Hewlett, MD.)

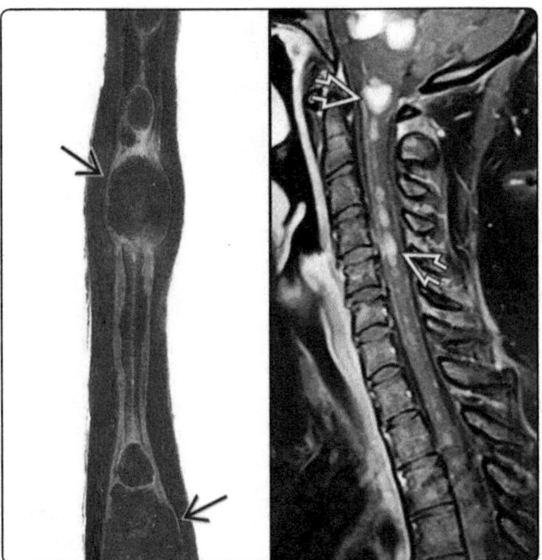

(39-15) Autopsy (L) shows intramedullary ependymomas ⇒. (Courtesy A. Ersen, MD.) (R) T1 C+ shows multiple cord ependymomas ➡ in NF2.

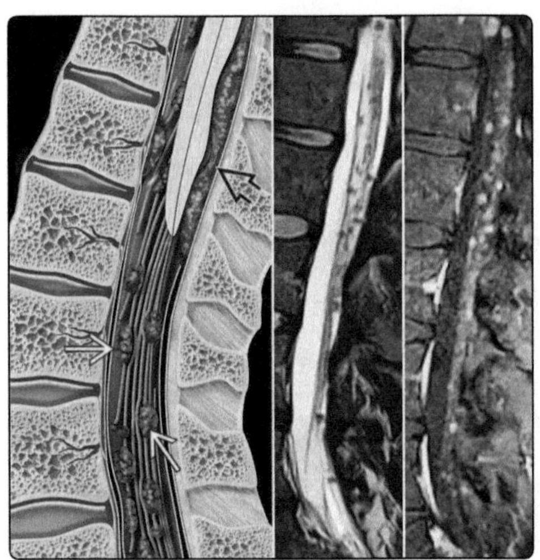

(39-16) NF2 graphic (L) depicts spinal "tumorlets" ➡, meningioma ⇒. T2 (middle), T1 C+ (R) show cauda equina schwannomas.

NF1 vs. NF2 vs. SCHWANNOMATOSIS

NF1

- Common (90% of all neurofibromatosis cases)
- Chromosome 17 mutations
- Almost always diagnosed by age 10
- Cutaneous/eye lesions common (> 95%)
  - Café au lait spots
  - Lisch nodules
  - Cutaneous neurofibromas (often multiple)
  - Plexiform neurofibromas (pathognomonic)
- CNS lesions less common (15-20%)
  - T2/FLAIR hyperintensities (myelin vacuolization; lesions wax, then wane)
  - Astrocytomas (optic pathway gliomas—usually pilocytic—other gliomas)
  - Sphenoid wing, dural dysplasias
  - Moyamoya
  - Neurofibromas of spinal nerve roots

NF2

- Much less common (10% of all neurofibromatosis cases)
- Chromosome 22 mutations
- Usually diagnosed in 2nd-4th decades
- Cutaneous, eye lesions less prominent
  - Mild/few café au lait spots
  - Juvenile subcapsular opacities
- CNS lesions in 100%
  - Bilateral vestibular schwannomas (almost all)
  - Nonvestibular schwannomas (50%)
  - Meningiomas (50%)
  - Cord ependymomas (often multiple)
  - Schwannomas ("tumorlets") of spinal nerve roots

Schwannomatosis

- Very rare; usually de novo mutation
- Multiple *nonvestibular* schwannomas; meningiomas less common
- *SMARCB1* (INI1) and *LZTR1* mutations

Other Common Familial Tumor Syndromes

Tuberous Sclerosis Complex

Terminology

Tuberous sclerosis complex (TSC) is a neurocutaneous syndrome characterized by the formation of nonmalignant hamartomas and neoplastic lesions in the brain, heart, skin, kidney, lung, and other organs. It is associated with autism, seizures, and neurocognitive and behavioral disabilities.

Etiology

Genetics. Approximately 50% of TSC cases are inherited and follow an autosomal dominant pattern while the other 50% represent de novo mutations. Two separate genes are mutated or deleted in TSC: *TSC1* and *TSC2*. The *TSC1* gene is located on chromosome 9q34 and encodes a protein called **hamartin**. The *TSC2* gene is localized to chromosome 16p13.3 and encodes the **tuberin** protein. Mutations in either gene are identified in 75-85% of patients with TSC.

The TSC protein complex functions as a tumor suppressor. Hamartin/tuberin inhibits the mTORC1 signaling pathway (mammalian target of rapamycin complex 1). Mutations that lead to increased mTORC1 activation promote cellular disorganization, overgrowth, and abnormal differentiation. *TSC2* mutations are associated with a more severe disease phenotype with more and larger tubers, more radial migration lines, and more subependymal nodules (SENs) compared with *TSC1*.

Pathology

The four major pathologic features of TSC in the brain are **cortical tubers, SENs, WM lesions**, and **subependymal giant cell astrocytoma (39-17)**.

Cortical Tubers. Cortical tubers are glioneuronal hamartomas and are found in over 90% of TS patients. They are firm, whitish, pyramid-shaped, elevated areas of smooth gyral thickening. Cortical tubers grossly resemble potatoes ("tubers").

Cortical tubers consist of giant cells and dysmorphic neurons. Balloon cells similar to those seen in Taylor-type focal cortical dysplasia (FCD type IIb) are also commonly found in tubers. Tubers do *not* undergo malignant transformation.

Subependymal Nodules. SENs are located immediately beneath the ependymal lining of the lateral ventricles, along the course of the caudate nucleus.

SENs appear as elevated, rounded, hamartomatous lesions that grossly resemble candle guttering or drippings. They often calcify with increasing age. SENs along the caudothalamic groove adjacent to the foramen of Monro may undergo neoplastic transformation into subependymal giant cell astrocytoma (SEGA).

White Matter Lesions. WM lesions are almost universal in patients with TSC. They appear as foci of bizarre dysmorphic neurons and balloon cells in the subcortical WM &/or fine radial lines extending outward from the ependymal ventricular surface toward the cortex. These radial migration lines often terminate in a tuber.

Subependymal Giant Cell Astrocytoma. SEGA is seen almost exclusively in the setting of TSC, occurring in 6-9% of patients. Grossly, SEGAs appear as well-circumscribed solid intraventricular masses located near the foramen of Monro. SEGAs are WHO grade I tumors that often cause obstructive hydrocephalus but do not invade adjacent brain. Although most SEGAs are unilateral, bilateral tumors occur in 10-15% of cases.

Clinical Issues

Epidemiology and Demographics. TSC is the second most common inherited tumor syndrome (after NF1). Almost 80% of cases are diagnosed before the age of 10.

Presentation. The classic clinical triad of TSC consists of facial lesions ("adenomata sebaceum"), seizures, and mental retardation. All cutaneous features are age dependent and may not become apparent until later in childhood. Hypomelanotic macules ("ash leaf") spots are seen in over 90% of cases and may be the first visible manifestation of TSC. Other common cutaneous findings, such as facial angiofibromas ("adenoma sebaceum"), and periungual fibromas usually do not appear until after puberty.

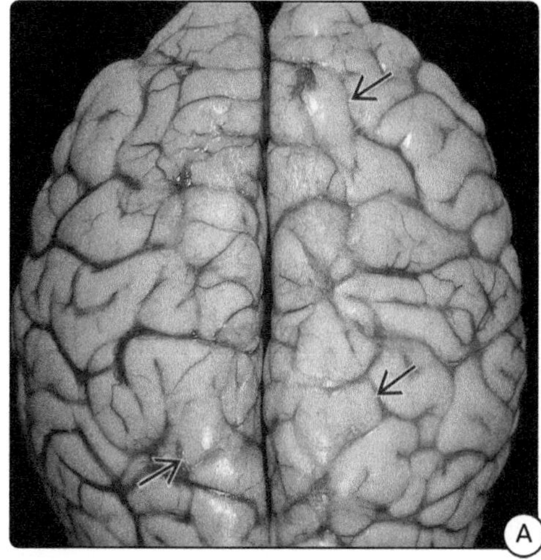

***(39-17A)** Autopsy of TSC shows multiple expanded gyri with the potato-like appearance characteristic of cortical tubers ⇒.*

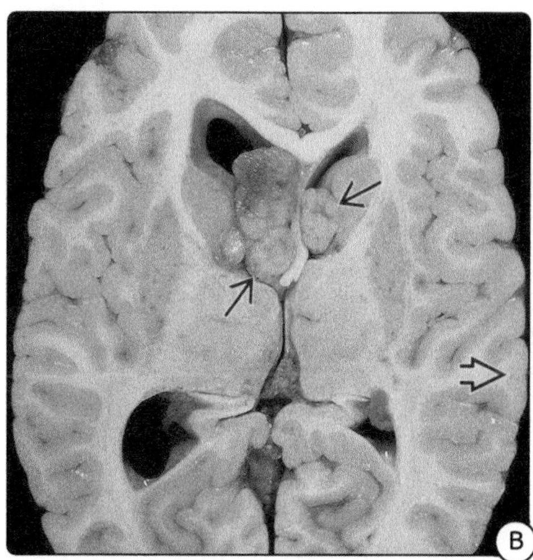

***(39-17B)** Axial cut section from the same case shows bilateral subependymal giant cell astrocytomas ⇒ and cortical tubers ⇒.*

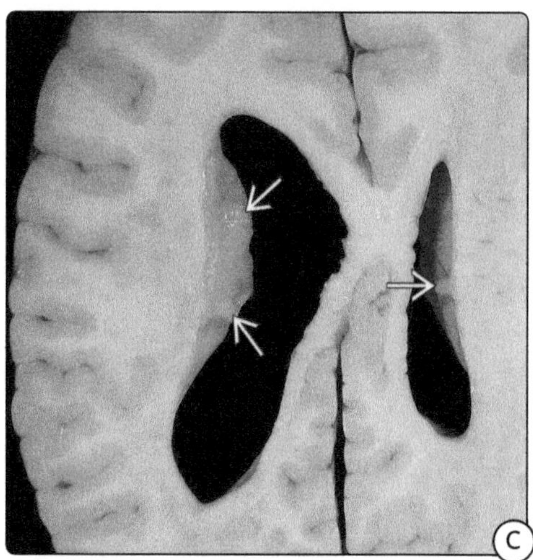

***(39-17C)** Note "heaped-up" subependymal nodules along the striothalamic groove ➡. (All 3 images courtesy R. Hewlett, MD.)*

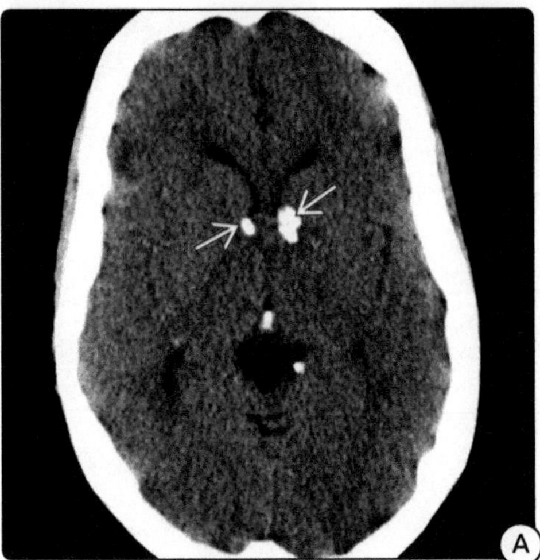

***(39-18A)** NECT in a 22-year-old woman with TSC demonstrates typical calcifications ➡ seen in subependymal nodules.*

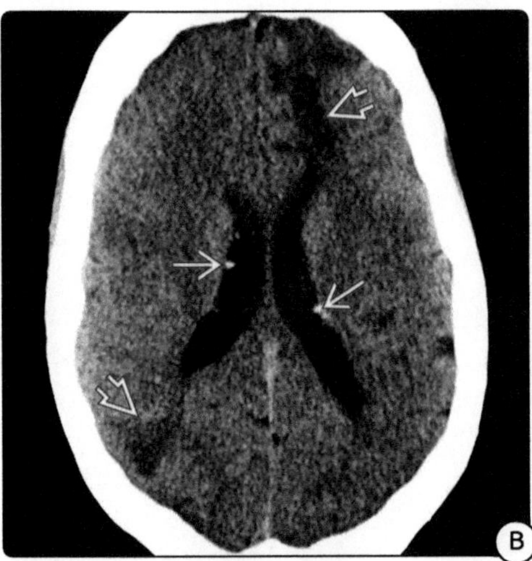

***(39-18B)** NECT scan shows additional calcified SENs ➡, wedge-shaped hypodensities ⇨ characteristic of the WM lesions in TSC.*

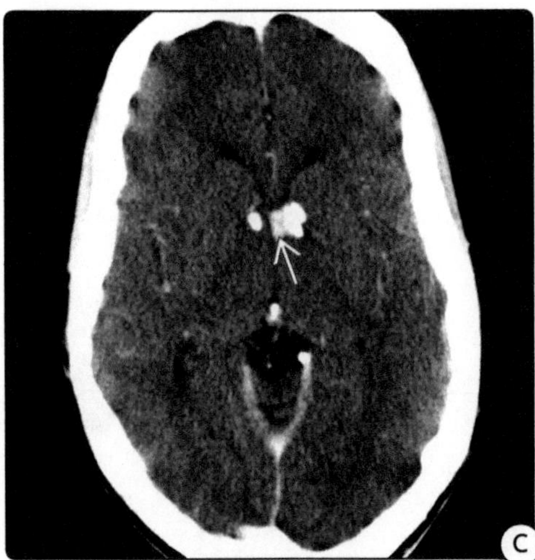

***(39-18C)** CECT shows enhancement ➡ adjacent to the foramen of Monro, suspicious for subependymal giant cell astrocytoma (SEGA).*

TSC: DIAGNOSTIC CLINICAL FEATURES

Diagnosis

- Definite TSC
  - 2 major features *or* 1 major + 2 minor
- Probable TSC
  - 1 major + 1 minor feature
- Possible TSC
  - 1 major *or* ≥ 2 minor features

Major Features

- Identified clinically
  - ≥ 3 hypomelanotic ("ash leaf") macules (97%)
  - Facial angiofibromas (75%) or forehead plaque (15-20%)
  - Shagreen patch (45-50%)
  - Ungual/periungual fibroma (15%)
  - Multiple retinal hamartomas (15%)
- Identified on imaging
  - Subependymal nodules (98%)
  - Cortical tubers (95%)
  - Cardiac rhabdomyoma (50%)
  - Renal angiomyolipoma (50%)
  - Subependymal giant cell astrocytoma (15%)
  - Lymphangioleiomyomatosis (1-3%)

Minor Features

- Identified clinically
  - Gingival fibromas (70%)
  - Affected 1st-degree relative (50%)
  - Pitting of dental enamel (30%)
  - Retinal achromic patch (35%)
  - Confetti-like skin macules (2-3%)
- Identified on imaging
  - WM hamartomas, radial migration lines (100%)
  - Hamartomatous rectal polyps (70-80%)
  - Nonrenal hamartomas (40-50%)
  - Bone cysts (40%)
  - Renal cysts (10-20%)

Natural History. Disease severity and natural course vary widely. Neurologic manifestations—primarily intractable seizures from brain hamartomas and obstructive hydrocephalus secondary to SEGA—are the leading cause of morbidity and mortality.

SEGAs are benign and usually slow-growing neoplasms. Although they can develop at any age, they are most frequent in patients between 5-19 years of age. Rapamycin inhibitors ("rapalogs"), such as everolimus and sirolimus, have been approved for the treatment of TSC-associated SEGAs in patients with TSC.

Imaging

CT Findings

Cortical Tubers. Neonatal and infantile cortical tubers are initially seen as hypodense cortical/subcortical masses within broadened and expanded gyri. The lucency decreases with age. Calcifications progressively increase with age. By 10 years, 50% of affected children demonstrate one or more globular or gyriform cortical calcifications.

Subependymal Nodules. SENs are a near-universal finding in TSC. Most are found along the caudothalamic groove. The walls of the atria and temporal horns of the lateral ventricles are less common sites.

SENs are rarely calcified in the first year of life. Like cortical tubers, SEN calcifications increase with age. Eventually, 50% demonstrate some degree of globular calcification **(39-18B)**. SENs typically do not enhance on CECT scans. An enhancing or enlarging SEN—especially if located near the foramen of Monro—is suspicious for SEGA **(39-18C)**.

Subependymal Giant Cell Astrocytoma. SEGAs show mixed density on NECT scans and frequently demonstrate focal calcification. Hemorrhage is rare. Moderate enhancement on CECT is typical.

MR Findings. In general, MR is much more sensitive than CT in depicting parenchymal abnormalities in TSC. Findings vary with lesion histopathology, patient age, and imaging sequence.

Cortical Tubers. In infants, tubers appear as thickened hyperintense cortex compared to the underlying unmyelinated WM on T1WI and become moderately hypointense on T2WI. "Streaky" linear or wedge-shaped T2-/FLAIR-hyperintense bands may extend from the tuber all the way through the WM to the ventricular ependyma **(39-20A)**.

Signal intensity changes after myelin maturation. Tubers gradually become more isointense relative to cortex on T1WI (unless calcification is present and causes T1 shortening). Occasionally, the outer margin of a tuber is mildly hyperintense to gray matter, while the subcortical component appears hypointense relative to WM.

Tubers in older children and adults demonstrate mixed signal intensity on T2/FLAIR. The periphery of the expanded gyrus is isointense with cortex while the deeper component is strikingly hyperintense **(39-19C)**. Between 3-5% of cortical tubers show mild enhancement on T1 C+ imaging.

Subependymal Nodules. SENs are seen as small (generally < 1.3 cm) nodular "bumps" or "candle gutterings" that protrude from the walls of the lateral ventricles **(39-19)**. In the unmyelinated brain, SENs appear hyperintense on T1WI and hypointense on T2WI. With progressive myelination, the SENs gradually become isointense with WM.

Calcified SENs appear variably hypointense on T2WI or FLAIR and are easily identified on T2* sequences (GRE, SWI). They can be distinguished from blood products on the SWI phase map, as Ca^{++} is diamagnetic and appears bright, whereas paramagnetic substances (blood products) are hypointense.

Enhancement of SENs following contrast administration is variable. About 1/2 of all SENs show moderate or even striking enhancement, which—in contrast to enhancement on CECT—does not indicate malignancy.

SENs are stable lesions. However, as SENs near the foramen of Monro may become malignant, close interval follow-up is essential. It is the interval change in size seen on serial examinations—not the degree of enhancement—that is significant. Some investigators suggest an increase of > 20% demonstrated on two consecutive MR scans as defining a SEGA.

White Matter Lesions. WM lesions are seen in 100% of cases. Even though they are considered a "minor" criterion for TSC, their appearance is highly characteristic of the disease. Streaky linear or wedge-shaped lesions extend along radial bands from the ventricles to the undersurfaces of cortical tubers **(39-20)**. In the unmyelinated brain, these linear foci (radial migration lines) appear mildly hyperintense to WM on T1WI. In older children and adults, they are hyperintense on T2/FLAIR sequences.

Small round cyst-like parenchymal lesions are seen in nearly 50% of TS cases. They are typically located in the deep periventricular WM **(39-20A)**. They are often multiple and resemble CSF, i.e., they suppress on FLAIR and do not enhance.

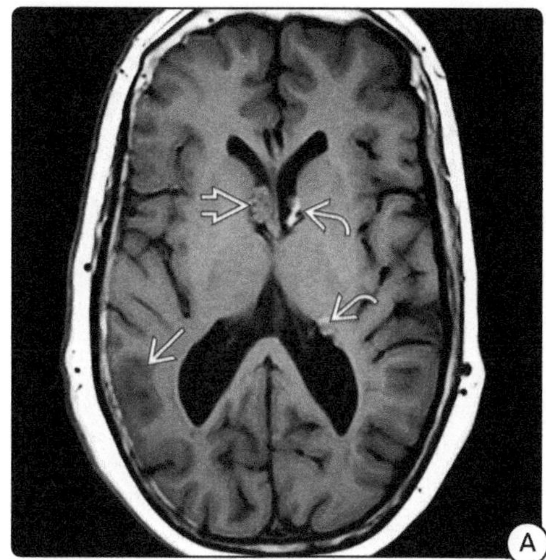

(39-19A) T1 MR shows hyperintense calcified SENs, R SEGA. Note poorly defined GM-WM junctions of typical cortical tubers.

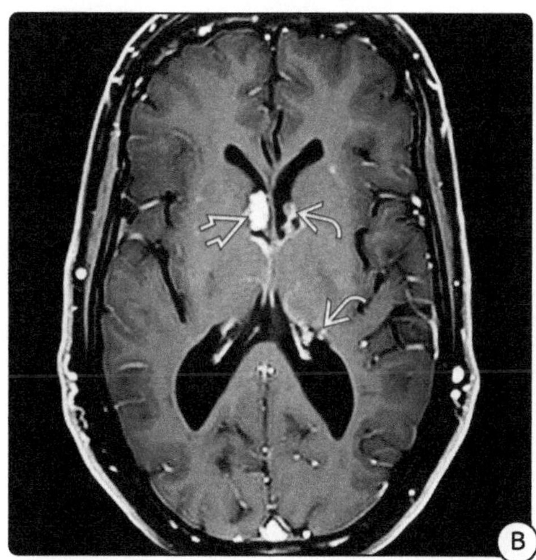

(39-19B) T1 C+ FS MR shows that the SEGA enhances intensely. The SENs also enhance moderately.

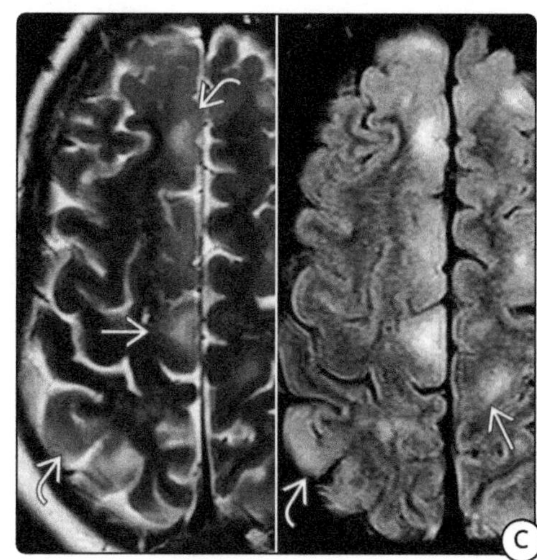

(39-19C) T2 (L), FLAIR (R) show tubers as expanded, hyperintense gyri with "flame-shaped" subcortical hyperintensities.

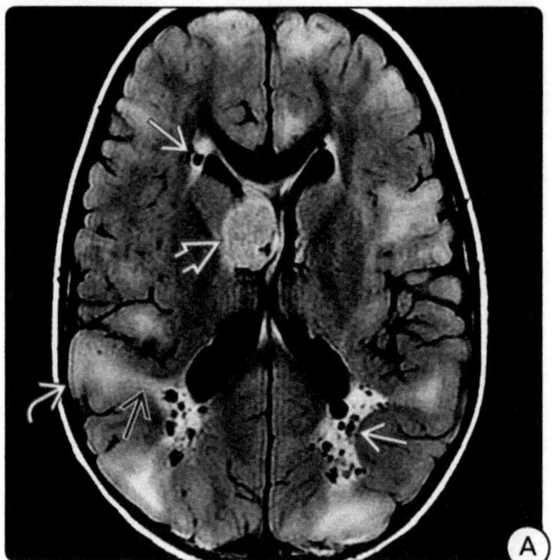

(39-20A) FLAIR in 5-year-old boy shows SEGA ➡, cortical tubers ➡ with WM band ➡, numerous CSF-like cysts in the deep periventricular WM ➡.

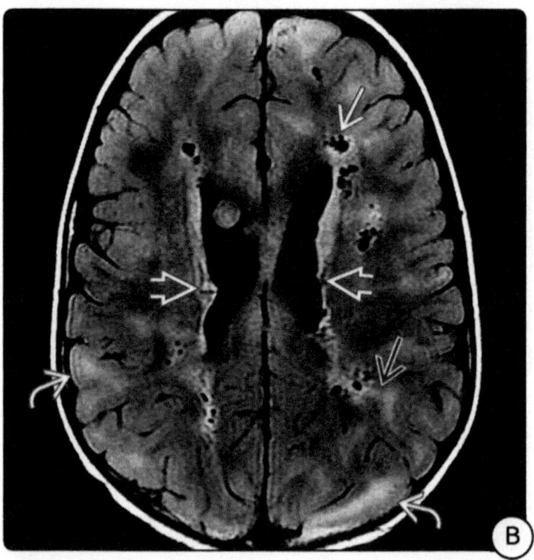

(39-20B) FLAIR MR shows multiple cortical tubers ➡, WM bands ➡, CSF cysts ➡, irregular "candle gutterings" ➡ of SENS.

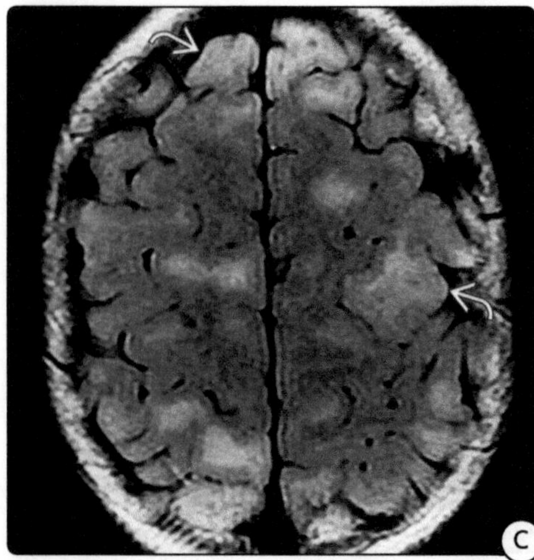

(39-20C) More cephalad FLAIR MR in the same case shows multiple hyperintense cortical tubers ➡ with poorly defined gray-white borders.

Subependymal Giant Cell Astrocytoma. Although SEGAs can occur anywhere along the ventricular ependyma, the vast majority are found near the foramen of Monro. SEGAs are of mixed signal intensity on both T1- and T2WI **(39-19)**. Virtually all enhance moderately strongly on T1 C+ scans **(39-19B)**.

SEGAs become symptomatic when they obstruct the foramen of Monro and cause hydrocephalus. Even large SEGAs rarely invade brain.

Miscellaneous CNS Lesions. Cerebellar tubers can be identified in 10-40% of cases and are always associated with supratentorial lesions. Other uncommon abnormalities include hemimegalencephaly, cerebellar malformations, and linear, clump-like, or gyriform parenchymal calcifications. Aneurysms (mostly fusiform aortic and intracranial) are seen in 1% of TSC.

Differential Diagnosis

Focal cortical dysplasia (FCD) can appear identical to cortical tubers on imaging studies, but lesions are typically solitary, whereas cortical tubers are almost always multiple. Foci of **subependymal heterotopic gray matter** can resemble SENs, but most SENs calcify and often enhance on T1 C+ sequences.

SEGAs can resemble other frontal horn/septum pellucidum lesions, such as **subependymoma**. Subependymomas are tumors of middle-aged and older individuals, and other TSC stigmata, such as cortical tubers and SENs, are absent.

TSC: IMAGING

Cortical Tubers
- Broad, expanded gyrus
- CT: Initially hypodense; Ca^{++} increases with age
  - 50% of patients eventually develop ≥ 1 calcified tuber(s)
- MR: Periphery isointense, subcortical portion T2/FLAIR hyperintense

Subependymal Nodules
- CT: Ca^{++} rare in 1st year; increases with age
  - 50% eventually calcify; do not enhance
- MR: T1 hyper-, T2 hypointense; 50% enhance

White Matter Lesions
- T2-/FLAIR-hyperintense radial lines/wedges
- CSF-like cysts in deep periventricular WM

Subependymal Giant Cell Astrocytoma
- CT: Mixed-density mass at foramen of Monro, moderate enhancement
- MR: Heterogeneous signal, strong enhancement

Miscellaneous Lesions
- Vascular (usually fusiform aneurysms), seen in 1% of cases
- Parenchymal calcifications

von Hippel-Lindau Disease

Terminology

von Hippel-Lindau disease (VHL) is also known as familial cerebelloretinal angiomatosis. VHL is characterized by retinal and CNS hemangioblastomas (HBs) **(39-21)**, endolymphatic sac tumors (ELSTs) **(39-27)**, abdominal neoplasms (adrenal pheochromocytomas, clear cell renal carcinomas), and pancreatic and renal cysts.

Etiology

Genetics. VHL is an autosomal dominant familial tumor syndrome with marked phenotypic variability and age-dependent penetrance. Mutations in the *VHL* tumor suppressor gene on chromosome 3p25.3 cause inactivation of the VHL protein (pVHL) and increased expression of factors, such as PDGF and VEGF, which in turn leads to angiogenesis and tumorigenesis. Approximately 20% of tumors in patients with VHL result from de novo germline mutations.

Two VHL phenotypes are recognized, distinguished by the presence or absence of associated pheochromocytoma. Type 1 has a *low risk* of pheochromocytoma and is caused by truncating mutations of the *VHL* gene. Type 2 is caused by missense mutations and has a *high risk* of developing pheochromocytoma. Type 2 VHL is subdivided into type 2A [low risk of renal cell carcinoma (RCC), 2B (high risk of RCC), and 2C (familial pheochromocytoma without either hemangioblastoma or RCC)].

VHL: GENETICS

Type 1 VHL

- Genotype = truncating mutations
- Phenotype
  - *Low* risk for pheochromocytoma (PCC)
  - Retinal angioma, CNS hemangioblastomas (HBs)
  - Renal cell carcinoma (RCC), pancreatic cysts, neuroendocrine tumors

Type 2 VHL

- Genotype = missense mutation
- Phenotypes
  - *All have high risk* of PCC
  - Type 2A (low risk of RCC); retinal angiomas, CNS HBs
  - Type 2B (high risk of RCC); retinal angioma, CNS HBs, pancreatic cysts, neuroendocrine tumor
  - Type 2C (risk for PCC only); no HB or RCC

Pathology

The great majority of VHL patients harbor significant CNS disease. The two most common VHL-related CNS neoplasms are craniospinal **HBs** (found in 60-80% of all VHL cases) and **ELSTs** (seen in 10-15% of patients).

Hemangioblastomas. HBs are well-circumscribed red or yellowish masses that usually abut a pial surface. The vast majority of intracranial HBs are infratentorial; the dorsal 1/2 of the cerebellum is the most common site followed by the medulla.

Approximately 10% are supratentorial; the most common site is the pituitary stalk (30% of all supratentorial HBs and 3% of those in patients with VHL). Most are asymptomatic and do not require treatment. Less common locations are along the optic pathways and in the cerebral hemispheres.

Nearly 1/2 of all VHL-associated HBs occur in the spinal cord. Intraspinal HBs are often multiple and are frequently associated with a syrinx.

Between 1/4 and 1/3 of HBs are solid; 2/3 are at least partially cystic and contain amber-colored fluid. One or more cysts together with a variably sized mural tumor nodule is the typical appearance. HBs are highly vascular with large arteries and prominent draining veins.

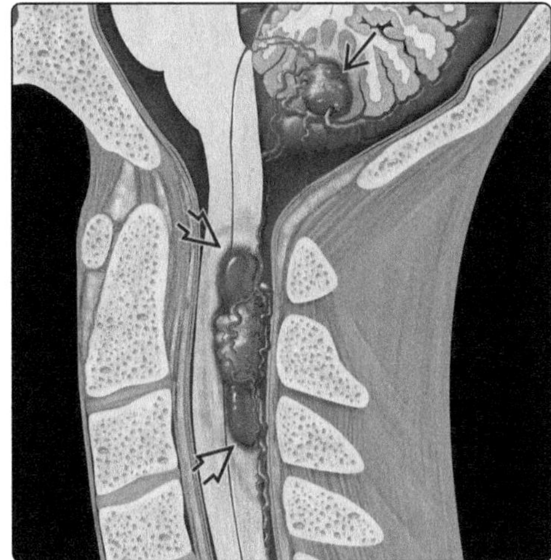

***(39-21)** Two HBs in VHL show spinal cord tumor has associated cyst ⇨, causing myelopathy. Small cerebellar HB ⇨ would be asymptomatic.*

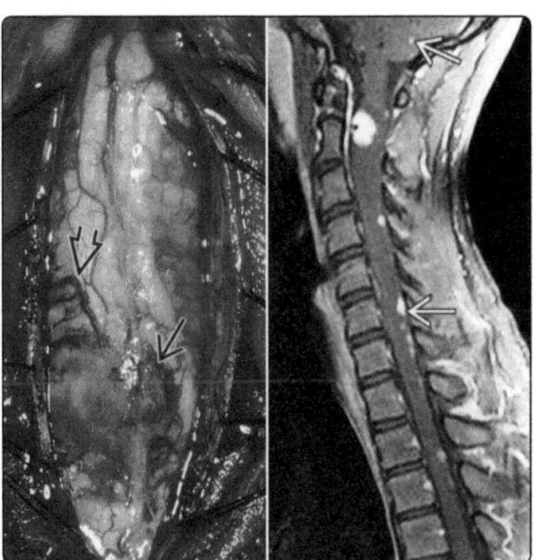

***(39-22)** (L) Surgical photo shows typical dorsal subpial location of HB nodule ⇨, prominent vessels ⇨. (R) T1 C+ MR shows multiple HBs ➡.*

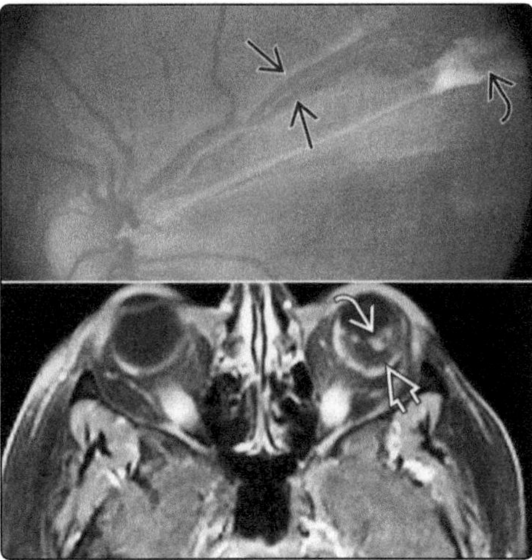

***(39-23)** (Top) Retinal angioma ⇨ supplied by prominent arteries ⇨. (Imaging in Neurology.) (Bottom) Angioma ➡, retinal detachment ➡.*

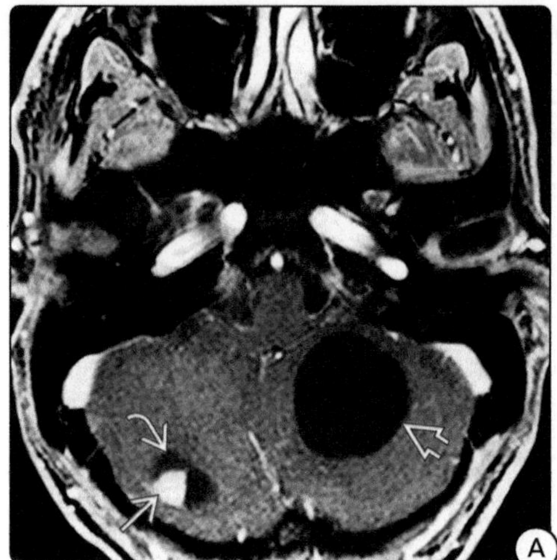

(39-24A) T1 C+ FS in VHL shows cystic left cerebellar mass ➡ and a smaller cyst ➡ with enhancing nodule ➡ in the right hemisphere.

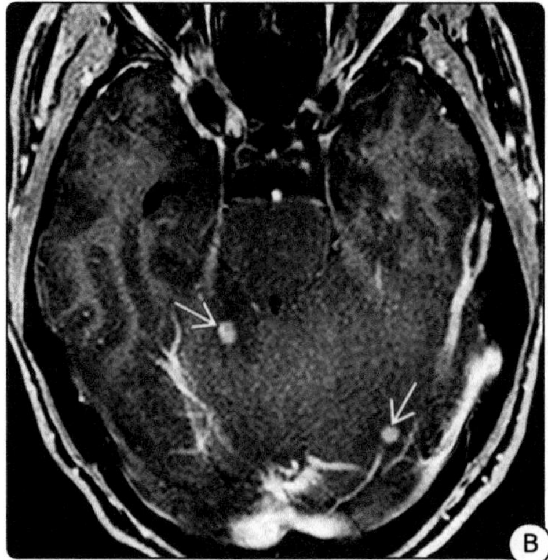

(39-24B) More cephalad scan in the same case shows 2 tiny enhancing nodules ➡.

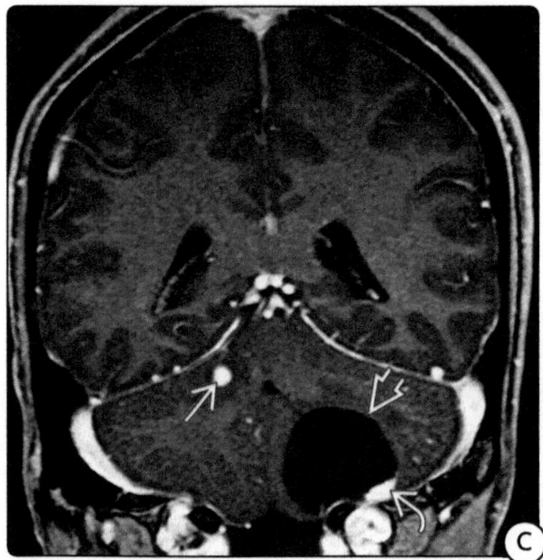

(39-24C) Coronal shows enhancing nodule ➡ abuts pial surface. Cyst wall ➡ does not enhance. Note separate enhancing nodule ➡.

Retinal Hemangioblastomas ("Angiomas"). Retinal capillary angiomas are the typical ocular lesions of VHL and are seen in 1/2 of all cases. Retinal angiomas are small but often multifocal, and almost 50% are bilateral.

Endolymphatic Sac Tumors. ELSTs are slow-growing, benign but locally aggressive papillary cystadenomatous tumors of the endolymphatic sac. Sporadic ELSTs are more common than VHL-associated tumors. Approximately 10-15% of VHL patients develop an ELST; of these, 30% are bilateral.

VHL: PATHOLOGY

CNS Neoplasms
- HBs (60-80%)
  - Retinal HBs ("angiomas") (50%)
- Endolymphatic sac tumors (10-15%)

Visceral Lesions
- Renal lesions (2/3 of all VHL patients)
  - Cysts (50-75%)
  - Clear cell renal carcinomas (25-45%)
- Adrenal pheochromocytoma (10-20%)
  - Hallmark of type 2 VHL
- Pancreatic cysts (35-70%), nonsecretory islet cell tumors (5-10%)
- Epididymal cysts, cystadenomas (60% of male patients, often bilateral)
- Broad ligament cystadenomas (female patients, rare)

Clinical Issues

Presentation and Clinical Diagnosis. Because all VHL-associated lesions can also occur as sporadic (i.e., nonfamilial) events, a clinical diagnosis of VHL disease in a patient without a positive family history requires the presence of at least two tumors (see box below).

Age at diagnosis varies. Although VHL can present in children and even infants, most patients become symptomatic as young adults. Painless visual loss from retinal angioma-induced hemorrhage is often the first symptom (mean: 25 years).

Tumors are the presenting feature in ~ 40% of cases. HBs, pheochromocytomas, and endolymphatic tumors typically become symptomatic in the 30s, whereas RCCs tend to present somewhat later. Mean age at diagnosis of symptomatic RCCs is 40 years, but asymptomatic tumors are frequently detected earlier on screening abdominal CT.

VHL: DIAGNOSTIC CLINICAL FEATURES

No Family History of VHL
- ≥ 2 CNS HBs *or*
- 1 CNS HB + visceral tumor

Positive Family History of VHL
- 1 CNS HB *or*
- Pheochromocytoma *or*
- Clear cell renal carcinoma

Natural History. VHL-associated HBs demonstrate a "saltatory" growth pattern characterized by quiescent periods (averaging slightly over two years) interspersed with periods of growth. Nearly 1/2 of all patients develop de novo lesions after the initial diagnosis of VHL.

The two major causes of death in VHL patients are RCC (50%) and HBs. Overall median life expectancy is 49 years.

Surveillance Recommendations. Imaging is crucial in the identification and surveillance of extra-CNS lesions. Identification of RCC is especially important because it is the major malignant neoplasm of VHL and one of the leading causes of mortality.

Patients with a family history of VHL should undergo annual screening (ophthalmoscopy, physical/neurologic examination) beginning in infancy or early childhood. Brain MRs are recommended every 1-3 years starting in adolescence. Abdominal MR or ultrasound screening for RCC and pancreatic tumors is recommended annually, beginning at age 16.

Methods for pheochromocytoma screening vary. Blood pressure should be monitored and 24-hour urine catecholamines obtained annually. More intense surveillance beginning at age 8 years should be considered in families at high-risk for pheochromocytoma (i.e., type 2 VHL).

Imaging

General Features. Two or more CNS HBs **(39-24)** or one HB plus a visceral lesion or concomitant presence of retinal hemorrhage (highly suggestive of intraocular HB) are the best imaging clues to the diagnosis.

Hemangioblastomas. Approximately 2/3 of HBs are cystic; 1/3 are solid or mixed solid/cystic lesions. NECT scans typically demonstrate a hypodense cyst with isodense mural nodule that abuts a pial surface of the cerebellum. The tumor nodule enhances intensely on CECT.

The cyst is slightly to moderately hyperintense to CSF on T1WI and iso- to hyperintense on T2/FLAIR. Signal intensity of the nodule is variable; large lesions may show prominent "flow voids." Hemorrhage is common, and peritumoral edema varies.

Tumor nodules enhance strongly on T1 C+ **(39-25)**. Enhanced scans often demonstrate several tiny nodules in the cerebellum &/or spinal cord **(39-22)**. Supratentorial HBs are uncommon; most occur in the pituitary stalk (the most common supratentorial site) **(39-25B)** or along the optic tracts. Disseminated leptomeningeal hemangioblastomatosis, seen as multiple tumor nodules with diffuse pial enhancement of the spinal cord **(39-25A)** &/or brain, is a rare, late manifestation of VHL.

DSA demonstrates one or more intensely vascular masses with prolonged tumor "blush" and variable arteriovenous shunting **(39-26)**.

Retinal Hemangioblastomas ("Angiomas"). Retinal angiomas (actually small capillary HBs) are usually visualized as hemorrhagic retinal detachments that are hyperdense compared with normal vitreous on NECT. Tiny enhancing nodules can sometimes be identified on T1 C+ MR **(39-23)**.

Endolymphatic Sac Tumors. ELSTs are located along the posterior petrous temporal bone between the internal auditory canal and the sigmoid sinus. The imaging hallmark of ELST is that of a retrolabyrinthine mass associated with osseous erosion. Bone CT shows an infiltrative, poorly circumscribed, lytic lesion with central intratumoral bone spicules **(39-28A)**.

MR demonstrates T1-hyperintense foci in 80% of cases. Signal intensity is mixed hyper- and hypointense on T2WI. Heterogeneous enhancement is seen following contrast administration **(39-28B)**. ELSTs are vascular lesions that may demonstrate prominent "flow voids" on MR and prolonged tumor "blush" on DSA.

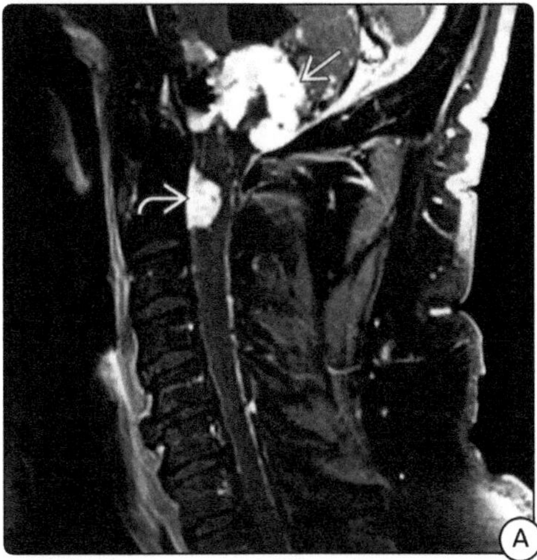

***(39-25A)** Sagittal T1 C+ MR in a 38-year-old man with VHL shows multiple HBs in the cerebellum ➡ and cervical spinal cord ➡.*

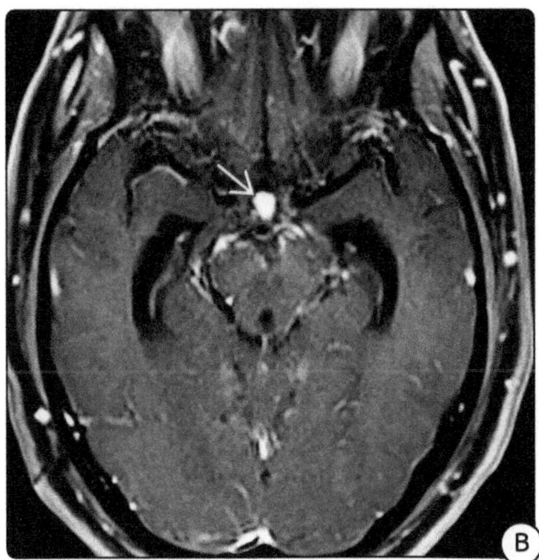

***(39-25B)** Axial T1 C+ FS MR in the same patient demonstrates an enlarged enhancing pituitary stalk ➡.*

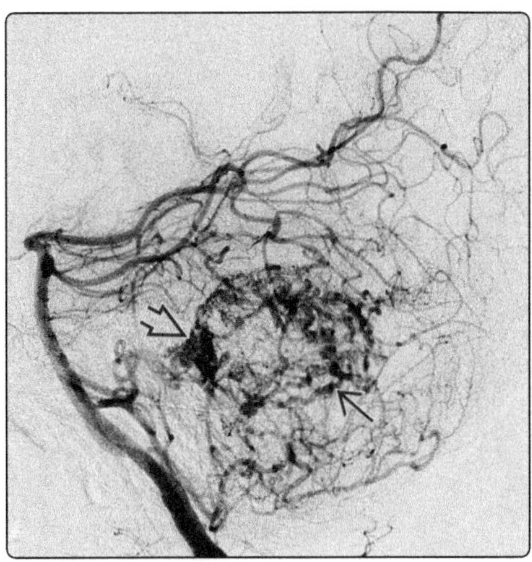

***(39-26)** DSA of HGBL shows vascular "stain" ➡ and striking neovascularity with tortuous, irregular-appearing vessels ➡.*

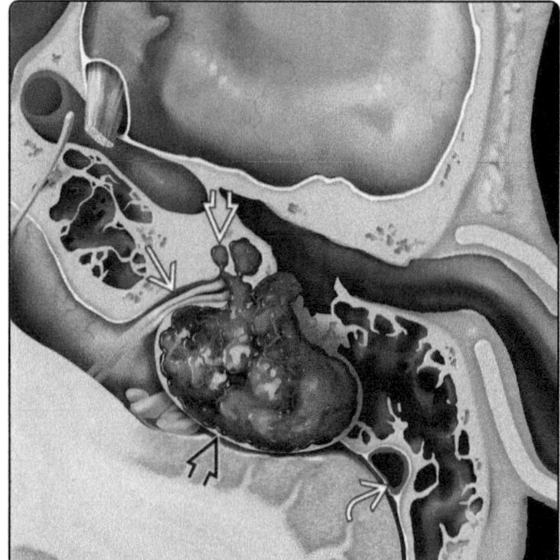

***(39-27)** ELST ➩ is a lytic, vascular, hemorrhagic mass between IAC ➡ and sigmoid sinus ➨. Note tendency to fistulize inner ear ➩.*

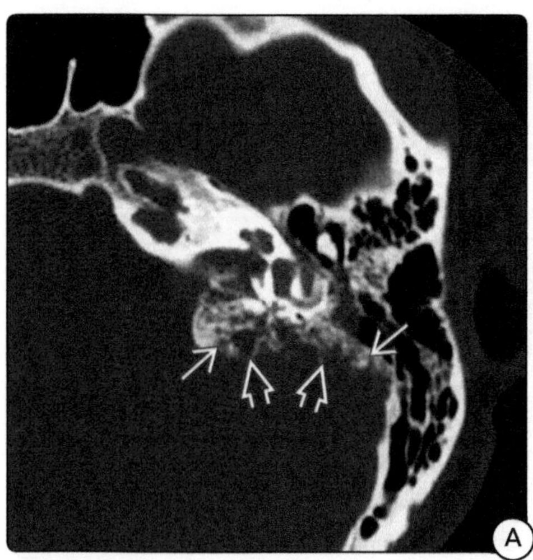

***(39-28A)** Lytic infiltrative lesion ➡ with preserved bond "spicules" ➩; location between the IAC, sigmoid sinus is characteristic for ELST.*

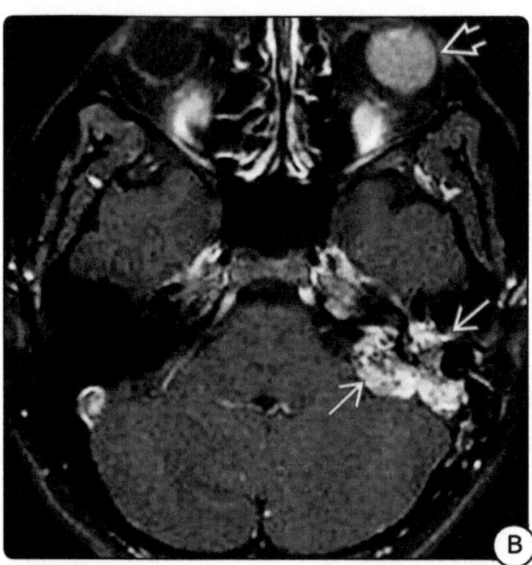

***(39-28B)** T1 C+ FS MR shows lesion ➡ enhances intensely but heterogeneously. Hyperintense retinal hemorrhage ➩ + ELST = VHL.*

VHL: IMAGING

Multiple Hemangioblastomas (Diagnostic of VHL)

- 2/3 cystic, 1/3 solid
- Nodule abuts pia
- 50% in cord (dorsal > ventral surface)
  - Multiple tiny "tumorlets" along cord common
  - Disseminated leptomeningeal hemangioblastomatosis

Retinal "Angiomas"

- Hemorrhagic retinal detachment
  - V-shaped hyperdense posterior globe
- With or without enhancing "dots" (tiny HBs)

Uni- or Bilateral Endolymphatic Sac Tumors

- Dorsal T-bone
  - Between IAC, sigmoid sinus
- Infiltrative, lytic, intratumoral bone spicules
- T1 iso-/hyperintense; T2 hyperintense
- Strong enhancement

Differential Diagnosis

- Solitary HB
- Vascular metastases

Differential Diagnosis

The major differential diagnosis of VHL in the brain is **sporadic non-VHL-associated hemangioblastoma**. Between 60-80% of HBs are sporadic tumors *not* associated with VHL. Multiple HBs &/or supratentorial lesions are highly suggestive of VHL.

Vascular metastases can mimic multiple HBs but are rarely isolated to the cerebellum &/or spinal cord.

Other neoplasms that commonly have a cyst + nodule configuration include **pilocytic astrocytoma** and **ganglioglioma**. PAs are solitary tumors of childhood whereas HBs are rarely seen in patients younger than 15 years. In contrast to HB, the tumor nodule in pilocytic astrocytoma typically does not abut a pial surface.

Ganglioglioma is typically a tumor of the cerebral hemispheres. While hemispheric HBs can occur, they are rare. When present, they are typically found along the optic pathways.

Selected References: The complete reference list is available on the Expert Consult™ eBook version included with purchase.

Vascular Neurocutaneous Syndromes

A number of syndromes with prominent cutaneous manifestations occur without associated neoplasms. Many of these are disorders in which both cutaneous and intracranial vascular lesions are the predominant features.

Some vascular neurocutaneous syndromes (e.g., Sturge-Weber syndrome) are present at birth (i.e., congenital) but are *not* inherited. Others, including hereditary hemorrhagic telangiectasia, have specific gene mutations and known inheritance patterns.

Capillary Malformation Syndromes

In the updated classification scheme adopted by the International Society for the Study of Vascular Anomalies, port-wine stains and associated syndromes [e.g., Sturge-Weber syndrome (SWS) and others] are grouped under the heading of capillary malformations.

Sturge-Weber Syndrome

SWS is one of the very few neurocutaneous syndromes that are sporadic, i.e., not familial and not inherited. It is also one of the most disfiguring syndromes, as a prominent nevus flammeus ["port-wine birthmark" (PWB)] is seen in the vast majority of cases.

Terminology

SWS is also known as **encephalo-trigeminal angiomatosis**. Its hallmarks are variable combinations of (1) a dermal capillary-venular malformation (the PWB) in the sensory distribution of the trigeminal nerve, (2) retinal choroidal angioma (either with or without glaucoma), and (3) a cerebral capillary-venous leptomeningeal angioma.

Etiology

GNAQ mutations cause a spectrum of vascular and melanocytic birthmarks. Depending on when they occur, they can lead to differing dermal phenotypes, either vascular alone (SWS), pigmentary alone (extensive dermal melanocytosis), or both.

Pathology

A tangle of thin-walled vessels—multiple enlarged capillaries and venous channels—forms the characteristic leptomeningeal (pial) angioma. The

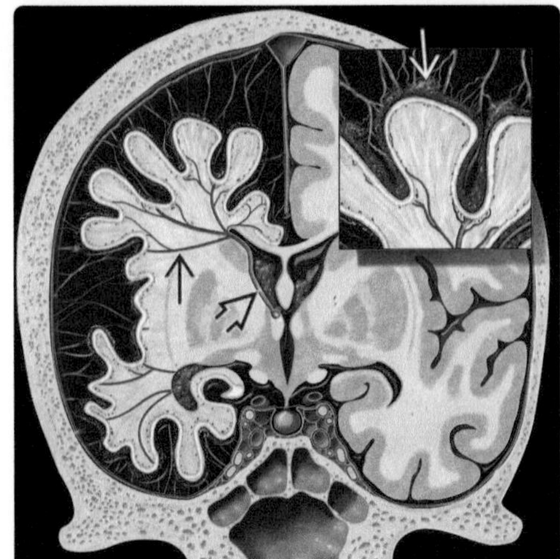

***(40-1)** SWS shows pial angiomatosis, deep medullary collaterals, enlarged choroid plexus, and atrophy of the right cerebral hemisphere.*

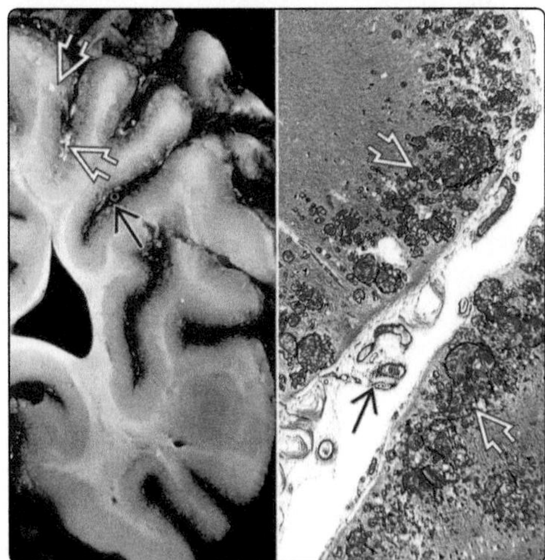

***(40-2)** Gross image (L), photomicrograph (R) of SWS show cortical atrophy, calcifications, and pial angioma within sulci. (AFIP Archives.)*

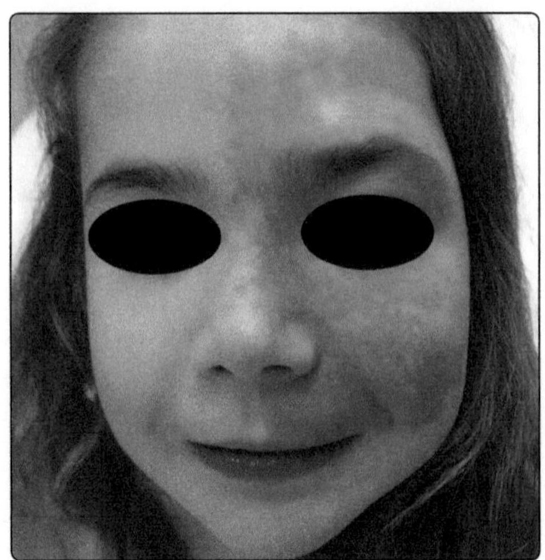

***(40-3)** Photograph shows the classic CNV1-V2 nevus flammeus characteristic of SWS.*

angioma covers the brain surface, dipping into the enlarged sulci between shrunken apposing gyri **(40-1)**.

The most common location is the parietooccipital region followed by the frontal and temporal lobes. Part or all of one hemisphere can be affected. SWS is unilateral in 80% of cases and is typically ipsilateral to the facial angioma. Bilateral involvement is seen in 20% of cases. Infratentorial lesions are seen in 11% of cases.

Dystrophic laminar cortical calcifications are typical **(40-2)**. Frank hemorrhage and large territorial infarcts are rare.

Clinical Issues

Presentation. The vast majority of SWS patients exhibit a nevus flammeus—formerly termed a facial "angioma" or "port-wine stain"—that is plainly visible at birth. It can be uni- (63%) or bilateral (31%) and is distributed over the skin innervated by one or more sensory branches of the trigeminal nerve. CNV1 (forehead &/or eyelid) or a combination of CNV1-V2 (plus cheek) are the most common sites **(40-3)**. All three trigeminal divisions are involved in 13% of cases. Approximately 1/3 of patients have ocular or orbital abnormalities, such as a diffuse choroidal hemangioma ("tomato catsup fundus"), congenital glaucoma with an enlarged globe (buphthalmos), and optic disc colobomas.

Occasionally, the facial vascular malformation involves the midline and may even extend to the chest, trunk, and limbs. *No facial nevus flammeus is present in 5% of cases,* so lack of a visible port-wine nevus does not rule out SWS!

Similarly, the presence of a PWB is *not* sufficient in and of itself for the definitive diagnosis of SWS. Patients with PWBs in the CNV1 distribution have only a 10-20% risk of SWS, although the risk increases with size, extent, and bilaterality of the nevus flammeus.

Seizures developing in the first year of life (75-90%), glaucoma (70%), hemiparesis (30-65%), and migraine-like headaches are other common manifestations of SWS.

Occasionally, children with SWS also have extensive cutaneous capillary malformations, limb hypertrophy, and vascular &/or lymphatic malformations. These children are diagnosed as having **Klippel-Trenaunay syndrome** (KTS), which is also known as angioosteohypertrophy or hemangiectatic hypertrophy. SWS and KTS most likely represent phenotypic variations within the same spectrum.

Natural History. SWS-related seizures are often medically refractory and worsen with time. Progressive hemiparesis and stroke-like episodes with focal neurologic deficits are common.

Imaging

General Features. Neuroimaging is used to identify the intracranial pial angioma and the sequelae of longstanding venous ischemia. This enables the radiologist to (1) establish or confirm the diagnosis of SWS and (2) evaluate the extent and severity of intracranial involvement.

Sequential examinations of SWS patients show progressive cerebral cortical-subcortical atrophy, especially during the first years of life. *Findings may be minimal or absent in newborn infants, so serial imaging is necessary in suspected cases.*

CT Findings. Dystrophic cortical/subcortical calcifications are one of the imaging hallmarks of SWS **(40-4B)**. (Note that the calcifications are in the

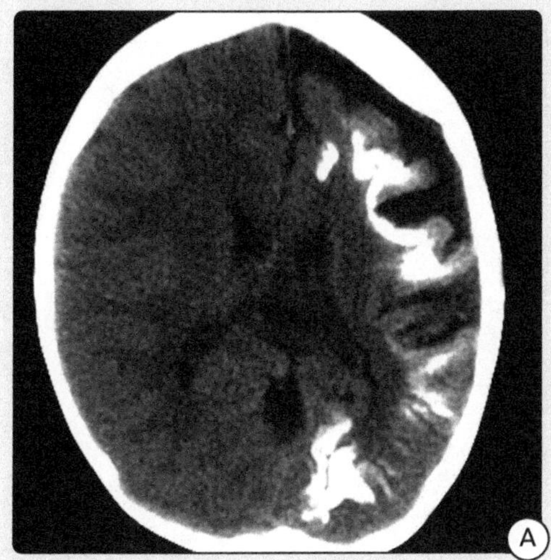
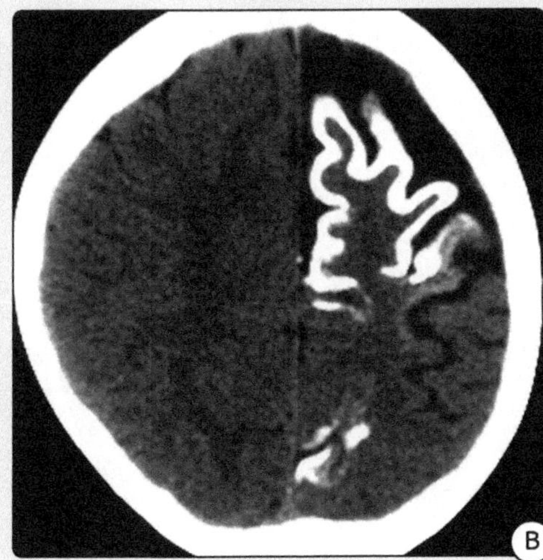

(40-4A) NECT in an 8-year-old girl with SWS shows striking cortical atrophy and extensive calcifications in the cortex and subcortical WM throughout most of the left cerebral hemisphere. ***(40-4B)*** *More cephalad NECT in the same patient shows the typical serpentine gyral calcifications together with significant volume loss.*

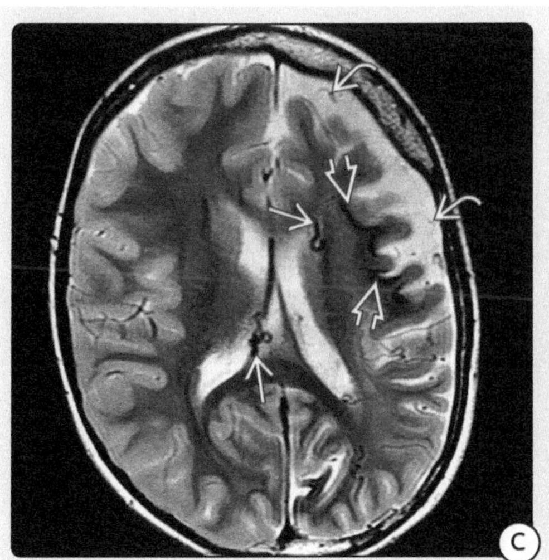
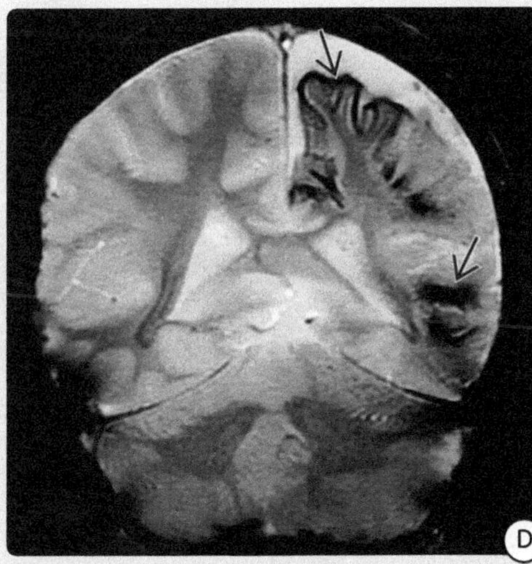

(40-4C) T2WI in the same patient shows atrophy with thinned cortex, extensive curvilinear hypointensity in the GM-WM interface ➡. Note the prominent "flow voids" in the subependymal veins ➡. The CSF in the enlarged subarachnoid space appears somewhat "dirty" with enlarged traversing trabeculae and veins ➡. ***(40-4D)*** *Coronal T2* GRE scan shows "blooming" of the extensive cortical/subcortical calcifications ➡.*

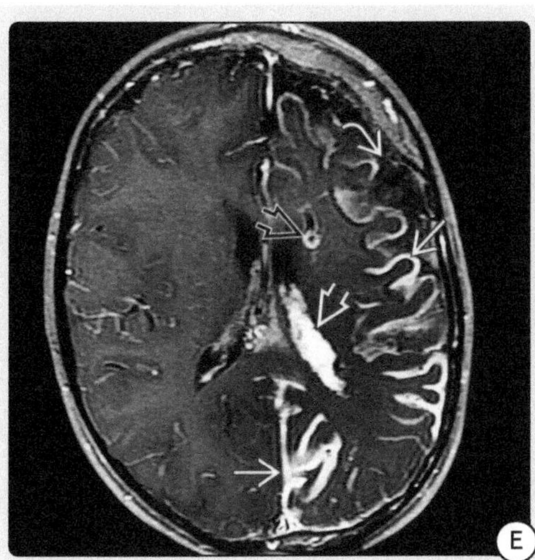
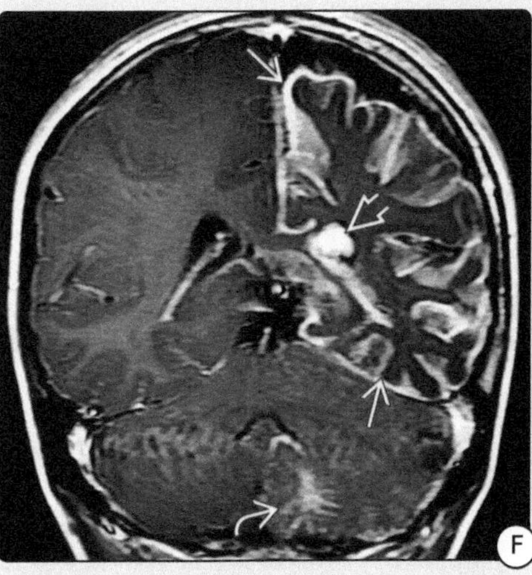

(40-4E) T1 C+ FS MR shows serpentine enhancement covering gyri, filling sulci ➡ with grayish "dirty" CSF ➡. Note enlargement, enhancement of ipsilateral choroid plexus ➡ and draining subependymal vein ➡. ***(40-4F)*** *Coronal T1 C+ MR shows pial angioma ➡ and enlarged choroid plexus ➡. Developmental venous anomaly is seen in the left cerebellar hemisphere ➡.*

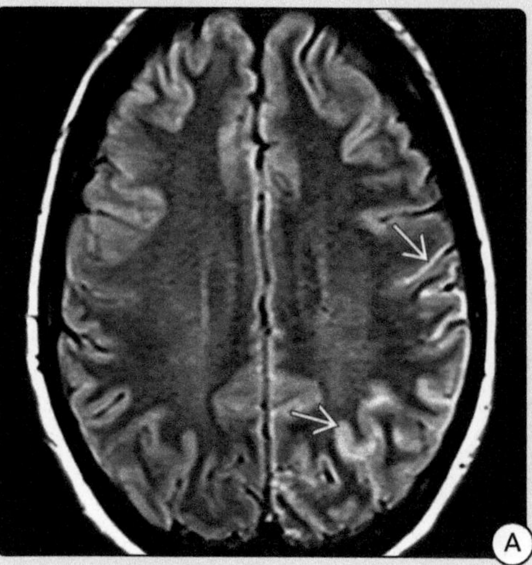

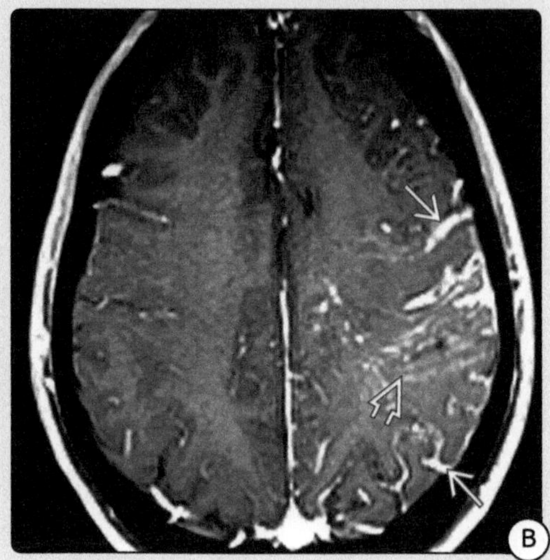

***(40-5A)** Axial FLAIR MR in a 25-year-old woman with seizures and SWS shows left parietooccipital sulcal hyperintensity ("ivy" sign) ➔. **(40-5B)** T1 C+ FS MR in the same patient shows that the enhancing pial angioma fills the affected sulci ➔. Note the linear enhancing foci caused by enlarged medullary veins ➔ that provide collateral venous drainage into the subependymal veins and galenic system.*

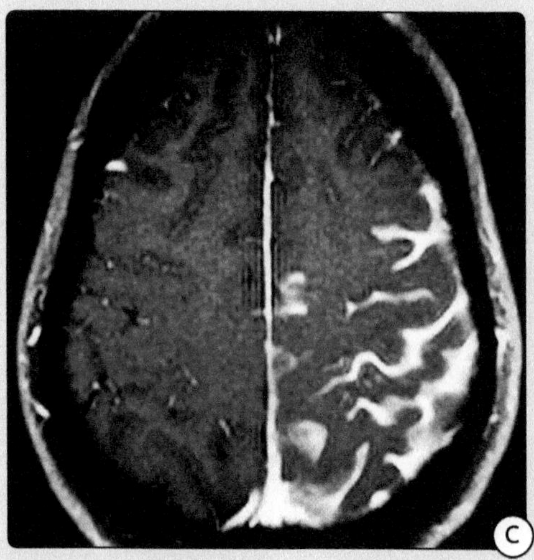

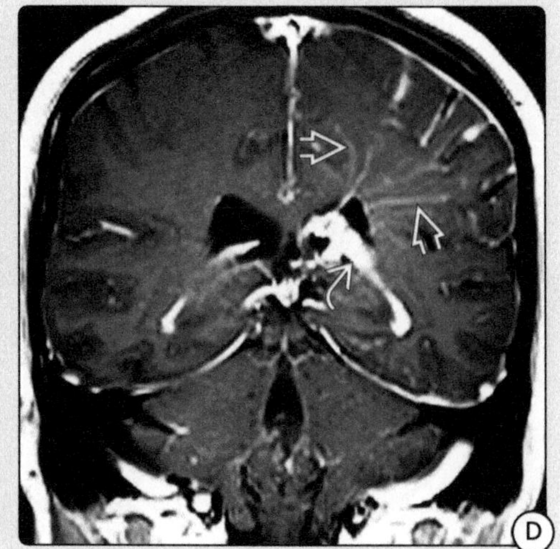

***(40-5C)** More cephalad T1 C+ MR in the same patient shows that the sulci and subarachnoid spaces are enlarged, completely filled by the enhancing pial angioma. **(40-5D)** Coronal T1 C+ MR nicely demonstrates the prominent enhancing medullary veins ➔ as they drain through the hemispheric white matter to converge on the subependymal veins that line the lateral ventricles. The ipsilateral choroid plexus ➔ is markedly enlarged.*

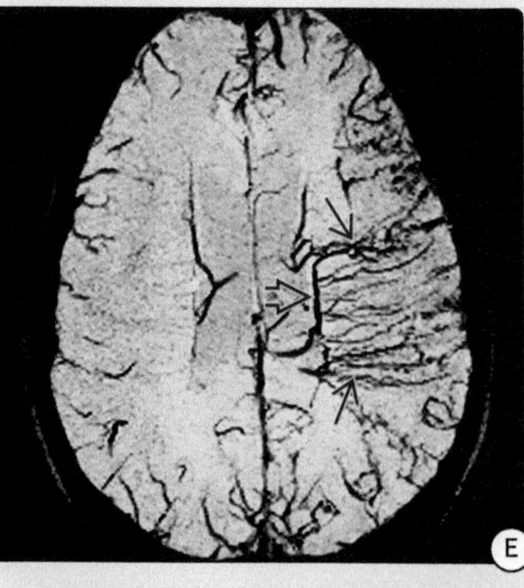

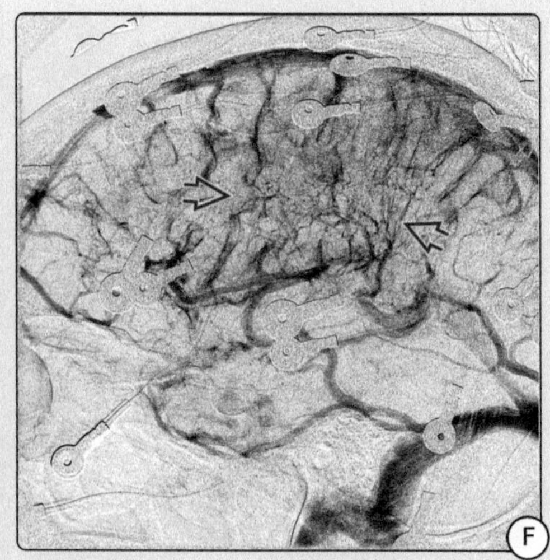

***(40-5E)** Axial T2* susceptibility-weighted image (SWI) demonstrates deoxyhemoglobin in the enlarged, tortuous medullary veins ➔ that are slowly draining into enlarged subependymal veins ➔. **(40-5F)** Venous-phase DSA in the same patient performed as part of a Wada test for language localization shows a paucity of normal cortical veins with a prolonged vascular "blush" caused by contrast stasis in multiple enlarged medullary veins ➔.*

underlying brain, not the pial angioma). Cortical calcification, atrophy, and enlargement of the ipsilateral choroid plexus are typical findings in older children and adults with SWS.

Bone CT shows thickening of the diploë and enlargement with hyperpneumatization of the ipsilateral frontal sinuses.

MR Findings. T1 and T2 scans show volume loss in the affected cortex with enlargement of the adjacent subarachnoid spaces **(40-4C)**. Prominent trabeculae and enlarged veins often cross the subarachnoid space, making the CSF appear somewhat grayish or "dirty" **(40-4)**.

Dystrophic cortical/subcortical calcifications are seen as linear hypointensities on T2WI that "bloom" on T2* (GRE, SWI) **(40-4D)**. SWI scans often demonstrate linear susceptibility in enlarged medullary veins **(40-5E)**. FLAIR scans may demonstrate serpentine hyperintensities in the sulci, the "ivy" sign **(40-5A)**.

T1 C+ shows serpentine enhancement that extends deep into the sulci and sometimes almost completely fills the subarachnoid space **(40-5C)**. Enlarged medullary veins can sometimes be identified as linear enhancing foci extending deep into the hemispheric white matter **(40-5D)**. The ipsilateral choroid plexus is almost always enlarged and enhances intensely **(40-4E)**.

Angiography. DSA typically demonstrates a lack of superficial cortical veins with corresponding dilatation of deep medullary and subependymal veins **(40-5F)**. The arterial phase is normal.

STURGE-WEBER SYNDROME

Etiology
- Congenital but sporadic, not inherited
- Postzygotic (i.e., somatic) mutation in *GNAQ*
  - Causes both SWS, nonsyndromic "port-wine birthmarks" (PWBs)

Pathology
- Pial (leptomeningeal) angioma
- Cortical venous ischemia, atrophy
- Parietooccipital > frontal

Clinical Issues
- Unilateral facial nevus flammeus
  - a.k.a. PWB
- Usual cutaneous distribution = CNV1, CNV2 > CNV3
  - Can be bilateral or even absent

Imaging
- CT
  - Atrophic cortex
  - Ipsilateral calvarium thick, sinuses enlarged
  - Cortical Ca^{++} (*not* in angioma!) increases with age
- MR
  - Cortical/subcortical hypointensity on T2
  - Ca^{++} "blooms" on T2*
  - Angioma enhances (unilateral 80%, bilateral 20%)
  - Ipsilateral choroid plexus enlarged
  - Enlarged medullary veins

Klippel-Trenaunay Syndrome

Klippel-Trenaunay syndrome (KTS)—also called Klippel-Trenaunay-Weber syndrome—is characterized by (1) capillary malformation, seen in 98% of patients either as cutaneous hemangiomas or port-wine stains, (2) limb overgrowth, which may include the underlying bones and soft tissues, and (3) venous varicosities. **KTS** shares overlapping features with SWS. Intracranial lesions, i.e., pial angiomas, are rare. When present, they are often bilateral.

Other Vascular Phakomatoses

Hereditary Hemorrhagic Telangiectasia

Terminology

Hereditary hemorrhagic telangiectasia (HHT) is a.k.a. **Osler-Weber-Rendu** or Rendu-Osler-Weber syndrome. HHT is an autosomal dominant monogenetic disorder characterized pathologically by multisystem angiodysplastic lesions.

Etiology

Mutations in two genes (*ENG* and *ACVRL1*/ALK1) cause most HHT cases. *ENG* (endoglin) gene mutations cause **type 1 HHT** and are associated with mucocutaneous telangiectases, early onset of epistaxis, pulmonary arteriovenous fistulas (AVFs), and brain arteriovenous malformations (AVMs). *ACVRL1*/ALK1 mutation causes **type 2 HHT**, is associated with milder disease, and presents primarily as GI bleeds and pulmonary arterial hypertension.

HEREDITARY HEMORRHAGIC TELANGIECTASIA: ETIOLOGY AND PATHOLOGY

Etiology
- Type 1 HHT
  - Endoglin (*ENG*) mutation
  - Mucocutaneous telangiectases, epistaxis, pulmonary AVFs/brain AVMs
- Type 2 HHT
  - *ACVRL1*/ALK1 mutation
  - Milder; predominantly GI bleeds

Pathology
- Neurovascular malformations 10-20%
  - > 50% multiple
- 2 main types (~ 50:50)
  - "Nidal" brain AVMs
  - Capillary vascular malformations
- Other intracranial vascular malformations
  - Developmental venous anomaly: 12%
  - Cavernous malformations: 2-4%
  - Capillary telangiectases (mucocutaneous common; rare in brain 1-3%)
  - Pial AVF: < 1%

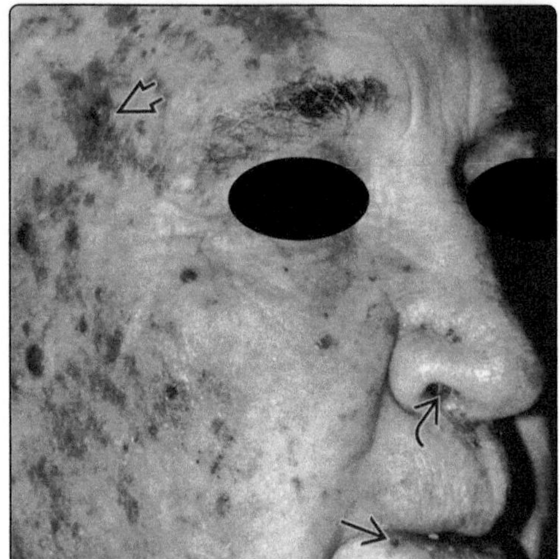

***(40-6)** Patient with HHT shows multiple mucocutaneous telangiectasias of the scalp ⇒, nose ⇒, and lips ⇒.*

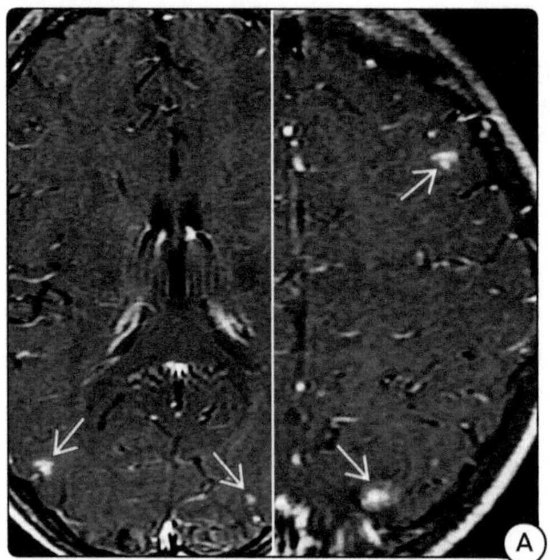

***(40-7A)** Axial T1 C+ FS MRs in an 11-year-old girl with HHT show multiple foci of fluffy "stain-like" enhancement ⇒.*

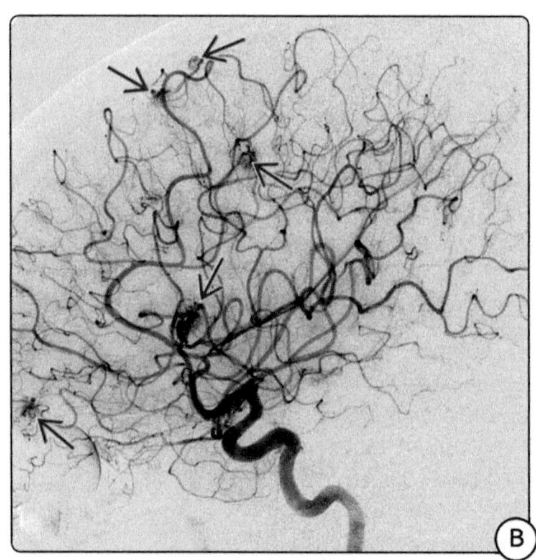

***(40-7B)** Lateral DSA in a 54y woman with HHT shows 5 small capillary vascular malformations ⇒ in the left cerebral hemisphere.*

Pathology

Between 10-20% of patients with a diagnosis of definite HHT have brain vascular malformations. Two main types are common: (1) Nidus-type AVMs and (2) capillary vascular malformations. AVFs—common in the lung—are rare in the brain. Nonshunting lesions in HHT include developmental venous anomalies, capillary telangiectasias, and cavernous malformations.

"Nidal" brain AVMs account for slightly less than 1/2 of all HHT neurovascular manifestations and are found in 10% of all patients. Nearly 60% are solitary, whereas multiple lesions are present in 40%; ~ 80% are supratentorial, whereas 20% are infratentorial.

Capillary vascular malformations account for slightly over 1/2 of all neurovascular manifestations of HHT. They are typically supratentorial (86%), are often peripherally located in the brain, and are almost always < 1 cm.

Capillary telangiectasias are distinct from capillary vascular malformations and consist of numerous thin-walled ectatic capillaries interspersed in normal brain parenchyma. Feeding arteries are absent, although sometimes a draining vein can be identified. Brain capillary telangiectasias are relatively rare in HHT (2-4%). They are typically found in the pons or medulla and are occult on DSA.

Other manifestations of HHT include pial AVFs and nonshunting lesions, such as **developmental venous anomalies** (12%) and **cavernous malformations** (3-4%). **Pial AVFs** are rare, accounting for just 1% of all HHT-related brain vascular malformations. **Malformations of cortical development**—usually perisylvian polymicrogyria—are found in 12% of HHT cases.

Clinical Issues

Presentation. The most common features of HHT are nosebleeds and telangiectases on the lips, hands, and oral mucosa **(40-6)**. Epistaxis typically begins by age 10, and 80-90% have nosebleeds by age 21. The onset of visible telangiectases is generally 5-30 years later than for epistaxis. Almost 95% of affected individuals eventually develop mucocutaneous telangiectases.

The diagnosis of HHT is considered "confirmed" in an individual with three or more of the following: (1) Nosebleeds, (2) mucocutaneous telangiectases, (3) visceral AVM, and (4) a first-degree relative in whom HHT has been diagnosed. HHT patients should be screened for cerebral vascular malformations at least once during their clinical evaluation.

Natural History. HHT displays age-related penetrance with increasing manifestations developing over a lifetime; penetrance approaches 100% by age 40. Epistaxis increases in frequency and severity and, in some cases, can require multiple transfusions or even become life threatening.

Although most HHT-associated brain AVMs are small and have a low Spetzler-Martin grade, 20% present with rupture, and nearly 50% are symptomatic.

Shunting of air, thrombi, and bacteria through pulmonary AVMs can cause TIAs, strokes, and cerebral abscesses.

Imaging

Brain MR without and with contrast enhancement is the recommended screening procedure for patients diagnosed with HHT and, when possible, should be obtained within the first six months of life. Molecular diagnostics may obviate further imaging. In adults, if no AVMs are detected on initial MR scans, further screening for cerebral AVMs is unnecessary.

Although some HHT-associated **AVMs** are large, nearly 90% are small (Spetzler-Martin ≤ 2) **(40-7B)**. Large lesions can demonstrate prominent "flow voids" on T2WI; smaller lesions are seen as "speckled" enhancing foci on T1 C+ studies.

Capillary vascular malformations do not show "flow voids" on MR and are defined by a "blush" of abnormal vessels on the late arterial/capillary phase on DSA **(40-7B)** or an area of fluffy "stain-like" enhancement on T1 C+ MR **(40-7A)**. A dilated feeding artery that empties directly into a draining vein is typical of an **AVF**.

Capillary telangiectasias are most common in the pons and are usually invisible on T2/FLAIR. A faint "brush-like" area of enhancement is seen on T1 C+, whereas T2* sequences show decreased signal intensity.

HEREDITARY HEMORRHAGIC TELANGIECTASIA: IMAGING

Capillary Vascular Malformations
- Slightly > 50% of HHT vascular malformations
- No "flow voids" on MR
- "Blush" of fluffy, "stain-like" enhancement on T1 C+

Arteriovenous Malformations
- Slightly < 50%
- Most are Spetzler grades ≤ 2
  - Multiple AVMs: 40%
- Large lesions rare
  - "Flow voids" on T2WI
- Small lesions show "speckled" enhancement on T1 C+
- Feeding artery, nidus, draining vein on DSA
- Other vascular malformations less common
- Perisylvian polymicrogyria: 12%

PHACE Syndrome

PHACE syndrome is an acronym for **p**osterior fossa malformations, **h**emangioma, **a**rterial cerebrovascular anomalies, **c**oarctation of the aorta and cardiac defects, and **e**ye abnormalities (sometimes called PHACES with the addition of the less common **s**ternal clefting or **s**upraumbilical raphe).

PHACE is characterized clinically by a large infantile hemangioma (IH) **(40-8)** that is associated with developmental defects. A definitive diagnosis of PHACE is determined when a **craniofacial hemangioma** is present together with one or more characteristic extracutaneous anomalies.

Hemangiomas are—by definition—found in 100% of PHACE patients. Hemangiomas are true vascular neoplasms and are the most common benign tumor of infancy, occurring in 2-3% of neonates and 10-12% of children under 1 year of age. The majority are sporadic, nonsyndromic lesions; only 20% meet the diagnostic criteria for PHACE.

MR is the best technique to evaluate the presence and extent of craniofacial hemangiomas and to delineate coexisting intracranial malformations **(40-9)**. T1 scans depict callosal dysgenesis and cerebellar anomalies. Gray matter heterotopias are best seen on T2WI. Proliferating hemangiomas appear hyperintense on T2WI and may exhibit prominent internal "flow voids." Intense homogeneous enhancement following contrast administration is typical.

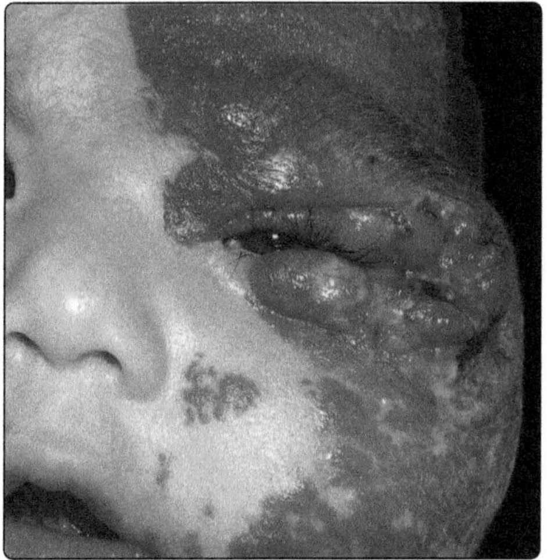

***(40-8)** Clinical photograph of a patient with PHACES shows a typical facial infantile hemangioma. (Courtesy S. Yashar, MD.)*

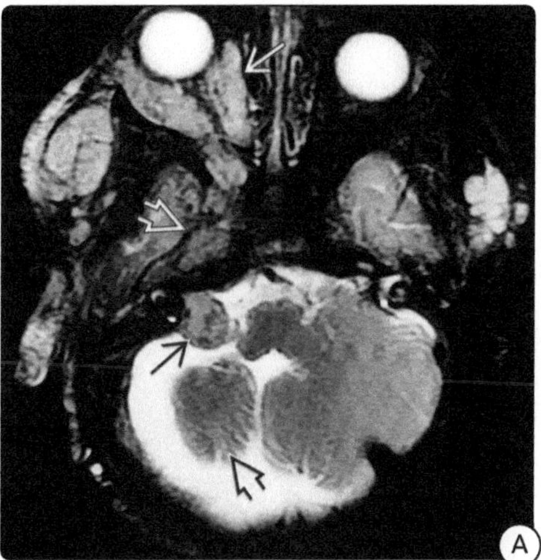

***(40-9A)** T2 MR in PHACES shows orbital ➡, cavernous sinus ➡, CPA hemangioma ➡. Ipsilateral cerebellum hypoplasia ➡.*

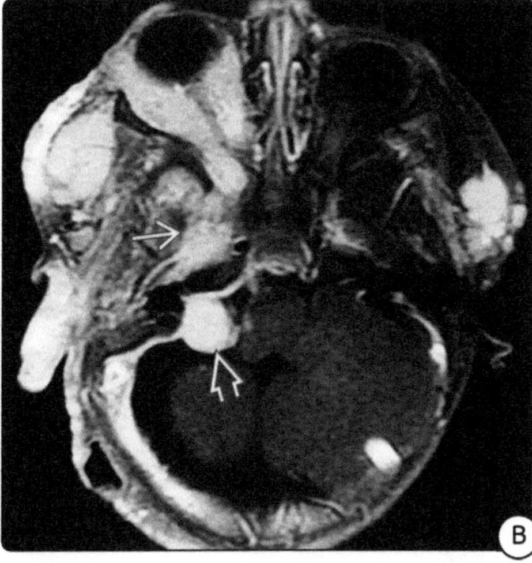

***(40-9B)** T1 C+ FS MR shows intracranial extension of the hemangioma into the cavernous sinus ➡ and cerebellopontine angle cistern ➡.*

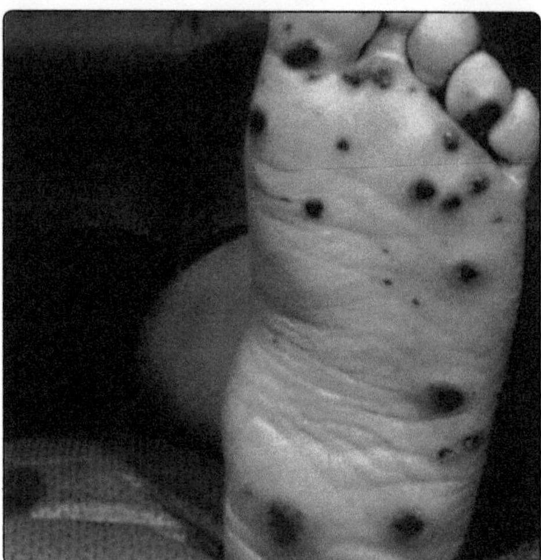

(40-10) *Photo of a patient with BRBNS shows multiple elevated and bluish skin "blebs" on the foot. (Courtesy AFIP Archives.)*

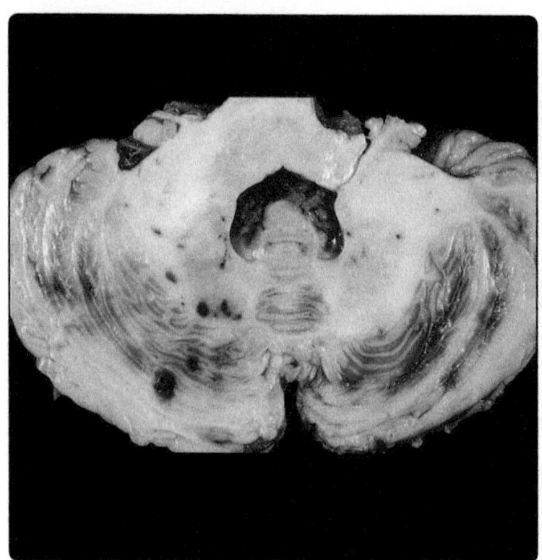

(40-11) *Axial cut section through the cerebellum shows multiple developmental venous anomalies (DVAs) characteristic of BRBNS. (R. Hewlett, MD.)*

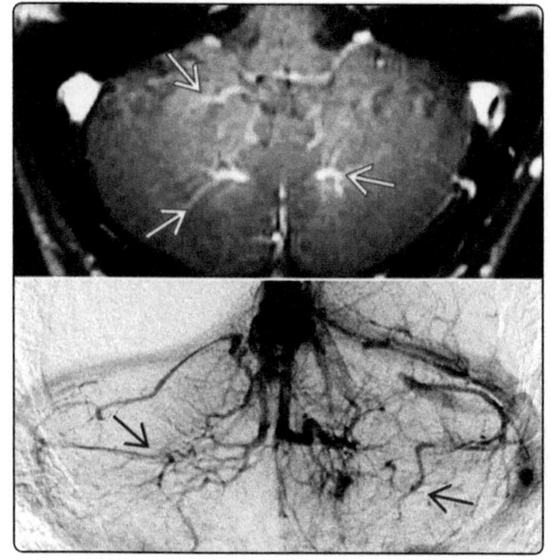

(40-12) *(Top) T1 C+ FS MR in a patient with probable BRBNS shows bilateral enhancing DVAs ➡. (Bottom) AP DSA shows bilateral DVAs ➡.*

PHACE(S) SYNDROME

Terminology

- **P**osterior fossa malformations
- **H**emangioma
- **A**rterial cerebrovascular anomalies
- **C**oarctation of the aorta and cardiac defects
- **E**ye abnormalities
- ± **s**ternal clefting or supraumbilical raphe

Pathology

- Hemangiomas (vascular neoplasm, not malformation)
- Ipsilateral cerebellar hypoplasia
- Posterior fossa cystic lesions (e.g., Dandy-Walker) common
- Arterial stenoses/occlusions, saccular aneurysms, aberrant vessels

Clinical Issues

- Hemangiomas proliferate, then involute

Imaging

- T1 C+ FS MR to delineate hemangiomas
- CTA/MRA to evaluate for vascular anomalies

Blue Rubber Bleb Nevus Syndrome

Blue rubber bleb nevus syndrome (BRBNS) is a rare disorder characterized by multiple venous malformations. BRBNS is caused by a somatic mutation in the receptor tyrosine kinase or *TEK*, the gene encoding TIE2. *TEK* is a controller of endothelial cell assembling and remodeling that organizes the vascular network and recruits the perivascular cells necessary for stabilizing vessel walls. The same mutation also occurs in sporadic multifocal venous malformations.

BRBNS usually affects the skin, oral cavity, and gastrointestinal tract. Small raised bluish, compressible rubber- or "bleb-like" nevi are the clinical hallmarks of this disorder **(40-10)**. The most common presentation is iron deficiency anemia caused by intestinal bleeding.

CNS lesions occur in 15-20% of cases. Reported imaging manifestations include an extensive network of developmental venous anomalies with or without sinus pericranii **(40-11)** **(40-12)**.

Wyburn-Mason Syndrome

Wyburn-Mason syndrome, a.k.a. congenital unilateral retinocephalic vascular malformation syndrome, is a rare nonhereditary neurocutaneous syndrome that presents with unilateral AVMs of the brain, orbit, and face. Craniofacial vascular malformations can involve the eyelids and orbits as well as the retina and optic nerve. Lesions range from barely visible to large tangles of dilated, tortuous vessels. Patients with extensive retinal AVMs are at high risk for visual loss, whereas patients with brain AVMs are at risk for parenchymal hemorrhage.

Selected References: The complete reference list is available on the Expert Consult™ eBook version included with purchase.

Anomalies of the Skull and Meninges

Anomalies of the skull and meninges represent maldevelopment of the embryonic mesenchyme. These include cephaloceles, congenital calvarial defects, and other meningeal malformations, including lipomas.

Cephaloceles

"Cephalocele" is a generic term for the protrusion of intracranial contents through a calvarial or skull base defect. Cephaloceles that contain herniations of brain tissue, meninges, and CSF are called **meningoencephaloceles**. If the meninges and accompanying CSF are herniated *without* brain tissue, the lesion is termed a **meningocele**. An **atretic cephalocele** is a small defect that contains just dura, fibrous tissue, and degenerated brain tissue.

Cephaloceles can be congenital or acquired. The most common congenital cephaloceles are occipital, frontoethmoidal, parietal, and skull base cephaloceles.

Cephalocele imaging has four goals: (1) Depict the osseous defect, (2) delineate the sac and define its contents, (3) map the course of adjacent arteries and determine the integrity of the dural venous sinuses, and (4) identify any coexisting anomalies.

Occipital Cephaloceles

Occipital cephaloceles account for 75% of cephaloceles in European and North American Caucasians and are usually recognized at birth as a variably sized occipital or suboccipital soft tissue mass.

Bone CT with 3D reconstruction delineates the osseous defect well, and multiplanar MR best depicts the sac and its contents. The herniated brain—which can derive from both supra- and infratentorial structures—is always abnormal, appearing dysmorphic, disorganized, and dysplastic. Depending on the size of the cephalocele, severe traction and distortion of the brainstem and supratentorial structures can be present.

Dura and CSF-filled structures (including the fourth ventricle and sometimes part of the lateral ventricles) are often contained within the sac. In addition to delineating the sac and its contents, identifying the course and integrity of the dural venous sinuses is essential for preoperative planning.

At least 1/2 of all patients with occipital cephaloceles have associated abnormalities, such as callosal dysgenesis, Chiari 2, Dandy-Walker spectrum disorders, and gray matter heterotopias.

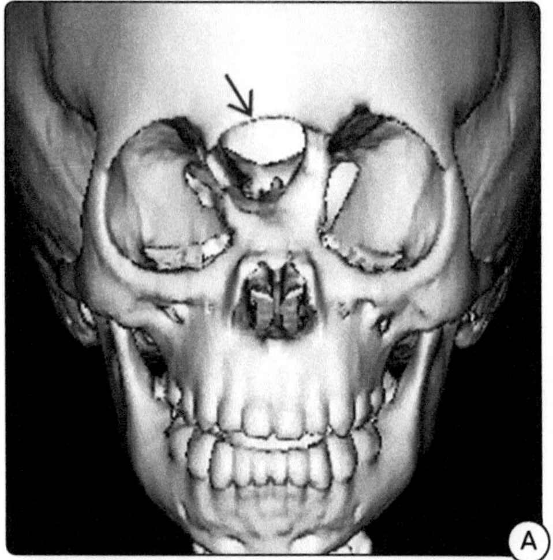

(41-1A) 3D reformatted bone CT shows a well-delineated frontonasal bony defect ➔ just above the bridge of the nose.

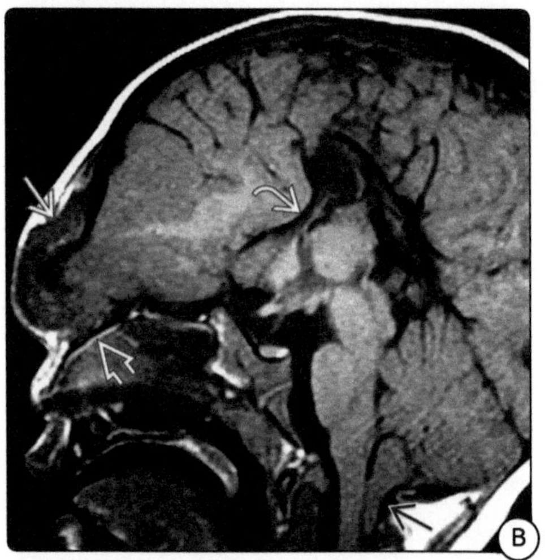

(41-1B) Sagittal T1WI shows soft tissue mass ➔ protruding through a patent fonticulus frontalis ➔. Note absent corpus callosum ➔, Chiari 1 ➔.

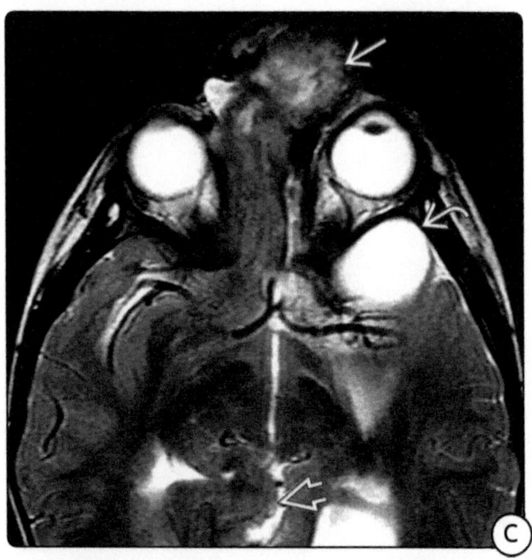

(41-1C) T2WI shows cephalocele is mostly dysplastic brain ➔. Note arachnoid cyst ➔, polymicrogyria ➔. (Courtesy M. Michel, MD.)

Frontoethmoidal Cephaloceles

Frontoethmoidal cephaloceles are the most common type of cephalocele seen in Southeast Asia. Brain parenchyma herniates into the midface, typically the forehead or dorsum of the nose.

Frontonasal cephaloceles represent 40-60% of frontoethmoidal cephaloceles. Brain herniates into the forehead between the frontal bones above and the nasal bones below **(41-1)**. In **nasoethmoidal** cephaloceles (30%), the sac herniates through a midline foramen cecum defect into the prenasal space. The cribriform plate is deficient or absent; the crista galli may be absent or bifid.

NECT scans show a well-demarcated, heterogeneous, mixed-density mass that extends extracranially through a bony defect. MR shows a soft tissue mass in direct contiguity with the intracranial parenchyma.

Parietal Cephaloceles

Parietal cephaloceles comprise just 5-10% of all cephaloceles. Most have underlying brain and vascular anomalies, such as a persistent falcine sinus or sinus pericranii.

MR best delineates cephalocele contents. Defining the position of the superior sagittal sinus and adjacent cortical draining veins with MRV, CTV, or DSA prior to surgery is essential.

Atretic cephaloceles (APCs) are small lesions that typically present as midline scalp masses near the posterior vertex **(41-2)**. They are often associated with a persistent falcine sinus and frequently split the superior sagittal sinus **(41-3)**.

Skull Base Cephaloceles

Skull base cephaloceles account for 10% of all cephaloceles. MR of skull base cephaloceles is essential to delineate the sac contents. The pituitary gland, optic nerves and chiasm, hypothalamus, and third ventricle can all be displaced inferiorly into the cephalocele. Associated anomalies, such as corpus callosum dysgenesis and an azygous anterior cerebral artery, are common.

CEPHALOCELES

Occipital Cephaloceles
- Most common in European/North American Caucasians
- 75% of cephaloceles
- Typically contains dysplastic brain

Frontoethmoidal Cephaloceles
- Southeast Asian predominance
- 10-15% of cephaloceles
- Frontonasal (40-60%) = forehead
- Nasoethmoidal (30%) = nose

Parietal Cephaloceles
- 5-10% of cephaloceles
- Most are atretic ± falcine sinus, sinus pericranii

Skull Base Cephaloceles
- 10% of cephaloceles
- Brain anomalies common (e.g., callosal dysgenesis)

Craniosynostoses

Craniosynostosis Overview

Craniosynostoses are a heterogeneous group of disorders characterized by abnormal head shape. Craniosynostosis can be nonsyndromic (70-75% of cases) or syndromic and may affect a single suture or multiple sutures.

The cranial sutures form relatively late (at around 16 weeks of gestation). As long as the brain grows rapidly, the calvarium expands. As brain growth slows, the sutures close.

The normal order of closure is metopic first, followed by the coronal and then the lambdoid sutures. The sagittal suture normally closes last. Craniostenosis occurs when osseous obliteration of one or more sutures occurs prematurely.

Nonsyndromic Craniosynostosis

Nonsyndromic craniosynostoses (NCSs) are genetically determined lesions that occur in the absence of a recognizable syndrome. The genetic component is suture specific (e.g., sagittal craniostenosis and *BMP2).*

Approximately 60% of all single-suture craniosynostosis cases involve premature fusion of the sagittal suture followed in frequency by those that involve the coronal (22%) and metopic (15%) sutures. Lambdoid craniosynostosis is very rare, causing just 2% of all cases.

Craniosynostosis is generally classified by head shape as **scaphocephaly** or dolichocephaly (long and narrow), **brachycephaly** (broad and flattened), **trigonocephaly** (triangular at the front) **(41-4)**, or **plagiocephaly** (skewed).

Gross examination shows fibrous or bony sutural "bridging." Focal synostosis or diffuse bony "beaking" along the affected suture are typical findings.

Head shape generally predicts which suture(s) will be abnormal, but CT is required to determine whether part or all of the affected suture(s) is fused. Thin-section CT scans with multiplanar reconstruction and 3D shaded surface display (SSD) are invaluable for detailed evaluation and preoperative planning.

MR is helpful to rule out coexisting anomalies. Hydrocephalus, corpus callosum dysgenesis, and gray matter abnormalities may be present but are more common in syndromic craniosynostoses. MRA or CTA is useful to delineate venous sinus drainage prior to surgical intervention.

CRANIOSYNOSTOSIS

Normal Suture Development
- Late (16 weeks' gestation)
- Metopic closes first, sagittal closes last

Pathology
- Location
  - Sagittal (60%): Scaphocephaly
  - Coronal (22%): Brachycephaly
  - Metopic (15%): Trigonocephaly
  - Lambdoid (2%)
  - Multiple (5%)
- Gross pathology
  - Suture obliterated by diffuse or focal bony "beaking"

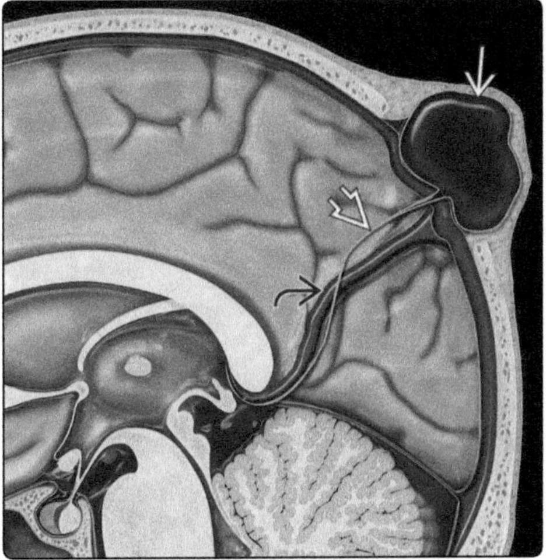

***(41-2)** Skin-covered atretic parietal cephalocele ➡ is associated with a dura-lined sinus tract ➡ and a persistent falcine sinus ➡.*

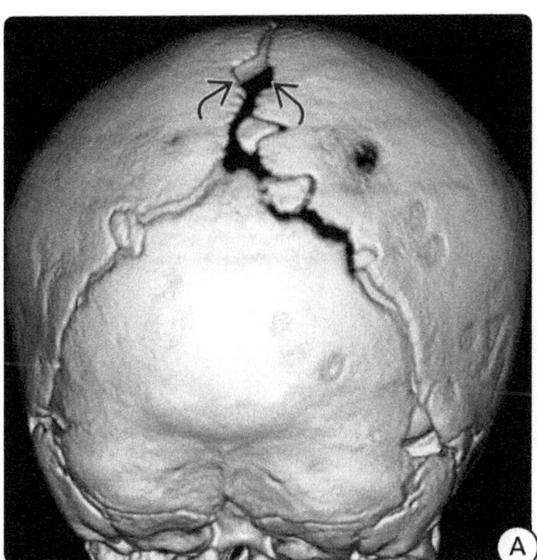

***(41-3A)** 3D-rendered bone CT in a child with an atretic parietal cephalocele demonstrates a small, well-demarcated midline skull defect ➡.*

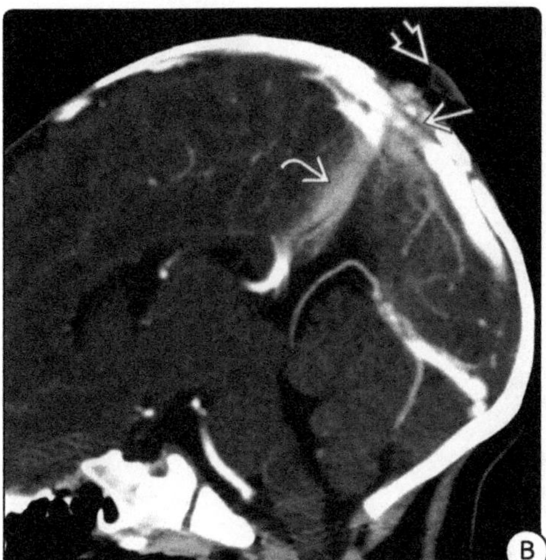

***(41-3B)** CTA shows persistent falcine sinus ➡ and atretic cephalocele ➡ passing between the split superior sagittal sinus ➡.*

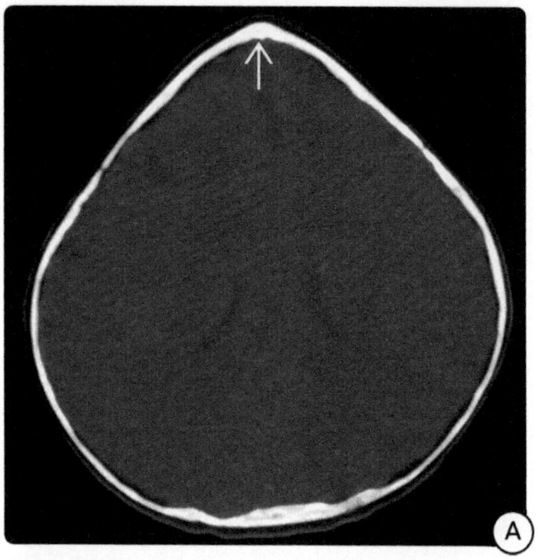

(41-4A) *Bone CT of trigonocephaly shows triangular anterior pointing of the skull ➡. In the transverse plane, calvarium appears widened.*

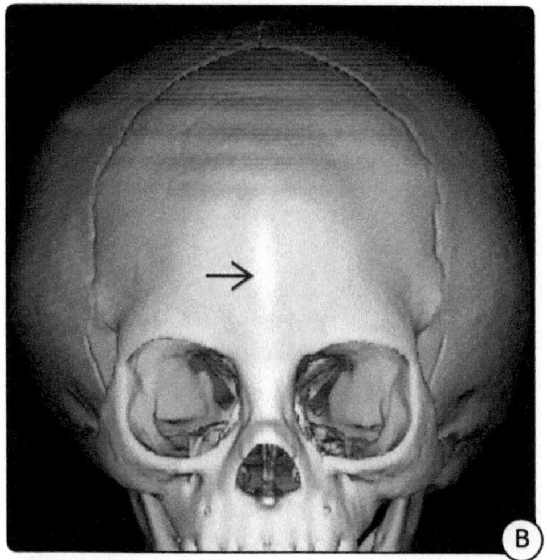

(41-4B) *AP 3D SSD in the same patient shows premature metopic suture synostosis with a distinct vertical ridge of bone ➡.*

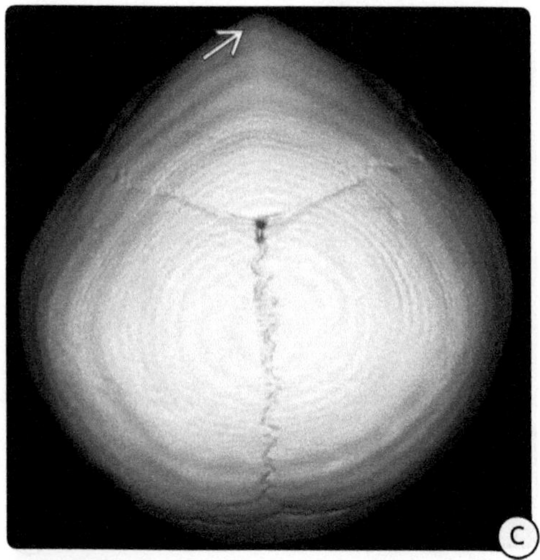

(41-4C) *Vertex view shows distinct triangular shape ➡ of trigonocephaly secondary to metopic suture synostosis.*

Syndromic Craniosynostoses

Syndromic craniosynostoses account for just 25-30% of all cranial stenoses but are much more likely to be associated with additional craniofacial or skeletal anomalies. These include limb abnormalities, dysmorphic facial features, and skull deformity. In addition, brain malformations are common, and developmental delay is more frequent. In contrast to nonsyndromic craniosynostoses (in which the sagittal suture is most often affected), bilateral coronal synostosis is the most common pattern in these patients.

Examples of syndromic craniosynostoses include Apert syndrome (a.k.a. **acrocephalosyndactyly type 1**). Bilateral coronal synostosis is the most common calvarial anomaly. Hypertelorism, midface hypoplasia, and cervical spine anomalies are common.

Of all the syndromic craniosynostoses, patients with Apert syndrome are most severely affected in terms of intellectual disability, developmental delay, CNS malformations, hearing loss, and limb anomalies. Intracranial anomalies occur in > 1/2 of all cases and include hydrocephalus, callosal dysgenesis, and abnormalities of the septi pellucidi (25-30% each).

Meningeal Anomalies

Anomalies of the cranial meninges commonly accompany other congenital malformations, such as Chiari 2 malformation. **Lipomas** and **arachnoid cysts** are two important intracranial abnormalities with meningeal origin. Arachnoid cysts were considered in detail in Chapter 28. We therefore conclude our discussion of congenital anomalies by focusing on lipomas.

Lipomas

The 2016 WHO places intracranial lipomas in the mesenchymal, nonmeningothelial CNS neoplasms under "Other Mesenchymal Tumours" but also notes that "whether these various lesions (i.e., lipomas and complex lipomatous lesions) are neoplasms or malformative overgrowths is yet to be determined."

We include lipomas in this chapter rather than in the discussion of intracranial neoplasms because of their frequent association with other congenital malformations.

Fat—adipose tissue—is not normally found inside the arachnoid. Therefore, any fatty tissue inside the skull or spine is abnormal. Because fat deposits commonly accompany congenital malformations, such as callosal dysgenesis or tethered spinal cord, imaging studies should be closely scrutinized for the presence of additional abnormalities.

Terminology

So-called ordinary lipoma is the most common of all soft tissue tumors and is composed of mature adipose tissue. "Complex lipomatous lesions" may contain other mesenchymal tissues, such as striated muscle, and have sometimes been referred to as **choristomas**.

Etiology

Lipomas were once thought to be congenital malformations of the **embryonic meninx primitiva** (the undifferentiated mesenchyme). The primitive meninx normally differentiates into the cranial meninges, invaginating along the choroid fissure of the lateral ventricle. Maldifferentiation and persistence of the meninx was thought to result in deposits of mature adipose tissue, i.e., fat, along the subpial surface of the brain and spinal cord and within the lateral ventricles.

Recent fluorescence in situ hybridization (FISH) and comparative genomic hybridization (CGH) studies have identified clonal cytogenetic aberrations in nearly 60% of ordinary systemic lipomas.

Pathology

Location. Nearly 80% of intracranial lipomas are supratentorial, and most occur in or near the midline. The interhemispheric fissure is the most common overall site (40-50%). Lipomas curve over the dorsal corpus callosum, often extending through the choroidal fissures into the lateral ventricles or choroid plexus.

Between 15-25% are located in the quadrigeminal region, usually attached to the inferior colliculi or superior vermis **(41-5)**. Approximately 15% are suprasellar, attached to the undersurface of the hypothalamus or infundibular stalk. About 5% of lipomas are found in the sylvian fissure.

Approximately 20% of lipomas are infratentorial. The cerebellopontine angle cistern is the most common posterior fossa site (10%).

Lipomas are generally solitary lesions that vary from tiny, barely perceptible fatty collections to huge bulky masses. Most are < 5 cm in diameter.

Gross Pathology. Lipomas appear as bright yellow, lobulated soft masses. They usually adhere to the pia and underlying parenchyma. At least 1/3 encase adjacent vessels &/or cranial nerves. Lipomas are composed of mature, nonneoplastic-appearing adipose tissue with relatively uniform fat cells.

INTRACRANIAL LIPOMAS: ETIOLOGY AND PATHOLOGY

Etiology
- 2 theories
  - Maldifferentiation of embryonic meninx primitiva
  - Genetic aberration

Pathology
- Usually solitary
- Supratentorial (80%)
  - Interhemispheric fissure (40-50%)
  - Quadrigeminal (15-25%)
  - Suprasellar (15%)
- Infratentorial (20%)
- Gross appearance: Lobulated, yellow
- Microscopic: Mature, nonneoplastic adipose tissue

Clinical Issues

Lipomas are relatively rare, accounting for < 0.5% of intracranial masses. They can be found in patients of all ages.

Lipomas are rarely symptomatic and are usually incidental findings on imaging studies. Headache, seizure, hypothalamic disturbances, and cranial nerve deficits have been reported in a few cases. Lipomas are benign lesions that remain stable in size. Some may expand with corticosteroid use.

Lipomas encase vessels and nerves, so they are generally considered "leave me alone" lesions. Surgery has high associated morbidity and mortality.

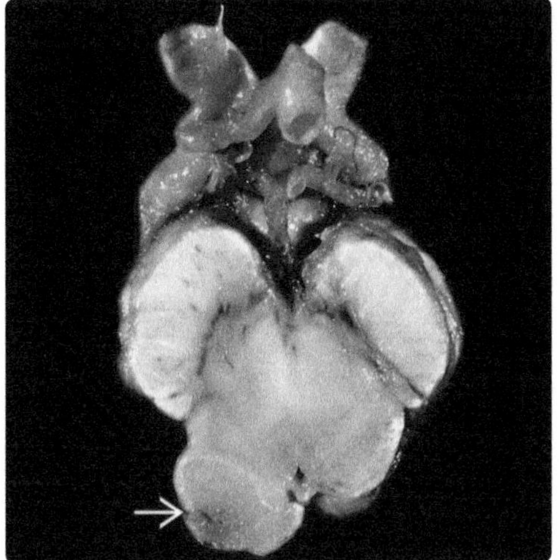

***(41-5)** Autopsy case demonstrates subpial lipoma ➡ attached to quadrigeminal plate. (Courtesy E. T. Hedley-Whyte, MD.)*

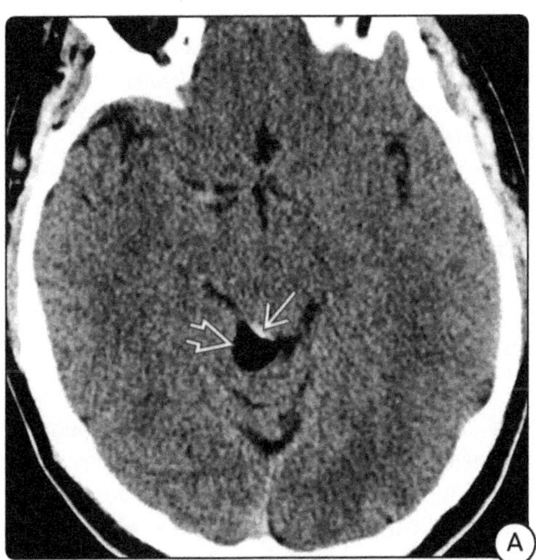

***(41-6A)** NECT shows hypodense (-75 HU) lipoma ➡ attached to the quadrigeminal plate. Some calcification is present ➡.*

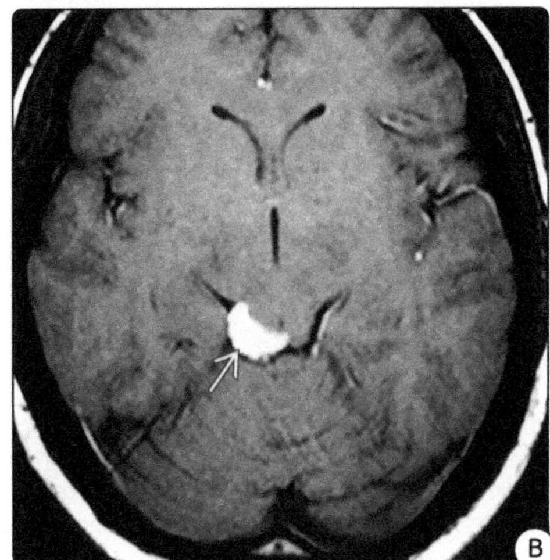

***(41-6B)** T1 MR shows hyperintense lipoma ➡ is attached to the quadrigeminal plate without a distinct medial border.*

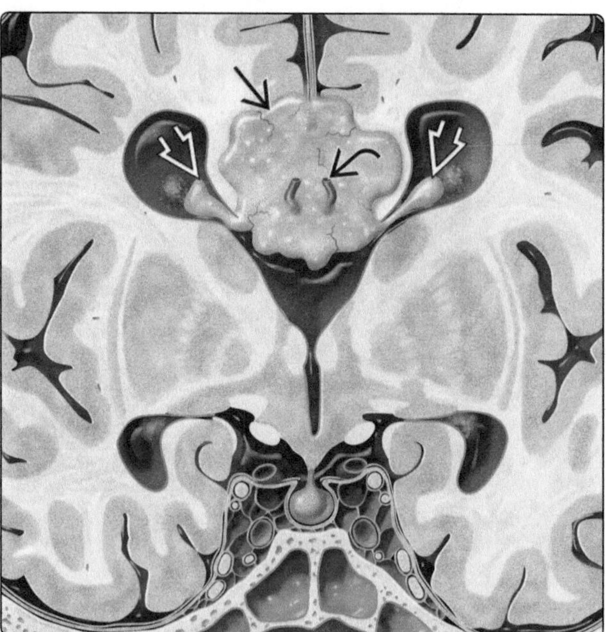

(41-7) CC agenesis with interhemispheric lipoma ➡ encases ACAs ➡ and extends through choroidal fissure into both lateral ventricles ➡.

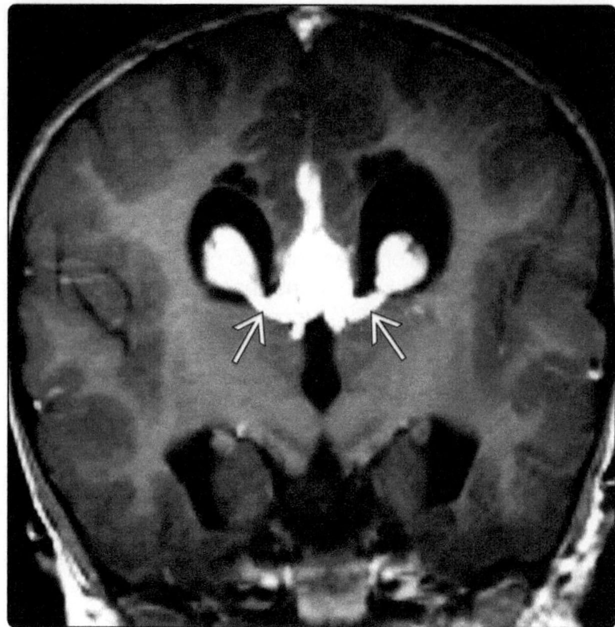

(41-8) Coronal T1 MR shows lipoma with extension through choroidal fissures into both lateral ventricles ➡ and the choroid plexi.

Imaging

General Features. Lipomas are seen as well-delineated, somewhat lobulated extraaxial masses that exhibit fat density/signal intensity.

Two morphologic configurations of interhemispheric fissure lipomas are recognized on imaging studies: A **curvilinear** type (a thin, pencil-like mass that curves around the corpus callosum body and splenium) and a **tubulonodular** type (a large, bulky interhemispheric fatty mass). Dystrophic calcification occurs in both types but is more common in tubulonodular lesions.

CT Findings. NECT scans show a hypodense mass that measures -50 to -100 HU. Calcification varies from extensive—nearly 2/3 of bulky tubulonodular interhemispheric lipomas are partially calcified—to none, generally seen in small lesions in other locations **(41-6A)**. Lipomas do not enhance on CECT scans.

MR Findings. Lipomas follow fat signal on all imaging sequences. They appear homogeneously hyperintense on T1WI **(41-6B)** and become hypointense with fat suppression. Lipomas exhibit chemical-shift artifact in the frequency-encoding direction.

Signal on T2WI varies. Fat becomes hypointense on standard T2WI but remains moderately hyperintense on fast spin-echo studies because of J-coupling. Fat is hypointense on STIR and appears hyperintense on FLAIR. No enhancement is seen following contrast administration.

On SWI, lipomas show hyperintensity surrounded by a low signal intensity band along the fat-water interface that is more prominent than seen on T2* GRE sequences.

Other CNS malformations are common. The most frequent are corpus callosum anomalies. These range from mild dysgenesis (usually with curvilinear lipomas) to agenesis (with bulky tubulonodular lipomas) **(41-7)** **(41-8)**.

Differential Diagnosis

Although fat does not appear inside the normal CNS, it *can* be found within the dura and cavernous sinus. **Metaplastic falx ossification** is a normal variant that can resemble an interhemispheric lipoma. Dense cortical bone surrounding T1-hyperintense, fatty marrow is the typical finding.

The major DDx of intracranial lipoma is unruptured **dermoid cyst**. Dermoids generally measure 20-40 HU, often calcify, and demonstrate more heterogeneous signal intensity on MR.

INTRACRANIAL LIPOMAS

Clinical Issues
- < 0.5% of intracranial masses
- Usually found incidentally; "leave me alone" lesions

Imaging
- NECT: -50 to -100 HU
  - Ca^{++} rare except in tubulonodular lesions
- MR: "Just like fat"
  - Other intracranial malformations common
  - Often surrounds, encases vessels/nerves

Differential Diagnosis
- Dermoid cyst
- Falx ossification

Selected References: The complete reference list is available on the Expert Consult™ eBook version included with purchase.

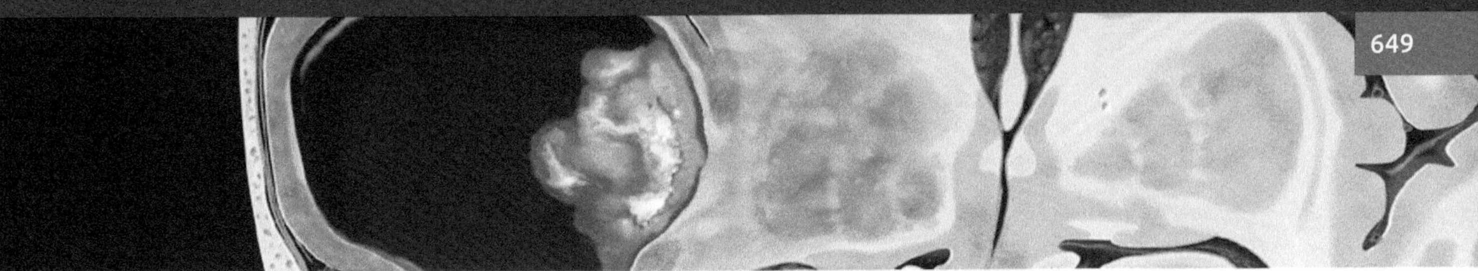

A

Index

B

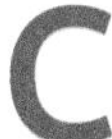

Index

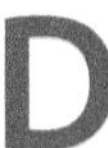

Index

E

Index

F

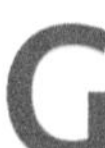

Index

H

Index

J

K

L

M

N

P

Index

Index

Index

T

Index

U

V

W

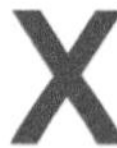

Z